# Regenerative Medicine in China

Xiaobing Fu
Editor

# Regenerative Medicine in China

長江出版傳媒
湖北科学技术出版社

Springer

*Editor*
Xiaobing Fu
PLA General Hospital
Beijing
China

ISBN 978-981-16-1181-0 ISBN 978-981-16-1182-7 (eBook)
https://doi.org/10.1007/978-981-16-1182-7



Jointly published with Hubei Science and Technology Press Co., Ltd.
The print edition is not for sale in China (Mainland). Customers from China (Mainland) please order the print book from: Hubei Science and Technology Press Co., Ltd.


This Springer imprint is published by the registered company Springer Nature Singapore Pte Ltd.
The registered company address is: 152 Beach Road, #21-01/04 Gateway East, Singapore 189721, Singapore

# Foreword 1

Severe trauma and tissue repair and regeneration are among the oldest medical problems. Treatment needs are significant in modern society. In recent years, much work has been carried out in this field at home and abroad. There have been many new discoveries in basic research, but some of the results have begun to be translated into clinical applications. In addition, a number of academic leaders with important influence have emerged in this field at home and abroad, and a number of innovative teams with development potential have been formed. Many research bases with great influence have been built. Therefore, trauma and tissue repair and regeneration are not only hotspots in the field of biomedicine, such research also hopes to make major breakthroughs in theory and technology and provide theoretical and technical support for the final solution of tissue repair and regeneration.

The Severe Trauma and Tissue Restoration and Regenerative Medicine Innovation Group, led by Academician Xiaobing Fu, is the only innovative group in the field of trauma, burns, critical illness and emergency medicine in National Nature Science Foundation of China. In recent years, the group has made outstanding achievements in the following areas: discovering the phenomenon of dedifferentiation of epidermal cells and related mechanisms, basic research and clinical treatment of stem cell differentiation and sweat gland regeneration, new tissue engineering skin development with appendages, new features of chronic refractory wounds on the surface and innovative theory and key measures of preventions. The group has had high-level achievements, represented by the First Class Prize for The State Science and Technology Progress Award, and has been highly praised by peers internationally. The regeneration of sweat glands has been called "milestone research" by international peers, and the innovative achievements of prevention and control of chronic refractory wounds are highly evaluated by internationally important peers who are "looking to the east". These achievements show that the team's work partially solves the major needs of the country in the field and also has a wide international impact. It is one of the outstanding achievements in the field of trauma medicine and tissue repair and regenerative medicine in China.

As a prominent representative of outstanding young and middle-aged people in the field of trauma and tissue repair and regenerative medicine in China, Academician Xiaobing Fu took the lead in writing and submitting the advice to the senior leaders of the central government about the prevention of injury, to promote the industrialization of stem cell and regenerative medicine technology and products and other major recommendations were highly recognized. At the same time, under Dr. Fu's suggestion, we co-organized three Xiang Shan Science Conferences on the theme of "regenerative medicine", published *Regeneration Medicine: From Basic to Clinical Research*, *Regeneration Medicine: Basic and Clinical Research* and *Regeneration Medicine: Transformation and Application* as well as three large-scale academic monographs and participated in the formulation of the Chinese Academy of Engineering's development plan for Chinese regenerative medicine. All of this work shows that Xiaobing Fu and his team have played an important role in promoting the development of trauma medicine, stem cell and tissue repair and regenerative medicine, and biotherapeutics in China, in addition to important innovations in scientific research.

Hubei Science and Technology Press has published *Regenerative Medicine in China—A Team's Work of Xiaobing Fu*, which is a full affirmation of the academic team's outstanding achievements in this field for Dr. Fu and his team. This monograph reflects the fruitful results of trauma and tissue repair and regenerative medicine in recent years. It has both original theoretical findings and partial clinical treatment results. At the same time, there is also an exploration of the discipline construction and talent training model in the field of trauma and tissue repair and regeneration. It is an academic monograph with distinctive characteristics and important reference value. I warmly congratulate Dr. Xiaobing Fu in writing a preface for the publication of this important monograph with great pleasure.

Zhengguo Wang, Professor
Academician of Chinese Academy of Engineering
(Division of Medicine and Health)
Daping Hospital
Army Medical University
Chongqing
China

# Foreword 2

I knew Professor Xiaobing Fu earlier, before he was elected as an academician of the Chinese Academy of Engineering. At that time, there were mainly academic exchanges. My true understanding of him began when we assessed the National Key Laboratory as invited experts in 2001. At the time, he told me about some of the findings of dedifferentiation of epidermal cells. After I carefully studied his basic experimental process, related results and evidence, I thought his observation method was correct and his findings were of great value, and I encouraged him to publish in international journals as soon as possible. At the same time, I emphasized that in basic scientific research, we must adhere to the principle of seeking truth from facts but also seize the opportunity to occupy the commanding heights of academic frontiers; although new ideas may cause some criticisms, we must be brave enough to break through the traditional concepts. Later results confirmed the various reactions and doubts of this discovery at home and abroad. Fortunately, he did not sink but persevered. In the end, his original discovery of epidermal cells transformed into epidermal stem cells through dedifferentiation pathways has been highly recognized by domestic and foreign counterparts. At present, dedifferentiation has been shown to be an important cytological basis for tissue repair and regeneration.

Since then, Professor Xiaobing Fu has focused on the trauma and the basic, clinical and translational studies of tissue repair and regeneration after trauma and has made outstanding achievements in elucidating the mechanisms of dedifferentiation of epidermal cells, basic and clinical aspects of sweat gland regeneration, new features of chronic refractory wounds on the surface and innovative theory and key measures of prevention and control. These findings have been highly recognized by the academic community, and some of the results have been transformed and applied in clinical practice and achieved good therapeutic effects.

In recent years, under Professor Fu's initiative, we have organized three Xiang Shan Science Conferences on the theme of "regenerative medicine". We published *Regeneration Medicine: From Basic to Clinical Research*, *Regeneration Medicine: Basic and Clinical Research* and *Regeneration Medicine: Transformation and Application*, three major academic monographs in the field. We also participated in the formulation of China's regenerative medicine development plan organized by the Chinese Academy of Sciences and the Chinese Academy of Engineering and related societies. This body of work fully demonstrates that Professor Fu not only does his best but also leads the team in the frontiers of tissue repair and regenerative medicine. At the same time, as a prominent representative of outstanding young and middle- aged people, Professor Fu has been a very good leader, demonstrating and promoting a role in Chinese trauma and tissue repair and regeneration. I congratulate Academician Xiaobing Fu on his achievements and hope that he will achieve further success in his future work.

Zuze Wu, Professor
Academician of Chinese Academy of Sciences
Academy of Military Medical Sciences
Beijing
China

# Preface

In 2015, Guoxiang Huang, editor of Hubei Science and Technology Press, told me that the press has planned and is publishing a series of Academicians' monographs as a reference for science and technological innovation. They invited me to publish a monograph entitled *Regenerative Medicine in China—A Team's Work of Xiaobing Fu*. Originally, I have already declined because as a relatively young academician, my experience is not enough, and there is no need to participate in this activity. Later, the press repeatedly invited and proposed that in recent years China's tissue repair and regenerative medicine has achieved relatively great results. Our team has played an important role in this field; whether in basic research or clinical treatment, team building and academic exchanges at home and abroad both have been recognized to a certain extent. Under the guidance of this idea, I agreed to participate in this series of monographs. The main purpose is to reflect on the innovative achievements of our country, especially our team, in this field, and provide a communication platform for peers. At the same time, it also provides some useful reference materials for China's research in this field, which has contributed a little to the development of tissue repair and regenerative medicine in China.

After accepting the mission, how to accomplish this work with high quality is a difficult point. First of all, what is written? Scientific development has its own stage and more continuity. Regenerative medicine is no exception. It should reflect the main findings and important progress in this field at home and abroad, while at the same time avoids repeats of previous publications. Reproductive medicine monographs are too much crossover on the main content. Therefore, this monograph should focus on the research results of our team in this field, which requires further clarification and distinction on what to write. Second, who should write it? In the past, my teachers, Academician Zhengguo Wang, and Academician Zuze Wu and myself, edited and published three monographs on regenerative medicine. Most of the experts who participated in these monographs are famous scholars in the field in China. This monograph, named after the individual, should theoretically be based on the members of our team; that is, we need to clarify the concept of what our team is. Finally, how is it written? As a professional academic work, it is neither a summary report of a specific project study nor a personal autobiographical life summary. I believe that this monograph should be defined as a phased academic summary of my team in the field of trauma and tissue repair and regeneration. It should reflect the main progress and development direction of this field at home and abroad and should describe our own innovation and academic contribution and at the same time reflect the innovation process and the true meaning of the realization, thus drawing lessons for the younger generation.

With these considerations, I have identified the following writing principles: the writing content may be not comprehensive, but the major content is trauma and tissue repair and regeneration work that my team and myself are mainly engaged in, including scientific research, clinical treatment, epidemiology, policy advice, discipline construction, etc. My team is a relatively broad concept, including an innovative team from the PLA General Hospital (301 Hospital) and the First Affiliated Hospital of the PLA General Hospital (formerly 304 Hospital) that I led directly, including more than 20 years in the country. Under the"973", "863" projects, and the projects form National Natural Science Foundation of China, other units are involved in project completion, discipline construction, and personnel training and transformation of results, as well as closely connected teams and experts. These teams are from the Army Military Medical University and Shanghai Jiaotong University Affiliated Ruijin Hospital and Affiliated to the Ninth People's Hospital, The Second Affiliated Hospital Zhejiang University School of Medicine, Wenzhou Medical University and the People's Liberation Army 306 Hospital. The writing should reflect the characteristics of our team's disciplines in organizational rehabilitation and regeneration, including academic thinking, innovative cognition, struggle experience, innovative results, transformation of results and service clinical, discipline and team building, etc., not necessarily as comprehensive as textbooks. Taking the national "973", "863" projects, the new national key R&D plan project and the National Natural Science Foundation Innovation Group project as the traction, it reflects the national needs and will of the team engaged in regenerative medicine. It also reflects the related results finally obtained, such as theoretical discovery and innovation, product (technology) R&D and clinical applications, service-generating patient benefits, and access to national awards and international assessments.

After nearly a year of hard work, this monograph containing everyone's hard work resulted in the first draft. On the eve of its upcoming release, I am very excited and would like to give my thanks to Academician Ao Li, Academician Zhiyong Sheng, Academician Tianmin Cheng, Academician Shibi Lu, Academician Zuze Wu, Academician Zhengguo Wang, Professor Yinqiu Liu and other predecessors who gave me direct guidance and training during my growth and development. Without their guidance, I may not continue to explore without a goal in the academic ocean. It is impossible to achieve some achievements today without the careful guidance of Academician Zhengguo Wang. Thanks to Academician Zhengguo Wang and Academician Zuze Wu in their busy schedules, personally writing a preface for the publication of this monograph, fully affirming and encouraging the results achieved by my team. Thanks for giving me the opportunity to study abroad, so that I could study and understand the world in the early 1990s. I thank Prof. Pedro Cuevas Sanchez from the Hospital Ramon Y Cajal of the University of Madrid, Spain, and Prof. Gimenez-Gallego Guillermo, a member of the Spanish National Academy of Sciences, for helping me in the early days of my career. I also thank Dr. George W. Cherry, Professor Tan. Ryan, etc. from Churchill Hospital of Oxford University, UK. I am grateful to all the old colleagues and old friends who have worked with me at different stages after returning to China, especially Professor Xiaokun Li, associate senior technician Yaping Wang and technician Tongzhu Sun, who helped me in the early stages of my return. I am grateful to my students, especially a large number of previous students represented by Postdoctor Biao Cheng and Dr. Haihong Li. Your hard work has not only completed your studies but also promoted my development. You are also my friends. I am grateful for the specific assistance in the preparation of this monograph, especially the relevant experts who contributed different chapters and the press staff, especially associate senior editor Fang Guo of *Infection, Inflammation, and Rehabilitation*. With your specific work, this monograph can be published.

Finally, I would like to thank my family, especially my parents; when I was very young, they urged me to take time to learn and set a great goal; my wife, Ms. Xiaoling Wang, for her hard work and firm support; and my daughter Shanshan, her husband David H and their babies Charlotte and Catherine who have brought me joy. These are the foundations of a person's development, and the foundation of success is in dispensable.

Like other monographs, despite careful design and careful deployment, it still seems to have flaws in content organization, writing style and text expression. I hope that experts can educate us and make criticisms and suggestions so that we can correct and improve our future work.

Beijing, China　　　　Xiaobing Fu

# Contents

# Editor and Contributors

## About the Editor

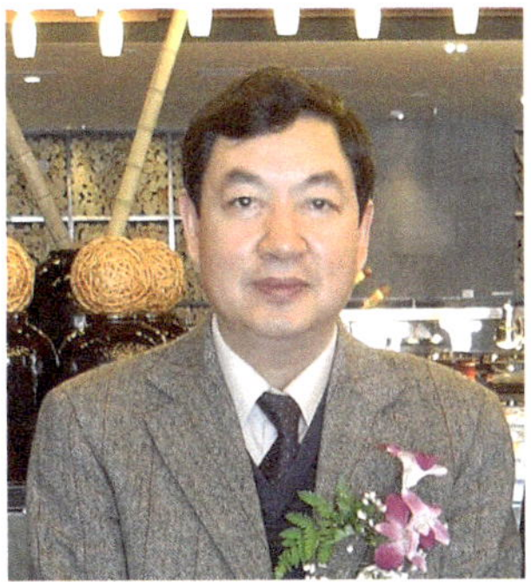

**Xiaobing Fu, MD, PhD** Academician of the Chinese Academy of Engineering (Division of Medicine and Health) and Chinese Academy of Medical Sciences, President of the College of Life Science, the PLA General Hospital, Director of the Key Laboratory of Wound Repair and Regeneration of PLA, PLA Medical College.

He has made great contributions on trauma, especially in growth factors and stem cell biology, tissue repair and regenerative medicine. His works were supported in part by the National Basic Science and Development Programme (973 Programme), National High-Technique Programme (863 Programme), Grant for National Distinguished Young Scientists and Grant for National Natural Science Foundation of China. He has published more than 600 scientific papers, including papers published in the Lancet (1998, 2001), and 28 books as the editor in chief, and won 25 international and national prizes of Sci-Tech Progress from 1989 to 2015.

He was the member of the Scientific Committee of the Third Joint Meeting of the European Tissue Repair Society and the Wound Healing Society held in Boudreaux in 1999, the Scientific Committee Member, Advisor or Member of the International Faculty from the First World Union of Wound Healing Societies (WUWHS) Congress to 5th WUWHS Congress, held in Melbourne in 2000, Toronto in Canada in 2008, Yokohama in Japan in 2012 and Florence in Italy in 2016. He was the Vice Chairman of Trauma and Burn Section of the International Conference on Life Science and Clinical Medicine in 2000.

He was the Chairman of Chinese Trauma Society from 2010 to 2013. Now, he is the Chairman of the Asian Wound Care Association (AWCA), the President of Chinese Society for Biomaterials, the President of the Chinese Tissue Repair Society (CTRS), President of the Chinese Tissue Repair and Regeneration Society (CTRRS) and the member of National Natural Science Foundation of China.

Professor Fu was awarded the International Lifetime Achievement Award in Wound Repair and Regeneration in 2008. He was selected as the Academician (Chinese Academy of Engineering, Division of Medicine and Health) in 2009, Chinese Academy of Medical Sciences in 2019 and the Foreign

Academicians of France Academy of Medicine in 2018 and National Academy of Engineering, USA in 2021. Also, he was selected as the fellow of American Institute for Medical and Biological Engineering (AIMBE) College in 2018 and International Union of Societies for Biomaterials Science and Engineering (IUSBSE) in 2019.

## Contributors

**Andong Zhao** The Chinese People's Liberation Army General Hospital, Beijing, China

**Biao Cheng** General Hospital of Southern Theater Command of Chinese People's Liberation Army, Guangzhou, China

**Bin Yao** The Chinese People's Liberation Army General Hospital, Beijing, China

**Ce Yang** State Key Laboratory of Trauma, Burns and Combined Injury, Research Institute of Surgery, Daping Hospital, Army Medical University, Chongqing, China

**Changyong Wang** Academy of Military Medical Sciences, Military Cognition and Brain Science Research Institution, Beijing, China

**Zhaoyang Yang** Department of Neurobiology, School of Basic Medical Sciences, Capital Medical University, Beijing, China

**Chiyu Jia** Xiang'an Hospital Affiliated to Xiamen University, Xiamen, China

**Chong Huang** General Hospital of Southern Theater Command of Chinese People's Liberation Army, Guangzhou, China

**Chunmao Han** The Second Affiliated Hospital of Zhejiang University School of Medicine, Hangzhou, China

**Chunmeng Shi** Army Medical University, Chongqing, China

**Cuiping Zhang** The Chinese People's Liberation Army General Hospital, Beijing, China

**Duyin Jiang** The Second Hospital of Shandong University, Jinan, China

**Xiaobing Fu** The Chinese People's Liberation Army General Hospital, Beijing, China

**Haisheng Li** State Key Laboratory of Trauma, Burns and Combined Injury, Research Institute of Surgery, Daping Hospital, Army Medical University, Chongqing, China

**Hong Li** Academy of Military Medical Sciences, Military Cognition and Brain Science Research Institution, Beijing, China

**Hongmei Duan** Department of Neurobiology, School of Basic Medical Sciences, Capital Medical University, Beijing, China

**Hongmin Gong** The Second Hospital of Shandong University, Jinan, China

**Hongwei Liu** The First Affiliated Hospital of Jinan University, Guangzhou, China

**Hongyu Zhang** Wenzhou Medical University, Wenzhou, China

**Hua Qin** The Chinese People's Liberation Army General Hospital, Beijing, China

**Huiqi Xie** West China Hospital, Sichuan University, Chengdu, China

**Jialiang Zhu** The Chinese People's Liberation Army General Hospital, Beijing, China

**Jianfu Li** Huatai International Hospital, Guang'an City, Guang'an, China

**Jiang Wu** Wenzhou Medical University, Wenzhou, China

**Jian Xiao** Wenzhou Medical University, Wenzhou, China

**Jianxin Jiang** State Key Laboratory of Trauma, Burns and Combined Injury, Research Institute of Surgery, Daping Hospital, Army Medical University, Chongqing, China

**Jing Liu** Xiamen University School of Medicine, Xiamen, China

**Jin Zhou** Academy of Military Medical Sciences, Military Cognition and Brain Science Research Institution, Beijing, China

**Jixun Zhang** The Second Hospital of Shandong University, Jinan, China

**Lei Liu** The Second Hospital of Shandong University, Jinan, China

**Min Xuan** General Hospital of Southern Theater Command of Chinese People's Liberation Army, Guangzhou, China

**Nanbo Liu** Southern Medical University, Guangzhou, China

**Peng Hao** Department of Neurobiology, School of Basic Medical Sciences, Capital Medical University, Beijing, China

**Qi Wang** The Ninth People's Hospital, Shanghai Jiaotong University School of Medicine, Shanghai, China

**Quanyi Guo** The Chinese People's Liberation Army General Hospital, Beijing, China

**Rungong Yang** The Chinese People's Liberation Army General Hospital, Beijing, China

**Sha Huang** The Chinese People's Liberation Army General Hospital, Beijing, China

**Shenglin Qian** General Hospital of Southern Theater Command of Chinese People's Liberation Army, Guangzhou, China

**Shuliang Lu** Ruijin Hospital, Shanghai Jiaotong University School of Medicine, Shanghai Burns Institute, Shanghai Wound Healing Institute, Shanghai, China

**Shuyong Wang** The Chinese People's Liberation Army General Hospital, Beijing, China

**Siming Yang** The Chinese People's Liberation Army General Hospital, Beijing, China

**Ting Xie** The Ninth People's Hospital, Shanghai Jiaotong University School of Medicine, Shanghai, China

**Wei Dong** The First Affiliated Hospital of Jinan University, Guangzhou, China

**Weimin Guo** The Chinese People's Liberation Army General Hospital, Beijing, China

**Wei Wang** The Second Hospital of Shandong University, Jinan, China

**Wen Zhao** Department of Neurobiology, School of Basic Medical Sciences, Capital Medical University, Beijing, China

**Xiaochuan Wang** The Second Hospital of Shandong University, Jinan, China

**Xiaoguang Li** Department of Neurobiology, School of Basic Medical Sciences, Capital Medical University, Beijing, China

**Xiaokun Li** Wenzhou Medical University, Wenzhou, China

**Xiaoning Yang** Academy of Military Medical Sciences, Military Cognition and Brain Science Research Institution, Beijing, China

**Xiao Wang** The Second Hospital of Shandong University, Jinan, China

**Xiaoyan Sun** The Chinese People's Liberation Army General Hospital, Beijing, China

**Ya Jiao** The Second Hospital of Shandong University, Jinan, China

**Yao Lu** The Chinese People's Liberation Army General Hospital, Beijing, China

**Yingkai Liu** Ruijin Hospital, Shanghai Jiaotong University School of Medicine, Shanghai Burns Institute, Shanghai Wound Healing Institute, Shanghai, China

**Yiwen Niu** Ruijin Hospital, Shanghai Jiaotong University School of Medicine, Shanghai Burns Institute, Shanghai Wound Healing Institute, Shanghai, China

**Yongjun Qi** The Second Hospital of Shandong University, Jinan, China

**Yudan Gao** Department of Neurobiology, School of Basic Medical Sciences, Capital Medical University, Beijing, China

**Yuehong Shen** The Second Affiliated Hospital of Zhejiang University School of Medicine, Hangzhou, China

**Yuesheng Huang** Shenzhen People's Hospital, The First Affiliated Hospital of Southern University of Science and Technology, The Second Clinical Medical College of Jinan University, Shenzhen, China

**Yufeng Jiang** The Chinese People's Liberation Army Strategic Support Force Characteristic Medical Center, Beijing, China

**Yunfang Wang** Academy of Military Medical Sciences, Military Medical Research Institute, Beijing, China

**Yu Zhang** Nanjing Drum Tower Hospital, Nanjing, China

**Zuguo Liu** Xiamen University School of Medicine, Xiamen, China

# 1 Introduction to the Repair and Regeneration of War Wound Tissue

Biao Cheng, Siming Yang, and Xiaobing Fu

## 1.1 A Brief History of the Development of War Wound Tissue Repair and Regenerative Medicine

Trauma is the oldest medical problem. Because since the birth of mankind, there has been a history of people fighting against nature. In order to survive, human beings will experience falls and various injuries during activities such as hunting and fruit picking. Trauma has become one of the earliest forms of human disease, and it has been used in the continuous exploration of such things as clay and charcoal. The hemostasis of wound, sputum wounds, chewing plants applied to the wound surface to accelerate healing and complete the most primitive wound healing prototype of human beings. With the development of mankind, wars began to emerge due to the emergence of classes and religions. Ambulance and healing wounded and sick became the origin of war trauma medicine. War became one of the important factors in promoting the theory and technology development of trauma treatment. The development and upgrading of war further promote the theoretical and clinical improvement of posttraumatic tissue repair and regeneration. Therefore, war wound and trauma are actually two areas under the big concept that are both interconnected and have certain connotations. Trauma is the general concept of injury, while war wound is a special form of trauma. Fourth century BC, war wounds were cold weapon wounds, and the treatment was very simple. From the fourteenth century, firearms gradually replaced cold weapons, and a large number of armed forces completely changed the nature of war wounds. In the sixteenth century, French surgeon Ambroise Paré (1510–1590) suggested that due to the large amount of peripheral tissue damage caused by firearm injuries, the wound should be incision when the wound is severe. The word "debridement" appeared in the seventeenth century. In the eighteenth century, the initial treatment of firearm injuries included incision, resection, and drainage. During the Napoleonic Wars, Dominique-Jean Larrey (1766–1842) set a precedent for regular and certain system of battlefield ambulances, transporting the wounded to safe areas for further treatment, and establishing aid station. The foundation for modern trauma repair medicine has been laid. During the First World War, the number of people killed on the battlefield was about 10 million, and the number of injured reached more than 20 million. During the Second World War, the belligerents lost a total of about 50 million people. The number of casualties far exceeded that of the First World War. This fully shows that the weapons are more and more advanced, and the killing power is getting bigger and bigger. In addition to the early field ambulance to save the lives of the wounded, millions of wounded in the later stage in order to reduce disability need to obtain ideal and fine repair and reconstruction treatment. Surgeons face a large number of tissues and organs that need to be repaired and reconstructed, such as cracked skulls, severe facial burns, crushed jaw bones, nose and lip gunshot wounds, etc. The type and severity of trauma is unprecedented. Past war statistics show that during the Second World War (1939–1945), the total number of US casualties reached 963,403, of which 291,557 (30%) died in combat. In the Vietnam War (1955–1975), the total number of casualties in the US military was 200,727, and the number of deaths in combat was 47,424 (24%). With the further improvement of transportation tools, communication means, medical and health equipment, as well as the improvement in the quality and technology of the rescue personnel, the fatality rate of war wounds has gradually declined. According to the statistics of the US Department of Defense on November 17, 2004, the number of casualties of the US military in the wars in Afghanistan and Iraq reached 10,726, of which 1004 were killed in combat, accounting for only 10%. Therefore, a lot of work is repair and functional reconstruction. In the era of peace, the number of deaths from traffic injuries caused

B. Cheng
General Hospital of Southern Theater Command of Chinese People's Liberation Army, Guangzhou, China

S. Yang · X. Fu (✉)
The Chinese People's Liberation Army General Hospital, Beijing, China



X. Fu (ed.), *Regenerative Medicine in China*, https://doi.org/10.1007/978-981-16-1182-7_1

by the rapid development of transportation has greatly increased, which has become one of the important causes of injury in modern society. In addition to the casualties caused by other factors, trauma has become the main cause of death in modern society. In 1966, the American Academy of Sciences published a programmatic document entitled *Injury Caused by Accidental Injuries, a Disease Neglected by Modern Society*, which changed people's perceptions of trauma, from "trauma is an accident" to "trauma is a disease that can be prevented and controlled," effectively promoting the development of modern trauma first-aid systems, basic research, technology research, and clinical treatment. The establishment of a trauma emergency center and a first-aid system is the basis for standardized treatment of trauma, and each state has established its own regional trauma emergency center. Since then, the developed countries, such as Britain, France, Germany, and Japan, have also established their own trauma emergency systems. After more than 30 years of development, developed countries have formed a relatively complete network of trauma emergency and formulated various corresponding normative documents. It significantly improved the success rate of trauma treatment. In Canada, for example, the ever-improving trauma emergency system has reduced the severe trauma mortality rate from 51.8% in 1992 to 8.6% in 2002. At present, the concept of war wound treatment has changed a lot. In addition to the wounded directly caused by the war, the treatment of wounded people in nonwar military operations (including major natural disasters, counterterrorism, and stability) is also included in the scope of war wound treatment. At the same time, war wound treatment is no longer a patent for army surgeon, and many nonmilitary hospitals have directly or indirectly participated in the treatment of war wounds. With the increase in the number of noncombatants injured in modern conflicts, the equipment and technology for traumatic treatment in peacetime cannot meet the requirements for treatment. Therefore, it is imperative to establish a complete war wound treatment system, linking the site, transshipment, hospital treatment, and later rehabilitation and regeneration to form a complete chain of treatment. In addition, due to changes in social development and disease spectrum, various tissue damages caused by diseases, such as the treatment of diabetic foot (the important complication of diabetes), have also been included in the scope of trauma treatment, which deserves everyone's attention.

### 1.1.1 A Brief Review of the Development of Traumatic Repair Medicine in the World War

As early as 3500 BC, the Mesopotamia region, one of the birthplaces of the four major civilizations, had records of doctors participating in war wounds. In ancient Egypt, there were 48 examples of how wounds were treated in 1600 BC, and they were similar to today's surgical treatment principles; there was also a mixture of gum, goat's milk, and human milk to treat burns. In 600 BC, Chinese people used tinctures or tea extracts rich in tannin to converge on the wounds, while the Romans used honey and exposed treatments for burns. In the decree of the Babylonian dynasty, there is also a record of "if the free man dies due to surgery, the surgeon's right hand must be cut off." There is still no systematic understanding of anatomy in this period, and there is still limited progress in surgical medicine to the Middle Ages (sixth–fifteenth century). In the era of the Roman Empire, from 30 BC to 38 AD, the highly educated Roman aristocrat Celsus had reconstructed the surgical repairs of the glans, face, lips, nose, and ears of the Roman soldiers. In Egypt, according to historical records, ancient Egyptians did not perform reconstructive surgery using living tissue transplantation as a means. In ancient India, there was a nose-cutting wind. The winner of the war could cut off the nose of his prisoners of war. The government could impose a cut-off sentence on the criminals to show punishment. Therefore, the lack of nose in this period is no shortage of people. Since the position of the nose is most prominent on the face, its deformity is very significant, so most people who lack the nose are eager to get a new nose. In order to meet this need, the Indian society invented the forehead midline flap for nasal reconstruction.

In the ninth century BC, the ancient Greek epics Iliad and Odyssey recorded some treatments for orthopedic diseases such as trauma. In the sixth century BC, the Indian Sushruta Samhita described a technique in detail in his related medical monograph *The Collection*, which is a reconstructive surgery for the repair of organ defects. At the same time, the book also describes the surgical suture and suture line in detail. From the fifth century BC to the fourth century BC, the ancient Greek famous doctor Hippocrates (460 BC–370 BC), regarded as the "father of medicine," explained the importance of hemostasis, bandaging, and providing cleaned equipment and the concept of "War is the only proper school of the surgeon" was presented. The school's principle of dealing with wounds is to keep the wounds quiet and minimize external stimuli. The careful docking can heal the broken tissues and bones. This is the prototype of the theory of surgical sutures and fracture repair. *The Hippocrates Collection* records manual reduction, external fixation of the splint can treat limb fractures, and dislocation of the joints. The Hippocratic Reduction for shoulder dislocation is still used in clinical practice. Later, Rome's most famous surgeon, Galen (130—200? AD), sutured the sword cut for the gladiator and tried the repair of muscles and nerves, laying the anatomical basis for the traumatic surgery of Western medicine. His work has influenced people's perceptions of soft tissue repair for centuries.

In the first century, the Celsus people mentioned the use of alcohol and myrrh (myrrh is a tropical resin, which can be used as a medicinal material) to make an antibacterial detergent to treat burns. Galen uses vinegar and wound exposure technique to treat burns.

In the seventh century (around 695), the nose of the Byzantine Emperor Justinian II was cut off in a mess. Because the forehead skin was used to repair the reconstructed nose to form a distinct scar, which did not meet the rules that the emperor could not have obvious physical defects at the time, he could not return to the throne of the emperor. In the thirteenth century, Theodoric had a new and deeper understanding of wound healing, especially delayed healing, and he made a significant contribution to the formation of modern concepts in military surgical wound healing. From 1337 to 1453, the Hundred Years' War between Britain and France was intermittently carried out for 116 years. In the war, a lot of new weapons emerged. Especially in the later period, the large-scale use of gunpowder and artillery by the French army not only rewrote the war process, but also brought a large number of wounded people with serious injuries or burns, which accelerated the development of trauma repair surgery. While saving the lives of soldiers, we should minimize the disability of injured soldiers, so that they can return to society. This becomes an important job in trauma repair surgery. In the fourteenth century, the surgeon of the Bavarian army, Pfolspreundt, described rhinoplasty, and the surgeon of the Alsatian army, Brunschwig, contributed to the gunshot wound. By the fifteenth century, Brancas used Italian-style nasal reconstruction to avoid facial scarring. In the sixteenth century, Copernicus's *On the Revolutions of the Heavenly Spheres* was published. Since then, the development of the natural science has dealt a heavy blow to religious theology. This is not only a revolution in the history of science, but also an ideological emancipation movement. Subsequently, the publication of Vesalius's *Structure of the Human Body* freed medicine from the idealistic theology and laid the foundation for modern anatomy. Ambroise Paré (1510–1590) was hailed as one of the founders of modern surgery for his great contribution to surgery. He first proposed the use of ointment burns. During the Renaissance, Gaspare Tagliacozzi (1546–1599), a well-known anatomist and surgical professor at the University of Bologna in Italy, used a single-armed flap to create a new nose for patients with nasal defects. This technique is described in great detail in his surgical monograph. In the seventeenth century, the rapid development of physics and mechanics quickly penetrated into the medical field, bringing unprecedented prosperity to medicine and laying the foundation for the rise of trauma surgery. In 1610s, the British anatomist Harvey reported "blood circulation and its structure of bone tissue," pioneered the anatomical physiology of bone tissue, and made human understanding of bone from macro to micro. In 1741, based on the development of anatomy and anatomical physiology, Nicholas Andre first proposed the scientific name of orthopedics at the University of Paris and was widely accepted, marking the rise of modern orthopedics. Because traumatic orthopedics is the essence of the initial orthopedics (because humans have a relatively shallow understanding of orthopedic infections, tumors, etc., traumatic orthopedics have not yet differentiated from the big family of orthopedics), so the rise of modern orthopedics also reflects the rise of trauma repair science. In 1812, Dominique-Jean Larrey first reported the trench foot. In the early nineteenth century, Dupuytren studied on 50 burn patient treated with bandage therapy and proposed a classification of burn depth. The Englishman Joseph Lister (1827–1912), the founder of the surgical disinfection method, contributed a lot to the treatment of trauma. He first proposed lacking disinfection is the main cause of infection after surgery. Since his publication in 1867, the postoperative mortality rate reduced from 45% to 15% in less than 10 years, saving hundreds of millions of lives. Later, the German surgical specialist Friedrich von Esmarch (1823–1908) invented the first-aid kit and the tourniquet in 1876.

During the American Civil War, Jones suggested a one-stage repair of damaged facial wounds and advocated retaining the skin as much as possible. The necessary trimming of the edges of the irregular wounds should be carried out. Plastic surgeons began to recreate eyelids, nose, cheeks, lips, moles, and chin. Buck completed the first major reconstruction of the total damage, nasal reconstruction with forehead flap. In 1832, the French army's gunner, Louis, in the Siege of Antwerp, was almost killed by the pieces of artillery shells. The left cheek and most of the upper lip were missing, and the right side involved a 1.25-cm earlobe. The soft palate was extensively torn to the upper esophagus, the tongue was extensively avulsed, the lower jaw was almost completely defected, and the four molars were broken. Only a small right side part of the mandible is still intact. His right forearm was a composite fracture with an extensive soft tissue damage caused by shrapnel. M. Louis was immediately taken to the Hoboken Battlefield Hospital, and some thought his death was inevitable. Dr. Forjet, as a surgeon in the Northern Army, completed a preliminary maxillofacial hemostasis and debridement surgery and bandaged him. After the wound healed, the entire mandibular bone defect caused the craniofacial deformity made him almost unable to eat and talk. At that time, no relevant doctors had the knowledge to solve the problem of reconstructing the chin. A silversmith used a mask to cover the missing face. The first to describe this incident was Ballingall, a professor of military surgery at Edinburgh. For almost a century, British and French soldiers masked their face deformities if they had severe facial damage.

In 1863, Gibson completed a complex orthopedic surgery during military service to repair the loss of the lower jaw and lower lip due to gunshot wounds. In the same year, Gouley completed a mandibular reconstruction with two rotating flaps. In 1868, the US military surgeon Prince pointed out that plastic surgery had a lot of uses in military surgery. As a medical inspector of the US military, Hamilton made an outstanding contribution to plastic surgery. That is the application of the transfer flap increased the local blood supply. On the 14th day, the cross-leg flap successfully broken ensured the flap survival rate.

The war has a significant role in promoting the development of modern trauma repair surgery. This can be seen from the incidence of bone trauma in war. In the Franco-Prussian War of 1870–1871, the incidence of limb injuries was 72.5%. In a short period of time, the emergence of a large number of casualties is not only a promotion for the development of traumatic orthopedics, but also provides a lot of practical opportunities and lessons worth summing up, so that the trauma orthopedics can be quickly promoted and developed. The plaster-fixing technique was invented by the Belgian military doctor Antonius Mathijsen during the war and quickly promoted.

In the middle of the nineteenth century, the Russian military doctor Pirogov made a major contribution to the treatment of war injuries. He focused on the systemic reaction of the wounded and fixed it with ether and plaster bandages. In the field of trauma care, an outstanding figure, Nightingale, who reduced the death rate of British soldiers from 50% to 2.2% in the Crimean War, is recognized as the founder and pioneer of modern nursing and nursing education.

In the twentieth century, the outbreak of the two world wars made the trauma repair surgery develop rapidly and was continuously subdivided and improved.

During the First World War, many new weapons, such as tanks and airplanes, were invented, which caused a large number of serious wound-burning patients. On the other hand, although the use of trenches and steel helmets had saved the lives of many warriors, it also brought a lot of facial and neck injuries, especially bone and soft tissue defects of the maxillofacial region. Nonfatal jaw and facial trauma accounted for 10% of the total body trauma, and these wounded were urgently required for advanced repair surgery. Take the German army as an example, the percentage of limb injuries was 63.3%. Therefore, doctors from the United Kingdom, France, Germany, and Russia faced such serious and numerous patients, and established teams of surgeons. The plastic surgery, trauma orthopedics (including hand surgery), and reconstructive surgery developed rapidly, and at the same time a large number of well-known trauma repair surgeons appeared, like Varaztad Kazanjian, Blair, Maliniac, and Gustave in the United States, Veau and Dufourmentel in France, Trueta in Spain, Lexer in Germany, Gillies and Rainsford Mowlem in the United Kingdom, Hâlit Ziyâ Konuralp and Cihat Borçbakan in Turkey, Risdon and Waldron in Canada, Henry Pickerill in New Zealand, Newland in Australia, etc. Blair of the United States and Kazanjian, a French dentist, returned to the United States to create plastic surgery and craniofacial surgery there. Kazanjian, who is revered as the "Western Line Legend," became the first professor of plastic surgery at Harvard University. In the 15th volume of the book *The Medical Department of the United States Army in the World War*, there are three chapters in the 11th volume that cover the craniofacial surgery. In 1917, surgeon Gorgas formed plastic surgery and oral surgery and assigned Blair to manage it. A dentist from Philadelphia, Ivy, was his assistant. Their primary task was to train general surgeons and dentists to work together on craniomaxillofacial wounds. In 1917, the initiative revised Blair's textbook *Surgery and Diseases of the Mouth and Jaws* in 1913. Some new information about gunshot wound treatment was compiled, and the plastic and oral parts were distributed to every hospital in the United States overseas. A summary of the latest articles on craniomaxillofacial surgery was published in the *Review of War Surgery and Medicine* and *Survey of Head Surgery*.

Captain Gillies, a New Zealand-born surgeon in the United Kingdom (later a major), made a significant contribution to the development of trauma repair surgery. His book, *Plastic Surgery of the Face*, described gunshot wounds, shell fragments, and some craniofacial damage that occurs in a car accident. Although Tagliacozzi had described the use of pedicle grafts to reconstruct the nose as early as in the sixteenth century, Gillies was not familiar with Tagliacozzi's classic surgery. He borrowed a book written by the German surgeon Lindemann, invited Morestin, the most famous French plastic surgeon at the time, to persuade medical authorities to form a special treatment center for craniofacial injuries. In less than a year, the Cambridge Hospital in Aldershot began work, and patients with facial injuries were sent to the new medical facility. Gillies took the £10 label written "the Faciomaxillary injury-cambridge hospital, Aldershot," to the hospital in France and pasted it on the injured person's chest. A total of nearly 2000 wounded people were sent there for treatment. He used the flap technique to reconstruct the nose, mouth, eyelids, and auricles, and filled the mandibular defects with ribs. Many complicated operations were original. For example, Gillies and his colleague the Royal dental specialist Valadier first attempted to reconstruct the anatomy and repair the mandibular defect with bone and other tissues, which is called the enlightenment of craniomaxillofacial surgery. The imagery of orthopedics is very important. Gillies asked Tonks to paint all the damage and surgery in picture. It still looks very rare today. Due to his contribution, Gillies was crowned by the British Empire after the war. After returning to the United Kingdom, he continued to work on plastic surgery. In his later book, *Principles and Art of Plastic Surgery*, Gillies left a large space for Millard to write the part of craniomaxillofacial surgery. There were many principles of emergency treatment for craniomaxillofacial surgery that occurred during the First World War, but perfected in the Second World War, combining dental expertise such as oral infections, injuries, and mandibular fractures, with the experience of ordinary surgeons. The treatment of patients with craniofacial and maxillofacial defects was completed by the designated hospital. He emphasized the need to initiate early treatment and make postrepair systematic. When there is a defect in the internal tissues of the mouth, the mandible, and the skin, it is desirable to immediately perform a good aesthetic substitution and restore normal function as soon as possible. The musculocutaneous flap and the free flap become the basic means of replacing the tissue, and many operations during this period have opened up a history. Filatov published a design on the tubular flap in 1917 to address chronic osteomyelitis. In addition to the skin tube, other important contributions of the First World War include: free cartilage graft reconstruction of the nose, double pedicle flap reconstruction of the lips, and repair of intraoral defects with cervical flap.

In the European theater of war during the Second World War, the 298th General Hospital in December 1942 established the first plastic surgery center, from then to Normandy landing on June 6, 1944, in just 18 months, the United Kingdom alone has 10 functionalities. The plastic surgery centers were located in Basingstoke, Gloucester, Birmingham, and Edinburgh. The African theater was located in Algiers and the Italian theater was in Naples. This allowed all the wounded to be effectively treated within a few hours of the injury. After the United States declared war on Japan and Germany, it sent troops from New York to England in October 1942. After landing in Liverpool, a burns hospital was established in November. The plastic surgery had a ward with 25 beds, and in May 1945, at the end of the European battlefield, there were three wards. Due to the use of aircraft and tanks, a large number of patients with burns and facial injuries appeared. In order to share the experience of treatment, the first plastic surgery magazine *The Brenthurst Papers* appeared in the United Kingdom, and it was also the first English plastic surgery journal. In the latter part of the war, nearly 11,572 craniofacial operations were performed at Queen's Hospital in Kent, England. The 4th Maxillofacial Surgery Unit in North Africa and Italy also handled nearly 5000 seriously wounded, including 3000 maxillofacial injuries and 1000 burn patients.

In the 1930s, there were only two plastic surgeons in the United Kingdom. At the beginning of the Second World War, there were four plastic surgeons in the United Kingdom, but by the end of the war, there were about 25 plastic surgeons. There were more than 150 plastic surgeons in the United States at this time. Davis even said that the development of plastic surgery in the United States was a gift from the Second World War to the United States. At the beginning of the Second World War, there were four plastic surgeons in Canada, of which Tilley handled hundreds of allied pilots who needed organ reconstruction for serious damage in the war. Some even joked that the wounded were like laboratory "guinea pigs," which brought Tilley and others back to Canada with a lot of experience in traumatic tissue repair. Even if the war was over, the war wound repair work had not stopped, and these "guinea pigs" continued to play their role.

If the First World War was only the initial establishment of craniofacial surgery, after the Second World War, the French plastic surgeon Tessier really created and developed the craniofacial surgery, with the help of neurosurgery colleague Guiot. A series of plastic surgeries were reformed according to the situation and used to correct facial deformities to bring them closer to normal facial contours. The Germans used mafenide acetate to treat open wounds during the Second World War. In addition, the true skin transplantation technology (first reported by German Bunger in 1823) was widely used and made breakthroughs by means of the treatment experience in the Second World War, and related tissue transplantations such as cartilage, fascia, fat, nerves, etc. appeared at this stage. Bunnel's professional training base for hand surgery has greatly improved the treatment of plastic surgery. At the same time, the psychological work of plastic surgery has also received great attention.

Before the Second World War, hand surgery was basically a blank field. In the 1930s, hand surgery was established in the United Kingdom, the United States, Germany, and Japan. With the advancement of human infection and control technology, hand surgery gradually progressed from the fingers/limbs/toes amputation to the fingers/limbs/toes salvage and put emphasis on functional recovery. In 1944, Sterling Bunnell published the first-hand surgery monograph *Surgery of the Hand*.

In the 1970s, debridement and other advances had significantly reduced mortality, and Andrew M. Munster began to focus on the quality of life of patients with severe burns. In 1979, the first published *Burn-Specific Health Scale* by him became an important work in modern burns research.

During the Korean War, Vietnam War, and Iran-Iraq War, with the development of microsurgery, vascular surgery had made tremendous progress, and the proportion of amputation had dropped to a very low level. At the same time, advances in vascular surgery have provided a strong guarantee for craniomaxillofacial surgery. Due to the impact of high-speed bullets, the damage to soldiers is often from outside to inside, accompanied by various tissue injuries such as skin, bones, and muscles, making the damage more serious and complicated, thus requiring higher repair. The iliac crests and fibulas have reliable vascular pedicles, and secondary deformities are few, often used as donor sites to repair composite tissue defects.

In short, the modern trauma repair surgery has evolved to the present, largely influenced by the two world wars of the first half of the twentieth century. Modern war weapons are rapidly updated. High-speed, high-killing weapons cause a high incidence of bone and soft tissue trauma, and the injury is more complicated. In addition, nerve and blood vessel damage, multiple injuries, and combined injuries are more and more. In the Malvinas War, the rate of limb injury was 67.5% and severe trauma accounted for 90%. How to reduce the health reduction, ensure the combat effectiveness of the troops, and adapt the trauma orthopedics to the needs of military medical support in modern warfare is an important research topic for trauma orthopedics.

After the Second World War, more than 200 local wars or armed conflicts occurred in the world, and new research topics were constantly raised in the tissue repair surgery of the wounds. Russia has conducted an in-depth research on the injury condition, category of wound, injury characteristics, and the organization and management of surgical treatment in local wars or armed conflicts, and introduced the concept of early specialist treatment.

The characteristics of the treatment on the wounded in local wars or armed conflicts are: the war is carried out in a limited area, the human and material resources are limited, and the number of casualties arriving at the rescue ladder is significantly less; due to the effective helicopter air transport, the time for the injured to reach the ladder rescue unit is obviously short; medical conditions improved, early specialist treatment is feasible; not many combat personnel, however, medical ambulance personnel have sufficient reserves, can continuously use to gather strength, and can widely use efficient battlefield surgical techniques. Accordingly, the Russian field surgery focused on the issue of the organization of the wounded in local wars. In the Afghan War and the Chechnya War, due to the widespread use of helicopter evacuation, reducing the level of stairs, shortening the time of specialist treatment, the death rate of the Afghan War was reduced to 4.7%, and the return rate reached 82%. In combination with the actual situation of the war, the study on a large number of mine blast injuries during the war in Afghanistan proposed measures to reduce the complications and casualties. In the treatment of firearm long bone fractures, they first used external fixation devices, first used temporary blood vessels during aortic injury. At the same time, in the treatment of the wounded, a two-step treatment mode was implemented, that is, after the first medical treatment, the wounded were directly sent to the first-step multispecialty hospital for specialist treatment, and new treatment techniques, such as external fixation, endoscopic, injury control techniques, and comprehensive treatment techniques for infection complications, were used in actual combat. In addition, with the development of science and technology and the application of telemedicine technology, it may have an important impact on the application of organization, service, and technology for trauma treatment.

In addition to the above brief historical review, since the beginning of the twentieth century, international scholars have made rapid progress in the basic research, product development, clinical treatment, and discipline construction of war wound tissue repair and regeneration, which has significantly promoted the discipline to a certain extent. It is mainly manifested in: the understanding of tissue repair and regeneration process is further deepened, from the traditional general, tissue, and cellular levels to the molecular and genetic levels. The representative event is the research of growth factors involved in tissue regulation and regeneration in the 1990s and the development of a genetic engineering drug represented by the basic fibroblast growth factor (bFGF) for wound burn wound treatment; the description of the connotation of the repair and regenerative treatment process from the past using three "Rs" (Resection, Repair, and Replacement) to summarize the disposal concept, and later added the fourth "R," that is, regeneration. Later, Xiaobing Fu and other experts recognized the important role of rehabilitation theory, techniques, and methods in tissue repair and regeneration, and proposed rehabilitation as the fifth "R" for perfect repair and regeneration, thereby damaged tissue repair and regeneration forming an organized whole [1, 2] in the treatment technology, the method of debridement of damaged tissue has been developed from the simple use of scalpel debridement to the use of protease debridement, ultrasonic debridement, and other methods to make debridement more precise and beneficial to post-tissue repair and regeneration; breakthroughs in the theory of wound wet healing have enabled many advanced dressings (revolutionary dressings) to be developed, produced, and used in clinical applications. Since then, the theory and technology of using dressings to promote wound healing have been initiated. It has played a major role in shortening the wound healing time, reducing the intensity of nursing, and improving the quality of patients. The technology of tissue engineering has enabled people to construct related tissue repair materials in vitro, thus changing or repairing the damaged tissue; with the breakthrough in genetic engineering technology, people can produce large quantities of proteins or peptides for tissue repair and regeneration to regulate the proliferation and differentiation of repair cells at the molecular and genetic levels; in addition, the establishment and development of negative pressure drainage techniques, physical or chemical methods, and tissue repair of sound, light, electricity, magnetism, oxygen, etc. The elaboration of the regenerative relationship has made many techniques and methods have been applied to the treatment of tissue repair and regeneration, and has become an important means of modern wound repair and tissue regeneration. In the discipline construction, it is proposed to treat wounds (especially various complicated and refractory wounds) as a large class of complex diseases caused by various reasons [3, 4]. In view of the characteristics of wounds, especially the rising incidence of various chronic refractory wounds, the more and more complicated pathogenesis, and the increasing difficulty of treatment, the authors put forward the idea of establishing a specialist for wound healing (center) and carrying out special treatment for wounds. At the same time, in order to shorten the hospitalization time of patients with chronic refractory wounds, a new model of two-way linkage between the wound treatment specialists of large hospitals and the wound treatment points of community health institutions was developed. Through advanced technologies such as "4G" and Wi-Fi, the hospital's wound treatment specialists are linked to the community to ensure the treatment of patients at the grassroots level. These theories have been validated in later clinical practice and have played an important role in improving wound healing speed and improving healing quality. Theories, techniques, and methods for these innovations will be described in detail in later relevant chapters.

### 1.1.2 A Brief History of the Development of Trauma Repair in Ancient China

Among the various diseases, the earliest and most experienced is surgery. It can be said that from the Stone Age, there has been a certain knowledge of healing damage. Traditional Chinese medicine surgery was initially formed in the Shang, Zhou, Qin, and Han Dynasties. In the Jin and Song Dynasties, relatively systematic surgery was performed, especially the theory of traumatology. At that time, the famous Gao Boji, Liu Juanzi, and others had worked for a great development of the principle, diagnosis, and treatment methods for carbuncle-abscess of the back, compared with what the *Lingshu* had said. At that time, the treatment methods such as trauma anastomosis and suture were different, but most of them have a great scientific value. For example, mulberry bark is used as suture for suturing wounds, bamboo curtains, splints, etc. can be used in fixed reduction, etc., and all these have achieved the desired therapeutic effect. In short, although the subject originated from the Hua Tuo in the second century AD, it was much later.

In the case of Jinchuang, there were two famous books, but unfortunately both of them were lost. Gan's hereditary family had a profound medical history and many writings, and left a glorious historical record in the history of traumatic science in China.

As for the masterpieces in surgery, there are endless streams. For example, "*Lingshu,*" "*Liu Juanzi Guiyi Fang,*" "*Yongjubu Dang zabing Jiyuan,*" "*Ge's Fang,*" "*Xiaopin Fang,*" "*Waike Zhengzong,*" "*Treatment of phlegm and blood stasis,*" etc., all provide a wealth of practical and theoretical guidance for future. Among them, the "*Liu Juanzi Guiyi Fang*" written by Gong Qingxuan in Nanqi is the earliest surviving surgical book in China with great practical value.

For a long time in the past, the Chinese have always believed that "the body is affected by the parents and does not dare to damage." In the oracle bones of the Shang Dynasty in the fourteenth century BC, there were records of the words "jie" and "sore." In the Zhou Dynasty (1046 BC–256 BC), surgery became an independent procedure, and surgeons called it the "drug medicine." The "drug medicine" recorded in "*Zhou Li*" is responsible for the treatment of "tumor, ulcer, golden ulcer, and ulcer." The term "golden ulcer" as used herein, that is, "Jinchuang" refers to the wound caused by the metal blade to damage the limb; "Folding and ulceration" summarizes the diseases such as bone fracture and bone injury caused by hitting, smashing, falling, and fluttering. The treatment methods are also relatively rich. In addition to oral administration of traditional Chinese medicine, there are also treatments such as dressing (giving medicine) and surgery (scrapping). At that time, although there was no monograph on traumatology, it was recorded in several of the oldest medical literatures in the same period. For example, in the "*Huangdi Neijing,*" there is a discussion of the symptoms, diagnosis, and treatment of bruises. There are dozens of drugs in the "*Shennong Bencaojing*" collected by the "Master Jin Chuang continued bones and bones." The "*Jingui Yaolüe*" contains the prescriptions for the treatment of "golden sores," Wangbuliuxing San, and the treatment of horses and some bone and bone injuries. It can be seen that traumatology had achieved certain development at that time. "*Lingshu·Jingshui*" pointed out: "If the husband of the eight-footer, the flesh is here, the outside can be measured, and it can be obtained by cutting it. The death can be dissected and viewed." "*Lingshu·Boneness*" through the measures of the length, size, and width of human skeleton, and divides the standard deviation according to the head, torso, and limbs. "*Lingshu·Jingjin*" discusses the muscle system attached to the first and second meridians. The development of anatomy and physiology has significantly promoted the development of traumatology. In the ninth century, the first traumatic orthopedics monograph "*Xianshou Lishang Xuduan Mifang*" came out, forming a treatment of fractures with the principle of "reconstruction, fixation, activity and internal and external medication," marking a human understanding of trauma orthopedics. Gradually deepened, the formation of the traumatic orthopedics.

During the Spring and Autumn Period and the Warring States Period, traditional Chinese medicine Surgery began to take shape. Ma Wangdui Han Tomb's book "*Mai Fa*" has long been used to treat sputum and purulent sputum, and the pus deep sputum shallow, pus shallow sputum deep, pus large sputum small, four kinds of situation and the size of the meteorite does not match "Four evils." "*Shan Hai Jing*" said: "The Mountain of Gao there are many meteorites." Guo Pu note: "Acupuncture needles, cure sputum." At that time, the needle was the tool to cut the pus and the earliest surgical instrument. The "*52 Bing Fang*" is another early medical literature that records various surgical diseases such as trauma and frostbite. The "*Lingshu·YongJu*" in the theoretical work "*Nei Jing*" records 17 kinds of surgical diseases and has a considerable understanding of the etiology and pathology of sputum. It must be soft, but the stone is born. "Stone" is the meaning of cutting stone, also known as phlegm or phlegm. Some chapters propose the use of toe surgery to treat gangrene, indicating that surgery has greatly improved from theory to practice.

The Han Dynasty (206 BC–220 AD) was the prosperous era of the traditional Chinese medicine. Hua Tuo, a well-known traumatic medical scientist in history, could treat diseases with prescriptions and acupuncture, and was better at surgery. Extremely high surgical skills have prompted him to use surgery for wound healing, elimination of purulent infections, and treatment of visceral diseases. Moreover, he used the "powder for anesthesia" anesthesia to perform surgery on patients, which is the earliest record of the use of general anesthesia for surgical treatment in the history of medical science in the world.

In the Jin Dynasty, Chen Yanzhi wrote "*Xiaopin Fang*" to record the earliest use of "fire needles" for surgical diseases, such as "attached bones, if not lost when the time is lost, use fire needles, cream, scattered." The book "*Liu Juanzi Guiyi Fang*" written in 499 AD is the earliest existing surgery monograph in China.

The main content is the differential diagnosis of sputum. It summerized many in the treatment of cold sore, phlegm, and skin diseases. Among them, Volume 4, "*Xiang Yongju Zhi Younong Ke Po Fa*," the use of the sputum needle to smash the "pum up the pus." The method of breaking the sputum "should be broken from the bottom, so that the pus easily." It is the pioneer of today's "low-level drainage" and "Where there is sepsis, all kinds of medicines are not broken, it is better to use a cooked copper needle on the oil fire, first use the ink pen to point to the head, then use the copper needle shallow needle, and the needle out of the pus, Shun also. If you do not pus with the needle, when using white paper for fine sputum, smash into the pinhole, lead to its sepsis, then swollen a few points will be good," this is the ancestor of the posterior sputum medicine line drainage method. Ge Hong's use of alpaca (e.g., wildflowers) and aconite as an anesthetic drug is an early stage in the development of surgical anesthetics, which is of great significance. At the same time, there are records of treatment of water and fire.

In the Sui Dynasty (581–618), Chao Yuanfang's "*Zhu Bing Yuan Hou Lun*" explored the source of various diseases, and the nine waiting items listed more than 1700 diseases, which was the first pathological monograph in China. The book "*Jinchuang Shangjing Duangu Hou*" states that after a tendon injury, it can cause circulatory disorders (the camp is impassable). Although the wound is healed, the symptoms of nerve palsy and dyskinesia can still be left behind, and the wound must be treated immediately after the injury. It introduced the correct point of stitching. Even the "8" suture method and continuous suture method are introduced in detail, and it is pointed out that if the suture is improper, it will cause infection. Once the infection occurs, the suture should be removed. For those with serious pollution, it is recommended to avoid suturing for drainage. The previous related treatment theories are more complete.

In the Tang Dynasty (618–907), Sun Simiao recorded the reduction method of temporomandibular joint dislocation in "*Qian Jin Fang*." "A person takes a finger and pulls it to gradually push it, then he re-enters the cockroach, pushes it out, and fears that the person is also hurting." And pointed out that after the restoration, wax therapy and hot compress can be used to help the recovery of joint function. This is the world's first method of treatment for the dislocation of the temporomandibular joint, which is still widely used until now. Sun Simiao also used cannabis as an anesthetic drug and studied the depth of anesthesia, the amount of use, and the rescue of poisoning. Wang Tao wrote "*Waitai Miyao*" and advocated using the felt as a moist heat to relieve the pain of the injured limb. Wang Tao's "*Waitai Miyao*" is treated with a bamboo tube. "Repeatedly boiled. And the hot out of the tube, the place where the cage ink is pressed for a long time. The knife is used to break the corner. Bring to a boil and repeat heavy angle. When the yellow and white waters are out, there are pus outs, and there are also insects. Counting such a horn, the evils are exhausted, that is, they are removed. The day is light and light." This is the most detailed drainage of the bamboo tube at that time. Lin Daoren wrote "*Xianshou Lishang Xuduan Mifang*," which is the first traumatic monograph in China. It describes the treatment principles of fractures for correct reduction, splinting, functional exercise, drug treatment, and fracture healing.

In the Song Dynasty (960–1279), surgery developed rapidly, and the incision and drainage technique was further developed. In the pathology, we pay attention to the relationship between the whole and the local. The treatment focuses on the combination of righting and stagnation, and internal and external treatment. The "*Sheng Ji Zonglu*" proposed "five good and seven evils," of which chapter 145 detailed the method of drainage. "*Taiping Shenghui Fang*" pointed out that the "five good and seven evils" should be identified, and the internal treatment methods such as internal elimination and Tori are summarized. The idea that the drainage should be cut in the treatment of pus is more positive than in the previous period. Chen Ziming's "*Waike Jingyao*" records multiple prescriptions of Tori's pus, which is still in clinical use.

In the Yuan Dynasty (1271–1368), the Mongolian people were good at riding and shooting, and they had considerable expertise in the traumatology department. Among the 13 subjects in the medical system, there were orthopedics. Wei Yilin's "*Shiyi Dexiao Fang*" has great achievements in the traumatology department. He believed that "the invading injury, the pain of the flesh and blood, the rectification is not allowed, first use the anesthetic clothes, until they do not know the pain, before they can start." The amount of anesthetic is determined according to the patient's age, physical condition, and bleeding, and then gradually increases or decreases according to the patient's anesthesia. "There is no need to take too much medicine." Wei Yilin is the first person in the world to treat spinal fractures by suspension reduction.

In the Ming Dynasty (1368–1644), there were 13 departments of large hospitals, among which there were orthopedics. Xue Ji wrote "*Zhengti Neiyao*," in which he pointed out: "If the limb is damaged, the qi and blood will be injured, the camp will be inconsistent, and the viscera will be disharmonious." The dialectical relationship between the local and the overall disease is clarified. This period is also an important stage in the development of TCM surgery, and the debridement and suturing has been further improved. In the Ming Dynasty, Chen Shigong, who is good at surgical treatment, clearly stated in the "*Waike Zhengzong*," "The person who has been necrotic cannot be resurrected, but only those who have not been necrotic in the future. But those who are not rotted, cut one by one." The understanding and elucidation of this issue is more thorough. Shen Douyuan in his book "*Waike Qi Xuan*" also said: "There is a necrosis, if the pain is difficult, get more rotten when it is considered to be urgent, the size of the necrosis or the method of cutting with a needle knife cannot be cured." Zhao Yizhen of the Ming Dynasty also pointed out, "If the pus is exhausted, use the cockroach to pick out the carrion and pus," in the "*Michuan Waike Fang*." Both have new supplements to the understanding on the removal of necrotic tissue and the severity of its problems, as well as treatment measures.

In the Qing Dynasty (1636–1911), the traumatology department had a new development. Wu Qian collected the great achievements of the traumatology department in the past and wrote "*Yizong Jinjian·zhenggu Xinfa Yaozhi*." This book systematically summarizes the experience of orthopedics before the Qing Dynasty. It described the bones, techniques, binding devices, and internal and external prescriptions of various parts of the human body. It is the most detailed book, both from theoretical and practical points of view, and has a picture and text. A more complete orthopedic book. In the late Qing Dynasty, Gao Wenjin wrote the "*Waike Tushuo*" (1856), which was an exegesis-based Chinese medicine surgery.

After the Opium War in 1840, China became a semicolonial and semifeudal country. With the cultural aggression of imperialism, Western medicine was introduced to China, and traditional Chinese medicine orthopedics was greatly devastated. During this period, there were very few books on orthopedics, and the extremely rich experience of traumatology was scattered among the older doctors and the public. It lacked finishing and improvement, and even almost lost.

In the 1920s and 1930s, some Chinese Western medicine orthopedic pioneers who received orthopedic training in Europe and the United States returned to China, and successively carried out orthopedic surgery in Shanghai, Beijing, Tianjin, and other big cities, opened Western medical orthopedic wards and orthopedic hospitals. The predecessors worthy of people's memory include Meng Jimao, Hu Lansheng, Niu Huisheng, Fang Xianzhi, Zhu Lvzhong, Ren Tinggui, Ye Yanqing, and others. In 1937, the orthopedic group was organized under the auspices of the Chinese Medical Association in Shanghai, which laid the foundation for the beginning of modern orthopedics in China.

After the founding of the People's Republic of China, the trauma department of traditional Chinese medicine has renewed its vitality. At the same time, Western medicine orthopedics has also developed rapidly in China. In the 1960s, Professor Fang Xianzhi and Shang Tianyu from Tianjin Hospital absorbed the advantages of traditional Chinese medicine orthopedics theory and Western medicine orthopedics. They proposed a new principle of fracture treatment including the combination of dynamic and static, both jin and bones, internal and external treatment, and doctor-patient cooperation, and published *Chinese and Western Medicine for the Treatment of Fractures* in 1966 to promote treatment experience in the country. In the 1950s, Beijing Jishuitan Hospital established a hand surgery specialty and opened a hand surgery ward. In 1960, Shanghai Huashan Hospital also established hand surgery. In 1978, China published the first classic of hand surgery *Hand Surgery*. In 1980, the Chinese Medical Association Orthopedics Society was established. After 1984, a number of professional groups were established. For example, in 1984, the Chinese Medical Association orthopedics branch established the Hand Surgery Group. In 1994, it was renamed the Chinese Medical Association Hand Surgery Society. In 1985, *the Journal of Hand Surgery* was officially launched. In 1993, it was renamed as *Chinese Hand Surgery Magazine*. In clinical work, the survival rate of replanted limbs (finger) was continuously improved, and famous surgeries, such as forearm flap (Yang Guofan), hand reconstruction (Yu Zhongjia), and replacement of C7 cervical nerve in the healthy side (Gu Yudong), were performed. In 1999, Professor Pei Guoxian of the Southern Hospital successfully carried out limb allograft (the third and fourth cases in the world). These achievements have made China's hand surgery a success.

Since the early 1960s, microsurgery in China has generally experienced three stages of initiation, development, and improvement/gradual maturity. From the early 1960s to the early 1970s, it was the initial stage of microsurgery in China. Design and improve microsurgical instruments, explore small vessel anastomosis, improve the patency rate of small blood vessel anastomosis, and carry out limb and finger replantation was the main progress at this stage. Professor Yang Dongyue explored boldly, pioneered, and innovated. In 1966 and 1973, he pioneered the second toe and free flap transplantation. In 1970, Gu Yudong first created a radial nerve transposition for the treatment of brachial plexus root avulsion, which made Chinese hand surgery rank first in the world of hand surgery. From the early 1970s to the mid-1980s, it was the development stage of microsurgery in China. Further improvement in the patency rate of small vessel anastomosis, extensive replantation of severed fingers, and expansion of the application field of microsurgical techniques are major advances in this phase. From the late 1980s to the present, it is in the improvement and gradual maturity stage of microsurgery in China. Microsurgical technology has matured and achieved fruitful results in basic and application fields. At the same time, it has gradually improved the theoretical aspect of the system and developed into an emerging clinical discipline. Chinese scholars have made important milestone contributions to the development of microsurgery [5, 6].

The real surgical treatment of burns in wound repair started in the 1950s in the War to Resist U.S. Aggression and Aid Korea, and a large number of burns of napalm and other burning weapons, which quickly cultivated professional rescue talents for early treatment and postplastic surgery in China. In the Great Leap Forward era, the whole country has set off a wave of treatment for burns. Medical universities, provincial/municipal/regional hospitals, and even grassroots hospitals have established burn departments or burn treatment groups. With the establishment of professional burn teams, burn surgery in China has flourished. The successful case of Qiu Caikang with 80% of the burn area, who was rescued in Ruijin Hospital affiliated to Shanghai Second Medical University, marked a breakthrough in the treatment of large-area burns in China. From the end of the 1960s to the end of the 1970s, it was the stage of burn treatment popularization, stable and further improvement in China. Due to the progress made in anti-shock and anti-infection, especially on the basis of the successful experience of cutting III degree eschar and intensive skin grafting to eliminate wounds as early as possible, the first large-scale staged batch removal of III degree eschar was carried out. The allogeneic skin opening was embedded in a small piece of autologous skin graft after full coverage of the wound method (German burn medical doctors call the Chinese method), in one fell swoop in the country and the world to break through the cure for the III degree burn area of 70% of the mark. This breakthrough is a great leap in the treatment of burns in China, and then it has further cured a large number of severely burned patients with.

III degrees of 90% or more than 95% in the country, making China's burn treatment level a world leader. It has been the basic theoretical research stage of burns since the end of the 1970s. The clinical treatment level of burns in China has been consistently ranked first in the world or is in the leading position. However, from the perspective of basic theoretical research, there is still a gap compared with the advanced countries in the world. How to use theoretical research results to guide clinical practice and improve the level of treatment and rehabilitation has become the key to the present [7].

The development of plastic surgery in trauma in China began around the first half of the twentieth century.

Ni Baochun (1899–1997) received his doctorate in medicine from Johns Hopkins University in 1925. In 1926, he studied under the famous plastic surgery expert John Davis. He returned to China in 1927. He served as the Acting President of St. John's University and the Dean of St. John's University School of Medicine. In 1952, he served as the Associate Dean of Shanghai Second Medical College. In 1929, Ni Baochun opened a plastic clinic at the Tongren Hospital of St. John's University School of Medicine (St. Luke's Hospital), where he served as the director of plastic surgery and is concurrently in the teaching faculty of anatomy and plastic surgery at the Shanghai Medical College. In the *Shen Kefei Surgery* published in the early 1950s, he wrote the chapter on "Plastic Surgery." According to the information that can be accessed now, Ni Baochun should be called the earliest pioneer of modern Chinese plastic surgery, and the first person to establish a modern Chinese plastic surgery discipline in medical colleges. During the same period, in the 1930s and 1940s, Shi Guanghai opened a cosmetic clinic with Yang Shuyin and others in Shanghai and Beijing before the founding of the People's Republic of China. After Ni Baochun established plastic surgery in Chinese medical colleges for 19 years, from September to December in 1948, J. Webster, a famous American professor of plastic surgery, held a plastic surgery class at Shanghai Zhongshan Hospital. Zhu Hongyin, Zhang Disheng, Song Ruyao, Wang Liangneng, Li Wenren, and other students took part in the class. They were predecessors of the later development of plastic surgery in China.

At the beginning of the founding of the People's Republic of China, especially after the War to Resist US Aggression and Aid Korea, the trauma repair surgery entered a stage of stable development. Taking maxillofacial surgery as an example, before the 1950s, China's oral and maxillofacial trauma and repair surgery had not been established. After 1949, with the treatment of war wounds and work injuries, traffic accidents and other accidental injuries increasing, the oral and maxillofacial trauma and repair surgery are constantly evolving. For example, during the Korean War, the volunteer medical teams in Shanghai and Tianjin, the Southwest Plastic Surgery Team, and later the Nanjing Medical Team participated in the rescue of maxillofacial trauma, and created the oral and maxillofacial trauma and repair surgery in China. Subsequently, a specialist ward was established in higher medical colleges and various types of specialist classes were held to train a large number of professionals. In 1955, the Ministry of Education of China hired Professor Kosh-he of the Soviet Union Molotov School of Stomatology to hold a national high-level teacher course in oral and maxillofacial surgery at Beijing Medical University, systematically introducing the Soviet Union in the rescue of oral and maxillofacial injuries in the Second World War. In the anti-self-defense counterattack against Vietnam in the late 1970s, in the process of treating maxillofacial wounds, the development of oral and maxillofacial trauma and repair surgery in China was further promoted.

Plastic surgery has also developed rapidly during this period:

(a) Song Ruyao, a student at the University of Pennsylvania School of Medicine in Philadelphia, is a student of Professor Avi, the founder of American Plastic Surgery. After returning from the United States in 1948, he became a professor of maxillofacial surgery and plastic surgery at Huaxi University. In the War to Resist U.S. Aggression and Aid Korea, the US military used a variety of modern weapons other than atomic bombs, causing injuries to the wounded among the volunteers, and these injuries were far more complicated and serious than those caused during the War of Resistance Against Japan and the War of Liberation. In 1951, when major medical colleges and universities across the country organized the medical team, Song Ruyao, a professor of plastic surgery at West China University, also organized a team of medical and surgical aids with the teachers and assistants of the medical school and the dentistry school to treat the wounded with plastic surgery and maxillofacial surgery. This time, the plastic surgery and maxillofacial surgery for the wounded are of great significance. First of all, it is the first large-scale official plastic surgery work in China. Secondly, it has made the people of the People's Republic of China fully aware of the importance of plastic surgery in war trauma. If there is no plastic surgery, many face and hand wounded or burned people will not be able to get the best treatment and will not be able to return to society. In the War to Resist U.S. Aggression and Aid Korea, the US air force used a large number of napalm bombs for low-altitude bombing. The volunteers had a large number of burns by napalm bombs. These wounded people were seriously injured and numerous. If routine treatment was used consistently, the treatment of a large number of casualties could not be completed. Therefore, they invented innovative treatments such as continuous getting skin, one operation to complete full face burn skin grafting and full hand burn skin grafting, which became an important stage in the enlightenment and development of burn surgery in China. In 1952, Song Ruyao became a professor of plastic surgery at Peking Union Medical College. In 1954, the "Chinese People's Liberation Army Plastic Surgery Hospital" was born, and Song Ruyao was appointed as Dean. In 1957, the General Logistics Department of the Chinese People's Liberation Army decided to merge the General Logistics Department Peace Hospital with the Peking Union Medical College Hospital. The Commander-in-Chief Zhu De autographed the hospital's title "Chinese People's Liberation Army Plastic Surgery Hospital." In 1958, the State Council decided to transfer seven military academies such as the "Chinese People's Liberation Army Plastic Surgery Hospital" to the Central Ministry of Health, belonging to the local leadership, and affiliated to the Chinese Academy of Medical Sciences.
(b) Professor Zhu Hongyin, graduated from the Department of Biology, Yanjing University in 1939, and received his doctorate in medicine from Union Medical College in 1943. He established a plastic surgery department at Beijing Medical College in September 1949. He has served as a professor at Beijing Medical College, Director of Plastic Department and Associate Dean of the Fourth Affiliated Hospital of Beijing Medical College, Director of Plastic Department and Associate Dean of the Third Affiliated Hospital of Beijing Medical College, Professor of Beijing Medical University, and Member of the Medical Science Committee of the Ministry of Health. After the founding of the People's Republic of China, he led the first plastic surgery delegation to the Czech Republic to participate in the International Plastic Surgery Academic Exchange Conference.
(c) Zhang Disheng and Song Ruyao had successively studied under the American plastic surgeon Ivy, and returned to China to carry out plastic surgery, and participated in the War Resist U.S. Aggression and Aid Korea.
(d) Chen Shaozhou after returning from the United States in 1948 was hired as a professor of oral and maxillofacial plastic surgery by Aurora University (Shanghai) and

concurrently at Shanghai Guangci Hospital (now Shanghai Jiaotong University Ruijin Hospital) as the director of the department. In 1951, he established plastic surgery at the Renji Hospital (now Renji Hospital affiliated to Jiaotong University).

(e) Wang Liangneng, who graduated from the National Central University School of Medicine in 1942, went to the United States to study in 1949. In September 1951, Professor Wang Liangneng, who was full of patriotism and enthusiasm, embarked on a journey back to the motherland, but was severely obstructed by the US government. When passing through Honolulu, the US Customs prevented him from leaving the country on the grounds that "wartime scientific and technical personnel were not allowed to leave the United States," causing his return to fail. In 1954, he took the opportunity to go to Hong Kong to take over his family and left the United States alone. With the help of the underground party organization of the Chinese travel agency in Hong Kong, he finally returned to the embrace of the motherland and created the first burn and plastic surgery department at the Fourth Military Medical University in the northwest.

(f) In the early years, Zhang Guangyan was first admitted to the Qilu University School of Medicine and then transferred to the West China Medical College. In 1938, he graduated from the medical school and was a school doctor. He graduated from the School of Dentistry of West China Medical College in 1941 and was recommended to study in the United States. He studied at Northwestern University in Chicago and majored in dentistry and plastic surgery. After the victory of the War of Resistance Against Japan in 1945, Professor Zhang Guangyan returned to China. He has developed and established plastic surgery at Beijing Medical College and Henan Medical College. In 1963, he established the first department of plastic surgery in Henan in the First Affiliated Hospital of Henan Medical College.

(g) Dong Shufen, graduated from Harbin Medical University in 1941, worked as a dentist in Changchun and Tianjin, worked in the Tianjin Medical Team of the War to Resist U.S. Aggression and Aid Korea in 1950, and went to the Institute of Stomatology of the Moscow University in 1954. After returning to China, he established the maxillofacial surgery in Xi'an in 1957 [8].

Hospitals with plastic surgery in the 1950s were mainly distributed in Beijing, Shanghai, and Xi'an, followed by Zhengzhou, Nanjing, Shenyang, Taiyuan, Dalian, Nanchang, Gansu, Urumqi, Fuzhou, Guangzhou, and Zhanjiang. In the 1970s, the Beijing Plastic Surgery Hospital compiled a total of seven lectures on "*Plastic surgery training*," which played an important role in cultivating the plastic surgery personnel in China. From 1949 to 1978, a variety of plastic surgery monographs were published, including Professor Zhang Disheng's *The Reconstruction of Cleft Lips and Splits* (1957), *Summary of Formal Surgery* by Zhu Hongyin, Wang Damei, Kong Fanhu, et al. (1959), Professor Song Ruyao's *Organic Surgery of Hand Trauma* (1962), Professor Kong Fanhu's *Practical Plastic Surgery* (1964), and Song Ruiyao's *Repair of Cleft Lips and Cleft Palate* (1965), which are important for the popularization and development of plastic surgery in China. Since 1966, due to the influence of the "Cultural Revolution," the development of plastic surgery in China had suffered setbacks. In 1978, according to statistics before the reconstruction of Beijing Plastic Surgery Hospital, there were only 170 doctors engaged in plastic surgery in China at that time.

In the Sino-Indian border, the Chen-pao Island, the Xisha Islands' self-defense counterattack, and the counterattack against Vietnam, the plastic surgery in China has made advances and explored some good experiences. In recent years, through the earthquake relief, the military health work has been further exercised, which is conducive to further improvement in the field of plastic surgery.

After the mid-1980s, the Chinese Medical Association Trauma Branch (including the tissue prosthetics group), the Chinese Medical Association Plastic Surgery Society, the Chinese Medical Aesthetic Surgery Society, the Chinese Reconstructive Surgery Society, the Chinese Hand Surgery Society, and the Chinese Microsurgery Society, academic organizations related to wound healing, tissue repair, and regeneration, have been established. At the same time, the corresponding professional academic journals have also been born. The military also established various professional committees. In 1962, the Army Burning Professional Team of the People's Liberation Army was formally established, and a military conference was held every 2 years, which played an important role in promoting the development of plastic surgery and trauma repair surgery in the new era. During this period, China's plastic reconstructive surgery and microscopic reconstruction surgery have entered the world's advanced ranks. In 2007, the Army Plastic Surgery Committee became independent from the Burn Professional Committee and became a separate academic organization. In addition, military traumatic academic organizations such as the Army Trauma Professional Committee have also been established.

In the new era, China's tissue repair and regenerative development benefited from the advancement of modern science and technology, the transformation of related therapeutic concepts, multidisciplinary collaboration, and the rapid transformation and application of new theories and new technologies.

Systematic and in-depth research and development of wound tissue repair and regeneration began in the 1980s, represented by the development and application of growth factors (cytokines), stem cells, and new dressings.

In 1986, with the Nobel Prize in Physiology or Medicine for growth factor research represented by nerve growth factor and epidermal growth factor, it was gradually recognized that various growth factors (cytokines) are important in regulating tissue repair and regeneration. Thus, traditional tissue repair begins with pathological descriptions and shifts to research at the cellular, molecular, and genetic levels. At that time, because the genetic engineering recombinant protein technology was not mature enough, many growth factors applied to tissue repair and regeneration could only be extracted from the organs of cattle and rats. This method took time, effort, and expense, and the amount of growth factors obtained was also very few, and could not meet the needs of basic research, let alone clinical applications. At the same time, a large number of scientific and technological workers had little understanding of the growth factor, and the treatment in this area was very limited. In the early 1990s, the People's Military Medical Press published a comprehensive monograph on growth factors and tissue repair and regeneration, published by Xiaobing Fu, *Growth Factor and Wound Repair*. This is the first international monograph devoted to growth factors and tissue repair and regeneration. The publication of this book helped domestic experts to comprehensively and systematically understand the basic knowledge of growth factor biology and growth factors involved in wound repair and tissue regeneration regulation. This book played a positive role in promoting basic research, new drug development, and clinical application in related fields on a large scale in China. Later, the publication of the first international *Molecular Trauma* led by Academician Wang Zhengguo further refined and improved the cellular, molecular, and genetic basis of trauma and wound treatment. China is in an advanced position in the fields of trauma and wound treatment in the world [4, 9].

At the same time, Professor Lin Jian from Jinan University of China began research on genetic engineering technology to recombine bovine basic fibroblast growth factor. The Zhuhai Bioengineering Co. Ltd., which was established at that time, quickly developed the first generation of recombinant bovine basic fibroblast growth factor (bFGF). Through close cooperation with researchers and clinical experts in many large hospitals, in 1998, the company obtained the new drug certificate of the State Food and Drug Administration and began clinical application. It became the first new drug in the country of genetic engineering for wound healing. The relevant research results were published in the internationally renowned medical journals *Lancet and Wound Rep Reg* [10, 11], which attracted the attention and positive evaluation of international peers, such as the Health Column of the British BBC: Bovine protein promotes wound healing. The Lancet commented in the Highlights: This is a time to promote wound healing. Later, recombinant human basic fibroblast growth factor (rhbFGF), recombinant human acidic fibroblast growth factor (rhaFGF), recombinant human epidermal growth factor (rhEGF), and platelet-derived growth factor (PDGF) were developed at home and abroad. These products have been used as a conventional drug for the treatment of wound burns and have achieved remarkable results.

The idea of traditional treatment is that in a relatively large open wound, in order to prevent bacterial infection, a dry method should be used for treatment. In the 1960s, British scientist Winter confirmed through animal experiments that if the wounds kept moist, not only did the bacterial infection rate not increase significantly, but the wound healing was also significantly faster than the control. This discovery has changed the basic understanding of the wound healing environment. According to this principle, various advanced dressings (revolutionary dressings) represented by moisturizing dressings were produced in the 1980s. A significant feature of this large class of dressings is the ability to provide a relatively moisturizing and slightly acidic healing environment for the wound, which facilitates the dissolution of necrotic tissue and the release of various growth factors associated with wound healing, while not significantly increasing the infection rate of bacteria. In addition, due to the translucent membrane, it is beneficial to the gas exchange between the wound surface and the external environment. At the same time, after using the dressing the patient's wound surface does not affect the daily work, labor, even bath and can be replaced weekly saving a lot of manpower and financial resources. Clinical applications have proven that these dressings significantly reduce patient suffering and, in general, save medical costs and labor costs. So far, various advanced dressings for moisturizing, antibacterial, dissolving necrotic tissue and damage tissue repair and regeneration have been widely used in the treatment of various acute and chronic wounds [12]. The dressing for wound treatment covers the wound from mere gauze, "insulates" the contact between the wound and the outside world, avoids the traditional concept that the wound is contaminated again, and promotes the "active" repair and healing of the wound with advanced dressing, which is completely benefited from wound treatment. The discovery of theory and the breakthrough of traditional concepts are a successful example of translational medicine. Although it is not an original work in the field of advanced dressings, it has significantly promoted the application of this technology and products in China through the introduction, digestion, and integrated innovation.

The basic research of stem cell and tissue engineering and related clinical application are important advances and development directions in the field of wound tissue repair and regeneration. At present, preliminary effects on chronic wound treatment, wound angiogenesis, and sweat gland regeneration have been observed by adult stem cell induction techniques. In particular, the innovative theory and key technologies for the induction of autologous bone marrow mesenchymal stem cells to regenerate sweat glands by the team led by Xiaobing Fu and Sheng Zhiyong of the General Hospital of the People's Liberation Army have broken through the international problem of sweat gland regeneration, and first realized the function in human wounds in the world. The sweat glands regenerated, and some cases followed up for 10 years proved to have a stable sweating function, and no adverse reactions were observed. The result was evaluated by international peers as a "milestone study." [13] At present, some tissue engineering skin, nerves, tendons, cartilage, etc. have begun preliminary clinical application, which proves that it has a good effect on warfare tissue repair and regeneration [14, 15].

In the 1990s, the main academic works related to tissue repair and regeneration were published in China: *Basic for Wound Repair* (Edited by Xiaobing Fu, Wang Dewen, People's Military Medical Press, 1997), *Wound Healing and Tissue Restoration* (Edited by Wang Zhengguo, Shandong Science and Technology Press, 1998), and *Modern Trauma Restoration* (Edited by Xiaobing Fu, Wang Dewen, People's Military Medical Press, 1999) have played a positive role in further expanding the academic influence and communication of tissue repair and regeneration.

Since the beginning of the twenty-first century, the epidemiology of trauma and wounds has undergone great changes. Related research by Xiaobing Fu et al. showed that in 1998, the main etiology of inpatients in China due to chronic refractory wounds was traumatic burns and infections, accounting for about 67%, while the chronic refractory wounds caused by diabetic foot accounted for only 4.9%. However, new research in 2008 after 10 years shows that after only 10 years, the main etiology of chronic refractory wounds in China has undergone a fundamental change, and diabetic foot has become the main cause of chronic refractory wounds accounting for about 36%, and chronic wounds caused by traumatic burns fell to about 20%. This result suggests that with the rapid development of China's economy and the continuous improvement of people's living standards, chronic refractory wounds have become one of the important chronic diseases affecting the Chinese people's physical and mental health and quality of life. The epidemiological characteristics are the same with developed countries in the West. The social economic burdens and consumption of medical resources that it caused should be highly valued by the whole society. During this period, the country began systematic research on the mechanism, treatment, and prevention of chronic refractory wounds. In terms of treatment, in addition to traditional surgical treatment, new techniques and drugs such as new dressings (also known as revolutionary dressings), growth factors, optical therapy, and vacuum suction have played a positive role in accelerating the healing rate of chronic refractory wounds and improving the quality of healing. In the field of academic publishing, he has edited *Modern High-tech and Trauma Repair* (Xiaobing Fu, Wang Zhengguo, People's Military Medical Press, 2002), *Modern Wound Dressing: Theory and Practice* (Xiaobing Fu, Wu Zhigu, Chemical Industry Press, 2007), and *Theory and Practice of Prevention and Treatment of Chronic Wounds* (edited by Xiaobing Fu, People's Medical Publishing House, 2008). Especially in medical undergraduate and postgraduate education, he has edited many textbooks, such as *Stem Cell and Regenerative Medicine* (Pang Xining, Xiaobing Fu, People's Medical Publishing House, 2014) and *Study on Stem Cell and Regenerative Medicine* (Pang Xining, Xiaobing Fu, People's Medical Publishing House, 2016). The textbook introduces stem cells and regeneration medical overview, clarifies the concept and research content of stem cells and regenerative medicine, the status of stem cells and regenerative medicine in life sciences, and the relationship between regenerative medicine and normal growth and development, and on this basis, introduces a brief history of stem cells and development of regenerative medicine. The textbook runs through the relationship between stem cells as a regenerative seed cell and regenerative medicine, and introduces the mechanism of regeneration, tissue level regeneration, new regeneration and deformation regeneration, physiological regeneration and pathological regeneration and its significance, and methods of regenerative medicine, including cell transplantation and biological artificial tissue and in situ regeneration induction. The key chapters describe the regeneration and regenerative medicine of skin, eye and cornea, nerves, cardiovascular, digestion, respiration, bone, cartilage, muscle, tendon and ligament, reproductive system, dental tissue, and appendage. In 2014, Academician Xiaobing Fu also edited the postgraduate textbook of the National Twelfth Five-Year Plan of the National Health and Family Planning Commission, *Wound, Burn and Regenerative Medicine* (published by People's Medical Publishing House). The book brings together more than 80 experts and scholars in the field of trauma, burns, and tissue repair and regenerative medicine.

In the publicity education and training of prevention and control of chronic refractory wounds, the hospital has established treatment specialists for complex chronic refractory wounds in Shanghai, Hangzhou, Xi'an, and Beijing (new or expanding previously established burn and trauma surgery), a new model for the treatment of complex chronic refractory wounds as a disease has been created. Its representative experts include Professor Lu Shuliang, Professor Han Chunmao, and Professor Xie Ting. At the same time, the Chinese Medical Association Trauma Branch Professional Reconstruction Committee (CTRS) and the World Diabetes Foundation (WDF) and the Access to Healthcare (Ath) work closely together to use the international fund to conduct propaganda and education of prevention and control of chronic refractory wounds in China for more than 3 years. By organizing high-level expert teams, writing different levels of training materials, and establishing training bases, at the completion of the project, training bases were established in nearly 60 hospitals in more than 20 provinces, municipalities, and autonomous regions across the country, a total of more than 10,000 doctors, nurses, and other related personnel were trained. This project achieved remarkable results.

In 2011, in order to promote the specification of diagnosis and treatment of chronic wounds, under the guidance of Xiaobing Fu, according to the relevant literature on chronic wounds at home and abroad, the first guide book on chronic wounds was edited and published in China——2011 edition of *Chronic Wound Diagnosis and Treatment Guide*, which has been welcomed by everyone. At the end of 2013, in order to further promote the standard of diagnosis and treatment of acute wounds in China, and in order to make the guidelines more in line with the characteristics of Chinese people, Academician Xiaobing Fu guided the establishment of a Chinese-based wound treatment guide based on relevant domestic literature and foreign-related guidelines. In the beginning of 2014, the guideline development team was established and the guideline development plan was officially launched. The guideline was developed based on the contents of clinical research papers published in China. The main purpose of the guideline is to develop guidelines that are consistent with China's national conditions, and it has practical guidance. This work was basically completed by consulting domestic literature and eight seminars. This document retrieval searches all papers about wound from January 1, 2004 to May 1, 2014, from the China National Knowledge Infrastructure (CNKI) and CNKI dissertation databases. After many researches and conference discussions by various experts for more than a year, the guide to China's wounds was finally born!

Perfect tissue repair and regeneration is the highest goal of war wound tissue treatment, and it has always been the main content and goal of research on science and technology workers in China. At the national level, relevant departments attach great importance to research in this field. In addition to the Chinese Academy of Sciences and the Chinese Academy of Engineering planning the organization of restoration and regeneration as the main research direction in relevant science and technology planning, since 1999, three National Basic Research Planning Projects ("973" Project) have been invested to study key scientific and technical problems in tissue repair and regeneration after trauma. The chief scientists are Academician Wang Zhengguo, Professor Jiang Jianxin, and Academician Xiaobing Fu. At the academic level, Academician Wang Zhengguo, Academician Wu Zuze, and Academician Xiaobing Fu successively organized and held three "Regenerative Medicine" Xiangshan Science Conferences on the theme of regenerative medicine. The major recommendations were launched that played an active role in further consolidating key scientific issues and organizing academics to tackle key problems and treating tissue repair and regeneration as a national strategic initiative. During this period, three large-scale academic monographs were published in succession *Regenerative Medicine: From Basic to Clinical Research, Regenerative Medicine: Basic and Clinical Research,* and *Regenerative Medicine: Transformation and Application.* These books have had a good influence on academia. The first one is *Regenerative Medicine: From Basic to Clinical Research*, published by Shanghai Science and Technology Press in 2008. The second one is *Regenerative Medicine: Basic and Clinical Research*, published by People's Medical Publishing House in 2013. The third one is *Regenerative Medicine: Transformation and Application*, published by People's Medical Publishing House in 2016. The three books can be called the trilogy of academic monographs on regenerative medicine in China [16–18]. In 2012, the internationally renowned academic journal *Science* also invited Prof. Xiaobing Fu to organize Chinese scientists to publish a series of *Regenerative Medicine in China* in the form of a supplement. After the publication, there was a good international response, in addition to the highly praised publications in the *Science* and its supplement, other international journals also commented, which has significantly expanded the international impact in the field.

### 1.1.3 The Promotion of Science and Technology Development in the Development of Trauma Repair and Tissue Regeneration

#### 1.1.3.1 Disinfection, Anesthesia, Hemostasis, and Blood Transfusion Provide a Good Foundation for the Establishment of Modern Trauma Repair Surgery

In the old days, infection, bleeding, and pain limited the development of surgery. Since the 1940s, the scope of surgery has been expanded and the safety of surgery has been greatly increased due to the problems of wound infection, surgical pain, hemostasis, and blood transfusion solved [19].

##### Infection

Wound "suppression" is one of the biggest problems faced by surgeons more than 100 years ago. The biggest achievement in war trauma surgery is the treatment of wound infections. At that time, the mortality rate after amputation was as high as 40–50%. Before the First World War, people cultivated and fertilized (animal feces) year after year, causing every soldier injured in the trenches to carry a different number of pathogens. At the time of the war front, sepsis was very common. Although many measures have been taken, these attempts have been in vain, and disinfection of infected wounds has proven to be an effective measure. Surgeons have tried countless disinfectant solutions as well as surgical dressings. Ultimately, trimming necrotic tissue and repeated rinsing stand out in the principles of wound management. Henry Dakin (1880–1952) was a British chemist and Alexis Carrel (1873–1944) was a French-American surgeon and Nobel laureate. These two are the main advocates of this method of wound treatment. In addition to the aseptic processing of wounds, the achievements of surgery are also reflected in the use of X-rays for the diagnosis of war injuries and the fine design of surgical operations. The latter have been obtained in the treatment of war wound facial reconstruction and war wounds.

Aseptic technique is an effective preventive method for the source and route of infection, and is the key to determining the effectiveness of the diagnosis and the success or failure of the operation. In 1864, Semmelweis of Hungary first proposed washing hands with bleaching solution before checking the parturient, which is the beginning of antibacterial technology. In 1867, British surgeon Baron Joseph Lister laid the foundation for antibacterial technology and was recognized as the founder of antibacterial surgery. In 1877, Bergmann of Germany invented the high-pressure steam sterilization and established the aseptic technique in modern surgery.

#### Pain

Surgical pain was one of the important factors that hindered the development of surgery. In 1846, Morton first used ether as a general anesthetic and assisted Warren in performing many major operations with ether anesthesia. Since then, ether anesthesia has been commonly used in surgery. In 1892, Schleich in Germany first advocated cocaine for local infiltration anesthesia. However, due to its high toxicity, it was soon replaced by procaine. Now, procaine is still a safe and effective local anesthetic. The three main stages of anesthesia development include:

(a) The stage of ancient anesthesia development——the discovery and germination of anesthesia.
(b) The stage of modern anesthesia development——the formation of clinical anesthesiology.
(c) The development stage of modern anesthesiology. Since the beginning of the First World War, due to the improvement of anesthesia technology, the surgical procedure can last for more than 12 h, and the safety is greatly improved, which greatly improves the success rate of tissue transplantation repair.

#### Bleeding

The earliest blood transfusion record was in 1667, when a French aristocrat transfused 280 mL of calf blood to a mentally disordered tramp, trying to heal his mental problems. The unfortunate patient experienced a severe immune reaction. After several times he almost died, but he survived miraculously and maintained a period of calm, so the blood transfusion therapy was accepted by some doctors with innovative ideas. For the next 300 years, transfusion therapy is still in the exploratory phase. Because there is no support of relevant knowledge (such as blood type), blood transfusions have caused many deaths, but doctors have also found that blood transfusions can sometimes save lives. It was not until 1912 that the Frenchman Alexis Carrel won the Nobel Prize for the creation of vascular anastomosis for blood transfusions, blood transfusion therapy gained a wide range of recognition. The person who really made blood transfusion a scientific and effective treatment was Karl Landsteiner, a pathologist in Vienna. He discovered the ABO blood type and agglutination of humans since 1901, providing a solid pathophysiological basis for modern blood transfusion. In the following 20 years, other doctors gradually invented blood anticoagulation and cross-matching techniques, making blood transfusion a routine and effective treatment. Landsteiner also won the Nobel Prize in Physiology or Medicine in 1930.

### 1.1.3.2 The Establishment and Development of Immunology Provide a Basis for Breakthroughs in Various Types of Transplantation

The so-called "immune" was originally derived from the Latin word "immunis." Its original meaning is "exception from charges" and also contains the meaning of "free of disease." Immunology is the biomedical science of studying immune response to antigenic substances and their methods. The immune response is the body's response to antigenic stimuli and is a biological process that identifies and excludes antigenic material. It is a physiological function in which the body recognizes "self" and "non-self" antigens, forms natural immune tolerance to autoantigens, and produces rejection of "non-self" antigens. Under normal circumstances, this physiological function is beneficial to the body and can produce anti-infective, anti-tumor, and other immune protections that can maintain physiological balance and stability. In some cases, it may become an obstacle to tissue transplantation.

The ancient and emerging discipline of immunology is developed by people in their constant exploration, summarization, and innovation in practice. After four periods of immunology, namely, the period of empirical immunology, the period of classical immunology, the period of modern immunology, and the period of contemporary immunology, tissue transplantation technology has been greatly improved, with allotransplantation and xenotransplantation making breakthrough progress. There have been many successful cases of "changing faces" around the world, and there have been reports of successful handovers.

#### 1.1.3.3 The Emergence of Microsurgery Provides a New Technical Means for Trauma Repair Surgery

In a broad sense, microsurgery is not unique to a specialist, but a surgical technique that can be used by all majors in the surgical discipline. It can even be a specialized subdiscipline from the profession, such as microsurgery in urology, microneurosurgery, etc. Some disciplines, such as surgical surgery, ophthalmology, and otolaryngology, have used surgical magnifier as a conventional surgical instrument for surgical dissection and suturing. However, in a narrow sense, the development of microsurgery itself has its own theoretical system. For example, small blood vessel anastomosis has many principle differences with large and medium blood vessel anastomosis. In the early stage, due to the lack of special small vessel anastomosis surgery, the principle of vascular anastomosis was borrowed, so the postoperative patency rate was not high. After the special rule of small vessel anastomosis was found, the postoperative patency rate was greatly improved. For example, in the past, the flap was limited to the inguinal flap, the dorsal flap, and the intermuscular flap. The larger musculocutaneous branch of the musculocutaneous flap was used as the main blood supply vessel of the flap, such as the anterolateral thigh flap. The use of limbs with blood vessel characteristics developed retrograde flap. These depend on the deepening of theoretical research to develop new methods. Therefore, microsurgery should, on the one hand, vigorously develop new surgical methods using microsurgical techniques in various surgical disciplines and improve the professional level from this aspect. On the other hand, it has its own disciplinary research, discovering its new theories and new laws, and promoting the development of disciplines. As for the research of microsurgical instruments and equipment, it is constantly improving, and the two complement each other.

The emergence of microsurgery provides a powerful means for wound repair and tissue regeneration, greatly expanding the indications for wound repair. Vascular repair is the best treatment for vascular injury. One of the most amazing techniques in the field of surgery is the replantation of the limbs, which is the successful replantation of fingers, hands, arms, or feet that are interrupted by the trauma or cut by the machine. To reattach a broken limb and reinstate it, you need to stitch the blood vessels, nerves, and skin and bones together. As early as 1912, there was a method of replanting a broken limb. At that time, Alexis Carrel invented a method of suturing large blood vessels. In 1952, microsurgery began to be used in the treatment of vascular warfare, reducing the amputation rate from 51.4% to 13.0%. The methods used include side-wall repair, vascular anastomosis, and intervening grafts. Nanobashvili et al. reported a direct anastomosis ratio of 38% after debridement, while approximately 56% of vascular injuries require an interstitial graft. In the 1960s, the advent of better microscopes, fine needles, and filaments made it possible to suture small blood vessels. But the reconstruction of the damaged peripheral nerves was reported only in 1967. In 1968, Kamachu and Tamayo used all the new technologies at the time to replant the broken thumb.

In the field environment, grafts for vascular repair often use autologous saphenous veins or artificial blood vessels. There is no consensus as to which of the two is better or worse. The autologous saphenous vein has a long history as a graft. The earliest in the Vietnam War, Rich et al. began to use it in vascular treatment of warfare trauma. However, the site and length of the autologous vein are limited, new wounds are added, the operation time is prolonged, and there are defects that the diameter of the repaired blood vessel does not match. In addition, although the early limb salvage rate of the autologous saphenous vein as the graft was higher than that of the artificial blood vessel, there was no significant difference in the patency rate and the limb salvage rate. Therefore, artificial blood vessels can replace autologous veins for emergency treatment or autologous veins are not available.

#### 1.1.3.4 The Application of Bioengineering and Various Materials Has Broadened the Field for Wound Repair

The two major leaps in cell biology and molecular biology in the field of life sciences in the twentieth century have made humans' understanding of the life essence reach an unprecedented height. With the development of science and technology, human beings regard the study of life sciences as a main line for their own survival and development, and continue to apply other modern science and technology. It gradually formed an interdiscipline of science, engineering, and medicine——bioengineering.

In 1949, the United States first published a prospective paper on medical polymers. The article, first introduced the use of polymethylmethacrylate as a human skull and joints and the use of polyamide fiber as a surgical suture in clinical treatment. According to incomplete statistics, as of 1990, more than 30,000 academic papers and patents on medical polymers were published in the United States, Japan, and Western Europe. It is predicted that in the twenty-first century, medical polymers will enter a new era. In addition to the brain, all parts of the body and organs can be replaced by polymer materials.

Tissue engineering is an emerging discipline that combines cell biology and materials science to construct tissues or organs in vitro or in vivo. It takes a small amount of living tissue from the body, separates the seed cells from the tissue with special enzymes or other methods, and cultures and expands them in vitro, and then mixes with the absorbable biological materials. Finally, cells adhere to the biological material forming a cell-material complex. The composite is implanted into the lesion site of the body. On the one hand, the biological material is gradually degraded and absorbed in the body; on the other hand, the implanted cells continuously proliferate in the body and secrete the extracellular matrix, and finally form corresponding tissues and organs, thereby achieving the purpose of trauma repair and reconstruction. Because tissue engineering has the potential to replicate "tissues" or "organs," some scholars say that tissue engineering is "a new era of regenerative medicine" or even "a far-reaching medical revolution." At present, bone, cartilage, muscle, tendon, ligament, skin, blood vessels, periodontal, peripheral nerves, etc. have been studied in tissue engineering, and some of them have begun clinical trials or have become commercially available products for clinical application.

#### 1.1.3.5 Information Network Builds a Platform for Improving the Level of Wound Repair

Telemedicine is a new medical service model that combines modern medicine, computer technology, and communication technology by applying telecommunication technique, interactive transmitting information, and carrying out long-distance medical services. Telemedicine services are available in a variety of forms, using a series of modern communication technologies such as satellite transmission, fiber-optic communication, and television transmission for point-to-point remote consultation and multiparty consultation. Doctors and patients can communicate face-to-face through remote video systems, can transmit and store patient data through the network, and accommodate multiple experts from different regions to consult the same patient at the same time. Medical information delivered in telemedicine includes data, text, video, audio, and images. Telemedicine can be divided into global, intercontinental, national, regional, hospital, community, and home telemedicine, depending on the scope of application. The value of the construction and development of military telemedicine for the military medical support work has become more and more concerned by the military of various countries with the successful application of the US military in military operations around the world.

The United States has developed the USAMRMC (US Army Medical Research Material Command) to solve critical medical problems for the frontline battlefields of the US military at home and abroad. The Telemedicine Strategic Project is part of the project, which includes the identification, development, and demonstration of relevant key technologies and biomedical-related technologies that address both medical and military barriers. Its main objectives are:

(a) Provides a fast and flexible way to develop the specialization of the military's important medical field and obtain relevant support.
(b) Integrates health awareness into the battlefield.
(c) Improves the skills and efficiency of medical service personnel.
(d) Improves the quality and collaboration of internal and surgical medical services throughout the battlefield.

The exploration of telemedicine in China since the 1980s has developed rapidly in recent years. In the late 1990s, China's telemedicine moved from theoretical exploration to practical application. The Ministry of Health, the China Medical Foundation, and the Ministry of Health of the People's Liberation Army successively launched the Jinwei Network Project, the China Medical Foundation Internet, and the Junwei II Engineering (Telemedicine Network). Some well-known medical colleges and hospitals have set up remote consultation centers and have carried out various forms of telemedicine work with hundreds of hospitals nationwide. Currently, they can implement real-time expert consultation for patients with acute and severe diseases, transmission of shared medical data, and pathological diagnosis. In the military, with the help of network coverage, our military's telemedicine information system has been equipped with front-line company and remote duty checkpoints. Make full use of existing resources, and take advantage of the comprehensive collection of experts and disciplines. At the same time, actively explore new operating modes and manage the rights by the server. Provide free information browsing services and hospital guide, consultation, initial diagnosis, inspection, treatment, and follow-up for trauma patients. Telemedicine has made the tissue repair of wounded more standardized and popularized.

Network technology is one of the most visible areas for achieving graded treatment, consultation, training, and education. Because wound treatment has the characteristics of intuitive shape and relatively low site requirements, it is suitable for development in grassroots and remote areas. Since 2010, we have used the "4G" and Wi-Fi system to carry out a two-way linkage between the wound healing center of large hospitals and the community health institutions in Shanghai and the two-way linkage with the wound healing specialty of Zhejiang Jinhua Wucheng District Hospital. The effect was highly praised by the internationally renowned peers for "looking in the East."

#### 1.1.3.6 Digital Medicine Provides Guarantee for Accurate Wound Repair

Medicine has also gone from ancient medicine, traditional medicine to today's digital medicine. Many new technologies have been or are being used in medical research and application. Digital human technology and digital medical technology derived from it are such new technologies that are increasingly focused and intensively researched. Professor Dai Kerong, an academician of the Chinese Academy of Engineering, defined in the eleventh Chinese engineering frontier *The Status and Future of Digital Medicine*: "Digital medicine is a discipline of applying digital technology to explain medical phenomena, solve medical problems, explore medical mechanisms, and improve the quality of life." It covers many areas of cross-disciplinary research in life science and information science, medicine and engineering, and its research methods and results benefit the implementation and popularization of precision surgery. At the same time, digital medical technology, as an important part of modern medicine, will also promote the development of modern medical technology in the direction of individualization, precision, microinvasion, and remoteness.

Digital medical technology is an extension of digital human research in medical application. It is a new cross-disciplinary research field integrating medical science, biomechanics, mechanics, materials science, computer graphics, computer vision, mathematical analysis, mechanical mechanics, robotics, and many other disciplines. Through modern computer technology (mainly virtual reality technology), a human body structure model for anatomy, a treatment effect model for restoration evaluation, a pathway model for surgical evaluation, a field model for surgical exercises, etc. are established. The research of digital human body has also evolved from the construction of the originally simple human dataset to digital anatomy and its practical application. Its research direction and focus are mainly on the acquisition of special human tissues such as nerves, lymph and tiny organs, image segmentation and reconstruction techniques, grid computing storage and data synchronization sharing, applications in medicine and related fields, and other fields.

#### 1.1.3.7 New Technologies and Methods of Regenerative Medicine Represented by Growth Factors, Stem Cells, and Gene Therapy Technologies Show a Bright Future for Wound Repair and Tissue Regeneration

In recent years, research on genetic engineering technology and stem cells has advanced by leaps and bounds, and many major advances have been made. As mentioned above, the development of genetic engineering technology has enabled a large number of growth factors to be obtained in clinical and basic research, and these growth factors or cytokines are important factors regulating wound repair and tissue regeneration. At present, epidermal growth factor (EGF) and fibroblast growth factor (FGF) approved by the State Food and Drug Administration (SFDA) have been applied in clinical medicine, which has a good effect on promoting wound repair and tissue regeneration. Relevant data showed that the healing time of acute wounds (such as the donor site, shallow II degree burn wounds, etc.) treated with growth factors was 2–4 days earlier than the control; while the cure rate of chronic refractory wounds increased from the previous 84% to about 94%, it has produced good social and economic benefits. Stem cells are the soul of the development of regenerative medicine. Stem cells and gene therapy are the most representative high-tech biotechnology of regenerative medicine. They have unlimited potential for treatment and repair of war wounds (trauma, burn). A large number of studies have found that mesenchymal stem cells (MSCs) with multidirectional differentiation potential can be transformed into epidermal cells, vascular endothelial cells, etc. by inducing differentiation in vitro and in vivo, directly involved in wound repair. At the same time, MSCs also have the potential to differentiate into sweat gland cells and sebaceous gland cells, providing an important biological basis for the future functional restoration of damaged skin. The gene therapy applied to wound repair mainly involves injecting the growth factor gene into the tissue repairing cells by transfection, and expressing it in the repairing cells to produce a certain amount of growth factors to promote wound healing. At present, scientists have successfully isolated and cultured stem cells from tissues and organs such as skin, bone, bone marrow, and fat, and tried to use these cells for tissue repair. Such as accidental injury and radiation damage in patients with skin grafting; nerve repair, repair of muscle, bone, and cartilage defects; vascular disease or replacement of blood vessels after injury; and removal of tissue or organ replacement. This technology has emerged in some areas and achieved some results, but there are still many difficult technical problems to be applied to the treatment and repair of war wounds (trauma, burn).

In military medicine, the status of regenerative medicine is equally important. In the past few years, the United States has not stopped launching wars of all sizes. More and more American soldiers have lost their arms or legs in battles or accidents. They have to endure the pain of great disability for the rest of their lives. Faced with this problem, US military scientists have challenged the human body limb regeneration technology, stepped up research, hope to speed up the treatment of injured soldiers, find the limb regeneration, and make the disabled soldiers become perfect. In March 2008, the US Department of Defense (DOD) announced that in the next 5 years, they will raise $250 million in the rapidly growing field of regenerative medicine to form the new Armed Forces Institute of Regenerative Medicine (AFIRM). The organization's research focus is on the regrowth of defective fingers, comminuted fracture regeneration, reconstruction of facial disability, and skin that matches the severely burned wounds. The American Academy of Regenerative Medicine (AFIRM) consists of 30 research institutes in two research consortia universities and hospital research centers. Alan Russell, a biochemist at the University of Pittsburgh, who led the McGowan Institute of Regenerative Medicine, will help lead AFIRM, making great efforts to develop regenerative treatments for bones, muscles, tendons, nerves, and blood vessels.

In China, the "biomedical treatment" project of war trauma led by Academician Xiaobing Fu of the PLA General Hospital has been launched. The implementation of this project will have a profound impact on military's application of stem cell technology to comprehensively treat the wounds and improve the medical support capabilities. The platform of "regenerative medicine and stem cell technology" under construction will lay a solid foundation for the comprehensive clinical application of stem cell technology and the wounding of officers and soldiers. At present, the phased results indicate that sweat gland tissue can be regenerated by stem cell-induced differentiation technology, and after 10 years of follow-up, these regenerated sweat gland tissues have stable sweating function. The three-dimensional (3D) bioprinting technology can construct the new tissue-engineered skin with skin attachment in vitro, providing important ideas and technical basis for the new generation of tissue engineering skin construction. Using ladder or cascade induction we can observe that mesenchymal stem cells can synchronize simultaneously differentiation into tissue cells in one culture system. These provide important clues for the simultaneous repair and regeneration of various tissues at the injury site. These preliminary results suggest that a new tissue repair and regeneration target, that is, the perfect repair and regeneration of damaged tissue at the injury site are about to come. Therefore, it can be predicted that the related basic and applied researches on stem cells, tissue engineering, and biological therapy in regenerative medicine will enable humans to realize the dream of repairing and manufacturing tissues and organs, which is an inevitable direction of the medical science development.

## 1.2 Posttraumatic Tissue Repair and Regenerative Medicine in Military Medicine

### 1.2.1 Overview

In the military, there were health organizations and doctors who treated officers and soldiers. However, for a long time, the military medicine was in the stage of experience medicine, and it was only after the nineteenth century that it became a scientific military medicine. Military medicine is the science of studying sanitary guarantee both in peacetime and wartime, by using general medical principles and techniques. Through the implementation of health services, we achieve the goal of maintaining the health of the troops, improving the field medical and epidemic prevention, and consolidating and enhancing the combat effectiveness of the troops. In the battle and training, the modern army often encounters many medical problems that are rare in society and needs special research and resolution, which promotes the development of military medicine [20].

Zeng Hengde's "*Xiyuan Lu Biao*" contains: "The gun hurts in the muscle, and the big magnet attracts the bullets." The book of "*Junzhong Yifang Beiyao*" also has this, but there is no way for the copper bullets, and surgery has to be used. This method was first seen in the "*Junzhong Yifang Beiyao*," in the "guns hurts" article said: "if the copper is hard to take out, it must be cut with a sharp knife, take care of it, use the child defecation to wash the wound, wash the dressing, use the Taiyi cream to protect it." The book also contains the method of taking anesthetic drugs to obtain bullets. The use of Chuanwu, Caowu, wildflowers, etc., as for the use of internal medicine to cure bullets, but it is a commonly used medicine. To treat guns and injuries.

Before the establishment of the New Army in the Qing Dynasty, there appeared to be no fixed military doctors in the army. In case of illness, the soldiers will be dispatched. According to the records of *Donghua Lu*, from the Qianlong to the Guangxu, when the senior general is wounded or sick, if the military affairs are urgent or the disease is mild, the emperor will send a doctor or medical officer to treat in the camp, or go to a nearby city or the provincial capital for medical treatment. If the condition is serious, the emperor will let them leave or return to Beijing for treatment. Injured or sick soldiers were nursed in the camp during the war and repatriated after the war. In this way, there are no fixed military doctors in the army, and there are no regular sanitation facilities. It can only temporarily deal with them and cannot solve the medical problems of the military.

After the nineteenth century, the development of general medicine and science and technology created conditions for the rapid development of military medicine. In the Franco-Prussian War, the Prussian army basically established a medical evacuation system from the ambulance to the rear hospital after the field hospital. During the First World War, Russian military doctor V. A. Opelli proposed the idea of ladder treatment. Although the surgery, anesthesia, medication, and treatment techniques have improved compared with the previous generation, they still lag far behind the needs of military medicine at that time. After the Second World War, the number of antibiotics increased, the knowledge of trauma ballistics increased, the development of microsurgery, and the use of helicopters to send the wounded directly to the hospital for treatment, which further reduced the wound infection rate, amputation rate, and death rate. The Soviet Red Army gradually implemented after the victory of the October Revolution, and in the Second World War, the wounded and sick directionally evacuated. The military of other countries also implemented graded treatment in the Second World War.

Russia is the first country to set up a specialized research institution for field surgery in the world, and there have also been many scholars who have made important contributions to the emergence and development of field surgery. At the same time, Russia has experienced numerous wars, large and small, and accumulated rich experience in field surgery, forming its own advantages and characteristics. In many aspects, our military field surgery has developed from Russia. Field Surgery is a discipline that studies the theory, technology, and organization of large numbers of wounded people under field conditions, especially early treatment. It is a branch of surgery and an important part of military medicine. The field surgery of our army was gradually formed in the practice of war wound healing in successive wars, and developed with the development of combat weapons, war forms, tactical changes, and general science and medicine.

In the next few decades, there has been great development in medicine, making tetanus toxoid, synthesizing sulfa drugs, various antimalarials and DDT, producing penicillin, successful researching fresh blood preservation techniques, advocating early trauma debridement and delayed anastomosis, and promoting gypsum blocking therapy for multiple fractures. The US military's death rate was lower in the Second World War, which was closely related to the tetanus.

The development of conventional weapons and the emergence of new weapons have produced traumas of a different nature or degree than in the past. It is necessary to study methods of treatment and protection to improve the treatment rate. For example, the increasing speed of the ball increases the injury; the cluster bombs cause multiple injuries; the widespread use of incendiary bombs causes a large number of severe burns; the nuclear weapons expand the scope of the killing and increase the radiation damage and compound injuries; the emergence of injuries caused by high toxic neurotoxic agents and infectious diseases caused by biological warfare agents, etc. The improvement of military equipment has put forward special physical and psychological requirements for the operators. It is necessary to medically study the special conditions of such soldiers in order to better grasp the new weapons and equipment. With the expansion of the scale of war, more seriously wounded need to be sent quickly. It is necessary to study the war wound pathology and war injury surgery, and implement the most reasonably graded treatment to minimize the death rate (incident mortality rate). The special conditions of the field require the development of lightweight, applicable, and portable medical technology equipment to meet the needs of the army's mobile operations.

Although the possibility of a global world war is small, regional wars or conflicts have continued. In addition, the usual trauma is also a major disease that endangers human health today. Therefore, tissue repair after trauma is always an important topic in clinical medicine and military medicine.

### 1.2.2 The Development of Tissue Repair and Regenerative Medicine After the Trauma of Our Military

In ancient China's war, in the era of cold weapons, the battlefields were dominated by fists, knives, lances, arrows, and halberds. In the treatment, "jinchuang zheyang" were the mainstay. Therefore, ancient military medicine has very few special works, and it is attached to the traumatology department. After the Song Dynasty, with the development of firearms, guns were used in warfare, and their lethality was 100 times higher than that of the sword and arrow era. But before 1840, there were not many applications of guns. Therefore, in ancient Chinese military medicine, the treatment was still similar to that of cold weapons.

In the early days of the army, the curriculum of war wound surgery and frequent disease prevention and control was set up in the health school of the Red Army. The period of the Agrarian Revolutionary War was the bud of the field surgery of our army. In the many anti-encirclement wars, it accumulated the experience of mass prevention work in difficult circumstances, and the ability to treat war wounds has been improved. On the basis of summing up the experience of war wounds in the battles and the experience and lessons of the medical organizations, our army's field surgery has gradually transited from disorder to order. In October 1927, the first Red Army Hospital was established in Jinggang Shan. It was divided into slight injuries, serious injuries, and patient departments. It unified the various health service systems, issued trauma treatments, and promulgated health regulations and health services outline above the division, making the health work institutionalized. It emphasized the concept of sterility, properly stop bleeding, dressing, fixation, and wound treatment, and paid attention to technical operations such as shrapnel removal and amputation. It relied on military and civilian efforts to use Chinese and Western medicine and took local materials to treat the wounded. Field hospitals have begun to pay attention to emergency surgery and early treatment of wounds. In terms of organization, an organization system with health workers in company, health centers in battalion, health teams in regiment, and health departments in division has been formed. A series of wounded rescue agencies have been set up from the front to the rear, and the relatively complete medical evacuation system from rescue team, the group bandages, the division army field hospital, the military station hospital to the rear hospital has been established.

During the War of Resistance Against Japan, due to the development of the anti-Japanese national united front, more medical personnel at home and abroad came to the base areas, especially the Canadian medical team led by Norman Bethune, which strengthened the health technology of our army. Because of the weak technical foundation and materials shortage, the development of field surgery was still subject to many restrictions. In terms of theoretical technology, extensive self-help and mutual rescue activities were carried out, and first aid in frontline was strengthened. The medical team and the surgical team were as close as possible to the position, and early debridement within 12 h was implemented, which significantly improved the treatment of fracture injuries. The scope of field surgery has been expanded, the dressing method has been changed, and traumatic shock, traumatic infection, and complications have been actively prevented and cured. Some units have adopted techniques such as blood transfusion and infusion, and have had preliminary experience in the prevention and treatment of poisonous injuries. In terms of organization, the tasks of organizations at all levels were stipulated. The health workers in company mainly rescue the wounded on the fire line, carry out dressing, hemostasis, fixation and handling, and educate the soldiers to learn to use first-aid kits and wrap knowledge in order to save themselves and rescue each other in an emergency. The rescue center in the battalion is responsible for bandaging and transporting the wounded. After the initial rescue of the wounded by the rescue center in the battalion, in addition to the short-term survivable, the others are sent to the division or the military hospital for treatment.

During the War of Liberation, we learned of the advanced experience of military health service in the countries of the Second World War and the techniques of war wound treatment. We established a regular ladder treatment system and continuously summarized the practical experience of war wound treatment. Field surgery has developed rapidly. In terms of theoretical technology, the study and application of new technologies for war wound treatment have been generally carried out. They emphasize the early implementation of early surgical treatment based on debridement, the implementation of plaster bandage therapy, and the prevention and treatment of special infections such as tetanus and gas gangrene, the correct method of dressing, comprehensive prevention, and treatment of shock. The Provisional Regulations on Field Ambulance Treatment, the Temporary General Rules for War Damage Treatment, and the War Damage Medical Regulations have been formulated one after another, which has enabled our military's basic technology of war wound treatment to be organized and institutionalized, marking our army's war wound treatment work to a new stage. In terms of organization, the Wartime Health Service Regulations and Interim Health Regulations were formulated, and the medical service organizations at all levels of the company, the battalion, the regiment, and the division were further improved. The organization, tasks, working principles, and requirements of the rescue agencies at all levels were made with clear provisions. This made the treatment of the wounded and sick from the frontline ambulance, regiment rescue center, the division (brigade) station to the column (military) hospital, forming a unified ladder treatment system with both divisions of labor and continuity.

After the founding of the People's Republic of China, the Department of Experimental Surgery was established by the Academy of Military Medical Sciences in 1952. In 1962, it was renamed the Institute of Field Surgery. In 1978, it merged with the Third Affiliated Hospital of the Third Military Medical University and was placed under the leadership of the Third Military Medical University. Among them, Shen Kefei, Sheng Zhiyong, and other experts have made outstanding contributions to the development of our military experimental surgery. In addition, the Field Surgery edited by Professor Wu Gongliang and Professor Zhao Lianbi in the early stage has played a positive role in promoting the development of trauma surgery and tissue repair and regenerative medicine in China. Later, Academician Wang Zhengguo also edited a new *Field Surgery*, which played an important role in inheriting and developing our military field surgery. Field Surgery was approved as a master's degree in 1984. In 1986, it was approved as a doctoral degree. In 1989, it was approved as a national key discipline. In 1994, it was approved as a postdoctoral research station. In 2005, it was approved as a key discipline of Army Project 2110.

In the new historical period, the concept, scope, and treatment techniques of war trauma surgery have undergone significant changes. It is imperative to write a series of new large-scale academic monographs reflecting the latest theories, techniques, and methods of modern war trauma. In 2014, Academician Xiaobing Fu, Academician Wang Zhengguo, and Professor Li Jianxian of Yangming University in Taiwan province as chief editors, the famous trauma medical workers in mainland and Taiwan province as authors, *The Chinese Trauma Medicine* was officially published. This large-scale academic monograph fully reflects the latest achievements in the fields of trauma epidemiology, trauma medicine, clinical treatment, trauma rehabilitation, etc. in the mainland and Taiwan province, especially more than 20 traumatologists in Taiwan province, China participating in it. The compilation has become an important achievement in the academic exchange of traumatic medicine between the two sides.

In order to better reflect the perfect combination of trauma medicine and military medicine, in 2016, Academician Wang Zhengguo, Academician Lu Shibi, Academician Cheng Tianmin, and Academician Sheng Zhiyong served as consultants, and Academician Xiaobing Fu was the chief editor of the large-scale academic monograph *Chinese Trauma* officially published. Different from the *Chinese Trauma Medicine* published in 2014, this large-scale academic monograph not only reflects the traumatic in peacetime, but also pays special attention to the latest developments and future directions in the field of war injury treatment in recent years. It summed up the experience of war wound healing from US military in Afghanistan War and Iraq war. The book contains a total of 11 volumes, including the general theory of war trauma, traumatic brain trauma, oral and maxillofacial trauma, eye trauma, otolaryngology-head and neck trauma, chest and abdomen trauma, limb spine and pelvic trauma, special causes of trauma, special environmental trauma, regeneration and rehabilitation, trauma care, and psychology, a total of 16.5 million words, composed of more than 500 Chinese traumatic medical experts. This series of monographs is the latest, most systematic, and comprehensive academic monograph in the field of traumatic medicine in China. It is believed that its publication will greatly promote the development of traumatic medicine in China.

Since the founding of the People's Republic of China, under the support of medical research, especially after the test of self-defense operations such as the War to Resist US Aggression and Aid Korea and the Sino-Indian border, Chenpao Island, Xisha Islands, and China-Vietnam border, our military's war wound treatment technology has shown new developments on the basis of perfection and improvement over the original treatment system. In 1982, our military listed ventilation and long-term use of hemostasis, dressing, fixation, and handling as five basic techniques for first aid. In 2006, in the new version of the war injury treatment rule, the basic life support technology was added to expand the first-aid technology to six. The cricothyroid membrane puncture, cricothyroidotomy, and hemostasis with peripheral blood vessels were added on the basis of what the original health workers should master.

In response to changes in weapons development, operational concepts, and operational styles, our military has conducted an in-depth research on nuclear weapon wounds, new concept weapon injuries, impact injuries, burns, crush injuries, and special environmental injuries. The principle of prevention and cure has greatly improved the level of wound treatment of our army and enriched the connotation of field surgery. Among them, the basic and clinical research on burns, impact injuries, and nuclear weapon wounds are at the internationally advanced level. In 1999, the Third Military Medical University established three military key (open) laboratories into a "combination laboratory for trauma, burn and combined injury." In 2001, as a key laboratory of the department, it entered the state key laboratory evaluation. In 2003, it was included in the state key laboratory construction plan by the Ministry of Science and Technology. In November 2005, it passed the acceptance of the Ministry of Science and Technology and officially became the first state key laboratory of the army. In August 2012, the seven military units including the Third Military Medical University, the Academy of Military Medical Sciences, the PLA General Hospital, and the China Academy of Engineering Physics, etc. established the first "Community Innovation Center for War-Wound Prevention and Control." The center is led by the Academician Wang Zhengguo. The high-level academic team with the "Talent Project" national-level candidates and the winners of the National Science Fund for Distinguished Young Scholars as the core backbone has undertaken a series of major project researches on the traumatic treatment of the military over the years. Relying on the established state key disciplines—Field Surgery, Burn Surgery, Military Preventive Medicine, and the State Key Laboratory of Trauma, Burn and Combined Injury, which have been functioning well, the center has confirmed four research directions including the innovative theory of war wound prevention and cure, the key technology of war wound prevention and cure, the research of field health equipment, war wound treatment equipment and drug, and the conversion of war trauma theory, technology, equipment, and drug.

Especially in the field of burn wound tissue repair, our military research work has achieved fruitful results. In the early 1990s, the National Natural Science Foundation's first major project involved burn wounds and posttraumatic wound repairs, led by Professor Shi Jixiang of Ruijin Hospital of Shanghai Second Medical University and Professor Li Ao of Southwest Hospital of the Third Military Medical University. The focus is on the pathophysiological mechanism of burn wound repair. In 1999, the field of trauma medicine was funded by the National Major Project "973." The chief scientist was Academician Wang Zhengguo. Later, Professor Jiang Jianxin and Academician Xiaobing

Fu successively assumed the National "973" Trauma and tissue repair and regeneration project as the chief scientist. This series of research has made breakthroughs in "Basic Research on Severe Trauma Treatment and Injury Tissue Repair." Focusing on the two core issues of improving the level of severe trauma treatment and the quality of damaged tissue repair, we work together and carry out a series of studies on vascular reactivity, permeability, and "shock heart" related to the occurrence of ischemia and hypoxia in traumatic shock, and found a new regulatory target. According to the mutual regulator control of neuroendocrine, immunoregulatory cells and immunosuppressive molecules, we proposed a new mechanism of posttraumatic immune dysfunction. According to the aspects of genetic background differences, immune molecules, and immune cell phenotype changes, a series of biological indicators for early detection of traumatic complications have been proposed and a series of comprehensive measures to antagonize pathogen infection, enhance the body's own anti-injury ability, and early prevention and treatment of traumatic complications have been established. This further confirms the important biological phenomenon of dedifferentiation of epidermal cells, and by inoculating transplanted stem cells, the tissue structure resembling sweat glands is cultivated to solve the problem of perspiration in patients with deep burns. From the clinical perspective, the long-term mild hypothermia treatment of patients with severe brain injury better than short-term mild hypothermia therapy has been proved. Breeding more than 10 kinds of mice with transgenic or gene knockout for traumatic research, we found a new target to promote fracture healing. We first proposed the concept of activated Schwann cells and found that activated Schwann cells are more conducive to the repair of peripheral nerve defects, providing a new method for the treatment of peripheral nerve injury. We revealed that the microenvironment of wounds promotes the regulation mechanism of adult stem cell repair and has created a variety of key technologies for adult stem cells to repair damaged tissue. In addition, great progress has been made in the research of chronic wound repair, damage mechanism, and prevention methods of skin soft tissue blast injury and seawater immersion injury, and new techniques for the treatment of traumatic facial deformity.

The related research in the field of tissue repair and regeneration has been highly recognized by the state, and the first class prize of The State Science and Technology Progress Award is taken as an example. It can be seen that the innovation and transformation application in this field promote clinical treatment. In the repair of facial injuries, with the widespread use of high-explosive weapons, the proportion of facial warfare increased from 3.4% in World War II to 23% in the Iraq war. Its repair and treatment is an internationally recognized military medical problem. Professor Zhao Yimin's research team of the Fourth Military Medical University, after 20 years of hard work, formed autologous transplantation repair—"face," allograft repair—"face change," prosthetic simulation repair—"prosthetic face," tissue regeneration repair— "face regeneration" as one of the serious face warfare wounds and deformed morphological repair and functional reconstruction technology system, which can meet the needs of a variety of facial injuries. In 2011, the country selected a total of 20 first class prizes for scientific and technological progress, including "Severe Face Warfare, Wound Defect and Morphological Repair and Functional Reconstruction" as a military-specific project, which stood out from 863 declaration projects and finally won the national first class award.

In the aspect of repairing chronic refractory wounds on the surface of the body, the team of Academician Xiaobing Fu of the People's Liberation Army General Hospital won the first class prize of The State Science and Technology Progress Award in 2015, for the study of the innovative theory and key measures for the new characteristics and prevention of refractory wounds in Chinese human body. This is the unique first class prize of The State Science and Technology Progress Award in China's clinical medicine field in 2015.

Through fruitful collaboration, after more than 10 years of research, the project has achieved four innovations:

(a) Two new characteristics of wound epidemiology were discovered. Through the large-scale multicenter epidemiological study of 1.48 million inpatients, it is the first time in the world that the main cause of refractory wounds in Chinese human body has been changed from trauma and infection 10 years ago to diabetic foot and complications of senile chronic diseases. Based on this, the high-risk factors and wound characteristics of diabetic foot in China were identified through the investigation of 3000 cases of diabetic foot, which pointed out the direction for scientific prevention.
(b) Three special mechanisms for the treatment of diabetic foot and radioactive wounds were first proposed. They are, the "hidden damage" mechanism of cell or matrix dysfunction caused by accumulation of toxic substances such as high sugar and advanced glycation end products (AGEs) in diabetic skin; glycosylation of growth factors and macrophage chemotaxis and abnormal phagocytosis—the difficult immune mechanism; the mechanism of radioactive wounds' "network disorders of healing factors with cell damage as the key link," providing innovative theories for establishing key control measures.
(c) Based on previous treatments, four key prevention measures were created. The first use of photon technology to reduce the "hidden damage" caused by wound glycation products, the use of regulating the internal environment to reduce the "progressive damage" of repair cells, the recruitment of cells, and the provision of scaffold mate-

rials to promote wound healing and the first international adoption of "4G" to realize that complex wounds are treated under the same standard at different levels of medical institutions, so that the cure rate of difficult wounds is significantly improved. The overall cure rate for a typical unit increased from 60% to around 94%. In this achievement, the total amputation rate of diabetic foot was 7.2%, and the large amputation rate was 4.0%. In the same period, the corresponding indicators in Europe reported 22% and 5%, respectively, the difference was very significant (Fig. 1.1).

(d) We innovated treatment mode for the characteristics of refractory wounds with preventable control, large outpatient, and small ward. We also advocated the establishment of more than 50 wound treatment specialists (centers); created a new scientific prevention and treatment model for the two-way linkage and referral of single disease between wound treatment specialists and community medical institutions; established a new strategy by cooperation with international and domestic funds to develop early stage prevention and control education of refractory wounds.

The discipline construction and talent cultivation in the field of trauma and wound repair and tissue regeneration in China have also achieved rapid development. Talents are the key to the development of disciplines. China's trauma medicine has not only a large number of talents, but also qualified successors. There are many founders and pioneers of the older generation of disciplines, such as Academician Li Ao, Academician Sheng Zhiyong, Academician Cheng Tianmin, and Academician Wang Zhengguo. In recent years, a large number of innovative people have emerged. The excellent young and middle-aged generation is not only based on their own work, but also with an international outlook. According to preliminary statistics, there were eight members who served as members of the Chinese Medical Association Trauma Branch and later became academicians of the two academies (Li Ao, Sheng Zhiyong, Cheng Tianmin, Li Jieshou, Wang Zhengguo, Gu Yudong, Zhou Liangfu, Xiaobing Fu). There were nine members who served as members of the Chinese Medical Association Trauma Branch or the Academic Group, or participated in the National "973" Trauma and Tissue Repair and Regeneration Project, and has won the National Science Fund for Distinguished Young Scholars for basic research and clinical treatment of wound healing (Xiaobing Fu, Xia Zhaofan, Huang Yuesheng, Jiang Jianxin, Yao Yongming, Jiang Baoguo, Liu Liangming, Chen Lin, Zhao Min). In particular, the establishment of the State Key Laboratory of Trauma, Burns and Combined Injury at the Third Military Medical University and the "Repair and Regenerative Medicine" innovation research group of the PLA General Hospital was funded by the National Natural Science Foundation of China in 2011, marking the overall level of the field to have been recognized by the state. During the "Eleventh Five-Year Plan" period, Xijing Hospital Plastic Surgery and Changhai Hospital Plastic Surgery have successively become the All-Army Plastic Surgery Research Institute and Plastic Surgery Center. The plastic surgery of the three military medical universities has entered the ranks of national key disciplines. In the field of international wound repair, in 2008, in Toronto, Canada, Professor Xiaobing Fu was awarded the "International Wound Healing Research Lifetime Achievement Award" for "International Discovery in the Field of Tissue Repair and Regeneration and the Role of These Discoveries in Promoting Clinical Therapy."

In the course of decades of development, our military field surgery has grown from scratch, from weak to strong, providing theoretical support and technical services for the research and clinical treatment of postwar tissue repair in our army. It has maintained the health of the officers and soldiers of the army, improved the combat effectiveness of the troops, and made great contributions to the cause of national defense and health. However, the trauma care of our country is still far from the most advanced treatment system in foreign countries. In the future, we should further improve

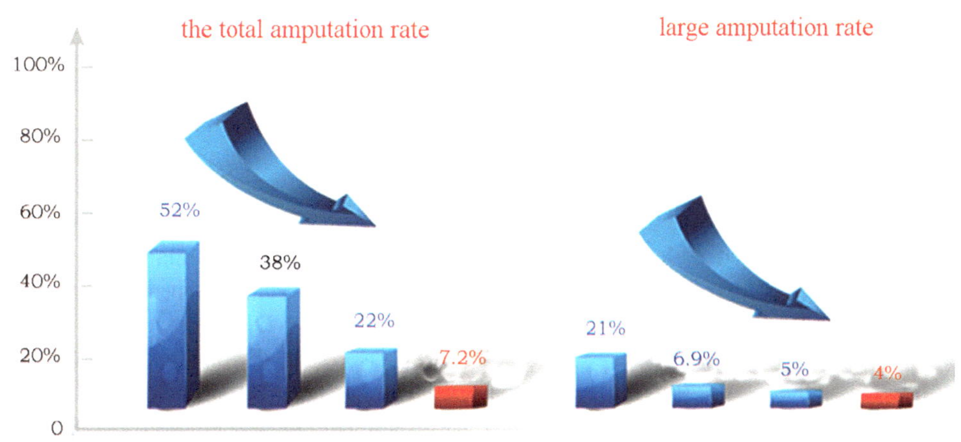


**Fig. 1.1** Compared with developed countries, the total amputation rate and large amputation rate of diabetic foot in China are significantly lower

the medical emergency network, standardize first-aid organizations, emergency personnel, medical equipment, transportation and communication equipment, etc., especially strengthen on-site first-aid and transportation, and strive to achieve a coordinated process of prehospital care and hospital treatment.

### 1.2.3 The Future Development of Posttraumatic Tissue Repair and Regenerative Medicine

Under the new situation of rapid advancement of medical science and technology, new military reforms, and military health preparations, the traumatic treatment and posttraumatic tissue repair in field surgery face severe challenges and major opportunities. The mission is lofty and has a long way to go. I look forward to the writing of a new chapter by the vast number of field surgeons.

Expand the research field of weapon traumatology. In the future war, the increase in the types of new weapons and the killing factors will increase the proportion of nonfirearms war wounds, and the form of warfare that is not directly contacted by air strikes and anti-air strikes will increase. Therefore, first of all, it is necessary to study the injury effects and injury mechanisms of various new killing weapons. Secondly, we must strengthen the study of explosive weapon injuries. From the local wars that have occurred in recent years, explosive weapons are gradually becoming the main killing weapons in modern warfare. Explosive weapons not only have great killing power, but also have many damage factors. The damage caused is characterized by multiple injuries, combined injury and serious injury increasing. It is predicted that under the conditions of high-tech local war in the future, the following characteristics may occur in war injuries.

(a) Increased impact injuries: With the application of high-explosive weapons and burning air bombs, shock waves will play a more important role in killing factors. If the enemy uses a tactical nuclear weapon with strong shock wave bombs, the killing effect of the shock wave will be more prominent, and the resulting impact injury will be more and more serious.
(b) Increased mechanical injuries and multiple injuries: Under the action of strong shock waves, a large number of houses collapsed and the fortifications destroyed. The masonry and wooden blocks from the destroyed building will hit human body in the form of secondary projectiles. There will be many mechanical injuries such as crush injuries and multiple injuries.
(c) Increased burns: Buildings, woods, etc. are often on fire after being hit by bombs. If the enemy uses flaming weapons, anti-tank weapons, or fuel-air bombs, it is more likely to cause fires. In this case, burns will inevitably increase.
(d) Increased combined injury: Two or more of the killing factors simultaneously or successively acting on the human body, the injury is called combined injury. In future wars, weapons with different injury factors may be used at the same time. The same weapon may sometimes have multiple killing factors, so the number of combined injuries will increase. The research on the characteristics of explosive weapons and the treatment should be strengthened, especially the study on the combined effects of punching, burning, fragmentation, and crush. If a tactical nuclear weapon is used, radioactive combined injury may also occur.
(e) Increased psychic trauma: With the suddenness and cruelty of the war, some people who lack experience in warfare, especially young soldiers with poor stability of psychology and spirit, are prone to combat stress reactions caused by tremendous mental stress. If there are other war injuries at the same time, the condition will be heavier.
(f) Other new weapon injuries: Laser damage, microwave damage, infrasound damage, etc., which have never been seen before on the battlefield, may occur under certain local war conditions. Based on these characteristics, research emphasis on tissue repair and clinical applications should be adjusted. Strengthen research on war injuries under special environmental conditions. Under the conditions of high cold, high heat, high altitude, sea, etc., the characteristics of various war wounds and the treatments are obviously different.

Although the injury factors are various and can occur in various parts of the body, after any kind of trauma, the body's systemic reaction and the repair of the damaged tissue have a common law. Strengthening the basic research of war trauma and clarifying these common problems are of great significance for guiding the early treatment of various war wounds and the later tissue repair. In the war-wounded patients who died, at least 50% died of postinjury complications, except that the vital organs were directly injured and immediately killed. Most tissues are structurally repairable after damage, but functional repairs are poor. For example, large-area burn wounds are healed, but there are a lot of scars, especially the lack of skin attachments, so there are still serious disabilities. Therefore, only by further strengthening the basic research of war trauma medicine can we better improve the level of war wound healing.

Early systemic damage, visceral complications, and damaged tissue repair are the common problems of various types of war wounds. The basic laws can guide the treatment of various types of trauma.

(a) Pay attention to the mechanism and prevention of wound infection. Traumatic infections are mainly endogenous infections caused by displacement of the resident bacteria and their toxins in the body. Decreased immune function, mucosal barrier damage, and dysbacteriosis in the body during severe trauma are important mechanisms leading to endogenous infection after trauma.
(b) Focus on the intrinsic relationship between early neurological, endocrine, immune response, and posttraumatic complications in severe trauma, and explore the interaction between injury and anti-injury. In severe trauma, not only is the injury response very serious, but the body's anti-injury reaction and endogenous protection mechanism are also significantly weakened. The serious imbalance between the two is an important basis for further damage after trauma.
(c) Deeply understand the complex mechanisms of tissue repair and regeneration. The contents include the changes in the biological behavior of repair cells and extracellular matrix and their effects on the repair and regeneration of tissue repair, and the role of various repair cells, growth factors, genes, and microenvironment changes in wound healing and regeneration. Combining the research of developmental science and comparative biology, it shows a new understanding of scar healing and delayed healing of tissue, and proposes the scientific hypothesis and research goal of achieving simultaneous repair and regeneration of damaged tissue at the injury site, to achieve perfect repair and regeneration of damaged tissue.
(d) Pay attention to the repair research of bone, peripheral nerve, central nerve, etc. On the one hand, it helps to study the regularity of self-regeneration and repair or cellular and molecular basis of these tissues after damage, and the factors affecting their regeneration and repair. On the other hand, it is used to explore measures to artificially promote the repair of these tissues, mainly including various biological factors (recombinant growth factors, etc.) and physical factors (acoustic, optical, electrical, magnetic field stimulation, etc.).
(e) The application of high-tech biotechnology in wound repair and tissue regeneration is mainly reflected in new intelligent biomaterials, tissue engineering, and stem cell research. Tissue engineering is a new technology in the field of wound repair. It is important to research and develop new biomaterials and tissue substitutes and fillers with better biocompatibility. Using tissue engineering principles and techniques it is possible to construct tissue-engineered tissues and organs. The clinical exploration and basic research of allograft (xenograft) composite tissue transplantation, although far from the clinical application, have initially shown their broad application prospects [21].

In short, paying attention to the research on the repair and regeneration of damaged tissue after trauma is of great significance to improve the level of war wound treatment and enhance the morale of the army. Its position in military medicine is irreplaceable.

## 1.3 Wound Tissue Repair and Regeneration Concept

Although trauma is an ancient medical problem, it is also a social issue that deserves attention at the same time. According to foreign data, more than 50% of the people wounded by explosions and earthquakes have skin and soft tissue damage. With the development of social productivity, the improvement of industrialization level, and the improvement of medical care level, the incidence of trauma has not only decreased, but has also continued to increase. Trauma has become one of the leading killers of death in both developed and developing countries.

Regardless of the size of the wound, there is a problem of tissue repair. The traditional understanding of wound repair mainly stays at the general and cellular level, which is mainly based on the level of understanding of people in different eras and the limitations of research methods at that time. Since the 1980s, the development of science and technology has enabled people to have the ability to re-recognize the basic processes of wound healing at the molecular and genetic levels, thus laying a good foundation for further basic theoretical research and clinical treatment.

In general, the wound itself initiates the repair process. Posttraumatic tissue repair begins with coagulation and is coordinated by a number of cells, extracellular matrices, and regulatory factors. Initially, platelets, neutrophils, and macrophages enter the wounded area in large quantities to remove the damaged tissue and contaminating microorganisms. Platelets and macrophages also secrete some growth factors associated with fibroblasts and endothelial cells. The fibroblasts and endothelial cells then gradually replace the damaged matrix. At the same time, epithelial cells also grow inward from the wound margin until they cover the wound. Therefore, the speed of wound repair depends on the speed at which the above cells enter the wound and proliferate there, and the entry and proliferation of the cells are dependent on the regulation of chemokines and growth factors.

Chemokines are usually peptides, proteins, and protein fragments that cause cells to move in a certain direction, such as from low to high concentrations. The response of a cell to a chemokine depends on the number of corresponding growth factor receptors. Different cells respond differently to different chemokines. Chemokines are produced in the coagulation process, and aggregated platelets are their main source. Therefore, some cytotoxic drugs that reduce the number of circulating platelets can also affect the wound healing process, such as anti-macrophage antibodies. In addition, macrophages, fibroblasts, and endothelial cells themselves produce some chemokines and cleavage factors.

Growth factors are also proteins or peptides that act alone or in combination with several growth factors to induce DNA synthesis and cell division. There are dozens or even hundreds of growth factors that have been discovered, but there are more than 10 kinds of researches that can be used as basic and clinical. The representative factors are platelet-derived growth factor (PDGF), acidic or basic fibroblast growth factors (FGFs), epidermal growth factor (EGF), transforming growth factor (TGF), insulin-like growth factor (IGF), etc. They participate in wound repair mainly through mechanisms such as autocrine and paracrine. At low concentrations, the responsiveness of cells to growth factors depends on the presence of corresponding growth factor receptors on the cells. For example, PDGF acts only on fibroblasts, whereas FGF has effects on both fibroblasts and endothelial cells. It should be pointed out that some growth factors also have chemotaxis, and this dual action has special significance for wound healing. Therefore, they are sometimes referred to as split chemokines. This dual action factor is required for intercellular action in the early stages of wound healing, and in the later stages, such as DNA synthesis, chemotaxis is no longer needed. Studies have confirmed that these growth factors can show significant effects on treatment without obvious side effects. The basic research and clinical application of growth factors are currently in a positive development stage. Although genetic engineering drugs represented by growth factors have shown unique effects on wound healing, they are still only one of the ways to promote repair, and cannot replace the basic treatments such as debridement, anti-infection, and skin grafting. Therefore, the application of growth factors can only be better if they are based on surgical treatment. Because the growth factor repairs the wound, it is still scar repair, lacking structures such as sweat glands, sebaceous glands, and hair follicles, and even nerve endings. These problems in the recovery and reconstruction of healing tissue function, as well as the adverse reactions that may be caused by the application of growth factors in local wounds, and the regulatory relationship between growth factors and wounds are the focus of current attention and research.

It has a long history of adding certain substances extracted from tissues to the wound site to promote healing. In the past 20 years, with the deepening of research on growth factors, especially the development of genetic engineering technology, people can mass produce such genetic engineering products in vitro. Therefore, there have been many reports on the use of growth factors to promote acute and chronic wound healing. However, some people believe that due to the local addition of growth factors, the effective concentration is difficult to maintain due to the wound environment (including enzymes, salts, and pollution), and it is often necessary to give large doses of growth factors. To solve this problem, a genetically modified approach can now be used to solve this problem. This method uses technology such as gene gun and micro-planting to transfer the target gene into the site to be healed by in vivo and in vitro methods, so that the factors that promote repair can be continuously produced in the wound site. However, since the safety and methodology are not completely solved, this method is not yet practical. The safety and long-term effects of topical application of growth factors remain the focus of attention. Platelet-rich plasma (PRP) is a plasma containing platelets that exceed several times the physiological concentration. It is mainly used to repair by various high-concentration growth factors (such as PDGF, FGF, TGF, and IGF) and has become a research focus in recent years, with a relatively positive effect, it has become one of the new therapies to promote wound healing.

The size of the scar tension depends on the synthesis and deposition of collagen. The latter is related to the number of fibroblasts and to wound oxygen tension, vitamin levels, and nutritional status. Growth factors promote collagen synthesis by enhancing cell division. Most growth factors also promote the production of collagenase, which in turn enhances collagen degradation. In contrast, although TGF-β also promotes collagen synthesis, it also inhibits collagen degradation. Therefore, it is believed that TGF-β may be involved in the development of certain fibrotic diseases.

With the improvement of people's living standards, the past repair mode that aims to achieve the anatomical repair of wounds has been difficult to adapt to people's needs, especially in large-area burn patients. The wounds of scar repair have no sweat glands and hair follicles. It is physiologically difficult to adapt to changes in the environment, and psychologically cannot return to society. Therefore, the transformation of wounds from anatomical repair to functional repair is receiving increasing attention.

It can be predicted that the damage and repair of important internal organs caused by severe trauma and disease will become the focus of further research. On the one hand, it is the active repair after the important organ injury caused by ischemia-reperfusion. On the other hand, it is the excessive repair after the organ damage caused by some diseases, that is, the prevention and treatment of fibrosis. With the deepening of research, both issues are expected to be resolved. The replacement of depleted organs with artificial organs is also a direction that people are working hard.

Stem cell technology, cloning technology, and tissue engineering technology are some of the research contents of wound repair and tissue regeneration, while others provide the basis and conditions for wound repair and tissue regeneration research, which is an important part of trauma repair research in the twenty-first century. They should be taken seriously. Medical workers should work closely with experts in biology, tissue engineering, and materials science to collaborate, so that multidisciplinary collaboration is likely to break through.

The biggest feature of high-tech local warfare is sudden and rapid advancement. If officers and soldiers cannot quickly adapt to the battlefield environment or be deterred by high-tech weapons and equipment in a short period of time, there may be a series of psychological obstacles and even psychological collapse.

Strengthening research on the prevention and control of battlefield stress and mental illness is the focus of attention in recent years. Our military still has some blind spots in military psychological training. For the battlefield stress and mental illness, and their impact on the ability of wound repair, there is still a lack of in-depth systematic research, so it needs to be further strengthened.

### 1.3.1 Repair and Repair "Out of Control"

Repair is a series of pathophysiological processes that actively repair wounds by proliferation or regeneration, or affect the wound repair by manual intervention after tissue defect due to trauma or other disease, such as through surgical techniques to transfer the flaps to repair wounds. Therefore, the concept includes both the healing process of the organism itself and the impact of human factors on wound healing. There are two types of repair: the repair by the surrounding cells of the same kind is called regeneration; the repair by the fibrous connective tissue is called fiber repair.

Repair "out of control" is an academic concept that needs further clarification. In theory, the growth, development, and repair of organisms is an orderly biological process. After the tissue is damaged, the wounds should be fully recovered by anatomy and function. But this goal is often difficult to achieve after the birth of the human body. At present, the repair outcome of a wound that is unhealed (hard to heal) or repair of excessive hypertrophic scars or keloids for some reason is called repair "out of control" (Fig. 1.2).

Scar tissue is mainly composed of collagen and fibroblasts. In the wound with a small defect, neat wound edge, no infection, and good wound, the scar tissue is not obvious, like a line, and has no effect on function. In wounds with large defects, incomplete wounds, or infections, scars often form large and high out of wounds, which not only affect the tissue function, but also unsightly. According to histopathology, scar tissue can be divided into the following categories: normal scars and pathological scars. The general skin scars gradually heal in a few weeks, may show redness and hardening, but will automatically disappear within 6 months to 2 years, leaving a normal color scar. Pathological scars can be divided into hypertrophic scars, keloids, and unstable scars. These pathological scars differ in morphology, pathology, and biological behavior and the treatment methods are quite different.

The role and impact of scar tissue:

1. The beneficial side of the body: The formation of scar tissue can permanently connect the damaged wound or the defected tissue and maintain the integrity and firmness of the tissue and organs.
2. Adverse effects on the body:
   (a) Due to poor elasticity of the scar tissue, the strength of the tensile force is weak. If the local pressure is

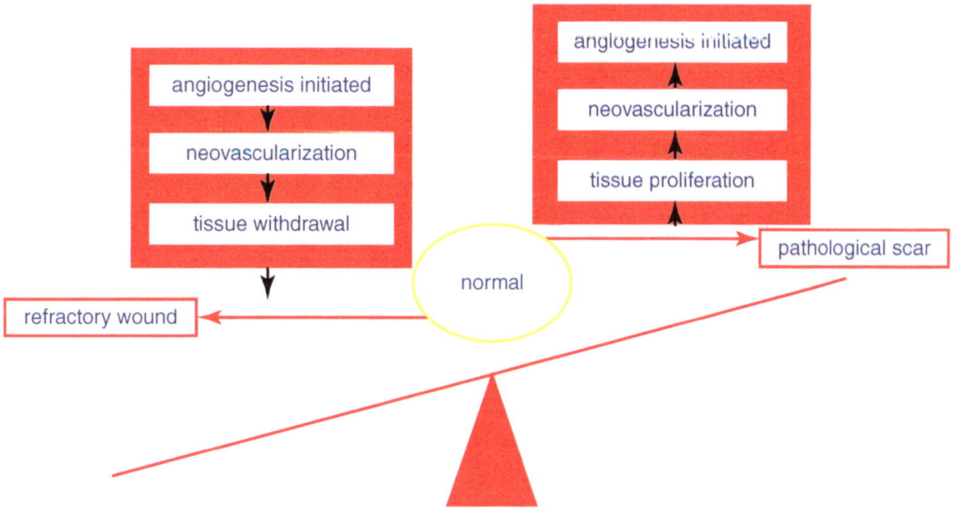


**Fig. 1.2** Microvascular formation may have a relationship with different healing outcomes
Note: Various factors cause damage to the microvascular formation of the wound, resulting in insufficient material and energy necessary for tissue repair or failure to remove the metabolites in the wound, which will interfere with the normal procedure of wound repair and abnormal repair outcomes (over and under), including hyperplasia of scars, keloid formation, diabetic microangiopathy, and venous stasis ulcers

excessively applied, the healing scar tissue can bulge outward. Just as the abdominal wall scar due to abdominal pressure increased can form abdominal wall hernia, the scar formed by myocardial infarction protrudes outward to form a ventricular aneurysm.

(b) Scar tissue can contract, which can lead to luminal stenosis, joint movement disorder, organ adhesion, or hardening.

(c) A small number of patients with hyperplasia of scar tissue to form a raised plaque, called keloid. After a long period of time, the collagen fibers in the scar tissue are decomposed and absorbed under the action of collagenase, so that the scar shrinks and softens. Collagenase is mainly derived from macrophages, neutrophils, and fibroblasts.

#### 1.3.1.1 Hypertrophic Scar

Hyperplastic scars, also known as hypertrophic scars, occur mostly in the depth of injury that affects only the dermis. The pathological difference between a hypertrophic scar and a normal scar is only due to the thickening of collagen fibers in the deep scar, which is characterized by an irregular arrangement, or wavy, or wound into a rope. Hypertrophic scars often occur after wound healing in deep burns. Reticular hypertrophic scars are also common in sutures after skin grafting of the III degree burn wound. In addition, any incision scar after suturing is also included in this type. Hypertrophic scars are characterized by prominent surfaces, irregular shapes, uneven heights, flushing and congestion, firmness and toughness, burning, and itching. Excessive hyperplasia is higher than the wound, but is still limited to the wound. There will be obvious atrophy and lightening in the 2 years after the scar is formed.

#### 1.3.1.2 Keloid

Keloid refers to hypertrophic scars that infiltrate the surrounding skin beyond the wound area itself. It is more common in the chest and limbs, and has a higher incidence of colored people (especially black and yellow races). Skin scars continue to proliferate during healing and spread to the surrounding area, like the shape of the foot or butterfly, become hard and are accompanied by red pain. These scars are often called keloids. Keloids are common in the anterior chest, scapular, earlobe, and upper arm, and are highly prevalent in women. The physique of those who are prone to keloids is called scar physique. Some mast cells are common around the blood vessels in the keloid, so it is believed that due to persistent local inflammation and hypoxia, the mast cells are promoted to secrete various growth factors, and the granulation tissue is excessively grown, thereby forming keloids. The current study found that the etiology and pathogenesis of keloids are also related to many factors. Among them are the combination of cytokines and extracellular matrix collagen metabolism, the role of nuclear transcription factor NF-κB signaling pathway in skin physiology, and the family genetic factors. Only a clearer understanding of the pathogenesis of keloids may provide a basis for the clinical treatment of keloids and bring breakthroughs.

#### 1.3.1.3 Scar Ulcer or Unstable Scar

Scar ulcer or unstable scar, also known as chronic wounds, is defined by the International Society for Wound Healing as a state of the wound failing to achieve anatomical and functional integrity through normal, orderly, and timely repair. These wounds often delay healing or even nonhealing, and have specific causes such as diabetes, ischemia, stress, etc. Clinically, chronic wounds refer to wounds formed by various reasons after 1 or 3 months (time is not completely absolute) treatment fails to heal and there is no tendency to heal. It covers a variety of factors such as the size of the wound, the cause of the disease, and the general health of the individual. One type of ulcer is due to unstable scarring. In the early stage of scar formation, fibroblast proliferation, and capillary dilatation, the appearance of redness and thickening is observed, showing a strong proliferation phenomenon; then the scar tissue continues to shrink; after a period of time, the scar tissue enters a stable stage, at which point the scar becomes soft and thin. In some areas (one third of the lower leg, joints, etc.), some are easy to rupture, resulting in chronic ulcers. In particular, some of them can develop into malignant ulcers, namely, marjolin ulcers.

#### 1.3.1.4 Scar Cancer

In 1828, French surgeon Marjolin first described the "warty ulcer" that occurred on the scar and called it "cancroidal ulcers" (also known as "ulcer canchroides"). Later, Dupuytren and Robert Smith made it clear that the scar can be cancerous and called the ulcer "warty ulcers of Marjolin," the Markov ulcer. From scarring to carcinogenesis, the length of time varies, the shortest is 6 weeks, whereas the elderly can reach more than 30 years. The older the patient, the more likely it is to become cancerous. Marjolin ulcers occur in one third of the lower leg, the heel, the joints of the limbs, and other wearable parts, the scalp and trunk are also good sites. The current treatment is still based on surgery.

### 1.3.2 Compensation and Remodeling

#### 1.3.2.1 Compensation

Compensation refers to the process in which the structure of an organ or tissue is damaged, the metabolism and function are impaired, the organ, the normal part of the tissue, or other organs and tissues are replaced and compensated. There are three main types of compensation: metabolic compensation, functional compensation, and structural compensation.

(a) Metabolic compensation refers to a kind of compensation in the body during the course of the disease, in which the substance metabolism changes adapting to the new situation of the body is the main manifestation. That is, the metabolism of the three major nutrients is strengthened or slowed down.
(b) Functional compensation refers to a compensatory form of the body to compensate for the dysfunction and damage of the diseased organ through the enhancement of organ function.
(c) Structural compensation refers to the body's function enhancement, accompanied by changes in morphological structure to achieve compensation, mainly as the parenchymal cells of organs or tissues volume increased (hypertrophy) or number increased, or both. Structural compensation is divided into two kinds of compensation: physiological hypertrophy and pathological hypertrophy.

#### 1.3.2.2 Remodeling

Remodeling refers to the fact that after the change in the functional burden of organs and tissues, in order to adapt to new functional needs, its morphological structure changes accordingly. It is mainly divided into three types: remodeling of blood vessels, remodeling of bone tissue, and remodeling of connective tissue.

### 1.3.3 New Concepts Involved in Wound Repair

#### 1.3.3.1 Growth Factor

Growth factor (GF) refers to a polypeptide or protein that is widely present in living organisms and regulates the growth and development of organisms, such as epidermal growth factor (EPF), fibroblast growth factors (FGFs), and platelet-derived growth factor (PDGF), which are closely related to wound repair and tissue regeneration. Growth factor, also known as growth hormone, is an important area of medical and molecular biology research in the past 30 years and one of the milestones in modern medical research. In 1986, biologist Levi-Montalcini and biochemist Cohen were awarded the Nobel Prize in Physiology or Medicine for research on nerve growth factor (NGF). There are about 50 growth factors that have been found to promote cell growth and differentiation. There are a large number of growth factor (GF) receptors on the cell surface. The essence of the GF receptor is a glycoprotein or a simple membrane protein with a molecular weight of 130–170 ku. Its composition is generally divided into three parts:

(a) A ligand-affining site outside the cell.
(b) The tyrosine kinase binding site inside the cell.
(c) The junction of the cell membrane.

The combination of various growth factors with their respective receptors may occur in the following three ways.

(a) GF intracellular migration: After GF binds to the receptor, the cells endocytose it to form a receptorsome, which acts on the nucleus and causes an effect.
(b) Tyrosine phosphorylation: GF binds to the receptor and directly causes this process to have an effect.
(c) Through the second messenger mediated by cyclic adenosine monophosphate (cAMP) and cyclic guanosine monophosphate (cGMP): GF binds to the receptor, causing an increase in the concentration of cAMP to cause an effect.

#### 1.3.3.2 Cytokine

Cytokine is a group of hormone-like regulatory molecules that are extremely small in the human body and function at the level of pictogram (pg.). They act locally mainly by autocrine and paracrine, that is, on secretory cell itself or the adjacent tissue cell. In the past, it was divided into lymphokines and monocyte factor according to its source. In recent years, studies have found that many cytokines can be produced by different types of cells (immune cells and nonimmune cells). To avoid confusion, the name cytokine is now used more. Cytokines produce biological effects by transmitting signals into cells by binding to corresponding receptors on target cells. Many cytokines can act on the same target cell to mediate the same or similar effects, while the same cytokine can act on different target cells, producing different effects. For example, interleukin-1 (IL-1), in addition to regulating the immune system, can also act on different sites of the hypothalamic-pituitary-adrenal axis (HPA) to produce neuroendocrine effects. A network is formed between different cytokines, and mutual regulation produces and exerts effects. In addition to being regulated by the immune system, cytokines are also regulated by the neuroendocrine system. Cytokines can be roughly divided into five groups: interferon (IFN), interleukin (IL), colony-stimulating factor (CSF), tumor necrosis factor (TNF), and transforming growth factor (TGF).

#### 1.3.3.3 Gene Therapy

Gene therapy refers to a method in which a genetic technique is used to introduce a specific foreign gene into a cell and obtain expression, thereby obtaining or enhancing its specific function for therapeutic purposes. For a long time, skin has been one of the most suitable organs for gene therapy. A large number of studies have confirmed that in the process of wound healing, a therapeutic gene with a certain regulatory effect is selected and introduced into cells by the gene transfection technology, which can promote the repair of wounds. The problems that restrict clinical application mainly include safety, transfection efficiency, and economical practicability. At the same time, in vitro isolation and culture of cells, introduction of the target gene, and then transplantation to the wound surface by the in vitro transfection method require a long preparation time. Therefore, exploring safe and effective methods of transfection in vivo is also an important direction of current research. In addition, since wound healing is a multifactorial process, it is not realistic to hope that a single gene transfection will improve the healing process of wounds. Gene therapy methods that explore the comprehensive treatment of multiple growth factors should be able to more effectively regulate the microenvironment of the wound surface to maximize their biological effects. The use of cytokine gene therapy, apoptosis gene regulation, suicide gene, and other treatment of pathological scars is also an important direction in wound repair.

#### 1.3.3.4 Cell Therapy

Cell therapy, also known as live cell therapy, involves the repair of damaged tissue by living cells. Cell therapy has been around for hundreds of years, dating back to the fifteenth–sixteenth centuries, and was proposed by the Aureolus Paracelsus (1493–1541) in the Philippines. In 1912, German doctors used cell therapy for the first time to treat "hypothymism and hypothyroidism in children." In 1930, Paul Niehans (1882–1971) became a famous doctor of cell treatment for skin rejuvenation, known as the "father of cell therapy." Cellular treatment classification is given as below:

(a) Cell replacement therapy (fibroblasts, chondrocytes, pigment cells, keratinocytes, osteoblasts, skeletal muscle cells, macrophages, renal epithelial cells, bladder cells).
(b) Cell stimulation therapy (cell regeneration and regenerative medicine). Both types are applied during the wound repair process.

#### 1.3.3.5 Stem Cell

The general concept is that the body exists to self-renew and produce one or more undifferentiated and nonspecific cells with special functions. According to its developmental stage, it can be divided into embryonic stem cells and adult stem cells. According to its differentiation potential, it can be divided into totipotent stem cells, pluripotent stem cells, and special stem cells. With the continuous development of regenerative medicine and the deepening of human understanding of stem cells, the role of stem cells in the treatment of diseases has received more and more attention. In theory, when any tissue or organ of the body is damaged, the stem cells can repair or even replace the tissues and organs that have lost function. The main advantage of using self-stem cells to replace tissues and organs that have lost function is that the source is sufficient, the materials are convenient, and the immune rejection caused by foreign transplant organs and a series of chronic syndromes can be avoided.

#### 1.3.3.6 Tissue Engineering

Tissue engineering (TE) was originally used to describe the theory and technology of constructing tissues or organs in vitro. Now its connotation is expanding, and all methods and techniques that can guide tissue regeneration have been included in the tissue engineering category. Tissue engineering is considered to be a new milestone and a far-reaching medical revolution in the history of life sciences following cell biology and molecular biology. Its scientific significance is not only to propose a new treatment, but more importantly, to propose a new concept of copying tissues and organs, so that regenerative medicine faces major opportunities and challenges. It includes the principles of applied cell biology and engineering to research and develop new medical fields for tissue repair, maintenance, or enhancement of the morphology and function of human tissues and organs. Using the principle of bionics, biodegradable cells are combined with the carrier using a degradable polymer to form a complex having a specific three-dimensional structure and being biologically active. Thereafter, the complex is cultured in vitro or in vivo to finally form a target organ or tissue. At present, there are three main types of tissue-engineered artificial skin produced at home and abroad:

(a) Substitutes only containing cellular components, represented by Epicel.
(b) Substitutes only containing extracellular matrix, represented by Integra, Pelnac.
(c) A composition consisting of cell and extracellular matrix, represented by Dermagraft.

#### 1.3.3.7 Regenerative Medicine

Regenerative medicine (RM) refers to the use of biological and engineering theoretical methods to promote the body's self-repair and regeneration, or to construct new tissues and organs to repair, regenerate, and replace damaged tissues and organs. This technical field covers many modern bioengineering technologies such as stem cell technology and tissue engineering, and seeks to explore the possibility of tissue and organ regeneration and functional reconstruction from all levels. And its content is still expanding, including cell and cytokine therapy, gene therapy, and micro-ecological therapy. Its core content and ultimate goal is to regenerate a tissue or organ that was the same as the pre-traumatic.

#### 1.3.3.8 Others

1. Biotherapy: A method of treating damage and disease using biotechnology, biotechnology products or methods. It mainly includes immunocytotherapy, tissue engineering and product therapy, stem cell technology and product therapy, and gene therapy technology and product therapy. The application and development of biotherapeutics in tissue repair has always been at a leading position.
2. Skin substitutes: Skin wound covers that have been commercialized for clinical include epidermal grafts, dermal grafts such as allogeneic dermis, synthetic omentum, acellular collagen sponge, and complex skin grafts such as collagen gel skin substitutes.
3. New type dressings: With the in-depth study of the pathophysiology of the wound healing process, people's understanding of the wound healing process has become more and more profound, which has promoted the continuous improvement and development of wound dressings. Today, new types of wound dressings have revolutionized the situation relative to the early days, and a variety of different performance dressings are available to clinical caregivers. New dressings were born with the concept of wet wound healing. There are two factors driving the development of such products, namely, the medical industry's in-depth study of wound healing and management processes and the continuous advancement of materials technology. So far, the domestic new dressing market is rich in variety. Several major new medical dressings include foam dressings, hydrocolloid dressings, alginate dressings, antibacterial dressings, composite dressings, hydrogels, etc.

## 1.4 Classification of Wound Tissue Repair and Regeneration

War wounds are a kind of special injury to the body. Because the environment, types of damage, and treatment methods of wounds are different from the usual traumas, our army has divided various types of wounds, but the concept of damage classification has not been proposed. Classification is based on certain characteristics of things, according to certain rules. Taxonomy is a method of grouping and combining things according to certain external or intrinsic characteristics of things. It is the preliminary work of statistics and analysis. It is an effective means to understand the law of the development of things and to study the nature of things. Putting forward the criteria for classification of war injuries can make the classification of injuries scientific, standardized, and normalized, which is of great significance.

### 1.4.1 The Classification of Wounds

For the classification of wounds, the standards used at home and abroad are different due to different classification purposes. The characteristics and meanings of injuries are also different, and there are differences and overlaps between them. The commonly used classification criteria mainly include the injured part, the cause of injury, the mechanism of injury, the type of wound, whether the body cavity is open, the condition of injury, the need for delivery, operation or not, the recovery, and the outcome. If only a few simple criteria are used for classification, they will not fully reflect the nature, current situation, and characteristics of wounds, nor can they meet the needs of modern wound diagnosis, first aid, and treatment. However, if the standard is too complicated and repetitive, it will be difficult to adopt in the process of classification and treatment in front line.

Therefore, the classification of wounds is based on certain characteristics. According to certain rules, the similar wounds are grouped and become an orderly combination. By classifying wounds, we can effectively study the nature of wounds.

Our 2000 version of the injury ticket is classified according to the injury part, injury category, injury condition, injury type, and injury severity. The injury category is essentially the cause of injury, and the injury condition and injury type often cause confusion and even lead to errors in the clinical treatment. The classification of scientific injury should not only comprehensively reflect the nature, condition, and characteristics of wounds, but also meet the needs of early diagnosis, first aid, evacuation, and treatment. Therefore, the new classification of war injuries highlights the principles of science, conciseness, and practicality, and classifies war injuries according to the four aspects: injury part, the cause of injury, injury type, and injury severity. The new classification method can basically describe the characteristics and conditions of the part, the nature, characteristics, and extent of the injury, and the medical staff slightly specifically describe on the basis of the basic frame of the injury severity + injury part + the cause of injury + injury type, forming a relatively complete clinical diagnosis of injury, which can meet the needs of rapid diagnosis and treatment in the early stage of wounds.

#### 1.4.1.1 Injury Part

At present, the classification of the wounded departments varies from department to department. For example, modern war wound surgery and our army's 2000 version of the injury ticket, the injury part of the brain, maxillofacial, neck, chest (back), abdomen (waist), pelvis (perineum), spine, upper limbs, lower limbs, internal organs, etc. 10 parts. At present, the clinical trauma at home and abroad is mostly based on the classification and adoption of the American Affordable

Trauma Score (ais) classification. The injured part is the head, face, neck, chest, abdomen and pelvis, spine, upper limbs, lower limbs, skin, and others. Wait for 9 parts. Ais has detailed description and differentiation of the anatomy, damage properties, and injury scores of the wound, which has been widely recognized and adopted by scholars at home and abroad. Taking into account the distinction between the function of the body and the characteristics of the region, the treatment and research, and the long-term development of war injuries, as well as the international integration and communication, the new classification of war injuries has been wounds into the head, face, neck, and chest (back). 9 parts of the Ministry, abdomen (waist) and pelvis (perineum), spinal cord, upper limbs, lower extremities, other and multiple injuries. The head injury includes craniocerebral injury; the facial injury includes jaw injury; the spinal cord injury includes cervical vertebra, thoracic vertebrae, lumbar vertebrae, and corresponding spinal nerve injury; neck, chest (back), and abdominal (waist) injuries do not include corresponding parts. Spinal and spinal cord and nerve damage; other injuries mainly include electric shock, hypothermia, ionizing radiation injury, microwave damage, etc. It is difficult to determine the damage of specific wounds; multiple injuries refer to the simultaneous or sequential movement of the body under the same injury factor. Two or more anatomical lesions have occurred.

#### 1.4.1.2 Cause of Injuries

According to the different factors of injury, the classification of injuries is a characteristic part of the classification of war injuries. In the past, the classification of injuries (formerly known as injuries) was mainly based on injuries, but because modern weapons are developing very rapidly and the types are increasing, it is almost impossible to enumerate their injuries. Therefore, the new classification method of war damage is to use the injury factor of the weapon as the classification basis, and divide it into injury, bullet wound, blade wound, crush injury, impact injury, impact injury, burn, frostbite, poison injury, ionizing radiation damage, biological weapon injuries, laser damage, microwave damage, other, and composite injuries. For the damage factors of new concept weapons that are not yet weaponized and have no clear effect on personnel injury, they are not included in the cause of war injury and can be included in other. According to the injury factor and the wounded weapon, different types of war wounds are distinguished. According to the type of injury factors: the injury is divided into single injury and composite injury, according to the number of injury factors. The damage caused by single factor is burn, impact injury, radiation injury, injury, gunshot wound, crush injury, frostbite, poisonous injury, etc.; two or more injuries caused by the combination of injuries, including burning, burning, burning, and combined injury. The types of injuries are classified into five categories: conventional weapon injuries, nuclear weapon injuries, chemical weapons injuries, biological weapon injuries, and new concept weapon injuries.

##### Gunshot Wound

The incidence of gunshot wounds in a conflict depends on the type and intensity of the battle. The proportion of gunshot casualties in large-scale wars is generally lower than that of low-intensity wars or asymmetric warfare. The causes of gunshot wounds are: direct damage to important structures in the injured area, stretching of tissues (cavities) causing rupture of blood vessels and tissue inactivation, secondary pollution. The nature and extent of ballistic damage depends on the energy delivered by the bullet to the body's tissues and is also related to the characteristics of the affected tissue. The bullet causes damage to the body by transferring its energy to the tissue, and the energy transfer is related to the type of bullet. The hollow bomb and the dam can transfer their energy to the maximum. The high-speed bullets fired by military rifles have more energy and have greater damage potential than pistols. However, if the bullet only penetrates the limbs without damaging the bone, this reduces the energy it transmits to the body and causes less damage.

##### Impact Injury

Explosions such as rockets, aerial bombs, mortars, grenades, etc. can cause impact injuries. A small volume of explosives can generate a large amount of gas in a short time after the explosion, which causes a high pressure at the explosion point, causing the gas molecules to rapidly transfer from the explosion point to the surroundings, thereby forming a so-called shock wave. Its front edge is called the shock wave front. The characteristics of the impact injury are as follows.

(a) Primary impact injury: It is the most common type of injury near the explosion point. It is caused by the interaction between the shock wave front of the explosion and the gas-containing organs in the body (such as the middle ear, lung, intestine, etc.).
(b) Secondary impact injuries: Explosive stimuli impact damage caused by the body, such as prefabricated metal fragments contained in modern weapons. Due to the lack of aerodynamic characteristics, the flying speed of the shrapnel decreases rapidly, so it is mainly caused by low-energy transmission.
(c) The third type of impact injury: The victim is thrown into a fixed object such as a wall and other damage after being subjected to the shock wave.

(d) The fourth type of impact injury: Due to the impact of shock waves, secondary damage is caused by the collapse of various buildings. Shockwave victims often have multisystem injuries, and the types of injuries are complex, such as blunt injuries, penetrating injuries, and burns.

#### Thermal Injury and Chemical Injury Wound

Thermal and chemical damage is caused by cold or heat, tissue damage rays, acids or alkalis. Skin damage depends on the duration of the injury, the intensity and extent of the action. Thermal injury such as burns, etc., are divided into I degree, shallow II degree, deep II degree, and III degree. Frostbite can also be divided into I–IV grades: erythema in grade I; blister formation in grade II; necrosis in grade III; thrombosis in IV grade, and occlusion of blood vessels.

#### Combined Wound

Such wounds may be caused by blunt force injuries of penetrating wounds, or by thermal or mechanical injuries, such as large-area soft tissue injuries, open fractures with severe crushing injuries, and avulsion injuries. In the case of combined injuries, there is another important problem, secondary injury, which is mainly caused by ischemia, reperfusion, or vascular injury caused by the compartment syndrome. It is often difficult to distinguish between penetrating wounds and composite wounds.

### 1.4.1.3 Injury Type

According to the characteristics of the injury of the injured tissue, it can clearly reflect the nature and characteristics of the local injury, which is helpful for the judgment of the injury and the choice of treatment measures. Because the classification criteria of single tissue damage characteristics are difficult to reflect the characteristics and nature of various tissue damages, the purpose and basis of different classification methods are different, which may lead to some overlap between the different types of injuries. If burns and crush injuries are usually classified according to the characteristics of tissue damage, they are repeated with burns and crush injuries in the classification of injuries. The new classification method of war damage can not only reflect the damage characteristics of war wound tissue, but also minimize the overlap between different types of injuries by summarizing and synthesizing the classification criteria. The new war wounds are divided into penetrating wounds, non-through wounds, tangential wounds, skin and soft tissue injuries (scratches, contusions, lacerations, avulsions), fractures, broken limbs and broken fingers (toe)), and others. Since most of the war injuries are mechanical injuries, they are classified by the type of injury. According to the presence or absence of entrance and exit of the injured road, it is divided into: through injury, non-through injury, tangential injury, and rebound injury. The above four types of injuries and closed injuries were classified as injuries in our current injury ticket. Because they are classified according to the characteristics of the projectile producing the wound in the body, it basically reflects the characteristics of local histological damage. For example, penetrating injury refers to the injury that causes the wound to penetrate the body cavity (the cranial cavity, the spinal membranous cavity, the pleural cavity, the peritoneal cavity, the joint cavity, etc.) and causes the body cavity to communicate with the outside. It has distinctive features in the emergency treatment of war wounds. Important position; skin and soft tissue injury (scratch, contusion, laceration, avulsion injury), the injury type basically reflects the type and characteristics of skin soft tissue injury; fracture, broken limb, and broken finger (toe) reflect bone and limb damage The characteristics of the injury type; for other rare nonmechanical injuries (ionizing radiation damage, etc.) and those that cannot be classified, they are classified into other injuries.

### 1.4.1.4 Injury Severity

In the past, injuries were classified into minor, moderate, and severe, and the classification was based on the length of treatment required after the injury and whether or not there was a disability. Because the length of treatment and the prognosis and outcome are not only related to the degree of injury, but also closely related to the nature of the injury, whether it gets timely and reasonable treatment, and the level of medical treatment, the uncertainty is great. So, the new classification method of war injury is based on accurate data reflecting the severity of the damage to the human tissues and organs, life risk and prognosis. The new classification divides injuries into four categories, namely minor, moderate, severe, and critical. The degree of danger to life can be judged by the vital signs of the wounded, which is conducive to timely and accurate classification and determination of first-aid measures.

### 1.4.1.5 Others

#### Divided by Different Operational Environments

Under different conditions, war wounds have their own particularities. Therefore, they are divided into five categories: war wounds in the plateau, war wounds in desert areas, war wounds in alpine regions, war wounds in mountain jungles, and urban war wounds.

#### Divided by the Anatomy System

The tissues and organs of various parts of the human body have their structural and functional characteristics. The pathological changes after injury are different and can be divided into skin system, exercise system, digestive system, respiratory system, genitourinary system, cardiovascular system, endocrine system, nerve system, sensory (visual, hearing) injury, multiple system organ injury, and 10 types of war wounds.

#### Others

In addition, according to the time of injury, it can be divided into acute wounds and chronic wounds. According to the depth of the skin involved in the injury, it can be divided into partial cortical damaged wounds and full-thickness wounds. According to the cause of injury, it can be divided into mechanical or traumatic wounds, thermal injury wounds, chemically damaged wounds, ulcerative wounds, and radiation-damaged wounds. Depending on the color, they can be divided into red, yellow, black, and mixed wounds.

1. Acute wounds: It refers to a wound that forms suddenly and heals quickly. This type of wound healing usually involves I stage healing, such as elective surgical incision, II degree burn wound, superficial skin trauma, acute radioactive I degree injury, II degree pressure sore, and other wounds.
2. Chronic wounds: Skin tissue injury caused by various reasons, the healing process is more than 8 weeks, such as ulcerative wounds (III degree and IV degree pressure sore, diabetic foot ulcer, venous lower extremity ulcer, arterial lower extremity ulcer, chronic radioactive II degree and III degree damage), deep burns or burns, granulation wounds formed by trauma, etc.
3. Partial cortical damaged wounds: Wounds involving the epidermis and dermis, such as II degree burns and II degree pressure sores.
4. Full-thickness wounds: It refers to wounds that spread from the epidermis and dermis to subcutaneous fat, sometimes deep into the fascia and muscles, and even invade the tendons and bones, measuring the depth, most of which are at least more than 1 cm, such as III degree and IV degree pressure sores, III degree burns, off-skin avulsion, and so on.

## 1.4.2 Classification of Wound Healing and Regeneration

### 1.4.2.1 Classification of Wound Healing

Wound healing is a complex biological process involving bleeding and coagulation, inflammatory exudation, formation of vascular and granulation tissue, reepithelialization, fibrosis, and tissue remodeling. Various growth factors in this series of biological activities play an important role. According to pathology the healing situation can be divided into:

#### First-Stage Healing

First-stage healing generally refers to the process in which the wound is healed by the newly formed epidermal cells, capillary endothelial cells, and connective tissue on both sides of the wound in a short time. It is the simplest form of wound healing and is also a direct combination of tissues. This type of healing occurs mainly in surgical incisions that have fewer tissue defects, neat wound edges, no infection, and by suture or adhesion. The basic process is that after tissue damage, the blood forms a blood clot on the wound surface, connecting the two ends of the broken end, and protecting the wound surface. The specific pathological manifestations are: early postinjury (within 24 h), the changes in wounds are mainly inflammation, exudation, and dissolution of blood clots. Afterward, the infiltrating macrophages remove fibrin, red blood cells, and cell debris from the wound. From the third day after the injury, it can be seen that the capillary germ grows from the edge and bottom of the wound at a rate of 2.0 mm per day, forming a new blood circulation network. At the same time, adjacent fibroblasts proliferate and migrate into the wound, producing matrix and collagen. One week after the injury, collagen fibers can cross the wound and connect the wound. Then the collagen in the wound continues to increase and is engineered to increase wound tension. In the past, this type of healing has long been thought to be caused by the nascent epidermal cells, capillary endothelial cells, and connective tissue crossing the wound over a short period of time, without the formation of granulation tissue. Recent studies have shown that this process also involves granulation tissue, which is similar to other soft tissue injury repairs, except that the wound edge is lightly damaged, the inflammatory response is weak, and the amount of granulation tissue produced is small, leaving only one linear scar after repair.

### 1.4.2.2 Second-Stage Healing

Second-stage healing generally means that the healing process of wound is first filled with granulation tissue, followed by the neonatal epidermal cells. Of course, some studies have suggested that such healing is preceded by epidermal cell regeneration, followed by stimulating granulation tissue formation and proliferation, or granulation formation in parallel with epidermal cell regeneration. This process begins with a variety of growth factors (TGF, FGF, etc.) that stimulate the vascular endothelial cells at the bottom of the wound or the "dormant" of the wound edge, activate it, and then generate new capillary germs through "germination" to communicate with each other. The capillary network in the new granulation tissue is formed. Compared with the first-stage healing, the healing by second intention is characterized by the following aspect: due to the large defect of the wound, and the more necrotic tissue, usually accompanied by infection, the time to start regeneration of the epithelium is delayed. Due to the large wound surface, the more granulation tissue, thus forming scars that are large, often have a certain influence on the appearance. Due to the influence of large wounds, infections, etc., the healing time is longer, and usually takes 4–5 weeks. Healing by second intention is mainly seen in wounds with large defects or infections.

#### Healing Under Scab

Healing under scab is a wound healing process under a special condition. It mainly refers to the second-stage healing process under a layer of dark brown hard scab formed by the exudate, blood, and necrotic material, such as the healing process of leather-like hard scab after deep II degree or III degree burn. The healing process also starts with the epidermal basal cell proliferation of the wound edge, which migrates to the center of the wound while growing under the scab, and the granulation tissue of the wound also proliferates. The healing speed of the under scab is slower than that of the non-scab wound, and the time is longer. The formation of hard scab has the effect of protecting the wound surface, and also hinders the outflow of the wound exudate, which is easy to induce infection and delay healing. Therefore, it is often necessary to adopt the "escharectomy" or "tangential excision" surgery in clinical treatment to expose the wound and facilitate the repair.

### 1.4.2.3 Classification of Regeneration

Regeneration can be divided into physiological regeneration and pathological regeneration, according to the condition of tissue regeneration. Physiological regeneration refers to the process in which some cells and tissues are aging and depleted during physiological processes, and then supplemented by the same type of cells to maintain the original structure and function. For example, the surface keratinocytes of the epidermis often fall off and are supplemented by the continuous proliferation of the basal cells of the epidermis; the endometrium periodically falls off and is repaired by basal cell proliferation; after blood cell aging and disruption, it is also necessary to continuously export a large number of new cells from the lymphoid hematopoietic organs. Pathological regeneration refers to regeneration that occurs after tissue and cell defects in a pathological state. It can be divided into complete regeneration and incomplete regeneration. Complete regeneration refers to the proliferation and replenishment of cells after necrosis, and the regenerated tissue completely restores the structure and function of the original tissue. Incomplete regeneration (i.e., fibrous repair) means that the defect cannot be repaired by the original tissue, but replaced by granulation tissue, and finally forming scars, also known as scar repair.

The basic process of physiological regeneration is similar to pathological regeneration, in which cells reenter the cell cycle for division and proliferation. A cell cycle refers to the process from the end of the last mitosis to the end of the next mitosis. It consists of G1 phase (pre-synthesis phase), S phase (DNA synthesis phase), G2 phase (pre-division phase), and M phase (division phase). Among them, it can be divided into two categories: physiological regeneration (one-time physiological regeneration, periodic physiological regeneration, continuous physiological regeneration) and pathological regeneration (complete pathological regeneration and incomplete pathological regeneration).

#### Physiological Regeneration

During normal physiological processes, some tissues and cells are continuously consumed, aged, and disappeared, and are constantly supplemented by the same type of cell division and proliferation. This process of regeneration is called physiological regeneration. It is characterized, in that the regenerated cells and tissues can completely maintain the original structure and function, such as the periodic shedding of the endometrium and the continuous renewal of the skin, so it is also called complete regeneration.

#### Pathological Regeneration

In the pathological state, regeneration of cells or tissues after damage is called pathological regeneration. If the damage is mild, it can be proliferated by the same kind of cells and maintain the original structure and function. This type of regeneration is called complete pathological regeneration. If the damage is serious, the damage can only be filled by another tissue and the original structure and function are lost. It is called incomplete pathological regeneration.

According to the strength of regenerative capacity, human tissue cells can be divided into three categories.

(a) Labile cells: These cells are constantly proliferating to replace dead or damaged cells, such as epidermal cells, respiratory and digestive tract mucosal cells, covered cells of the male and female reproductive organs, lymphoid cells and hematopoietic cells, mesothelial cells, etc. The regenerative capacity of these cells is quite strong.
(b) Stable cells: Under physiological conditions, this type of cell proliferation is not obvious, it seems to be in the stationary phase (G0) during the cell proliferation cycle, but when stimulated by tissue damage, it enters the early stage of DNA pre-synthesis phase (G1), showing a strong ability to regenerate. This kind of cells includes parenchymal cells of various glands or adenoid organs, such as epithelial cells of the liver, pancreas, parotid gland, endocrine glands, sweat glands, sebaceous glands, and renal tubules; and also includes primitive mesenchy-

mal cells and their differentiated cells. Not only do they have a strong regenerative capacity, but the primitive mesenchymal cells also have a strong ability to differentiate into many specific mesenchymal cells. For example, when the fracture heals, the mesenchymal cells proliferate and differentiate into the chondrocytes and osteoblasts. The smooth muscle cells also belong to stable cells, but generally their ability to regenerate is weak.

(c) Permanent cells: Cells belonging to this class include nerve cells, skeletal muscle cells, and cardiomyocytes. Regardless of the central nervous cells and the ganglion cells of the peripheral nerves, they cannot divide and proliferate after birth. Once they are damaged, the defects become permanent. However, this does not include nerve fibers. Under the premise of nerve cell survival, damaged nerve fibers have an active ability to regenerate. Although myocardium and striated muscle cells have a weak ability to regenerate, it has little meaning for postinjury repair, and they are basically repaired by scars.

## 1.5 Characteristics of Repair and Regeneration of War Wound Tissue

Through rapid conversion of chemical energy such as gunpowder burning and explosives' explosion into mechanical energy, the projectiles, shrapnel, marbles, and other objects are thrown at high speed and hit the human body, causing firearm injuries. Generally speaking, the targets of light weapons such as bullets are mostly individual, while the targets of heavy weapons such as shells and missiles are mostly groups. Therefore, the former is often referred to as point-killing weapons, while the latter is called surface-killing weapons. However, modern light weapons are not only powerful, high precision, but also have the characteristics of combining point and surface. Therefore, the abovementioned point- and surface killing are just a relative distinction between weapons.

By studying the local wars in the Gulf, the Balkans, and Afghanistan, it can be seen that due to the development of high technology, weapons' performance and damage factors have undergone tremendous changes. The form of war has evolved from a conventional, comprehensive war to a small-scale regional armed conflict that uses high-tech weapons and equipment, that is, local wars under high-tech conditions. The war is multilayered, all-round, and without front and rear boundaries. It is sudden, concealed, destructive, and cruel. To this end, these types of war wounds and treatment system have also begun to take shape.

### 1.5.1 The Main Features of Tissue Repair After Trauma

#### 1.5.1.1 Characteristics of Modern War Wounds

Due to the improvement of modern weapons and the improvement of performance, the injury factors are superimposed and compounded, especially the simultaneous or alternate use of nuclear weapons, biological and chemical weapons, resulting in burn-blast, blast-poison compound injuries and blast injuries increasing. Shock waves can cause pulmonary edema, pulmonary hemorrhage, lung rupture, hearing and gastrointestinal damage, with external light internal weight, rapid development, and complex injuries. At the scene of the explosion, there was no obvious trauma while in a state of shock, or large areas of burns were mostly combined injuries based on impact injuries. Multiple injuries refer to the same injury factor directly or sequentially resulting in injuries of more than two anatomical sites. Polytraumas refer to wounds with more than two lesions in the same anatomy or organ. In the Gulf War, the wounded had an average of more than nine injuries. The head, chest, heart, liver, and spleen accounted for 20%, 73.3%, 10%, 43.3%, and 6.7%, respectively. The wound is heavily polluted, the infection rate is high, the severe and extremely severe injuries are more, and the shock rate is high. The mutual influence in the treatment is large, involving multiple specialist theories and techniques, and the on-site first aid is time-sensitive.

Large vascular injury, combined injury, mostly causes extensive damage, strong systemic reaction, significant contusion symptoms, central nervous disorders, unconsciousness, and focal softening of the brain. Heart contusion accounted for 45.6% and lung contusion accounted for 22.8%. Forty-two percent of the wounded were treated in the division hospital. As much as 74.5% of the mine injury was accompanied by shock. One out of six patients died on the operating table. The shrapnel was prominent, with more fractures (33.3%) and more non-penetration injuries (92.7%). In modern local wars, various explosive weapons are still the main strategic and tactical weapons. The power of the explosion has increased greatly, and the shrapnel has increased. It can be fanned or stereoscopically projected, and the killing area is enlarged and the target is accurate. Forty percent in the Vietnam War, 56% in the Middle East War, and 74% in the Gulf War were shrapnel or shrapnel compound injuries. The shrapnel enters the body at an initial velocity of 1360 m/s, large amount, high energy, and high density. Due to different tissue morphologies, densities, and elasticities, the resistance varies. The shrapnel is flipped and scattered in the tissue to form a multidirectional secondary blind tube and multiple fractures, which may be accompanied by a residual cavity of up to 2000 mL and down to 50 mL, and residual foreign matter. The rate of disability and death is high. Battlefield deaths accounted for 50% of all deaths, and most of them died within 6 h of injury. The proportion of casualties: The Second World War 3.1: 1, Korean War 4.1: 1, Malvinas War 3.6: 1, and Vietnam War 3.7: 1. In the Second World War, 6% is maimed by war wounds, the Vietnam War is 12.4%, the self-defense counterattack against Vietnam is 29.8%, and Afghanistan War is 30%. Disability and mental disorders increase. With the changes in modern local war forms and methods of warfare, the use of high-tech laser, infrasound, and electromagnetic nonlethal weapons can lead to no obvious wounds, normal visceral function, but combat capability and technical effectiveness play poorly and lack of concentration, etc. The incidence of psychological disorders and even mental abnormalities increases, which is one of the more prominent features of local warfare under high-tech conditions.

In short, the typical characteristics of war injuries are:

(a) The wound has been contaminated.
(b) Injured tissues involving multiple body cavities.
(c) The same patient often has multiple injury sites.
(d) Seventy-five percent injured the limbs.
(e) Symptoms are often heavy.

The development of high-tech weapons and usage in some local wars have led to significant changes in the types and characteristics of war injuries. Limb injuries have increased dramatically, reaching 96.0%, while 70–87% are various blast injuries which are more complicated. The proportion of blast injuries and burns is obviously increased, resulting in an increase in the large defects of soft tissue on the surface, and the damage is more extensive. The negative pressure formed by the damage caused by fragments causes bacteria, foreign bodies, etc. in the surrounding environment invading into the wound cavity deeper and more. Combined with extensive and serious tissue damage, it makes the infection very serious. The incidence of disability and residual deformity increases, and is more serious. High-energy explosion injury can cause damage to distant organs.

In the future war, new concept weapons such as electromagnetic guns, nuclear pulses, lasers, and microwaves may be used. These weapons, known as super killers, make the treatment of the wounded more difficult. We must start from the characteristics of complex electromagnetic environment in the future battlefield, study the characteristics of war wounds in complex electromagnetic environment, and explore new diagnostic methods, classification standards, and treatment plans, so as to do the trauma treatment and repair work in a complex electromagnetic environment.

#### 1.5.1.2 Characteristics of Modern War Wound Tissue Repair

The injury assessment is a guarantee that the organization will be accurately and reasonably repaired After the wounded recover, a thorough examination from head to toe is required. While checking for a penetrating wound with a torso, you cannot ignore the back, buttock, perineum, and armpits. Every wound must be evaluated and recorded. The assessment of the injury included: location and size, cavities or not, degree of contamination, anatomical structural peripheral blood flow, fractures or not, and whether the limb damage is so severe that it cannot be reconnected.

##### Debridement Is the Basis of Later Tissue Repair

Debridement involves the removal of necrotic or contaminated tissue, if this tissue is left over, it will become the vector of infection. If there are limb injuries, an inflatable tourniquet should be used to reduce blood loss. The first step in debridement is to cut the skin along the longitudinal axis to achieve decompression of the wound and to protect the damaged tissue from swelling. However, such a cut must not cross the joint along the longitudinal axis. When the decompression is completed, the contaminated tissue and the nonviable tissue must be removed. Because the skin tissue is elastic, the incision can be as small as possible, and it is typically done around the edge of the wound. Although all foreign objects in the wound should be removed, it is not worthwhile to remove the small metal foreign objects that are farther away from the wounded path, so as not to damage the healthy tissue too much. At the same time, necrotic and contaminated tissue in the wound should be completely removed, but it is often difficult to determine the extent of necrotic or contaminated tissue. Necrotic muscle tissue usually has a dark red color, no bleeding when cut, and no contraction when clamping muscle fibers. For bone fragments that are completely free from soft tissue, they should be removed. If left, they will cause infection or osteomyelitis. Damaged nerves and tendon tissue should be marked with sutures for delayed repair. After the debridement process is completed, the wound is repeatedly washed with a large amount of physiological saline, then the wound is opened without being sutured and covered with a large amount of dry sterile gauze. Some low-energy wounds, such as pistol wounds, do not require extensive debridement and tissue resection. In some cases, these wounds may not be surgically treated. There is no ideal treatment for the multiple small injuries caused by secondary impact injury. Due to the large number of small wounds, it is not feasible to debride each wound one by one. Moreover, the irregularly flying shrapnel that causes these damages has lower energy and poor penetrability, so the damage is often lighter and the cavity is not formed. Therefore, the appropriate treatment is to wash the wound as thoroughly as possible under general anesthesia, and to remove the main wounds with a lot of pollution or large necrotic tissue by surgical treatment.

#### Delayed Closure of the First Phase After Debridement Is the Principle of Repairing Wound Tissue

After debridement, the wounded are sent to the ward to continue the monitoring and analgesic treatment. The wound should always be wrapped with dressing until the delayed closure operation. The International Committee of the Red Cross recommended an observation of delayed wound closure for a period of 5 days, but in practice, the developed country tends to shorten the observation time to 2–3 days. Before the end of the observation period, if there is sepsis or an unpleasant smell from wound dressings, it is an indication of reoperation, and the common cause of sepsis is incomplete debridement. The removal of dressings from the wounded should be carried out in the operating room under appropriate anesthesia. If there is no sign of infection, necrosis, or residual contamination, the wound can be sutured or skin grafted. However, there are also patients who need multiple debridements. According to the statistics of the International Committee of the Red Cross, after the first debridement, only 45% of the wounds can be closed, 33% need to be debrided again, and 22% need multiple debridements. If the wound tends to close, it is necessary to ensure that the wound is not strained to facilitate the repair of the wound.

#### Accurate Amputation Level Is the Feature of War Wound Tissue Repair

Some ballistic injuries, especially mine injuries, sometimes require amputation. Of course, other severe limb injuries may also require amputation. The decision to amputate is made at the time of injury assessment. The scoring system of limb injury is less correlated with the severity of ballistic injury, while the lack of sensation and blood supply of the distal limb is an important indication for amputation. Getting the consent of other surgeons is helpful in deciding whether to amputate. Skin and bone have a relatively large blocking function to impact on shrapnel conduction, while muscle tissue has a weaker blocking function, so contamination may continue to spread across the fascia. The extent of contaminated or inactivated tissue is usually much larger than that seen in the initial appearance. Military surgeons are accustomed to traditional amputation that cuts off skin, muscles, and bones at the same level. Although this method is simple and fast, the wound is difficult to close and the amputation level is often higher than the actual needs. Most humanitarian surgical organizations recommend flap formation prior to amputation, which preserves more residual limbs and facilitates wound closure, and the use of muscle-containing flaps to cover amputation stumps is strongly advocated. In order to reduce blood loss, tourniquet should be used to stop bleeding during amputation. The surgical strategy of injury amputation is similar to other war injuries: debridement removes contaminated and necrotic tissue, determines the optimal amputation level of limb function, and constructs the flap. The wound should remain open and covered with a large amount of dry sterile dressings until the delayed first phase closed surgery.

### 1.5.2 The Characteristics of Posttraumatic Tissue Repair Research in the Modern Warfare of Foreign Military

Since 2001, the US military has been conducting military operations, so the research on trauma treatment is very important. The US Army Surgery Research Institute is the main institution for studying the trauma of the war in the US military. Its research covers the whole process of self-rescue and mutual rescue, treatment at all levels, and rehabilitation. The progress of the Institute in the field of limb trauma and regenerative medicine, pain management, clinical trials, and transformation studies in the US military is briefly described below.

#### 1.5.2.1 Limb Trauma and Regenerative Medicine

Trauma of the extremities and head and neck has the highest incidence in war injuries, reaching 55% and 30%, respectively. Trauma of the extremities is mainly soft tissue penetrating injury and open fracture. Infection, delayed fracture healing, and muscle dysfunction or loss are the most common complications. The limb trauma and regenerative medicine research team evaluated the injury, prognosis, and complications, and established a military orthopedic trauma database to identify the causes of poor clinical outcomes after fractures, such as combined soft tissue defects, nerve damage, infection, different fixed types, etc. At present, skeletal muscle injury has been identified as the main cause of incomplete functional recovery after fracture. In addition, preclinical studies of treatment method evaluation were conducted. Using traumatic animal models we can evaluate treatment options and technical methods for infection, soft tissue, and bone injury. Clinical guidelines for the treatment of contaminated wounds have been established, and animal models of fascia compartment syndrome, large contaminated defects, and large muscle defects have been constructed. An implanted bone material has been developed for the dual purpose of promoting regeneration and preventing infection. At the same time, the Institute is also conducting research on regenerative medicine projects for the treatment of skin, muscle, and bone injuries by the combination of stem cells and biomaterials. On this basis, the

Institute's clinical trial research in the field of trauma treatment, through the Orthopedic Extremity Trauma Research Program (OETRP), and other military hospital orthopedics for multicenter clinical trials, will promote the use of military medical resources and talent development. In addition, the Army Surgery Institute has established a partnership with the Army's Institute of Regenerative Medicine and other internal and external agencies through the OETRP, and plans to significantly improve the prognosis of limb injuries within the next 5 years.

Anthony Atala, an organ engineer and AFIRM researcher in Wake Forest University, is building an "inkjet printer" that prints the entire organ on demand, in order to replace the severely damaged liver, kidney, and even the heart. The "inkbox" of the device contains a special mixture containing cells from the corresponding organs, auxin, and special nutrients. The printer prints the required organs one layer at a time under computer control. Now, it is possible to initially print out a complex organ like a rat heart. Atala plans to develop a portable version for the battlefield in the next 5 years to print the skin directly into the deep wounds. For surface injuries, such as burns, the American Academy of Regenerative Medicine is working on a handheld spray can, like a cosmetic hair spray, that sprays a thin layer of immature skin cells called keratin to the wound. These cells are extracted from the patient's own skin and stimulate the healing of the wound. Recent clinical trials have been very confident: all 16 burn patients showed "good healing" in 1–3 weeks. Another major focus is the "fascia compartment syndrome": internal muscle damage or other injuries, resulting in rapid swelling of the upper or lower limb, compressing nerves and blood vessels. If you don't deal with it quickly, muscle will die, and amputation is usually necessary. By regenerative medicine to regrow your fingers and toes is a dream that people chase.

#### 1.5.2.2 Pain Management

Acute and chronic pain are considered to be the primary problems faced by US casualties, and 71% of those admitted to the emergency department at levels 2 and 3 have experienced severe pain of grade 5 or above (classified from 0–10). Pain usually combines multiple diseases, including post-traumatic stress disorder (PTSD), anxiety, and depression. Chronic pain and PTSD are often concomitant occurrences and interact. The Institute's pain study covers all pain management studies from battlefield to rehabilitation, such as the molecular mechanisms of new targets and pain pathways, as well as field pain and analgesia for acute and chronic pain syndromes, PTSD incidence, and the influence of long-term prognosis in mentality pathology. Current research focuses on the effects of analgesics on short-term prognosis, the mechanism of PTSD, addiction and tolerance of opioids, and chronic pain. The US military also conducted a "virtual reality" technology assessment to control acute pain to reduce the demand for opioids, improve analgesic effects, increase the level of conscious, and cooperate with daily rehabilitation training. By entering the virtual cold world, the wounded reduce pain, anxiety, and mental stress during trauma and burn dressing change. Other ongoing research projects include:

(a) Assessing the role of rapid opioid detoxification agents in reducing the anesthetic intake and opioid dependence in burn patients.
(b) A standardized electronic prescription system and guideline developed for the anesthetic ketamine significantly improved the use of the drug in burns.
(c) Developed a nasal spray preparation that can be used as an analgesic device for battlefield soldiers.
(d) In the severe burn operation, the use of intravascular temperature control to reduce the incidence of low temperature shock.

#### 1.5.2.3 Clinical Trials and Transformation Studies

Under the responsibility of the Clinical Trial Department of the US Army Surgery Research Institute, it proposes the best treatment plan for the current law of casualties on the battlefield, and transforms relevant research from preclinical research to clinical therapeutic applications, such as testing the performance of dressings, assessing the recovery strategy of burn wounds, etc. Clinical studies include local and remote ambulance equipment and rehabilitation programs, protective equipment, continuous renal replacement therapy, blood loss control in the operating room of the burn, nutrition supplementation during inpatient, ICU, outpatient, and rehabilitation. In addition, the US Army Surgery Research Institute, as the only burn center certified by the American Burns Federation, which belongs to the Ministry of Defense, received all the severely burned from the Iraqi and Afghan battlefields and studied the causes of burns. At the same time, in order to deal with a large number of hand burns, an equipment research plan for fire-resistant gloves was developed. For the thermal damage of the trunk part that the body armor covered, improved protective clothing was developed. The standardized clinical path of burn rehabilitation was carried out to ensure a good prognosis.

### 1.5.3 The Characteristics of Wound Ballistics in Modern Warfare and the Principle of Postinjury Tissue Repair

#### 1.5.3.1 The Characteristics of Modern War Wounds in Wound Ballistics

Trauma ballistics is a branch of science that studies the movement law, injury effect, and mechanism of projectiles such as warheads and fragments in the body. It is not only an integral part of the terminal ballistics, but also an important part of field surgery, and it is the theoretical basis for guiding the treatment of modern firearm injuries. In theory, there are firearms in the case of firearm wounds, and firearm wounds can be treated. However, the so-called firearm wounds treatment before the First World War was only a simple record of injury type, injury part, injury condition, and projectiles by some medical personnel and very primitive and simple surgical treatment. Before and after the Second World War, due to the establishment and development of wound ballistics, people had a systematic and in-depth understanding of firearm injuries. Especially since the American M16 automatic rifle (launched M193 type 5.56 mm projectile, initial velocity 970 m/s) was introduced in 1962 and put into the Vietnam War, the research on wound ballistics has been greatly developed from both technology and theory, which not only deepens people's understanding of modern firearm injuries, but also makes the treatment of modern firearm injuries more correct and standardized under the guidance of theory. For example, in mastering the characteristics of firearm injuries, it is recognized that the damage effect of the projectile is not only related to its quality, but also depends on its speed, shape, and structure, and also closely related to the structural characteristics of the injured tissue. In terms of treatment, people have enhanced the awareness of debridement and formulated the principle of early debridement and delayed suture. In the judgment of the scope of firearm injury, the obvious and repeated pulsation of the temporary cavity has deepened people's understanding of the scope of damage. At the same time, it is also aware of the inevitability and seriousness of contaminated wound caused by firearms. The extensive and serious systemic reaction makes people deeply understand the importance and necessity of the overall inspection and treatment of the wounded.

The blast injuries have broadened the research content of wound ballistics and firearm injuries. Due to the introduction of precision guidance technology, explosive weapons have been widely used in modern warfare, resulting in a large number of explosive wounded. The main physical factors of explosive weapon injuries are fragments and shock waves, so the content of wound ballistics and firearm injuries must be broadened. As far as the fragment is concerned, the shape of the fragment is different, and the resistance coefficient, the speed attenuation, the energy release, the energy transmission, and the like are also different, so the damage characteristics are different. The triangular and square fragments have a fast decay rate, but the energy transfer rate is high, so they often form a wound with a large entrance and a small exit, or a non-penetrating injury without an exit. The surface of the spherical fragment is smooth, so that on the one hand, it has low resistance, slow decay, penetrating the tissue deep, but the energy transfer rate is relatively low. On the other hand, when encountering different densities of tissues in the body, it often changes the direction of the ballistic, forming twists and turns complex wound tract, thus injuring multiple organs. Cylindrical fragment damage occurs between the triangle and the spherical fragment. The shape of the fragments is different, and the volume of the wound cavity formed is also different. When the speed and shape are the same, the triangular fragment has the largest volume of wounds, which in turn is square, cylindrical, and spherical. Because different materials have different specific gravities and structural characteristics, the energy transfer and physical state when hitting the tissue are also different, so the damage must be different. The constituent material of the fragment itself is also one of the important factors affecting the damage ability of the fragment. In terms of shock waves, previous research on impact injuries mainly focused on the relationship between physical parameters and injury effects and the mechanism of impact injuries. In terms of dose-effect relationship, the peak pressure, positive pressure action time, pressure rise time, and negative pressure damage have been studied intensively, and many protection standards have been developed based on it. In the mechanism of impact injury, it is revealed under the direct action of positive pressure and negative pressure, the body can be injured by hemodynamic changes, implosion effect, fragmentation effect, inertia effect, and pressure difference between different parts, thus summing up the impact damage has on the characteristics of external light internal weight, complex injury, and rapid development. As far as the combination of fragmentation and shock wave is concerned, it is characterized in that not only is the local damage range large, the tissue defect is large, the wound is heavily polluted, the injury tract is complicated, and the combined injury is more, the multiple injuries are more, the associated injury is more, and the complications are more. Therefore, the explosion wounded have a high rate of death, a high rate of injury, and a high rate of disability. Fragments and shock waves also have the effect of aggravating each other.

Environmental factors have increased the research direction of wound ballistics and firearm injuries. Military struggles are not always carried out in the normal environment according to people's wishes. Military struggles often occur in special environments such as plateaus, cold regions, hot regions, deserts, islands, etc. Especially when political, economic situations and certain beliefs are mutated and cannot be solved by peaceful means, a particular environment becomes a highly sensitive area where war occurs. The special meteorological conditions in different geographical environments and the unique atmospheric physical characteristics will inevitably affect the ballistic characteristics of the projectile and the local injury, overall response, and injury outcome after the firearm injury. Therefore, the principle of firearm injury treatment in a special environment is inevitably different from the conventional environment. Based on these considerations and needs, domestic research on wound ballistics and treatment has been carried out since the 1990s on firearm injuries in high altitude, high cold, high temperature, and high humidity, and seawater conditions. For example, when the plateau is damaged by the same projectile and distance as the plain, the degree of damage to the animal is much more serious. In addition, because the plateau climate is cold, dry, and strong in ultraviolet rays, the infection rate of firearm wounds is also relatively low, but the systemic reaction is heavy, and complications such as pulmonary edema and cerebral edema are prone to occur. Another example is the firearm wound after seawater immersion, because we cannot use the usual 4C (color, consistency, contractility, capillary bleeding) as surgical criteria to judge the inactivation of muscle tissue in firearm injury, but only 3C methods other than color.

There are many kinds of modern weapons, and the purpose of weapons is increasing. Although weapons have a lot of generality, different weapons and weapons with different combat objectives must have their own characteristics and mechanisms of injury. Therefore, the principles and methods of treatment must be different. The injury characteristics and mechanisms of special bombs such as multiheaded, arrow-shaped, hollow, and shell less bombs should be studied. The injury characteristics and treatment methods of personnel in closed combat weapons should also be confirmed through research, especially with earth penetration bombs continuing to be put into combat, and the personnel in the shelter and underground fortifications are no longer safe. Although the rescue equipment is not a professional content of wound ballistics, its development is inseparable from the theoretical guidance of wound ballistics, such as the principle of early treatment of firearm injuries as far as possible is directly from the research results of firearm injuries. Although the research on the damage of new concept weapons such as laser, microwave, infrasound, gene, kinetic energy, and particle beam is largely unlisted in the category of firearm injuries, there is no doubt that it is the object of concern for weapon trauma. Weapon traumatology solves not only damage and treatment problems, but can also assess the combat capabilities of the troops at the military command level.

#### 1.5.3.2 Tissue Repair of Ballistic Wounds

Unlike the principle of conventional wounds repair, the principle of conventional tissue repair is to reduce or cover the wound, prevent reinjury and promote tissue regeneration, and recover from anatomical and functional levels. In 2002, Sibbald and other scholars dedicated to wound repair at the 14th International Wound Healing Society Annual Meeting proposed the TIME principle of wound bed preparation based on the current understanding of wound healing mechanisms and the experience of wound healing. TIME is the abbreviation of the first English letter of four wound bed preparation principles in the wound treatment process, that is, T refers to the removal of necrotic tissue (tissue); I refers to the control of inflammation, infection (infection/inflammation); M refers to keeping the wound under normal moisture creating conditions for the growth of the granulation tissue and the epithelialization (moisture); and E refers to the removal of the damaged epidermis (epidermis, nonmigrating). The four principles of wound treatment were first published in the form of a table in *Wound Repair Regeneration* in early 2003, and revised in September 2003, changing "epiderm is" to "edge of wound."

War wounds are often caused by high-energy explosion, which is characterized by severe and extensive tissue defects, ischemia, complications, and high mortality. Such soft tissue defects place new demands on wound repair surgery. The traditional view is that blast injury is extensive, and it is difficult to completely debride at one time. The wound is easy to be infected and the failure rate of vascular anastomosis at early stage is high. Repair surgery should be performed after the wound is clean and the granulation is good.

Leininger et al. believe that high-energy projectiles can produce hollowing and impact effects, resulting in a tissue ischemic area similar to the "stagnation zone" in burns. There is no obvious abnormality during the initial debridement, but it will show progressive embolization and tissue inactivation in 24–72 h after injury, so wound closure at the time of initial debridement is dangerous. According to the modern view, due to the use of highly effective antibiotics, wounds can be repaired in advance under the premise of thorough debridement and wound improvement. It has been reported in the literature that the early repair of common wounds is conducive to the recovery of patients. Explosive wounds cause extensive wound damage, and the damaged tissue and necrotic tissue are alternately existing. Simply relying on debridement cannot prevent secondary infection. The wound loses the barrier function of the skin, leading to the loss of water and protein, the rate of bacterial infection increasing, causing hypermetabolism and sepsis. The blood supply and anti-infective ability of the wound tissue after injury is poor, so it is very important to reconstruct the physiological barrier of the wound. Early closure of the wound can save more reversibly damaged tissue, use "bioscavenging" to remove necrotic tissue and bacteria, reduce the proliferation of pathogenic microorganisms, prevent infection, and promote healing. In recent years, more and more war injury experts have emphasized the importance of early repair and have studied the repair of soft tissue blast injuries. By comparing the characteristics of the injuries in the Iraq War and the Vietnam War, it was found that the chest, abdomen, head, and neck of the combatants were well protected by protective equipment, but the limbs were prone to injury and the injuries were relatively heavy. Compared with the oral and maxillofacial region, the blood supply of the extremities and the trunk is poor, and the anti-infective ability and repair ability are weak. Domestic and foreign scholars have conducted related research. Lerner et al. performed limb salvage surgery on 18 patients with severe limb injury, and tissue flap repair after 5–7 days. These patients have a good functional recovery after surgery. The flaps and myocutaneous flaps have good blood supply, strong anti-infective ability, and wide indications. The blast injury has a wide range of tissue damage, and it is generally impossible to perform local flap transplantation. It is necessary to choose free flap with vascular anastomosis or distal flap. Free flap transplantation has a long hospitalization period, and there are risks such as infection, embolism, and skin flap necrosis, secondary deformity in the donor site. The operation is difficult and the requirements for medical personnel are high. Therefore, the free flap transplantation is not suitable for the wound repair of a large number of wounded in the battlefield environment. The operation of distal flap transplantation is simple, but it takes a long time to fix the limbs, which is easy to cause adhesion and rigidity of the joints. Patients with war wounds often have fractures. Early activities are very important, so there is less choice for distant flap. The operation of the skin graft is simple, deformity in the donor site is light, and the impact on the patient's activity is not obvious. The mesh skin graft is elastic, which can reduce the swelling after operation. The permeability is good, and the tissue fluid is easy to be taken out. And the early closure of the wound can reduce the infection. Regarding the skin graft repair after soft tissue blast injury, some field surgery experts believe that the survival rate of early skin graft is low, and advocate delayed skin grafting. It has been reported that two cases of gunshot wounds were immediately taken for debridement and foreign body removal after injury, and the fascial space syndrome appeared on the second day. After relieving tension, the reticular skin graft was performed and good results were obtained.

The improvement of wound preparation method provides conditions for skin graft of soft tissue blast injury. In recent years, negative pressure wound therapy (NPWT) has been gradually applied to the treatment of war wounds, achieving good results and broadening the indication of skin graft. The wounds in war are seriously damaged, often accompanied by serious pollution. Evacuating the wounded has to go a far distance and takes a long time. The characteristics of negative pressure drainage determine that it is suitable for the treatment of such wounds, which can isolate the wound surface from the battlefield and the ward, and can effectively maintain wound cleaning and reduce wound infections, as well as washing the wounds. For patients with huge soft tissue defects caused by explosion and combined with tendon and bone exposure, Helgeson et al. combined NPWT and Integra artificial skin for wound preparation, after the wound condition is improved, taking the skin graft. The postoperative effect is good, avoiding complicated skin flap transplantation and reducing the risk of donor deformity and skin flap necrosis. Sharony et al. summarized the experiences of treating wounded in the Second Lebanon War, emphasizing the application of the NPWT and Ilizarov external fixation system. It is believed that NPWT can be used almost at all stages of wound healing, can close multiple subcutaneous sinus, and strengthen the attachment of tissue flaps with the periphery of the wound surface and the base, for the preparation of the wound or covering the wound of the donor site. Soft tissue blast injury is the most common cause of injury to military personnel in the battlefield. Because of the threat of terrorist bombs, the probability of these injuries appearing among civilians is also increasing. The key to the repair of high-speed high-energy soft tissue blast injury is early, timely, and thorough debridement, removal of necrotic tissue, adequate drainage, attention to dressing fixation, rational use of antibiotics, elective repair of bone and soft tissue defects, delayed wound coverage or closure, postoperative enhancement of rehabilitation exercises, and patient education. There are a variety of causes of explosive injuries and the injury conditions are different, we must thoroughly study and have a comprehensive understanding of the damage mechanisms of soft tissue blast injuries and the characteristics of injury conditions. That is a prerequisite for effective treatment of soft tissue defects after blast injury. On this basis, clinicians actively use surgical procedures and combine new methods and techniques, to reconstruct damaged tissues and organs, improve deformity, and restore function.

Academician Xiaobing's Fu key laboratory for wound healing in the whole army has conducted research on the negative pressure wound treatment of contaminated wounds after blast injury. It confirmed that on the first day after treatment, the negative pressure wound treatment group showed more fibroblasts and vascular endothelial cells, which have no obvious edema, and the number of vascular endothelial cells is also significantly increased. The main reason is that negative pressure drainage can help reduce the edema of the peri-wound. At the same time, it can reduce the bacterial load in the infected wounds, thereby reducing the range of secondary necrosis of explosive wounds, quickly starting the wound repair process of infected wounds, and shortening the time for the granulation tissue to fill the wound.

## 1.6 The Basic Process of Repair and Regeneration of War Wound Tissue

### 1.6.1 The Basic Pathophysiological Process of Wound Healing

The development of modern high-tech biotechnology has revealed many mysteries of wound healing from the cellular, molecular, and even genetic levels. However, traditionally, people describe the pathophysiological process of tissue repair in the field of pathology, although different scholars have different stages/deletion methods in the stage of wound healing. Generally speaking, the more commonly used staging method is still to roughly divide the basic pathophysiological processes of wound healing into four stages: early bleeding and coagulation, inflammatory response, granulation tissue proliferation, and scar formation. Of course, there is no clear dividing line between them, they are interconnected and characterized.

#### 1.6.1.1 Bleeding and Coagulation Process

From the moment of the formation of the wound surface, the first reaction of the body is its own hemostasis process. This process involves some very complex biological reactions: first, small blood vessels, capillaries around the wound cause reactive contractions to reduce the local blood flow, followed by the exposure of collagen fibers to attract platelets forming blood clots. Later platelets release vasoactive substances such as 5-hydroxytryptamine and prostaglandins, which cause further contraction of blood vessels, slowing of blood flow, and release phospholipids and ADPs to attract more platelets. Finally, endogenous and exogenous coagulation processes start. After the end of the coagulation process, the body begins the next stage of wound healing.

#### 1.6.1.2 Inflammatory Response Period

The posttraumatic inflammatory response period occurs mainly from 48 h after injury. In the first few minutes, after a short period of contraction of the blood vessels in the injured area, thrombosis begins in the damaged blood vessels. Locally unclosed small blood vessels dilate. Platelets interact with the damaged vascular endothelium and exposed collagen to form an embolus that blocks the damaged blood vessel. The complement system is activated and stimulates a range of inflammatory responses including: the local hemagglutination system, the fibrinolytic system, and the kallikrein system. Fibrin deposition and dissolution occur locally in the wound and release many inflammatory mediators, especially bradykinin, free radicals, hydrogen peroxide, and histamine. During this period, various mediators produced by the inflammatory reaction increase the permeability of the blood vessels, causing the liquid, protein, and enzymes in the normal blood vessel to leak into the extracellular space through the blood vessel wall to cause local edema and redness. At this time, the inflammatory cell infiltration is mainly neutrophils, and after 3 days, the macrophage becomes the dominant cell for performing immune function in the wound area.

In the process of inflammation, on the one hand, inflammatory cells such as monocytes and mast cells phagocytose and remove harmful substances such as bacteria in the vicinity of the wound, and at the same time release inflammatory factors and growth factors to coordinate with each other to promote repair and healing of the damaged tissue. On the other hand, it shows an increase in vascular permeability. Due to the destruction of vascular endothelial integrity and permeability changes, a large amount of protein-rich fluid exudes outside the blood vessels, forming inflammatory edema. Local tissue edema can dilute toxins, reduce the damaged effect of toxins on local, bring nutrients to the locally infiltrated white blood cells, and transport metabolites. The antibodies and complement contained in the exudate help to eliminate pathogens and create favorable conditions for wound healing. If the inflammatory response is too strong, cellular immunity and humoral immunity cause degeneration and necrosis of cells and tissues, and vascular permeability increasing, including a large number of neutrophils and protein-rich fluids exuded outside the blood vessels, causing tissue edema and suppurative lysis disruption, delaying wound healing. Therefore, the inflammatory response is a double-edged sword for wound healing. The proper inflammatory response is beneficial to wound healing, while too strong inflammatory reaction and exudation are unfavorable for wound healing.

The latest research shows that the essence and core of the inflammatory response period is the regulation of growth factors and their results. After tissue injury, various growth factors such as PDGF, FGF, and TGF-β released during bleeding and coagulation can play the following roles during the inflammatory response phase:

(a) As a chemotactic agent, neutrophils, macrophages, etc. aggregate to the wound surface. A variety of proteolytic enzymes are released to dissolve the necrotic tissue, and these inflammatory cells themselves release new growth factors, further regulating the inflammatory process of the wound.
(b) Chemotaxis and direct stimulation to fibroblasts, vascular endothelial cell division and proliferation, laying the foundation for later repair.

It should be pointed out that at this stage, the aggregation of inflammatory cells and a large amount of local exudation can play the following roles:

(a) The aggregated leukocytes can phagocytose and remove foreign bodies and cell debris.
(b) Local exudates can dilute local toxins and irritants.
(c) Antibodies in plasma can specifically neutralize toxins.
(d) The exuded fibrin solidifies to form a local barrier.
(e) Activated macrophages not only release a variety of growth factors, but also further regulate the inflammatory response, and also affect the formation of collagen in granulation tissue. In short, this phase of change is the basis for the later restoration.

### Immune Response

The body has an acute inflammatory response period after the wound. On the one hand, the contracted small arteries near the wound expand under the action of vasoactive substances such as histamine, 5-hydroxytryptamine, and kinin, which increases the blood perfusion of the wound and strengthens the local metabolism to help in the removal of harmful substances. At the same time, the wound exposes the nerve endings, and a large amount of inflammatory mediators such as bradykinin, etc. stimulate the wound and cause local pain. On the other hand, cell phagocytosis and immune response run through the whole process. In addition to coagulation and hemostasis, platelet lysis during inflammation also produces platelet-activating factor (PAF) and platelet-derived growth factor (PDGF). These cytokines have the chemotaxis of granulocytes and macrophages to promote the accumulation of these immune cells to the wound. After the phagocytic cells move into the wound, they recognize foreign bodies, then move and adhere to the foreign bodies. Finally, the pseudopods are extended to envelop foreign bodies, phagocytose them. Phagosomes and lysosomes form a phagolysosome, and finally the foreign bodies are digested, this process is called the first cleaning of the wound. The migration of white blood cells lasts about 3 days until the wound is "clean." The proper inflammatory response is beneficial to wound healing. However, if the infection occurs during the inflammatory phase and the inflammatory response is strong, the white blood cells continue to migrate and the phagocytic activity is strengthened. The inflammatory period is prolonged and the wound is delayed in healing.

Peripheral white blood cell count increasing is another typical manifestation of inflammatory response, especially when inflammation is caused by bacterial infections. The increase in white blood cell count is mainly due to the accelerated release of leukocytes from the bone marrow pool caused by interleukin-1 (IL-1) and tumor necrosis factor-α (TNF-α), and an increase in the proportion of relatively immature rod-shaped neutrophils. This phenomenon is called "nuclear left shift." Therefore, most of the researches at home and abroad have selected specific cytokines, such as IL-6, IL-8, TNF-α, etc., as indicators of the degree of inflammation. Controlling the degree of inflammatory response plays a crucial role in the wound healing, so infection prevention and anti-inflammatory are particularly important in promoting wound healing.

### Vascular Permeability

In the inflammatory response induced by wounds, inflammatory cells release a large number of inflammatory mediators and oxidation products. The accumulation of these substances can lead to dysfunction of vascular endothelial cells, the main manifestations are: permeability of endothelial cells increasing, abnormal expression of adhesion molecules, the adhesion of endothelial cells and inflammatory cells increasing, and vascular dysregulation leading to localized edema. Local inflammatory edema contributes to wound healing, but excessive blood and protein exudation cause excessive tissue edema, which can delay the wound healing. Therefore, in the study of promoting wound healing, attention to vascular permeability is particularly important.

Increased vascular permeability is mainly mediated by two pathways: the cell-through pathway and the paracellular pathway. The cell-through pathway is achieved by the "vesicle-vacuole organelles" (VVOs). VVOs are a string of glucose-like unencapsulated vesicles and a variety of vacuoles formed by the endothelium membrane internalized, which are composed by vesicle-vacuole fusion. It is surrounded by three layers of unit membranes, each membrane and the endothelium membrane interconnected by small pores, macromolecular tracers (such as ferritin, horseradish peroxidase, etc.) can rapidly exude from the venules to the outside of the blood vessels through VVOs. Using continuous high-level ultrathin sections, transmission electron microscopy, three-dimensional reconstruction, and other techniques, an acute inflammatory state is formed under the action of high heat, high-pressure, vascular endothelial growth factor (VEGF), etc., and it is found that endothelial cells have openings through cells. These openings are not located in the endothelium. However, it is located in the peripheral part of the endothelial cells itself, which may be the cell passage formed by the intracellular vesicles fuse, thereby increasing the permeability of the blood vessels. In addition, inflammatory mediators (such as TNF-α) cause the formation of perforating cell channels, while also shrinking the endothelial cytoskeleton, thinning the cytoplasm, and promoting the formation of channel openings, which is also a factor that increases the permeability of the cell-through pathway. Another pathway for increased vascular permeability is the paracellular pathway, which is an important pathway for increased vascular permeability and macromolecular material exudation. Studies have shown that when endothelial cells are subjected to various endogenous or exogenous stimuli, endothelial cells are affected by exogenous signaling pathways, opening the intercellular junctions and forming fissures between endothelial cells, resulting in increased permeability. SP in neuropeptides can cause an increase in tracheal vascular permeability, the mechanism of which is accomplished by the paracellular pathway. There is an overlap of 1–2 μm in the interstitial junction of normal venules, and there is no fissure. At the time of inflammation (1 min after injection of substance P), 48% of the junctions of endothelial cells showed fissures, indicating that the inflammatory response disrupted the tight junction of endothelial cells. The paracellular pathway increases vascular permeability. The integrity and tightness of vascular endothelial cell connections directly affect the permeability of blood vessels. The structure that maintains its tightness relies on vascular endothelial junctions and their associated proteins, including tight junctions and adhesion junctions between endothelial cells-cells, and adhesion junctions between endothelial cells and basement membranes. Vascular endothelial cadherin (VE-cadherin) is the main structural protein of vascular endothelial cell adhesion and connection. Its essence is a transmembrane protein, and its extracellular N′ end and adjacent cell VE- cadherin N′ end are interconnected, allowing VE-cadherin to aggregate into clusters at the junction between cells. Thereby allowing the endothelial cells to closely adhere together to form a selective semipermeable membrane, forming a barrier between the blood and the tissue, and controlling the material exchange on both sides of the vessel wall. When an inflammatory response occurs, under the influence of inflammatory mediators, the function and structure change, causing dissociation, and the gap between the cells is increased, resulting in an increase in vascular permeability. In the inflammatory response, inflammatory cells and inflammatory mediators eventually lead to the disintegration of the VE-cadherin complex through different pathways, resulting in the breakdown of endothelial cell junctions and increased endothelial permeability.

#### 1.6.1.3 Granulation Tissue Proliferative Phase

On the third day after injury, with the regression of inflammatory response and the gradual proliferation of tissue repair cells, the pathophysiological process of granulation tissue hyperplasia and epidermal cell proliferation was observed. At this time, histomorphology is characterized by capillary germ formation and fibroblast proliferation, and produces a large amount of extracellular matrix called granulation tissue.

The growth of granulation tissue in proliferative phase is the key link in the process of wound repair and healing. The quality of new granulation tissue directly affects the repair, healing degree, and prognosis of wounds. The granulation tissue is composed of fibroblasts, endothelial cells, and new capillaries. Its formation can fill and repair the tissue defects of the wound, which is beneficial to the anti-infection and absorption of the wound, and the removal of necrotic tissue. At the same time, granulation tissue shrinks the wound, which is good for wound healing and creates the necessary conditions for epithelial crawling. The growth rate and growth amount of granulation tissue are directly proportional to the healing rate of the wound. The growth of granulation tissue is closely related to the degree of vascularization of the wound. The angiogenic activity is enhanced, and the granulation tissue is easy to grow. On the contrary, if the angiogenic activity is lowered, the granulation tissue is not easy to grow and the wound is not easy to heal. Therefore, the growth of granulation tissue is largely determined by vascularization.

Newborn capillaries are formed primarily by "germination." First, a variety of growth factors act on the bottom of the wound or the vascular endothelial cells (especially the venous endothelial cells) in the "dormant" state, causing them to "activate" and generate capillary germs. After the formation of capillary germs, they grow into the wounded area with a loop shape and get mutually connected to form a capillary network. The capillaries grow at a rate of 0.1–0.6 mm per day, and their directions are mostly perpendicular to the wound surface. Since there is no nerve in the granulation tissue, there is no feeling. However, the basement membrane of these neovascular vessels is incomplete, very fragile, and prone to leakage. Capillary endothelial cells secrete a collagenase that degrades the collagen secreted by fibroblasts and facilitates the movement of capillary endothelial cells. Capillaries formed in this way can participate in the formation of large blood vessels or stop functioning in the future and then degeneration and disappearance.

Angiogenesis refers to the process of new microvessels existing from the mature vascular sprouts. It begins at 24–48 h after wound formation and reaches its peak on the fifth day, playing an important role in wound repair. Microvessels are mainly composed of lining endothelial cells and peripheral pericytes. Angiogenesis involves important processes such as differentiation, proliferation, migration, and interaction of these two kinds of cells. According to previous studies, angiogenesis is initiated after the balance of pro-angiogenic factors and inhibitors is broken in the absence of oxygen. First, endothelial cells activate to form an angiogenic phenotype, while the matrix metalloproteinase activates to degrade the basement membrane and extracellular matrix. Therefore, endothelial cell migration is possible. Endothelial cells proliferate and migrate to form neovascular sprouts. Thereafter, the vascular buds form lumen under the impact of blood flow, and the pericytes in the interstitial adhere to the neovascularization, completing the shape of new blood vessels. Angiogenesis is an important part of wound repair, and a variety of cells and regulatory factors are involved in this process. A mouse skin injury model study showed that angiogenesis in neonatal granulation tissue is most pronounced at 5 days, and the measurement of neonatal microvessel density is consistent with the pathological observation. When the wound has hemorrhage, necrosis, and inflammatory reaction, the local pro-angiogenic factors are increased, such as VEGF, PDGF, transforming growth factor-β (TGF-β), basic fibroblast growth factor (bFGF), etc. Growth of vascular bud of surrounding tissues and transformation of precursor cells of vascular constitutive cells initiate angiogenesis. At the same time, mesenchymal stem cells in the stroma are activated and converted into fibroblasts, myofibroblasts, etc., together forming granulation tissue to repair the wound.

VEGF plays an extremely important role in the process of promoting wound vascularization and wound healing. It is the most potent angiogenic growth factor found so far. VEGF can promote cell proliferation and migration, vascular endothelium growth and wound vascularization, enhance vascular permeability, and improve the ability of glucose to transfer into endothelial cells, so that the high energy required by angiogenic cells is supplemented accordingly. Many aspects promote the healing of wounds. Immunohistochemistry confirmed that neutrophils near the wound began to express VEGF on the first day after wound formation in rats and were detected in macrophages, fibroblasts, and endothelial cells on 3rd–7th days after injury. And its expression in wound tissue is much higher than those in surrounding normal tissues. At the same time, by RT-PCR (reverse transcription polymerase chain reaction), the expression of VEGF on the first day is much higher than those on the third day and the seventh day after injury, confirming that VEGF expression is mainly produced by inflammatory cells in the early stages of wound healing. Therefore, promoting VEGF expression in the early stage is considered to be an important way to promote wound healing. VEGF is widely recognized as an angiogenic substance, and it was found to have mitogenic function of ROS in addition to pro-angiogenic function 10 years ago. A large number of studies in the last 5 years have pointed out that VEGF expression has a close relationship with endogenous H2O2 and VEGF signaling factors. These new findings provide a large number of new theoretical bases for the development of drugs and treatments for the promotion of angiogenesis.

Another kind of vascular endothelial growth factor with strong promotion and high specificity is bFGF, which is also a multifunctional cytokine, which has a strong role in promoting cell division and blood vessel growth. Its biological functions during tissue repair include promoting capillary angiogenesis and reconstruction of capillary structures, promoting the growth and proliferation of endothelial cells, fibroblasts, smooth muscle cells, and the like. During the inflammatory response phase, bFGF stimulates the directional migration of fibroblasts and endothelial cells, initiating the formation and vascularization of fibrous tissue. During the granulation tissue formation stage, bFGF activates fibroblasts to migrate to the edge of the wound, proliferate and synthesize new intercellular substances (such as collagen), and also induces capillary endothelial cell migration and proliferation to form vascular sprouts, and causes new blood vessels extending to the wounded regional matrix to provide nutrients to local cells and improve the excretion of local metabolites, thus creating conditions for promoting wound healing. Experiments have confirmed that bFGF can accelerate the proliferation of epithelial cells and promote wound healing. bFGF promotes angiogenesis in vivo and in vitro, and synergizes with VEGF to upregulate VEGF production by regulating VEGF gene expression, thereby affecting angiogenesis.

The extracellular matrix is mainly composed of hyaluronic acid, chondroitin sulfate, collagen, and acid mucopolysaccharide, and its main component is derived from fibroblasts. Fibroblasts produce collagen fibers which are formed by stepwise polymerization of three peptide chains with glycine, hydroxyproline, and hydroxylysine as basic components. Collagen fibers have a high degree of toughness, which increases the tensile strength of the wound. The formation of collagen fibers peaked on 14th–21st days. The clinical manifestations are scarred red, slightly elevated, often itchy, and the texture is hard and tough.

The significance of granulation tissue formation is to fill the wound defect, protect the wound to prevent bacterial infection, reduce bleeding, mechanized blood clot, necrotic tissue, and other foreign bodies, provide nutrients for the newborn epithelium, and create further conditions for reepithelialization. The reepithelialization process is generally performed in synchrony with granulation tissue proliferation, mainly by proliferation, differentiation, and migration of epidermal cells (including stem cells) remaining at the edge or the bottom of the wound. Under the influence of a series of regulatory factors, the new epidermis of the wound crawls to the center of the wound in a "crawling" manner, eventually covering the wound.

#### 1.6.1.4 Scar Formation Period

The formation of scars is one of the final outcomes of soft tissue wound repair. The stage of granulation tissue transformed into scar tissue and collagen tissue continuously forming lasts several months. Fibroblasts are transformed into myofibroblasts to contract the wound, collagen tissue is produced in large amounts, and keratinocytes cover the wound surface by epithelialization.

The proliferation, differentiation, and migration of epithelial cells exert new epithelium on the edge of the wound skin until it covers the entire wound. This process is also accomplished by a variety of cells and regulatory factors, of which keratinocyte growth factor (KGF) is widely considered to be a more potent and highly specific one. As an epithelial-specific growth factor, KGF can promote the proliferation, migration, and differentiation of epidermal cells, which is closely related to skin wound healing and can improve the quality of wound healing. Fibroblasts at the basal part of the skin wound are capable of synthesizing and releasing KGF, inducing proliferation of epidermal cells around the wound, and migrating to the wound. In addition, KGF, insulin-like growth factor-1 (IGF-1), and their composite cDNA can significantly increase the expression of IGF-1, KGF, FGF, VEGF, and type IV collagen, accelerate neovascularization, enhance dermal and epidermal regeneration, accelerate reepithelialization, and promote the migration of keratinocytes from the edge of the wound to the wound matrix. Experiments have confirmed that fibroblasts are capable of producing and releasing KGF and promoting the proliferation and migration of epidermal cells through KGF, thereby promoting wound healing.

KGF-2 is another highly specific growth factor that promotes epithelial cell proliferation. The experiment confirmed that the specific target cell of KGF-2 is epithelial cell. Its main physiological role is to undertake signaling between mesenchymal cells and epithelial cells, promote proliferation of keratinocytes and epithelial cells, and stimulate regeneration, differentiation, and migration of epithelial cells around the wound, thereby promoting wound healing. At the same time, it has no direct effect on fibroblasts and endothelial cells, and can reduce the formation of scar tissue during wound healing.

There are many factors affecting the formation of scars. If the wound defect is small, the alignment is neat, and no infection occurs (such as a clean surgical incision), the repair (healing) can be completed 2–3 weeks after the injury. At this time, the scar is not obvious, and the function has no effect. For wounds with large defects, irregularities, or infections, it usually takes 4–5 weeks to heal. At this time, the scar is wide, affecting the appearance and even causing dysfunction. The morphological features of scars are the deposition of a large number of fibroblasts and collagen fibers, and their biochemical and molecular biological characteristics are caused by abnormal collagen metabolism in fibroblasts. Studies have shown that the ratio of type I and type III collagen precursor mRNA in abnormal scar fibroblasts is as high as 22:1, while normal skin is only 6:1, indicating that the transcription selectivity of type I collagen precursor mRNA is enhanced. These genetic changes are associated with changes in local wound growth factors (TGF, TNF), local immunity (IgG, IgA, IgM). The formation and regression of scars often depend on the balance between collagen fiber synthesis and catabolism. In the early stage of wound healing or in the stage of fibroproliferation, local collagen fibers will increase due to the predominance of synthesis. When the synthesis is balanced with catabolism, there is no change in the size of the scar. When collagenase is dominant in the decomposition and absorption of collagen, the scar will gradually soften and shrink, and the time varies depending on the size of the scar, which usually takes several months. The study found after skin damage, there is no scar healing in early embryo, but scar healing in the postembryonic development and after birth.

### 1.6.2 The Characteristics and Repair of Gunshot Wounds

The damage caused by bullets is the process of releasing a large amount of energy in a very short time. The physical factors involved include the mass, speed, shape, and flight state of the bullet. It is also related to the characteristics of the target tissue, such as density, elasticity, viscosity, and toughness. Traditionally, there are three types of bullet injury mechanisms.

(a) Direct damage: It mainly refers to the tear effect, similar to cold weapons. It is the tissue breaking and tearing caused by the projectile passing through the tissue. For the low-speed bullet with a speed of not more than 340 m/s, the tearing effect is the main effect; while for the high-speed bullet, the tearing effect is in a secondary position. The tearing effect does not transfer much energy to the surrounding tissue.
(b) Instantaneous cavity effect: The pressure wave generated after the bullet entering the soft tissue pushes the tissue around the injured road forward and outward in a few milliseconds or even microseconds to form an instant cavity which is several times or even tens of times larger than the diameter of the primary wound. The cavity is timed and repeatedly contracted and expanded. The rapid change of pressure in the cavity causes the tissues and organs around the wound to be compressed and pulled in a very short time. Extensive tears and contusions have occurred.
(c) Pressure wave effect: When the bullet injures the body, part of the energy is transmitted to the surrounding tissues and organs in the form of pressure waves and shock waves, causing damage.

Chinese scholars have earlier noted the importance of pathological observation and zoning of injured tissues, and realized that reasonable pathological zoning can provide a scientific basis for determining the scope of debridement and clinical treatment. In the early 1980s, Wang Zhengguo suggested that the gun wounds and surrounding tissues can be divided into the primary wound zone, the contusion zone, and the oscillation zone. The primary wound zone is the cavity caused by the bullet passing through; the contusion zone is the tissue necrotic zone closed to the primary wound zone; outside the contusion zone is the oscillation zone.

The North Atlantic Treaty Organization (NATO) 1975 version of the War Damage First-Aid Manual has clearly stated that gunshot wounds caused by high-speed bullets must be extensively debrided. Because the instantaneous cavity effect of such a bullet can cause all tissues within

30 times its diameter to be inactivated. However, the 1988 edition of the manual corrects this. In a war environment, rescuers often tend to adopt methods similar to the removal of malignant tumors. All necrosis, injury, and suspected tissue are removed, which may result in greater damage than the gunshot itself, but it is reasonable and necessary from a military medical perspective. The wounds on the battlefield are often heavily polluted, the wounds are not treated in time, and the objective conditions such as the large number of wounded, limited medical resources, and insufficient doctor experiences make it easy for people to adopt a thorough debridement method. The experience of previous war treatments also suggests that incomplete debridement often leads to higher infection rates and mortality, leading to unnecessary waste of medical resources. However, in the past two or three decades, more and more people have advocated conservative treatment. It has been found that the cavity effect is only the tissue displacement caused by mechanical traction. If the decompression and infection are controlled in time, the damaged skeletal muscle may recover.

#### 1.6.2.1 Characteristics of Gunshot Wound

(a) Often it occurs in multiple parts, in the brain, maxillofacial, thoracic cavity, abdominal cavity, and limbs and can have unique characteristics.
(b) Often it is accompanied by bone, joint, nerve, and soft tissue damage, heavy pollution, and severe damage to blood vessels, nerves, and adjacent soft tissue beds.
(c) Except the tissue and vascular damage directly caused by firearm injury, the range of shock waves and thermal indirect damage are larger than those of the naked eye, and the edge of the defect is not neat.
(d) High-energy damage in the local area of the wound causes severe embolization of the damaged blood vessel, damage and defects of the intima.
(e) Warheads or metal foreign objects are embedded in the damaged blood vessels. There is no major bleeding before surgery, but you should be alert.

#### 1.6.2.2 Repair Principle of Gunshot Wound

Due to the different characteristics of each part, the repair is very different (refer to the introduction of each specialist). Usually gunshot wounds include the primary wound zone, the contusion zone, and the oscillation zone. Due to their unique pathological changes, the surgical field should be fully exposed, and nerves, blood vessels, and tendons should be routinely explored to determine the presence or absence of nerve and blood vessel damage, and the location, nature, and extent of the injury. Look for damaged blood vessels, thoroughly debride and remove foreign bodies, and repair and reconstruct according to the order of bones, blood vessels, nerves, and soft tissues. At the same time, look for vigorous muscle nearby to cover, and if necessary, move adjacent muscles to provide a good tissue bed for repair or the reconstruction of blood vessels. In the case of defective blood vessel transplantation, the vessel should be cut to the normal endometrium. Otherwise, thrombosis may occur and the operation may fail. If the patient's general condition is extremely poor, the amputation should be decisive to save the life. If there is no condition for the amputation, the vascular end should be found and ligated, and the operation is terminated immediately after effective hemostasis.

### 1.6.3 Soft Tissue Blast Injury

Blast injuries are the most common cause of injury to military personnel on the battlefield.

#### 1.6.3.1 Classification of Modern Soft Tissue Blast Injuries

Explosion is a phenomenon of instantaneous release of energy. The explosion effect is divided into the following four types:

(a) Type 1 blast injury. The damage comes from the overpressure and negative pressure caused by the shock wave. The target organs are the hollow organs like ear, lung, and intestine.
(b) Type 2 blast injury. The injury comes from penetrating damage caused by projectiles.
(c) Type 3 blast injury. The collapse of buildings and fragments of vehicles caused by explosion, leading to crush injury, contusion, traumatic amputation of fractures, opened or closed head injury.
(d) Type 4 blast injury. It includes burns, asphyxia, and toxic gas damage. Explosive weapons generate a large amount of high-pressure gas, heat, shock waves, and scattered fragments at the moment of explosion, forming a variety of damage factors such as fragments, impact, burns, etc., which jointly cause damage to the human body.

#### 1.6.3.2 Clinical Features of Blast Injury

##### Multiple Sites, Multiple Organs, Multiple Tissue Damage

There are many types of explosive weapons, and the methods of injury are varied, the sites and extents are different. Peleg et al. analyzed 1155 terrorist-related injuries in the Israeli National Trauma Registry from October 1, 2000 to September 30, 2002, and compared the differences between gunshot wounds and explosive wounds. They concluded that the explosive wounded have more injury sites, 62% of them combined with multiple site injuries, while gunshot wounds 47%; and patients with blast injuries are in a more serious condition, 17.3% of blast injuries with Injury Severity Score (ISS) > 25 points, while gunshot wounds just 14.9%.

#### Severe Soft Tissue Defect

The pressure wave propagates in different density media, causing various effects such as spallation, explosion, polymerization, acceleration, deceleration, and pressure difference, resulting in tearing and blast injury of the tissue, severe damage of soft tissue, and deep tissue exposure. In recent years, suicide bombings have brought new changes to the characteristics of blast injuries. A variety of foreign bodies have been added to explosives, resulting in an increase in damage sites, aggravation of soft tissue damage, and more retention of foreign bodies. The US military conducted statistics on the causes of injuries from the wounded in Iraq, and the roadside homemade improvised explosive devices ranked first. Such explosions often cause damage to the chest and limbs through the unprotected sub axillary area, which causes crush injury of the limbs, which is manifested by severe damage to the soft tissues, bones, and blood vessels of the extremities, and the potential fatality rate is high. According to Geiger, lower extremities are more likely to be damaged than upper limbs, with lower limb injuries accounting for 61.76% and upper limbs accounting for 29.4%; lower extremity injuries are wide, the defect degree of muscle and neurovascular are different, and the former is significantly more damaged than the latter.

#### Complex Infection, Difficult to Handle

Explosive soft tissue defects are serious. There are foreign bodies such as sediment, debris, and hair around the wound and deep surface, which aggravate the wound pollution, and the infection rate is high. The disease develops rapidly, and the immune response is inhibited after severe damage to various tissues. It is susceptible to infection and other complications. In the modern war wounds, the spectrum of infected bacteria has changed significantly. The multidrug-resistant *Acinetobacter baumannii* infection in the Iraqi warfare has shown an upward trend. Analysis of the results shows that it may be related to the use of drugs and the colony of the soldiers. According to statistics, 50% of the wounds are positive for bacterial culture and 57% of them are infected with *Acinetobacter baumannii.*

#### High Limb Damage Rate, Heavy Functional Impact, Difficult to Repair

The blast injury is severely damaged, the soft tissue and bone are extensively deficient, the vascular and nerves in the deep and injured areas are damaged. The joints, bones, and tendons are exposed, which seriously affects the function. The surgical repair is difficult, and some of the wounded are eventually amputated. The main reason for the failure of limb salvage is the presence of other organ damage, life-threatening severe blood loss, and sepsis.

#### E. Delayed Delivery, Delay the Best Treatment Opportunity

Under the conditions of war, the number of wounded people is large and the injuries are complicated.

Medical treatment is limited by various factors such as medical environment, instruments, and human resources. Coupland and Samnegaard counted 18,877 civilian wounded admitted to the International Red Cross Hospital, and only 2012 wounded were delivered to the hospital within 6 h after injury. The delayed delivery causes the injured to miss the best treatment opportunity. The bacteria in the injured wounds multiply and the infection rate increases. Some reversibly damaged tissues develop ischemic necrosis or inflammation progresses, resulting in increased damage and eventually tissue necrosis. Some wounded fail to get timely first-aid resuscitation treatment and eventually die.

### 1.6.3.3 Repair of Explosive Injuries

The key to the repair of high-speed and high-energy soft tissue blast injury is early, timely, and thorough debridement, removal of necrotic tissue, adequate drainage, attention to dressing fixation, rational use of antibiotics, elective repair of bone and soft tissue defects, delayed wound coverage or closure, postoperative enhancement of rehabilitation exercises, and patient education.

The traditional view is that blast injury is extensive, and it is difficult to completely debride at one time. The wound is easy to be infected. The failure rate of early anastomosis is high. Surgery should be performed after the wound is clean and the granulation is good. Negative pressure wound treatment (NPWT) has been gradually applied to the treatment of war wounds, achieving good results and broadening the indications for skin graft repair. The wounds in war are seriously damaged, often accompanied with serious pollution. The wounded are sent far away and have a long time. The characteristics of NPWT determine that it is suitable for the treatment of such wounds, which can isolate the wound from the surrounding battlefield and the environment of the hospital, effectively maintain the wound clean, and reduce wound infection while washing the wound. For patients with huge soft tissue defects caused by explosion and combined with tendon and bone exposure, Helgeson et al. combined the application of NPWT and Integra artificial skin for wound preparation, and when the wound condition is improved, skin graft repair is performed and the postoperative effect is good. This method can avoid complicated skin flap transplantation and reduce the risk of donor deformity and skin flap necrosis. Sharony et al. summarized the experiences of rescuing the Second Lebanon War wounded and emphasized the application of NPWT and external fixation systems. It is believed that the NPWT can be used in various stages of wound healing, which can close multiple subcutaneous sinuses, strengthen the adhesion of tissue flaps and wound periphery and basement, ready for wound preparation or cover the donor site.

Explosive injury causes are various and injury conditions are different. It is necessary to conduct an in-depth research on them and comprehensively understand the damage mechanisms and injury conditions of soft tissue explosive wounds. This is the prerequisite for an effective treatment of soft tissue defects after a blast injury. On this basis, clinicians actively use surgical procedures and combine new methods and techniques to reconstruct damaged tissues and organs, improve deformity, and restore function.

## 1.7 Progress and Prospects of Research on Repair and Regeneration of War Wound Tissue

In the past 20 years, with the continuous development of science and technology, the research of molecular biology, materials science, tissue engineering, and other aspects has been deepened, and the overall level of wound healing has been greatly improved. The goal of wound healing and regeneration has also gradually changed from the pursuit of healing speed to the emphasis on healing quality, from the repair of a single tissue component to the simultaneous repair of multiple tissue components, from local tissue repair to the whole body, paying more attention on how to solve psychological, functional repair problems, etc.

### 1.7.1 Posttraumatic Tissue Repair Research from Local Tissue Repair to Overall (Whole Body) Repair

The human body is a harmonization of the whole composed of multilevel structures. The life movement of the human body is an advanced movement in the natural world. The internal and the body with the external environment are always in the process of dynamic contradictory movement. The scientific view of the human body will guide people to better reveal the laws of movement of human life activities. People are the product of long-term differentiation in nature. The human body contains more than 60 chemical elements, which are basically consistent with the chemical composition of the Earth's surface, and are mostly light and even elements in the top 20 of the element periodic table. From microscopic to macroscopic, the human body can be summarized into: quantum→molecular→subcellular→cell→tissue→organ→system→body. The high level is composed of low levels, but the high level is not a simple accumulation of low levels. Different levels have different morphological structures and functional activities. The organic connection between different levels forms the whole of the human body system and forms an ecosystem with the external environment. Therefore, the overall unity of the human body is mainly manifested in the unity of morphological structure and functional activities, the unity of the local and the whole, and the unity of the body and the environment. Firstly, the unity of structure and function. In the human body, the unity of material and movement is the unity of morphological structure and functional activity. Morphological structure is the material basis of functional activities, and certain functional activities are the performance of certain morphological structures. Therefore, the morphological structure and function are mutually restricted. Different organs perform different functional activities in different morphological structures. The certain morphological structure of each organ is expressed as a certain functional activity. Different systems composed of individual organs have different functional roles. The morphological structure of the cells is consistent with the functional activity. Just as muscle cells with a fusiform and long cylindrical shape, rich in myofibrils, are suitable for contraction and relaxation. Nerve cells with axons and dendrites are suitable for stimulation, conduction excitation, and so on. At the molecular level, the strict ordering of linear primary structures of nucleic acids and protein molecules determines the specificity of their functional activities. If the structure of an organ, cell, or biomacromolecule changes, it will affect the corresponding functional activity. Conversely, functional activity also affects morphological structure. The morphological structure of various organs of the body is actually the result of continuous evolution of the body under the influence of the environment, with the adaptation of functional activities. Secondly, the unity of the local and the whole. The human body is composed of numerous cells, tissues, and organs. There are complex interactions between local and whole, local and local, which constitute a unity of the whole and the local. The overall function is accomplished by the coordination and cooperation of various local activities. In the unified whole of the human body, any local change is not isolated, it will affect other parts later or early, more or less, and eventually lead to overall changes. The functional activities of various systems and organs of the human body are accomplished through the neurohumoral regulation. Thirdly, the unity of the body and the environment. The human body is an open system, a dissipative structure that constantly links with the external environment. Input various substances, energies, and information, and output processed materials, energies, and information to the environment through changes in the internal environment of the body. The external environment includes climate, water, soil, sunlight, air, and working conditions, spiritual life factors, they are intertwined, intricate, and constantly changing.

On the basis of modern science and technology, medicine is rapidly developing in both micro- and macro directions. The deepening of the microscopic is not only a deepening from the subcellular, molecular, to the quantum level, but also a deepening of intrinsic mechanism for the activities of life and disease. The expansion to the macro is not only an extension of the human body, people, and the ecological environment, but also an increasingly close combination of medicine and sociology. The social functions of medicine are continuously strengthened. The deep development of modern medicine in these two directions, combined with each other, penetrates each other and crosses each other to form a trend of comprehensive research and development. To the micro level, it is the requirement of the development of life science and medical science itself, and it is also an objective requirement that medical practice is increasingly urgently proposed. With the development of molecular biology and the penetration into medicine, molecular physiology, molecular pathology, molecular pharmacology, molecular genetics, molecular immunology, etc. have been formed, which directly promoted the medical research from the description of the phenomenon into the analysis of the internal mechanism. Understanding this holistic and partial concept will contribute to the study of tissue repair in trauma and postinjury.

At present, the development of modern medicine is increasingly characterized by a combination of micro and macro. The deepening of the microscopic level enables people to explain the complex changes and interrelationships of various parts of the overall connection, forming a qualitative description of the overall complex system. The study of macroscopic phenomena in life activities reveals the premise of local changes and the interrelationships in the reality, driving the discussion of microscopic changes. Therefore, micro-in-depth and macro-level researches are mutually reinforcing, and the combination of the two is objective and inevitable. Complex life activities are the results of the regular integration of various parts according to certain relationships. The combination of micro and macro in modern medicine will lead to a leap in the understanding of the nature of life activities.

The effects of nerve, endocrine, and hormonal changes on skin repair and regeneration have recently received great attention. From an anatomical point of view, with the deep understanding of subcutaneous tissue and skin attachments, especially fat cells and mesenchymal cells, the adipose tissue has not only been regarded as an energy storage organ, but also as a metabolic organ of sex hormones and endocrine organ. Adipose tissue is capable of producing a large number of bioactive peptides, including adipokines and leptin, which act in an autocrine and paracrine form in combination with specific receptors on the surface of adipocytes in local. Functionally, the function of the skin among mammalian populations is more or less different. Among them, human skin functions mainly include maintaining endogenous homeostasis, such as regulating body temperature and body fluid equilibrium; participating in substance metabolism, such as vitamin D synthesis; performing sensory afferent; blocking external damage such as infection, mechanical damage, and ultraviolet rays' irradiation. In addition, it is also the most initial and basic part of the body's immune system. Except these previously discovered functions of the skin, more and more evidence shows that the skin is a highly active "biological plant" capable of synthesizing or participating in the metabolism of many biologically active substances (e.g., structural proteins, glycoproteins, lipids, and signaling molecules). People's understanding of skin function has become clearer and more complete. The immune-nerve-endocrine system cross-talk has opened up many new fields for the research of skin tissue repair and regeneration, which has led to many new ideas.

### 1.7.2 Posttraumatic Tissue Repair Research from Passive Repair to Active Repair

People have paid more and more attention to the damage caused by trauma, surgery, organ transplantation, and other serious diseases and consequences, and they are competing to carry out research on its mechanism and prevention. The traditional treatment method is mainly based on "guarantee," that is, the self-repair of the damaged organ is dominant, waiting for the metabolism of the damaged organ to self-heal. This passive repair method not only prolongs the treatment time, but also leads to a series of adverse complications, and also increases the psychological and economic burden of the patient, which is extremely unfavorable for treatment. In the 1980s, the research on the effect of growth factors on wound repair caused fundamental changes in the concept of modern wound repair. Firstly, the connotation of repair has expanded from simple surface wound repair to internal organs and the whole body. Secondly, with manual intervention, the natural process of wound healing can be somewhat "promoted" or "accelerated." Under the guidance of this modern understanding, research on the role of growth factors in wound repair has become a hot topic in the field of tissue repair in the past 10 years. The theoretical basis for the active repair of damaged tissue by growth factors is derived from the interdependence and interaction of growth factors and systemic organs in biological processes such as embryogenesis and tissue growth. Studies have shown that in tissues such as liver, pancreas, and gastrointestinal tract in early embryonic development, epidermal growth factor (EGF), insulin-like growth factor (IGF), hepatocyte growth factor (HGF), and transforming growth factor (TGF) have been found to show the gene expression increasing, and with organ embryo development, levels of above growth factor mRNA increasing. The above facts indicate that growth factor is one of the intrinsic components of these organs. It not only participates in the process of embryogenesis of organs, but also plays an important role in the maintenance and repair of mature organs.

### 1.7.3 Posttraumatic Tissue Repair Research from Anatomical Repair to Functional Restoration

The ideal wound healing and tissue regeneration repair should enable the injured tissue to achieve complete repair in anatomical structure and physiological function. This phenomenon can only be seen in fetal skin repair. In clinical work, a large number of tissue repair results are that the anatomical structure of the injured tissue is basically restored, and its physiological function is only partially restored, and some scar tissue is left in the affected part. In addition, there are two kinds of repair anomalies, which we call repair out of control, which is the main problem we are facing and need to solve. One is the healing of scars after extensive full-thickness skin burns. Although patients have preserved their lives, there are no skin appendages such as sweat glands, sebaceous glands, and hair follicles in large areas of scars, so these patients cannot regulate their body temperature by sweating. The physiological dysfunction reduces the quality of life. In addition, due to scar hyperplasia and/or keloids, it seriously affects the physical and mental health of patients, and some cannot even integrate into social life, resulting in a significant decline in the quality of life. The other is insufficient wound healing or difficulty in healing, leading to the formation of chronic ulcers. Chronic refractory ulcers and scar hyperplasia are two different manifestations of repairing out of control. Although the repair out-of-control does not cause death as quickly as cancer, but because they occur on the surface, long course, difficult treatment, and high cost, they do cause great pain to the patient and seriously affect the quality of life of the patient. In order to solve the problem of repair out-of-control, we advocate vigorously carrying out basic research on tissue repair from anatomical repair to functional repair. On the one hand, it is hoped that medical scientists will pay attention to the functional rehabilitation of patients in the early stage of trauma treatment, and try to avoid loss of function; on the other hand, it is hoped to achieve breakthroughs through in-depth and meticulous basic research, laying a groundwork for a revolution in clinical therapeutics. At present, the research on the functional repair of wound tissue has been paid enough attention at home and abroad. The focus of the research is mainly on exploring the mechanism of tissue regeneration and how to transform high-tech biotechnology in the field of tissue regeneration and repair into clinical treatment and other aspects. In particular, our goal of "achieving the simultaneous repair and regeneration of multiple damaged tissues at the injury site" marks the formation of a new research direction in this field, with more specific goals and a better future.

### 1.7.4 Posttraumatic Tissue Repair Research from the Emphasis on Basic Research to Clinical Transformation and Precision Treatment

Translational Medicine first appeared in the literature in 1993, also known as the clinical translational research (CTR). In 2003, the National Institutes of Health (NIH) developed a long-term plan for the development of biomedicine. In 2004, an initial investment of $125 million was made. In 2009, the total investment reached $2 billion. One of the most important goals is to cultivate a new research team with different professional backgrounds, who can collaborate on basic research and clinical work. By 2012, 60 Clinical and Translational Science Centers (CTSCs) were established in the United States. In the field of burn wound research, translational medicine has received extensive attention from researchers. In September 2010, the 218th Young Scientists Forum of China Association for Science and Technology was held in Chongqing. The theme was "Thinking and Countermeasures of Translational Medicine Leading Burn Research." At the meeting, the translational prospects in research areas, such as burned clinical nutrition, sepsis, wound repair, stem cells, and diabetes wounds, were discussed in depth. At the 8th National Burn Treatment Symposium on the theme of "Regeneration Medicine and Translational Medicine" held in June 2011, Academician Sheng Zhiyong emphasized the importance of translational medicine and affirmed the transformation significance of the major burns from clinical to basic research to the clinical. Many experts have made an in-depth interpretation of the importance of the "bench to bedside and bedside to bench" (B2B). Reproductive medicine has been listed as a major research direction in the scientific and technological planning of the Chinese Academy of Sciences' *China's Population Health Science and Technology Development Roadmap to 2050* and the Chinese Academy of Engineering's *China's Engineering Technology Medium and Long-term Development Strategy Research*. The Ministry of Health has organized the *Regulations for the Management of Tissue Engineering Tissue Transplantation Therapy (Trial)* and classified stem cell technology into "Third Class Medical Technology" for management. Recently, the relevant departments have further strengthened the management of stem cell therapy. At the same time, the academic community held three "Reproductive Medicine" Xiang Shan Science Conferences in 2005, 2010, and 2015, fully discussing the concept, scope, key breakthrough directions, technical routes, and the key scientific issues that need to be solved for the development of regenerative medicine in China. These have laid a good foundation for the future development of Chinese regenerative medicine and provided relevant guarantees. Academician Xiaobing Fu pointed out that China's tissue repair and regeneration is not only actively in line with the international mainstream direction, but also highlights its own innovative features and unique research ideas. This is the idea of using the results of basic research through the concept of translational medicine, in some key field realizes theoretical and technological breakthroughs, applies relevant results to various fields of tissue repair and regeneration as soon as possible, and hopes to benefit patients with injuries as soon as possible. Of course, the existing problems are also quite prominent. On the one hand, there are not many original things, especially some innovative ideas and research directions that can lead the trend; on the other hand, the efficiency of conversion is still relatively low, and the advantages of the overall research are not very prominent, which need further attention and enhancement. In general, through further research, in the future, China's regenerative medicine may make substantial progress and breakthroughs in stem cell differentiation and simultaneous repair and regeneration of multiple damaged tissues, the construction of large organs in tissue engineering, tissue engineering products from basic research to large-scale application, further establishment and improvement of systems and regulations involving regenerative medicine and the large-scale construction of regenerative medicine transformation bases.

Precision medicine comes from the State of the Union Address of US President Barack Obama in early 2015. Its core philosophy is no strange. It aims to incorporate individual differences into the strategies of disease prevention and treatment. It is based on DNA sequencing and genomics analysis to better tailor the body for more targeted treatment. In general, precision medicine is still mining data, looking for evidence, and targeting the more microscopic genes, trying to use big data to find evidence that has not been discovered in the past, and using it for more targeted treatment of the diseases.

In the field of trauma, how to apply these new concepts and theories to guide the trauma treatment in a scientific, normative, and more rational way is a question that everyone should consider. As mentioned earlier, translational medicine has a good practice in the field of war wounds and tissue repair and regenerative medicine. Many new treatment techniques, methods, and products are derived from the practice of transforming the innovative theory into clinical treatment. At the same time, precise debridement and precise suturing of wounds are actually the practice and application of precision medicine in the field of trauma treatment. At present, although the occurrence of war trauma has certain genetic factors, especially the complications may involve the participation of some genes. In general, precision medicine is a systematic process in the field of wound healing and tissue repair and regeneration. It is not necessary to pin the success rate of the treatment on the genetic changes. It should be noted that traditional trauma treatment often focuses on the treatment of specific parts and specific mechanisms. However, referring to multiple injuries involving multiple organs, multiple mechanisms, and multiple levels of regulation, the treatment, prognosis, and clinical practice are often weak. The important role of translational medicine in the clinical practice of trauma will be reflected in the following aspects:

(a) Prognosis of multiple injuries and critical injuries. Establish a more sensitive and efficient early warning diagnosis technique for high-risk patients and detect early patients with a poor prognosis.
(b) Reevaluate the existing diagnosis and treatment techniques with the system biology orientation and screen a more targeted and specific diagnosis or treatment combination.
(c) Damage repair and regeneration. Combine new materials and new technologies to develop repair techniques for central nervous system damage, large-area tissue defects, and complex wounds.

China's trauma research and practice must actively participate in this wave of translational medicine, which is the only way to gain a place in the fierce competition with international counterparts in future. In the next few decades, research and research institutions that further integrate medical practice with laboratories to produce clinically usable outcomes will emerge in the field of trauma, thereby greatly improving the service level of traumatic care. As the country with the largest population, the number of traumas and critically wounded people also top in the world, we should grasp the trend and create a group of internationally advanced trauma-transforming medical research institutions to make greater contributions to human health.

## References


1. Xiaobing F. Rethinking the development of tissue regeneration and regenerative medicine. Chin J Burns. 2011;27(1):1–2.
2. Xiaobing F, Cheng B, Jinshu T. Chinese war trauma medicine: war wound repair, regeneration and rehabilitation. Zhengzhou: Zhengzhou University Press; 2016.
3. Xiaobing F, Cheng BIAO. Progress and prospects of research on several important areas of wound repair and tissue regeneration. Chin J Traumatol. 2005;21:40–4.

4. Xiaobing F. Organizational regeneration: dreams, hopes and challenges. China Eng Sci. 2009;11(10):122–8.
5. Chunlin H. Development of microsurgery in China. Chin J Trauma Orthop. 2005;7(1):16–8.
6. Guangtai M. Trauma orthopedics and microsurgical repair. Ningxia Med J. 2013;35(8):673.
7. Xiaobing F, Yang S. Regenerative medicine and burn treatment in China. Chin J Burns. 2013;29(2):102–4.
8. Guo E. History and prospects of plastic surgery in China. J Second Mil Med Univers. 2005;26(1):2–3.
9. Xiaobing F, Cheng B, Zhiyong S. Application of growth factors in clinical wound repair: a major progress and prospects in the past decade. Chin J Rep Reconstr Surg. 2004;18(6):508–12.
10. Fu X, Shen Z, Chen Y, et al. Randomised placebo-controlled trial of use of topical recombinant bovine basic fibroblast growth factor for second-degree burns. Lancet. 1998;352(9141):1661–4.
11. Fu X, Li X, Cheng B, et al. Engineered growth factors and cutaneous wound healing: success and possible questions in the past 10 years. Wound Repair Regen. 2005;13(2):122–30.
12. Xiaobing F, Zhiyong S. New dressing and wound repair. Chin J Traumatol. 1998;14(4):247–9.
13. Sheng ZY, Fu XB, Cai S, et al. Regeneration of functional sweat gland-like structures by transplanted differentiated bone marrow mesenchymal stem cells. Wound Rep Reg. 2009;17(3):427–35.
14. Fu XB, Han B, Cai S, et al. Migration of bone marrow-derived mesenchymal stem cells induced by TNF-α and its possible role in wound healing. Wound Rep Reg. 2009;17(2):185–91.
15. Fu XB, Li HH. Mesenchymal stem cells and skin regeneration: possibility and questions. Cell Tissue Res. 2009;335:317–21.
16. Xiaobing F, Wang Z, Wu Z. Regenerative medicine: basic and clinical research. Beijing: People's Medical Publishing House; 2013.
17. Xiaobing F, Wang Z, Wu Z. Regenerative medicine: from basic to clinical research. Shanghai: Shanghai Science and Technology Press; 2008.
18. Xiaobing F, Wang Z, Wu Z. Regenerative medicine: transformation and application. Beijing: People's Medical Publishing House; 2016.
19. Wang Z. Review and prospect of surgery development. J China Med Univers. 2013;42(4):289–92.
20. Wang Z. Surgery and field surgery. Beijing: People's Military Medical Press; 2007. p. 3.
21. Xiaobing F. Bacterial biofilm formation and chronic refractory wounds occur. J Traumatic Surg. 2008;10(5):416–7.

# Cellular Basis for Tissue Regeneration: Cellular Dedifferentiation

# 2

Hua Qin, Andong Zhao, Xiaobing Fu, and Cuiping Zhang

## 2.1 The Prevalence of Cellular Dedifferentiation and the Significance of Tissue Repair and Regeneration

### 2.1.1 Tissue Regeneration: From Lower Animals to Mammals and Cellular Dedifferentiation

Tissue repair and regeneration are ubiquitous phenomena and are required for the long-term survival of animals in the natural environment. However, the ability of tissue repair and regeneration in different animals varies widely. Some lower invertebrates (such as polyps and worms) can regenerate a new individual. Lower vertebrate animals such as newt can regenerate limbs, retina, lens, spinal cord and tail. Zebrafish can regenerate heart and fins [1, 2]. Higher vertebrates, such as mammals, cannot completely regenerate tissues and organs, and can only undergo simple healing and fibrotic repair [1, 2].

The differences in the regenerative ability of different animals are related to the cellular mechanisms of regeneration. There are two main types of regeneration: morphallaxis and epimorphosis [2]. Morphallaxis relies on the differentiation of existing stem cells into the desired cells in the tissue, which does not require cell division and proliferation. Epimorphosis relies on dedifferentiation by mature cells, which divide, proliferate, and re-differentiate, eventually replacing the cells that have been damaged. Morphallaxis of the polyps and worms are mainly due to the large number of totipotent or pluripotent stem cells in their bodies [2]. The regeneration of newt and zebrafish rely on the dedifferentiation of mature cells [1]. In mammalian adults the number of stem cells remaining in various tissues and organs is extremely small, and therefore repair and regeneration after injury cannot be spontaneously achieved.

In mammals, some mature cells are found to dedifferentiate to participate in tissue repair and regeneration. After peripheral nerve injury, Schwann cells dedifferentiate, proliferate, migrate, and re-differentiate into new Schwann cells, which support the regeneration of peripheral axons [3]. When the kidney suffers from acute injury, the proximal tubular epithelial cells dedifferentiate, proliferate and migrate to the injured site, and participate in the repair of the damaged renal tubules [4]. Unfortunately, mature cells in most tissues and organs of mammals cannot spontaneously dedifferentiate into proliferative stem cells after an injury. Therefore, inducing dedifferentiation of mature cells is an important way to promote tissue repair and regeneration in mammals.

This section outlines the prevalence of cellular dedifferentiation after injury and its role and significance in the repair and regeneration of various tissues and organs.

### 2.1.2 The Definition of Cell Dedifferentiation

Mature cells have their own morphology, function, and physiological characteristics. In general, mature cells are very stable and cannot divide and proliferate. Dedifferentiation refers to a state in which mature cells return to an undifferentiated or immature state. In terms of morphology, the specific morphology of the original cells is lost, the cells become smaller, and the proportion of nucleus to plasma increases. In terms of gene expression, the expression of differentiation-related genes decreases and gene expression related embryonic development rises. In terms of cell cycle, cells re-enter the cell cycle, undergoing division and proliferation.

The result is that the potential of proliferation and differentiation is regained by dedifferentiation.

H. Qin · A. Zhao · X. Fu (✉) · C. Zhang
The Chinese People's Liberation Army General Hospital,
Beijing, China



X. Fu (ed.), *Regenerative Medicine in China*, https://doi.org/10.1007/978-981-16-1182-7_2

### 2.1.3 Epidermal Cell Dedifferentiation and Skin Regeneration

The skin is the largest organ in the body. Epidermal stem cells exist in the basal layer of the epidermis. Under normal conditions, epidermal stem cell proliferate and differentiate to keratinocytes, maintaining the dynamic balance of the epidermis. When the skin is severely wounded, a large number of epidermal stem cells are destroyed and are insufficient in number to rebuild new skin. Therefore, obtaining epidermal stem cells is the key to skin regeneration. In 2001, Xiaobing Fu et al. were the first to report the phenomenon of epidermal cell dedifferentiation in Lancet [5]. The patient's leg wound ulcer was treated with recombinant human epidermal growth factor (rhEGF), and tissue biopsy was performed for immunohistochemistry. The authors found that β1-integrin and CK19, the markers of epidermal stem cells, were detected in the spinous and granular layers of the new epidermis. However, in normal skin, the cells in the spinous and granular layers are already differentiated, and these two layers do not express β1-integrin and CK19. This study demonstrates that differentiated epidermal cells dedifferentiate to form new epidermal stem cells under skin injury conditions. Mannik et al. provided strong evidences to confirm the dedifferentiation of epidermal cells [6]. They used the Cre/lox tracing technique to track differentiated epidermal cells after transplantation onto the fascia of mice. In the early stages of transplantation, they found that epidermal cells dedifferentiated. The dedifferentiated epidermal cells subsequently re-differentiate to form epidermis, hair follicles, and sebaceous glands. Therefore, promoting the dedifferentiation of epidermal cells is an important way to improve skin regeneration.

### 2.1.4 Renal Cell Dedifferentiation and Kidney Regeneration

Acute kidney injury (AKI) is a clinical syndrome of acute renal secretion loss. The disease is often caused by ischemic or toxic irritation, such as vasoconstrictor drugs, contrast agents, hypotension caused by sepsis, surgery, or traumatic bleeding [7]. In these cases, local hypoxia and massive metabolite accumulation lead to damage of renal proximal tubular epithelial cells.

The kidneys of mammals such as humans and mice can return to normal function after mild ischemic or toxic damage. Cell lineage tracing techniques reveal that dedifferentiation of surviving proximal tubular epithelial cells is a major source of regenerating tubular epithelial cells [4, 8]. Surviving tubular epithelial cells dedifferentiate under the stimulation of injury and become proliferative and undifferentiated cells (Fig. 2.1). Normal tubular epithelial cells are columnar or elliptical with rich adhesive connections. After dedifferentiation, the cells lose their apical–basal polarity, become flat and long, and lack tight junctions between cells. At the gene expression level, dedifferentiated tubular epithelial cells re-express the renal mesenchymal cell marker vimentin, while vimentin is not expressed in normal renal tubular epithelial cells [9]. The neural cell adhesion molecule (NCAM) expressed by the renal mesenchymal cells is also re-expressed after injury [10]. After kidney injury, the embryonic transcription factor Pax2 is re-expressed in renal tubular epithelial cells [11]. In addition, dedifferentiated tubular epithelial cells also express undifferentiated markers such as Kim1, Annexin A3, CD44, CD133, and CD24 [4]. After dedifferentiation, renal tubular epithelial cell migration ability is enhanced. The cell proliferation ability is also enhanced, and the expression of proliferation markers PCNA and Ki67

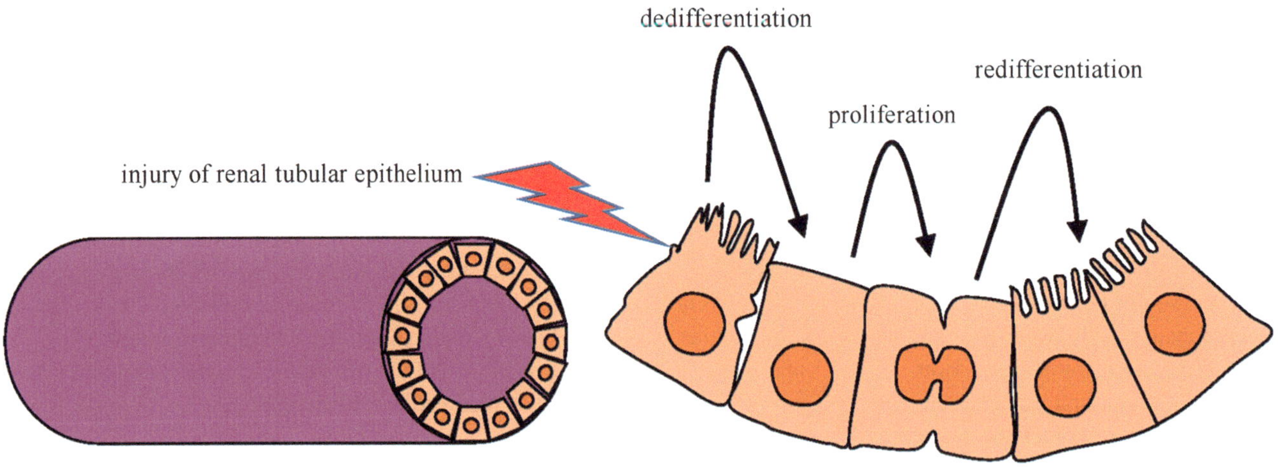


**Fig. 2.1** Dedifferentiation of renal tubular epithelial cells

are detected [11]. Dedifferentiated renal tubular epithelial cells migrate to the necrotic or apoptotic area, and then differentiate into functional tubular epithelial cells. Therefore, enhancing the dedifferentiation of renal tubular epithelial cells will benefit patients with acute kidney injury.

### 2.1.5 Cardiomyocyte Dedifferentiation and Heart Regeneration

Mammalian heart regeneration is weak, and the infarcted myocardium is basically not regenerated. However, the zebrafish perfectly regenerates the heart. When the ventricle of the zebrafish heart is removed by 20%, the remaining cardiomyocytes near the wound re-grow the lost cardiomyocytes [12]. The zebrafish heart is completely regenerated 60 days after injury (Fig. 2.2). Studies have found that the strong regenerative capacity of the zebrafish heart is attributed to the dedifferentiation of cardiomyocytes [13]. Normal zebrafish cardiomyocytes have well-ordered sarcomere and clear Z-line. After the cardiac injury, the cardiomyocytes near the injury are separated from each other, the sarcomere is dissociated, the Z-line is missing, and the morphology of altered cardiomyocytes is similar to that of the embryonic period. Consistent with this, sarcomere-associated gene expression is downregulated [13]. It is further found that these dedifferentiated cells become more proliferative and expressed proliferation markers such as phosphorylated H3 and PCNA [14]. At the same time, dedifferentiated cardiomyocytes re-express the genes such as Gata4 that is involved in embryonic cardiac development [14]. The expression of the Hand2 gene in embryonic heart is also upregulated, which is beneficial to the proliferative response of dedifferentiated cardiomyocytes [15]. Cre/lox lineage tracing techniques show that proliferative cardiomyocytes are derived from already differentiated cardiomyocytes [13]. These results indicate that differentiated cardiomyocytes undergo dedifferentiation and regain proliferation and differentiation potential, which is the cellular basis for zebrafish heart regeneration.

Adult mammals lose their ability to regenerate their heart, but neonatal mice can regenerate their heart [16]. However, this ability to regenerate is lost 1 week after birth. The study found that the gene Gata4 related to cardiac development, is highly expressed on day 1 after birth, but decreased sharply on the 7th day after birth, corresponding to the period of cardiac regeneration ability lost. Introduction of Gata4 by adenovirus significantly improved the regenerative capacity of the mice heart 7 days after birth [17]. Although mammalian adult cardiomyocytes do not spontaneously initiate dedifferentiation after heart injury, it is found that a very small number of cardiomyocytes re-enter the cell cycle and proliferate under normal physiological or injured conditions [18, 19]. Recently, epicardial cells have been found to contain Follistatin-like 1 (Fstl1) protein that promotes heart regeneration [20]. The human Fstl1 protein is applied to the myocardial infarction by epicardial patch, which can stimulate the survived cells around the infarction to dedifferentiation, ultimately improving heart regeneration. However, this protein is not expressed after myocardial infarction injury, maybe it is an important cause of mammalian loss of myocardial regeneration. Therefore, enhancing dedifferentiation of mammalian cardiomyocytes may improve the ability of heart regeneration.

### 2.1.6 Visual Cell Dedifferentiation and Retinal Regeneration

Vision is the most important sensory system. The retina is the most important organ for inputting visual information, and it is also the most vulnerable to trauma and diseases such as glaucoma, diabetic retinopathy, and macular degeneration. Death of retinal neurons will severely impair vision and even lead to total blindness.

Mammalian retinas lack the ability to regenerate after injury, but lower animals, such as zebrafish, amphibians, and reptiles, can completely regenerate retinal neurons and restore vision after retinal damage.

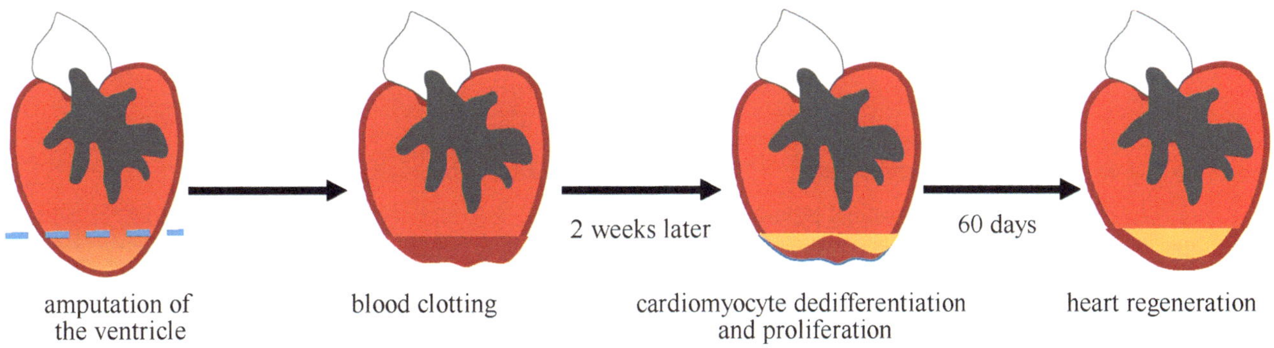


**Fig. 2.2** Zebrafish heart regeneration and cardiomyocyte dedifferentiation

The retina of the newt can completely regenerate a new retina after surgical removal, which relies mainly on dedifferentiation of retinal pigmented epithelial cells (RPEC) [21]. When the entire retina is removed, RPEC are separated from each other, re-synthesizing DNA and entering the cell cycle. Reentry of RPEC into the cell cycle is associated with activation of the MEK-ERK pathway after injury [22]. Then, RPEC lose the pigment and begin to express retinal progenitor cell markers. Dedifferentiated RPEC acquire the potential for proliferation and differentiation, then divide along the Bruch membrane and differentiate to form new epithelial cells, including neural retinal progenitor cells and RPEC [23, 24]. The outer cells stop dividing, synthesize pigments, reconstruct the retinal pigment epithelial layer, and the inner cells continue to proliferate and differentiate into various retinal neuronal cells, and finally regenerate the functional retina (Fig. 2.3).

The retina of the zebrafish can also regenerate after injury, mainly relying on dedifferentiation of retinal Müller cells. After surgical removal, neuronal toxic damage, genetic or photodamage, Müller cells can dedifferentiate, proliferate and re-differentiate, regenerating various neurons in the retina. During dedifferentiation, firstly Müller cells decrease expression of glial cell markers and begin to express retinal progenitor cell markers. The Müller cell-specific gene Rlbp1a decreases sharply within 4 h after acute photodamage, completely disappears 1 day after injury, and the glial cell marker GFAP expression is downregulated [25]. In contrast, after 1 h of thermal injury or photodamage, Müller cells begin to express the neural stem cell marker Blbn and the pluripotent retinal progenitor cell marker Rx1 [26, 27], and Müller cells also re-express the retinal progenitor markers Pax6 and Vsx2 [28]. Six3 is a transcription factor which is responsible for the development of vertebrate eyes. After acute photodamage, Müller cells express Six3b and it is found that the expression of Six3b is beneficial to the proliferation of progenitor cells derived from Müller cells [29]. Olig2 is expressed in progenitor cells derived from Müller cells after photodamage [30]. The expression of Olig2 controls the differentiation of retinal progenitor cells into photoreceptor cells and amacrine neurons. Dedifferentiated Müller cells have significant pluripotency and can differentiate into various retinal nerve cells (Fig. 2.4).

Similar to zebrafish, retinal regeneration in neonatal chicken also relies on dedifferentiation of Müller cells. In the N-Methyl-D-aspartate (NMDA)-induced retinal damage model, chicken retinal Müller cells re-enter the cell cycle and proliferate, at the same time, express embryonic retinal progenitor markers Gash-1, Pax6, and Vsx2 [31]. Dedifferentiation-derived retinal progenitor cells migrate to the inner and outer nucleus of the retina, some differentiate into retinal neurons.

The dedifferentiation ability of mammalian retinal Müller cells is even weaker. Generally, after retinal injury, Müller cells can only be activated to form glial scars. The loss of retinal regeneration in mice has recently been found to be associated with the inability of Pax6-positive Müller cells to re-enter cell cycle and proliferate after photoreceptor cell injury [32]. However, when cultured in vitro, after treatment with bFGF, Müller cells are able to form neurospheres and express neural stem cell markers Sox2, Nestin, and Musashi, and also express retinal progenitor markers Pax6 and Rx1 [33].In a mouse or rat model treated with NMDA in vivo, the retina is treated with bFGF or retinoic acid, Müller cells can proliferate and express the progenitor cell marker Pax6, and a small number of dedifferentiated progenitor cells can re-differentiate into bipolar cells, rod-shaped visual receptor cells or amacrine cells [34, 35]. This demonstrates that mam-

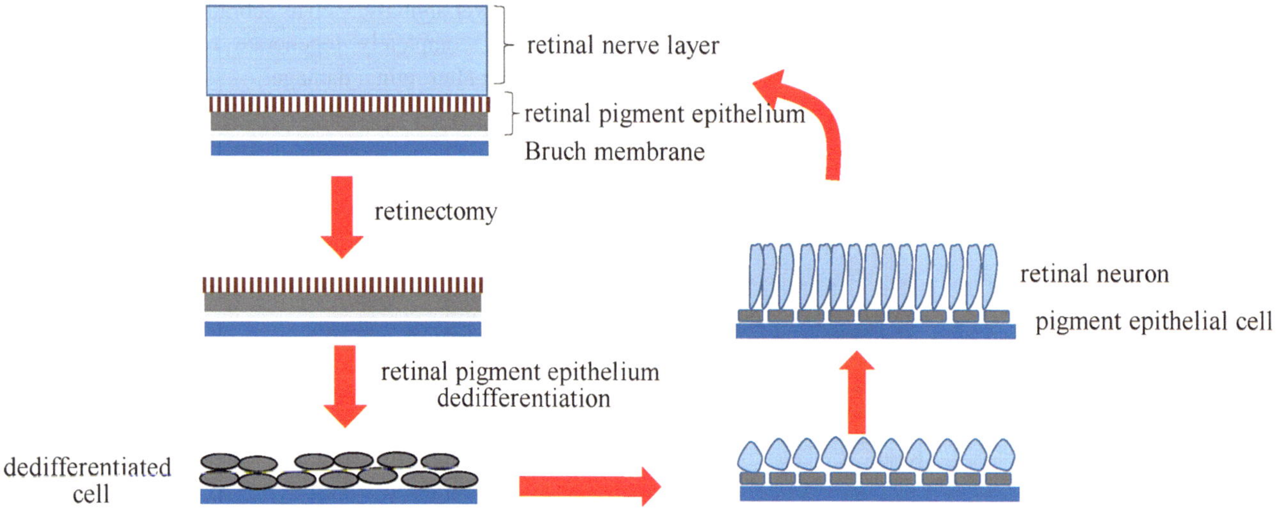


**Fig. 2.3** Newt retinal regeneration and dedifferentiation of retinal pigment epithelial cells

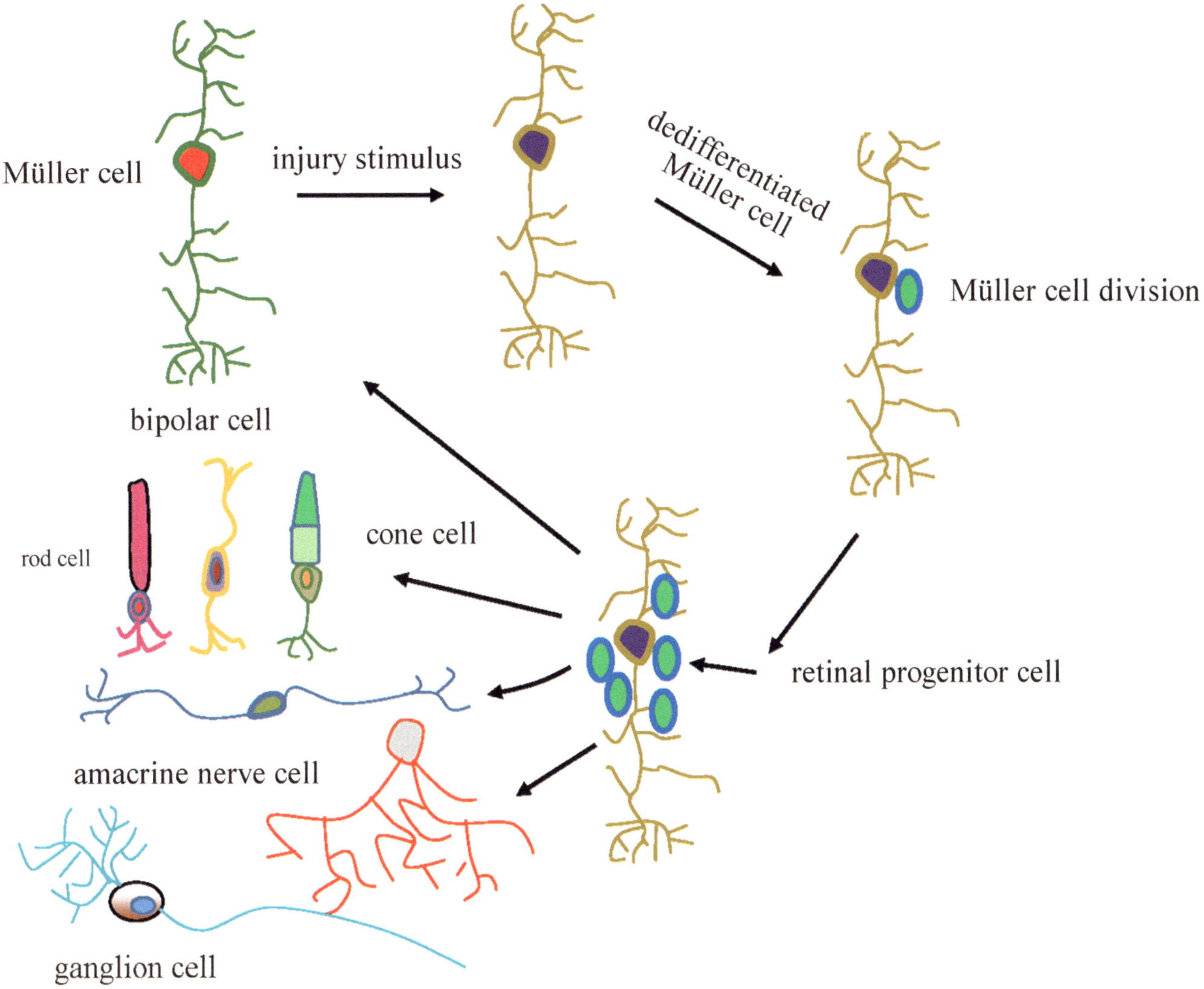


**Fig. 2.4** Dedifferentiation of zebrafish, neonatal chicken and mouse Müller cells involved in retinal regeneration

malian Müller cells still retain low levels of dedifferentiation. In vitro, glutamate and alpha-aminoadipate stimulate Müller cells to dedifferentiate into retinal progenitor cells [36]. Subretinal injection of glutamate and alpha- aminoadipate can also induce Müller cells to become retinal progenitor cells in vivo. Similarly, human Müller cells can also dedifferentiate into cells expressing neural stem cell markers and retinal progenitor cell markers after being treated with bFGF or retinoic acid in vitro [37]. In vitro, transfection of the transcription factor Ascl1 or Lin28b into mouse or rat Müller cells also induces dedifferentiation of Müller cells into retinal progenitor cells [38, 39]. In vivo, transfection of the Ascl1 into mouse Müller cells can induce retinal regeneration after retinal damage [40]. Therefore, promoting dedifferentiation of Müller cells will likely improve mammalian retinal regeneration.

### 2.1.7 Dedifferentiation of Bone Cells and Muscle Cells and Musculoskeletal Regeneration

Mammal limbs cannot be regenerated after amputation, but lower animals such as zebrafish and newt can completely regenerate limbs. The important components of the limb are bones and muscles. The repair of mouse bones mainly depends on the differentiation of bone marrow mesenchymal stem cells into osteoblasts, and bone healing can only be achieved within a certain range of damage. However, the bone components of the zebrafish fins can be completely regenerated, mainly relying on osteoblast dedifferentiation (Fig. 2.5). When the fins are cut off, the mature osteoblasts in the proximal end change in morphology and express cell proliferation markers, suggesting that osteoblasts dedifferen-

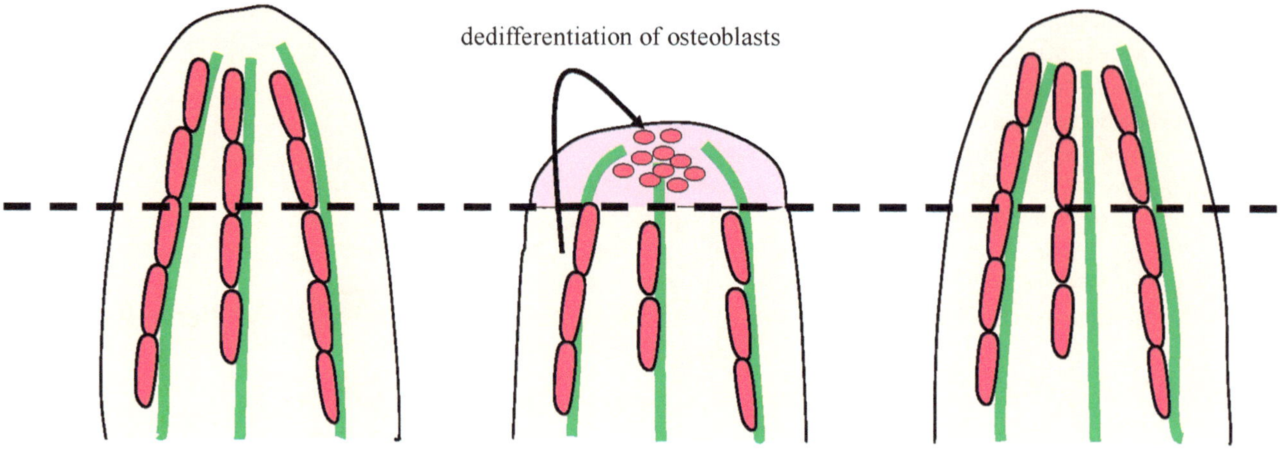


**Fig. 2.5** Regeneration of zebrafish fins and dedifferentiation of osteoblasts

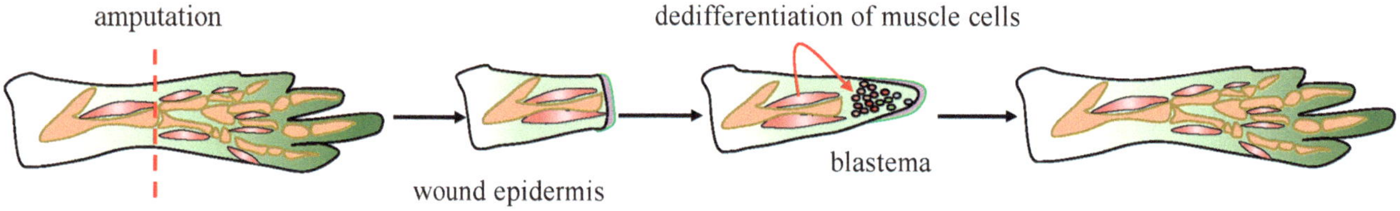


**Fig. 2.6** Newt limb regeneration and muscle dedifferentiation

tiate. Knof et al. use lineage tracing techniques to label mature osteoblasts and find that when fins are amputated, the mature osteoblasts downregulate markers associated with osteoblast differentiation such as osteocalcin and the osteoblast-specific transcription factor Osterix, and upregulate precursor osteoblast markers such as Runx2b and Tenascin, demonstrating that osteoblasts undergo dedifferentiation after amputation of fins and become osteoblast progenitors [41]. Dedifferentiated osteoblasts participate in the formation of the blastema of the fin, and then differentiate into osteoblasts, regenerate new bone spurs [42]. These suggest that osteoblast dedifferentiation is the major cellular mechanism for the regeneration of the bone components of zebrafish fins.

During the regeneration of adult newt limbs, the regeneration of muscle components also depends on muscle cell dedifferentiation (Fig. 2.6). Muscle cell dedifferentiation participates in muscle regeneration during the regeneration of adult newt. In vivo fluorescent labeling of individual muscle fibers showed that multinucleated muscle fibers near the amputated plane of the limb dedifferentiated to form monocytes [43]. More convincing evidence comes from experiments by Sandoval Guzman et al. Using Cre/lox tracing technology, they found that multinucleated myofibers break into proliferating Pax7 (a marker of muscle stem cells) negative monocytes, and that these cells are involved in the blastema formation [44]. These dedifferentiated sources of muscle cells then proliferate and differentiate into new muscle fibers, regenerating the muscle parts of the limbs. Interestingly, in different developmental stages, the regeneration of newt limb muscles depends on different ways [45]. In the larval stage of the newt, the muscle regeneration depends on the proliferation and differentiation of muscle stem cells (satellite cells); when the newt is deformed, muscle regeneration depends on dedifferentiation of muscle cells. This may be due to the presence of sufficient muscle stem cells in the body at the larval period. With development, muscle stem cells gradually decrease, and adult newt do not rely on muscle stem cells, instead rely on muscle dedifferentiation.

### 2.1.8 Schwann Cell Dedifferentiation and Peripheral Nerve Regeneration

Peripheral nerve damage often results in partial or total loss of motor, sensory, and autonomic function. Despite this, mammalian peripheral nerves have a degree of regenerative capacity after injury. When the peripheral nerve is damaged, the axons can be slowly regenerated, generally 1–3 mm per day [46]. In patients with brachial plexus injury, damaged neurons must grow more than 1 m of axons to innervate the muscles and sensory organs of the hand, which can take several years [47].

After peripheral nerve injury, the axons at the distal end of the injury dissociated from the proximal neuron, and

Wallerian degeneration occurred. Schwann cells and macrophages are activated to dissolve and clear distal axons and myelin debris, creating a microenvironment that facilitates nerve regeneration [48]. Activation of Schwann cells plays an important role in peripheral nerve regeneration. As the distal axon dissociates, the nearby Schwann cells lose contact with the axons, and the Schwann cells dedifferentiate and lose the myelinating properties, becoming an undifferentiated repairing cell (Fig. 2.7). Dedifferentiated Schwann cells can phagocyte myelin and myelin-associated glycoproteins, secreting cytokines to attract macrophages to function in the nerve stump. Dedifferentiated Schwann cells provide scaffolding and nutritional support for the new axons. When the axon regeneration is over, the Schwann cells contact with the new axons again, encapsulating the new axons to form the myelin sheath, and restoring the electrophysiological conduction of the axons.

During the dedifferentiation of Schwann cells, a series of changes take place in morphology, phenotype, and function. First, the normal morphology of the Schwann cells is lost. At the same time, the characteristic markers of myelinated Schwann cells such as myelin proteins P0, MBP, and Periaxin are downregulated [49]. Dedifferentiated Schwann cells can proliferate and secrete a variety of neurotrophic factors and neurotropic factors [50]. For example, the secreted neurotrophic factors NGF, BDNF, NT-4, GDNF, and IGF-1 promote axonal regeneration; neurotropic factors such as Fibronectin, Laminin, and Tenascin provide matrix support for axonal elongation.

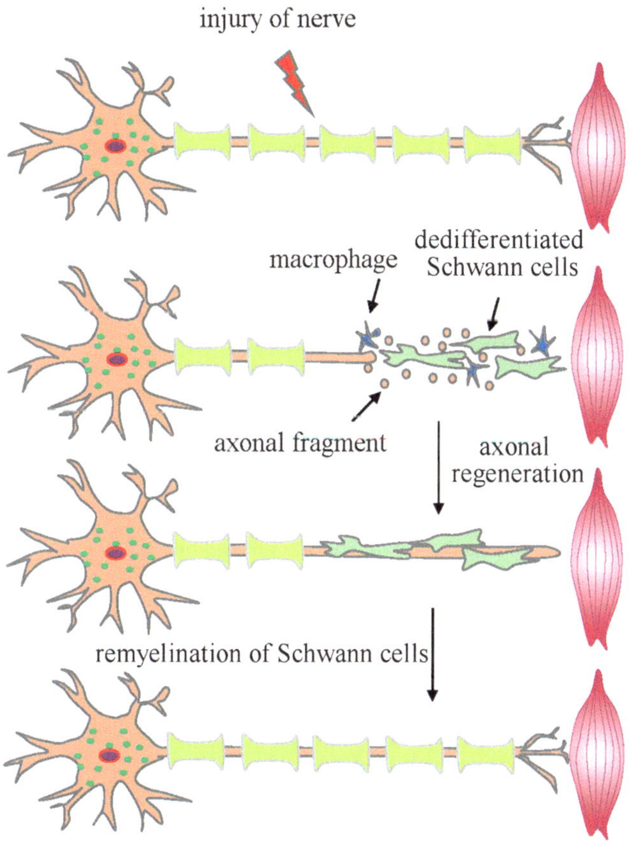


**Fig. 2.7** Schwann cell dedifferentiation and peripheral nerve regeneration

## 2.1.9 Dedifferentiation or Reprogramming of Somatic Cells into Pluripotent Stem Cells

In 2006, Japanese scientists induced the dedifferentiation of fibroblasts in the skin into embryonic stem cell-like cells, namely induced pluripotent stem cells (iPSCs) [51]. The study introduced four pluripotency-related transcription factors into the fibroblasts through the virus, activating the genetic program of pluripotent stem cells. This process of dedifferentiation to the pluripotent stem cell state is also known as somatic cell reprogramming. Inspired by this research, other somatic cells such as epidermal cells, epithelial cells, mesenchymal stem cells, liver cells, and gastric cells can all be completely dedifferentiated into iPSCs [52]. In addition, non-gene integration methods such as microRNAs, episomal vectors, recombinant proteins, and small molecule compounds can be used to induce iPSCs [53] (Fig. 2.8). iPSCs avoid the ethical issues faced by embryonic stem cells. Currently, iPSCs have been widely used in medical research and clinical treatment, and have rapidly promoted the development of regenerative medicine.

## 2.1.10 Perspectives

Adults have very few residual stem cells in various tissues and organs, which are insufficient to compensate for the large number of cell loss caused by injury, resulting in the loss of normal function of tissues and organs. Replenishing stem cells is the key to tissue regeneration. Dedifferentiation of differentiated cells that have survived in the damaged site into stem cells is the best source of stem cells, being more compatible with local tissues. Lower animals have significant regenerative capacity due to their strong dedifferentiation potential. Mammalian cells have weak dedifferentiation potential and cannot compensate for cell damage caused by injury. Therefore, how to enhance the dedifferentiation potential of local viable cells in the injured environment is of great significance for the in situ regeneration of tissues. At present, some tissue cells can induce dedifferentiation by biological, physical or chemical stimulation in vitro. How to induce dedifferentiation of mature somatic cells in vivo is challenging in regenerative medicine research. Studies have been conducted to induce in vivo dedifferentiation by transgene, growth factors, or small molecule compounds.

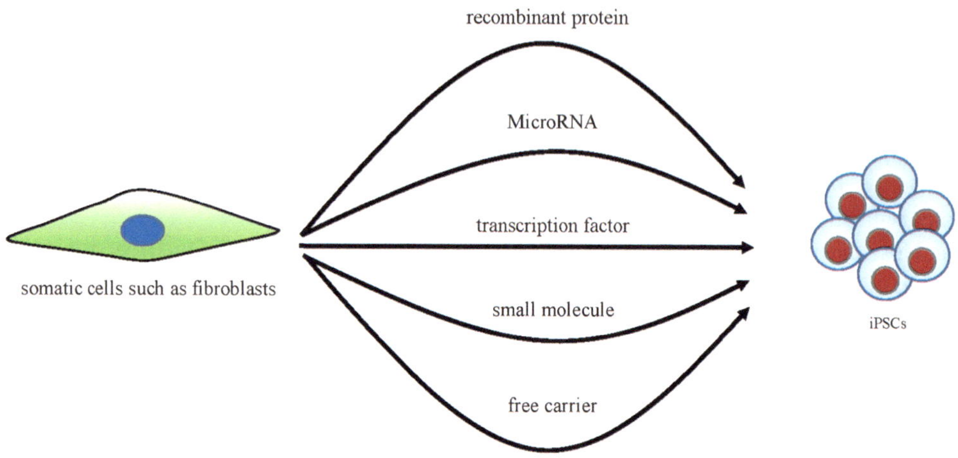


**Fig. 2.8** Method of reprogramming somatic cells to induced pluripotent stem cells (iPSCs)

In the regenerative animal model, a variety of tissue cells have the potential to dedifferentiate. Studying their dedifferentiation mechanisms will have important insights for inducing dedifferentiation of mammalian cells. We believe that in the future, by promoting dedifferentiation, it will help to improve the mammalian regeneration.

## 2.2 Dedifferentiation of Epidermal Cells and Sweat Gland Regeneration

In 2001, during the research of tissue repair and regeneration, we accidentally discovered an important biological phenomenon that skin cells can be reversed into stem cells under the stimulation of certain factors during wound healing [54], which is academically called dedifferentiation and finally confirmed by hard work. On this basis, with the help of the basic biological law of dedifferentiation, we have transformed the human bone marrow mesenchymal stem cells (BM-MSCs) into sweat gland cells for the first time in the world, and successfully regenerated sweat glands in human bodies. After nearly 10 years of follow-up of typical cases, we proved that local wounds have stable and sustained sweating function, and no adverse reactions are observed, thus establishing an innovative method for sweat gland regeneration and providing important innovation theories and key technologies for solving the post-treatment problems of patients with severe trauma and burns.

### 2.2.1 A Huge Controversy Brought by an Accidental Discovery

In 2000, we cooperated with related gene pharmaceutical companies to study the mechanism of skin wound healing promoted by growth factors. When observing some tissue sections by microscope stained with the markers of epidermal stem cells, we found that the positive cells appeared in areas where epidermal stem cells should not appear. At that time, we felt that this phenomenon was difficult to explain with conventional knowledge, because the classical view was that epidermal stem cells should be located in the basal layer of the epidermis. But our result showed that the positive cell cluster appeared in the prickle cell layer above the basal layer of the epidermis, so we called it "stem cell island."

In 2001, the results of the study titled "Dedifferentiation of epidermal cells to stem cells in vivo" were published in Lancet (2001, 358: 1067–1068), the internationally renowned medical journal. After that, it caused a relatively large response at home and abroad. About 5% of the experts considered it to be a very important discovery, and suggested further researches. About 85% of scholars disagreed with this discovery and the existence of this phenomenon. The common question at that time was "How can old cells become younger?" Even about 10% of people thought that it was pseudoscience and opposed it.

### 2.2.2 Giving a Correct Explanation to the Academic World through Hardship

On the basis of the success in the wound model of the nude mice, we have demonstrated the prevalence of this dedifferentiation phenomenon in animal skin and human skin respectively, and also reproduced it in vitro by growth factors and UV stimulation at the cell level. At the same time, we also have basically cleared up the three aspect questions.

First, what signaling pathway induces the dedifferentiation of these cells into stem cells? Through literature research, we found that Wnt [55] and ERK pathways play an important regulatory role in the dedifferentiation of mature cells and maintenance of skin stem cells. It was found that repairing factors in the wound microenvironment can promote the expression of Wnt-1 and Wnt-7α, thereby increasing intranuclear transfer and deposition of β-catenin, then promoting transcription and expression of its target genes Cyclin D1 and c-Myc. We used transgenic technology to obtain epidermal cell lines with high expression of Cyclin D1. After 5 days of culture in vitro, the morphology, phenotype and functional properties of most cells were similar to those of epidermal stem cells. In addition, we also detected the activation of the ERK signaling pathway. This signaling pathway cooperates with Wnt/β-catenin to regulate the dedifferentiation process of the epidermal cells.

The second is whether these epidermal stem cells derived from dedifferentiation have the same or similar biological characteristics of normal epidermal stem cells. Through a series of analysis of cell morphology, structure and phenotypic characteristics, we have found that the morphological characteristics, ultrastructural and phenotypic characteristics of the dedifferentiated epidermal stem cells are consistent with those of normal epidermal stem cells [56].

The third is whether these epidermal stem cells derived from dedifferentiation have the same biological functions as normal epidermal stem cells. Under the condition of in vitro culture, these dedifferentiated cells have a high colony-forming efficiency and long-term proliferative potential. Under the condition of three-dimensional culture, these cells can form a three-dimensional skin that is similar in structure to that constructed by normal epidermal stem cells. Thus, it is confirmed that these dedifferentiated epidermal stem cells can be used as seed cells for skin tissue engineering as well as normal epidermal stem cells to form the relevant skin structure.

In 2006, Cell, the internationally renowned magazine, reported that skin cells were reprogrammed into pluripotent stem cells (iPS) by transfecting Oct4, Sox2, Klf4, and c-Myc [51], which provided direct evidences for the dedifferentiation of epidermal cells into epidermal stem cells by growth factors. Especially, the special review written by Professor T. M. Beardsley, editor of BioScience in 2007, highly appraised our research on dedifferentiation of epidermal cells.

### 2.2.3 The Original Discovery of Cellular Dedifferentiation Is Used to Guide the Clinical Research on Sweat Gland Regeneration

We know that after several generations of burn medical experts in China, the current success rate of burn treatment in China has reached more than 98%, but unfortunately many skin wounds of rescued patients are repaired by scar without skin attachments, especially sweat glands. Due to the lack of sweat glands, the living and working of many rescued patients are seriously affected and it is difficult to return to society. Based on clinical problems, we have carried out a new round of research on transformation application from basic theory discovery to sweat gland regeneration and achieved the goal of innovation and transformation in 10 steps.

In the first step, we found out the process and regularity of sweat gland development before and after human birth from the perspective of development and summarized the causes of difficulty in regeneration of sweat glands after severe burns in clinical practice. From the point of embryogenesis, the sweat glands are formed by the germinal cells, epidermal stem cells, in the epidermis derived from the ectoderm, which grow into the mesenchyme by developing a cylindrical cell cord. The study finds that human sweat glands appear about 12 weeks, peak around 24 weeks, and end around 36 weeks of embryo. After the scar healing, the non-perspiration function of the wound does not mean that there is no sweat gland tissue in the scar. Studies have shown that in the scar tissue, the presence of CK19 and CK14 positive cells can be detected, the CK19 expression is mainly located at the junction of the deep dermis and the normal subcutaneous tissue at the base of the scar, and the CK14 positive cells are scattered in the scar tissue, showing concentric circles. We need to remove scars, plant sweat gland cells or transplant tissue-engineered skin containing sweat gland cells to solve the sweating problem of severely burned patients. However, the patient's own sweat gland cells have been severely damaged, so it is necessary to promote sweat gland regeneration by exogenous methods, especially by the induced differentiation of stem cells.

In the second step, we confirmed the feasibility of BM-MSCs as seed cells for regeneration of sweat glands. Since epidermal stem cells and sweat glands have a common origin in auxology, it is possible to induce epidermal stem cells to differentiate into sweat gland cells and regenerate sweat glands. However, the key to the problem is that when a large area of severe burns occurs, the epidermis of the patient is destroyed, and the source of autologous mature epidermal cells or epidermal stem cells is lacking. BM-MSCs, under appropriate conditions, can not only differentiate into mesenchymal tissue cells homologous to mesoderm, but also break through the boundaries of germ layers and differentiate into ectodermal tissue. Therefore, we consider the use of BM-MSCs (or umbilical cord mesenchymal stem cells) as seed cells for the regeneration of sweat glands. Our previous research also found that under severe trauma and burn conditions, the mesenchymal stem cells in circulating blood have actually participated in the repair process of the wound. Recently, we have been able to directly induce fibroblasts into sweat gland cells, which provides a new source of seed cells for sweat gland regeneration and has great clinical application value.

In the third step, we confirmed the feasibility of inducing the BM-MSCs into sweat gland cells by a new generation of in vitro co-culture system [57] and established key induction differentiation techniques. By exploration, we initially established a direct co-culture system of heat shock sweat gland cells and mesenchymal stem cells. This system can successfully induce mesenchymal stem cells into sweat gland-like cells, but the cells obtained from the induction system are heterogeneous, and may contain some residual sweat gland cells. In order to solve this problem, we established an indirect co-culture system of heat shock sweat gland cells and mesenchymal stem cells. This method adopts the transwell culture model. The heat shock sweat gland cells are in the lower chamber, and the mesenchymal stem cells are in the upper chamber, and the active components in the culture system can pass freely, thus effectively solving the problem of heterogeneous cells. With the deepening of research and continuous improvement of induction conditions, we have successfully established a new generation of induction system of sweat gland regeneration, which is composed of the indirect co-culture induction system adding a series of sweat gland lineage development-specific proteins or factors (e.g., EDA-A1 and EGF). This new system effectively improves the trans-differentiation efficiency of mesenchymal stem cells into sweat gland-like cells. Phenotypic analysis showed that 40–60% of the induced cells expressed CEA, CK7, CK8, and CK19, the markers of original sweat gland cells.

In the fourth step, we confirmed the safety and effectiveness of BM-MSC transdifferentiation into sweat gland-like cells under in vitro co-culture conditions. The safety of cell co-culture is a concern for everyone and a prerequisite for regenerating sweat glands. It is also a question that must be answered. In the experiments, we co-cultured sweat gland cells with cells from different germ layers, observed changes in cell behaviors and related indicators, and focused on changes in apoptotic rate and karyotype. Finally, we demonstrated that there is no abnormal change in sweat gland-like cells under co culture conditions.

In the fifth step, we further confirmed that the sweat gland-like cells transdifferentiated from BM-MSCs have similar electrophysiological properties with sweat gland cells. The electrophysiological index is another indicator for evaluating whether sweat gland-like cells have the characteristics of sweat gland cells. By patch-clamp technique, we confirmed that the induced MSCs have unique ion channels (CFTR Cl- channels and Amiloride-sensitive Na+ channels) and the potential of sweat gland cells, whereas non-induced MSCs do not have this characteristic potential, which further confirmed that the induced MSCs are transformed into sweat gland cells from the electrophysiological point of view.

In the sixth step, we initially identified the signaling pathways that may be involved in the transdifferentiation of BM-MSCs into sweat gland-like cells. In the study on transdifferentiation, we first discovered the role of ERK signaling pathway. During the transdifferentiation of MSCs into sweat gland-like cells, EGF can significantly increase the transdifferentiation rate and the ERK pathway blocker PD98059 can partially block the transdifferentiation of MSCs, which means that there may be other regulatory pathways beside the ERK pathway during this process. Our follow-up studies have also found that the EDA-A1/ EDAR signaling pathway is also involved in the transdifferentiation process of sweat gland regeneration. In the process of transdifferentiation of stem cells into sweat gland-like cells, we found that high expression of EDA-A1 could successfully induce transdifferentiation of BM-MSCs into sweat gland-like cells, and the increase of EDA-A1 and EDAR expression was also observed during the process of UC-MSC transdifferentiation into sweat gland-like cells. In addition, we found that NF-B is the downstream pathway of EDA/EDAR to transfer signals into the nucleus, and promote the expressions of a series of genes that regulate the repair and regeneration of sweat glands, such as Shh and cyclin D1.

In the seventh step, after transplantation of the induced BM-MSCs into the paws of the nude mice, we observed the sweat gland-like structure which had sweating function. We made deep II degree burn wounds on the paws of nude mice, followed by multiple point injection of BrdU-labeled BMSCs at the injured site. After 2 weeks, the wound healing was observed and the iodine-starch sweating experiment was performed. The results showed that the sweating test was positive in the wounds injected with the induced BM-MSCs, while the control was negative. When the sweat-positive site was taken for histological examination, we found the relatively intact sweat gland-like structures in the tissue sections and these sweat gland structures were derived from transplanted induced BM-MSCs.

In the eighth step, on the basis of the success of experiments in vitro and in vivo, we performed the first clinical research on sweat gland regeneration by autologous BM-MSCs with the approval of the ethics committee and informed consent of the patient. This case was burned in 2006 due to careless work, and the area and depth of burns in both upper limbs were basically the same. We used the left upper limb of the patient as a control and the right upper limb as a test. The induced autologous BM-MSCs were transplanted into the right upper limb wound using the method described above, and the left upper limb wound was treated as well as the right upper limb except for the stem cell transplantation. A sweating test was performed 2 months after transplantation. The results demonstrated that the wounds where the induced BM-MSCs were transplanted had sweating function, and the iodine-starch test was positive, while the control was negative for the iodine-starch test. Furthermore, the sweating test at 12 and 24 months after transplantation showed that the wounds had a stable sweating function.

In the ninth step, after the successful regeneration of the sweat glands, another question to be answered is whether the sweat-positive test sites have sweat gland-like structures and whether the sweat produced by transplanted area is consistent with the sweat produced by normal skin. To this end, we conducted in-depth research on these issues. The biopsy specimen of transplanted area was taken for histological examination after informed consent of the patient. We found that there were positive cells stained by the markers of sweat gland cells and cell clusters similar to sweat glands (but did not form the complete structure of sweat glands including secretions and ducts). Furthermore, neuronal-like structures and the capillary structures were found around the sweat gland-like structures, which suggested that the sweat gland-like structures were active and functional. In 2009, the results of the clinical study were published in the form of the cover story and research paper in the Wound Rep Reg [58], an important journal in the field of repair and regeneration. Professor Patricia A. Hebda, editor-in-chief of the magazine, wrote a special review that highly praised the sweat gland regeneration as a "landmark study."

### 2.2.4 The Perception and Experience Gained from the Experiment in the Past Ten Years

From the discovery of dedifferentiation of epidermal cells to the initial clinical application of sweat gland regeneration, a total of about 10 years of research was conducted. This experience of 10 years is how we can confirm the discovery in the course of scientific research, how to perfect the discovery and how to turn this discovery into an application process. The main experience can be summarized as follows:

1. Some accidental phenomena and casual discoveries may be the basis of a major innovation. Never give up because of arbitrariness. And whether you can seize this momentary opportunity lies in whether you are ready in the early stage, whether you have a wealth of knowledge accumulation and a correct judgment.
2. To prove these accidental phenomena and discoveries is a long and very difficult process, which involves science and other aspects and is affected by many factors. We must be prepared to be questioned and answer various questions.
3. The final aim of the basic discovery is the application to practice. In terms of medical research, basic discovery should be applied to create new clinical treatment technologies that ultimately benefit patients.
4. From the discovery of basic theory to the establishment of major new technologies for clinical treatment, the key to the success is the grasp of theoretical discovery and innovation and the understanding of clinical treatment needs and difficulties.
5. From the discovery of basic theory to the application of clinical treatment, it is a cyclical process. In this process, clinical needs put forward requirements for basic theoretical research and basic theory innovation provides the possibility to solve these needs. The combination of the two provides a way for this successful transformation.

Scientific research needs constant innovation, and the results of innovation need to be transformed and applied and then its value will be realized. Therefore, we believe that in scientific research, the research without innovation is nonsense, and the research without application is done for nothing. An excellent researcher can neither do nonsense nor do for nothing. This is the true meaning of scientific research.

## 2.3 Cellular Dedifferentiation and Synchronized Repair and Regeneration of Complex Tissues In Situ

### 2.3.1 Difficulties and Breakthroughs in Repair and Regeneration of Complex Tissues: Cellular Dedifferentiation

With the development of life science and medicine, significant improvements have been made in the repair and regeneration of single tissues, such as bones, blood vessels, nerves, and muscles. However, multiple tissues cannot be regenerated at the same time. For instance, when the limbs are traumatized, the wound undergo scar healing, without regeneration of distal damaged tissues.

Synchronized repair and regeneration of multiple tissues has more challenges compared to a single tissue. A single tissue, such as the skin, can regenerate the epidermis as long as there are enough epidermal stem cells. However, the complex structure of the limb, including bones, blood vessels, nerves, and connective tissue, requires a variety of tissue-specific stem cells or progenitor cells [59]. Although it is possible to amplify these cells in vitro, these cells are difficult to regrow complex tissues in vitro or spontaneously regrow complex tissues in vivo after transplantation. However, terminally differentiated cells can dedifferentiate into an immature progenitor cells or stem cells in a damaged environment. Lower animals such as salamander and zebrafish lack stem cells in their adult stages, but mature cells have strong potential to undergo cellular dedifferentiation and can provide sufficient stem cell sources for regeneration of complex tissues [1]. By contrast, the potential for cellular dedifferentiation in mammals is very weak, and after tissue damage, mature cells cannot provide stem cells or progenitor cells by regenerating damaged tissues [1]. Therefore, how to induce the dedifferentiation of various mature cells is a key issue to achieve in situ synchronized regeneration of multiple tissues.

Current methods of using transgenes and small molecule compounds can induce adult cells to dedifferentiate into stem cells in vitro [52, 53, 60]. If this technology can be achieved in vivo, it is possible to induce mature cells to become progenitor cells in situ, providing a source of stem cells for regeneration.

The following sections describe animal models with synchronized regeneration of multiple tissues, focusing on the important role of cellular dedifferentiation and the molecular mechanisms underlying dedifferentiation.

## 2.3.2 The Study Model of In Situ Synchronized Regeneration of Complex Tissues

### 2.3.2.1 The Fin Regeneration of Zebrafish

Zebrafish is an animal model for studying the regeneration of complex tissues [61]. Zebrafish can regenerate complex tissues, such as the heart and fin, after injury. The fin is a complex limb appendage, like human limbs, containing multiple tissue components such as fish bones, mesenchymal cells, nerve fibers, and blood vessels; 10–14 days after the fins are amputated, the zebrafish can completely regenerate new fins in situ [62]. At the proximal end of the amputated fin, epidermal cells surrounding the wound area migrated to the wound surface, forming a wound epidermis (Fig. 2.9). A mass of proliferating cells is formed under the wound epidermis, called fin blastema. The cells of fin blastema can continue to proliferate and differentiate under the guidance of the wound epidermis, and regrow the distal end of the amputated fins. Because zebrafish is easy to perform genetic manipulation and its genetic spectrum is clear, it is a typical model to study the synchronized regeneration of multiple tissues.

### 2.3.2.2 Salamanders Limb Regeneration

Salamanders, such as axolotl and newt, are capable of regenerating various organs and tissues [59]. Unlike mammals, their limbs can be completely regenerated after amputation. Along the long axis of the limb, amputation at any position can perfectly regenerate the distal end (Fig. 2.10). The limbs are derived from various germ layers. The epidermis and peripheral nerve tissue are derived from the embryonic ectoderm, and the internal tissue components (such as dermis, muscle, bone, and blood vessels) are derived from the embryonic mesoderm [63]. Therefore, it is necessary to restore the original organized structure of various tissue cells for regeneration. A group of proliferating cells, namely limb blastema, is formed under the wound epidermis. The cells in the limb blastema then grow all the tissue components of the limb. Therefore, salamanders are also important biological models for studying limb regeneration in vertebrates.

### 2.3.2.3 Mouse Toe Tip Regeneration

Mammalian limbs do not have the same ability to regenerate as zebrafish fin and salamander limbs. After trauma, the limb undergoes wound healing and cannot grow the lost distal part. Although the mammal loses the ability to regenerate the entire limb, the distal toe tip can be completely regenerated

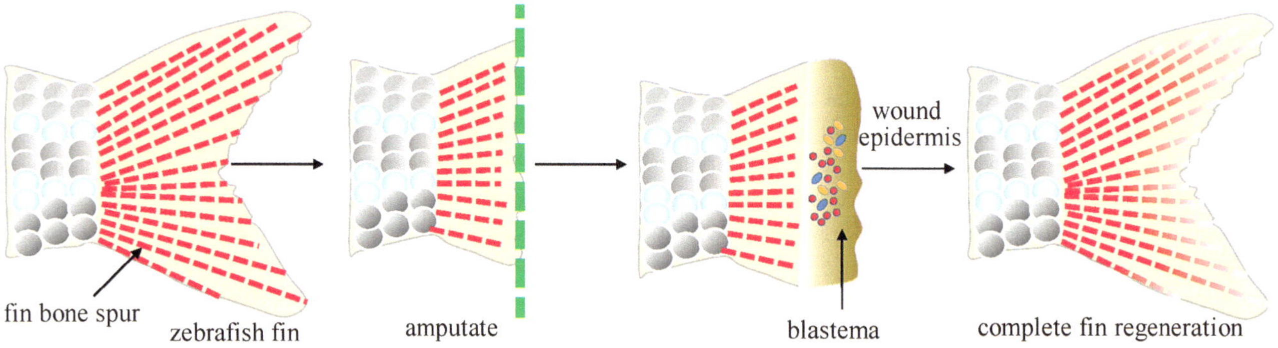


**Fig. 2.9** Regeneration pattern of zebrafish fin after truncation

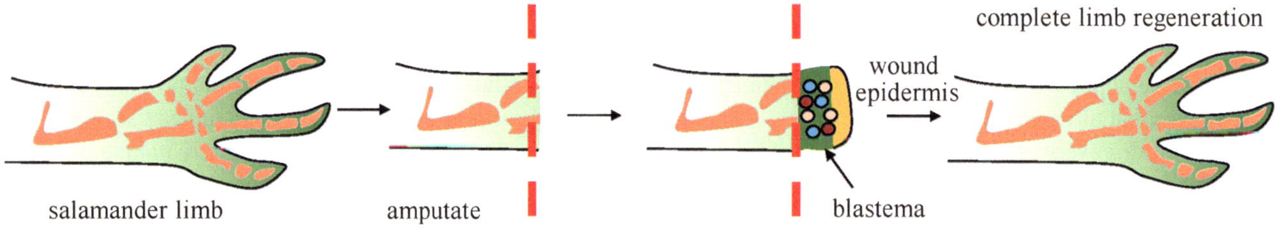


**Fig. 2.10** Regeneration pattern after the salamander limb is cut off

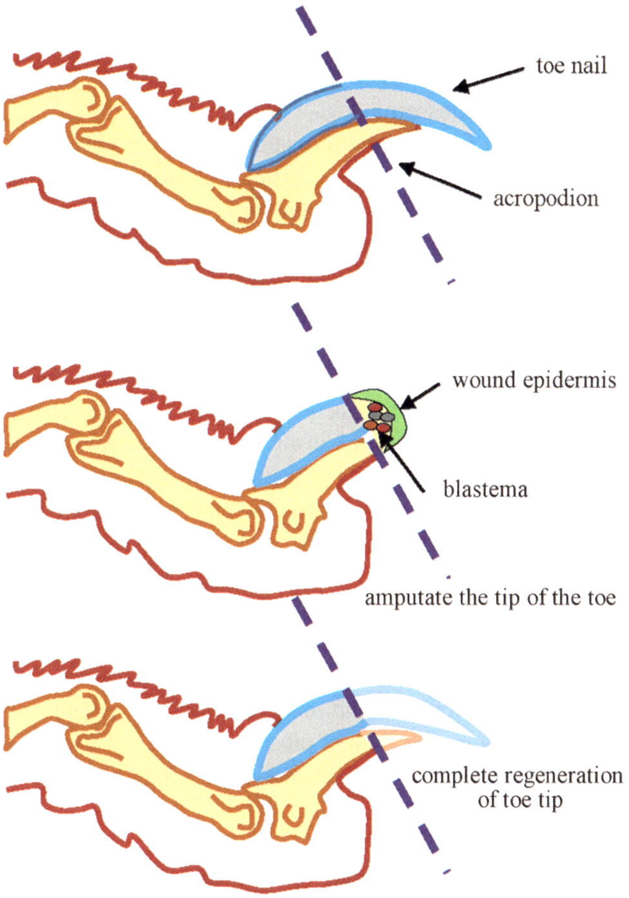


**Fig. 2.11** Regeneration pattern after the toe tip of the mouse is cut off

[64, 65]. It is clinically found that the tip of the finger and the nail can be regenerated after the finger tip of the child or adult is cut off. Similarly, both neonatal mice and adult mice regenerate the toe and nail after amputation of the distal third toe (Fig. 2.11). It is worth noting that the second toe and the proximal end cannot be regenerated, indicating that the mammalian limb regeneration ability is very limited [66]. The blastema is formed under the wound epidermis and regenerate the toe tip [64]. Therefore, the mouse toe tip regeneration model is an important model for studying the complex tissue regeneration of mammalian limbs.

### 2.3.2.4 Zebrafish and Neonatal Mouse Heart Regeneration

The mammalian heart lacks the ability to self-repair and regenerate after injury. However, zebrafish have a strong heart regenerative potential [12]. When the ventricles are surgically cut by 20%, the cardiomyocytes near the wound undergo dedifferentiation and proliferate, and about 60 days after amputation, the zebrafish heart can be completely regenerated (Fig. 2.11). This fully demonstrates that zebrafish heart has a strong ability to regenerate and is a classic biological model for studying the heart regeneration.

Adult mammals generally lose the ability to regenerate the heart, but neonatal mice within 1 week of birth can fully regenerate the heart after removal of the apex (Fig. 2.12) [16]. But after the first week, the mouse heart gradually loses its ability to regenerate. This indicates that the mammalian heart retains some of its ability to regenerate early in life.

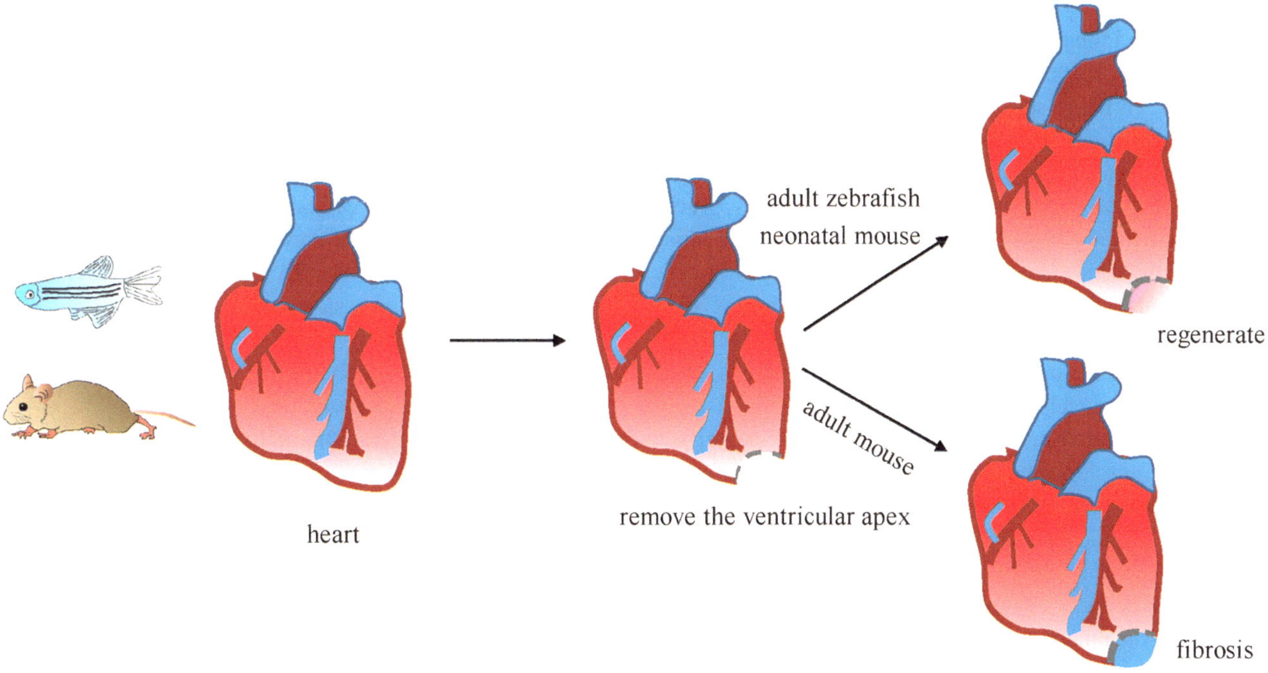


**Fig. 2.12** Schematic diagram of zebrafish heart and mouse heart regeneration

Therefore, using the mouse heart as a model for regenerative research can help reveal the mechanisms that regulate cardiac regeneration in mammals.

### 2.3.3 The Cellular Basis of Limb Regeneration: Blastema and Cellular Dedifferentiation

The regeneration of the appendages, from lower animals to mammals, shares similar cellular mechanisms. The epidermal cells around the wound cover the wound and form a wound epidermis. Below it, a cell mass having proliferative activity is formed, that is blastema. The blastema is the cellular basis of limb regeneration, and it will proliferate and differentiate all tissue cells of the limb. The blastema formation depends on dedifferentiation of mature cells. Therefore, cellular dedifferentiation is the core mechanisms for limb regeneration.

#### 2.3.3.1 Cellular Dedifferentiation: The Basis of Blastema

The development of cell-lineage tracing techniques provides a powerful tool for studying the cell fate and revealing the cellular mechanisms underlying the blastema formation.

##### Salamander Limb Blastema Formation

By using cell-lineage tracing method, Krag et al. revealed the cellular mechanism of Salamander blastema formation. They designed a clever experiment to transplant a transgenic salamander donor expressing GFP into a GFP-negative recipient embryo, such that various tissues express GFP in the limb of the recipient embryo [63]. The limbs expressing GFP were amputated and found that the labeled muscle cells can regenerate new muscles but not cartilage or skin, dermal cells can regenerate cartilage and connective tissue, and Schwann cells can only regenerate Schwann cells. This study demonstrates for the first time that existing tissues in the limb provide their own tissue-specific progenitor cells during regeneration, and then these progenitor cells differentiate into their own cells and do not become other types of cells. However, this study did not demonstrate whether these lineage-specific progenitor cells derive from dedifferentiation of mature cells or activation of resident stem cells. Using Cre/loxP tracing technology, Sandoval-Guzman et al. found that multinucleated myotubes cleave into Pax7-negative (a marker of muscle stem cells) monocytes with proliferative ability, and that these monocytes are involved in the blastema formation of adult newt limbs [44]. Recent studies have found that in the larval stage of the newt, limb muscle regeneration depends on Pax7-positive satellite cells [67]. Therefore, the muscles of the newt rely on muscle stem cells during the larval stage, and rely on the dedifferentiation of muscle cells during the adulthood [45]. In contrast, muscle regeneration in axolotl relies on muscle stem cells participating in the blastema formation [44]. The regeneration of peripheral nerves in the limbs relies on the dedifferentiation of Schwann cells into immature Schwann cells.

##### Zebrafish Fin Blastema

The zebrafish fin blastema formation depends mainly on the cellular dedifferentiation mechanisms, but also includes stem cell activation. For the bone component of the fin (i.e., bone spur), Knopf et al. confirmed that the mature osteoblasts undergo transient dedifferentiation, gain proliferative capacity, migrate and participate in the blastema formation, and then proliferate and differentiate to form new osteoblasts [41]. Interestingly, zebrafish can also regenerate fin spurs by de novo osteoblasts [68]. When all of the fin osteoblasts are destroyed by genetic damage, those surviving are still able to re-grow osteoblasts and bone spurs. The authors believe that when osteoblasts are present, the bone regeneration of the fin mainly depends on the dedifferentiation of osteoblasts, and when osteoblasts are absent, the de novo osteoblasts support regeneration. For muscle components, in the larval stage of zebrafish, it was found that the muscle regeneration of the fins was mainly dependent on the activation of satellite cells, and no dedifferentiation of muscle cells was found [69]. In adult zebrafish, there is no reliable evidence that the regeneration of other components of the fins is realized by cellular dedifferentiation or stem cell activation.

##### Mouse Toe Blastema

During the toe tip regeneration, the tracing technique shows that the mesoderm bone, tendon, dermis, nail bed, blood vessels are derived from mesodermal progenitor cells or stem cells, while the ectoderm epidermal cells and sweat glands are derived from ectoderm cells [70]. Are the progenitor cells derived from the activation of residual stem cells in the tissues or the dedifferentiation of mature cells? There are toenail stem cells in the mouse toenail, and when the toe tip is amputated, the toenail stem cells depend on the activation of the Wnt pathway to differentiate and regenerate [71]. The regeneration of the toe tip depends not only on the activation of the toenail stem cells, but also on the cellular dedifferentiation (Fig. 2.13). Schwann cell precursors dedifferentiate and secretes oncostatin M and platelet-derived growth factor AA (PDGF-AA) to promote the continuous expansion of the blastema [72].

#### 2.3.3.2 Molecular Mechanisms of Cellular Dedifferentiation, Proliferation, and Blastema Formation

After injury, the damaged microenvironment will release various factors to activate signaling pathways, induce resident to dedifferentiate, proliferate, re-differentiate, and participate in the regeneration and repair of tissues. The microenvironment mainly includes growth factors, cytokines, and extracellular matrices. Among them, growth factors are the most critical components in the microenvironment. Growth factors and related signaling pathways play an important role in the regeneration of complex tissues. The signaling pathways is as follows (Fig. 2.14).

**Fig. 2.13** Cytological mechanism of regenerated bud in the appendages of zebrafish, salamander, and mouse

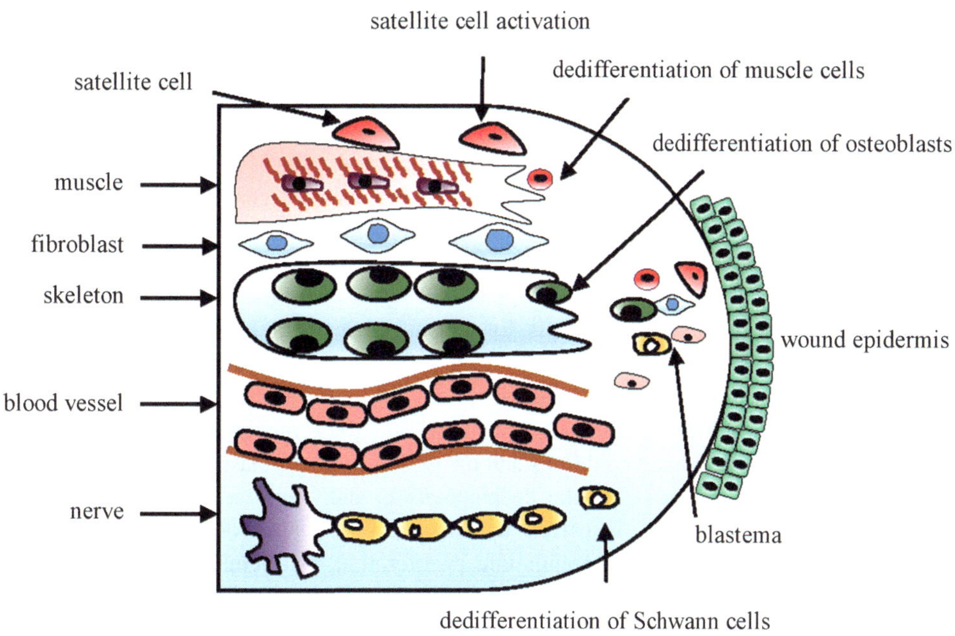


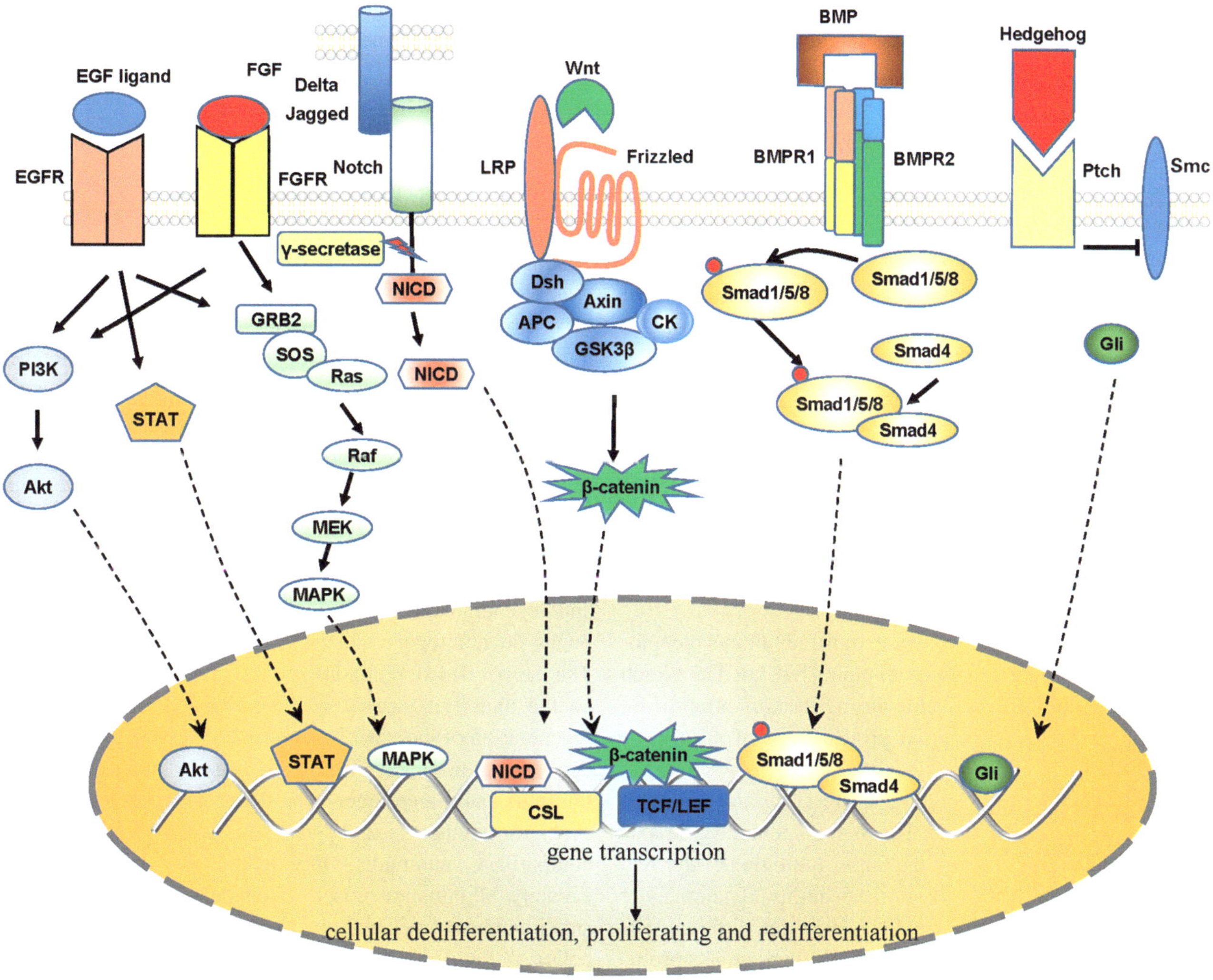


**Fig. 2.14** Conduction pattern diagram of common signal pathways involved in regeneration

The epidermal growth factor (EGF) binds to the epidermal growth factor receptor (EGFR) and activates downstream signaling pathways to cause expression of target genes. Neuregulin 1 is a member of the EGF family and its expression is significantly increased after the amputation of zebrafish fins [73]. Neuregulin 1 activates the EGFR and PIK/Akt signaling pathways, promoting the proliferation and migration of dedifferentiated progenitor cells to form blastema [73].

Fibroblast growth factor (FGF) acts by activating the four-transmembrane FGF tyrosine kinase receptor (FGFR). During the regeneration of zebrafish fins, it was found that FGF20a is critical for the regeneration of fins [74]. FGF20a was expressed near the wound epidermis and the mesenchymal space within 6–12 days after the fin amputation, and then FGF20a was gradually restricted to the blastema. FGF20a may promote cell dedifferentiation, proliferation, and blastema formation. FGF3/10a expressed in the late blastema regulates the proliferation of blastema progenitor cells [75]. During the regeneration of the salamander limbs, the wound epidermis and peripheral nerves produce FGF1 and FGF2, which promote the blastema formation [76]. FGF2 also promotes the proliferation of the blastema progenitor cells during the mouse toe tip regeneration.

Bone marrow morphogenetic protein (BMP) is a member of transforming growth factor-β (TGF-β) that binds to transmembrane type 1 BMP receptor and type 2 BMP receptor (BMPR). After amputation of zebrafish fins, BMP2 expression was significantly upregulated, and BMP2 was able to induce dedifferentiated osteoblasts to redifferentiate and form spurs [77]. BMP is a growth factor essential for mouse toe regeneration. After the toe tip was amputated, BMP2, BMP4, and BMP7 were upregulated in the stump and blastema. By using exogenous BMP4 to treat Msx-1 mutant mice (gene-deficient mice with loss of regeneration ability of toe tip), the ability to regenerate toe tip can be restored [78]. It cannot be regenerated after the proximal end of the toe tip is cut off, but when exogenous BMP2 and BMP7 magnetic beads are embedded in the proximal end, the regeneration of the proximal part can be promoted [79].

The Notch protein is a single transmembrane receptor that possesses the intracellular domain (NICD). The Notch signal is continuously activated during the formation of fin blastema, which promotes the proliferation of progenitor cells [80].

Wnt protein binds to the Frizzled receptor and promotes nuclear transfer of β-catenin. The Wnt/β-catenin signal axis regulates the regeneration of the limbs. Inhibition of the Wnt signaling pathway will result in the inability of salamander and zebrafish fins to regenerate [81]. However, different Wnt proteins play an opposite role, such as Wnt8 promotes proliferation of blastema progenitor cells, whereas Wnt5b inhibits proliferation [82]. Therefore, different Wnt proteins can coordinate with each other to form a negative feedback loop that regulates the regeneration process of the limb. The expression of Wnt is increased in the wound epidermis of the toe and guides the differentiation of the toenail stem cells [71]. Similarly, the Wnt pathway regulates the proliferation and further differentiation of osteoblast progenitor cells into osteoblasts during the toe tip regeneration [83].

Hedgehog proteins include Sonic Hedgehog (Shh), Desert Hedgehog (Dhh), and Indian Hedgehog (Ihh). The Hedgehog signal regulates the patterning of limb development. Shh and Ihh expression increased during salamander limb regeneration [84]. Blocking the Hedgehog pathway severely impedes limb regeneration. This is because the Hedgehog pathway regulates polarity and promotes proliferation and outgrowth of blastema. Shh and Ihh are activated to regulate the proliferation and growth of fin blastema progenitors [85]. The spurs of zebrafish fins are segmented and bifurcated, and this structural pattern is regulated by the Shh signaling pathway [86]. Before the spur bifurcation, the Shh expression in the fin epidermis is divided into two regions. This expression pattern regulates the proliferative activity of osteoblasts and bifurcations of the regenerated spur. Destroying the expression pattern of Shh, the fins cannot be bifurcated when they are regenerated.

### 2.3.4 Differences in Cellular Dedifferentiation Potential and Regeneration

Salamander and zebrafish have strong regenerative capacity, mainly due to high dedifferentiation potential of mature cells. However, the dedifferentiation potential in mammals is much lower than that of lower animals such as salamander and zebrafish. To some extent, the dedifferentiation potential reflects the strength of animal regeneration.

Salamander and zebrafish regenerate limbs and fins, and their strong regenerative capacity is closely related to their high degree of dedifferentiation. The terminally differentiated osteoblasts dedifferentiate, regain their proliferative capacity, migrate and differentiate into newly formed osteoblasts, and regenerate fin bone spurs [41]. However, mammalian bones do not regenerate truncated parts after amputation. The lack of dedifferentiation in mammalian osteoblasts may be the underlying cause of weak bone regeneration. The regeneration of the newt limb muscle is related to the strong dedifferentiation potential of the muscle cells. Its mature multinucleated myotubes can dedifferentiate into monocytes, form blastema, and participate in regeneration [87]. In comparison, mammalian muscle has weaker regenerative capacity. Mammalian muscle regeneration relies mainly on a small number of residual muscle satellite cells (muscle stem cells), rather than the dedifferentiation of muscle fibers. However, mammalian muscle fibers can be induced to dedifferentiate to form proliferative progenitor cells. The introduction of the gene msx1 expressed in the blastema of salamander limbs into the muscle fibers of the mouse can turn the mouse muscle fibers to progenitor cells [88]. In addition, the muscle fibers of the mice treated with the substances extracted from the salamander regenerated limbs can also induce dedifferentiation [89]. Even small molecule compounds can induce dedifferentiation of mouse muscle fibers [90]. These studies demonstrate that mammalian muscle cells retain their intrinsic dedifferentiation potential, but this potential cannot be activated by itself after injury and requires external stimulation. Strengthening the dedifferentiation of muscle cells may promote the regeneration of mammalian muscles and various tissues of the limbs.

The zebrafish mature cardiomyocytes rapidly dedifferentiate after injury, re-enter the cell cycle, and regenerate the lost cardiomyocytes. Human has a very small number of mature cardiomyocytes that can re-enter the cell cycle and produce new cardiomyocytes. During normal aging, only 0.0006–1% of cardiomyocytes can re-enter the cell cycle [19]. From this, it can be seen that the dedifferentiation potential of human cardiomyocytes is much weaker than that of zebrafish cardiomyocytes. The heart of the neonatal mouse in the first week has the ability to regenerate [16]. One week later, the mouse heart also lost its ability to regenerate, most likely due to a decrease or loss of cardiomyocyte dedifferentiation. Enhancing the dedifferentiation potential of mammalian cardiomyocytes may be an effective strategy to promote cardiac regeneration.

Although most tissue cells in mammals have lost the potential to dedifferentiate, some tissue cells still have this natural ability. A classic example is that human Schwann cells can be regenerated by dedifferentiation [48]. When the peripheral nerve is injured, the mature Schwann cells dedifferentiate into immature Schwann cells with proliferative capacity. Immature Schwann cells migrate and redifferentiate to new Schwann cells, providing structural and nutritional support for axonal regeneration. Another example is the repair and regeneration of the kidneys after an acute kidney injury [91]. Toxic kidney damage often leads to necrosis of proximal tubular epithelial cells. The renal tubular epithelial cells that survived the injury can dedifferentiate, proliferate and regenerate the necrotic epithelial cells, and reconstruct the integrity of the glomerulus [4]. These indicate that the regenerative capacity is closely related to the dedifferentiation potential.

### 2.3.5 Cellular Dedifferentiation Potential and Cell Cycle

Why are lower animal cells more likely to dedifferentiate and re-enter into the cell cycle? Although this mechanism has not been fully understood, there is evidence that cell cycle regulators can partially explain the differences in dedifferentiation. In theory, the cell cycle needs to be strictly controlled, otherwise it is carcinogenic. With biological evolution, the more perfect the cell cycle inhibition mechanism develops, the more difficult it is for mature cells to enter the cell cycle again. For example, pocket proteins (Rb, p107, p130) block the transition from G1 to S phase, and p53 blocks the transition from G2 to M phase [92]. Most cancer cells have mutations in Rb or p53 to obtain unlimited proliferation [93]. Salamanders can spontaneously inhibit the expression of cell cycle inhibitors, undergo dedifferentiation, and re-enter the cell cycle [94]. Under normal conditions, the differentiation of muscle cells requires the expression of the tumor suppressor Rb protein, which inhibits cell cycle entry. Although the Rb protein is also retained in the mature myotubes of salamander, the serum released by limb amputation induces the expression of cell cycle-dependent kinase 4 and 6 (CDK4/6) that can phosphorylate Rb and make it inactive [95]. The result is to allow cell cycle-related genes to be re-expressed. In stark contrast, mammalian myotubes cannot phosphorylate Rb protein and cannot re-enter the cell cycle. However, when the Rb gene is knocked out from mature myotubes of mammals, serum can induce dedifferentiation and re-entry into the cell cycle [96]. From this, it can be seen that the mammalian muscle cells cannot be dedifferentiated because the cell cycle inhibitor is not automatically removed after the injury. Interestingly, in mature cardiomyocytes of mammals, tumor suppressor Rb and p130 were also found to block the expression of cell cycle genes and maintain the state of mature cardiomyocytes. Knocking out Rb and p130, mature cardiomyocytes enter the cell cycle again and gain proliferative capacity [97]. During the regeneration of salamander limbs, the expression of tumor suppressor p53 decreases in the early stage of injury, promoting the dedifferentiation of mesenchymal cells and the blastema formation [98]. The expression of p53 increased in the late stage, promoting the differentiation of blastema progenitor cells and regenerating limbs. The homeodomain transcription factor Meis1 is expressed in mouse mature cardiomyocytes, causing cardiomyocytes to exit the cell cycle. When Meis1 was knocked out in mature cardiomyocytes, the cardiomyocytes regained proliferative capacity [99]. Therefore, the elimination of cell cycle inhibitors helps to increase the dedifferentiation potential of mammalian mature cells. The relationship between cell cycle regulation and cellular dedifferentiation is as follows (Fig. 2.15).

### 2.3.6 Inducing Cellular Dedifferentiation to Promote In Situ Synchronized Regeneration of Complex Mammalian Tissues

Mammals mostly lose the dedifferentiation potential, resulting in weak regenerative capacity. To achieve regeneration of complex tissues, the ideal way is to mimic lower animals,

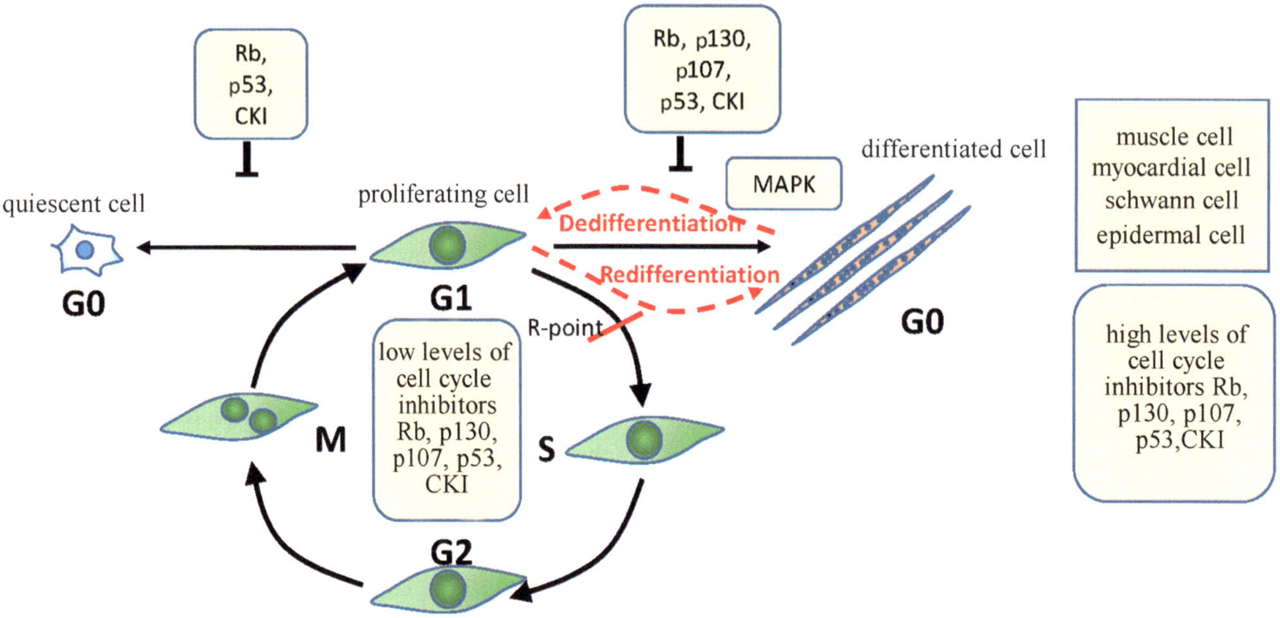


**Fig. 2.15** Relationship between cell cycle regulation and cell dedifferentiation

inducing the dedifferentiation of mature cells. It is much more difficult to induce dedifferentiation in the local injury than in vitro culture environment. Currently, based on cell reprogramming technology, reintroduction of exogenous transcription factors in vivo has been found to alter the fate of cells [53, 60]. For example, three transcription factors (Ngn3, Pdx1, and Mafa) are introduced into exocrine cells in the mouse pancreas, and the exocrine cells are reprogrammed into insulin-producing β cells in vivo [100]. The three transcription factors Gata4, Mef2c, and Tbx5 were introduced into the ischemic infarcted myocardium to induce myocardial fibroblasts to cardiomyocyte-like cells and participate in the regeneration of myocardium [101]. In the brain, transcription factors or miRNAs can reprogram astrocytes or radioactive glial cells to participate in neuronal regeneration [102, 103]. The introduction of exogeous gene induces liver myofibroblasts into liver cells in vivo, which reduces liver fibrosis [104]. In addition, the combination of small molecule compounds can induce fibroblasts to dedifferentiate into induced pluripotent stem cell (iPSC), neurons, neural stem cells, or cardiomyocytes [53]. The addition of small molecules SB431542 and XAV939 in vivo increases the efficiency of transcription factors in reprogramming cardiac fibroblasts to cardiomyocytes [105]. If it is effective to use small molecules instead of transcription factors in vivo to induce dedifferentiation of tissue cells in situ, it is possible to achieve in situ regeneration of complex tissues. Accordingly, it is expected to induce in situ dedifferentiation of tissue cells in mammals to achieve the repair and regeneration of complex tissues.

## References

1. Zhao A, Qin H, Fu X. What determines the regenerative capacity in animals? Bioscience. 2016;66(9):735–46.
2. Tanaka EM, Reddien PW. The cellular basis for animal regeneration. Dev Cell. 2011;21(1):172–85.
3. Chen Z-L, Yu W-M, Strickland S. Peripheral regeneration. Annu Rev Neurosci. 2007;30:209–33.
4. Kusaba T, Lalli M, Kramann R, et al. Differentiated kidney epithelial cells repair injured proximal tubule. Proc Natl Acad Sci U S A. 2014;111(4):1527–32.
5. Fu X, Sun X, Li X, Sheng Z. Dedifferentiation of epidermal cells to stem cells in vivo. Lancet. 2001;358(9287):1067–8.
6. Mannik J, Alzayady K, Ghazizadeh S. Regeneration of multilineage skin epithelia by differentiated keratinocytes. J Invest Dermatol. 2010;130(2):388–97.
7. Bellomo R, Kellum JA, Ronco C. Acute kidney injury. Lancet. 2012;380(9843):756–66.
8. Berger K, Bangen J-M, Hammerich L, et al. Origin of regenerating tubular cells after acute kidney injury. Proc Natl Acad Sci U S A. 2014;111(4):1533–8.
9. Witzgall R, Brown D, Schwarz C, Bonventre JV. Localization of proliferating cell nuclear antigen, vimentin, c-Fos, and clusterin in the postischemic kidney. Evidence for a heterogenous genetic response among nephron segments, and a large pool of mitotically active and dedifferentiated cells. J Clin Invest. 1994;93(5):2175–88.
10. Abbate M, Brown D, Bonventre JV. Expression of NCAM recapitulates tubulogenic development in kidneys recovering from acute ischemia. Am J Phys. 1999;277(3):F454–63.
11. Imgrund M, Gröne E, Gröne HJ, et al. Re-expression of the developmental gene Pax-2 during experimental acute tubular necrosis in mice 1. Kidney Int. 1999;56(4):1423–31.
12. Poss KD, Wilson LG, Keating MT. Heart regeneration in zebrafish. Science. 2002;298(5601):2188–90.

13. Jopling C, Sleep E, Raya M, et al. Zebrafish heart regeneration occurs by cardiomyocyte dedifferentiation and proliferation. Nature. 2010;464(7288):606–9.
14. Kikuchi K, Holdway JE, Werdich AA, et al. Primary contribution to zebrafish heart regeneration by gata4(+) cardiomyocytes. Nature. 2010;464(7288):601–5.
15. Schindler YL, Garske KM, Wang J, et al. Hand2 elevates cardiomyocyte production during zebrafish heart development and regeneration. Development. 2014;141(16):3112–22.
16. Porrello ER, Mahmoud AI, Simpson E, et al. Transient regenerative potential of the neonatal mouse heart. Science. 2011;331(6020):1078–80.
17. Malek Mohammadi M, Kattih B, Grund A, et al. The transcription factor GATA4 promotes myocardial regeneration in neonatal mice. EMBO Mol Med. 2017;9(2):265–79.
18. Senyo SE, Steinhauser ML, Pizzimenti CL, et al. Mammalian heart renewal by pre-existing cardiomyocytes. Nature. 2013;493(7432):433–6.
19. Bergmann O, Bhardwaj RD, Bernard S, et al. Evidence for cardiomyocyte renewal in humans. Science. 2009;324(5923):98–102.
20. Wei K, Serpooshan V, Hurtado C, et al. Epicardial FSTL1 reconstitution regenerates the adult mammalian heart. Nature. 2015;525(7570):479–85.
21. Mitsuda S, Yoshii C, Ikegami Y, Araki M. Tissue interaction between the retinal pigment epithelium and the choroid triggers retinal regeneration of the newt Cynops pyrrhogaster. Dev Biol. 2005;280(1):122–32.
22. Mizuno A, Yasumuro H, Yoshikawa T, et al. MEK-ERK signaling in adult newt retinal pigment epithelium cells is strengthened immediately after surgical induction of retinal regeneration. Neurosci Lett. 2012;523(1):39–44.
23. Islam MR, Nakamura K, Casco-Robles MM, et al. The newt reprograms mature RPE cells into a unique multipotent state for retinal regeneration. Sci Rep. 2014;4:6043.
24. Susaki K, Chiba C. MEK mediates in vitro neural transdifferentiation of the adult newt retinal pigment epithelium cells: is FGF2 an induction factor? Pigment Cell Res. 2007;20(5):364–79.
25. Fimbel SM, Montgomery JE, Burket CT, Hyde DR. Regeneration of inner retinal neurons after intravitreal injection of ouabain in zebrafish. J Neurosci. 2007;27(7):1712–24.
26. Nagashima M, Barthel LK, Raymond PA. A self-renewing division of zebrafish Müller glial cells generates neuronal progenitors that require N-cadherin to regenerate retinal neurons. Development. 2013;140(22):4510–21.
27. Raymond PA, Barthel LK, Bernardos RL, Perkowski JJ. Molecular characterization of retinal stem cells and their niches in adult zebrafish. BMC Dev Biol. 2006;6:36.
28. Thummel R, Enright JM, Kassen SC, et al. Pax6a and Pax6b are required at different points in neuronal progenitor cell proliferation during zebrafish photoreceptor regeneration. Exp Eye Res. 2010;90(5):572–82.
29. Qin Z, Barthel LK, Raymond PA. Genetic evidence for shared mechanisms of epimorphic regeneration in zebrafish. Proc Natl Acad Sci U S A. 2009;106(23):9310–5.
30. Hafler BP, Surzenko N, Beier KT, et al. Transcription factor Olig2 defines subpopulations of retinal progenitor cells biased toward specific cell fates. Proc Natl Acad Sci U S A. 2012;109(20):7882–7.
31. Fischer AJ, Reh TA. Müller glia are a potential source of neural regeneration in the postnatal chicken retina. Nat Neurosci. 2001;4(3):247–52.
32. Joly S, Pernet V, Samardzija M, Grimm C. Pax6-positive Müller glia cells express cell cycle markers but do not proliferate after photoreceptor injury in the mouse retina. Glia. 2011;59(7):1033–46.
33. Das AV, Mallya KB, Zhao X, et al. Neural stem cell properties of Müller glia in the mammalian retina: regulation by notch and Wnt signaling. Dev Biol. 2006;299(1):283–302.
34. Ooto S, Akagi T, Kageyama R, et al. Potential for neural regeneration after neurotoxic injury in the adult mammalian retina. Proc Natl Acad Sci U S A. 2004;101(37):13654–9.
35. Karl MO, Hayes S, Nelson BR, et al. Stimulation of neural regeneration in the mouse retina. Proc Natl Acad Sci U S A. 2008;105(49):19508–13.
36. Takeda M, Takamiya A, Jiao J-W, et al. Alpha-Aminoadipate induces progenitor cell properties of Müller glia in adult mice. Invest Ophthalmol Vis Sci. 2008;49(3):1142–50.
37. Lawrence JM, Singhal S, Bhatia B, et al. MIO-M1 cells and similar muller glial cell lines derived from adult human retina exhibit neural stem cell characteristics. Stem Cells. 2007;25(8):2033–43.
38. Zhao C, Tao Z, Xue L, et al. Lin28b stimulates the reprogramming of rat Müller glia to retinal progenitors. Exp Cell Res. 2017;352(1):164–74.
39. Pollak J, Wilken MS, Ueki Y, et al. ASCL1 reprograms mouse Muller glia into neurogenic retinal progenitors. Development. 2013;140(12):2619–31.
40. Ueki Y, Wilken MS, Cox KE, et al. Transgenic expression of the proneural transcription factor Ascl1 in Müller glia stimulates retinal regeneration in young mice. Proc Natl Acad Sci U S A. 2015;112(44):13717–22.
41. Knopf F, Hammond C, Chekuru A, et al. Bone regenerates via dedifferentiation of osteoblasts in the zebrafish fin. Dev Cell. 2011;20(5):713–24.
42. Blum N, Begemann G. Osteoblast de- and redifferentiation are controlled by a dynamic response to retinoic acid during zebrafish fin regeneration. Development. 2015;142(17):2894–903.
43. Echeverri K, Clarke JD, Tanaka EM. In vivo imaging indicates muscle fiber dedifferentiation is a major contributor to the regenerating tail blastema. Dev Biol. 2001;236(1):151–64.
44. Sandoval-Guzmán T, Wang H, Khattak S, et al. Fundamental differences in dedifferentiation and stem cell recruitment during skeletal muscle regeneration in two salamander species. Cell Stem Cell. 2014;14(2):174–87.
45. Tanaka HV, Ng NCY, Yang Yu Z, et al. A developmentally regulated switch from stem cells to dedifferentiation for limb muscle regeneration in newts. Nat Commun. 2016;7:11069.
46. Sunderland S. Rate of regeneration in human peripheral nerves; analysis of the interval between injury and onset of recovery. Arch Neurol Psychiatr. 1947;58(3):251–95.
47. Chen YY, McDonald D, Cheng C, et al. Axon and Schwann cell partnership during nerve regrowth. J Neuropathol Exp Neurol. 2005;64(7):613–22.
48. Scheib J, HÖke A. Advances in peripheral nerve regeneration. Nat Rev Neurol. 2013;9(12):668–76.
49. Navarro X, Vivó M, Valero-Cabré A. Neural plasticity after peripheral nerve injury and regeneration. Prog Neurobiol. 2007;82(4):163–201.
50. Allodi I, Udina E, Navarro X. Specificity of peripheral nerve regeneration: interactions at the axon level. Prog Neurobiol. 2012;98(1):16–37.
51. Takahashi K, Yamanaka S. Induction of pluripotent stem cells from mouse embryonic and adult fibroblast cultures by defined factors. Cell. 2006;126(4):663–76.
52. Qin H, Zhao A, Zhang C, Fu X. Epigenetic control of reprogramming and Transdifferentiation by histone modifications. Stem Cell Rev. 2016;12(6):708–20.
53. Qin H, Zhao A, Fu X. Small molecules for reprogramming and transdifferentiation. Cell Mol Life Sci. 2017;74(19):3553–75.
54. Fu X, Sun X, Li X, et al. Dedifferentiation of epidermal cells to stem cells in vivo. Lancet. 2001;358:1067–8.
55. Zhang C, Chen P, Fei Y, et al. Wnt/β-catenin signaling is critical for dedifferentiation of aged epidermal cells in vivo and in vitro. Aging Cell. 2012;11(1):14–23.

56. Zhang C, Fu X, Chen P, et al. Dedifferentiation derived cells exhibit phenotypic and functional characteristics of epidermal stem cells. J Cell Mol Med. 2010;14(5):1135–45.
57. Li H, Fu X, Ouyang Y, et al. Adult bone marrow derived mesenchymal stem cells contribute to wound healing of skin appendages. Cell Tissue Res. 2006;326(3):725–36.
58. Sheng Z, Fu X, Cai S, et al. Regeneration of functional sweat gland-like structures by transplanted differentiated bone marrow mesenchymal stem cells. Wound Rep Reg. 2009;17(3):427–35.
59. Nacu E, Tanaka EM. Limb regeneration: a new development? Annu Rev Cell Dev Biol. 2011;27:409–40.
60. Qin H, Zhao A, Fu X. Chemical modulation of cell fates: in situ regeneration. Sci China Life Sci. 2018;61(10):1137–50.
61. Gemberling M, Bailey TJ, Hyde DR, Poss KD. The zebrafish as a model for complex tissue regeneration. Trends Genet. 2013;29(11):611–20.
62. Tu S, Johnson SL. Fate restriction in the growing and regenerating zebrafish fin. Dev Cell. 2011;20(5):725–32.
63. Kragl M, Knapp D, Nacu E, et al. Cells keep a memory of their tissue origin during axolotl limb regeneration. Nature. 2009;460(7251):60–5.
64. Fernando WA, Leininger E, Simkin J, et al. Wound healing and blastema formation in regenerating digit tips of adult mice. Dev Biol. 2011;350(2):301–10.
65. Borgens RB. Mice regrow the tips of their foretoes. Science. 1982;217(4561):747–50.
66. Masaki H, Ide H. Regeneration potency of mouse limbs. Develop Growth Differ. 2007;49(2):89–98.
67. Morrison JI, LÖÖF S, He P, Simon A. Salamander limb regeneration involves the activation of a multipotent skeletal muscle satellite cell population. J Cell Biol. 2006;172(3):433–40.
68. Singh SP, Holdway JE, Poss KD. Regeneration of amputated zebrafish fin rays from de novo osteoblasts. Dev Cell. 2012;22(4):879–86.
69. Rodrigues AMC, Christen B, Martí M, Izpisúa Belmonte JC. Skeletal muscle regeneration in Xenopus tadpoles and zebrafish larvae. BMC Dev Biol. 2012;12:9.
70. Rinkevich Y, Lindau P, Ueno H, et al. Germ-layer and lineage-restricted stem/progenitors regenerate the mouse digit tip. Nature. 2011;476(7361):409–13.
71. Takeo M, Chou WC, Sun Q, et al. Wnt activation in nail epithelium couples nail growth to digit regeneration. Nature. 2013;499(7457):228–32.
72. Johnston APW, Yuzwa SA, Carr MJ, et al. Dedifferentiated Schwann cell precursors secreting paracrine factors are required for regeneration of the mammalian digit tip. Cell Stem Cell. 2016;19(4):433–48.
73. Rojas-Muñoz A, Rajadhyksha S, Gilmour D, et al. ErbB2 and ErbB3 regulate amputation-induced proliferation and migration during vertebrate regeneration. Dev Biol. 2009;327(1):177–90.
74. Whitehead GG, Makino S, Lien C-L. Keating MT. fgf20 is essential for initiating zebrafish fin regeneration. Science. 2005;310(5756):1957–60.
75. Shibata E, Yokota Y, Horita N, et al. Fgf signalling controls diverse aspects of fin regeneration. Development. 2016;143(16):2920–9.
76. Giampaoli S, Bucci S, Ragghianti M, et al. Expression of FGF2 in the limb blastema of two Salamandridae correlates with their regenerative capability. Proc Biol Sci. 2003;270(1530):2197–205.
77. Stewart S, Gomez AW, Armstrong BE, et al. Sequential and opposing activities of Wnt and BMP coordinate zebrafish bone regeneration. Cell Rep. 2014;6(3):482–98.
78. Han M, Yang X, Farrington JE, Muneoka K. Digit regeneration is regulated by Msx1 and BMP4 in fetal mice. Development. 2003;130(21):5123–32.
79. Yu L, Han M, Yan M, et al. BMP signaling induces digit regeneration in neonatal mice. Development. 2010;137(4):551–9.
80. Grotek B, Wehner D, Weidinger G. Notch signaling coordinates cellular proliferation with differentiation during zebrafish fin regeneration. Development. 2013;140(7):1412–23.
81. Kawakami Y, Rodriguez Esteban C, Raya M, et al. Wnt/beta-catenin signaling regulates vertebrate limb regeneration. Genes Dev. 2006;20(23):3232–7.
82. Stoick-Cooper CL, Weidinger G, Riehle KJ, et al. Distinct Wnt signaling pathways have opposing roles in appendage regeneration. Development. 2007;134(3):479–89.
83. Takeo M, Hale CS, Ito M. Epithelium-derived Wnt ligands are essential for maintenance of underlying digit bone. J Invest Dermatol. 2016;136(7):1355–63.
84. Singh BN, Doyle MJ, Weaver CV, et al. Hedgehog and Wnt coordinate signaling in myogenic progenitors and regulate limb regeneration. Dev Biol. 2012;371(1):23–34.
85. Iovine MK. Conserved mechanisms regulate outgrowth in zebrafish fins. Nat Chem Biol. 2007;3(10):613–8.
86. Zhang J, Jeradi S, Strähle U, Akimenko M-A. Laser ablation of the sonic hedgehog- a-expressing cells during fin regeneration affects ray branching morphogenesis. Dev Biol. 2012;365(2):424–33.
87. Wang H, Simon A. Skeletal muscle dedifferentiation during salamander limb regeneration. Curr Opin Genet Dev. 2016;40:108–12.
88. Odelberg SJ, Kollhoff A, Keating MT. Dedifferentiation of mammalian myotubes induced by msx1. Cell. 2000;103(7):1099–109.
89. Mcgann CJ, Odelberg SJ, Keating MT. Mammalian myotube dedifferentiation induced by newt regeneration extract. Proc Natl Acad Sci U S A. 2001;98(24):13699–704.
90. Duckmanton A, Kumar A, Chang Y-T, Brockes JP. A single-cell analysis of myogenic dedifferentiation induced by small molecules. Chem Biol. 2005;12(10):1117–26.
91. Guo J-K, Cantley LG. Cellular maintenance and repair of the kidney. Annu Rev Physiol. 2010;72:357–76.
92. Bertoli C, Skotheim JM, De Bruin RAM. Control of cell cycle transcription during G1 and S phases. Nat Rev Mol Cell Biol. 2013;14(8):518–28.
93. Sherr CJ, McCormick F. The Rb and p53 pathways in cancer. Cancer Cell. 2002;2(2):103–12.
94. Tanaka Em GAA, Gates PB, Brockes JP. Newt myotubes reenter the cell cycle by phosphorylation of the retinoblastoma protein. J Cell Biol. 1997;136(1):155–65.
95. Tanaka EM, Drechsel DN, Brockes JP. Thrombin regulates S-phase re-entry by cultured newt myotubes. Curr Biol. 1999;9(15):792–9.
96. Schneider JW, Gu W, Zhu L, et al. Reversal of terminal differentiation mediated by p107 in Rb−/− muscle cells. Science. 1994;264(5164):1467–71.
97. Sdek P, Zhao P, Wang Y, et al. Rb and p130 control cell cycle gene silencing to maintain the postmitotic phenotype in cardiac myocytes. J Cell Biol. 2011;194(3):407–23.
98. Yun MH, Gates PB, Brockes JP. Regulation of p53 is critical for vertebrate limb regeneration. Proc Natl Acad Sci U S A. 2013;110(43):17392–7.
99. Mahmoud AI, Kocabas F, Muralidhar SA, et al. Meis1 regulates postnatal cardiomyocyte cell cycle arrest. Nature. 2013;497(7448):249–53.
100. Zhou Q, Brown J, Kanarek A, et al. In vivo reprogramming of adult pancreatic exocrine cells to beta-cells. Nature. 2008;455(7213):627–32.
101. Qian L, Huang Y, Spencer CI, et al. In vivo reprogramming of murine cardiac fibroblasts into induced cardiomyocytes. Nature. 2012;485(7400):593–8.
102. Guo Z, Zhang L, Wu Z, et al. In vivo direct reprogramming of reactive glial cells into functional neurons after brain injury and in an Alzheimer's disease model. Cell Stem Cell. 2014;14(2):188–202.
103. Niu W, Zang T, Zou Y, et al. In vivo reprogramming of astrocytes to neuroblasts in the adult brain. Nat Cell Biol. 2013;15(10):1164–75.
104. Song G, Pacher M, Balakrishnan A, et al. Direct reprogramming of hepatic Myofibroblasts into hepatocytes in vivo attenuates liver fibrosis. Cell Stem Cell. 2016;18(6):797–808.
105. Mohamed TMA, Stone NR, Berry EC, et al. Chemical enhancement of in vitro and in vivo direct cardiac reprogramming. Circulation. 2017;135(10):978–95.

# Molecular and Genetic Basis for Tissue Repair and Regeneration

3

Jian Xiao, Jiang Wu, Xiaokun Li, Xiaoyan Sun, Biao Cheng, and Xiaobing Fu

## 3.1 Genes Involved in Tissue Repair and Regeneration

Scientists all over the world are working hard to find genes for tissue repair and regeneration, and hope to achieve the goal of regeneration and repair by regulating several genes. At present, many laboratories in this field have achieved breakthrough results, including Nobel Prize-level results. Chinese scientists, including the team of Xiaobing Fu, have also made important contributions in this field. The important genes involved in tissue repair and regeneration are described below.

### 3.1.1 The Four Genes of iPS Cells

Academician Xiaobing Fu first reported the reverse differentiation of epidermal cells in the internationally renowned medical journal *Lancet* published on September 29, 2001. In the study of the histological features of healing wounds treated with epidermal growth factors, the academician team found that there were some scattered cell mass positive for β1 integrin and keratin 19 staining in the prickle cell layer and granular layer of the regenerated epidermis. It has an island structure, small cells, few organelles, and no direct histological association with basal stem cells. Therefore, it is preliminarily determined that these β1 integrin and keratin 19 double-stained positive cells in the prickle cell layer and granular cell layer are epidermal stem cells or cells with epidermal stem cell characteristics. On this basis, they conducted a series of identification studies from development, histology, and methodology, and finally confirmed that this stem cell island phenomenon exists only in wounds healed by epidermal growth factor therapy. It is preliminarily proved that the stem cells in the prickle cell layer and granular layer of the regenerated epidermis are reversed by epidermal cell growth factor and is the result of reverse differentiation of differentiated epidermal cells into epidermal stem cells. The publication of this paper has aroused strong repercussions in the academic community. Many researchers in the academic circles thought that the reverse differentiation of mature somatic cells into stem cells was unthinkable until the discovery of induced pluripotent stem cells. It is confirmed that the reverse differentiation of mature somatic cells into stem cells is not only an objective fact, but also a milestone impact on the development of regenerative medicine.

Induced pluripotent stem cells (iPS) are a kind of cells that are reprogrammed to be similar to embryonic stem cells in terms of cell morphology and cell proliferation by introducing pluripotent genes into mature somatic cells or embryonic cells. At present, iPS has been differentiated into various cells such as nerve cells, cardiomyocytes, and cerebral cortical cells. iPS successfully avoided the ethical controversy involved in the study of embryonic stem cells (ESCs) and solved the problem of immune rejection, which is a landmark discovery of stem cell research.

The establishment of iPS cells mainly involves the introduction of several pluripotency-related foreign genes into the differentiated cells, that is, host cells, by virus-mediated or other means. Under suitable culture conditions, these differentiated cells will be transformed into iPS cells. In 2003, Mitsui K et al. found that 20 genes expressed more in embryonic stem cells than in pluripotent cells. Based on this research, in 2006, Shinya Yamanaka of the University of Tokyo in Japan used retrovirus to introduce 24 candidate genes into mouse embryonic fibroblasts and rat tail fibroblasts, and selected four genes Oct4, Sox2, c-Myc, and Klf4 through experiments. These four genes were introduced into

J. Xiao · J. Wu · X. Li
Wenzhou Medical University, Wenzhou, China

X. Sun · X. Fu (✉)
The Chinese People's Liberation Army General Hospital, Beijing, China

B. Cheng
General Hospital of Southern Theater Command of Chinese People's Liberation Army, Guangzhou, China


X. Fu (ed.), *Regenerative Medicine in China*, https://doi.org/10.1007/978-981-16-1182-7_3

mouse embryonic fibroblasts, and induced pluripotent stem cells were successfully obtained. The cells are highly similar to mouse embryonic stem cells in terms of cell morphology and cell proliferation ability.

#### 3.1.1.1 Introduction of iPS Cell Gene Function

##### Oct4 Gene Function

Octamer-binding transcription factor 4 (Oct4) is a member of the POU transcription factor family and is one of the most important transcription factors involved in regulating embryonic stem cell self-renewal and maintaining pluripotency and cell proliferation. It is also the most important factor in the process of inducing pluripotent stem cell recoding. The human Oct4 gene is located on chromosome 6, and there are 11 subtypes encoding 7 proteins.

Oct4 is a key gene that maintains ESC totipotency and self-renewal and is expressed in unfertilized oocytes. When Oct4 is mutated or knocked out, the embryo cannot form an inner cell mass, the embryoid body undergoes apoptosis, and the embryo loses totipotency in cell. When the Oct4 gene is silenced, mouse and human ESCs differentiate into trophoblast cells. Oct4 forms a network regulatory pathway with Nanog and Sox2 to regulate the totipotency of embryonic stem cells. These three genes maintain embryonic stem cell totipotency and inhibit differentiation through feedforward systems, self-regulatory networks, and other signal transduction pathways.

##### Sox2 Function

The Sox2 gene is a member of the Sox family, a transcription factor associated with the sex determination gene (SRY) superfamily, and is widely found in the animal kingdom. Sox2 is located on chromosome 3 and is a single exon structure. Sox2 is randomly dispersed throughout the genome and does not form a gene cluster.

The Sox2 gene is one of the important genes for cell reprogramming. It participates in cell formation, maintains embryonic stem cell totipotency and self-renewal, and determines the process of animal gender, nervous system development, and eye development. During embryogenesis, the levels of Oct4 and Sox2 are gradually reduced. As a synergistic gene of Oct4 gene, Sox2 mutation may cause mutation of Oct4 gene and lead to stem cell loss of totipotency. The loss of Sox2 causes the embryo to die shortly after implantation, unable to form trophoblast cells and neuroectoderm.

##### Klf4 Function

Klf4 is located on human chromosome 4 and has five exons. It is a member of the Klf family and has a multiple tandem zinc finger structure involved in the regulation of cell proliferation and differentiation. Klf4, together with Oct4, Sox2, and c-Myc, regulates stem cell self-renewal and maintains totipotency and participates in the process of human or mouse somatic cells reprogramming.

High expression of Klf4 promotes the increase of Nanog expression and reduces the differentiation ability of cells. Knockout or low expression of the Klf4 gene does not cause embryonic apoptosis, nor affect self-renewal and embryonic development, but can lead to genetic diseases. In ESCs, knocking out Klf4 and Klf2 or Klf4 and Klf5 at the same time results in a decrease in ESC self-renewal ability, but knocking out a gene alone does not change similarly. After the embryo is formed, knocking out Klf2 may cause fatal bleeding and death of embryo in 12–14 days. In the absence of Klf5, the embryo will die due to a lack of trophoblast. Therefore, Klf4, Klf2, and Klf5 are involved in maintaining embryonic development and embryonic stem cell self-renewal. The mechanism of maintaining ESC self-renewal may be related to Toll-Akt pathway, ERK1 and ERK2 enzymes. ERK1 and ERK2 enzymes activate Klf4 gene and phosphorylate Klf4 on Ser123 protein. Phosphorylated Klf4 inhibits Klf4 activity, leading to differentiation of embryonic stem cells.

##### C-Myc Function

The c-Myc gene is an important member of the cell oncogene, involved in cell proliferation and differentiation regulation, and plays an important role in mouse somatic cells reprogramming and regulates the self-renewal and differentiation of hemopoietic stem cells. The product of c-Myc gene is a 62 kD phosphorylated protein p62c-Myc, a protein consisting of 439 amino acids co-encoded by exons 2 and 3 of the C-one gene, which is located in the nucleus and is a nuclear protein. According to the c-Myc encoded product and functional classification, the c-Myc oncogene is a nuclear protein gene, which has the ability to transform cells and has the characteristics of binding to chromosomes and DNA, and plays a role in regulating cell growth, differentiation, and malignant transformation.

During embryonic stem cell culture, c-Myc expression is reduced when LIF is absent in the culture medium. When c-Myc is highly expressed, ESCs are delayed in differentiation. The mechanism of cell differentiation is related to the LIF-STAT3 pathway. High expression of c-Myc can inhibit the expression of GATA6 gene and reduce the multidirectional differentiation ability of cells. Tomoaki Hishida et al. found that c-Myc, N-Myc, and L-Myc synergistically reduce cell death rate and maintain stem cell totipotency. Maintaining embryonic stem cell totipotency is associated with MAPK and GSK3β pathways, independent of Myc/Max complex. Nakagawa et al. found that knocking out c-Myc during mouse somatic cells reprogramming can increase reprogramming rate and reduce the incidence of tumors.

The Oct4 and Sox2 genes play an important role in the maintenance of pluripotency of embryonic stem cells and are essential for inducing the reconstruction of iPS cells. These two transcription factors maintain the pluripotency of human iPS cells, while the role of Klf4 and c-Myc is to change the structure of chromatin, thus facilitating the binding of Oct4 and Sox2 and improving the efficiency of induction success. Therefore, Oct4 may be the only independent factor in the reprogramming process, and other factors may only play a synergistic role.

## 3.1.2 Development-Related Genes

The genes involved in tissue repair and regeneration are closely related to development. Many development-related genes discovered by developmental biologists are used in the research of regenerative medicine. Therefore, we believe that genes related to development are also the focus of regenerative medicine. The academician team believes that developmental biology is the foundation of regenerative medicine. In fact, the repair and regeneration process after tissue damage is also the process of redevelopment of damaged tissues and organs. However, due to changes in seed cells and environmental factors, the repaired and regenerated tissues cannot fully achieve the same structure and function as before the damage.

### 3.1.2.1 Homeobox Gene

In 1984, the homeobox was discovered, which enabled the important fields of developmental biology and molecular biology to be mechanically combined: regulation of gene transcription can control development. Homeobox gene is a kind of gene closely related to developmental biology. It regulates the growth and development of organisms in time and space. During embryonic development, it gives spatial specificity to the cells in different parts of the body's anterior-posterior axis, thus affecting cell differentiation.

In the following, an important class of homeobox gene Pax family is taken as an example to introduce the close relationship between homeobox gene and tissue repair and regeneration.

The homology of Pax1 and Pax9 is as high as 98%, which plays an important regulatory role in the growth and development of the spine, thymus, parathyroid gland, the third and fourth pharyngeal pouch and their derivatives, and embryonic bone tissues. The effect of these genes on skeletal development are mainly achieved by the following mechanisms: in embryonic development, Bapx1 is widely expressed in the tissue cells of sarcomere and vertebral developmental, Pax1 and Pax9 are essential regulators for the activation of Bapx1 transcription. Knocked out the Pax1 and Pax9 genes during the spinal formation of mouse embryos were completely unable to observe, during development, and the single gene-deficient subjects showed spinal deformity of different degrees.

The Pax2 gene is closely related to the development of kidney. It is one of the earliest genes expressed in the early stage of kidney development. It mainly regulates the proliferation of nephron precursor cells and the formation of mesonephric duct in the early stage. Under ureteric bud induction, Pax2 is continuously expressed in the metanephros interstitial and is active in the metanephros concentrate and epithelial derivatives surrounding the ureter. Pax2 mutant mice can also initially form a ureter, but then the ureter is rapidly decomposed. However, overexpression of Pax2 can accelerate cell proliferation, leading to renal carcinogenesis. Pax8 also has a certain regulatory effect on kidney development.

Pax3 plays an important role in the development of both neural crest cells and melanocytes. Neural crest cells (NCCs) are located on the dorsolateral side of the ectodermal neural tube. They are stem cells with multiple differentiation potential in development. According to their different migration and differentiation directions, they can be roughly divided into nervous system structural cells and melanocytes. Pax3 plays an important role in the development of both types of cells. Pax3 acts as a transcriptional regulator directly regulating the transcription of the melanin-specific gene MITF. The mutation of Pax3 single allele forms Splotch (Sp) mice which white spots on its abdomen due to the loss of melanin. Except for melanin deficiency, the heart, muscle, neural tube, and intestinal nerve center of the homozygous mutant Sp mice are not well developed. Congenital genetic diseases, Waardenburg syndrome (WS) type I and III, are also caused by mutations in the Pax3 gene. Symptoms include shallow hair color, poor hearing, and muscle atrophy of the extremities.

Pax3 and Pax7 are commonly expressed in the early stage of somite development, and then only appear in the skeletal muscle cells of the sarcomere. When the muscle cells differentiate into sarcoplasmic proteins, the expression levels of Pax3 and Pax7 are downregulated; later, Pax3 is strongly expressed in the lateral somites. Both MyoD and MyfS belong to myogenic differentiation factors (MDFs), most of which are active in skeletal muscle precursor cells. RNAi is used to reduce the RNA content of Pax3 and Pax7 in mouse embryos, and the activity of Myf5 and MyoD is inhibited, leading to muscle malformation. Experiments with Sp mice have shown that Pax3 mutation directly affects the formation of muscles in the limbs. Upregulation of the expression of Pax7 can compensate for the loss of Pax3 function within a certain extent, but it cannot play a substitute role.

When Pax7 is knocked out, the mice have normal muscle tissue during embryonic development and birth, and it is seen that Pax7 plays a minor role in muscle formation. In skeletal muscle satellite cells, Pax7, by inhibiting the expression of MyoD and sarcoplasmic protein genes, makes them stay in the stem cell state, so as to redifferentiate in sudden events such as muscle damage. Pax3 only plays an auxiliary role. It is speculated that Pax3 is essential for the formation of muscle cells, while Pax7 focuses on the self-repair and regeneration of muscles.

The Pax5 protein, also known as B-cell-specific activator protein (BSAP), is a transcription factor unique to B cells. By binding to B cell development-related genes, it can affect B cell proliferation, homotypic transformation, immunoglobulin gene transcription, and final differentiation.

#### 3.1.2.2 MicroRNA and Development

miRNA is a type of endogenous noncoding protein RNA, a single-stranded small molecule of 20–25 nucleotides in length, widely expressed in multicellular organisms and viruses. After binding to target mRNA, it plays a regulatory role by affecting its translation or degradation. At present, there are more than 2000 miRNAs found in the human body, accounting for 1% of the human genome, regulating 30% of gene expression, finely regulating the expression of target genes of a specific cell and tissue. They are not only involved in the regulation of normal physiological processes in the body, such as cell proliferation, differentiation, development, apoptosis, etc., but also closely related to the occurrence and development of tumors, heart diseases, and neurological diseases. It is predicted that miRNA regulates 30% of human protein-coding genes.

##### MicroRNA Is Involved in Tissue Development

MicroRNA and lung development studies have demonstrated that it plays a crucial role in many aspects of normal lung development. In 2005, Lu et al. found that the Dicer and AGO protein families are selectively expressed in mouse fetal lung branches, which indirectly indicates that microRNA may be involved in lung development. In 2006, Harris et al. selectively knocked out the Dicer enzyme gene in the endoderm of mice initial lung bud, causing lung dysplasia. MicroRNA was first proposed to play an important role in lung development. In 2010, Dong et al. systematically analyzed the expression profiles of microRNA, mRNA, and protein at different stages of lung development in mice. They found that during lung development, microRNA regulates genes expression mainly by inhibiting translation independent of mRNA degradation.

##### MicroRNA and Heart Development

With the in-depth study of microRNA, it has been found that microRNAs regulate heart development. MicroRNAs related to cardiac development are mainly microRNA-1 and microRNA-133. Zhao et al. used Cre homologous recombination technology to make mouse heart tissue-specific lack of Dicer, which is necessary for microRNA processing. Mouse heart has many developmental defects, and embryos die early, indicating that microRNA is necessary during heart development. Among them, muscle-specific microRNA expression is affected. miR-1 has two subtypes: miR-1-1 and miR-1-2. miR-1-1 is mainly present in the ventricle. In order to further study the role of miR-1-2 in heart development, the team constructed a mouse model of miR-1-2 knockout and found that miR-1-$2^{-/-}$ mice are prone to large-area ventricular septal defect and die soon after birth. Studies by Lin et al. found that miR-133 plays an important role in regulating cardiac gene expression and function. Experiments show that absence of miR-133a-1 and miR-133a-2 in mouse models causes fatal ventricular septal defect in about half of embryos or suckling mice; surviving mice still develop dilated cardiomyopathy and die of heart failure or sudden death.

##### MicroRNA and Nervous System Development

miR-124 is one of the most abundantly expressed miRNAs in mature neurons and is widely expressed in neurons of brain, retina, and spinal cord, but is extremely low in undifferentiated neural progenitor cells. Krichevsky et al. found that the phase in which miR-124a began to express was consistent with the phase in which neuronal precursor cells transformed into neural cells and astrocytes and confirmed that miR-124a can change the proportion of cultured embryonic stem cells differentiated into neurons and glial cells. The mature miR-124 sequence is completely conserved from worms to humans. There are three miR-124 genes on different chromosomes in the human and mouse genomes. Overexpression of miR-124 in HeLa cell lines can decrease the expression of more than 100 genes. Krichevsky et al. also found that miR-9 is highly expressed in neurons similar to miR-124a, and experiments have shown that miR-9 can also change the proportion of cultured embryonic stem cells differentiated into neurons and glial cells. Zhao et al. found that the introduction of miR-9 into the embryonic brain by electroporation triggered the early differentiation of neurons. The mechanism by which miR-9 promotes neuronal differentiation is at least partially achieved by inhibiting the nuclear receptor protein TLX. Experiments have confirmed that miR-9 can inhibit the expression of TLX and thus negatively regulate the proliferation of neural stem cells and accelerate the differentiation of neurons.

#### 3.1.2.3 Development-Related Genes and Tissue Repair

##### Wnt Gene

The epidermis is the outermost layer of the skin and is composed of stratified epithelial tissue. It plays an important role in the defense of animals against external stimuli such as pathogens and water loss. During embryonic development, the role of this barrier has been established, and monolayer epithelial cells differentiate into different stratum corneum. Many human genetic diseases have the characteristic of epidermal destruction, with at least 1 in every 5 patients. Skin regeneration and future treatment require a thorough understanding of the molecular mechanisms of the epithelial stratification process. Wnt ligand protein plays an important role in the process of inducing skin hair follicles and in the self-renewal of epidermal stem cells between adult hair follicles. However, during embryonic development, we know little about the role of Wnt signaling in epithelial stratification. In the research of Professor Zhang Zunyi's team, by using the mouse genetic model to block the secretion of Wnt signal in the epidermis during embryonic development, it was found that the Wnt signal generated by the epidermis can activate the dermal BMP-FGF signal axis, and the latter re-feedback regulated the stratification of the epidermis. The findings of this study identified a genetic hierarchy of signaling that plays a necessary role in epidermal-dermal interactions and promotes understanding of mammalian skin development.

#### Lin28a Gene

Professor George of Harvard Medical School reported on *Cell* that by reactivating a latent gene called Lin28a, hair, cartilage, skin, and other soft tissues of model mice can be regenerated. Lin28a can partially enhance tissue repair by enhancing mitochondrial metabolism, which provides new insights into the development of novel regenerative therapies. Lin28a was first discovered in worms. It is abundant in embryonic stem cells and is particularly strongly expressed during early embryogenesis. It has been used to reprogram skin cells into stem cells, and can also bind to RNA to regulate gene expression. In order to better understand the role of Lin28a in promoting tissue repair, the researchers observed which specific RNAs can bind to Lin28a and subsequently discovered a small RNA, Let7, which promotes cell maturation and aging. Lin28a enhances the production of metabolic enzymes in mitochondria and stimulates tissue to regenerate by altering the metabolism of mitochondria to produce more energy. Since Lin28a is difficult to introduce into cells, tissue repair can be achieved by directly activating mitochondrial metabolism. Direct activation of mitochondrial metabolism by using a small molecule compound can also enhance the healing rate of the wound, which suggests that tissue regeneration can be induced by some tissue repair drugs. However, Lin28a does not induce regeneration of all tissues, and Lin28a may be a key factor in the composition of healing compounds.

#### Smed-Prep Gene

The worm has an extraordinary ability to regenerate when it is cut off, and these parts even include the head and brain. Professor Aziz Aboobaker of the University of Nottingham in the UK reported on *PLoS Genetics* that a homeobox gene called Smed-prep plays an important role in the regeneration of worms. This study may make it possible to regenerate aging or damaged human organs and tissues. Smed-prep is an essential factor for the proper differentiation and localization of the cells that make up the worm's head and is the key to determining the position of the head. Although the emergence of Smed-prep is the determining factor to keep the head and brain in the correct position, worm stem cells will form brain cells under the influence of other irrelevant genes. Without Smed-prep, the relevant cells cannot organize themselves to form a normal brain.

### 3.1.3 Tumor-Related Genes

In the paper *Developmental biology and comparative biology: the important research fields in wound repair and regeneration*, Fu Academician pointed out: from the perspective of biological processes, wound repair and tumor formation are both the results of cell proliferation, differentiation, and angiogenesis; only the former is controllable and the latter is out of control. In the past, it was suggested that the formation of tumor is a result of overexpression and action of proto-oncogenes such as c-fos and c-jun caused by some gene mutations. However, many studies have suggested that proto-oncogenes or their proteins are also highly expressed or their activities are upregulated in different stages of embryonic development and in some important organs and tissues, and these tissues have no tumor formation. Conversely, during the rapid proliferation of such cells, the healing of the wound is scar-free. Therefore, the high expression of these proto-oncogenes in embryonic tissues without scars, cancer, and tumorigenesis also suggests that there may be similar and different regulatory mechanisms in normal cell proliferation and differentiation, uncontrolled cell proliferation and differentiation (such as uncontrolled growth of cancer cells), embryonic development, and postnatal repair. An understanding of these regulatory mechanisms may help us find a switch that regulates wound healing. Therefore, tumor-related genes, especially proto-oncogenes and tumor suppressor genes, are also closely related to tissue repair and regeneration.

#### 3.1.3.1 Proto-Oncogene

Proto-oncogene is a gene that controls cell growth in cells. It is a normal gene related to cell proliferation under normal conditions. It can stimulate cell growth to meet the requirements of cell renewal. It is highly conserved in evolution, and its expression products are extremely important for the physiological function of cells. More than 100 proto-oncogenes have been identified. When the structure or regulatory region of the proto-oncogene is mutated and the gene expression product is increased or the activity is enhanced, the cell will continue to grow or protect the cell from death without receiving the growth signal and finally cause cell carcinogenesis.

The proteins encoded by proto-oncogenes are known to be involved in many factors regulating cell growth, and these factors are involved in the regulation of cell growth, proliferation, and differentiation pathways. Proto-oncogene expression products are classified into the following four categories according to their role in the cellular signaling system.

#### Extracellular Growth Factor

Extracellular signals include growth factors, hormones, neurotransmitters, drugs, etc., which act on the receptor system on the cell membrane or are directly delivered to the cell, and then activated by various protein kinases to phosphorylate the transcription factor, triggering transcriptional activation of a range of genes. It is through this pathway that the Sis gene works. It is known that P28 protein encoded by v-Sis gene and human c-Sis gene is homologous to the β-chain of platelet-derived growth factor (PDGF). When the Sis gene expression forms a dimer like PDGF, it acts on the PDGF receptor and makes phosphatidylinositol in the cell membrane catalyzed by the corresponding kinase to form phosphatidylinositol-4, 5-bisphosphate (PIP2). Under the action of phospholipase C, PIP2 is hydrolyzed to generate diglyceride (DG) and inositol triphosphate (IP3), activate protein kinase C, transform the recipient cells, and stimulate intracellular receptor synthesis. It is indicated that the Sis gene is related to PDGF and its function is very similar. In addition, C-Sis expression protein P28 promotes vascular growth in the same way as PDGF.

#### Transmembrane Growth Factor Receptor

Another type of proto-oncogene product is a transmembrane receptor that accepts extracellular growth signals and transmits them into the cell. The transmembrane growth factor receptor has a cytoplasmic structural region and has tyrosine-specific protein kinase activity. Many proto-oncogene products also have this enzyme activity, such as c-src, c-abl, and the like. The kinases encoded by other proto-oncogenes (c-mos and raf) phosphorylate serine and threonine residues rather than tyrosine. By this phosphorylation, its structure is changed, the activity of the kinase on the substrate is increased, and the intracellular transmission of the growth signal is accelerated.

#### Intracellular Signalosome

After the growth signal reaches the intracellular, a series of intracellular information transmission systems are used to transmit the received growth signal from the intracellular to the nucleus to promote cell growth. Most of these transmit system members are products of proto-oncogenes, or affect the second messenger (cAMP, diglyceride, $Ca^{2+}$, etc.) by the action of these gene products. Oncogene products as intracellular signalosome include non-receptor tyrosine kinases (c-src, c-abl, etc.), serine-threonine kinases (c-ras, c-mas), ras proteins (H-Ras, K-ras and N-ras, etc.), and phospholipase (crk product).

#### Nuclear Transcription Factor

It is known that certain proto-oncogene expression proteins (such as myc/fos, etc.) are localized in the nucleus, and they bind to regulatory elements of the target gene to directly regulate transcriptional activity as a transcription factor. These proteins are usually expressed rapidly when cells are stimulated by growth factors, promoting cell growth and division. It is now widely accepted that c-fos is an immediate-early gene (IEG).Under the action of growth factors, phorbol esters and neurotransmitters, c-fos acts as the third messenger to transmit information and can be expressed instantly and transiently.

### 3.1.3.2 Tumor Suppressor Gene

A tumor suppressor gene or an anticancer gene is a type of gene that can inhibit the activity of proto-oncogene. When it is activated, it inhibits cell proliferation and plays an important role in regulating cell development, growth, and differentiation. When various reasons such as mutation cause gene inactivation or the product is inactivated, the inhibition disappears, which may lead to tumor formation and canceration.

Since the study on isolation and identification of tumor suppressor genes is later than proto-oncogenes, only the mechanism of Rb and p53 is well understood.

#### Retinoblastoma Gene (Rb Gene)

The Rb gene was the first tumor suppressor gene discovered in children's retinoblastoma; hence, it is called Rb gene. Under normal circumstances, retinal cells contain active Rb gene, which controls the growth and development of retinal cells and the differentiation of visual cells. When the Rb gene loses function or congenital deletion, retinal cells proliferate abnormally and form retinoblastoma. Inactivation of Rb gene is also common in many tumors such as osteosarcoma, small cell lung cancer, and breast cancer, indicating that the anticancer effect of Rb gene has a certain extent.

The Rb gene is relatively large, located in human chromosome 13q14, contains 27 exons, transcribes 4.7 kb mRNA, and encodes protein P105. The protein is located in the nucleus and has two forms of phosphorylation and non-phosphorylation. The non-phosphorylation form is called active type and can promote cell differentiation and inhibit cell proliferation. Experiments have shown that after the introduction of Rb gene into cells of retinoblastoma or osteosarcoma, the growth of these malignant cells was inhibited. Significantly, the phosphorylation of Rb protein is closely related to the cell cycle. For example, lymphocytes in quiescent state only express non-phosphorylated Rb protein. Under the induction of mitogen, lymphocytes enter S phase, and Rb protein phosphorylation level is increased. Terminally differentiated monocytes and granulocytes only express high level of non-phosphorylated Rb protein. Even under the induction of growth factors, Rb protein did not phosphorylate, and cells did not divide. It is suggested that cell growth stops, Rb protein is at a low phosphorylation level, and tumor cells in proliferation only contain phosphorylated Rb protein. It indicates that the phosphorylation modification of Rb protein plays an important role in regulating cell growth and differentiation.

#### P53 Gene

The human p53 gene is located at 17P13, has a full length of 16 ~ 20 kb, contains 11 exons, and transcribes 2.8 kb mRNA. The encoded protein is p53, which is a nuclear phosphorylation protein. The p53 gene is the most associated with human tumors. In the past, it has been regarded as an oncogene. It was not until 1989 that mutant p53 was known to play the role of oncogene. Later, it was confirmed that wild-type p53 is a tumor suppressor gene. The p53 gene expression product p53 protein consists of 393 amino acid residues and exists as a tetramer in vivo with a half-life of 20–30 min.

Under normal conditions, the p53 protein content in cells is very low, and because its half-life is short, it is difficult to detect. However, in the growing and proliferating cells, it can be increased by 5–100 times. Wild-type p53 protein plays an important role in maintaining normal cell growth and inhibiting malignant proliferation, and is titled "Geneguard." The p53 gene constantly monitors the integrity of the gene. Once the DNA of the cell is damaged, the p53 protein binds to the corresponding part, acts as a special transcription factor, activates the transcription of the p21 gene, arrests the cell in the G1 phase, inhibits the activity of the unwinding enzyme, interacts with replication factor A, and participates in DNA replication and repair. If repair fails, p53 protein initiates a programmed death process to induce cell suicide and prevent the formation of cancer-prone mutant cells, thereby preventing cell malignant transformation.

## 3.2 Protein Molecules Involved in Tissue Repair and Regeneration Regulation

### 3.2.1 Growth Factor Protein

As early as 1991, Academician Xiaobing Fu and his team began the leading research on modern wound repair, edited and published the first book on *growth factors and wound repair* in the world, Growth Factor and Wound Repair. Since the 1990s, Academician Xiaobing Fu led the team to systematically carry out research on growth factor-regulating wound healing in China and first reported the epidemiological characteristics of chronic refractory wounds on human body in China.

Academician Xiaobing Fu pointed out: "Studying the molecular biological mechanism of wound healing and applying growth factors to wound repair and treatment is a major advance in trauma medicine since the 1980s. It not only leads to a profound change in the concept of wound treatment, but also brings revolutionary breakthrough in wound healing." Professor Li Xiaokun, a leading scientist in the development of new growth factor drugs in China and a distinguished professor of Changjiang Scholars, has been working closely with the Academician Fu's group since the 1990s to lead the largest research team of fibroblast growth factor in China. They found out the way to engineering growth factor gene drugs, which made China the first country in the world to develop fibroblast growth factor into clinical drugs, and made outstanding contributions to accelerating the development of new biological drugs with China's independent intellectual property rights.

#### 3.2.1.1 FGF—Fibroblast Growth Factor

As one of the most important regulatory factors in the repair of tissues such as skin, hair follicles, and sweat glands, it is of great clinical and social significance to develop fibroblast growth factor as an innovative drug that shortens the healing time of wounds and improves the quality of wound healing.

In 1996, Professor Li's team solved a series of engineering and technical problems that have long restricted the industrialization of FGF. They are the first to develop FGF series of innovative drugs in the world, which are widely used in the treatment of burn, trauma, and diabetic complications. The team's main contributions to FGF drug development are as follows.

#### Establish FGF-Efficient Secretion Expression System

Before the 1990s, genetic engineering drugs have long faced a series of engineering and technical problems such as low protein expression, misfolding, easy formation of inclusion bodies, difficulty in large-scale preparation and purification, poor stability, and short half-life, which severely restricted the development and transformation of protein drugs. The team screened and obtained the SecB gene of *E. coli* secretion factor, which was used as a molecular chaperone for FGF secretion expression vector, constructed the recombinant expression plasmid pT7-SecB-FGF, established a high-efficiency secretion expression system of FGF, and realized the soluble expression of protein [1]. The expression reached more than five times the international level in the same period.

### The First Structural Transformation of FGF Successfully Solved the Technical Problems of Large-Scale Production Process

FGF2 easily forms intermolecular disulfide bonds, and it is easy to form dimers or polymers during expression to cause precipitation. Through structural analysis, Cys78 and Cys96, which are not in the active region, were mutated to Ser, and the highly expressed human mutant rhFGF2 was successfully constructed. Its expression level and stability were significantly higher than wild-type rhFGF2. The bioinformatics technique was used to analyze the mRNA of full-length FGF1, and it was found that it was easy to form a hairpin loop structure in the ribosome binding site, which affected the initiation of translation and resulted in a low expression level of full-length FGF1. Based on the interaction characteristics between protein and receptor, the 19 amino acids at N-terminal were knocked out on the basis of the retained protein activity, and the genetically engineered strain with high soluble expression of rhFGF1135 was successfully constructed, and the expression amount reached 108 mg/L, which satisfied the industrial production demand.

### Created FGF Large-Scale Preparation Process and Quality Standards

The growth and expression patterns of *E. coli* engineered bacteria loaded with FGF plasmid were found, and the production technology of fed batch high-density fermentation was established [2]. The high-efficiency two-step separation and purification process was established based on the characteristics of the specific binding of FGF and heparin. The purity of the target protein reaches 99%, and the protein recovery rate is increased by 50%. For the defects of poor stability and short half-life of the recombinant protein in vitro and in vivo, a specific affinity fixed-point solid phase modification technology was developed to form a standardized technical system for industrial production of FGF, and a standard activity assay for the determination of FGF-promoting cell proliferation by NIH3T3 cell line/MTT method was established. The FGF production and quality control technical standards were included in the third part of the 2005 edition of *Chinese Pharmacopoeia*, which is the first production and verification regulation for growth factor genetic engineering drugs.

### Developed the First Drug-Loaded Class III Implantable Medical Device that Combines FGF with Tissue Engineering Materials

A variety of drug-loading materials were screened, and the rhFGF2-collagen composite active material suitable for fistula, bedsore, uterine erosion, and the like was successfully developed for the first time. The production process and activity standard of the biomaterials were first established, and the sponge-like freeze-drying molding technology was optimized. The material was selected into the catalogue of foreign international assistance of the Ministry of Commerce of the People's Republic of China and the catalogue of war storage of the entire military. It is used for national defense and military first-aid equipment, and became an important strategic military product with independent intellectual property rights in China.

At the same time, Professor Li Xiaokun's team has carried out a lot of pioneering work around the development and mechanism of new endocrine FGF subfamily innovative drugs. It is the first report that the upregulation of FGF21 in diabetic patients through clinical practice, further reveal that FGF21 plays a role in the metabolism of glucose and lipid by activating FGFR and PPAR-adiponectin, and systematically elucidate the role of FGF21/FGFR in fatty liver and atherosclerosis. It has internationally firstly analyzed the complex structure of FGFR phosphorylation substrate PLCγ. Based on the above research, a series of high-level academic papers have been published in the international authoritative magazines such as *Cell Metab*, *Circulation*, *Mol Cell*, *JACC*, *J Hepatol*, *Biomaterials*, *Diabetes*, etc. as corresponding authors, in which the research on the role of FGF in metabolism was selected as one of the top ten breakthroughs of *Cell Metab* in the past 10 years. The above basic research work lays a theoretical foundation for screening, designing, and developing new growth factor drugs.

FGF series proteins can significantly accelerate the healing rate of burn wounds, bedsore, diabetic ulcers, flap transplantation, fistula, and other wounds, can significantly inhibit scar formation, reduce epidermal water loss, reduce skin cuticle thickness, and promote the wound skin accessory organs such as sweat glands, hair follicles, and nerve regeneration and repair. The long-term follow-up observation on the clinical application of FGF new drugs showed no adverse reactions such as hyperplasia and abnormal hyperplasia. Clinical application showed that FGF new drugs have changed the traditional treatment methods based on anti-infection in the process of wound repair and provided a safe and effective new treatment of active repair and functional repair for wound repair and tissue regeneration.

Through the above-mentioned series of technological innovations, Professor Li's team has taken the lead in solving the series of genetic engineering technical problems in the process of FGF family protein pharmaceutical production in the world. The team has developed a new class of bioproducts with independent intellectual property rights, namely, bovine bFGF fusion protein, human bFGF, aFGF modifier, together with a class III implantable medical device containing FGF, which provides new therapeutic drugs for severe trauma, ulcer, and diabetic complications with a cumulative output value of over 4 billion yuan. And the team has established the first National Engineering Research

Center for genetic engineering drugs, which promoted the improvement of engineering technology in related fields in China.

#### 3.2.1.2 PDGF—Platelet-Derived Growth Factor

Platelet-derived growth factor (PDGF) is a basic protein normally stored in platelet alpha granules, which is secreted by various cells, such as macrophages chemotactic to the damaged site, smooth muscle cells at the damaged vessel, and vascular endothelial cells in the damaged area. PDGF has many important roles in embryonic development, cell differentiation, and response to tissue damage. It is one of the early growth factors in wound healing. In particular, it has significant healing effects on some chronic refractory wounds, such as diabetic ulcers, chronic venous ulcers, bedsores, and radiation ulcers.

Becaplermin (recombinant PDGF-BB) is currently the only growth factor drug approved by the FDA for the treatment of diabetic foot ulcers. In addition, rhPDGF-BB developed by a company has entered clinical phase III trials for pressure ulcers and venous ulcers. After more than 10 years of market application, rhPDGF-BB has been clinically proven to be safe and effective. rhPDGF-BB has a significant effect on the repair of pathological deep ulcer wounds and the promotion of skin vascular regeneration [3].

#### 3.2.1.3 NGF—Nerve Growth Factor

In the 1960s, Levi-Montalcini and Cohen isolated and purified a soluble protein that promotes nerve growth and named it nerve growth factor (NGF). The discovery of NGF has led to the recognition that in the development of the nervous system, some factors that promote the development and growth and maintain the activity of neurons are needed, thus opening up a new field of neurobiology. These two scholars won the Nobel Prize in Physiology or Medicine in 1986. The current clinical use of NGF is taken from the submandibular gland of mice. Numerous basic and clinical trials have confirmed that NGF plays an important role in the treatment of TBI and stroke.

NGF exerts neuroprotective effects by blocking the cascade of secondary damage to nerve cells. Its neuroprotective mechanism is as follows:

(a) Antagonizing the toxicity of excitatory amino acids: the increase of excitatory amino acids such as glutamate can lead to calcium overload, activate the apoptotic signaling pathway to allow neurons to enter the apoptosis program. NGF can inhibit the increase of glutamate, block calcium overload, and prevent neuronal apoptosis.
(b) Reducing oxygen free radicals: NGF can increase the activity of oxygen free radical scavengers such as catalase and superoxide dismutase, and reduce the peroxidation damage of neurons.
(c) Reducing the cytotoxicity of nitric oxide (NO): NO can inhibit the activity of oxidative phosphorylation enzyme, thereby inhibiting the respiratory function of cells. NGF reduces the cytotoxicity of NO by reducing the activity of NO synthase.
(d) Stabilizing intracellular Ca2+ concentration: NGF can regulate protein expression and function related to calcium influx, stabilize Ca2+ concentration, and inhibit neuronal damage caused by calcium overload.
(e) Inhibition of apoptosis protein activity: NGF can inhibit the activity of apoptosis proteins, inhibit the activity of pro-apoptotic proteins and apoptosis-executing proteins, and then inhibit neuronal apoptosis.

### 3.2.2 Important Proteins Involved in the Regulation of Tissue Regeneration Found in Lower Organisms

The tissues of various organisms on the earth have different regenerative abilities. This varying degree of tissue regeneration is formed after the long-term evolution of the organism. In general, the regeneration ability of lower biological tissues is stronger than that of higher organisms. Tissues with lower differentiation have stronger regeneration ability than tissues with higher differentiation. Tissues that are usually vulnerable to damage and tissues that are frequently updated under physiological conditions have strong regeneration ability. On the contrary, the regeneration ability is weak or lacking. In general, lower organisms (including plants) have a strong ability to regenerate. Higher organisms, such as humans, have weaker ability to regenerate, and generally only heal wounds and cannot reproduce a certain limb or an organ. Humans also have a certain ability to regenerate, but extremely limited. Some of the lower organisms have a strong ability to regenerate: the tail of the gecko, the limbs of the salamander, the foot of the crab can be reformed after being lost, and the sea cucumber can form all the internal organs. In contrast, human regeneration capacity is very limited.

#### 3.2.2.1 Pax6 Gene Regulatory Proteins and Lens Proteins Found in the Lens

The expression order of related proteins in the lens regeneration of the *Bufo raddei* tadpole is similar to that of the salamander. The expression order of proteins is β-crystallin, γ-crystallin, and α-crystallin, and the latter two proteins are expressed almost simultaneously. In the early stage of *Bufo raddei* tadpole regeneration, the pigment cells in the dorsal and ventral edge of the iris undergo dedifferentiation and cell proliferation, and Pax6 gene is expressed in the dorsal and ventral edge of the iris. During the differentiation of the regenerated lens cells, the Pax6 gene is expressed in the lens epithelial cells. In the process of lens regeneration, Pax6 gene is expressed in the retina, ciliary body region, cornea, and lens epithelium, and is mainly expressed in the ganglion cell layer, the inner nuclear layer, and the outer nuclear layer of retina. The expression of Pax6 gene is closely related to the regulation of lens regeneration. βB1 lens protein is an important structural protein distributed in the lens of animals. Both Pax6 and Prox1 can regulate the expression of βB1 lens protein. The expression of βB1 lens protein was detected by immunofluorescence technique after 21 days of lens regeneration in *Bufo raddei* tadpole. The experimental results further confirmed that the lens regeneration of *Bufo raddei* tadpole experienced dedifferentiation, cell proliferation, and cell redifferentiation of pigment epithelial cells on the dorsal edge of iris. In the process, both the regenerated lens and the normal lens expressed the βB1 lens protein. This research suggests that lens-associated proteins play a crucial role in the lens regeneration of lower organisms.

#### 3.2.2.2 Genes and Proteins Related to Nerve and Spinal Cord Regeneration

The zebrafish's nervous tissue has a strong ability to regenerate. Studies have shown that throughout the life of the zebrafish, its retina and other nerve tissues have been continuously undergoing metabolism of new and old cells, which means precursor cells with neurogenesis ability are always present in zebrafish. Regeneration of the retina and optic nerve was first used to study the regeneration of the zebrafish nervous system. During the regeneration of the retina, Muller glia cells play a huge role. And for the molecular signaling pathways that activate the cells, researchers have discovered numerous genes such as hspd2, msp1, mdka, mdkb, stat3, and signaling pathways such as Wnt, Notch, and FGF all play an important role in it. In recent years, studies on the regeneration of zebrafish spinal cord have been gradually carried out. In the regeneration of spinal cord, the difference in the regenerative capacity of different brain nuclei is obvious, and this difference depends on the location of spinal cord injury, suggesting the molecular mechanism controlling its regeneration is complex. Studies have found that cell adhesion proteins L1.1, GAP-43, cAMP, and other factors play a major role in spinal cord regeneration.

#### 3.2.2.3 HP1-1-Related Proteins and Mcm5 Pathway Regulate the Related Proteins of the Planarian Regeneration

Freshwater planarian also has a strong ability to regenerate, and when the body is cut to 1/279, it can still regenerate an intact individual. The regeneration potential of the planarian is mediated by its abundant adult stem cells, which initiate proliferation, migration, and directional differentiation to participate in the regeneration after the damage of the planarian. Scientists have discovered the role and function of 205 epigenetic factors in the regeneration of planarian, 12 new stem cell regulatory factors, and revealed that the epigenetic regulation mechanism of adult stem cells of the planarian is highly similar to that of higher organisms. They found that the heterochromatin protein HP1-1 is specifically expressed in the planarian stem cells and maintains self-renewal of stem cells. After the injury, HP1-1 promoted the regeneration and proliferation of stem cells. Unlike the previous reports of major involvement in heterochromatin formation and gene silencing, the molecular mechanism of Hp1-1 involved in the regeneration is mainly through promoting transcription elongation, and Mcm5 is an important downstream target gene, which is highly enriched and expressed in the stem cell group of planarians. HP1-1 can bind to the proximal promoter region of Mcm5 like the activated RNA polymerase after injury, thereby activating Mcm5, leading to upregulation of Mcm5, which is beneficial to the regeneration of planarians.

### 3.2.3 Tumor-Associated Tissue Regeneration Regulatory Proteins

With the research on tissue regeneration regulatory proteins, some tumor-regulated tissue regeneration regulatory proteins, including paxillin, focal adhesion kinase (FAK), midkine (MK), mammalian target of rapamycin (mTOR), have been discovered. They also play an important role in the regulation of tissue repair.

#### 3.2.3.1 Paxillin

Paxillin is a cytoskeletal protein involved in actin-membrane attachment at the site of adhesion (adhesion) of extracellular matrix cells. Paxillin plays an important role in the signaling of integrin, and the reorganization of cytoskeleton mediated by integrin requires phosphorylation of the paxillin tyrosine residues. Paxillin is phosphorylated by focal adhesion kinase (FAK) at its 118th tyrosine residue. Due to its special structure and function, paxillin has gradually attracted the attention of researchers. Many studies have shown that paxillin as a junction in cells can bind to a series of structural proteins and signal proteins and participate in cell migration activities associated with damage repair, embryo development, and tumor metastasis. Paxillin not only participates in the assembly of focal adhesions, but also plays an important role in cell morphological change, movement, adhesion, and cell signal transduction.

#### 3.2.3.2 Midkine

The midkine (MK), a heparin-binding growth factor, is a low molecular weight protein. MK is widely distributed in tissues during embryonic period, but it is limited to certain specific sites in adults. There are many kinds of MK receptors and the complex signaling pathways, which determine the diversity of MK functions. It can promote the growth, survival, differentiation, and migration of many cell types, and has antiapoptotic effects. It is not only closely related to tumorigenesis, but also involved in the development of many tissues and the repair and regeneration process after injury. A large number of MK expression can be detected in the early stages of tissue damage and repair processes such as cerebral infarction, peripheral nerve injury, spinal cord injury, fracture, myocardial infarction, and skin damage.

MK is not expressed in normal adult bone tissue. When the mouse's tibia fractures, MK expression can be detected during bone repair. After transfection of MK cDNA into ATDC5 chondrocytes, MK was overexpressed in the cells. As a result, most of the transfected cells showed stronger cartilage-forming ability, and they synthesized more sulfated mucopolysaccharides, aggrecan, and type II collagen. These results indicate that MK not only participates in bone formation and repair after injury, but also plays an important role in cartilage formation.

#### 3.2.3.3 Mammalian Target of Rapamycin

Mammalian target of rapamycin (mTOR) belongs to the phosphatidylinositol kinase-associated kinase (PIKK) superfamily and is a class of evolutionarily highly conserved protein kinases widely present in various biological cells. mTOR is an effect protein downstream of the phosphatidylinositol-3 kinase (PI3K)-Akt signaling pathway. It plays a key role in cell survival and participates in various biological processes such as gene transcription, protein translation initiation, and apoptosis under the activation of various factors. The main functions of the PI3K-Akt-mTOR signaling pathway can be summarized as the regulation of the synthesis of various proteins, cell growth, proliferation, and apoptosis. The signal from the mTOR protein is essential for the unique tissue regeneration of the planarian, which is common in humans and most mammals. The flatworm has the ability to regenerate cells, and the inactivation of mTOR protein prevents the regeneration of flatworms. This also indicates that inactivation of mTOR protein in mutant cells can also inhibit the growth of cancer cells.

## 3.3 Stem Cell Niche

In addition to self-renewal, adult stem cells produce daughter cells that maintain homeostasis by constantly producing and replacing short-lived and highly differentiated cells in blood, skin, midgut, nerves. Whether the stem cells are self-renewing or differentiation, this decision process is carefully controlled. If too many progeny cells begin to differentiate, the stem cells will decrease. In another case, unregulated self-renewal will increase the number of cells with proliferative function and partial differentiation, and their secondary mutations may increase, which may lead to tumorigenesis. If we can learn more about how stem cells are selected between differentiation and renewal, it will help to increase the number of stem cells and maintain their main characteristics, which is also a key step for transplantation and gene therapy by using stem cell potential.

### 3.3.1 Stem Cell Niches

Stem Cell Niche have the ability to self-replicate, and under certain conditions, they can differentiate into various functional cells. The directed differentiation of stem cells requires a relatively fixed, regulated microenvironment and tissue, which is called the stem cell niche [4]. Stem cell niches are composed of tissue cells and extracellular matrix which contain one or more stem cells and control the self-renewal of stem cells and the production of progeny cells [5]. It allows the distance between cells to be adapted to the interaction between cells and the production and transmission of short-range regulatory factors. Stem cells must proliferate in the niches to maintain self-renewal properties [6]. Adult stem cells are present in a special microenvironment in tissues and are strictly protected by structures such as surrounding cells and matrix [7].

Stem cells are present in the niches [8]. Once required physiologically or pathologically, surrounding cells or factors will send mobilization signals to stem cells to proliferate and differentiate, rapidly replenishing or repairing damaged tissue. Since it is difficult to manipulate stem cells and their surroundings in vivo, currently it is not possible to explicitly study the structure and function of any stem cell niches. In recent years, stem cell niches such as gonads, blood, skin, midgut, nerves, and kidneys have become hotspots in stem cell research [9–11]. A clearer study is the functional stem cell microenvironment of drosophila reproductive stem cells.

### 3.3.2 Drosophila Reproductive Stem Cell Niches

The gonads of drosophila have been used as a model system for studying stem cell niches, as the drosophila gonads have many advantages in the study of stem cell niches. First, the gonads of drosophila are relatively simple, and their structure has been studied clearly. Secondly, the drosophila gonads contain a single activated germ cell, and their supporting cells are accurately determined. Finally, drosophila germline stem cells (GSCs) produce two progeny cells by asymmetric division. One keeps stem cell characteristics in the stem cell niche, and the other leaves the niche and begins to differentiate.

#### 3.3.2.1 Structure and Characteristics of Drosophila Reproductive Stem Cell Niches

**Structure of Drosophila Ovary Stem Cell Niches**

The ovary of drosophila is a tubular structure, and reproductive stem cells and their niches are located at the blind end of the apex of the tubular structure. The drosophila ovary tube is a functional unit of ovary containing two to three reproductive stem cells at the apex of the ovary tube. Drosophila has 16 ovary tubes, so the production capacity of them is amazing. The front end of the drosophila ovary contains three different types of cells: terminal filament cells, cap cells, and inner germinal sheath cells (IGSs). Drosophila ovary stem cell niches are composed of these cells [12]. In addition, there is another stem cell, somatic stem cells (SSCs) in the niche [13].

**The Niche Structure of GSCs in Drosophila Testis**

The testis of drosophila is also a tubular structure [14]. In the testis of adult drosophila, hub cells, germ cells, and proto-encapsulated cells constitute the niches of testis stem cells. Among them, SSCs are in contact with hub cells and are also involved in the formation of niches. The testis stem cells divide in a similar manner to the ovary and in an asymmetric manner. The hub cells in the niches play a major role in signaling pathway. There exist two kinds of stem cells in the drosophila testis niches, namely GSCs and SSCs, just like ovarian.

### 3.3.3 Stem Cell Niches in Mammalian Tissues

Stem cells are a class of undifferentiated cells or primitive cells that have self-renewal and high proliferative capacity, and can differentiate into at least one mature cell in the body, which is one of the key factors for maintaining the morphology, function, and internal balance of tissues and organs. In recent years, with the development of stem cell research, people have paid more and more attention to the influence of living environment (niches) of stem cells in organism. The microenvironment around the stem cells (also known as stem cell niches or stem cell nests) maintains the characteristics of stem cells, the number of stem cells, and the fate of stem cells by direct and/or indirect interaction between their components (niche cells, extracellular matrix, related cytokines, and signal transduction molecules) and stem cells. In this chapter, we describe the structure of mammalian stem cell niches and their effects on stem cell self-renewal and biological characteristics by taking stem cell niches in germ cell lines, hematopoietic cell lines, epidermis, and small intestinal epithelium as examples.

#### 3.3.3.1 Testicular Germ Stem Cell Niches

**Testicular Germ Stem Cells and Their Niches**

The testis is an organ that produces sperm and secretes androgen [15]. The surface of the testis is covered with a serosa, and the inner membrane is a white membrane composed of dense connective tissue. The white membrane is thickened at the posterior edge of the testis to form the mediastinum testis, and radiated into the testis parenchyma. The testis is divided into about 250 conical lobules, each containing 1–4 seminiferous tubules. The seminiferous tubules are composed of spermatophytic epithelium. The spermatogenic epithelium is composed of spermatophytic cells and Sertoli cells, which are sites of spermatogenesis in the testis. At the fourth week during embryogenesis, there exist many large round cells derived from endoderm located near the posterior wall of the yolk sac, called primord germ cells. Primordial germ cells migrate to the gonadal ridge in the sixth week and enter the primary sex cord. Therefore, the seminiferous tubules in the embryonic period are solid cell cords, which contain two types of cells, namely, Sertoli cells differentiated from primary sex cord and spermatogonium differentiated from primord germ cells. In adults, the order of the seminiferous tubules from the basement membrane to the lumen is spermatogonia or spermatogonial stem cells (SSC), primary spermatocytes, secondary spermatocytes, spermatoblast, and spermatozoon.

The Sertoli cells mainly support and nourish the spermatogenic cells and promote the production of sperm and the movement of spermatogenic cells to the surface of the seminiferous tubules. Adjacent Sertoli cells are closely connected on the side near basal membrane to divide the spermatogenic epithelium into two parts: the basement compartment and the abluminal compartment. There are spermatogonia in the basement compartment, so the number of Sertoli cells limits the expansion of the number of spermatogonia. At the same time, the Sertoli cells, the basement membrane closely connected with spermatogenic epithelium and myoid cells, constitute the microenvironment (testis germ stem cell niches) for the growth of the testis germ stem cells (Fig. 3.1). The biological behavior of spermatogonial stem cells in the niche is affected by both their own factors and the niche microenvironment. They are slowly renewed or accelerated to keep their population constant, and at the same time produce a large number of differentiated spermatogonia to maintain organ function.

**The Role of Testis Germ Stem Cell Niches**

Testis germ cell niches provide a specific developmental environment for the self-renewal and survival of spermatogonia. Stem cells in the niche have strong ability to divide and proliferate, and maintain their undifferentiated state.

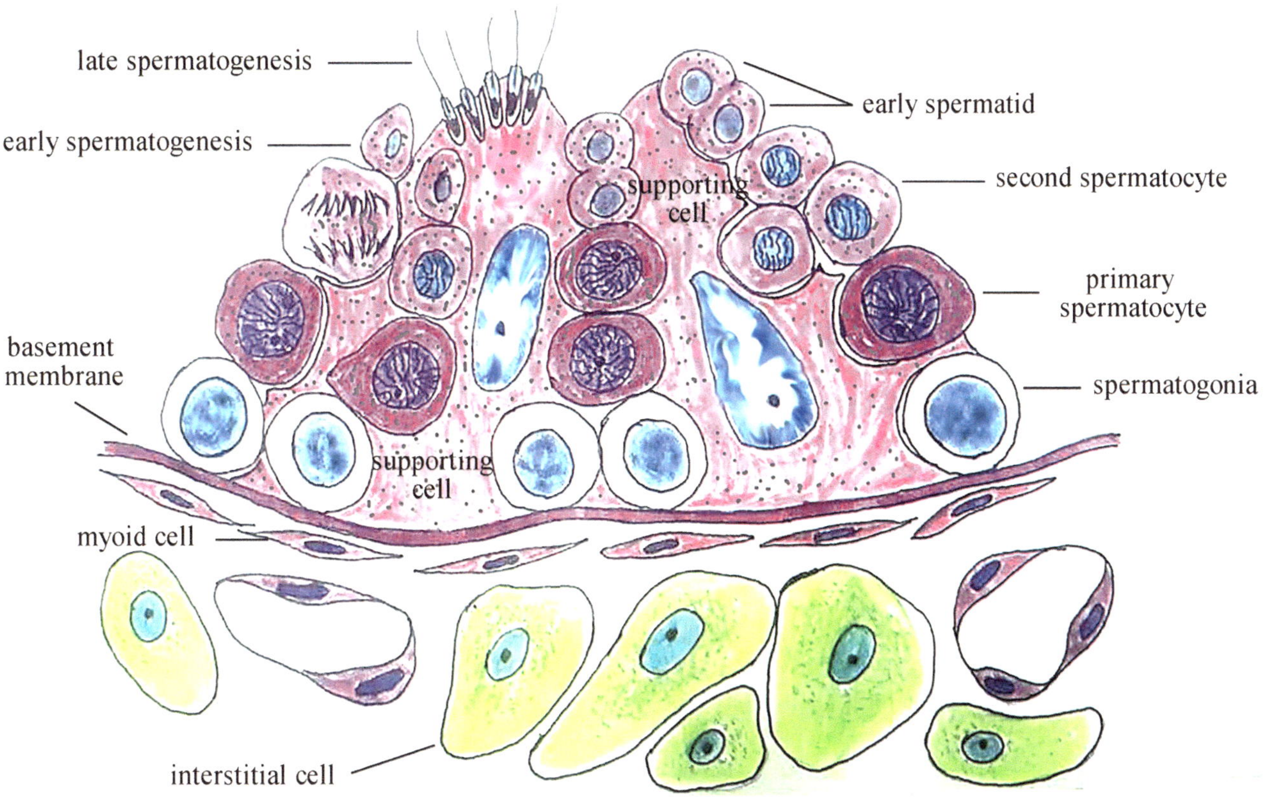


**Fig. 3.1** Schematic diagram of testis germ stem cell niche

Studies have shown that when spermatogonial stem cells were transplanted into the seminiferous tubule epithelium of immunodeficient mice, these exogenous germ stem cells could cross the tight junctions of multiple spermatogenic cells and Sertoli cells, search and migrate to the stem cell niches of basal compartment, form progeny clones, and perform biological functions [16].

#### Related Cytokines in Testis Germ Stem Cell Niches

On the one hand, the biological characteristics of stem cells are the results of their own pre-programming; on the other hand, they are affected by the microenvironment, that is, niches. Niches not only provide a specific developmental environment for stem cell self-renewal and survival, but also shield other factors that induce stem cell differentiation and help stem cells maintain their undifferentiated naive state. Current studies have shown that factors closely related to the differentiation and phenotypic maintenance of testis germ stem cells include c-Kit receptor and its ligand SCF, leukemia inhibitory factor (LIF), vitamin A (vitamin A, VA), epidermal growth factor (EGF), and glial cell line-derived neurotrophic factor (GDNF) [17–21].

### 3.3.3.2 Bone Marrow Hematopoietic Stem Cell Niches

#### Location and Concept of Bone Marrow Hematopoietic Stem Cells

Hematopoietic stem cells (HSCs) occur very early. Embryonic stem cells produced by several divisions of fertilized eggs begin to differentiate into hematopoietic stem cells while differentiating into embryo and extraembryonic structures. In the extraembryonic structure, hematopoietic stem cells are first seen in the extra-embryonic yolk sac blood island, which is a cell plexus formed by the primordial germ cells (PGCs) of the extraembryonic mesoderm on the yolk sac wall. The outer cells differentiate into vascular endothelial cells, which gradually become longer and connect to each other to form the original vascular network. The inner cells of the blood island remain round, free from the developing primitive vascular network, and differentiate into the earliest blood stem cells. During 16–19 days of gestational period, there are blood stem cells in the extra-embryonic tissues such as the yolk sac wall, body stalk, and chorion, and some stem cells develop into red blood cells. This period is called the hemopoietic period of yolk sac. During this period, the establishment of blood circulation inside and outside the embryo provides conditions for cell migration. The primordial germ cells present at the base of the extraembryonic allantoic sac begin to migrate to the para-aortic splanchnopleura (PAS) of the embryo and it further developed the aorta-gonad-mesoneph site (AGM), part of which is differentiated into blood stem cells in PAS/AGM. The blood stem cells formed in the embryo migrate to the liver primordium, making the liver the main hematopoietic organ in the fetal period, and also migrate to the spleen, thymus, and bone marrow, providing the most primitive blood stem cells for the formation of hematopoietic organs during fetal development. The yolk sac hematopoiesis terminates at the sixth week of embryonic development and is replaced by fetal liver hematopoiesis into the liver hematopoietic phase. In the 3- to 5-month-old fetal liver, there are about 50% immature red blood cells, only a small number of immature granulocytes and megakaryocytes. During this period, lymphocytes develop mainly in the thymus, spleen, and lymph nodes. Liver hematopoiesis begins to decline at the sixth month of embryonic development and ends at birth, replaced by bone marrow hematopoiesis. The bone marrow is a lifelong hematopoietic organ.

Hematopoietic stem cells have a high degree of self-renewal. Its basic characteristics are as follows:

(a) It has a strong proliferative potential, and can repeatedly divide under certain conditions and proliferate in large quantities, but under normal physiological conditions, most cells are in the G0 quiescent state.
(b) It has a multidirectional differentiation potential. Under the influence of some factors, it can differentiate into different progenitor cells.
(c) It has the ability of self-replication, that is, the daughter cells after cell division still have the original characteristics, so hematopoietic stem cells can maintain a constant amount for life. In hematopoietic tissue, hematopoietic stem cells are difficult to distinguish from other monocytes in morphology. In recent years, due to advances in monoclonal antibody technology, the application of flow cytometric sorting (FACS), research on the surface markers of hematopoietic stem cells has made great progress. It is currently believed that the surface markers of human hematopoietic stem cells are $CD34^+$, $CD38^-$, $HLA^-$, $DR^-$, $Lin^-$, Thy-$1^+$, c-$Kit^+$, Sca-$1^+$, LFA-$1^-$, $CD45RA^-$, $CD71^-$, Rhodull, and so on.

### Bone Marrow Hematopoietic Stem Cell Niches and their Effects

During physiological development, blood stem cells are mainly distributed in hematopoietic tissues. The hematopoietic inductive microenvironment is extremely important, which is the internal environment for growth and development of hematopoietic cells. The hematopoietic inductive microenvironment is a connective tissue composed of bone marrow nerve components, microvasculature system, fibers, matrix, and stromal cells. It is a "niche" for blood stem cells to maintain the best functional state (Fig. 3.2). Stromal cell is an important component in hematopoietic stem cell niches, including reticular cells, fibroblasts, sinusoidal endothelial cells, macrophages, and adipocytes. Bone marrow stromal cells not only support hematopoietic cells, but also secrete cytokines and regulate the proliferation and differentiation of hematopoietic cells. The distribution of various blood cells in the hematopoietic tissue during development has certain regularity. Immature red blood cells are often located near the sinusoids, and they are embedded in the surface of macrophages to form the erythroblastic islet (Fig. 3.3). As the cells mature, they are close to and pass through the sinusoidal endothelium, and their nuclei are removed to become reticulocytes. The immature granulocytes are far away from the sinusoids. When they develop into metamyelocytes and have the ability to move, they approach and penetrate the sinusoids by their amoeboid movement. The megakaryocytes are often attached to the endothelial space of the blood sinusoid, and extend the cytoplasmic processes into the sinus cavity to form platelets after falling off. This distribution indicates that different parts of the hematopoietic stem cell niche have different induction and regulation effects on hematopoietic cells.

### Related Regulatory Factors in the Bone Marrow Hematopoietic Stem Cell Niche

Blood circulation ensures the formation of embryonic and fetal hematopoietic organs and the evolution of multistage hematopoietic centers. Similarly, after hematopoietic stem cell transplantation, exogenous hematopoietic stem/progenitor cells migrate, recognize, and locate from peripheral blood to bone marrow through complex molecular interaction. This multistep process is called homing. Hematopoietic stem cells cannot develop normally in the peripheral blood circulation or non-hematopoietic organs. Only after they return to a certain position of the hematopoietic organs through blood circulation, that is, homing, can they exercise their physiological functions. The Wnt signaling pathway, the Notch signaling pathway, and the homeobox (HOX) transcription factor family have all been proven to be closely related to the development and renewal of hematopoietic stem cells, regulating the behavior of hematopoietic stem cells from different levels [22–24].

The self-renewal capacity of HSC is limited, and continuous transplantation can eventually lead to exhaustion of HSC. The senescence of human adult cells is associated with the lack of expression of telomerase and shortening of telomere length. The low level of telomerase activity in

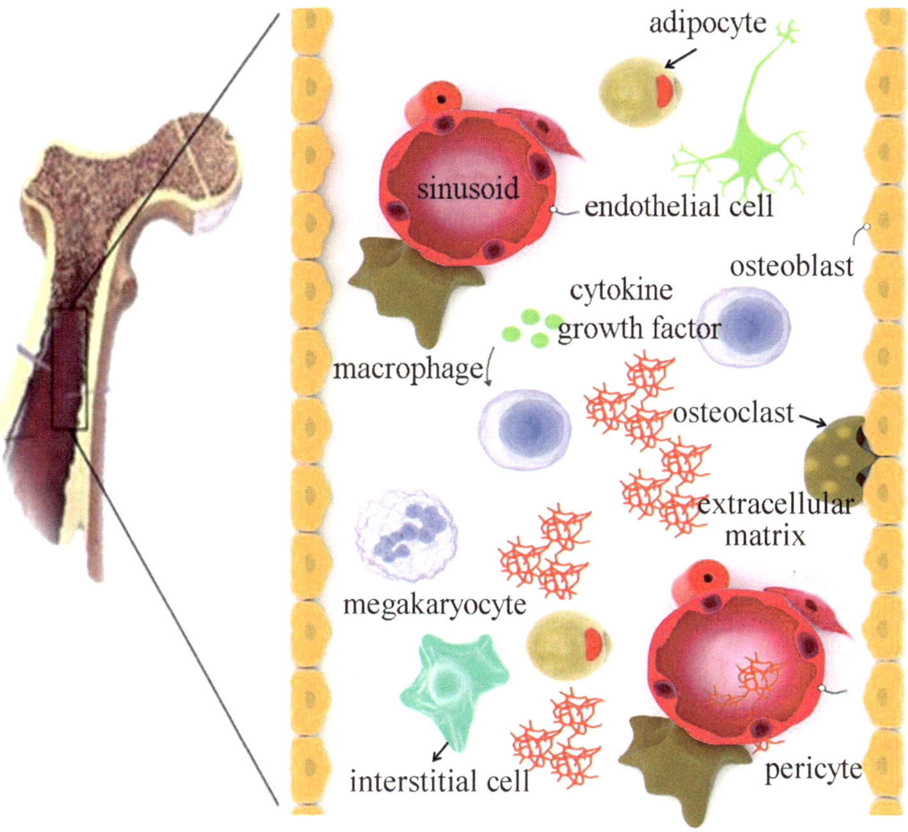


**Fig. 3.2** Schematic diagram of the hematopoietic inductive microenvironment of the red bone marrow

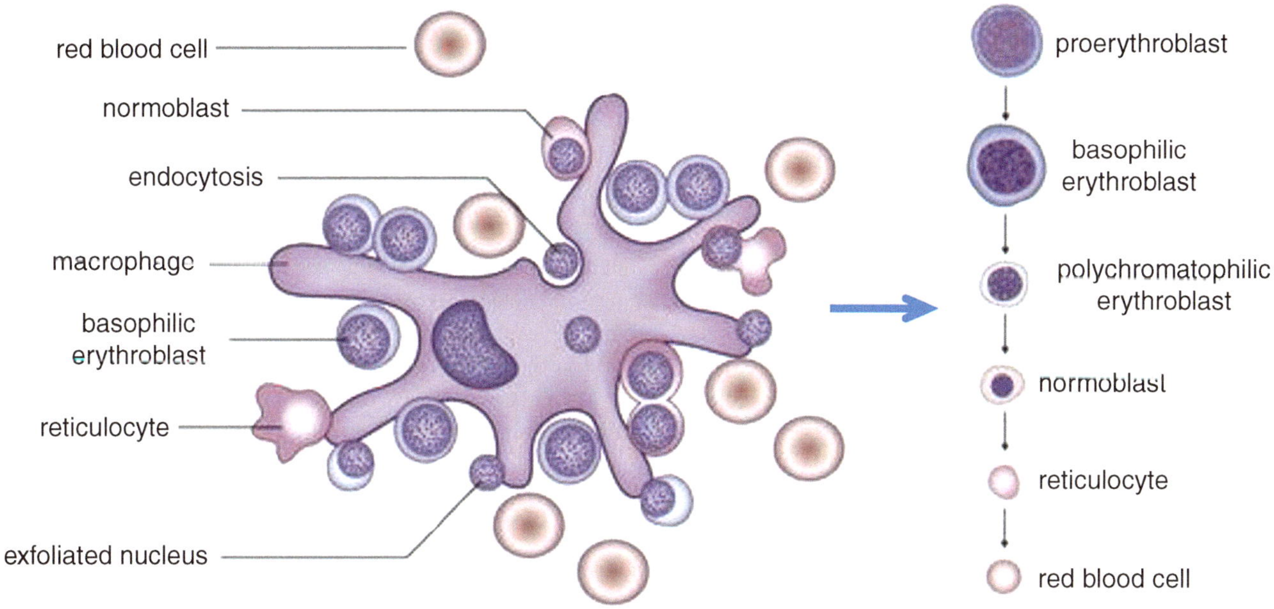


**Fig. 3.3** Ultrastructural diagram of bone marrow erythroblastic islet

HSC is not sufficient to inhibit HSC telomere shortening, so it is speculated that HSC overexpression of telomerase or its components can enhance HSC self-renewal ability. However, Allsopp et al. found that telomerase reverse transcriptase (TERT) overexpression inhibited the shortening of telomere length of HSC in continuous transplantation, but the hematopoietic reconstitution ability of HSC in transgenic mouse was not different from that of wild type [25]. Overexpression of the antiapoptotic gene bcl-2 in HSC can increase the number of HSCs, indicating that antiapoptotic signals are involved in the regulation of HSC self-renewal. Cyclin-dependent kinase inhibitor (CKI) p21 controls stem cells into the cell cycle and is an important factor in maintaining HSC in quiescence.

In the absence of HSC, activation into the cell cycle and self-renewal ability are impaired. P18 specifically acts on the early G1 of the cell cycle and binds to cyclin-dependent kinase (CDK) 4/6 to inhibit phosphorylation of retinoblastoma protein (Rb) and arrest cell cycle progression [26]. At present, the relationship between Wnt signaling pathway, Notch signaling pathway, and HOX transcription factor family regulating HSC self-renewal and CKI is still unclear, and further research is needed [27].

#### 3.3.3.3 Skin Stem Cell Niches

##### Location and Concept of Skin Stem Cells

Skin stem cells, that is, keratinocyte stem cells, are mainly located in the basal layer of the epidermis, the periphery of the sebaceous glands, and the bulge of root sheath outside the hair follicle [28]. Skin stem cells self-renew through asymmetric division, and at the same time form a new daughter cell, transit-amplifying cells (TA cells) [29]. The transit-amplifying cells continue to divide, expand, and move up to form other cell layers such as granular cell layer, prickle cell layer, and the like. With the passage of time, the granular cells and spinous layer cells mature and perform the tissue function, gradually aging and losing their organelles, which are replaced by the keratin secreted by the cells themselves to form a transparent layer or a stratum corneum until falling off. This process can be called anagen, catagen, and telogen. The epidermis is following this continually recurrent physiological process, self-renewal, and self-healing.

Like other stem cells, keratinocytes have the following characteristics: the cell morphology is naive, maintaining a relatively undifferentiated state; it has strong self-renewal ability; in normal state, the cell cycle of stem cells is slow, but it can also respond to external stimuli, rapidly enter cell division cycle, and maintain the integrity of organ or tissue morphology and function. Potten used 3H-thymidine absorption method to measure skin stem cells. It was found that the cells with slow metabolism of 3H-thymidine were mainly located in the basal layer of the epidermis, while the cells with active metabolism were located in the suprabasal layer. Jones and Watt found that epidermal stem cells can express integrins β1. Later, Kaur study found that keratinocytes can also express integrins α6. The cells with strong positive expression of these integrins β1 and α6 not only showed strong proliferative ability, but also showed different adhesion ability to extracellular matrix. In 1980, Fuchs and Green reported for the first time that skin stem cells can express keratin 19 (K19) [30].

There are many types of keratin, which are widely expressed in skin tissues. The occurrence and development of skin are closely related to the programmed expression of keratin gene. K5 and K14 are mainly expressed in the basal layer and upper basal layer of the primary epithelium of the embryonic mouse. After 9.5 days of embryonic development, K5 and K14 are only expressed in the basal layer of the epidermis and downregulated. K1 and K10 are mainly expressed in the granular cells and spinous layer cells. In the process of studying the expression of cytokeratin in skin, Li Haihong found that K7 is mainly expressed in the outer root sheath of hair follicles in fetal period, and has no obvious expression in adult stage. K7 can be used as an indicator to study the development and maturity of hair follicles. K10 is mainly expressed in the basal layer, which can be used as a marker for terminal differentiation of epidermal cells. K14 is strongly expressed in the basal layer and skin appendages. Bokis Risek found that the expression time, expression level, and expression site of the gap junction gene-encoding products α1 and β2 connexin are related to the directional differentiation of skin stem cells. The intermediate filament protein Nestin, which is abundantly expressed in neuroepithelial cells in early embryonic development, can also be strongly expressed in hair follicle precursor cells. In 1996, Thierry Magnaldo reported that CD24 cDNA is abundantly expressed in the cytoplasm of keratinocyte colony-forming cells (K-CFCs), which are mainly distributed in the bulge, one-third of outer root sheath and the end of the hair ball. As the hair follicle matures, CD24 cDNA expression also showed relative displacement changes. Although CD24 does not directly act on the self-renewal of keratinocytes, it provides a reference for distinguishing keratinocytes from differentiated cells at the molecular level. In 2000, Hiroaki successfully isolated stem cells from TA cells by using in vivo cell dynamic analysis and fluorescent living cell tracer technology and demonstrated that mouse epidermal stem cells have high-level expression of α6 integrin and low-level expression of transferrin receptor (CD71), so it is also called α6bri/CD71dim cells; the TA cells are positive for α6 integrin and CD71, so it is called α6bri/ CD71bri cells.

##### Skin Stem Cell Niches and their Effects

Skin stem cells play an important role in maintaining the balance, renewal, and repair of the internal environment of tissues and organs. Under normal circumstances, skin stem cells proliferate and differentiate according to a certain probability and mode. When the body is damaged, the proliferation and differentiation mode of skin stem cells will change to meet the needs of the body. Therefore, the proliferation and differentiation behavior of skin stem cells are preprogrammed on the one hand; on the other hand, they are regulated by the microenvironment of skin stem cells (also known as skin stem cell niche). Nowadays, more and more studies have shown that hair follicle bugle is one of the concentrated areas of skin stem cells, where cells not only have strong proliferative capacity, but also have the potential of multidirectional differentiation, so bulge is also known as hair follicle stem cell niche (Fig. 3.4). In 1990, Cotsarelis first proposed the "bulge activation hypothesis" (Fig. 3.5). Subsequently, Taylor and Oshima confirmed the localization of hair follicle stem cells through experiments, and proposed the "hair follicle stem cell migration hypothesis." The hypothesis is that during the periodic growth of hair follicles, the cells in the bugle migrate down to the hair ball after being induced by some factors, transform into proliferative hair matrix cells, and then proliferate and differentiate into hairs upward and inward. When the cells in bugle receive some unknown signal and stop producing new stem cell individuals, the growth phase ends. In 2000, Commo et al. proposed the "hair follicle stem cell reservoir hypothesis" by studying K19 staining in the outer root sheath of hair follicles. They speculated that the outer root sheath of the hair follicle contained two stem cell regions, one migrated down with the newborn hair follicle and the other was fixed at the bulge of the hair follicle. Although there is still much controversy in this hypothesis, it explains the origin of trichoepithelioma and the reasons for the growth and regeneration ability of the hair follicles after being removed.

The stromal cells surrounding the dermal papilla in the decline period stop dividing and expanding, the hair follicles

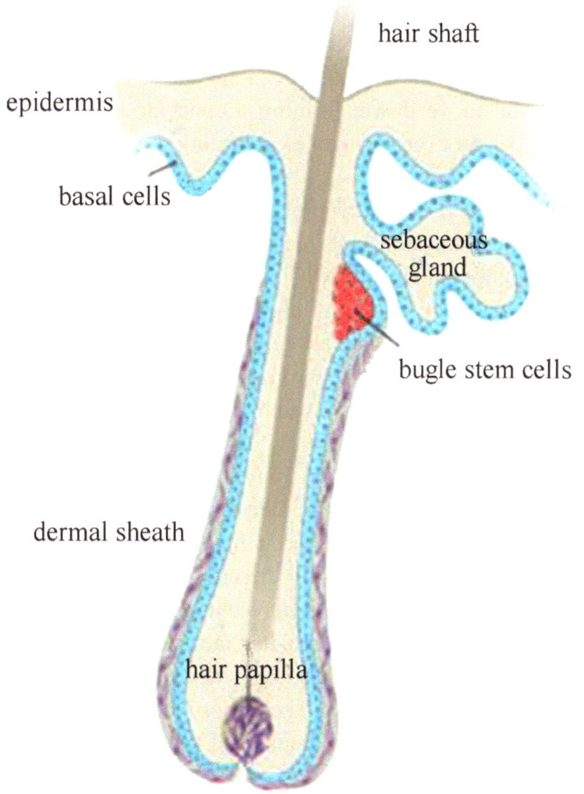


**Fig. 3.4** Schematic diagram of hair follicle stem cell niche

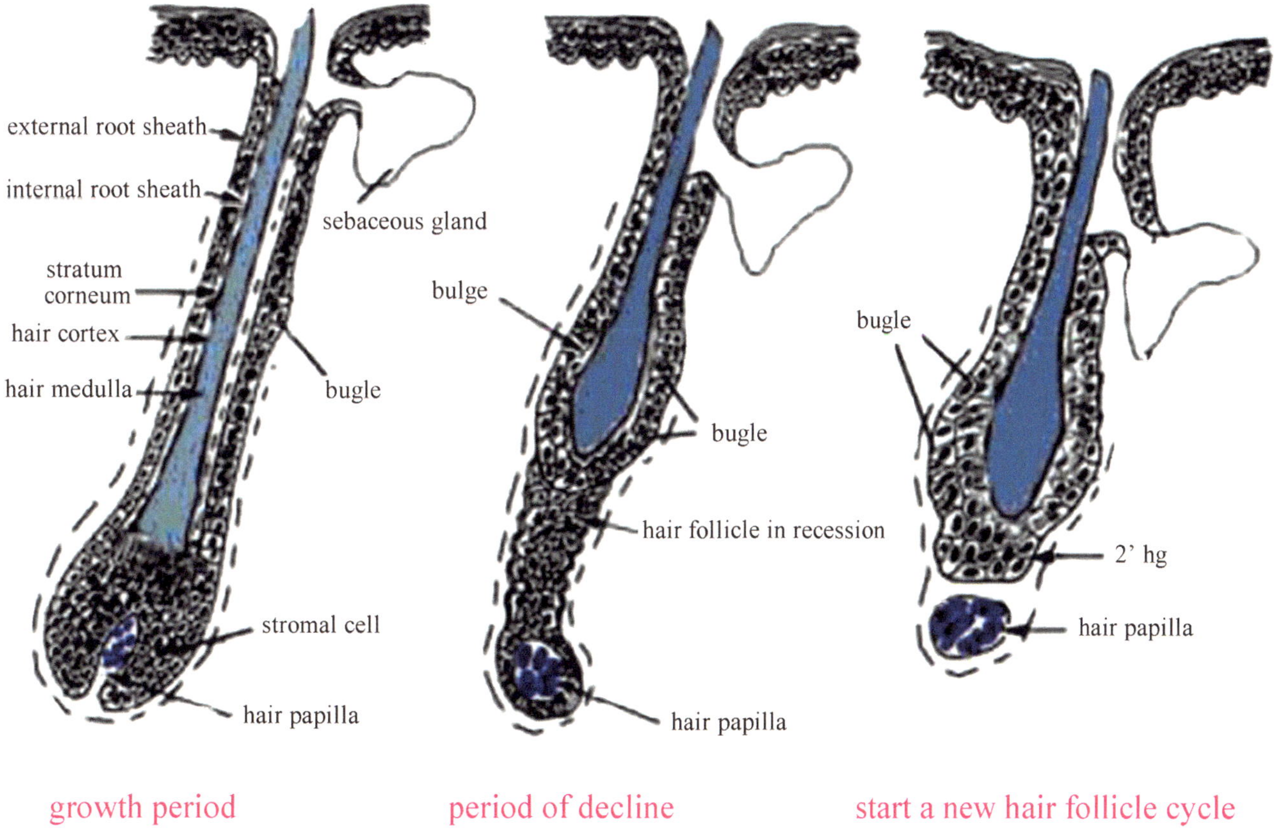


**Fig. 3.5** Bulge activation hypothesis

no longer grow, and the bottom is degenerated; then the DP cells move up to the outer root sheath to enter the stationary phase; the dermal papilla interacts with the bulge cells to induce stromal cells and outer root sheath cells to divide, expand, and move down, forming a concentric circle-like IRS and hair root (growth stage) according to a certain spatial structure.

Skin stem cell niches regulate the proliferation and differentiation of skin stem cells mainly through cells and cells, cells and extracellular matrix [7]. Cytokines play an important role in the transmission of information between cells and extracellular matrix, cells and cells [31, 32]. Extracellular matrix components such as fibronectin, laminin, and different types of collagen are involved in the maintenance of epidermal stem cell characteristics and the regulation of biological processes such as proliferation and differentiation. The gap junction between the epidermal stem cells, as one of the information channels between niches and the outside world, limits the differentiation direction of the epidermal stem cell community. In addition, recent studies have shown that many signal transduction-related factors are involved in the regulation of keratinocyte self-renewal, division, and proliferation, such as lymphoid enhancer factor/T cell factor (LEF/TCF), tumor necrosis factor (TNF), transcription factor Myc, and T lymphocyte differentiation regulator GATA-3.

#### Skin Stem Cell Niche-Related Signaling Regulators

At present, it has been found that the signaling pathways that maintain and regulate epidermal stem cell status are mainly MAPK, Wnt, Notch, BMP, and Shh. In addition, there are many other signal pathways to be discovered.

(a) Mitogen-activated protein kinase (MAPK) [33]: MAPK is a class of protein kinase with serine/threonine residues, which is widely distributed in cells and a group of important signal-regulating enzymes that are closely related to membrane surface receptors and decisive genes expression. The MAPK pathway is an important nuclear activation transcription factor response pathway involved in the regulation of various physiological and pathological processes such as growth, differentiation, division, death, and synchronization of cell functions.

(b) Wnt signaling pathway [34]: Wnt gene encodes a variety of secretory signaling molecules, which are related to the occurrence and development of many tissues and organs, such as brain, nerve, spinal cord, bone, retina, and kidney. A variety of Wnt proteins such as Wnt3, Wnt3a, Wnt4, Wnt5a, Wnt7a, Wnt7b, Wnt10a, Wnt10b, Wnt11, and Wnt16 can be expressed in the skin. Wnt10a and Wnt10b are expressed in the primordial primordium of hair follicles, and Wnt3, Wnt3a, Wnt4, Wnt5a, Wnt10a, Wnt10b, and Wnt11 are expressed in hair follicle anterior cortex cells.

(c) Notch signaling pathway [35]: The Notch signal transduction pathway regulates the fate specification of embryonic and terminally differentiated tissue cells through local cell-cell interactions, and is mainly involved in promoting the differentiation of root sheath keratinocytes in hair follicles.

(d) Bmp signal transduction pathway [36]: Bone morphogenetic protein-4 (BMP-4) can induce the expression of LEF1 in mesenchymal cells at the early stage of hair follicle primordium formation. Bone morphogenetic protein and bone morphogenetic protein inhibitors regulate the expression of LEF1 by regulating the homeostasis between them, thereby determining the response of mesenchymal tissue cells, epithelial precursor cells, and hair follicle progenitor cells to Wnt signaling pathway.

(e) Shh signal transduction pathway: Shh is mainly expressed in stromal cells at the end of hair follicles during the growth phase and is involved in the regulation of hair follicle stem cell migration and differentiation during hair follicle growth and regeneration. When the Shh function is blocked, the hair follicles stop growing, and the ectopic expression of the Shh target gene can cause the occurrence of hair follicle tumors.

### 3.3.3.4 Intestinal Stem Cell Niches

#### Intestinal Stem Cells and Their Niches

Mammalian intestinal mucosal epithelium is the most active place of the body's metabolism. The intestinal mucosal epithelial cells undergo continuous self-renewal throughout the life, which is mainly driven by pluripotent stem cells located at the bottom of the small intestine crypt. The stem cells located at the bottom of the small intestine crypt maintain a strong proliferation and differentiation ability [37], and there is a dynamic balance between the cells with apoptosis and damage necrosis and stem cell with proliferation and differentiation. Therefore, intestinal stem cells play an important role in maintaining the structural and functional integrity of the intestinal barrier and repairing after injury. The epithelium of the small intestine consists of monolayer columnar cells, such as absorptive cells, goblet cells, M cells, Paneth cells, and a small number of endocrine cells. The intestinal epithelium of human, mouse, and rat can be functionally divided into two discrete units: the villus differentiation unit and the crypt proliferation unit. The small intestinal stem cells proliferate and differentiate to form oriented progenitor cells, and the oriented progenitor cells rapidly differentiate into Paneth cells, goblet cells, M cells, absorptive cells, and endocrine cells. Paneth cells migrate down to the bottom of the crypt, and the remaining four cells migrate toward the intestinal lumen to supplement the mucosal epithelial cells which shed from the top of the villi. The entire migration process takes 3–5 days. The main characteristics of small intestinal stem cells are as follows:

(a) Stem cell markers are relatively clear and can express surface marker proteins such as musashi-1, Sca-1, keratin-6, integrinβ1, Hes1.
(b) With radiation hypersensitivity, small dose irradiation can induce apoptosis.
(c) Small intestinal stem cells selectively isolate chromosomes to retain the characteristics of the parental stem cells and maintain the stability of the genetic material.
(d) Small intestine crypts and adjacent villi in adult are monoclonal sources.

In addition, the proliferation and differentiation of small intestinal stem cells is achieved by the division of crypts. The small intestinal stem cells are located in the fourth to fifth layer from the bottom of the small intestine crypt, above the Paneth cells. Each crypt has 4 to 6 actual stem cells and about 30 potential stem cells. Small intestinal stem cells maintain a stable number of stem cells in the crypt by symmetric and asymmetric divisions. Which way is the main one depends on the internal environment in which the stem cells are located. Under normal physiological conditions, small intestinal stem cells of adult mice generally undergo proliferation and differentiation processes by asymmetric division. Therefore, supporting cells, extracellular matrix, and secretory cytokines derived from supporting cells in the small intestine crypt constitute stem cell niches that affect the proliferation and differentiation behavior of small intestinal stem cells (Fig. 3.6).

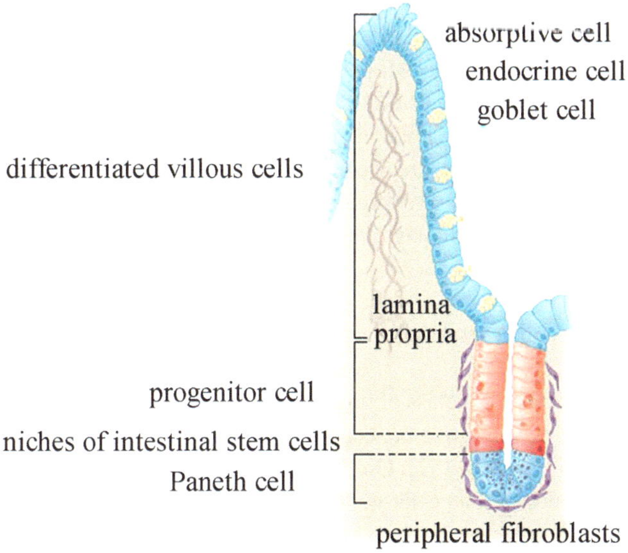


**Fig. 3.6** Schematic diagram of intestinal stem cell niche

As shown in the figure, the small intestine stem cells are located in the fourth to fifth cells from the bottom of the small intestine crypt, above the Paneth cells; the supporting cells, the extracellular matrix, and the secretory cytokines derived from the supporting cells in the small intestine crypt constitute microenvironment for the proliferation and differentiation of small intestinal stem cells.

#### Intestinal Stem Cell Niche-Associated Regulatory Molecules

Small intestinal stem cell niches provide a material basis for the proliferation and differentiation of intestinal stem cells, in which cytokines play an important role in affecting the proliferation and differentiation of stem cells, such as basic fibroblast growth factor (bFGF) [38], transforming growth factor-β (TGF-β), EGF, TNF, IGF-1, and the like [39]. In addition, many apoptosis-related genes such as p53 [40], Bcl-2 [41], p38, c-Fos, and c-Jun have also played an important regulatory role in the proliferation and differentiation of intestinal stem cells.

#### Intestinal Stem Cell Niche-Related Signal Transduction Pathway

As for the effects of small intestinal microenvironmental signal transduction on stem cell maintenance and differentiation, the current research focuses on the Notch and Wnt/β-catenin signaling pathways; the former determines the fate of stem cells differentiation, and the latter determines the maintenance of stem cell status [1, 42].

### 3.3.3.5 Neural Stem Cell Niches

#### Neural Stem Cells and Their Niches

In 1992, Reynolds et al. isolated stem cells from the corpus striatum of rat brain, which can continuously proliferate in vitro and have potential to differentiate into neurons and astrocytes [43]. Since then, the isolation, culture, identification, and research in vitro of neural stem cells have made gratifying progress. Neural stem cells (NSCs) are specific primitive nerve cells in the nervous system that can proliferate and differentiate into neurons and glial cells. They have the characteristics of high self-renewal ability, multipotential differentiation, migration function, and good tissue fusion [44]. NSCs are widely distributed in the central nervous system of mammalian embryos, including the cerebral cortex, corpus striatum, hippocampus, olfactory bulb, cerebellum, spinal cord, etc. In adult, NSCs are limited to the hippocampal dentate gyrus and subependymal zone. At present, the specific surface marker proteins of NSCs are still not well defined, and Nerns is commonly used as a detection marker to identify NSCs [45]. Nestin belongs to the class VI intermediate filament protein and is abundantly expressed in the neuroepithelial cells in the early stage of embryonic development. However, in recent years, it has been found that Nestin is not only expressed in neural stem cells, but also expressed in many tissues, such as pancreatic precursor cells, hair follicle precursor cells, human umbilical cord blood mononuclear cells, bone marrow stromal cells, pancreatic vascular endothelial cells, etc. Other neural stem cell markers such as Vimentin, RNA binding protein Musashi-1, CD133, glial fibrillary acidic protein (GFAP), etc. are less used due to relative lack of specificity.

The proliferation and differentiation of neural stem cells are affected by the surrounding microenvironment [46, 47]. The state and the microenvironment of the stem cells determine whether the stem cells are in the resting or dormant state, whether they differentiate or mature, and which type of cells they are going to differentiate [3]. For example, in mammals, only the neural stem cells of the subventricular zone (SVZ) and the subgranular zone (SGZ) of the hippocampal dentate gyrus can differentiate into neuronal cells in vivo, while in other regions neural stem cells can only differentiate into glial cells in vivo. If the stem cells of the neurogenesis area are transplanted into a non-neurogenic region, these stem cells can only differentiate into glial cells, and stem cells derived from non-neurogenic regions can differentiate into neurons after being transplanted into the neurogenesis region [48]. The microenvironment surrounding the neural stem cells is also called neural stem cell niche or neural stem cell nest, which mainly includes nearby supporting cells, extracellular matrix, microvascular network, cell regulatory factors, and neurotransmitter mediators. These components interact to form a complex regulatory network that affects the biological characteristics and behavioral outcomes of neural stem cells.

#### Neural Stem Cell Niche-Related Regulatory Molecules

The effects of neural stem cell niches on the differentiation of NSCs are mainly reflected in the following four aspects:

(a) The effect of cytokines on the differentiation of NSCs: Cytokines play a key role in the growth and differentiation of NSCs. Currently, growth factors can be used to separate NSCs from brain tissue, which can make stem cells further proliferate and differentiate in vitro, so as to provide a large number of seed cells for the study of biological characteristics of stem cells and stem cell transplantation. Among them, FGF and EGF are widely studied.

    In addition, in vitro experiments have also observed that brain-derived growth factor (BDNF), insulin-like growth factor-1 (IGF-1), and retinoic acid can promote the differentiation of NSCs into neuron phenotypes. The neurotrophic factor NGF has the ability to induce the differentiation of NSCs into cholinergic neurons and promote the growth and thickening of differentiated neuronal processes. Platelet-derived growth factor (PDGF) and retinoic acid can induce hippocampal NSCs to differentiate into neurons.

(b) The effect of intercellular interaction on NSCs differentiation: The supporting cells of the neural stem cell nest mainly include astrocytes, ependymal cells, and radial neuroglia cells. When NSCs are in different cellular environments, their differentiations are not the same. Intercellular interactions affect NSC differentiation and maturation [49].

(c) The effect of extracellular matrix on neural stem cells: Extracellular matrix (ECM) is composed of various glycoproteins, mucins, neuroadhesion factors, etc., which is an important part of neural stem cell nest in space. ECM can play the role of microenvironment signal amplifier by adjusting adhesion and signal molecule aggregation [50].

(d) The effect of Notch signal transduction pathway on NSCs differentiation [2]: Although many foreign signals play an important role in stem cell development and differentiation, it does not negate the role of stem cell expression in regulating differentiation and development. There is evidence that the diversity of neural cell development may be related to the expression of various transcription factors in stem cells, and the expression of different transcription factors leads to the differentiation of different lineages. Gene regulation of NSCs involves both positive and negative dual regulation. Negative regulation keeps NSCs in their undifferentiated state, increasing the number of NSCs by symmetric division, mainly including Notch signaling pathway; positive regulation promotes NSCs differentiation by asymmetric division, and bHLH (basic helix loop helix) transcription factors include Mash1, NeuroD, Neurogenins (Ngn1/Ngn2), and the Mash family. The Notch signaling pathway, which conducts the Mash signal of interaction between cells, precisely regulates the behavior of cells in each lineage through signal transmission between adjacent cells and plays a key role in cell differentiation [51].

### 3.3.4 Summary

Stem cells are a class of undifferentiated primitive cells with strong proliferative capacity and multidirectional differentiation potential [52]. On the one hand, the biological characteristics of stem cells are the results of self-preprogramming; on the other hand, they are affected by the microenvironment. Stem cell niches can exert multiple biological effects through direct and/or indirect effects between its components (niche cells, ECM, and the cytokines secreted by niche cells) and stem cells. The functions of stem cell niches are summarized below.

(a) Anchoring stem cells and regulating their presence in the G0 phase: This ability of stem cell niches is related to the expression of adhesion molecules by their components. Cadherin- and integrin-mediated cell adhesion are ubiquitous. The mechanism of anchoring stem cells in niches is that the integrin on the surface of stem cells can mediate the adhesion between stem cells and ECM, so that stem cells can settle in the niches. In addition, stem cell niches can also recruit new stem cells and make them migrate back into the niches, which are the "homing" phenomenon of stem cells.
(b) Maintaining the balance between self-renewal and differentiation of stem cells: Stem cell function is dual. It is necessary to maintain the self-renewal of stem cells as well as the differentiation of stem cells. Stem cells generally self-renew through asymmetric division and produce daughter cells at the same time; or maintain the balance between self-renewal and differentiation by alternate symmetrical proliferation and differentiation. The niche structure is asymmetrical, and this asymmetry may be combined with the mechanism of stem cell division to determine the division mode of stem cells and affect the fate of the daughter cells.
(c) Regulating stem cell fate: Stem cell niche provides a protective microenvironment for stem cells, shielding the influence of externally induced differentiation factors on stem cells and maintaining the undifferentiated state of stem cells. Niche components: niche cells, extracellular matrix, and soluble factors derived from niche cells can regulate stem cells by direct or indirect interaction with stem cells. The change of niche signals can cause changes in stem cell fate. A variety of growth factors related to niche, such as interleukin, Wnt protein, EGF, and its family members, IGF, TGF-β, LIF, etc., are closely related to the proliferation and differentiation of stem cells. In addition, multiple signaling pathways such as Wnt, BMP, MAPK, Notch, Shh, and Tie2/Ang-1 interweave into a network to control the behavior of stem cells [53].

At present, stem cells have become a hotspot in life science research, which makes people see the hope of conquering diabetes, Parkinson's disease, tumor, and other clinical diseases that are still difficult to cure. With the further study of stem cells and their surrounding microenvironment, people can control the self-renewal and differentiation of stem cells through regulation of stem cell niches, which can provide new research strategies for the treatment of tumors and other degenerative diseases and the development of regenerative medicine.

## 3.4 Signals Involved in Tissue Repair and Regeneration

Wound repair and tissue regeneration refer to a series of complicated and orderly pathological and physiological processes that local tissues complete repair and reconstruction through regeneration and replacement after tissue loss due to the role of wound causing factors. It is a cascade reaction involving local inflammatory cells, extracellular matrix, damaged site cells, blood-derived cells, growth factors/cytokines, and even nervous system, immune system, and endocrine system. The process mainly includes the inflammatory phase, the proliferative phase, and the remodeling phase. A series of biological activities involve the transmission of cellular signals to complete all biological effects.

### 3.4.1 Mitogen-Activated Protein Kinase

Mitogen-activated protein kinase (MAPK) is a kind of serine/threonine protein kinase widely distributed in animal cells and plant cells. Its main function is to transmit extracellular stimulation signals into cells and nuclei to cause cellular biological reactions (proliferation, differentiation, stress, apoptosis, etc.). Multiple parallel MAPKs signaling pathways have been identified. Different extracellular stimuli activate different MAPKs signaling pathways to mediate different cellular biological responses. Four different MAPKs pathways have been discovered in mammals: the extracellular signal-regulated kinase (ERK) pathway, the JNK/SAPK pathway, the p38/MAPK pathway, and the ERK5 pathway. These four pathways are activated by independent (sometimes interactive cross-talk) signal cascades.

#### 3.4.1.1 Extracellular Signal-Regulated Kinase

Extracellular signal regulated protein kinases (ERKs) are a class of protein kinases that are distributed in the cytoplasm and have the dual phosphorylation ability of serine and tyrosine. They are important members of the MAPK family. ERK includes five families: ERK1/ERK2, ERK5, ERK3/ERK4, of which ERK1/ ERK2 is the first cloned member of the MAPK family. Mitogen can activate ERK1 and ERK2 in almost all mammalian cells. ERK1 and ERK2, also known as p44MAPK and p42MAPK, have relative molecular masses of 4400 and 4200, respectively, and are downstream signaling proteins of various growth factors (EGF, bFGF, NGF, PDGF, IGF, etc.). The basic signal transmission steps follow the three-stage enzymatic cascade of MAPKs, that is, upstream activating protein → MAPK kinase kinase (MAPKKK) → MAPK kinase (MAPKK) → MAPK. The signaling pathway it mediates involves the core of the signaling network that regulates cell growth, development, and division. ERK can also be phosphorylated (p-ERK) by activation of ion beam irradiation and hydrogen peroxide, enter the nucleus to act on transcription factors such as c-Myc, AP-1, NF-κB, and promote the transcription and expression of certain genes, which are related to the process of cell death and transformation.

Skin acts as the largest organ of the body, and the maintenance of the structure and function of the epidermal layer is mainly dependent on the basal cells of the epidermis. The cells at this site are composed of epidermal stem cells and transient expansion cells. Stem cells rapidly divide and proliferate, form short-expanded cells, and further differentiate, producing a large number of cells with different structures and functions. During the migration of these cells to the epidermal layer and dermal layer, on the one hand, they have supplemented apoptotic or necrotic cells; on the other hand, they form new structures and tissues that cause thickening of the epidermis and dermis. The transition of stem cells from proliferation to differentiation occurs in the G1 phase of the cell cycle. The conversion of cells from the resting phase to G1 phase requires the involvement of the ERK1/ERK2 signaling pathway. Observation of hypertrophic scar tissue showed a higher rate of positive cells for Ras and phosphorylated ERK1/ERK2. This may be related to the rapid division, proliferation, and differentiation of skin stem cells by activation of ERK1/ERK2 pathway to form terminally differentiated cells with special structure and function, especially fibroblast, which is one of the mechanisms of hypertrophic scar formation and maturation.

#### 3.4.1.2 C-Jun N-Terminal Kinase (JNK) Signaling Pathway

JNK signal transduction pathway is a member of the MAPK superfamily. It is originally named for its phosphorylation of c-Jun (a transcriptional regulator, a member of the leucine zipper family), N-terminal active regions Ser63 and Ser73. JNK signal transduction pathway can be activated by tumor necrosis factor (TNF), epidermal growth factor (EGF), interleukin (IL) and other growth factors/cytokines, and some guanylate-binding proteins (G-protein)-coupled receptors and stress, and participate in cell proliferation and differentiation, cell morphology maintenance, skeleton construction, programmed cell death, cell malignant transformation, and other biological reactions.

The typical JNK signal transduction pathway is activated by the MAP3K, MAP2K, and JNK three-stage enzyme chain reactions. During this process, MAPKK4 and MAPKK7 are double-phosphorylated and activate Thr and Tyr in the characteristic modular structure of Thr-proline-tyrosine. JNK in the cytoplasm moves into the nucleus and activates the phosphorylated substrate of JNK. The regulation mechanism of JNK signal transduction pathway is complex, in addition to phosphorylation regulation; it is also regulated by signal component modularization, ubiquitin, and signal crosstalk.

JNK is a major signal transduction molecule in cells. It can induce apoptosis in stress response after injury and is closely related to cell proliferation. Studies have shown that in hypertrophic scar tissue, p-JNK is present in the basal layer and part of fibroblasts, while in normal skin, p-JNK is localized in the basal layer of the epidermis. Studies even found that p-JNK was expressed by polymorphonuclear granulocytes, monocytes, and fibroblasts in the healing process of mouse skin wounds. p-JNK has a regulatory effect on the apoptosis of these cells and then affects wound healing.

##### JNK Signal Transduction Pathway Regulates Migration and Repair Process of Epithelial Cells and Fibroblasts

During the process of EGF-induced migration of human corneal epithelial cells, JNK signal transduction pathway is activated, and paxillin (Pax) Ser178, Tyr31, and Tyr118 sites are phosphorylated. Inhibition of RhoA activity or JNK inhibitors delays ActB-induced wound healing. Further experiments confirmed that ActB promotes epithelial wound healing through the RhoA-Rho-related rho-associated coiled-coil protein kinase (ROCK)-JNK-c-Jun signal transduction pathway. Studies have shown that ActB can promote muscle tension fibers formation and bone marrow mesenchymal stem cells migration by activating JNK and ERK signaling pathways, thereby promoting bone marrow mesenchymal stem cells-mediated wound healing.

Studies have shown that the JNK signal transduction pathway is involved in the fibroblast migration process. Retinoic acid-related orphan receptors-2 (ROR-2) associates with filamin A (FLNa) and protein kinase C (PKC) during mouse embryonic fibroblasts migration induced by wingless-type mice mammary tumor virus integration site family (WNT) 5a, then activates JNK at the wound edge to promote cell polarity and migration. However, inhibition of JNK or PKC signaling pathways can inhibit WNT5a-induced JNK activity and microtubule tissue center relocalization. ROR-2 is required during WNT5a-induced cell migration, and the mechanism by which FLNa and PKC regulate JNK activity and how activated JNK in turn regulates cell polarity and migration needs further study. Tan Zhen et al. found that the PI3K-Rac1-JNK signal transduction pathway plays an important role in bFGF regulation of fibroblast migration. Wang et al. found that JNK is involved in WNT5a regulation of adhesion and migration of human dental papilla cells, and that WNT5a may or may not rely on the RhoA signal transduction pathway to activate the JNK pathway. The results suggest that the migration of human dental papilla cells is inhibited after inhibition of the JNK signal transduction pathway, and the mechanism may be related to the inhibition of focal adhesion formation.

#### JNK Signal Transduction Pathway Regulates Cell Migration Process in Inflammatory Environment

Macrophage migration inhibitory factor (MIF) is a chemokine-like multi-effect pro-inflammatory cytokine. In T-cell and fibroblasts, MIF can trigger the 4-CD74-SRC-PI3K axis of cysteine-X-cysteine chemokine receptor to activate JNK signal transduction pathway rapidly and temporarily upregulate the gene expression of inflammatory factor cysteine-X-cysteine chemokine ligand 8. Catestatin (a neuroendocrine antimicrobial peptide) induces mast cell migration and degranulation, and produces cytokines and chemokines. Catestatin-mediated mast cell activation is regulated by GBP, phospholipase C, and MAPK-ERK signaling pathways. In MAPK signal transduction pathway, both ERK and JNK are phosphorylated (p38 is not activated), and ERK-specific inhibitor U0126 almost completely suppresses the production of cytokines and chemokines stimulated by the catestatin, whereas JNK inhibitor SP600125 does not. The JNK signal transduction pathway is involved in the activation of mast cell mediated by catestatin, but its role is not necessary, and its regulatory mechanism needs further study. A variety of pro-inflammatory stimuli, such as IL-1, IL-6, TNF-α, and lipopolysaccharide, can activate the JNK signaling pathway and regulate cell migration. Studies have shown that TNF-α- and IL-1-induced or transforming growth factor β-induced nuclear factor-κB (NF-κB) inhibits the activation of protein kinase and JNK-AP1 signal transduction pathway.

Xiaobing's Fu team used 18 cases of full-thickness skin on the back of the fetus whose pregnancy was terminated due to unexpected factors such as trauma [54]. The embryo gestational age (EGA) was 13 to 32 weeks, including 2 cases of EGA 13, 15, 17, 21, 23, 25, 28, 30, and 32 weeks, respectively. According to the different periods of fetal development, the fetal skin specimens were divided into three categories: early pregnancy fetal skin (EGA 13–17 weeks), mid-pregnancy fetal skin (EGA 21–25 weeks), and late pregnancy fetal skin (EGA 28–32 weeks). The corresponding six cases of children's skin were normal skin of the back or upper limbs due to plastic surgery, aged 4–12 years. The total RNA from fetal and children skin of different gestational ages was extracted, and the quality and concentration of the extracted total RNA were detected by ultraviolet spectroscopic analysis and gel electrophoresis. The mRNA was isolated and purified according to the PolyATtract mRNA Isolation System, and its purity was analyzed by ultraviolet spectrometry. The RT-PCR products of the JNK-1 and JNK-2 genes were 267 and 308 bp, respectively. The expression level of the JNK-1 gene rises to the highest in the fetal skin of the second trimester and then gradually decreases. During fetal skin development, the expression of JNK-2 gene gradually increased. In children's skin, the gray density of the expressed product was 2.1 times that of early fetal skin, and the gene expression was significantly enhanced ($P < 0.01$). In the skin tissues of early pregnancy, the expression level of JNK3 gene was low, and the expression of this gene was significantly increased in the skin of late pregnancy and children ($P < 0.05$).

### 3.4.1.3 p38 Mitogen-Activated Protein Kinase

The first discovered p38 MAPK member is p38α, a 38 ku protein whose tyrosine site was rapidly phosphorylated by LPS stimulation. This protein is a target of pyridazoles, which can inhibit the production of inflammatory factors such as interleukin-1 (IL-1) and tumor necrosis factor (TNF) in LPS-stimulated monocytes. In addition, the protein can activate MAPK-activated protein kinase 2 (MK2) when the cells are subjected to heat shock, arsenite, or IL-1. Three other homologs of p38α were also found, namely p38β, p38γ (SAPK3, ERK6), and p38δ (SAPK4). The four members of the p38 family are encoded by different genes and expressed differently in different tissues. P38α and p38β are expressed in almost all tissues, p38γ is mainly present in muscle tissue, and p38δ is mainly expressed in testis, pancreas, and small intestine. The active substrates of these members have partial overlaps, but each also has its own specific substrate.

The biological roles of p38 mitogen-activated protein kinases include cell differentiation, migration, cell cycle regulation, and inflammatory responses. Schematic diagram of the p38MAPK signaling pathway is shown in Fig. 3.7 [55]. In the skin tissue, the experimental results showed that the expression of p-p38MAPK was observed in the epidermal layer, sarcolemma, hair follicle, and sebaceous gland of the normal skin of mice, which was related to the physiological function, distribution, and the maintenance of skin homeostasis of p38MAPK. P38σ regulates the activity of the involucrin during differentiation of keratinocytes. It has been reported that under normal conditions, tyrosine 323 site is autophosphorylated, and p38MAPK expression in T lymphocytes is activated by T cell receptor (TCR), but not in B lymphocytes. In the process of skin damage repair, it mainly divides into inflammatory phase, fibroproliferative phase, and tissue remodeling phase. In these three consecutive processes, neutrophils, monocytes, and fibroblasts play a major role, and signal is involved in cell migration, inflammatory response, and cell cycle regulation. In the early stage of skin injury, neutrophils infiltrate the damaged area, and then neutrophils undergo apoptosis, which is cleared by macrophages. In the past, it was thought that neutrophil apoptosis was related to Fas/FasL and ROS. Other studies have shown that p-p38MAPK is always expressed during neutrophil apoptosis, without activation of ERK and JNK proteins. The apoptotic effect of p38MAPK on neutrophils is not necessarily achieved by activation of Fas/FasL and ROS. At least two pathways mediate neutrophil apoptosis, one is p38MAPK and the other is Fas/FasL, and eventually may

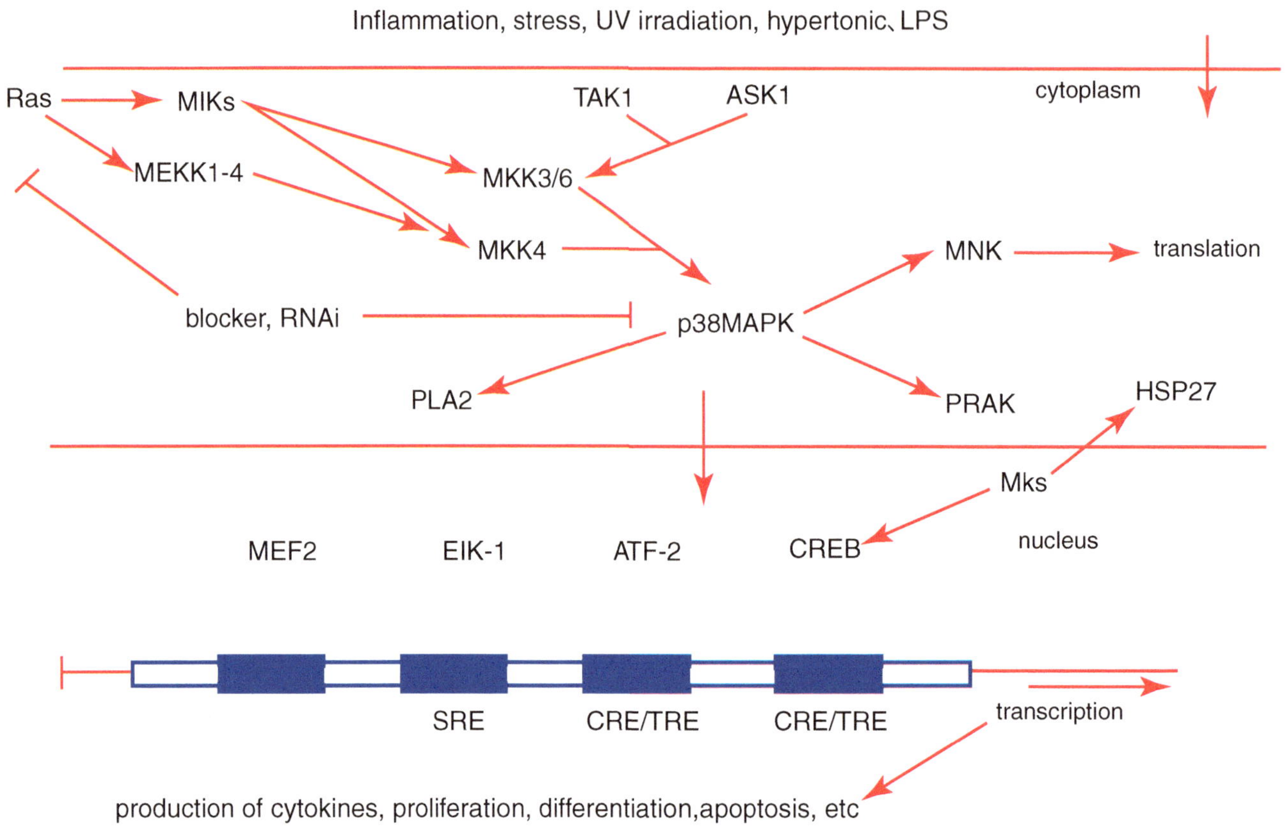


**Fig. 3.7** Schematic diagram of the p38MAPK signaling pathway (Extracted from Zhang Qi, Bai Xiaodong, Xiaobing Fu. Progress in p38MAPK signaling pathway. Infection, Inflammation, Repair, 2005, 6(2): 121–123)

undergo apoptosis through caspase. Studies have shown that the number of neutrophils infiltrated from 0 to 12 h gradually increases, and the number of cells and the rate of positive cells reach the peak, suggesting that after skin damage, the body's defense system was started, and the number of apoptotic neutrophils was also gradually increasing. At 12 h, p38MAPK-mediated neutrophil apoptosis was the most, which may be related to the stimulation of inflammatory factors, leading to rapid apoptosis of neutrophils. The number of neutrophils decreased significantly in 1 to 3 days, the number of monocytes increased gradually, and a large number of fibroblasts proliferated, indicating that the tissue could eliminate too many neutrophils by phagocytosis of monocytes/macrophages to avoid tissue damage. The positive cell rate was relatively high in 1 ~ 5 days, the highest in the third day, indicating that this may be the peak of monocyte apoptosis. And studies have shown that the peak of caspase-3 expression is also on the third day after skin injury. Other studies have confirmed that both mononuclear macrophages and fibroblasts express Fas/FasL during skin injury healing, and some cells co-expressing Fas/FasL have apoptosis. The expression of p-p38MAPK was found during the apoptosis of macrophages, and it was found that transforming growth factor (TGF-β) and inducible NO synthase (iNOS) can activate p38MAPK through different pathways, and then initiate exogenous cell death pathway Fas/FasL and endogenous cell death pathways p53 and Bax, and finally induce macrophage apoptosis through caspase-3. In addition, studies have shown that the differentiation and chemotaxis of monocytes in serum is also mediated by the activation of p38MAPK. This indicates that p38MAPK can transmit different signals to regulate the function of monocytes. Under normal circumstances, 5 days after injury, monocytes decreased and fibroblasts increased gradually. In this stage, the number of cells was small and the tissue entered the reconstruction stage. After 5 ~ 14 days, the positive expression of fibroblasts increased first and then decreased gradually. Finally, the expression of positive cells and the content of p38MAPK approached normal skin. At this stage, the ERK pathway plays an important role in accelerating wound healing, and p38MAPK may mediate fibroblast apoptosis via Fas/FasL and may be based on dephosphorylation of the ERK pathway. In addition, in proliferative scar tissue, the protein expression of p38MAPK is higher than that of normal skin. This may be that after stimulating cells by inflammatory factors, p38MAPK can upregulate the expression of c-Jun gene, induce the synthesis and secretion of basic fibroblast

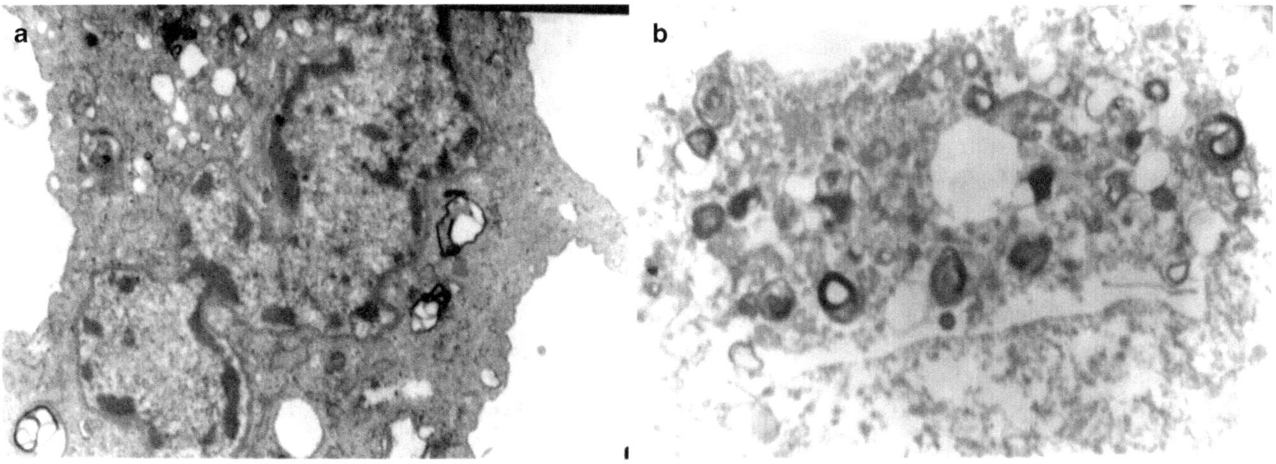

**Fig. 3.8** (**a**) Nuclear chromosome collected and aggregated to form a crescent (transmitted electron microscopy) (**b**) Apoptotic bodies formed after thermal damage (transmitted electron microscopy)

growth factor (bFGF) and other factors, and promote the excessive proliferation and fibrosis of granulation tissue.

The team led by Xiaobing Fu first explored the activation of MAPK signaling pathway in apoptosis induced by thermal injury in vitro [56]. First, a scale model of fibroblasts in vitro was made. The primary human fibroblasts were cultured by subculture (selecting cells from 6 to 8 generations). When the density of inoculation reaches $10^5$–$10^6$/mL, the DMEM medium with 10% serum concentration was changed to the DMEM with 5% serum concentration. The culture was continued for 24 h at 37 °C, 5% CO2, and saturated humidity. The cultured fibroblasts were placed in water baths at 43 and 45 °C for 10, 30, and 40 min, respectively. The apoptosis characteristics were most obvious after incubation in constant temperature water bath at 45 °C for 10 min. Under the inverted microscope, the cells of the normal control group were fusiform, with full body and smooth and bright membrane; after the thermal damage, some cells became round and appeared protuberance on the surface, that is, bubble phenomenon. DNA gel electrophoresis showed that the cells were incubated in water at 37 °C for 30 min (the normal control group) without any bands, and the heat-damaged group had DNA fragments, which showed typical ladder-like markers of apoptosis. Under the fluorescence microscope of Hoeschst33258, the living cell nucleus showed diffuse and uniform fluorescence, while the apoptotic cells, the nucleus, and cytoplasm showed dense particle fluorescence, especially 3–4 fluorescent fragments, which is considered to be typical apoptotic cells. Under transmission electron microscopy, the nuclear chromosomes of apoptotic cells were collected and aggregated to form a crescent. Some cells had pyknosis, increased electron density, irregular nuclear shape, and uneven nuclear membrane surface. Some cells underwent nuclear fragmentation, and multiple electron density-enhanced nuclear fragments appeared in the cytoplasm (Fig. 3.8). Some cells became smaller in size, the cytoplasm was concentrated, the organelles were well preserved, or slightly hyperplasia, the number of mitochondria was slightly increased and mildly swollen, the cytoplasmic vacuoles were increased, the cell membrane was preserved intact, and the surface microvilli and pseudopods were reduced or disappeared, and the bubble phenomenon of cell membrane can be seen. In the late stage of apoptosis, apoptotic bodies with intact organelles and nuclear fragments can be seen.

Using the above studies to make cell damage in vitro, it was observed that ERK1/2 changed after the simple injury, and the change of ERK1 was more significant. At 30 min, ERK1/2 expression reached the peak, and after 180 min, expression was almost complete. With bFGF stimulation, the expression level of each phase was enhanced, which was significantly higher than that of the control group. At 30 min, ERK1/2 expression was the strongest, peaked, and then began to diminish. The ERK pathway was specifically blocked in advance, and ERK expression was decreased after adding PD98059. Phosphorylated ERK expression: The phosphorylated ERK at each phase was lower than the total expression. When bFGF stimulator was added, the peak value of ERK at 30 min was significantly higher than that in the simple injury group, especially the expression of ERK-2. After blocking with the blocker PD98059, the phosphorylated ERK1/2 protein was not expressed at 0 ~ 180 min.

After induction of scald in vitro, the expression of proto-oncogene c-Fos in cultured fibroblasts increased gradually (0–30 min), decreased after 60 min, and weakened after 180 min. When adding exogenous growth factor bFGF, its expression increased and lasted for 180 min. Use ERK-specific blocker ahead of time PD98059, c-Fos expression was not significantly reduced compared with the simple scald-induced group, and the duration of sustained expression was prolonged. However, c-Fos expression was significantly reduced after blocking both ERK and p38MAPK pathways with PD98059 and SB203580 antagonists.

In vivo, the team led by Academician Xiaobing Fu did the following study [57]. Twenty-six male Wistar rats weighing 160 ~ 190 g were purchased from the Institute of Laboratory Animals Science, CAMS & PUMC (license number: SCXK11000006). The diabetic rat model was prepared by the Institute of Materia Medica Chinese Academy of Medical Science. One week before the experiment, the rats were fed in the laboratory, and on the day of experiment, they fasted. Under the condition of ketamine and SU-XIN-MING compound anesthesia, the hair on the back was cleaned, with an area of 9.0 cm × 8.0 cm. After disinfection, 4 round wounds were cut on both sides of the back spine with a diameter of 1.8 cm and an area of 2.54 $cm^2$ by a special wound causing device (perforator). After hemostasis, 52 wounds were selected (the rest of the wounds were reserved for other purposes). They were randomly divided into two groups:

(a) Control group (group A), dressing with sterile gauze, feeding in single cage, and changing gauze once a day until the wound healed.
(b) rhPDGF treatment group (group B): rhPDGF is REGRANEX produced by a company in the United States, and the dosage of wound surface is 7.0 $\mu g/cm^2$. The rhPDGF was evenly applied to the corresponding wound surface with a syringe according to the experimental design dose, wrapped with sterile gauze, fed in a single cage, and changed dressing once a day until the wound healed. The blood glucose level of the tail vein was measured by a portable blood glucose meter on the 3rd, 7th, and 14th day after the injury. The granulation formation, collagen deposition, re-epithelialization rate, and inflammatory cell infiltration were observed on the 3rd, 7th, and 14th day after injury, the expression of extracellular signal-regulated kinase 1/2 (ERK1/2) was detected by immunofluorescence technique, and proto-oncogene c-Fos, proliferation cell nuclear antigen (PCNA), focal adhesion kinase (FAK) changes were detected by immunohistochemistry technique. Histological examination showed that there were a large amount of inflammatory cells infiltrated in the wound treated with rhPDGF, the number of capillary germ and fibroblasts were significantly higher than those in the control group, collagen deposition was obvious, granulation tissue grew actively, and wound contraction was significant (Fig. 3.9). Immunological studies showed that the expression of ERK1/2 and c-Fos was significantly increased in the rhPDGF-treated group 3 days after injury, ERK1/2 and c-Fos were further enhanced at 7th day, and began to weaken after 14 days. The expression of PCNA and FAK in the repaired cells of rhPDGF-treated group was significantly stronger than that of the control group. It can be seen that the early use of rhPDGF can induce the expression of ERK1/2 in repair cells (including fibroblasts, vascular endothelial cells, and keratinocytes), thereby increasing the transcription and expression of proto-oncogene c-Fos. According to the rule of experimental wound healing and the role of influencing factors, the researchers speculated that ERKs control the expression of downstream genes by regulating the activity of AP-1. AP-1, as a transcription factor for FAK and PCNA expression, affects the biological activities of various repair cells, including fibroblasts, microvascular endothelial cells, and keratinocytes, especially the proliferation, migration, and differentiation of

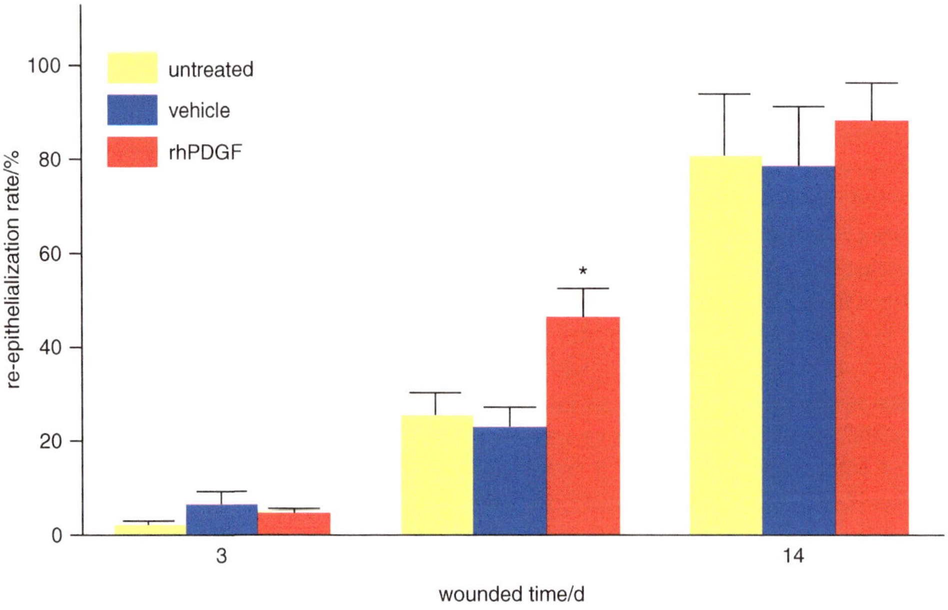


**Fig. 3.9** Effect of PDGF on the rate of re-epithelialization in diabetic rats

repair cells, and finally accelerates the collagen deposition, blood vessel formation, and re-epithelialization in granulation tissue, and promotes wound healing process. PDGF is a strong mitogenic agent, which induces the migration of wound vascular smooth muscle cells, the proliferation and migration of endothelial cells, and the formation of vascular lumen, and is beneficial to the oxygen supply of tissues; it promotes the proliferation of fibroblasts and increases the composition of extracellular matrix to facilitate tissue contraction; it promotes proliferation and migration of keratinocytes, and contributes to the re-epithelialization of wounds. In conclusion, rhPDGF-induced chemotaxis and migration of repair cells is an important component of the wound healing response. The ERK signal transduction pathway is the main pathway for PDGF to stimulate angiogenesis in granulation tissue. Fos protein is a key product involved in signal cascade. Further elucidation of the regulation mode and network characteristics of PDGF in the MAPKs signaling pathway will play an important role in understanding the mechanism of wound healing.

HE staining of wound tissue sections showed that the amount of inflammatory cells infiltrated in the control group of diabetic rats was much less than that in the rhPDGF-treated group on the 3rd day after injury. After treatment with rhPDGF, the inflammatory infiltration zone of wound was obvious, and a large number of inflammatory cells (macrophages, monocytes, and neutrophils) appeared in the injured area. The wounds in different groups showed different degrees of granulation tissue proliferation on the 7th day after injury. The collagen deposition in the wounds treated by rhPDGF was more, and the number of capillary germ and fibroblasts increased significantly (Table 3.1). On the 14th day after injury, the wound contraction was significant after rhPDGF treatment, and re-epithelialization was almost completed, while other groups were still not completely healed. Further observation of their changes in ERK1/2 expression revealed that phosphorylated ERK1/2 positive markers appeared in repair cells (fibroblasts, microvascular endothelial cells in the wound, and keratinocytes in the basal layer of wound edge epithelium) on the 3rd day after injury. Expression increased on the 7th day and remained high on the 14th day. The expression of ERK1/2 was enhanced after treatment with rhPDGF in group B. The number of ERK1/2 positive cells was significantly increased compared with the diabetic control group on the 3rd day after injury. There were still a large number of ERK1/2 positive cells in 7–14 days after injury. The study on the expression of proto-oncogene c-Fos revealed that the expression of proto-oncogene c-Fos in various repair cells of rats increased gradually after injury, and the number of positive cells reached the peak on the 7th day after injury; there are still a large number of positive cells on the 14th day. After rhPDGF was applied to the wound, the number of positive cells at each time point increased further, exceeding the diabetic control group. The general condition and pathological observation of diabetic rat skin defect wound treated by external rhPDGF shows the healing mechanism of the study.

**Table 3.1** Comparison of wound volume at different time points after treatment with different methods

| Group | 3 d | 7 d |
|---|---|---|
| Diabetic rats control | 0.21 ± 0.06 ($n$ = 29) | 0.07 ± 0.05 ($n$ = 25) |
| PDGF | 0.18 ± 0.04 ($n$ = 12)* | 0.03 ± 0.03 ($n$ = 11)* |

Compared with the diabetic control group: *$P < 0.05$; $n$ is the number of wounds

Subsequently, the team led by Xiaobing Fu further explored the expression of phosphorylated extracellular signal-regulated kinase 1/2 (ERK1/2), phosphorylated stress-activated protein kinase (p-SAPK), and phosphorylated p38MAPK (p-p38MAPK) during the formation and maturation of hypertrophic scars after wound healing [58]. 16 cases of hypertrophic scars were collected from hospitalized patients, including nine males and seven females, aged from 16 to 47 years old. The materials included five cases of the back, one case of the buttock, three cases of the maxillofacial and upper limbs, respectively, and two cases of the chest and inner thigh, respectively. The hypertrophic scar specimens were divided into two groups, 8 in each group:

(a) Hypertrophic scar in active growth period with formation time less than 1 year (including 1 year).
(b) Mature hypertrophic scar with formation time more than 1 year. Eight cases of normal skin were taken from normal skin of patients with hypertrophic scar resection. It was found that p-ERK1/2, p-SAPK, and p-p38MAPK were positively expressed in normal skin, among them p-ERK1/2 and p-SAPK were less expressed, and the protein particles were mainly distributed in the cytoplasm and nucleus of keratinocytes in the basal layer of the epidermis. The expression of p38MAPK protein is strong, and the positive staining signal is mainly located in keratinocytes, vascular endothelial cells, hair follicles and sweat gland epithelial cells, and some fibroblasts. In hypertrophic scars, the expression of all three proteins was enhanced, and the protein particles of p-ERK1/2 and p-SAPK were mainly localized in epidermal keratinocytes and a small number of fibroblasts; p-p38MAPK was strongly expressed, mainly in epidermal cells and fibroblasts. Studies have shown that in hypertrophic scars, the expression of p-ERK1/2 protein is significantly higher than that in normal skin, and positive signals were mainly distributed in epidermal basal cells, which were mainly epidermal stem cells and transiently expanded cells. This suggests that in hypertrophic scars,

extracellular signals can activate the signal transduction pathway mediated by ERK1/2 phosphorylation, causing rapid proliferation of epidermal stem cells and transiently expanded cells, and at the same time a large number of terminally differentiated cells are formed. As these cells synthesize and secrete extracellular matrix such as collagen, hypertrophic scars continue to expand and mature. In the active hypertrophic scar, the p-SAPK protein content was not significantly different from normal skin, but in the mature hypertrophic scar, the p-SAPK positive cell rate was significantly higher than that of normal skin, and mainly located in the epidermal basal cells and parts of fibroblasts. This suggests that as hypertrophic scars mature, extracellular stress signals (such as hypoxia and nutrient deficiency) increase, activating the SAPK signaling pathway, thereby slowing cell division, partial fibroblast apoptosis, and ultimately leading to the balance of proliferation and apoptosis of scar-forming cells, and hypertrophic scars are in a relatively stable state. In the active hypertrophic scar, the expression of p-p38MAPK protein was significantly higher than that in normal skin, and its mechanism may be related to the strong inflammatory reaction and the high content of proinflammatory cytokines in the early stage of hypertrophic scar formation. The specific binding of extracellular signals and receptors on the cell membrane can activate p38MAPK signaling pathway, upregulate c-Jun gene expression, induce the synthesis and secretion of factors such as bFGF, promote hyperplasia and fibrosis of granulation tissue, and form hypertrophic scars. In mature hypertrophic scars, the expression of p-p38MAPK protein is decreased compared with that in active scars, but it is still higher than normal skin. The mechanism of this change may be related to the decrease of inflammatory cells and inflammatory response in mature hypertrophic scars. The p38MAPK signaling pathway may play an important regulatory role in the maintenance of mature hypertrophic scars.

## 3.4.2 Phosphatidylinositol-3-Kinase Signaling Pathway

### 3.4.2.1 Structural Characteristics and Activation Regulation of PI3K

Phosphatidylinositol-3-kinase (PI3K) is a heterodimer composed of a catalytic subunit p10 and a regulatory subunit p85. It has lipid kinase activity and protein kinase activity, and the p85 regulatory subunit is a phospholipid protein substrate of many receptor tyrosine kinases. According to the PI3K structure, it can be divided into three types (type I, type II, and type III): PI, phosphatidylinositol-4-phosphate (PIP) and phosphatidylinositol-4,5-diphosphate (PIP2) are used as substrates for type I PI3K; PI and PIP are used as substrates for type II PI3K, including PIK3C-α, PIK3C-β, and liver-specifically expressed isoform PIK3C-γ; type III PI3K consists of catalytic subunit Vps34 and regulatory subunit p150, and PI is the substrate, mainly involved in the regulation of cell growth and survival. Currently, the most widely studied is type I PI3K, which is activated by cell surface receptors. Type I PI3K is divided into two subtypes, I A and I B, which transmit signals from tyrosine protein kinase-coupled receptor and G-protein-coupled receptor, respectively. I A type PI3K has dual activities of phosphatidylinositol kinase and serine-threonine protein kinase. It is a heterodimer composed of catalytic subunit p110 and regulatory subunit p85. The catalytic subunits include p110α, p110β, and p110δ, which are encoded by PIK3CA, PIK3CB, and PIK3CD genes, respectively. Studies have shown that the PI3K/Akt pathway is independent of PKC, PKA, and MAPK, and is involved in the regulation of various tissue activities including angiogenesis, and plays a crucial role in cell proliferation, differentiation, and apoptosis.

The activation of PI3K is largely involved in substrates close to the inside of its plasma membrane. A variety of growth factors and signal transduction complexes, including fibroblast growth factor (FGF), vascular endothelial growth factor (VEGF), and insulin, all initiate the activation of PI3K. These factors activate the receptor tyrosine kinase (RTK), which causes autophosphorylation. The phosphorylated residue at the receptor provides a docking site for the heterodimerized PI3Kp85 subunit. In some cases, receptor phosphorylation mediates the recruitment of an adaptor protein. When integrin is activated, focal adhesion kinase (FAK) acts as an adaptor protein, anchoring PI3K through its p85. However, in each of the above cases, the SH2 and SH3 domains of the p85 subunit bind to the adaptor protein at a phosphorylation site. Phosphorylation of various PI intermediates is initiated after PI3K recruits activated receptors.

### 3.4.2.2 The Relationship Between PI3K/Akt and Various Growth Factors Related to Wound Healing

PDGF is mainly derived from platelet alpha particles, which can cause proliferation and migration of various cells such as fibroblasts, smooth muscle cells, and monocytes. It is an important growth factor and plays an important role in wound healing, especially angiogenesis. Studies have confirmed that PDGF promotes the proliferation of vascular smooth muscle cells by activating the Akt/FoxO1/3a signaling pathway.

FGF-2 antagonizes apoptosis induced by oxidative stress by activating the PI3K/Akt signaling pathway. In mouse ESCs, FGF activates ERK signaling pathway to promote

ESC differentiation, and inhibits ERK signaling pathway to promote self-renewal of mouse ESCs. Enzyme-linked immunosorbent assay (ELISA) analysis showed that bFGF can activate the Wnt pathway. RNA sequence analysis of β-catenin knockdown fibroblasts showed that β-catenin was positively regulated by bFGF and FGF21. In addition, FGF21 activates Akt and JNK, and its effect of accelerating fibroblast migration is similar to bFGF. Furthermore, ELISA analysis indicated that bFGF and FGF21 autocrine were regulated by stimulation of the Wnt pathway. In conclusion, in skin fibroblasts, β-catenin is involved in the regulation of bFGF (FGF21) and Wnt signaling in dermal fibroblasts.

EGF promotes proliferation of epithelial cells, fibroblasts, glial cells, and smooth muscle cells. EGF induces the phosphorylation of EGFR on the cell surface and activates Akt in the PI3K/Akt pathway of inositol triphosphate kinase, which is closely related to cell proliferation. Matrix metalloproteinases (MMPs) are a group of proteolytic enzymes that are required for cell-mediated contraction in cell migration and wound healing. It has been reported that matrix contraction and cell migration can be reduced by inhibiting the activity of MMPs. After activation, gelatinase A (MMP-2) secreted by connective tissue cells can degrade one or more collagens and proteins. It has the property of degrading denatured collagen gelatin and has certain effects on fibronectin and elastin. Studies have shown that EGF induces overexpression of MMP-2 in cultured human lens epithelial cells (HLECs) in a time-dependent manner and completes cell migration, which can be blocked by EGFR and Akt inhibitors. These results indicate that PI3K/Akt channel is a necessary condition for EGF to stimulate MMP-2 expression.

Transforming growth factor (TGF) is divided into TGF-α and TGF-β. The former amino acid sequence is 33–44% homologous to EGF, which can bind to EGF receptor and exert the same or similar effects. The latter effect on fibroblasts and smooth muscle cells proliferation varies according to its concentration: low concentration induces PDGF synthesis and secretion, which is an indirect mitogen; high concentration inhibits PDGF receptor expression and inhibits its growth. Many studies have shown that TGF-β and PI3K/ Akt signaling pathways interact at multiple levels and multiple steps to achieve fine-grained regulation of cells in specific environments.

Vascular endothelial growth factor (VEGF) is a highly selective and potent mitogen for endothelial cells. Previous studies have suggested that it can specifically act on vascular endothelial cells, induce the expression of matrix metalloproteinases and collagenases, promote the degradation of extracellular matrix, and facilitate the migration of endothelial cells, thereby inducing the migration of endothelial cells and preparing for the generation of new blood vessels. Hypoxia-inducible factor-1 (HIF-1) acts as a mediator of transcription activation during hypoxia. Growth factors, cytokines, etc. stimulate the synthesis of HIF-1α by activation of PI3K or MAPK. HIF-1 promotes the generation of new blood vessels by binding to the VEGF promoter hypoxia-responsive element (HRE) to regulate the expression of VEGF and the transcription of its receptor. Overexpression of PI3K or Akt increased VEGF mRNA expression, while LY294002 inhibited VEGF mRNA expression, but overexpression of PI3K or Akt restored inhibition. This suggests that PI3K may induce angiogenesis by regulating the expression of HIF-1 or VEGF.

Insulin-like growth factor 1 (IGF-1) is a single-chain polypeptide produced and secreted mainly by hepatocytes. It induces the expression of growth factors such as basic fibroblast growth factor, promotes the synthesis and secretion of extracellular matrix such as fibronectin, polyglucosamine, and collagen, and affects the remodeling of tissue after wound repair. It can stimulate the mitosis of the mother cell by binding to the specific IGF-1 receptor. Studies have suggested that plasma IGF-1 levels in diabetic patients are significantly lower than in normal controls, while IGF-1 levels in patients with high risk of diabetic foot ulcers are lower than those in patients without risk and low risk, that is, with the increase of the risk of diabetic foot ulcer, the level of plasma IGF-1 gradually decreases, indicating that the change of plasma IGF-1 level is closely related to the occurrence and development of diabetic foot ulcer. Ulcer healing in diabetic patients is slower than normal, indicating that IGF-1 plays an important role in the healing process of ulcers. Many studies have demonstrated that IGF-1-mediated multiple cellular functions may be primarily implemented through the PI3K/ Akt signaling pathway. The binding of IGF-1 to the IGF-1 receptor leads to the activation of two signaling pathways, namely mitogen-activated protein kinase (MAPK) and phosphatidylinositol-3-kinase/protein kinase B (PI3K/Akt), while activating the PI3K/Akt signaling pathway can affect cell apoptosis. The mechanism of PI3K/Akt signaling pathway interfering with apoptosis mainly includes the following aspects:

(a) Direct regulation. Activated Akt can phosphorylate the Ser136 site of Bad, effectively block Bad-induced apoptosis, inactivate the caspase-9 Ser196 site, and inhibit its pro-apoptotic effect.
(b) Play a role in cell survival regulation by directly or indirectly affecting the transcription factor family (Forkhead, NF-κB, p53, etc.).
(c) Influence cell proliferation by regulating cell cycle.
(d) Prevent mitochondria from releasing apoptotic factors. The protective effect of IGF-1 on cardiomyocytes is mainly through activating PI3K/Akt pathway. The PI3K/ Akt pathway is a classical pathway that mediates survival.

### 3.4.3 Wnt Signaling Pathway and Tissue Repair

In 1973, Sharma et al. first discovered the wingless gene in the study of drosophila embryo development. In 1982, Nusser et al. discovered a protein that can transmit proliferation and differentiation signals between cells when studying mouse breast tumors. At that time, it was called Intl. Later, it was found that the wingless gene of drosophila is a Wnt-like gene, which is later named Wnt1 gene.

At first, Wnt gene family was composed of wingless gene (Wg) products and the secreted glycoprotein Wnt1 gene. Wnt glycoprotein regulates homeostasis and development by binding to the Frizzled-low density lipoprotein receptor-associated protein complex. The Wnt signaling pathway is evolutionarily conserved and is a highly complex signaling pathway. It is also the key for cell development, differentiation, and maintenance of homeostasis. It is an important signaling pathway for controlling embryonic development and morphogenesis of tissues and organs. A total of 19 Wnt genes have been discovered, which are expressed in a variety of tissue cells. They act by activating the membrane receptor in an autocrine or paracrine manner. The Wnt protein encoded by the Wnt gene, its receptor, and regulatory proteins, together form a complex signaling pathway called the Wnt signal transduction pathway. The Wnt signal transduction pathway has the following two pathways:

(a) Classical Wnt-β-catenin-LEF/TCF pathway: After activation, this pathway will recruit β-catenin in cells, activate and transfer it into the nucleus, and activate the transcription of specific genes together with transcription factor LEF/TCF. β-catenin was first discovered by German cell biologist Walt Birchmeier in 1980 as a component of the cell adhesion connection. It is a member of the cytoskeletal protein family. The β-catenin protein contains three important functional regions: the N-terminal domain, the intermediate linking arm repeat region, and the C-terminal domain. The amino terminus contains about 150 amino acids. It is the phosphorylation site of β-catenin by glycogen synthase kinase 3β (GSK3β) and also a binding site to α-catenin. Among them, several serine/threonine residues can be phosphorylated by GSK3β and CK1α, and phosphorylated β-catenin can be recognized and ubiquitinated by β-transducin repeat-containing proteins, and finally degraded in the proteasome. It is one of the important mechanisms regulating the stability of β-catenin. The intermediate repeat region is a sequence with the same structure, which is the most conserved region and the main binding site with ligand, including β-catenin and cadherin, Axin, lymphoid enhancer factor (LEF), etc., thereby activating the T-cell factor (TCF) family transcription factor binding site at the carboxy terminus of the classical Wnt signaling pathway, and activating downstream target genes to play the role of transcription after binding to a transcriptional activator.
(b) Nonclassical Wnt signaling pathway: With the deepening of Wnt signaling pathways, more and more Wnt nonclassical signaling pathways have been discovered, including Wnt-PCP signaling pathway, Wnt-cGMP signaling pathway, Wnt/$Ca^{2+}$ signaling pathway, Wnt-PAP signaling pathway, etc. The study of PCP pathway and $Ca^{2+}$ pathway is clear in these pathways.

Under normal circumstances, Wnt gene of adult is in a relatively static state. After skin injury, TGF-β increases β-catenin expression in the wound. TGF-β activates β-catenin-mediated transcription of human epithelial fibroblasts via the Smad3 and p38 MAPK pathways, and TGF-β also induces upregulation of Wnt/β-catenin signaling pathway in hypertrophic scars and keloids. β-catenin is continuously increased in the nucleus of dermal fibroblasts, which is beneficial to the proliferation and migration of fibroblasts, and at the same time, it can feedback to activate TGF-β signaling pathway. The enhanced Wnt/β-catenin signaling pathway plays a negative feedback role in the transformation of normal skin from fibroblasts to myofibroblasts induced by TGF-β1, which is the key to wound healing.

The interaction between endothelial cells is an important factor affecting the vascular proliferation and vascular function of wounds. Studies have shown that VEGF and placental growth factor promote vascular proliferation through the receptor VEGFR-1, and the two have a synergistic effect. Blocking Wnt/$Ca^{2+}$ signaling pathway by siRNA or Wnt5a antagonist can inhibit endothelial cell proliferation and migration, and the addition of VEGF can reverse this phenomenon. It is suggested that Wnt5a-mediated nonclassical Wnt pathway (Wnt/$Ca^{2+}$) plays a positive role in endothelial cell proliferation and migration.

Wnt signaling pathway is activated after skin injury and is involved in every process of wound healing from inflammation control to apoptosis. The relationship between Wnt signaling pathway and wound healing is illustrated in the following aspects.

#### 3.4.3.1 Inflammatory Cells

Inflammation-related studies in wound healing have found that interferon-γ (IFN-γ) and lipopolysaccharide (LPS), as two potent inflammatory stimulators, can significantly upregulate Wnt5a. Studies on the relationship between macrophages and Wnt signaling pathways suggest that direct evidences of macrophage-stimulating Wnt signaling pathways include the following: macrophages can stimulate the remodeling of vitreous vessels, and Wnt7b secreted by macrophages is a very important protein involved in the entire process. Moreover, Wnt5a can promote macrophages to produce cytokines with proangiogenic effects, such as IL-6, IL-8, and the like.

#### 3.4.3.2 Fibroblasts

Zheng Fang et al. found that the proliferation and secretion of fibroblasts is beneficial to the repair of wounds, and Wnt signaling is involved in the proliferation of fibroblasts during wound healing, especially through the Wnt/β-catenin signaling pathway. Carre et al. found that the classical Wnt signaling pathway is significantly increased in the wound surface of newborn mice. After Wnt signaling pathway is activated, it could promote the proliferation of mouse fibroblasts after birth and increase the expression of HAS1 and Hyal2 genes in postnatal mouse fibroblasts, thereby significantly increasing the expression of type I collagen. β-catenin is involved in the proliferative phase of wound repair in rats and humans. It is believed that β-catenin plays a regulatory role in the movement of fibroblasts, while abnormal β-catenin can cause excessive fibrous tissue and scar formation. The phosphorylation of β-catenin, its accumulation in the cytoplasm, the transfer into the nucleus, and the regulation of target gene transcription can cause fibroblast proliferation, migration, and collagen deposition. The changes of β-catenin level in fibroblasts can regulate wound contraction, tensile strength, and TGF-β.

#### 3.4.3.3 Angiogenesis

New blood vessels provide adequate blood oxygen supply and nutrition for wound healing, which is conductive to granulation growth and wound healing. Therefore, the effect of Wnt signaling pathway on angiogenesis deserves attention. Studies have shown that the Wnt signaling pathway is involved in the regulation of vascular endothelial cell proliferation and plays an important role in maintaining the function of endothelial cells and endothelial progenitor cells. Wnt1, Wnt3a, and Wnt5a can control the proliferation, migration, and differentiation of endothelial cells. Endothelial cell proliferation and migration are inhibited by Wnt antagonist or siRNA blocking Wnt signaling pathway, which may be reversed by the addition of vascular endothelial growth factor (VEGF). It has been reported that Wnt can induce the expression of matrix metalloproteinases, promote the degradation of extracellular matrix, and facilitate the recognition and establishment of connections of sophisticated cells. In vitro experiments with vascular smooth muscle cells have shown that it can promote the degradation of β-catenin/cadherin complex at the adhesion junction and affect the migration of endothelial cells into new blood vessels.

#### 3.4.3.4 Epidermal Regeneration and Hair Follicle Regeneration

Epidermal regeneration and hair follicle regeneration play a very important role in the repair of wounds, and Wnt is involved in many processes of skin development, from dermogenesis to skin appendage formation. Fathke et al. [59] pointed out Wnt classical signaling pathway can promote the proliferation of hair follicle stem cells and promote hair follicle stem cells into the cell cycle and differentiate into corresponding cells according to different regulatory signals. Hair follicle stem cells have multidirectional differentiation potential and can differentiate into epidermis, sebaceous glands, and hair follicles. Wnt/β-catenin is essential for the development of hair follicles during embryogenesis and contributes to the differentiation of hair follicles after birth. Wnt signaling plays an important role in hair follicle regeneration after injury. For example, Langton et al. found that rats with tail skin damage and lack of hair follicles still had re-epithelialization, but this process was delayed. Inhibition of Wnt signaling in skin lesions will prevent the formation of skin appendages, including hair and sweat glands, which can cause permanent scar formation.

#### 3.4.3.5 Stem Cells

The Wnt signaling pathway affects stem cell proliferation and self-renewal, which is closely related to wound healing. These stem cells are important for tissue repair and regeneration. The Wnt signaling pathway regulates the recruitment and differentiation of stem cells during wound repair. Interstitial progenitor cells also contribute to the repair of wounds. Mesenchymal progenitors at different stages of differentiation are regulated by Wnt signaling pathway, and the differentiation of these cells can be affected by the change of signaling pathway activity, thus affecting the differentiation of these cells. The dermal papilla is the expression area of many genes related to hair growth. Many experiments have demonstrated that Wnt proteins and growth factors can stimulate the dermal papilla by promoting stem cell migration. Small doses of Wnt can induce differentiation of mesenchymal stem cells, while large doses of Wnt inhibit differentiation of mesenchymal stem cells. The terminally differentiated cells that do not migrate accumulate around the wound to hinder epithelialization. Blocking of the Wnt signaling pathway reduces the recruitment of stem/progenitor cells in the damaged area and affects the proliferation of the healing process. Whyte speculated that it might be due to changes in oxygen concentration, and speculated that HIF-1 might be the target of injury and Wnt signaling activation.

#### 3.4.3.6 The Role of Wnt/β-Catenin Signal Transduction Pathway in Pathological Scar Formation

The Wnt/β-catenin signal transduction pathway plays an important role in the healing process of skin wounds and is closely related to human fibrotic diseases. Emily et al. found that the expression of β-catenin was increased in keloid tissue. It is speculated that dermal hyperplasia is caused by the interaction of β-catenin with dermal cells, which is highly expressed in the epidermis. It is confirmed that β-catenin is involved in various stages of wound healing at multiple levels. Li et al. found that Wnt/β-catenin signaling pathway is closely related to cell carcinogenesis and tumor invasion. Pathological scars can be identified as a benign skin fibrotic tumor with tumor biological properties. Igota et al. found that the levels of Wnt5a mRNA β-catenin and protein in keloid fibroblasts were higher than those in normal skin fibroblasts. Domestic scholars have confirmed that β-catenin, which is highly expressed in pathological scars, activates the Wnt/β-catenin signal transduction pathway and promotes the formation of scars. Yasuniwa et al. found that Wnt10A has the effect of promoting tumor angiogenesis. Later, some scholars found that keratinocytes of keloids may induce the high expression of R-spondin2 in fibroblasts, and R-spondin2 cooperates with Wnt3a through the classical Wnt/β-catenin signal transduction pathway. O-gawa et al. believe that skin tension is an important factor in triggering scar formation. Reducing skin tension around wounds or scars is an effective measure to prevent and treat pathological scars. The formation and development of pathological scars may be related to local skin tension. Stretched cells migrate faster and farther than unstretched cells, with no proliferation and reduced apoptosis, and at the same time, the synthesis of collagen is unchanged and the degradation is increased. These biological effects are mediated by integrin and Wnt signaling pathway.

The team led by Xiaobing Fu explored the effects of Wnt/β-catenin signaling pathway activation on human epidermal cell phenotype changes [60]. They used differential adherence method to separate human mature epidermal cells and divided the cells into control group and induction group. The induction group was further divided into lithium chloride (LiCl, 20 mmol/L) induction group and GSK-3β inhibitor (15 μmol/L) induction group. The morphological changes of the cells were observed after 6 days of induction, the expression level of β-catenin in epidermal cells was detected by Western blot, and the expression of surface markers such as CK10, CK14, CK19, and β1 integrin were detected by immunohistochemistry. The results showed that the expression of β-catenin in human epidermal cells induced by LiCl (2.15 ± 0.54) and GSK-3β inhibitor (2.58 ± 0.65) was 2 and 2.5 times higher than that in the control group (0.71 ± 0.23), respectively ($P < 0.01$). Moreover, after induction, the cell volume became smaller and rounder and the ratio of nuclei and cytoplasm became larger. The results of immunohistochemistry showed that CK10 was highly expressed in epidermal cells before induction, and CK14, CK19, and β1 integrin expression were negative in some cells. After induction, there were no CK10 positive cells, some CK14 positive cells, and the expression of CK19 and β1 integrin was strongly positive. This indicated that Wnt/β-catenin pathway activation can cause dedifferentiation of human mature epidermal cells, and Wnt/β-catenin pathway may be the key link regulating human epidermal cell dedifferentiation.

If the molecular mechanism of regulating epidermal stem cell proliferation and differentiation is further clarified, it is possible to precisely regulate the limited proliferation and directed differentiation of epidermal stem cells by changing different gene signals in the Wnt pathway, thus providing new ways and means for the research of skin regeneration medicine and tissue engineering.

### 3.4.4 TGF-β/Smads Signal Transduction Pathway

#### 3.4.4.1 TGF-β Structure, Secretion, and Activation

To date, at least six subtypes of TGF-βs have been found, namely TGF-β 1 ~ 6, and three subtypes have been found in mammals, namely TGF-β1, TGF-β2, and TGF-β3. These three factors have similar biological activities, inhibit proliferation of most types of cells, induce apoptosis of epithelial cells, but stimulate the proliferation of mesenchymal cells to produce extracellular matrix, and induce various tissue fibrosis reactions in vivo. TGF-β must be activated after secretion to exert its effect, that is, the TGF precursor molecule LTGF must be activated into mature TGF-β (TGF-β1, TGF-β2, TGF-β3) forms to connect with the receptor, and then activate signal transduction pathway. Unlike most other hormones, mature TGF-β remains covalent bond to its propeptide after secretion, and this complex form of mature TGF-β cannot be recognized by signal receptors, so it is called TGF-β propeptide. TGF-β signaling molecules conduct signal through transmembrane receptor complexes, which are widely present on a variety of cell surfaces. Their cell effects include extracellular matrix deposition, cell growth inhibition, and apoptosis. Extracellular matrix deposition involves stimulation of matrix proteins and inhibition of proteases.

The Smad protein family is a signal mediator molecule that transmits signals produced by the binding of TGF-β to its receptor from cytoplasm to nucleus. Numerous different Smad proteins have been found in mammals. These proteins can be divided into three different subfamilies: receptor-regulated Smads (R-Smad), common-partner Smads (C-Smad), and inhibitory Smads (I-Smad). All Smads proteins consist of three parts: the highly conserved MH1 and MH2 domains at the amino and carboxy termini, and the proline-rich spacer linker (L). The MH1 region is a highly conserved amino terminus. In the ground state, the MH1 region of Smad2, Smad3, and Smad4 automatically inhibits the MH2 region and maintains it in an inactive state.

In the basic process of Smad-mediated TGF-β signaling transduction, TGF-β signaling is delivered to the nucleus in a non-amplified stoichiometric manner, requiring two single transmembrane serine/threonine receptors and Smad proteins. The dimeric ligand of the TGF-β superfamily has a high affinity for type I.

and type II receptors on the surface of the cell membrane to form a heterotetramer. In this complex, type II receptor phosphorylates autonomously, and it can phosphorylate the GS domain of type I receptor to activate it. Activated TGF-βR I phosphorylates two serine residues in the R-Smad SSxS region and combines with Smad 4 to form a heterotrimer or heterotetramer into the nucleus, and synergizes with a number of coactivators and coinhibitors to regulate transcription of the target gene.

#### 3.4.4.2 The Role of TGF-β/Smads Signal Transduction in Wound Healing

As a multifunctional cytokine, TGF-β is closely related to wound healing. The team led by Academician Xiaobing Fu found that the biological functions of the three isoforms of TGF-β in the body were different [61]. Compared with TGF-β2 and TGF-β3, TGF-β1 is most closely related to wound healing. At the same time, the team found that TGF-β1 protein content in the central tissue of the ulcer decreased compared with normal skin and ulcer margins, and positive signals were only found in epidermal basal cells and macrophages. The contents of TGF-β2 and TGF-β3 protein were significantly increased, and TGF-β2 was expressed in almost all cells, especially in hair follicle cells; while TGF-β3 was rarely expressed in hair follicle cells, and it was obvious in epidermis, sweat glands, and vascular endothelial cells. Therefore, the reason of delayed wound repair may be the decrease of TGF-β1 content in the ulcer, and the increased expression of TGF-β2 and TGF-β3 protein, causing slow growth of granulation, insufficient blood supply, imbalance of matrix fibrin metabolism, etc., eventually leading to the occurrence of ulcer, but the specific mechanism still needs further study. At the ulcer wound, the content and distribution of receptor I protein were not abnormal compared with normal tissues. It can be seen that the occurrence of ulcer may be independent of the expression and distribution of TGF-βR protein.

TGF-β can promote the synthesis of extracellular matrix (ECM), which mainly contains collagen types 1 to 4. In the process of TGF-β promoting ECM synthesis, Smad regulates this process by interacting with COL1A1, 3A1, 5A2, 6A1, 6A3, and TIMP-1 genes. In addition, non-Smad-dependent pathways such as the JNK pathway have also been discovered. At the same time, it was found that Smad3 can promote type I collagen synthesis in human skin fibroblasts. From the above studies, it is concluded that Smad3 and its family are involved in collagen synthesis. But does collagen synthesis involved in Smad3 and its family play a role in wound healing? If collagen synthesis is inhibited by inhibiting Smad3 and its family, the effect of this inhibition on wound healing remains to be demonstrated. In conclusion, this signaling pathway plays an extremely important role in tissue repair and regeneration regulation.

### 3.4.5 Slit-Robo Signal Pathway

Slit is a secreted extracellular matrix protein discovered in 1984 by Nusslein-Volhard et al. in drosophila. It is encoded by gene 4p15.2 and has a molecular weight of about 200 ku (2.0 × 105). The Robo family is the receptor family of Slit, which is a single-channel transmembrane receptor. There are four members of the family in mammals, Robo1/Dutt1, Robo2, Robo3/Rig-1, and Robo4/Magic Roundabout. Slit binds to the Ig1-2 region of Robo via the N-terminal D2 region (second leucine repeat region). HSPGs is a co-receptor of Slit and Robo, which can combine with Slit2 and Robo to form a ternary compound (Slit- Robo-heparin) to stabilize the binding of Slit and Robo. Early studies have found that the Slit-Robo signaling pathway is the neuronal axon guidance factor, the neuronal migration-rejecting factor, and the inhibitor in leukocyte chemotaxis. It has been found that it plays an important role in cell migration, apoptosis, and angiogenesis in recent years.

Neutrophils in the infected and injured areas are important components of the inflammatory response. Neutrophil chemotaxis, migration, and adhesion are important processes of inflammation, and various chemokines and chemical inducers can regulate leukocyte chemotaxis. Robo1-Slit2 has been proven to be an endogenous inhibitor of leukocyte chemotaxis and inhibits the migration of neutrophils, lymphocytes, and macrophages in the inflammatory response.

Slit2 inhibits VEGF-induced wild-type vascular endothelial cell migration, duct formation, and increased permeability, thereby blocking angiogenesis and vascular leakage. The Slit-Robo signaling pathway controls the integrity of vascular endothelial cells, and Slit2 may become a new drug for the treatment of neovascularization and increased vascular permeability. Slit mediates Robo4 activation to form the paxillin-GIT1 (ArfGAP) complex, which inactivates Arf6 and ultimately enhances vascular stability. Slit2 also induces angiogenesis through activation of mTORC2 (mammalian target of rapamycin)-dependent Akt and Rac.

### 3.4.6 Sonic Hedgehog

Sonic hedgehog is an important signaling pathway involved in growth, development, and injury repair, but it is well studied in tumors. This pathway is also closely related to the biological function of the nervous system, which promotes neural development and regenerative axon guidance. In recent years, research on stress damage, especially in oxidative stress damage, has become a new hot spot.

#### 3.4.6.1 The Hedgehog Signal Transduction Pathway and its Member

The Hedgehog (Hh) gene is found in drosophila. There are three Hedgehog signaling proteins in mammals: Sonic hedgehog (Shh), Desert hedgehog (Dhh) and Indian hedgehog (Ihh), among which Shh is a comprehensive one. Ptch is a 12 transmembrane receptor and Hh signal transduction starts from Ptch. When there is no Hh signal, Ptch binds to Smo to prevent the movement of Smo to primary cilia and inhibit Smo activity, and downstream signaling pathway is inhibited. Ptch does not directly bind to Smo, but indirectly affects Smo by altering the distribution and concentration of certain small molecule inhibitors. Smo is a 7 transmembrane receptor protein in the Frizzle family and is a member of the G-protein-coupled receptor family. Its C-terminus is located in the cell, while the N-terminus located outside the cell has a glutathione-rich domain and a transmembrane structural fragment. SAG (Smo agonist) and cyclopamine (Smo inhibitor) bind to the extracellular N-terminal structure of Smo and play a role. Gli protein is a transcription factor in the Hh pathway. There are three subtypes: Gli1, Gli2, and Gli3. Gli1 plays a major role in transcriptional activation in the Hh pathway, Gli3 acts as transcriptional repression, and Gli2 has dual roles of transcriptional activation and inhibition. When Hh is activated, the Hh signal peptide binds to Ptch, which relieves Smo inhibition. Smo accumulates on the primary cilia in an active form, enters the cell and activates the transcription factor Gli to enter the nucleus, regulates the opening of downstream signaling pathway, and synthesizes downstream-related functional proteins such as N-myc and cyclin.

#### 3.4.6.2 Hh Nonclassical Pathway

However, in recent years, there have been some reports on nonclassical Hh pathway. These non-classical pathways are mostly divided into two categories: independent of receptor Smo or independent of transcription factor Gli. A nonclassical pathway that does not require the receptor Smo: a nonclassical Hh pathway that promotes apoptosis and anti-tumor through the interaction between Ptch1 receptor and the cyclin B1. A nonclassical pathway that relies on the Smo receptor but does not require the transcription factor Gli: a nonclassical pathway that relies on Smo to activate the Rho family small molecules GTPases RhoA and Rac1, that relies on Smo to activate src to regulate axonal-directed nonclassical pathways, and that relies on Smo to regulate calcium signaling pathways and membrane function.

In addition to the above two categories, the study reports that during spinal nerve growth, Shh signaling dependent on Smo changes a classical Shh pathway that activates Gli1 transcriptional activity into a nonclassical Shh pathway that inhibits Gli1 transcriptional activity by regulating $Ca^{2+}$-dependent electrophysiological activity and CREB/PKA pathway. These nonclassical pathways are complementary to the complex Hh signaling pathways.

Previous studies have suggested that the Shh signaling pathway is only expressed in malignant keratinocytes in which the signaling pathway is activated, but not in normal keratinocytes, suggesting that specific regulation of the Shh signaling pathway only affects tumor cells, but not normal cells. Some scholars found that Shh can induce HaCaT keratinocytes to produce EGF. At the same time, EGF can in turn regulate the expression of Gli-1, the target gene of Shh signaling pathway in keratinocytes. This indicates that the Shh signaling pathway is closely related to the EGFR signaling pathway, which is a direct upstream pathway of the MEK/ERK pathway, further suggesting that the MEK/ERK signaling pathway may play an important role in the regulation of the metabolism of keratinocytes by the Shh signaling pathway. There are also many reports that the Shh signaling pathway plays an important regulatory role in the proliferation, apoptosis, and matrix penetration of normal keratinocytes. It is fully demonstrated that the Shh signaling pathway plays an important role in the proliferation and apoptosis of normal keratinocytes, but its molecular mechanism has not yet been elucidated.

Sonic hedgehog also has the effect of inducing angiogenesis, and the diameter of the formed blood vessels is large. Studies have shown that this is mainly related to Sonic hedgehog's ability to induce the expression of endothelial growth factor I and II, and its ability to rapidly activate C-Fes/PI3K pathway and gene transcription and regulate endothelial capillary formation, in which NO plays an important role. Some studies have found that in the animal model of diabetes, activation of the Hedgehog signaling pathway can partially improve the complications of diabetes. Studies by domestic scholars have found that the Shh signaling pathway was impaired in the skin tissue of diabetic mice, and the treatment of Shh protein on the wound surface can significantly promote the healing of diabetic skin wounds.

### 3.4.7 Other Signals

In the past, when people studied the molecular signaling mechanism of self-renewal, growth, and differentiation of cells (including stem cells), they paid more attention to the biochemical signals generated by chemical substances or solution media, and often ignored the influence of some physical factors or biomechanical signals. In recent years, some studies have begun to pay attention to the role of mechanical signals generated by the mechanical microenvironment inside and outside the cell and the mechanical force generated by cellular mechanical forces in controlling cell morphology and function. Biomechanical and mechanical signals are involved in the process of cell self-renewal and differentiation.

#### 3.4.7.1 Extracellular Microenvironment and Biomechanics of Cells

**Extracellular Microenvironment**

Cell aggregation and intercellular connectivity are affected by the microenvironment of the extracellular matrix, which are mainly chemical soluble and physical signal networks composed of hydrated proteins and polysaccharides. The signal molecule specifically binds to the receptor on the cell surface, causing a series of complex intracellular signal responses, regulating the expression of the target gene, causing a change in the phenotype of the cell, which in turn leads to a series of biological reactions.

**Biomechanical Effects of Cells**

Cell Tension

The integrity structure of cell tension consists of a pressure-bearing member and a series of continuous tension members connected with each other. The stability of this structure depends on the maintenance of the internal structural integrity of cells, and it is also called tension integrity. Studies have shown that the structure of cells conforms to the principle of tension integrity, and the tension integrity of the cellular framework (CF) affects the shape and function of cells. In addition, the tension integrity of the cytoskeleton is a major determinant of cell deformation. Related studies have shown that DNA synthesis of flat cells are more vigorous than that of round cells, suggesting that cell deformation is an important part of information transmission. Under the action of mechanical stress, all components of the cytoskeleton undergo an overall rearrangement for dispersing tension and pressure, which will cause cell deformation and the regulation information of cell shape, is transmitted in the form of force. Therefore, the change of mechanical stress can affect the growth and biochemical properties of cells by changing the balance of forces in the cells and their skeletons.

Hydrostatic Pressure

For the Relatively static fluid state, due to its own gravity or other external force, there is a force perpendicular to the contact surface inside the fluid and between the fluid and the wall surface of the container, which is called the static pressure of the fluid. Current studies have shown that hydrostatic pressure plays an important role in regulating cartilage metabolism and maintaining the normal phenotype of extracellular matrix, in which static pressure stimulation reduces the synthesis of type II collagen and proteoglycans, while normal dynamic pressure stimulation promotes the synthesis of type II collagen and proteoglycans. Studies have found that the force that causes the cell shape to become round in mitosis depends not only on the cytoskeleton of actomyosin, but also on the cell's ability to respond to the change of "osmolality" (i.e., in order to represent the osmotic pressure of a solution, sometimes the molecular concentration of an isotonic nonelectrolyte solution is used, referred to as osmolality). Studies have shown that the force that causes the cell shape round is due to changes in osmotic pressure, and it is necessary for actomyosin cortex to resist the external forces to maintain cell rounding. The transient decomposition of the actomyosin cortex increases the cell volume, and the actomyosin cortex contraction stimulation causes a decrease in cell volume, indicating that the cells maintain the balance of osmotic pressure by intrinsically regulating the contraction of the actomyosin cortex. Thus, by modulating actomyosin-dependent surface tension locally and osmotic pressure globally, cells can control their own volume, morphology, and mechanical properties.

Fluid Shear Force

Some cells may be in a fluid flow environment for a long time, for example, endothelial cells and smooth muscle cells of blood vessels and lymphatic vessels, epithelial cells of the esophagus and intestinal tract, and osteoblasts and osteoclasts in bones. These cells are always exposed to the scour of blood, lymph, tissue fluids, or digested food debris, and the mechanical forces that such fluids exert on cells are called fluid shear forces. Studies have shown that fluid shear forces can regulate cell function. Fluid flow is currently considered to be divided into two main forms: laminar flow and turbulent flow. Recent studies have shown that fluid shear force is an important factor affecting tissue metabolism, especially bone tissue metabolism, and regulating bone cell function and morphology.

#### 3.4.7.2 Effects of Biomechanical Force and Mechanical Signal Transduction on the Self-Renewal and Differentiation of Stem Cells

In the study of stem cells, how to maintain self-renewal of pluripotent stem cells is an important part of the research. In addition, pluripotent stem cells can be induced or spontaneously differentiated into tissue-specific cells, such as nerve cells, skin cells, or muscle cells. But for a long time, researchers have added growth factors and small molecule compounds to maintain the pluripotency of pluripotent stem cells. Even so, in the long-term culture process, stem cells will enter different stages of differentiation, showing different gene expression pattern. Therefore, how to maintain the characteristics of pluripotent stem cells long-termly and effectively in vitro is still a subject worthy of further study.

### Basement Hardness Affects the Proliferation and Differentiation Fate of Stem Cells

The importance of extracellular matrix sensing elasticity has been demonstrated in studies of fibroblasts, mesenchymal stem cells, and epidermal stem cells. Engler et al. found that different matrix hardness has different effects on the fate of cell growth. When the cells are cultured in a soft matrix similar to brain tissue, the cells show a neuronal phenotype; when the cells grow in a medium hardness matrix similar to muscle tissue, the cells show myogenic properties; and when the cells grow in a hard matrix similar to bone collagen, the cells show osteogenic phenotypes. Researchers at the University of Michigan in the United States found that stem cells exert a certain amount of force on the cell matrix, and this force may be related to cell differentiation. For example, stem cells grow in a hard matrix and finally differentiate into osteoblasts, while growing in a soft matrix differentiate into adipocytes. In addition, a team led by Professor Wang Ning, a Chinese-American scientist at the University of Illinois in the United States, found that mouse embryonic stem cells (mESCs) tend to adhere together to form round clones, but those cells contact hard culture dishes at the edge of the clones are relatively easy and rapid to differentiate. Based on this phenomenon, the researchers focused their attention on the biomechanical rather than biochemical studies of mESCs and found that cells cultured on soft gels showed greater homogeneity and pluripotency. Even in the absence of LIF, cells can be cultured continuously for more than 3 months. This study shows that reducing the elasticity of the matrix and cells helps the cells maintain a pluripotent state. However, the molecular mechanism of the change of extracellular matrix elasticity in inducing stem cell-specific differentiation has been a problem in the field of biomechanics.

### Changes in the Shape of the Basement Affect the Proliferation and Differentiation of Stem Cells

The different shape of the bottom of the cell culture medium has an important influence on cell proliferation and differentiation. Nelson and Bissell found that cells proliferated fastest in the places with large tractive force, that is, the edge of the round dish and the four corners of the square dish. McBeath et al. found that mesenchymal stem cells cultured on a small substrate differentiated into adipocytes, whereas those cultured on a larger substrate differentiated into osteoblasts. In order to study the effects of basement geometry and biomechanics on the differentiation of mesenchymal stem cells, Li Zhenhan et al. found that the geometry and area of cell spreading were significantly associated with the proliferation, differentiation, and migration of bone marrow mesenchymal stem cells. When the cell spreading width was narrow, the proliferation of bone marrow mesenchymal stem cells could be inhibited; when the cell spreading area was limited, the cell migration was enhanced. Studies suggest that dexamethasone may play an important role in reducing cell proliferation and migration. In addition, the team further explored the effects of three biophysical parameters of matrix hardness, shape, and dimension on rat mesenchymal stem cells, indicating that matrix hardness or dimension plays a major role in proliferation and regulation of cells growing in harder, dimensionally unbalanced matrices. However, the matrix geometry plays an important role in controlling the shape and extension of the cells growing in the columnar matrix and forming globular rather than grooved cells. Studies have shown that although the softness of the matrix regulates rat mesenchymal stem cells to differentiate into bone cells or differentiate into neural cells, matrix geometry and dimensions also play a regulatory role in stem cell differentiation. Lü et al. used a polyacrylamide hydrogel to precisely process three kinds of topographical culture dishes (grooves, columns, and hexagons) to culture mouse embryonic stem cells and systematically analyze the morphology, proliferation, and dryness of the cells. Studies have shown that the topological topography of the substrate plays an important role in regulating the dryness of stem cells. The clones formed in the groove-like and cylindrical dishes are relatively flat, while the clones formed at the bottom of the hexagonal dish are more rounded.

### Changes in Cell Morphology Affect Stem Cell Proliferation and Differentiation Fate

The shape and morphological characteristics are altered during cell differentiation. Studies have shown that cell morphology has an important relationship with cell proliferation, survival, and differentiation. Can changing cell morphology alter the differentiation fate of human mesenchymal stem cells? Early studies have shown that changes in cell morphology affect the activity of GTPase in the Rho family. The study found that RhoA is involved in the process of cell deformation, and changes in RhoA activity mediate the different differentiation of human mesenchymal stem cells. Inhibition of RhoA activity induces the production of adipocytes in human mesenchymal stem cells. Instead, continuous activation of RhoA can turn cells into osteoblasts. In addition, changes in cell morphology affect multiple regulatory mechanisms of RhoA downstream signaling. Studies have shown that members of the Rho GTPase family need to be activated in lipid rafts, and this position will change with the change of cell shape. RhoA-ROCK (RhoA-dependent kinase)-tension signals affecting stem cell fate may be transduced by focal adhesion. Altering cell elongation will alter RhoA-mediated contraction of cytoskeleton, assembly of focal adhesions, and downstream signaling pathways of integrins. In summary, the interaction among cell morphology, biochemical signal, and skeletal contraction mentioned above demonstrates the importance of cell structure and mechanics in cell and tissue development, and it provides a molecular basis for cells and tissues to complete negative feedback regulation of stabilization mechanisms.

#### Effect of Biomechanical Force on Gene Expression and Differentiation Fate of Stem Cells

Fluid shear forces play an important role in the differentiation of embryonic stem cells and mesenchymal stem cells. In embryonic stem cell research, Yamamoto et al. found that compared with static culture, the number and proportion of cells in the S and G2 ~ M phases were significantly increased. In addition, shear forces significantly increased the protein level and RNA expression of vascular endothelial cell marker molecules FLK-1, FLT-1, VE (vascular endothelial)-cadherin, and PECAM (platelet endothelial cell adhesion molecular)-1. Adamo et al. have shown that fluid shear forces can promote hematopoiesis during embryogenesis. When mouse embryonic stem cells differentiate in vitro, the expression of Runx1 in CD41 and c-kit double-positive hematopoietic precursor cells increased under fluid shear stimulation. In addition, the elimination of NO signal may be one of the reasons why shear forces increases the ability of hematopoietic cell clone formation and increases the expression of hematopoietic marker molecules in mouse embryos. Toh and Voldman found that fluid shear specifically upregulated the ectodermal specific marker FGF5 (fibroblast growth factor 5). The mechanical perception of shear force in mouse embryonic stem cells may be mediated by extracellular heparin sulfate proteoglycans, thereby regulating FGF5 expression. In terms of mesenchymal stem cells, using DNA chip and reverse transcription real-time quantitative PCR analysis, Glossop and Cartmell found that different fluid shear strength and action time affected the expression of related genes in the mitogen-activated protein kinase (MAPK) signaling pathway of human bone mesenchymal stem cells (hBMSCs). Under stimulation of different shear strength and action time, different gene expression patterns appeared in the cells, but when comparing the cells with different mechanical strength and action time, it was found that regardless of the mechanical strength and action time, the shear force could consistently and significantly upregulate the expression of MAP3K8 and IL-1. This study suggests that MAP3K8 may be an important mediator of intracellular force transduction in hBMSCs. Other studies have shown that shear forces stimulate the phenotype of hMSCs to differentiate into osteoblasts without the induction of chemical factors. Horizontal tensile stress has an important influence on the differentiation of mesenchymal stem cells. The changes of mesenchymal stem cells after being stretched by uniaxial horizontal stress were detected by micro image beam. The results showed that horizontal stress caused an increase in the expression of the smooth muscle cell marker molecule calponin1, while the expression of the cartilage matrix marker molecule decreased. If the cells are placed in the vertical direction of stress stretching, the previous changes of gene expression disappear. These results indicate that mechanical stress plays an important role in gene expression and cell fate of mesenchymal stem cells. He Xueling et al. found that both osteogenic chemical inducers and stress stimulation can promote osteogenic differentiation of rat BMSCs, and they have synergistic effects. Lü et al. performed a kinetic study of lateral migration and transmembrane migration of human epidermal cells or human fibroblasts using a stretching device and a modified invasive chamber method. It was observed that when epidermal cells were cocultured with fibroblasts in a noncontact manner, epidermal cells had asymmetric migration. For example, the number of human epidermal cells which are distant from human fibroblasts or can migrate from bottom to top is significantly higher than those which are close to human fibroblasts or migrate from top to bottom. This asymmetric migration is primarily regulated by epidermal growth factor (EGF) secreted by fibroblasts. In addition, mechanical stretching can further affect the asymmetric migration of human epidermal cells by increasing EGF secretion of fibroblasts. High-frequency magnetic bead oscillation affects the proliferation and differentiation of stem cells. Chowdhury et al. placed micron-sized magnetic beads on the surface of embryonic stem cells and then applied a tiny oscillating magnetic field to oscillate the magnetic beads back and forth in the magnetic field. Studies have found that this continuous oscillation can stimulate the production of internal forces, such as the periodic movement of myosin. They also found that mouse embryonic stem cells are softer than other types of cells, and more sensitive to local periodic forces. A small local force can alter the expression of Oct3/4 genes in a single embryonic stem cell, and the expression of other genes can also be altered.

#### Effects of Mechanical Effects Produced by Rotational Culture on Stem Cell Proliferation and Differentiation

In recent years, it has been reported that the mechanical effects of rotation culture can affect the proliferation and differentiation of stem cells. Yuge et al. found that the cells expanded 14-fold after 1 week of culture, while normal gravity culture only expanded 4 times. In addition, cells expanded in a 3D-clinostat have the ability to differentiate into hyaline cartilage in vivo. In contrast, cells cultured under normal gravity lose this property. The study suggests that a 3D rotation culture environment may be an important tool for expanding stem cells, and that expanded cells can avoid some adverse effects after cell transplantation. Kawahara et al. found that in the absence of feeder layer, serum, and LIF, mouse embryonic stem cells can still maintain dry growth, and expanded embryonic stem cells has the potential to differentiate into three germ layers. A rotary bioreactor developed by the National Aeronautics and Space Administration (NASA) was used to culture human foreskin-derived epidermal stem cells. The results showed that under the 3D rotation culture condition, the proliferation of human epidermal stem cells was enhanced, and the expression of the stem cells terminal differentiation marker molecule involucrin was reduced. The expanded cells form a compact 3D structure. In addition, in the study of mouse embryonic stem cell differentiation, it was found that rotary suspension culture promoted cell differentiation into mesendoderm, and the main mechanism was upregulation of Wnt/β-catenin signaling pathway. Although the mechanical effects of rotation culture can affect cell proliferation and differentiation, the exact mechanism remains unclear and needs further study.

### 3.4.7.3 Possible Mechanisms of Biomechanical Stress Regulating Stem Cells

The process in which cells sense the elasticity of ECM is the process in which cells transform the perceived mechanical stimuli into biochemical information. This process is called cellular mechanical signal transduction. The cells adhere to ECM through the adhesion spots, which are composed of a series of signaling molecules and are connected to the actin cytoskeleton. These signaling molecules can produce conformational changes under mechanical stimulation, triggering a series of molecular events such as kinase activation, phosphorylation site exposure, intracellular transport of signaling molecules, and changes in receptor ligand binding strength.

#### Integrin Activity and Mechanical Regulation of Signals

More and more studies have shown that a key molecular mechanism of cellular stress perception is the deformation of integrins, focal adhesion proteins, and other related structural proteins. Integrin has the function of mechanical stress transduction, which focuses on the integrin focused adhesion zone and acts to convert mechanical signals into chemical signals. Friedland et al. reported that α5β1-integrin is a switch that Myosin II causes cytoskeletal stress fibers to be in a state of relax and tension. There is some evidence that α-actin, which mediates actin filaments and the cytoplasmic portion of integrin, is a key molecular structure that interferes with the formation of actin stress fibers and blocks signaling transmission to the nucleus. G protein is a key signal transduction molecule. The large G protein is anchored to the cell membrane by lipid modification of amino acid residues on subunits, thus providing a structural basis for receiving the structural signals of cell membrane. The small G protein receives extracellular mechanical signals through the extracellular matrix-integrin-cytoskeleton. Recently, Grashoff et al. have demonstrated that the recovery of focal adhesions in living cells and the transmission of force between focal adhesions are necessary for the stabilization of focal adhesions under stress conditions by using the tension biosensor of focal adhesions. Therefore, integrin activity and signaling mechanical regulation may determine the fate of stem cells.

#### The Role of RhoA/Rho-Kinase (ROCK) Signaling Pathway

RhoA is a GTP enzyme located in the cell. ROCK is an effector molecule downstream of RhoA that is activated by activated RhoA. ROCK phosphorylates myosin light chain kinase (MLCK) and myosin phosphatase to inhibit the activity. This plays a very important role in maintaining the integrity of the cytoskeletal tension fibers, increasing the stretchability of actin tension fibers, and regulating cell morphology, adhesion, and movement. Although RhoA plays an important role in the mechanical response of cells, its molecular mechanism has not been revealed. Guilluy et al. found that tension stimulated the activation of these two molecules and recruited them to the adhesion complex via integrin. Furthermore, the results revealed that LARG is activated by Src family kinase Fyn. The enhancement of GEF-H1 activity is catalyzed by the downstream cascade of extracellular-regulated protein kinases (ERK), including focal adhesion kinase (FAK) and rat sarcoma (Ras).

#### The Function of Mechanical Signal Super Long-Distance Transduction

Short-distance mechanical transduction and mechanism in living cells have been well studied. Force and energy can cross-membrane through the integrin, adhesion proteins, binding focal adhesions, and cytoskeletal networks to connect the nucleus, nuclear internal scaffold, and circular chromatin to signal transduction. The speed and precision of this intracellular mechanical signal response can be adjusted by altering the prestress of the cytoskeleton. Prestress changes can control the stiffness of the cytoskeletal microfilaments under tension, such as actin stress fibers and intermediate fibers with large span in the cytoplasm. The force acting on the nucleus may cause morphological changes, folding and kinetic changes of specific load-bearing molecules in the nucleus, and may also alter the high-level structure of chromatin, which may affect the self-assembly of nuclear proteins, gene transcription, DNA replication, and RNA processing. This long-distance transduction of mechanical signals in living cells is faster and more efficient than biochemical signal transduction generated by diffusion. Long-distance transduction of mechanical signals also helps to understand how mechanical forces alter the activity of multiple molecules at different locations in the cytoplasm and nucleus. This cellular response is critical for regulating cell behavior, tissue development, and the fate of stem cells.

#### The Role of Myosin II Regulating Stem Cells

Non-muscle myosin II (NMM II) is a class of actin-binding proteins that regulate cell contraction. Among the three different NMM II subtypes identified, NMM II A and NMM II B are found in almost all higher organisms. Knockout of NMM II A or NMM II B leads to fetal death in mice. NMM II is essential for early embryo development. The important role of NMM II in mechanical regulation of stem cells has been reported. Matrix elasticity and cell morphology determine the mesenchymal stem cell lineage, which depends on NMM II, and its specific molecular mechanism is still unclear.

E-cadherin is a key target molecule of NMM II A in human embryonic stem cells. NMM II-induced contraction is not only a function of reading extracellular signals, but also plays an important role in determining the production and transduction of stem cell signals.

With the deepening of research on the regulation of cell structure and function by mechanical stress in recent years, the response of cells to stress-induced strain and the mechanism of mechanical transduction have gradually been recognized. However, there are still many unknown details to be explored in this field, such as the dose-effect relationship between stress size, frequency and stem cell proliferation, differentiation, apoptosis, the effect of stress on the biological behavior of tissue-repaired stem cells, and the regulation of intracellular mechanical signal transduction and gene expression under stress. Therefore, there will be futher study on the relationship between mechanical stress, mechanical transduction pathway and cells, and explore a mechanical-biological coupling law of mechanical effects on the life activities of cells, which will help to understand the role of force in the pathogenesis and wound repair process of certain diseases and help to adopt new and more effective coping strategies for these mechanisms and processes. It is also important for the research of tissue engineering, gene therapy, stem cell regenerative medicine, space life, and space medicine.

#### AGEs-RAGE Signaling Pathway

Diabetic wound healing is a complex process of multifactor regulation such as inflammatory cells, repair cells, and cytokines. Abnormalities in any part can lead to difficult healing of wounds. Advanced glycosylation end products (AGEs) and related cell signaling pathways are research hotspots in the study of the mechanism of difficult wound healing in diabetic wounds.

AGEs and their receptors, RAGEAGEs, are a group of stable end products produced by condensation, rearrangement, cleavage, oxidative modification, and other complex nonenzymatic glycosylation reactions of various intermediates. Normal humans also have AGEs, but their formation takes several weeks or even months, and the production is very low. However, when protein half-life is long, protein turnover is delayed, persistent hyperglycemia (such as diabetes) and active carbonyl levels are elevated, AGEs will significantly accelerate synthesis, resulting in more production of AGEs than clearance, accumulation in the body, damaging cells and tissues. Persistent hyperglycemia causes nonenzymatic glycosylation of many structural proteins, functional proteins, and nucleic acid proteins in the human body, ultimately resulting in irreversible AGEs. The receptor pathway is the main pathway for the action of AGEs. Currently known AGEs receptors include RAGE, macrophage scavenger receptors I and II, oligosaccharyltransferase 48, and galactose-binding protein-3. RAGE is the most studied and in-depth one. RAGE is a polypeptide with a unique amino acid end sequence and a molecular weight of about 35 ku. It is a multi-ligand member of the immunoglobulin superfamily in cell surface molecules. Many cells, such as endothelial cells, monocytes-macrophages, and vascular smooth muscle cells, have RAGE expression on the surface. Therefore, these cells also act as sites for the physiological and pathological effects of AGEs and RAGE interactions. In the normal physiological state of mature individuals, the level of RAGE expression in cells is low. When diabetes, inflammation, and so on cause cells to be stressed, RAGE can be highly expressed.

Classical pathophysiological studies have shown that spontaneous ulcers or difficult wound healing in diabetic patients are closely related to angioneuropathy caused by disorders of glucose metabolism. However, from the perspective of mechanism research, angioneuropathy is the pathological outcome of the diabetes disease, and it is not the starting point of difficult wound healing. Studies have shown that in the case of undamaged skin tissue of diabetic patients, there have been changes in histology and cell biological behavior, which is a kind of "hidden damage" that does not cause skin tissue integrity and continuity damage.

Although this damage is endogenous, it does not cause visible damage to skin defects or fractures, changes in histology and cellular function may increase the vulnerability of skin tissue to exogenous damage. The "hidden damage" is caused by the high glucose environment of local skin tissue and the accumulation of AGEs, resulting in the cell or matrix dysfunction of the skin tissue. Therefore, the production and accumulation of AGEs is an important pathological basis for the damage of multiple tissues and organs such as nerves and blood vessels. Vascular endothelial cells and fibroblasts are the main cells involved in repair during wound healing. The integrity of their structure and function is the main influencing factor of diabetic wound healing. Under normal conditions, endothelial cells express only a small amount of RAGE; in diabetic state, with the increase of AGEs in circulating and subendothelial matrix, the expression of RAGE in endothelial cells is enhanced and the interaction of AGEs with RAGE changes the function of endothelial cells. AGEs can significantly affect the morphology and proliferation of fibroblasts, inhibit the ability of fibroblasts to synthesize collagen, and affect wound healing. Studies have shown that AGEs exert biological effects primarily through two pathways: the non-receptor pathway (direct damage) and the receptor pathway. Non-receptor pathway: AGEs alter their structural functions by direct modification of proteins, lipids, nucleic acids, and the like. Receptor pathway: AGEs initiates a series of receptor signal transduction pathways by binding to RAGE, a specific receptor on cell membranes such as endothelial cells, to stimulate the formation and release of various cytokines, leading to pathological changes in the body's nerves and blood vessels. Among them, the receptor pathway is the main pathway of AGEs action, playing a more important role in the damage caused by AGEs.

(a) The combination of AGEs and RAGE promotes the increase of ROS production and induces oxidative stress. Abnormal oxidative stress leads to abnormal wound healing in diabetic skin. During wound healing, AGEs-RAGE effect is an important factor influencing the level of oxidative stress in diabetic wounds. The interaction of AGEs with its cell surface receptor RAGE is mediated by reduced coenzyme II (NADPH) oxidase, which increases ROS production, produces oxygen free radicals, causes cell membrane superoxide, impairs membrane protein function that maintains ion homeostasis, thereby causing calcium influx, increase of the intracellular calcium ion concentration, and finally lead to abnormal cell structure, function, metabolism, and induce oxidative stress reaction. In addition, when the ROS is excessive and exceeds the antioxidant capacity of the cells, it can directly activate or damage certain proteins, nucleic acids, lipids, etc. in the cells, affecting the function and integrity of the cells. Since ROS is produced in the mitochondria, mitochondria are most vulnerable. Oxidative stress promotes mitochondrial oxidative phosphorylation and also causes the formation of a large amount of peroxide, thereby inhibiting glyceraldehyde-3-phosphate dehydrogenase and causing accumulation of glycolysis intermediates. These intermediates further enhance the activity of aldose reductase and protein kinase C and in turn promote the production of AGEs, leading to nerve fiber dysfunction and damage.

(b) Activation of the nuclear transcription factor (NF-κB), triggering a cascade reaction that affects the healing of diabetic wound tissue. NF-κB is present in a variety of cells and is involved in various physiological and pathological processes such as immune regulation and inflammatory cell proliferation. NF-κB binds to the B cell-specific nuclear protein on the immunoglobulin κ light chain gene enhancer, exists in many types of cells, and controls the expression of various genes. The enhancers of these genes all contain binding site of NF-κB, which are the target genes regulated by NF-κB, including vascular cell adhesion molecule-1 (VCAM-1), intercellular adhesion molecule-1 (ICAM-1), endothelial cell adhesion molecule (ECAM-I), tissue factor (TF), monocyte chemoattractant protein-1 (MCP-1), nitric oxide synthase (NOS), and angiotensinogen gene. Activated NF-κB initiates transcription of these target genes, triggering abnormal inflammatory responses and autoimmune responses. In vivo, the activation-inducing response of NF-κB is transient and the system returns to baseline within a few hours. Diabetic patients have abnormal sustained NF-κB activation, and ligand-stimulatory RAGE activation can act as a switch to turn NF-κB short-term activation into long-term activation. AGEs interact with RAGE to cause oxidative stress and activate NF-κB by activating the proto-oncogene ras-encoded p38ms and mitogen-activated protein (MAP) kinase pathways. Activation of NF-κB stimulates the expression of numerous target genes, such as TF, P21, Has, and extracellular signal-regulated kinase 1/2 (ERK1/2), and the expression of RAGE. Activation of these pro-oxidative genes can increase the secretion of nitric oxide (NO), interleukin-1 (IL-1), interleukin-6 (IL-6), tumor necrosis factor-α (TNF-α), monocyte clone stimulating factor, VCAM-1, and ICAM-1. The release of a large number of pro-inflammatory cytokines (IL-6, TNF-α), growth factors (transforming growth factor-β, IGF), and adhesion molecules (VCAM-1, ICAM-1) can trigger uncontrolled systemic inflammatory cascade, forming a vicious circle, causing persistent cell damage and dysfunction, ultimately leading to the development of tissue damage.

The AGEs-RAGE signaling pathway is closely related to the repair of diabetic refractory wounds, involving many cytokines, oxidative stress, nerves, blood vessels, and many other aspects. The AGEs-RAGE signaling pathway is the initial stage of invisible lesions in diabetic wounds. If the upstream part related to the mechanism of difficult healing wounds can be intervened to terminate the occurrence or development of subsequent effects, it can provide effective and feasible preventive treatment. It is of great significance to improve the cure rate of difficult healing wounds, and also provides a solid theoretical basis for drug target intervention.

In summary, wound repair is a complex process involving many growth factors/cytokines and their signal transduction pathways. These pathways and growth factors/cytokines regulate each other to promote wound healing. This is a complicated process, and there are still many mechanisms that we need to explore.

## References


1. van de Wetering M, Sancho E, Verweij C, et al. The beta-catenin/TCF-4 complex imposes a crypt progenitor phenotype on colorectal cancer cells. Cell. 2002;111(2):241–50.
2. Tanigaki K, Nogaki F, Takahashi J, et al. Notch1 and Notch3 instructively restrict bFGF-responsive multipotent neural progenitor cells to an astroglial fate. Neuron. 2001;29(1):45–55.
3. Craig CG, Tropepe V, Morshead CM, et al. In vivo growth factor expansion of endogenous subependymal neural precursor cell populations in the adult mouse brain. J Neurosci. 1996;16(8):2649–58.
4. Mahoney MJ, Saltzman WM. Transplantation of brain cells assembled around a programmable synthetic microenvironment. Nat Biotechnol. 2001;19(10):934–9.
5. Spradling A, Drummond-Barbosa D, Kai T. Stem cells find their niche. Nature. 2001;414(6859):98–104.
6. Lemischka IR, Moore KA. Stem cells: interactive niches. Nature. 2003;425(6960):778–9.
7. Fuchs E, Tumbar T, Guasch G. Socializing with the neighbors: stem cells and their niche. Cell. 2004;116(6):769–78.
8. Watt FM, Hogan BL. Out of Eden: stem cells and their niches. Science. 2000;287(5457):1427–30.
9. Zhang J, Niu C, Ye L, et al. Identification of the haematopoietic stem cell niche and control of the niche size. Nature. 2003;425(6960):836–41.
10. Yamashita YM, Fuller MT, Jones DL. Signaling in stem cell niches: lessons from the drosophila germline. J Cell Sci. 2005;118(4):665.
11. Donovan PJ, Gearhart J. The end of the beginning for pluripotent stem cells. Nature. 2001;414(6859):92–7.
12. Kai T, Spradling A. Differentiating germ cells can revert into functional stem cells in Drosophila melanogaster ovaries. Nature. 2004;428(6982):564–9.
13. Lovell-Badge R. The future for stem cell research. Nature. 2001;414(6859):88–91.
14. Feng Z-Y, Pan M-H, Lu C. Drosophila germline stem cells and their microenvironment. Chin J Cell Biol. 2006;28(2):169–72.
15. Van Beek ME, Meistrich ML. A method for quantifying synchrony in testes of rats treated with vitamin a deprivation and readministration. Biol Reprod. 1990;42(3):424–31.
16. Rossi P, Sette C, Dolci S, et al. Role of c-kit in mammalian spermatogenesis. J Endocrinol Investig. 2000;23(9):609–15.
17. Vincent S, Segretain D, Nishikawa S, et al. Stage-specific expression of the kit receptor and its ligand (KL) during male gametogenesis in the mouse: a kit-KL interaction critical for meiosis. Development. 1998;125(22):4585.
18. Piquet-Pellorce C, Dorval I, Jégou B. Paracrine control of spermatogenetic stem cells: example of the leukemia inhibitory factor. Contracept Fertil Sex. 1997;25(7–8):565–8.
19. Nagano M, Avarbock MR, Leonida EB, et al. Culture of mouse spermatogonial stem cells. Tissue Cell. 1998;30(4):389–97.
20. Meng X, de Rooij DG, Westerdahl K, et al. Promotion of seminomatous tumors by targeted overexpression of glial cell line-derived neurotrophic factor in mouse testis. Cancer Res. 2001;61(8):3267.
21. Meng X, Lindahl M, Hyvönen ME, et al. Regulation of cell fate decision of undifferentiated spermatogonia by GDNF. Science. 2000;287(5457):1489–93.
22. Reya T, Duncan AW, Ailles L, et al. A role for Wnt signalling in self-renewal of haematopoietic stem cells. Nature. 2003;423(6938):409–14.
23. Thorsteinsdottir U, Mamo A, Kroon E, et al. Overexpression of the myeloid leukemia– associatedHoxa9 gene in bone marrow cells induces stem cell expansion. Blood. 2002;99(1):121–9.
24. Antonchuk J, Sauvageau G, Humphries RK. HOXB4-induced expansion of adult hematopoietic stem cells ex vivo. Cell. 2002;109(1):39–45.
25. Krosl J, Austin P, Beslu N, et al. In vitro expansion of hematopoietic stem cells by recombinant TAT-HOXB4 protein. Nat Med. 2003;9:1428–32.
26. Park IK, Qian D, Kiel M, et al. Bmi-1 is required for maintenance of adult self-renewing haematopoietic stem cells. Nature. 2003;423(6937):302–5.
27. Bhardwaj G, Murdoch B, Wu D, et al. Sonic hedgehog induces the proliferation of primitive human hematopoietic cells via BMP regulation. Nat Immunol. 2001;2(2):172–80.
28. Alonso L, Fuchs E. Stem cells of the skin epithelium. Proc Natl Acad Sci U S A. 2003;100(Suppl 1):11830–5.
29. Brouard M, Barrandon Y. Controlling skin morphogenesis: hope and despair[J]. Curr Opin Biotechnol. 2003;14(5):520–5.
30. Cotsarelis G, Kaur P, Dhouailly D, et al. Epithelial stem cells in the skin: definition, markers, localization and functions. 1999;8:1.
31. Fu X, Sun X, Li X, et al. Dedifferentiation of epidermal cells to stem cells in vivo. Lancet. 2001;358(9287):1067–8.
32. Fu X, Sun X, Sun T. Epidermal growth factor induce the epithelial stem cell island formation in the regenerated epidermis. Zhonghua Yi Xue Za Zhi. 2001;81(12):733–6.
33. Johnson G, Lapadat R. Mitogen-activated protein kinase pathways mediated by ERK, JNK, and p38 protein kinases. Science (New York, NY). 2003;298:1911–2.
34. Huelsken J, Vogel R, Erdmann B, et al. β-Catenin controls hair follicle morphogenesis and stem cell differentiation in the skin. Cell. 2001;105(4):533–45.
35. Artavanis-Tsakonas S, Rand MD, Lake RJ. Notch signaling: cell fate control and signal integration in development. Science. 1999;284(5415):770–6.
36. Kratochwil K, Dull M, Farinas I, et al. Lef1 expression is activated by BMP-4 and regulates inductive tissue interactions in tooth and hair development. Genes Dev. 1996;10(11):1382–94.
37. Brittan M, Wright NA. Gastrointestinal stem cells. J Pathol. 2002;197(4):492–509.
38. Houchen CW, George RJ, Sturmoski MA, et al. FGF-2 enhances intestinal stem cell survival and its expression is induced after radiation injury. Am J Phys. 1999;276(1):G249–58.
39. Potten CS, Owen G, Hewitt D, et al. Stimulation and inhibition of proliferation in the small intestinal crypts of the mouse after in vivo administration of growth factors. Gut. 1995;36(6):864–73.
40. Kubbutat MHG, Jones SN, Vousden KH. Regulation of p53 stability by Mdm2. Nature. 1997;387(6630):299–303.
41. Zamzami N, Brenner C, Marzo I, et al. Subcellular and submitochondrial mode of action of Bcl-2- like oncoproteins. Oncogene. 1998;16(17):2265–82.
42. Batlle E, Henderson J, Beghtel H, et al. ??-catenin and TCF mediate cell positioning in the intestinal epithelium by controlling the expression of EphB/EphrinB. Cell. 2002;111:251–63.
43. Reynolds BA, Weiss S. Generation of neurons and astrocytes from isolated cells of the adult mammalian central nervous system. Science. 1992;255(5052):1707–10.
44. Rakic P. Adult neurogenesis in mammals: an identity crisis. J Neurosci. 2002;22(3):614–8.

45. Gritti A, Vescovi AL, Galli R. Adult neural stem cells: plasticity and developmental potential. J Physiol Paris. 2002;96(1–2):81–90.
46. Tropepe V, Sibilia M, Ciruna BG, et al. Distinct neural stem cells proliferate in response to EGF and FGF in the developing mouse telencephalon. Dev Biol. 1999;208(1):166–88.
47. Kuhn HG, Winkler J, Kempermann G, et al. Epidermal growth factor and fibroblast growth factor-2 have different effects on neural progenitors in the adult rat brain. J Neurosci. 1997;17(15):5820–9.
48. Lim DA, Alvarez-Buylla A. Interaction between astrocytes and adult subventricular zone precursors stimulates neurogenesis. Proc Natl Acad Sci U S A. 1999;96(13):7526–31.
49. Gage FH. Mammalian neural stem cells. Science. 2000;287(5457):1433–8.
50. Lim DA, Tramontin AD, Trevejo JM, et al. Noggin antagonizes BMP signaling to create a niche for adult neurogenesis. Neuron. 2000;28(3):713–26.
51. Gaiano N, Nye JS, Fishell G. Radial glial identity is promoted by Notch1 signaling in the murine forebrain. Neuron. 2000;26(2):395–404.
52. Moore KA, Lemischka IR. Stem cells and their niches. Science. 2006;311(5769):1880.
53. Kiger AA, Jones DL, Schulz C, et al. Stem cell self-renewal specified by JAK-STAT activation in response to a support cell cue. Science. 2001;294(5551):2542–5.
54. Lian YM, Ge SL. Expression and change of stress activated proteinkinases in fetal skin at different developmental stages. Chin J Tissue Eng Res. 2005;9(22):136–8.
55. Zhang Q, Bai XD, Fu XB. Research progress of p38MAPK signaling pathway. Infect Inflamm Repair. 2014;6(2):121–3.
56. Cheng B, Fu XB, Sheng ZY, et al. Cellular signaling pathway involved in fibroblasts isolated from thermal injury. Chin J Med. 2003;28(7):590–1.
57. Cheng B, Liu HW, Fu XB, et al. Recombinant human platelet-derived growth factor enhanced dermal wound healing by a pathway involving ERK and c-Fos in diabetic rats. J Dermatol Sci. 2007;45(3):193–201.
58. Chen W, Fu XB, Sun TZ, et al. Changes in phosphorylated mitogen-activated protein kinase protein expression in hypertrophic scars. Chin J Med. 2004;29(2):147–9.
59. Fathke C, Wilson L, Shah K, et al. Wnt signaling induces epithelial differentiation during cutaneous wound healing. BMC Cell Biol. 2006;11(1):95–104.
60. Zhang CP, Chen P, Fu XB, et al. Effects of Wnt/β-catenin signaling pathway activation on phenotypic changes of human epidermal cells. J Third Mil Med Univ. 2010;32(16):1716–9.
61. Chen W, Fu XB, Sun TZ, et al. Characteristics of transforming growth factor-β1,β2,β3 and their receptor expression in ulcerative and normal skins and their effects on wound healing. Chin Crit Care Med. 2002;14(2):93–5.

# Skin Development and Tissue Repair and Regeneration

# 4

Biao Cheng, Hongwei Liu, Jianfu Li, and Xiaobing Fu

## 4.1 Development of Skin Tissue

The skin consists of three parts: the epidermis, the dermis, and the subcutaneous tissue. In embryogenesis, the skin tissue is derived from the ectoderm and mesoderm of the embryo. When the egg is fertilized to form a zygote, the repeated cleavage begins, forming the solid cell mass, called morula, and the cells at center are called cell group or germ cells. When the morula reaches the uterus, a cavity is formed inside. This is called a blastocyst or blastula, and the inner cell group is on the inner side of the blastocyst. On the 15th day, the inner cell group differentiates into a blastodisc composed of three germ layers: endoderm, mesoderm, ectoderm. The organs and tissues of the human body are developed and differentiated from the three germ layers of the blastodisc. The epidermis (including the oral mucosa), the majority of the skin appendages, and the nerves are all developed from the ectoderm. Tissues, such as dermis, subcutaneous tissue, blood vessels, lymphatic vessels, and muscles, are derived from the mesoderm.

The development of epidermis, dermis, and neurovascular in the skin are coordinated. The visible skin development begins in the second month of the embryo and does not complete until several months after birth. At all stages of skin development, skin differentiation is controlled by many internal (genetic, metabolic) and external (microenvironmental) factors.

B. Cheng
General Hospital of Southern Theater Command of Chinese People's Liberation Army, Guangzhou, China

H. Liu
The First Affiliated Hospital of Jinan University, Guangzhou, China

J. Li
Huatai International Hospital, Guang'an City, Guang'an, China

X. Fu (✉)
The Chinese People's Liberation Army General Hospital, Beijing, China

### 4.1.1 The Development of the Epidermis

At the 3rd week of embryonic development, the epidermis is only simple cuboidal epithelium. At the 4th week, the epithelium proliferate into two layers. The inner layer of cells is cuboidal, called the germinal layer; the outer layer is relatively flat, called the periderm. At the 8th to 10th week, the germinal cells continue to divide, producing a layer of discontinuous cells on the surface, located between the periderm and the germinal layer, called the stratum intermedium. As the embryo develops, the germinal cells continue to divide and proliferate, forming two to three layers of intermediate cells and moving up. After the 12th week, the middle layer cells show processes, and mosaic to form stratum spinosum. After the 16th week, the granular layer appears, and the cells near the surface of the middle layer lose the nucleus and become keratinocytes. The cells located in periderm are keratinized and shed into the amniotic fluid. At 5 months of gestation, the base of the epidermis is corrugated, forming epidermal process with the dermal papilla. After 6 months, the epidermis is similar to the newborn, and the basic structure is close to that of adults (Figs. 4.1–4.3).

The skin of normal adults consists of the epidermis and dermis. The epidermis is keratinized stratified squamous epithelium, and the dermis is composed of dense connective tissue (Fig. 4.4).

During embryonic development, the skin of the fetus has its typical tissue structure. In the early embryonic period (at 11th to 13th week), the skin of the fetus is composed of only two to three layers of epidermal cells, without skin appendages. At the beginning of the 15th week, the skin of the fetus begins to sprout from the basal layer and extends to the stroma below. At the 17th week, the epidermal cell group begins to differentiate into hair follicles, extending to the deep skin. After the 21st week, the skin of the fetus begins to thicken, and skin appendages such as sweat glands, hair follicles, and sebaceous glands are visible. After the 28th week, the skin continues to thicken, the number of sweat glands,


X. Fu (ed.), *Regenerative Medicine in China*, https://doi.org/10.1007/978-981-16-1182-7_4

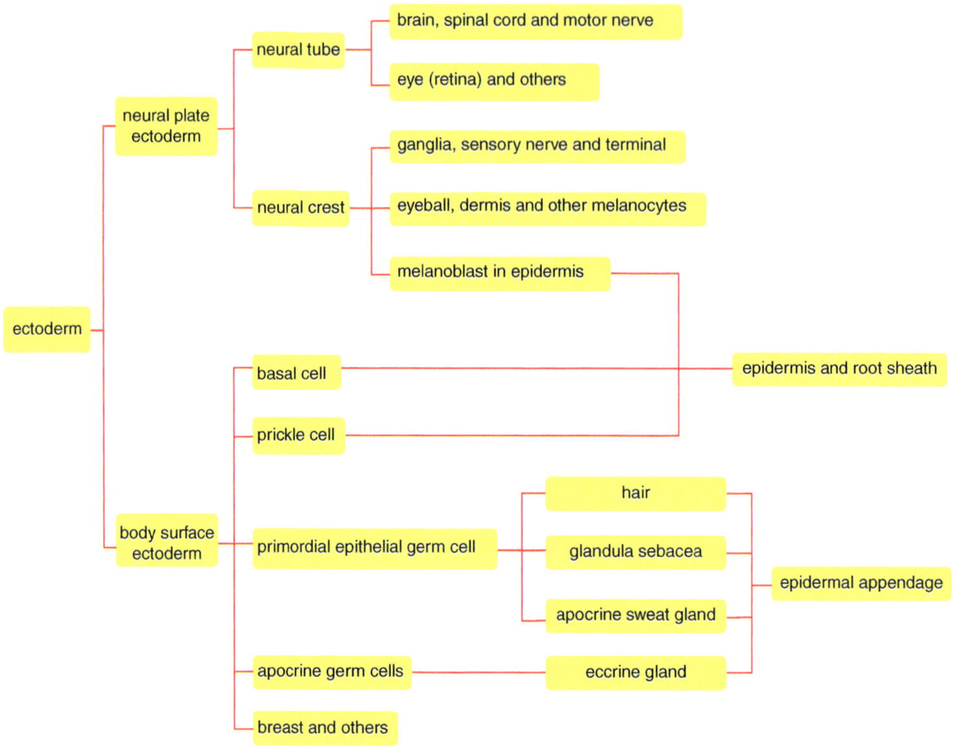


**Fig. 4.1** Relationship between ectoderm development and skin

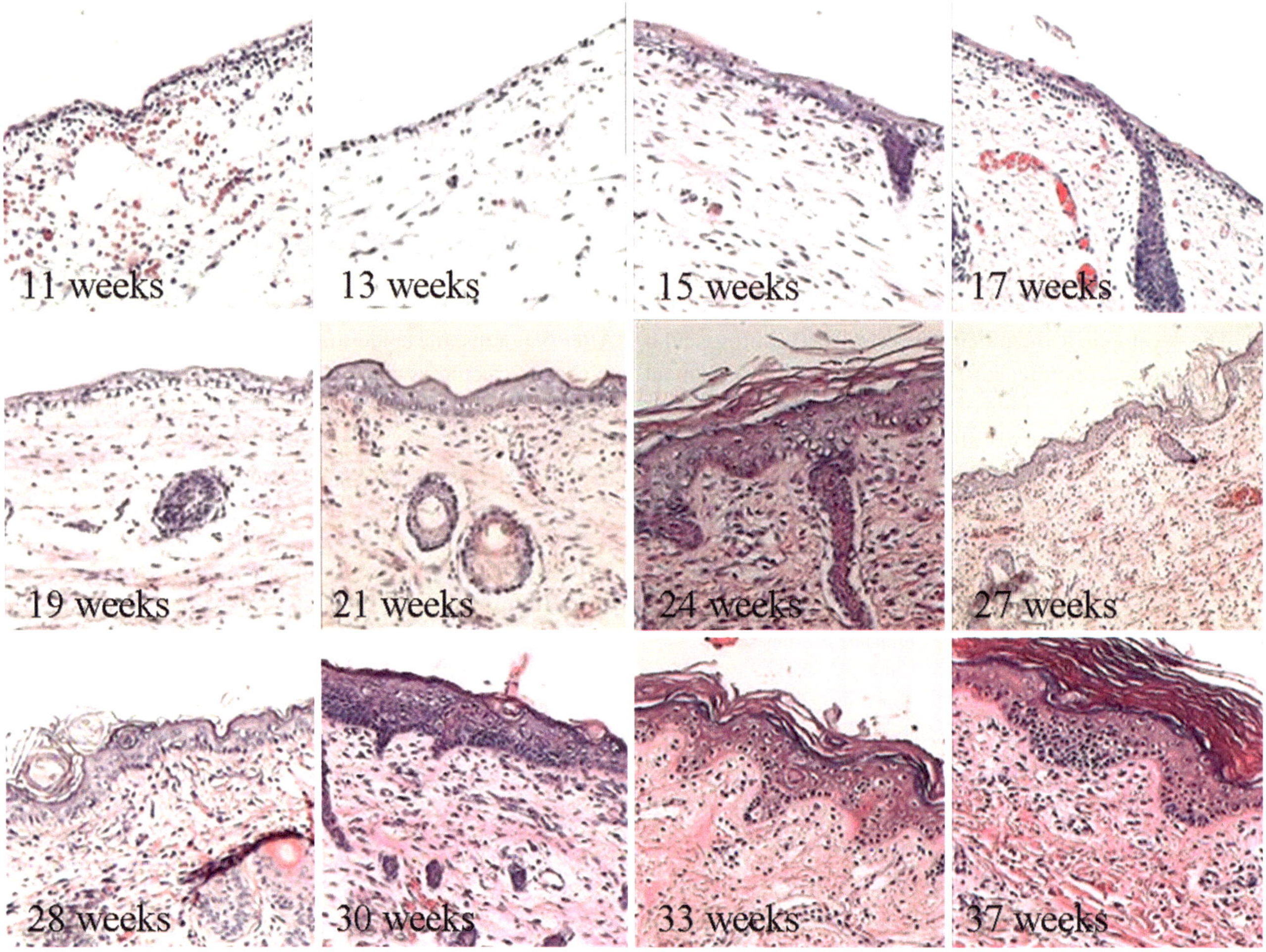


**Fig. 4.2** Histological changes in human embryonic skin development

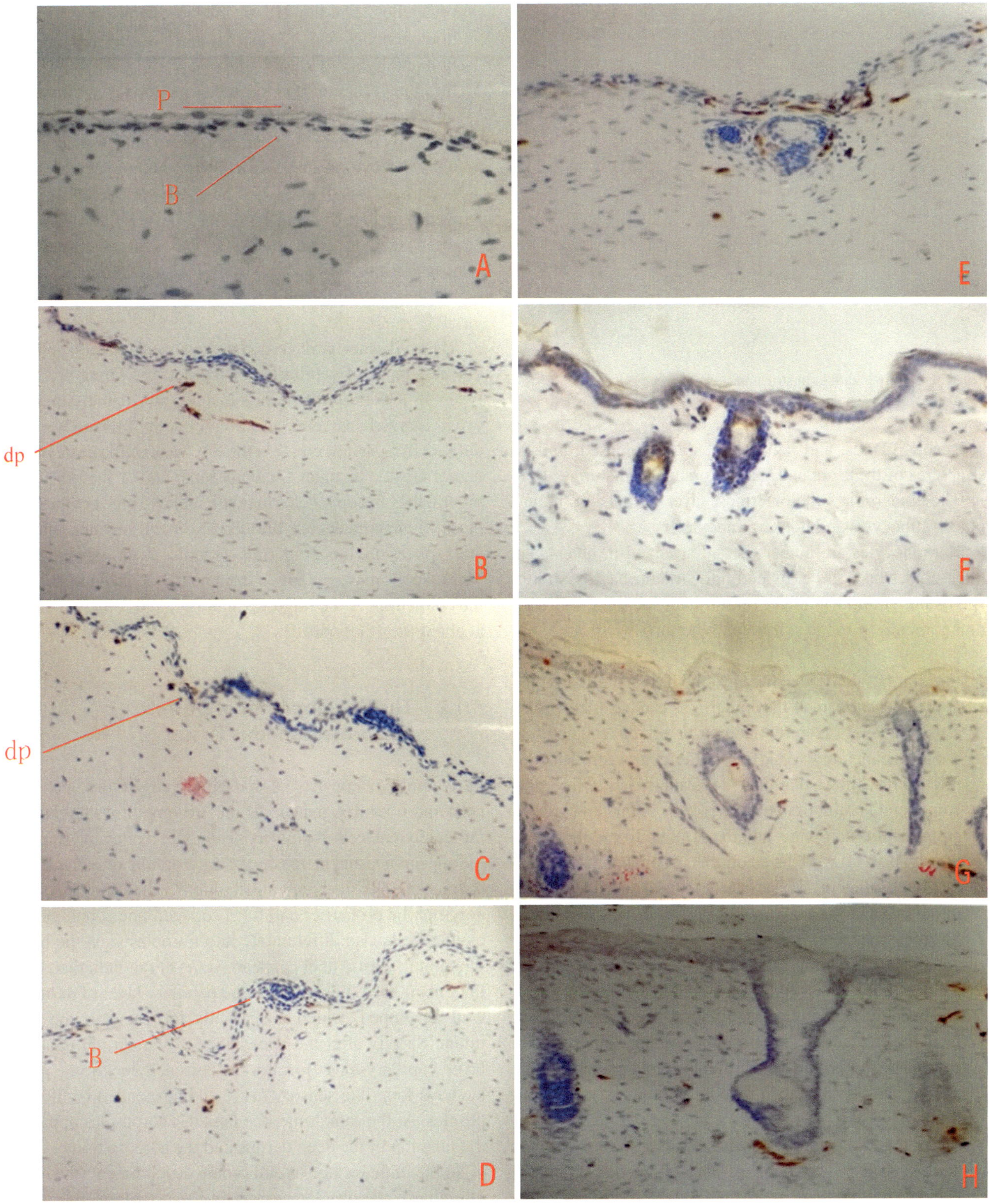


**Fig. 4.3** Development of epidermis and skin appendages. (**a**) At about the 8th and 9th week, the periderm(P) is seen in the section of embryo epidermis; (**b**) At about the 10th and 11st week, stratified cells begin to appear; (**c**) mesenchymal cells (dp) appear and aggregate at the appendages; (**d**) basal cells grow downward; (**e**) basal cells grow further downward; (**f**) forms primary skin appendages structures; (**g**) basically forms appendage structures; (**h**) peripheral innervation tends to be normal

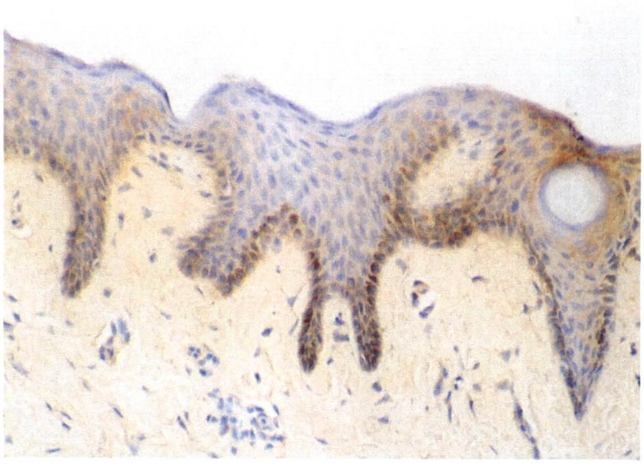

**Fig. 4.4** Normal adult skin structure

sebaceous glands, and hair follicles are increased, and the structures of these appendages are gradually matured.

The epidermis is the outermost layer of the skin, including keratinocytes and nonkeratinocytes.

Keratinocytes are numerous and arranged in layers. The thick epidermis can be divided into stratum basale, stratum spinosum, stratum granulosum, stratum lucidum, and stratum corneum from the substrate to the surface.

1. Stratum basale: It is adhered to the basement membrane, at the deepest part of the epidermis. The basal layer consists of a layer of short columnar or cubical cells with an ovoid nucleus and weak basophilic cytoplasm. Electron microscope shows that the cytoplasm is rich in free ribosomes and keratin filaments. The cells in this layer have a strong ability to divide, and the proliferative cells continuously move toward the epidermis to supplement the cells that have fallen off the surface, so it is also called the germinal layer.
2. Stratum spinosum: It consists of 4–10 layers of polygonal cells. The cell body is large, the nucleus is round and located in the center of the cell, and the cytoplasm is rich and weakly basophilic. Many short processes protrude from the cell surface. Electron microscope shows that the cytoplasm is rich in free ribosomes, bundled keratin filaments, and oval-shaped lamellar granules containing lipids.
3. Stratum granulosum: It consists of three to five layers of spindle cells. The nucleus and organelles gradually degenerate, and there are many large basophilic transparent keratohyalin granules in the cytoplasm. Under the electron microscope, the transparent keratohyalin granules are irregular, dense, and homogeneous, and the lamellar granules are obviously increased.
4. Stratum lucidum: It consists of several layers of flat cells. The cell boundary is unclear and there is no nucleus and organelles. On the HE stained sections, the cells are homogeneous and transparent, with strong light refraction and light red color.
5. Stratum corneum: It is located at the top layer, composed of several layers of keratinized squamous epithelial cells. The cell contour is unclear, there is no nucleus and organelle, the cytoplasm is filled with homogeneous acidic keratin, at this time the cell has been completely keratinized and is a dry and hard dead cell. Keratinized cells often shed to form dandruff. The stratum corneum is resistant to friction, has strong resistance to acid, alkali, and other stimuli, and has a strong protective function.

The epidermis has no blood vessels, and nutrition depends on the supply of capillaries in the dermis. There are three types of nonkeratinocytes in the epidermis, namely melanocytes, Langerhans cells, and Merkel cells. Melanocytes are derived from neural crest. At the 8th week of the embryo, the neural crest cells enter the epidermis, and at the 4th to 6th month, they become dendritic with melanosomes in the cytoplasm. Langerhans cells are derived from the bone marrow and appear in the epidermis together with melanocytes. Merkel cells may be derived from neural crest, and appear in the epithelium of the fingertip, nail bed, and follicular funnel at about the 4th month.

### 4.1.2 The Development of Dermis and Subcutaneous Tissue

Early embryo consists of loosely arranged mesenchymal cells and fiber-free matrix. At the 3rd month of the embryo, mesenchymal cells begin to synthesize collagen, showing the appearance and increasing of argyrophilic reticular fibers. As the reticular fibers aggregate into bundles, they lose their argyrophilic properties and form collagen fibers, and mesenchymal cells also differentiate into fibroblasts. At the 6th to 7th month, elastic fibers appear. At the 8th month, the elastic fiber net in the reticular layer and papillary layer of dermis is well developed, which is basically the same as the term infant. Shortly after the appearance of the dermal papillary layer, capillary loops form in the mesenchyme. Some papillae have loop-like sensory nerve endings, called tactile corpuscles. At the same time, the lamellar corpuscles appear at the junction of the deep dermis and the adipose tissue.

In the middle stage of embryonic development (the 4th to 6th month), fat droplets appear in the cytoplasm of mesenchymal cells in the loose connective tissue of the lower dermis, gradually differentiate into fat cells, and form a subcutaneous fat layer.

Normal adult dermis is 1–2 mm thick and consists of dense connective tissue, which can be divided into papillary layer and reticular layer. The dermis is rich in blood vessels, lymphatic vessels, free nerve endings, sensory bodies (tactile corpuscles, lamellar corpuscles, Merkel cell axon complexes), and other receptors, as well as sweat glands, hair follicles, and sebaceous glands.

(a) Papillary layer is located in the shallow layer of the dermis, adjacent to the basal layer of the epidermis. The connective tissue protrudes from the surface to form a papillary ridge, so it is called a dermal papilla. The papillae with abundant capillaries are called the vascular papillae, and the papillae with tactile corpuscles are called the nerve papillae.
(b) The reticular layer is located in the deep surface of the papillary layer, which is a thick and dense connective tissue. The collagen fibers are thick and interwoven into a net; it also contains a lot of elastic fibers, giving the skin greater toughness and elasticity. There are more blood vessels, lymphatic vessels, nerve fibers, and lamellar corpuscles in the reticular layer.

The deep layer of the dermis is the hypodermis, also known as the superficial fascia, which consists of loose connective tissue. The subcutaneous tissue connects the skin with the deep tissue.

### 4.1.3 The Development of Skin Appendages

#### 4.1.3.1 Hair

At the 3rd month of the embryo, the germinal layer of the epidermis proliferates focally and protrudes into the dermis to form a flower bud, which is called hair germ. The cells in the hair germ divide, proliferate, and grow obliquely downward to become a solid epithelial column, and the end is swollen into a hair bulb. At the 4th to 5th month, the mesenchyme under the hair bulb protrudes into the hair bulb to form the hair papilla, and the epithelium around the hair papilla becomes the hair matrix. It is the germinal cell of the hair follicle. The hair matrix cells differentiate and proliferate, forming a plurality of cell columns arranged in concentric circles. From the inside to the outside are hair cortex, hair cuticle, cuticle of internal root sheath, Huxley layer, Henle layer, and external root sheath. The mesenchyme around the hair follicle differentiates into a connective tissue sheath. As the hair forms and grows, the melanocytes from the neural crest invade the hair bulbs, gradually making the hair color darker. At the 17th week, the hair is first seen on the eyebrow and the head. After the 4th to 5th month, the hair gradually develops from head to sacrococcyx. At the end of the 6th month or the beginning of the 7th month, the hair is spread over the surface of the fetus. The arrector pilli muscle appears in the 4th to 6th month of the embryo.

#### 4.1.3.2 Sebaceous Gland

Most of the sebaceous glands are formed by the epithelial outer root sheath on the primordial side of the hair follicle and prolonged into the mesenchyme, which first appears on the scalp and face at the 4th month, then develops toward the end. Shortly after the appearance of these solid epithelial protrusions, they become lobular and form several vesicular acinus. The development of fetal sebaceous glands is affected by maternal estrogen, with larger glands and more secretion. Vernix caseosa can be seen on the body surface at birth.

#### 4.1.3.3 Nail

The nail is a special thickening zone of the epidermis. At the 3rd month, the epidermis of the palm surface of each finger (toe) has a thickened area called the original nail bed. The epidermis on both sides and the proximal end of each finger (toe) rises relatively, forming the lateral nail fold and the proximal nail fold. The germinal layer of the proximal nail fold proliferates, keratinizes, and hardens to form the nail plate. The thickened germinal layer of the proximal nail fold, called the nail matrix, is the source of the growing nail plate. Later nail plate growth accelerates. At the 8th month, the nail grows to the end of the finger, and the toenails reach the end of the toe at the 9th month.

#### 4.1.3.4 Sweat Gland

The eccrine sweat glands derive from the eccrine sweat gland germs of the germinal epidermal layer. Initially, it is a focal aggregation of germinal cells in the basal layer of the epidermis, and then vertically descends into the dermis with a slender column of epithelial cells, leading up to the epidermis. When the cell column is close to the subcutaneous tissue, its distal end is curved into a spherical shape. In the future, it develops into the secretory part of the sweat gland. The small sweat gland first appears in the palmar part. After 5 months, it begins to appear in other parts of the body, and a lumen consisting of two layers of cells gradually emerges. The secretory parts differentiate into secretory cells and myoepithelial cells, which are close to adult sweat glands at birth.

The apocrine glands originate from the buds at the top of the hair follicle. Initially it is a solid line, and later a lacunar-like structure appears, opening into the hair follicle above the sebaceous gland. In addition to specific parts such as the axillary, pudendal, and perianal, the apocrine glands that have developed with the hair during the embryonic period are degraded and disappeared.

### 4.1.4 The Development of Skin Nerves

The skin is rich in sensory nerves and motor nerves. The former comes from the cranial nerves, and the latter comes from the postganglionic fibers of the sympathetic nerves. The innervation of the skin is phased, but the adjacent segments overlap.

The skin nerve originates from the neural crest of the ectoderm and is formed by elongation of the axon of the neuron. After the 4th month of gestation, the nerve endings can reach the subepidermis and gradually develop and differentiate, and the Merkel tactile receptors are produced at the toes. At the end of the 5th month, the Krause body is formed at the finger. By the 6th month, the dermal papilla develops, and the peripheral nerve branches in the papilla in the form of reticular, filiform, or hoof. The Meissner corpuscles, Vater-Paccini corpuscles, and other nerve terminal organs are formed in the papillary dermis, deep dermis, and subcutaneous tissues.

### 4.1.5 The Development of Skin Blood Vessels and Lymphatic Vessels

The results of computer reconstruction technology and transmission electron microscopy show the vascular structures are found at 35–45 days of gestation. The embryonic skin blood vessels are composed of one or two vascular bundles parallel to the epidermis. At 35–40 days of gestational age, endothelial cells form a preliminary single vascular plane. Vascular endothelial cells have the same morphological size and functional structure as adults, but lack continuity. At 50–75 days of gestational age, the embryo develops two vascular planes, which are interwoven to form a preliminary vascular network. The vascular endothelial cells continue to proliferate and migrate to connect the shorter blood vessels, and the blood vessel wall is continuously thickened. By the gestational age of 60–80 days, four layers of microvascular networks parallel to each other and parallel to the epidermis are basically formed, and the continuity of blood vessels is improved.

1. Subcutaneous Vascular Plexus.
   The subcutaneous vascular plexus is located in the deep layer of subcutaneous tissue, with horizontal direction, and its branches can nourish various surrounding tissues. This is the largest vascular plexus in the skin, with many arteries and few veins.
2. Subdermal Vascular Plexus.
   The subdermal vascular plexus is located in the upper part of the subcutaneous tissue, and the branches nourish sweat glands, sweat ducts, dermal papilla, and sebaceous glands.
3. Subpapillary Vascular Plexus.
   The subpapillary vascular plexus is located in the lower part of the papilla, with horizontal direction, and branches nourish intradermal appendages. This plexus has many blood vessels, and has a blood storage function. The small arteries branch into blood vessels in the dermal papilla, nourish the epidermis, the descending branch of the blood vessels flows into the subpapillary venous plexus to merge into venules, and then merges with the deep veins.

The lymphatic vessels of the skin originate from the capillary lymphatic vessels of the dermal papilla, with a blind end at the beginning, composed of endothelial cells and a small amount of reticular fibers. The lower part of the papilla and the deep part of the dermis merge into superficial lymphatic vessels and deep lymphatic vessels respectively, with valves in the larger lumen. The pressure of capillary lymphatic vessel is lower than the osmotic pressure of the capillary and surrounding tissue space, and the excess tissue fluid can be recovered, which is an auxiliary system of blood circulation.

### 4.1.6 The Development of Skin Muscles

The muscles of the skin are mostly smooth muscles except for striated muscles in the face and neck. Except for myoepithelial cells of the sweat glands that are derived from the ectoderm, all smooth muscles, such as the arrector pili muscle and the smooth muscle of the scrotal sarcolemma, the nipple, the eyelid, and the blood vessel wall, are differentiated from mesodermal mesenchymal cells. At the site where the muscle tissue begins to appear, the astro-mesenchymal cells enlarge, gather together, and elongate in one direction, gradually becoming a spindle shape, forming myoblast, then myofibrils appear in the muscle, and the nucleus becomes rod shaped campanied with the change of cell morphology, located in the center of the cell, forming smooth muscle cells. Immature smooth muscles can be seen around the 5th month.

## 4.2 Understanding Skin Repair and Regeneration from Dermatological Development

### 4.2.1 The Development and Regeneration of the Epidermis

The epidermis of mammalian skin is a continuous, multilayered epithelium, and its regenerative ability is very strong. Under physiological conditions, the epidermis continues to senescence and shed, and at the same time, basal cells are constantly dividing and proliferating for replacement. In addition, several appendages, such as hair follicles, sebaceous glands, and sweat glands, are doped. The epidermis of interfollicular region and the associated sebaceous glands and sweat glands are called interfollicular epidermis (IFE).

The IFE is arranged in a column shape to form a so-called hyperplastic unit. The bottom of the columnar structure is a single layer of basal cells (basal layer), the middle are positively differentiated keratinocytes, spinous layer, and granular layer, and the top of the columnar structure is flat and keratinized cell layer, namely the stratum corneum. The structure of the epidermis constitutes a mechanical and physiological barrier, preventing moisture loss and the ingestion of harmful chemicals, and avoiding mechanical, chemical, and thermal damage.

The regeneration of the epidermis is maintained by epidermal stem cells (EpSC), which are mainly concentrated in the primary epidermis at the fetal stage, and distributed in sheets in the basal layer of the epidermis in adults. In the normal adult epidermal basal layer, there are mainly three cell subpopulations that maintain its metabolism: (a) Epidermal stem cells. (b) Progeny cells of epidermal stem cells—transient expansion cells (similar to committed progenitor cells). (c) Differentiated cells after mitosis. In vivo, approximately 40% of the cells in the normal epidermal basal layer are epidermal stem cells and transient expansion cells.

In addition to the two typical characteristics of all stem cells (slow cell cycling and self-renewal ability), EpSC also has adhesion properties to the basement membrane of the skin. Slow cell cycling is mainly characterized by retention of living cell markers. Self-renewal ability is characterized by clonal growth in vitro, such as continuous passage. Cells can undergo 140 divisions, which can produce $1 \times 10^{40}$ daughter cells. Stem cells mainly adhere to the basement membrane by expressing integrins, which is also the basic condition for stem cells to maintain their characteristics. Both EpSC and transient expansion cells in the normal epidermal basal layer express $\beta_1$ integrin ($\alpha_2\beta_1$, $\alpha_3\beta_1$ and $\alpha_6\beta_4$) at high levels. Although the expression intensity of EpSC is twice as high as that of transient expansion cells, it is difficult to distinguish by ordinary light microscopy alone, and the intensity of expression needs to be judged by confocal microscopy. In addition, the $\alpha6$ adhesion molecule, a member of the integrin family, and the surface marker mAb10G7 associated with proliferation can effectively distinguish EpSC from transient expansion cells. It is found that $\alpha_6(+)$ and 10G7(−) cells are stem cells; $\alpha_6(+)$ and 10G7(+) cells are transient expansion cells; $\alpha_6(-)$ cells that showed (+) keratin K10 expression are differentiated cells after mitosis. Telomerase activity is associated with cell proliferation, and some scholars have suggested that stem cells in normal tissues express telomerase. However, in the hair follicle, the high activity area of telomerase is located at the hair root where the proliferating cells are located, not the hair follicle bulge where the stem cells are located; in the epidermis of the hair follicle, the transient expansion cells with proliferating activity highly express telomerase. Therefore, telomerase cannot be used as markers for epidermal stem cells.

Keratin, a class of proteins specific to epidermis or epithelial cells, has at least 30 different types in the body. Keratin can be used as an indicator for epidermal stem cells, transient expansion cells, and differentiated cells after mitosis: epidermal stem cells (+) K8, K18, K19; transient expansion cells (+) K5, K14; differentiated cells after mitosis (+) K1, K10. It has been found that the epidermal stem cells of the hair follicle bulge express K15, but during the differentiation of stem cells, the decrease of K15 expression is earlier than that of K19 expression, the K15(−) and K19(+) cells may be "early" transient expansion cells, K15 may be more meaningful than K19 in identifying epidermal stem cells in the hair follicle bulge.

Although there are no specific markers for epidermal stem cells, it is generally accepted in the academic community that $\beta_1$ integrin, K19, and Bcl-2 are simultaneously expressed in cells, which can be considered as EpSC.

Angiotensin-converting enzyme (ACE) is a key enzyme in the synthesis of angiotensin II and has been found in the membrane of keratinocytes in the epidermis. Recently, the team led by Academician Xiaobing Fu has found in the preliminary study on the relationship between ACE and skin tissue damage repair and regeneration: the expression of ACE in human skin tissue is mainly concentrated in the basal layer of keratinocytes, hair follicle bulge, sweat glands, which seems to be consistent with the location of epidermal stem cells [1]. Subsequently, the characteristics of skin ACE expression during human embryo development have been studied. It is found that after the formation of epidermal whole layer structure, ACE expression is also localized on the cell membrane of epidermal basal layer, and is located almost in the same cell as the molecular markers of epidermal stem cells, such as β-integrin, K19, and p63 (Fig. 4.5). These findings suggest that ACE may be closely related to epidermal stem cells and may be used as a new marker to identify epidermal stem cells. In addition, ACE located on the cell membrane is conducive to the screening of living cells, which can provide a new technical mean for the identification and in-depth study of epidermal stem cells.

ACE expression is localized on the cell membrane of epidermal basal layer, and is located in the same cell as the molecular markers of epidermal stem cells, such as β-integrin, K19, and p63.

In epidermal stem cell niches, numerous cytokines regulate stem cell division, proliferation, differentiation, and migration by autocrine or (and) paracrine. The FGF and EGF families have been screened and studied in detail. FGF1, FGF2, FGF3 (including KGF), and their receptors play an important role in the lamellar structure of the skin. EGF receptors can be detected in the epidermal layering stage and increase in expression as the embryo ages. Therefore, EGF is an essential media supplement in the establishment of an in vitro culture model for epidermal stem cells. In vivo,

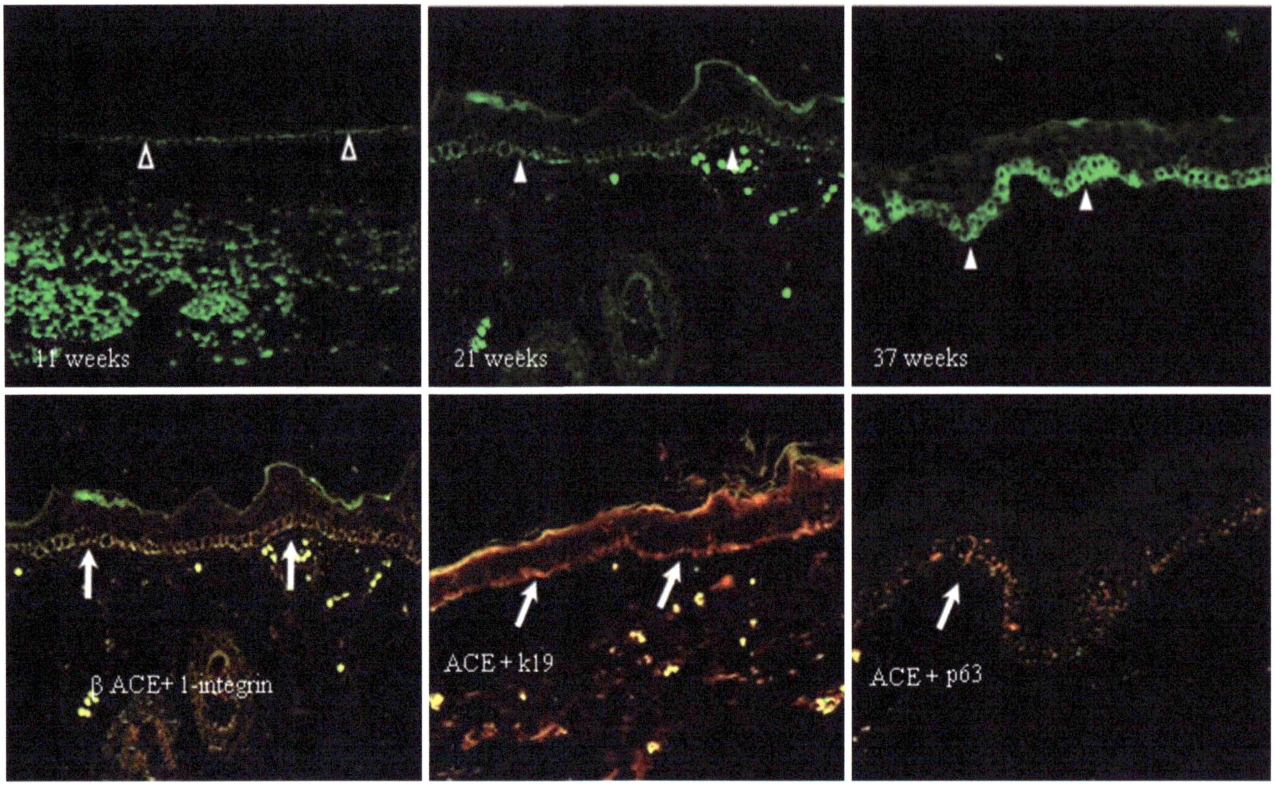


**Fig. 4.5** Expression of ACE in human fetal skin

exogenous EGF can also have certain effects on epidermal stem cells. For example, Xiaobing Fu treated human chronic skin ulcers with rhEGF and found that EpSC islands occurred in the granular layer and spinous layer of epithelialized wounds. It is thought to be derived from the reverse differentiation of mature epidermal cells. This finding deepens the theory that cytokines regulate EpSC [2].

Signal network systems are also important factors in regulating EpSC differentiation. Moles believes that EpSC expresses high levels of γ-catenin relative to other primary cells, while expressing low levels of E-cadherin and β-catenin, and downregulation of cadherin and β-integrin is a characteristic of cell-to-cell adhesion to terminal differentiation. β-catenin plays a signal transduction role in cell adhesion. The activation of β-catenin signaling pathway can produce a new epidermis in the skin. Overexpression of β-catenin in the epidermis can increase cell proliferation. In the cultured epidermal cells, increasing the expression of β-catenin can stimulate the proliferation of cells without affecting the adhesion between cells. In epidermal stem cells, β-catenin acts as a transcription factor that activates Tcf/Lef, which is more abundant than transient expansion cells. Its overexpression can increase the proportion of stem cells in vitro, and can cause keratinocytes transdifferentiation into pluripotent state in vivo. The interaction between β-catenin and Tcf/Lef can cause c-Myc expression, and the function of c-Myc is to promote cell proliferation, that is, the prerequisite for the initiation of cell terminal differentiation is to downregulate c-Myc expression. An important manifestation of EpSC detachment from the stem cell community into the differentiation phase is the induction of c-Myc with a decrease in the level of surface integrin, which de-adheres to the basement membrane. When the stem cell microenvironment changes, extracellular information can be transmitted to stem cells through integrin $\alpha_5\beta_1$, $\alpha_v\beta_5$, and $\alpha_v\beta_6$ to trigger transmembrane signal transduction and regulate cell gene expression. This process can not only change the way in which stem cells divide, but also activate the pluripotency of stem cells, allowing stem cells to produce one or more directed progenitor cells to meet the needs of the body. Therefore, integrin $\alpha_5\beta_1$, $\alpha_v\beta_5$, and $\alpha_v\beta_6$ are also referred to as emergency receptors during wound healing. The adhesion characteristics of stem cells caused by high levels of integrin expression may be necessary for maintaining stem cell populations. To further clarify this phenomenon, Watt transfected the $\beta_1$ integrin dominant negative mutant CD8$\beta_1$ into human epidermal cells cultured in vitro to interfere with the function of $\beta_1$ integrin and reduce the adhesion characteristics of $\beta_1$ integrin. The results showed that the surface level of $\beta_1$ integrin and the adhesion of cells to type IV collagen were significantly decreased, the activity of MAPK was decreased, the clonal ability of cells was decreased, the proliferative potential was lost, and the characteristics of transient expansion cells were observed. However, overexpression of wild-type $\beta_1$ integrin or activated MAPK can upregulate the expression of integrin and restore its adhesion and proliferative potential. Therefore, MAPK plays an important role in the signal transduction pathway of $\beta_1$ integrin regulating EpSC proliferation and differentiation.

Stem cell is one of the most interesting, complex, and attractive areas of biology in recent years. There are still many practical issues to be resolved, such as: a. EpSC replication. b. Development of stem cell proliferation and differentiation that has not been discovered under normal circumstances. c. Shortening the cell cycle to obtain more transient expansion cells proliferation. There is still a long way to go for clinical use as a source of mature stem cells. However, these initial achievements have opened up new avenues for the application of EpSC for large-scale deep skin trauma and burn wounds from anatomical repair to functional repair, and laid a certain foundation. With the advancement of research techniques, it is believed that it is not far to regulate the direct differentiation of EpSC into skin appendages, such as hair follicles and sweat glands, and realize the leap from anatomical repair to functional repair of skin burn wounds.

### 4.2.2 The Development and Regeneration of Hair Follicles

The hair follicles are epithelial catheters deep into the dermis. It has a unique property compared to other self-renewing tissues. The hair follicle proliferation has periodicity, which is through the anagen, catagen, and telogen. Therefore, it is inferred that hair follicles contain stem cells as well as other self-renewing tissues and are closely related to the hair growth cycle. At present, the location of hair follicle stem cells is not very clear. Traditionally it is thought to be in the hair bulb. According to the study of label restaining cells (LRCs) in rats, in 1990, the laboratory led by Cotsarelis proposed the "bulge-activation hypothesis" that human hair follicle stem cells may exist in the hair follicle bulge. This hypothesis can better explain the following points: (a) The growth cycle of hair follicles. (b) Why can the hair follicles regenerate after the whole hair bulb is removed. (c) The early stage of hair follicle growth is more susceptible to chemical carcinogens than telogen. (d) Why hair matrix cell culture is difficult to survive. Although there is no specific evidence that hair follicle stem cells are in the bulge. However, Cotsarelis observed in adult hair follicles in 1998 that the hair follicle bulge (the outer root sheath of the hair follicle between the opening of the sebaceous gland and the attachment of the hair follicle of the pilose muscle) is rich in stem cell-like cells, and K15 is proposed as a marker for such cells. Masashi observed the so-called stem cells with positive expression of $\beta_1$ integrin, E-cadherin, and α, γ-catenin in different stages of human embryo. It is found that these stem cells gradually migrate from the edge of the hair germ to the outer layer of the pile as gestational age increases, and then enter the differentiated fetal hair follicle, and finally concentrate on the outer layer and the bulge of the hair follicle outer root sheath. This procedural limitation is precisely where the positive expression of EGF receptor and K19 cells are located, and confirmed by electron microscopy that these cells have undifferentiated morphological characteristics, thus supporting the above viewpoints. In view of the current research status, the academic community basically recognizes that the bulge is the location of hair follicle stem cells. Based on Michael's study of corneal epidermal stem cells and transient expansion cells, Taylor observed the stem cells in the mouse hair follicle bulge by the double-labeled retention method and concluded that the mouse hair follicle bulge was the main habitat of skin stem cells. It not only plays a key role in the growth, remodeling, and metabolism of hair follicles but also is important for the repair of epidermal damage. Because the stem cells here form a group of transient expansion cell continuous lineages (TA1, TA2, TA3, Tan) that lack proliferative capacity, when the skin is traumatic, the early transient expansion cells (TA3 or TA4) migrate to the epidermis to participate in the repair, that is, the epidermal stem cells are the transient expansion cells mainly derived from hair follicles and a small amount of stem cells exist in the basal layer of skin (accounting for 1–10% of basal cells).

The mammalian hair follicle is a highly dynamic skin appendage that undergoes periodic cycles of growth, degeneration, and rest. Hair follicle stem cells play an important role in the morphogenesis and renewal of hair. When hair growth stops or the main structure of the hair follicle lower part changes, the keratinocytes that form more clones in the lower part of the hair follicle respond to morphogenesis or hair renewal signals, and the hair follicle stem cells migrate to the root of the hair follicle to participate in hair formation. Bull studied the expression of the transcription factor Myc superfamily, N-Myc, Max, Mad1, and Mad3, in the hair follicle growth cycle. Bull found that in the early and final stages of hair follicle growth, c-Myc was expressed in the basal and terminal differentiated upper basal layers of the hair follicle infundibular part (similar to the epidermis), while in the hair bulb, c-Myc was expressed both in the proliferating bud epithelial cells and terminal differentiated stromal cells that formed hair, but more strongly expressed in the outer root sheath bulge. He believes that members of the Myc superfamily fulfill different missions in different epithelial components of hair follicles and play an important role in the fate of hair follicle stem cells. The expression of c-Myc is associated with stem cells in the bulge, but not with the hair follicle growth cycle. Similarly, β-catenin also plays a key role in hair development. If β-catenin is deficient after hair follicle formation, hair will completely shed after the first hair cycle. β-catenin is essential for the fate of skin stem cells. In the absence of β-catenin, stem cells will not differentiate into hair follicle-forming cells, which alter epidermal fate. Studies on the developmental cycle of hair follicles showed that the bulge stem cells in the quiescent state continued to express Tcf3, and when transformed to express Lef1, the stem cells entered a differentiated state, forming a hairy embryo-like invagination in the epidermis, and some Tcf3-positive cells differentiated into the outer root sheath of the hair follicles, while others differentiate into the inner root sheath and hair shaft of the hair follicle; if the expression of Lef1/Tcf3 is out of control at this time, the hair follicle development will stagnate in an intermediate state, so during hair follicles development, Lef1/Tcf3 control the formation of intact hair follicles through the expression of different concentrations in different parts at different periods. In addition, in the in vitro culture of artificial hair follicle-like structures, some outer root sheath cells and hair bulb cells have appeared in the hairy embryo-like invagination structure, but no inner root sheath cells and hair shaft structures are formed. It is precisely due to the blockage of Lef1/Tcf3 expression that Tcf3 cannot be converted to Lef1, resulting in the inability of artificial hair follicles to continue to develop.

Sensory neuropeptides play an important role in inducing stem cell differentiation and regulating the hair follicle cycle. The distribution of nerve fibers and the concentration of sensory neuropeptides in the hair follicle bulge show periodic changes, that is, the concentration of sensory neuropeptides (SP, CGRP, etc.) around the hair follicles in the quiescent period is low, when entering the proliferative phase, the concentration is significantly upregulated. In this case, the sensory neuropeptide can induce the hair follicle to enter the next proliferation cycle. Exogenous SP can stimulate the hair follicle of the mouse from the quiescent phase to the proliferative phase. Therefore, sensory neuropeptides may play an important role in inducing the differentiation of hair follicle stem cells into hair follicles with intact function and normal structure.

In 2001, the third gene of the mouse keratin 6 (K6a, K6b) paired gene was discovered and named as the hair follicle keratin 6 gene (K6hf). The gene has a high homology with human K6hf and is believed to be closely related to the formation of hair follicles.

Hair tissue is mainly composed of epithelial hair follicles originating from ectoderm and connective tissue hair follicles originating from mesoderm. The interaction between them induces hair follicle development and reconstruction, but little is known about the biological characteristics and regulation mechanism of hair follicle epithelial (stem) cells.

#### 4.2.2.1 Regulation Mechanism of Hair Follicle Development

The dermal papilla cells located at the base of the hair follicle are a group of specific interstitial cells. During embryonic development of hair follicles, these interstitial cells with aggregation properties originate from dermal fibroblasts. Through the changes of extracellular matrix, dermal papilla cells play an important role in the morphogenesis of hair follicles and the periodic growth of adult hair follicles. The dermal papilla cells have different biological properties from the dermal fibroblasts. In vitro dermal papilla cells exhibit agglutinative growth characteristics when reached a certain concentration, while dermal fibroblasts do not exhibit this characteristic. In addition, the activity of dermal papilla cells is regulated by hair follicle epithelial cells, and unregulated dermal papilla cells will lose agglutinative growth characteristics and transform into fibroblasts. The agglutinative growth characteristics of the dermal papilla cells may be related to the biological properties that induce hair growth. Therefore, agglutinative growth of dermal papilla cells is closely related to the differentiation and functional status of hair follicle epithelial cells.

Regulation of multiple signaling pathways: Complex molecular signaling pathways are the basis of epidermal-interstitial interactions or hair follicle organogenesis, in which fibroblast growth factor, tabby/ downless, bone morphogenetic proteins (BMPs), epidermal growth factor (EGF) family, Wnt, β-catenin, Shh Patched, and Notch are involved in the regulation of hair follicle morphogenesis, hair cycle, and/or hair follicle differentiation. FGF10, also known as keratinocyte growth factor-2 (KGF-2), is released by mesenchymal cells under the skin substrate and stimulates the development of epidermis and hair follicles through BMPs, β-catenin, and other signaling pathways. Knocking out the FGF10 gene can cause hair follicle dysplasia in newborn mice. Abnormal human tabby/downless gene will result in hypohidrotic ectodermal dysplasia, that is, the inability to form organs such as teeth, hair follicles, and sweat glands. If the signal of Shh Patched is blocked, hair follicle development will stop midway; on the contrary, this signal overconduction can cause basal cell carcinoma. The latter has been confirmed in the Shh gene-deficient mice induced by the K14 promoter. The use of the K5 and K14 promoter Cre/lox P system to make keratinocyte-specific genetically altered mice is important for analyzing the function of such genes in the skin. Due to the early induction and activation of the K5 and K14 promoters, specific gene deletions occur in epidermal and hair follicle epithelial cells. The β-catenin deletion (−/−) mice produced by this technique may have hair cycle deficiency, but still form skin epidermis, suggesting that β-catenin must be involved in the formation of hair follicle structures by epidermal stem cells. It is also confirmed by β-catenin (−/−) mice that β-catenin present in the adherence junction (AJ) is located downstream of tabby/downless and upstream of BMP and Shh, moves to the nucleus via Wnt signaling, and then binds to Lef 1 to increase transcriptional activity. As the original hair buds grow into the dermis, the base of the distal epithelial cells expands and wraps the interstitial cells to form dermal papilla. This dermal papilla cells can induce the development of epithelial hair follicles even in adults. If the dermal papilla isolated from the rat whisker is transplanted into the dermis tissue of the plantar, the structure of the hair follicle formed by the epidermis can be observed. Similarly, transplanted cultured dermal papilla cells can also induce hair follicle regeneration and hair growth, but the Wnt signal provided by epidermal cells must be present in order to maintain this induced potential of cultured dermal papilla cells.

#### 4.2.2.2 The Biological Characteristics of Hair Follicle Stem Cells

Hair follicle stem cells are the main source of regeneration or repair of the epidermis and skin appendages. So what is the role of hair follicle stem cells in skin tissue? Hair cells that have been differentiated from hair follicle cells are thought to be stem cells of hair follicles. The bulge hypothesis of hair follicle stem cells has received extensive attention and support. In the case of skin damage, hair follicle stem cells are activated in addition to epidermal cells and participate in epidermal regeneration. c-Myc is a downstream gene of β-catenin, and its overexpression will overmobilize stem cells to transform into TA cells, eventually leading to stem cell depletion and skin ulceration. Stem cells can also cause a variety of epithelial tumors and skin diseases. It is speculated that skin epithelial stem cells may be important targets for the action of physical or chemical factors (including carcinogens) to damage the epidermis and hair follicle appendages, etc. In view of this, skin stem cells can be used as the first target for skin gene therapy in the future. Hair follicle stem cells are potentially important in the treatment of skin biology, pathology, and future dermatology. Not only hair follicle stem cells can participate in the repair of epidermal damage, but also in vitro and in vivo studies, adult multiple epithelial (stem) cells (such as keratinocytes, corneal cells), and bone marrow stromal cells have the potential to differentiate to the hair follicle sebaceous glands and other appendages. Just as the potential of transformation between hematopoietic stem cells and muscle stem cells depends on environmental stimuli. Adult epithelial cells can form skin appendages such as hair follicles under the appropriate dermal interstitial induction. These experimental results need to be confirmed by further basic and clinical studies.

#### 4.2.2.3 Developmental Regulation of Hair Follicles

With the improvement of high-throughput sequencing technology and the development of bioinformatics, the postgenome era provides a better way for miRNA research. miRNAs are a class of noncoding single-stranded small RNA molecules composed of 19–25 nucleotides discovered in recent years, which negatively regulate the expression of target genes by binding to the target gene 3'UTR. Recent studies have shown that the expression profile of miRNA is specific in hair follicle tissue and periodic development, and regulates the growth and development of hair follicles at the post-transcriptional level by interacting with signaling pathways and regulatory factors. The periodic development of hair follicles is a complex physiological and biochemical process involving multiple genes, closely linked and mutually restricted. miRNAs can play a role in the regulation and transformation of different developmental stages in the hair follicle cycle by targeting different signaling pathways and transcription factors. During the formation of hair follicles, FGF, Wnt, and BMP signaling pathways play important regulatory roles, and miR-31 can interfere with the activity of these signaling pathways by regulating the expression of keratin 14, 16, and 17 (essential components of the keratinocyte cytoskeleton). miR-31 regulates the cell cycle development. High expression of miR-31 may promote cell proliferation by downregulating CEBPA gene expression and promote cell transition from G2 to M phase. Studies have shown that miRNAs can also regulate the growth of hair follicles by indirectly regulating the development of hair follicle-related tissues. Increasing the vascularization level of the hair follicle during the development of the hair follicle cycle can increase the size of the hair follicle and promote the growth of the villus. miR-31 is considered to be a vascular-specific miRNA that acts as a negative regulator to regulate the growth and maturation of lymph and blood vessels.

Cultured primary and secondary hair follicle dermal papilla cells during the flourishing period of cashmere follicles also showed that many differentially expressed genes are involved in vascularization and signaling pathways, which are closely related to hair follicle morphogenesis. Thus, miRNA plays an important role in regulating hair fol licle growth and development and periodic regulation.

The miRNAs and miRNA families involved in the growth of different species and even different mammalian hair follicles are not the same. Some of the target genes for let-7b and miR-24 are associated with hair follicle growth and hair quality. It has been reported that miR-25 is related to the color of the hair and plays a regulatory role in the growth and development of the skin and hair. Studies have shown that miR-184 can interfere with miR-205, which may have the effect of inhibiting hair follicle growth and promoting decline. miR-18b inhibits TGF-$\beta_1$-mediated differentiation of human hair follicle mesenchymal stem cells into smooth muscle cells by regulating the target gene SMAD2.

A transcriptome is the sum of all RNA (including RNA encoding and noncoding proteins) transcribed by cells or tissues in a particular state. At present, transcriptome research techniques mainly include two types: DNA microarray based on hybridization technology and transcriptome sequencing technology (RNA- seq) based on sequencing technology. This technology not only focuses on the functional sites in the gene but also represents most of the adaptive sites in the genome, and can detect all the collections of all RNAs transcribed from a particular tissue or cell at a certain developmental stage or functional state. All of them are measured to study gene function and gene structure from an overall level, revealing specific biological processes and molecular mechanisms during disease development.

In recent years, studies on the mechanism of hair follicles at the transcriptome level indicate that many growth factors and their receptors are important links of endocrine coordination genes and environment in vivo, and play an extremely important role in the regulation of villus growth. These molecules shuttle between dermal cells and epithelial cells, mediating the interaction between the two cell populations, allowing the two cell populations to proliferate and differentiate in an orderly manner and eventually form intact hair follicles. In addition, it is found that some dermal papilla cells of hair follicles are derived from neural crest, and the development of hair follicles is very complicated.

A total of 161 molecules are known to be involved in hair follicle development. Using differential microarray analysis, Schellenberger et al. found that the cartilage oligomeric matrix protein (Comp) gene plays an important role in the biological properties of extracellular matrix and normal human hair follicles. The Comp gene is expressed during the resting and growing phases of hair follicle development and degenerates during the regression phase. Normal human connective tissue sheath fibroblasts are directly related to TGF-$\beta_2$ gene expression in connective tissue sheath fibroblasts by Comp gene selective autotranscription, regulated by TGF-β signaling. The study found that the IGF-1 gene plays a key role in maintaining linear hair growth during the primary stages of growth. In the growth of hair follicles, the expression of IGF-1 gene is associated with upregulation of PDGF-A and PDGF-B genes, and there is antiapoptotic regulation. Further validation revealed that IGF-1 gene increased the expression of platelet- derived growth factors PDGF-A and PDGF-B, confirming that IGF-1 gene is involved in upregulation of PDGF-A and PDGF-B genes in controlling hair growth. The Foxp1 transcription factor controls the initiation of hair follicle stem cells. The lack of Foxp1 gene in skin epithelial cells leads to premature activation of hair follicle stem cells, leading to a shortened resting period of hair follicles. Conversely, overexpression of Foxp1 in keratinocytes promotes cell cycle arrest and prevents cell proliferation. Studies have shown that Foxp1 transcription factors regulate the state of resting follicular stem cells (resting or proliferating) by regulating the expression of the Fgf18 gene in hair follicle stem cells.Br RNA inhibits hair expression by encoding a recognized transcription factor on the skin. Transcriptome sequencing revealed that in the hair follicle growth phase of normal mice, Br gene expression decreased, but increased significantly during hair development, and was upregulated in epithelial cells connected to the dermal papilla. The study found that in the hair follicle growth phase, the Br gene acts as a key factor regulating basic cellular processes (including hair formation, maintaining the integrity of dermal papilla cells, and keratinocyte apoptosis). In the study of the regulation of hair follicle degeneration, the researchers found that p53 gene controls apoptosis in the degeneration of mouse hair follicles. During hair growth, p53 may be an antagonist, which promotes the early entry of hair follicles into the regression phase. At present, although many genes that control the growth and development of hair follicles have been discovered, the regulation mechanism is still unclear and needs further study. Melatonin can promote the growth of cashmere goat fluff and change the fineness of fluff, which is widely used in the production of fluff. The hair follicles treated with melatonin were used as samples to perform transcriptome sequencing, and the changes of genes in the hair follicles after culture were detected, and the genes in hair follicle growth and development were excavated. Wnt, Shh, MAPK, NF-κB, TGF-β, JAK-STAT, and Notch hair follicle growth- and development-related signaling pathways were found in differentially enriched pathways in primary and secondary hair follicles. The role of most genes in hair follicle growth and development has not been reported, and their role as a candidate gene for melatonin-promoting hair follicle growth remains to be further studied.

It is unclear how many such signaling pathways or cytokines work in regulating hair follicle morphology. The identification of multiple transcription factors revealed that in addition to Lef1/β-catenin, a number of transcription factors are involved in the regulation of hair follicle differentiation and gene expression, the most important of which is the winged helix transcription factor Whn. This gene plays a regulatory role in the hairless phenotype in nude mice with phenotypic defects and in mouse and human zinc finger transcription factors. The regulation of the hair phenotype by the upstream and/or downstream genes of the Lef1/β-catenin and Whn targets remains to be studied in depth.

### 4.2.3 The Development and Regeneration of Sweat Glands

The apocrine glands are mainly distributed in specific parts of the body such as the armpits, areola, anus, umbilical fossa, and external genitalia. The formation of apocrine glands begins in the late 4th month of the fetus. Initially developed from the upper part of the hair follicle, a solid epithelial cord is formed, which protrudes perpendicularly to the long axis of the hair follicle into the mesenchyme around the hair follicle, and then grows downward through the developing sebaceous gland and the arrector pilli muscle. When it reaches the horizontal level of the sebaceous gland, the epithelial cord begins to form the lumen of the intradermal catheter. At the same time, the cavity in the hair follicle begins to form. At the 6th month of the fetus, the anterior end of the upper chorda of the apocrine gland is gradually coiled into a coil. At the 9th month, the inner layer differentiates into secretory cells. At birth, the myoepithelial cells around the apocrine gland are not recognized.

The eccrine glands are only found in the soles of mammals. From the view of germline development, except the human palms, the eccrine glands in other parts of the skin evolved later. Human eccrine glands are first seen in the palms and soles at the 4th month of the fetus. It is first seen in the armpits and other parts of the body at the 5th month. The eccrine gland germ begins with the accumulation of deep basophils in the basal layer of the epidermis and develops into a germ, but it is different from the hair germ, which is narrower and has fewer mesenchymal cells in its basal layer. It gradually protrudes into the dermis and grows vertically downward to form a cord-like shape with a rounded end. When reaching the subcutaneous tissue, the end portion is coiled into a spherical shape. Its upper end grows upward from the base of the epidermis and spirals through the epidermis to form cell cords. Like hair follicles, different stages of development of the eccrine glands are visible during this period. At the 16th week of the fetus, some eccrine glands in the palms and soles have begun to form coils, and some new eccrine gland germs are still forming in the epidermis. When the lumen of the eccrine gland is formed, a lumen composed of two layers of cells appears in the duct and secretion part of the dermis, the inner layer is composed of luminal cells, and the outer layer is composed of basal cells. However, the two layers of cells in the secretory part differentiate, and the luminal cells differentiate into high columnar secretory cells, which extend from the basement membrane to the free edge of the lumen, while the basal cells either differentiate into secretory cells or myoepithelial cells. At the 7th–8th month of the fetus, the glandular cavity is formed. The entire sweat gland consists of spiral sweat tubes or acrosyringium in the epidermis, straight sweat ducts in the dermis, coiled sweat ducts, and secretory parts. By birth, the shape of an infant's eccrine gland becomes similar to that of an adult.

The development of sweat glands is a very complicated process, and the mechanisms of morphogenesis, growth regulation, and expression of related genes have not yet been fully elucidated.

The team led by Academician Xiaobing Fu conducted a correlation study between epidermal stem cells and sweat glands in the full-thickness dorsal skin of the fetus of different embryonic ages [3]. It was found that from the 16th week of embryonic age, the basal cells of the primary epidermal ridge accumulated focally to form a mound-like sweat gland, and the terminal part of the cell cord was in a coiled shape and became the mature sweat gland at the 24th week of embryonic age (Figs. 4.6 and 4.7). A certain number of epidermal stem cells can be detected to persist in it (Figs. 4.8–4.11). Thus, it was confirmed the dynamic role of epidermal stem cells in the development of sweat glands. Recent studies have shown that the role of matrix metalloproteinases (MMPs), which are the enzymes of extracellular matrix (ECM), and cell movement are the two most fundamental processes of embryogenesis. The process is regulated by a series of growth factors, that is, the interaction between ECM, MMPs, and growth factors directly controls the differentiation of embryonic cells or affects its behavior. We performed dynamic observations on local ECM remodeling, MMPs, and EGF during embryonic sweat gland development [4]. It was found that mRNA signal and protein expres-

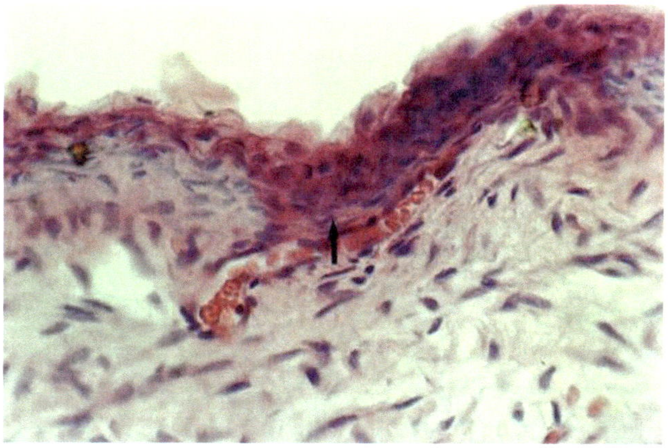

**Fig. 4.6** At the 16th week of embryonic age, the basal cells of primary epidermal ridge accumulated focally to form a mound-like sweat gland. HE×200

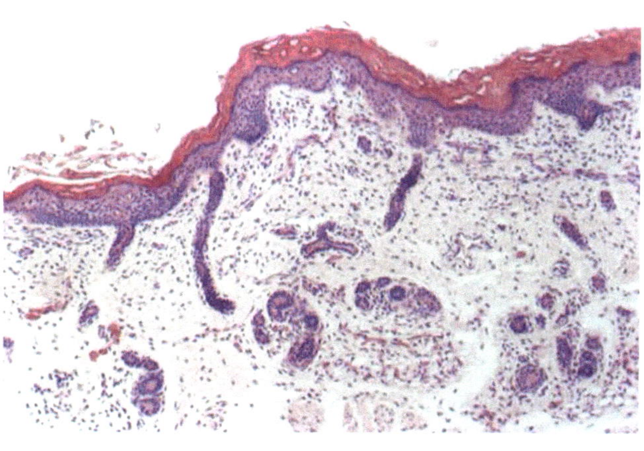

**Fig. 4.7** At the 24th week of embryonic age, myoepithelial cells can be seen in sweat duct, secretory part, and surrounding cells. HE×200

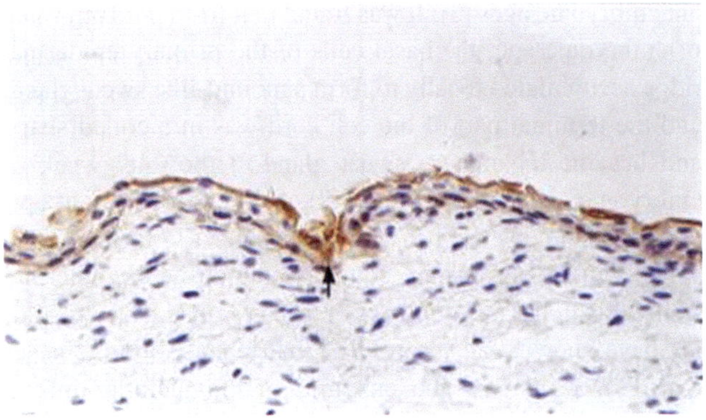

**Fig. 4.8** At the 16th week of embryonic age, the expression of $\beta1$ integrin in sweat gland primordial cells is positive. SP × 200

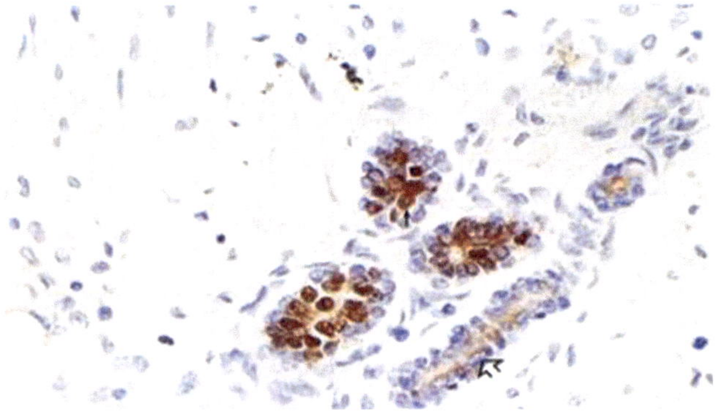

**Fig. 4.9** At the 22nd week of embryonic age, the expression of K19 in sweat gland cells is positive. SP × 200

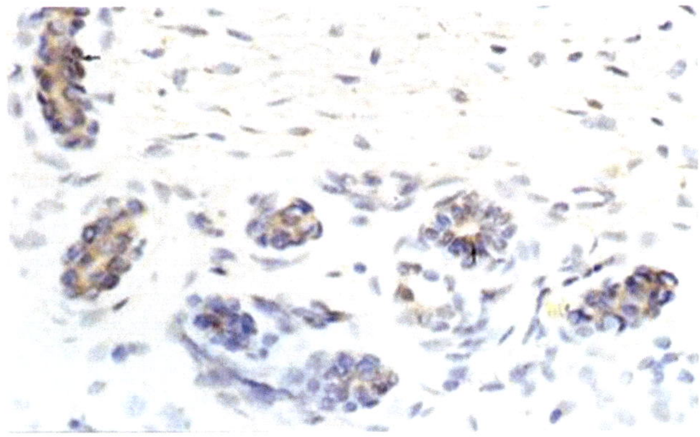

**Fig. 4.10** At the 24th week of embryonic age, the expression of K8 in sweat gland cells is positive. SP × 200

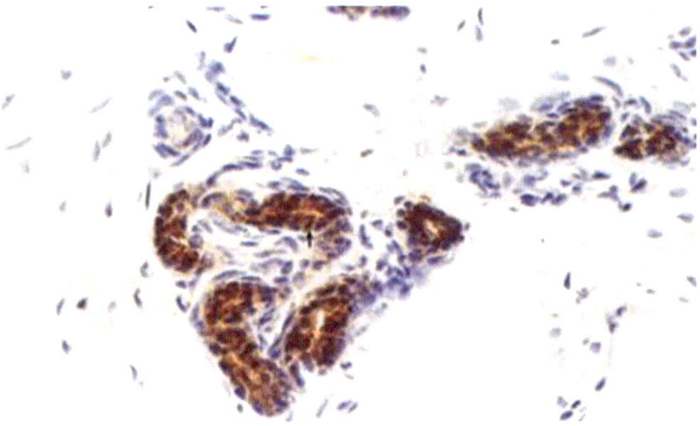

**Fig. 4.11** At the 24th week of embryonic age, the expression of $\beta_1$ integrin in sweat gland cells is positive. SP × 200

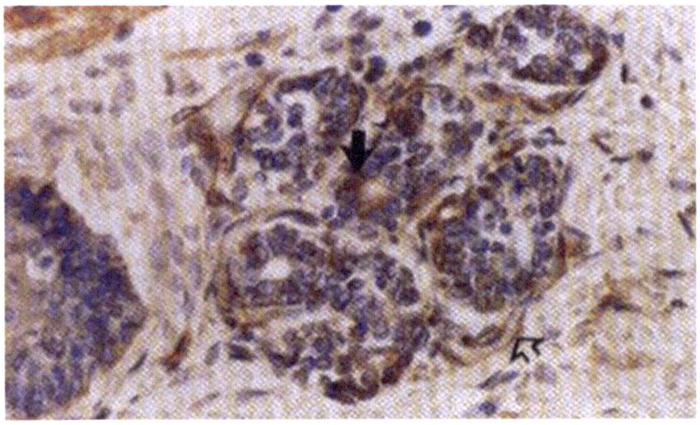

**Fig. 4.12** At the 18th week of embryonic age, MMP-2 is expressed in and around sweat gland cells

sion of MMP-2 and MMP-7 were present in the sweat gland primordia, and sweat gland cells matured as sweat gland germ cells penetrate into the dermis through the basement membrane. The mRNA signal and protein expression intensity of MMP-2 and MMP-7 were also significantly enhanced and localized in the sweat gland germ cells or sweat gland cells and their surrounding local matrix. Especially in the middle and late stages of sweat gland development (20–22 weeks of embryonic age), the mRNA and protein expression intensity of MMP-2 and MMP-7 peaked. After that, until the embryonic age was about 24 weeks, the sweat gland development was almost completed and matured, the mRNA signal and protein expression levels of MMP-2 and MMP-7 gradually decreased, but did not disappear. Therefore, it is speculated that the development of sweat glands is closely related to MMPs (including MMP-2 and MMP- 7). Both sweat gland germ cells and sweat gland cells can synthesize and secrete MMP-2 and MMP-7, and the ability to synthesize and secrete MMP-2 and MMP-7 increases with the development of sweat glands (Figs. 4.12–4.15). It is this programmed change that determines the appearance of sweat gland primordial cells, and due to the degradation of local ECM, while providing space, it guides the primordial cells whose differentiation direction has been determined to the sweat gland germ cells, and to the deep epidermis. In particular, because of the cleavage of FN, the main component of the basement membrane, and collagen VII, the main component of anchor fibers that support the true dermal-epidermal junction. Sweat gland cells break through the basement membrane area and cut into the dermis. In the

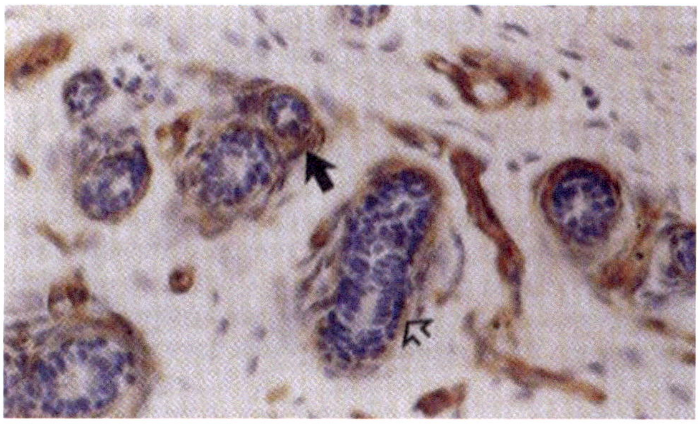

**Fig. 4.13** At the 22nd week of embryonic age, MMP-7 is expressed in and around sweat gland cells

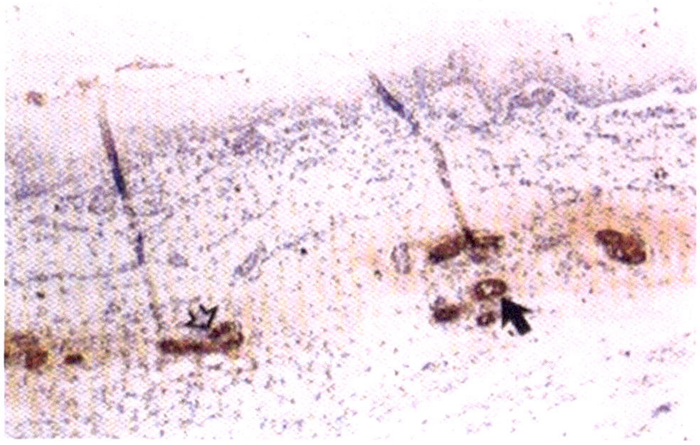

**Fig. 4.14** At the 22nd week of embryonic age, MMP-7 is strongly expressed in the sweat gland cells and its surrounding local matrix. SP × 200

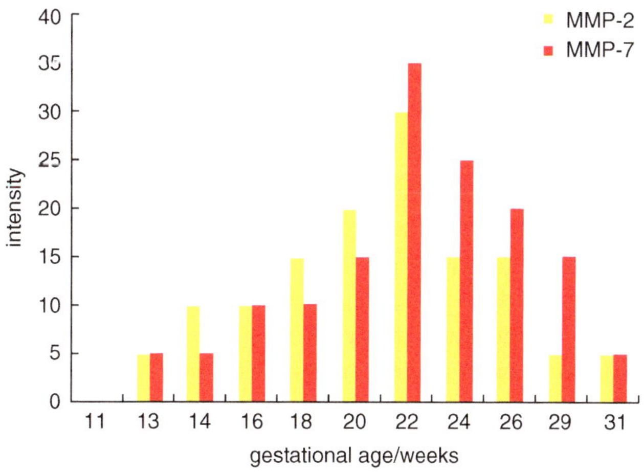


**Fig. 4.15** Positive signal intensity of MMP-2 mRNA and MMP-7 mRNA in each phase

whole process of sweat gland development, EGF is highly expressed, which provides some evidence for local ECM alteration, interaction between MMPs and EGF to induce sweat gland development (Figs. 4.16–4.18). The epithelium of the exocrine glands synthesizes and secretes cytokines, such as EGF, NGF, and interleukin family, and has homologous receptors to maintain its own development, growth, and stability. The epithelium of the exocrine gland also concentrates on the EGF receptor—tyrosine kinase receptor, and binding to the corresponding ligand activates multiple intracellular signaling pathways, which affect the development and function of the gland. From the appearance of sweat gland primordial cells to the maturation of sweat gland cells, the protein expression of EGF is localized to its cytoplasm and local matrix around the cells. The expression intensity increases with the development of sweat glands, and the expression intensity does not decrease significantly after maturity. EGF, as a mitogenic factor, can promote the development and maturation of sweat glands.

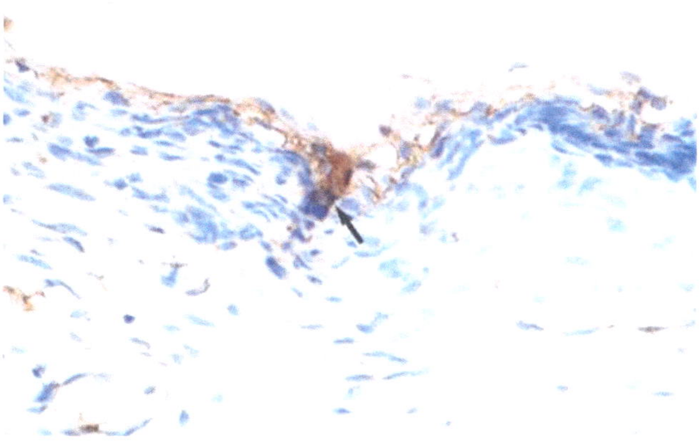

**Fig. 4.16** At the 13th week of embryonic age, LN is positively expressed in sweat gland germ cells. ISH × 200

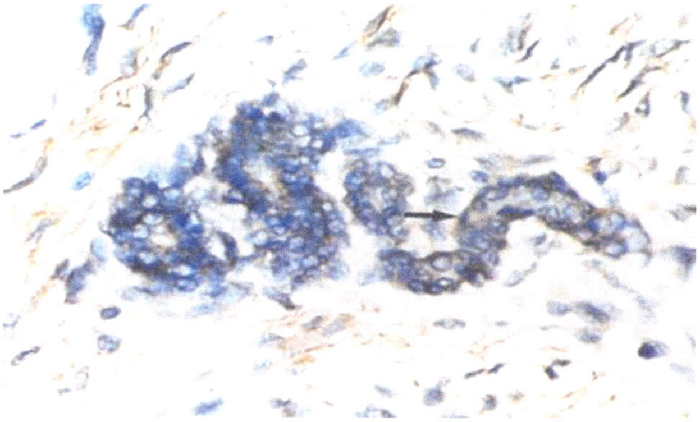

**Fig. 4.17** At the 24th week of embryonic age, FN is positively expressed in sweat gland cells. ISH × 200

Although Merkel cells are a member of the APDU and form a complex with nerve endings, they are also associated with the development of skin appendages. Its exocrine function has reached consensus in academia, such as Merkel cells in the epidermis secreting NGF—target cells of sensory nerve, and Merkel cells in the dermis expressing NGF recep-

**Fig. 4.18** Schematic diagram of the expression levels of EGF, MMP-2, and MMP-7 proteins in each phase

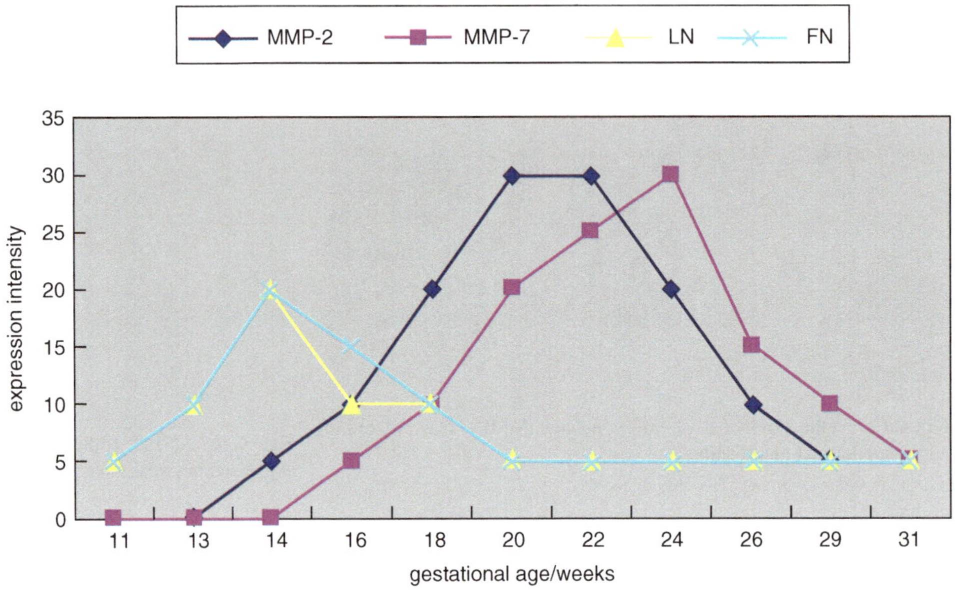


tors—acting on the neurogenesis of the plexus in the upper dermis. In addition, Merkel cells secrete vasoactive intestinal peptide (VIP), substance P, chromogranin A, calcitonin gene-related peptide (CGRP), neuron-specific enolase, and bombesin. Although there are no Merkel cells in the ductal cells and secretory cells of the sweat gland, and there is no direct evidence for the effect of Merkel cells on the sweat glands, the substances secreted by them are inextricably linked to the development of sweat glands. In order to confirm its relationship, Kim observed the appearance, distribution, and density of human fetal skin Merkel cells. Merkel cells in the hands and soles (without hair) appeared on the 56th day of gestational age, with a maximum density at the 80th–90th days; Merkel cells with hairy skin first appeared on the 75th day, reaching a high density at the 20th–24th weeks. The high concentration of Merkel cells is basically consistent with the initiation time of the two sweat glands, which may initiate the differentiation of the sweat gland primordial by paracrine effect. The appearance of Merkel cells in the funnel gland precedes the hair follicle bulge, where Merkel cells stimulate cell differentiation to develop toward structures close to the skin appendages, such as the nerves surrounding the follicles and the arrector pilli muscle. In addition, there are more Merkel cells in the adult hair follicle bulge, which can stimulate the viability of stem cells, and may also contribute to the differentiation of stem cells to the sweat glands. The sympathetic innervation of the sweat glands is a process from norepinephrine to cholinergic. In order to understand whether the differentiation behavior of sweat glands is related to the effects of neurogenic cytokines such as LIF, CNTF, CT-1, etc., Beth observed the differentiation behavior of sweat glands by blocking the receptors of LIF and CNTF through coculture of sympathetic neurons and sweat glands. It is believed that the differentiation behavior of sweat glands is consistent with the signaling pathway of neurogenic cytokines, which is associated with receptor phosphorylation and STAT-3 activation. Therefore, it is reasonable to believe that the development of sweat glands is associated with the nervous system, but the more detailed relationship, especially the regulation of the nervous system and epidermal stem cells needs to be further clarified.

### 4.2.4 The Development and Regeneration of Sebaceous Glands

#### 4.2.4.1 Tissue Development of Sebaceous Glands

Sebaceous glands are distributed in the skin except palms and dorsum of feet. They are composed of several epithelial lobules, which are concentrically differentiated. The outer surfaces of each sebaceous gland lobule are undifferentiated flat proliferating cells, similar to KC cells in the epidermal basal layer, with large nuclei and homogeneous, pale basophilic cytoplasm. The sebaceous gland duct connects the outer root sheath (ORS) of the hair follicle with the sebaceous gland, opens to the outer root sheath of the hair follicle or directly to the skin surface. The ductal epithelium is very thin, and the stratum corneum is closely arranged. The granular layer near the hair follicle is easy to see, but it is rarely seen near the sebaceous gland. Histologically, the hair follicle is divided into funnel and isthmus according to this boundary. The sebaceous gland is the apocrine gland. A small layer of naive cells around the acinus can produce new glandular cells. As the cells gradually increase, more and more lipid droplets form in the cytoplasm. Finally, the cells disintegrate, and the contents containing a large amount of sebum are excreted from the body. The secretion of sebaceous glands is sebum; of which more than 50% are free fatty acids, diglycerides, and triglycerides, and a small part are wax esters, squalene, cholesterol, and cholesterol esters. Only the sebaceous glands in the human body can produce wax esters and squalenes, which are characteristic substances of the sebaceous glands. The function of these secretions is to form a protective film on the surface of the hair to lubricate the hair and prevent the skin from dehydrating and drying. The free fatty acids on the surface of the skin have a moderate inhibitory effect on the growth of fungi and bacteria, and can prevent certain parasites from penetrating into the skin. Secretions also give the body a special odor. According to research, the mothers of the new baby may be related to this. The histogenesis of sebaceous glands begins at the 4th month of the embryo. The hair follicle develops earlier, which is expressed as the embryonic hair germ, that is, the basal cells of the epidermis are closely arranged to form the original bud-like hair germ, and the original hair germ rapidly enters the stage of the hair germ. At this time, the basal cells grow longer and become higher, and grow from the epidermis to the dermis. At the same time, the number of mesenchymal cells and fibroblasts under the hair germ increase, forming an early dermal papilla. The structure at this time is also called hairpeg. The outer cells of the hairpeg are arranged in a fence along the long axis, and then grow obliquely downward. The distal end is swollen and spherical, forming a spherical hairpeg. The hair bulb at the end contains a large number of hair matrix cells, gradually wrapping the dermal papilla. At the 16th week of human embryo, two epithelial-like enlargements appear in the posterior wall of the hair follicle at the globular hairpeg, and the bulge area below is the place where the arrector pilli muscle is attached. The bulge gradually decreases with the further development of the hair follicles. The sebaceous gland primordium is above, and the cell is filled with lipids. Through a catheter, they open to the outer root sheath at the upper end of the hair follicle, and finally develop into a sebaceous glands.

The hair follicle bulge area is continuous with the outer root sheath, which is located below the opening of the sebaceous gland duct and the attachment of arrector pilli muscle. As early as 1876, Unna et al. began the morphological study of the bulge area. In 1976, Al Barwari and Potten applied the $^{3}H$ labeling method to find that the $^{3}H$ marker appeared in the cells around the hair follicle tube and the upper part of the hair follicle with the damage of the epidermis, so it is speculated that potential stem cells are in the hair follicle. In 1990, Cotsarelis et al. showed that no stem cell indications were found in the hair follicles of mouse skin, eyelashes, and tentacles, but they were visible in the bulge area. On the contrary, the pulsed $^{3}H$ label was found to be covered with hair matrix, but not in the bulge area. According to this, it was first proposed that hair follicle stem cells were located in the bulge region of the upper hair follicle. Taylor used the $^{3}H$ and BrdU double-label method to continuously observe the skin and its appendages. It was found that the positive nucleus was only found in the bulge area, while the dermis, the upper part of the hair follicle, and the sebaceous glands were negative. After tracking, the ORS, MC, medulla, and other areas of the lower part of hair follicles were also found to have marker molecules, and positive cells were also found in the upper part of the hair follicles and the epidermis. Electron microscopy revealed that bulge cells showed the characteristics of large proportion of nucleoplasm and primitive cytoplasmic components. At the same time, bulge cells showed great proliferative potential in vitro culture. Moreover, the mixed culture of the upper part of hair follicles containing bulge and DP could regenerate the active hair follicles. In the renewal and maintenance of sebaceous glands after birth, there are several questions are not clear: for example, what is the source of stem cells? Does it come from single stem cells with multidirectional differentiation ability or from one of many stem cells that can strictly differentiate into their respective structures? The experimental results of mouse skin cell lines suggest that the embryonic hair follicles originate from multiple cell clones, that is, the orientation of epidermis, hair follicles, and sebaceous glands is determined in the embryonic stage, but the relationship between different clones in the differentiation process is unknown. Earlier radioisotope experiments found that the basal cells of the sebaceous glands easily bind to $^{3}H$. At that time, it was hypothesized that the sebaceous glands might have their own stem cells. The experimental phenomenon that intact hair follicles can still be regenerated after removal of the lower part of the hair follicle is usually interpreted as the result of bulge stem cell differentiation in the upper permanent part of the hair follicle, which Inaba et al. believe that this regeneration is derived from the sebaceous gland. Different staining results in different regions of the hair follicles suggest that there may be multiple progenitor cells acting on the formation of hair follicles, and after 37 weeks of labeling with β-galactosidase, the different performances of hair follicles the sebaceous glands also suggest that they may have their own stem cells, respectively. However, more experiments do not support the hypothesis that sebaceous glands contain pluripotent stem cells. The main bases are: (a) The organ culture of the sebaceous glands can be maintained for more than 2 weeks, during which DNA and protein synthesis remain unchanged, while lipid formation is progressively reduced. This suggests that although in vitro culture maintains normal cell division, newly formed cells do not differentiate into sebaceous glands. (b) The proliferative capacity of sebaceous gland cells in vitro is much lower than that of the upper part of the hair follicle. (c) After the sebaceous glands are destroyed, they can be regenerated from the upper ORS of the hair follicle. (d) No slow cycle cells are detected in the sebaceous glands. Therefore, most researchers have concluded that the stem cells of the sebaceous gland may be derived from other regions outside the gland. The cells with proliferative and differentiation ability in the sebaceous gland may not be the true stem cells, but the TA cells produced by stem cell division. Chase has speculated that there is a group of pluripotent stem cells in the outer root sheath of the hair follicle, which can not only form hair follicles but also form epidermis and sebaceous glands. It has been observed that there is no marker in the bulge area in the 3H radiolabeling experiment, but above and below the bulge area the cells are clearly labeled, showing the characteristics of TA cells. Especially mitotic phase can be seen in the lower part of the bulge area and in the isthmus and funnel of the hair follicles in the early growth stage and the approaching growth stage. This indicates that TA cells, the progeny cells of the stem cells, can not only grow down to form hair matrix cells but also grow upwards and play a role in maintaining normal epidermis and sebaceous glands. Based on the existing research results, Sun et al. proposed that epidermis, hair follicles, and sebaceous glands originate from a common stem cell population. Therefore, the three are unified into the epidermo pilosebaceous unit. In this hypothesis, all cell populations are derived from the bulge region, and the stem cells in the bulge region are pluripotent stem cells, which divide to produce a series of TA cells with progressively decreased proliferative capacity. Under the action of injury or chemical stimulation, $^{3}$H-labeled cells first appear in the isthmus, followed by sebaceous glands and epidermis, suggesting that the isthmus may store TA1 cells; in the funnel, the sebaceous gland basal layer cells and epidermal basal layer cells may represent further developed TA2, TA3 cells. Taylor believes that hair follicle stem cells may undergo two separate pathways of migration and differentiation, namely the bulge-epidermal pathway and the bulge-hair pathway. Using BrdU instead of $^{3}$H labeled skin, all the proliferating cells are stained with erythematous nuclei. After 8 weeks, the erythematous nuclei are found only in the bulge area, while the dermis, the upper part of the hair follicle, and the sebaceous gland are not seen, indicating that these parts do not contain stem cells. After 2 weeks of observation, it can be seen that many cells in the lower part of the hair follicle contain erythematous nuclei, which provides a direct evidence for the regeneration of hair follicles in the bulge area, and erythematous nuclei are also seen in the upper part of the hair follicle, and the migration of cells in the upper part of the hair follicle into the epidermis is observed. Since the hair follicle stem cells are located adjacent to the sebaceous glands and sebaceous basal cells are not label retaining cells (LRC), that is, there is no slow-cycle characteristic, it is speculated that bulge cells play an important role in the regeneration of sebaceous glands. Oshima et al. used the hair follicle microchimera experiment to obtain the same result. The bulge region of Rosa26 mice (β-galactosidase positive) was implanted into wild-type mice to form chimeric mice. The observation showed that β-galactosidase-positive cells could be seen in the sebaceous glands of the upper hair follicle, indicating that cells in the sebaceous gland are derived from the bulge region of Rosa mice. The HRS/J hairless mouse (Hr) experiment by Panteleyev et al. more directly illustrates the relationship between hair follicle bulge region and sebaceous gland regeneration. The hair follicles develop normally during the birth of Hr mice. The hair follicles degrade at the beginning of the first degeneration period, the hair follicle growth stops, and the hair disappears. However, this model can retain bulge cells and well-developed sebaceous glands. After treatment with dioxin, which only blocked the growth of sebaceous glands without affecting bulge cells, sebaceous glands disappeared completely after 9 days and due to degradation of hair follicles, bulge lost contact with the epidermis and was free from the subcutaneous. Sebaceous gland regeneration was seen in the bulge area after 2 days of dioxin withdrawal. Observation of mice not treated with dioxin revealed that the bulge was surrounded by sebaceous gland cells after 30 days of birth, and the poorly differentiated sebaceous gland cells were close to the bulge, and the highly differentiated sebaceous gland cells were away from the bulge. These cell dynamics experiments indicate that bulge-derived cells have the ability to differentiate into sebaceous gland cells under normal conditions.

#### 4.2.4.2 Several Regulatory Pathways for Sebaceous Gland Growth

Sebaceous glands self-renew and maintain under the regulation of hair follicles, and some molecules are also found to promote sebaceous gland differentiation through other pathways besides hair follicle cell differentiation induction, such as related genes and proteins in Wnt signaling pathway. In fact, because these molecules have a significant role in fat metabolism and hair follicle biology, they may also contribute to the differentiation of hair follicle stem cells in bulge region into sebaceous glands. The Wnt signaling pathway is a key pathway in cell development and regulation of growth, and plays an important role in embryonic development and adult morphogenesis and function under normal conditions. β-catenin is an important component of the Wnt pathway, often combined with E-cadherin to form a complex, even in the cytoplasm with only a small amount of β-catenin, it can also bind to APC complex protein. The latter can activate the activity of enzymes to degrade β-catenin in the cytoplasm. Wnt signaling is transmitted to the cell membrane surface to bind to the corresponding receptor, inhibits GSK-3β kinase activity and prevents β-catenin degradation. After accumulating in the cells, it can enter the nucleus, thereby activating transcription factors and stimulating cell proliferation. The Wnt signaling pathway is critical during embryonic development. Recently, it has been reported that stable β-catenin is expressed in the skin of transgenic mice. These mice continue to form new hair follicles and sebaceous glands after birth, indicating that β-catenin can cause mature epithelial cells to divide into active hair follicles and sebaceous glands. The process generally only occurs in the skin of the embryo. The proto-oncogene c-Myc acts as a transcription factor affecting cell cycle, cell differentiation, and tumor formation. Experiments have shown that c-Myc plays an important role in the formation and regeneration of sebaceous glands. Fusion of the c-Myc gene into the hormone-binding domain of the estrogen receptor in mutant mice (ERTM), due to the lack of activation activity of ERTM, it only responds to the OHT of synthetic steroids and is ineffective against estrogen, thus lacking OHT-Myc-ERTM means inactivation. After the transgenic mice and wild-type mice were treated with OHT for 4 weeks, it was found that the number of sebaceous gland cells in the transgenic mice was significantly increased, the differentiated sebaceous glands continued to proliferate, the lipid formation increased, the epidermis thickened, the hair follicle structure changed abnormally, and then the hair was removed, while the wild-type mice were not affected by OHT and their tissue phenotype was normal. The effect of c-Myc gene on sebaceous gland differentiation was further studied by red oil O staining. It was found that the sebaceous gland cells in the transgenic mice were significantly increased, almost filling abnormal hair follicle tissue. Another evidence for the promotion of sebaceous glands by c-Myc gene comes from the study of the tarsal gland. The tarsal glands of transgenic mice are significantly enlarged, and some differentiated sebaceous gland cells continue to proliferate, and sebaceous gland cells migrate from the hair follicle to the epidermis. These are characteristics of the development of sebaceous gland carcinoma. The activity of the c-Myc gene is to activate the proliferative activity of quiescent stem cells, resulting in the production of TA cells, which in turn leads to terminal differentiation in one direction. Of course, this process is not specific to the c-Myc gene and is regulated by other factors. Another important regulator of sebaceous gland differentiation is the transcription factor peroxisome proliferator-activated receptor (PPARγ). PPARγ is mainly found in adipose tissue and the immune system and can be activated by fatty acids and exogenous peroxisome proliferators to regulate the expression of certain enzymes involved in lipid metabolism. PPARγ binds to the ligand and forms a heterodimer with the retinoic acid receptor (RXR), and then binds to specific sites on the DNA to activate transcription. PPARγ has adipose tissue specificity and is induced before transcriptional activation of many adipocyte genes, which plays an important role in cell differentiation. In vitro studies, induced differentiation of embryonic stem cells into adipocytes is dependent on PPARγ, and PPARγ is required for differentiation of sebaceous gland cells in PPARγ-positive chimeric mice and wild-type mice. It is difficult to achieve the desired effect by inducing sebaceous gland differentiation with androgen in vitro, which may be due to the lack of a differentiation promoting factor.

At present, the clinical requirements for the primary healing and functional recovery after severe trauma are also higher. Rather than simply healing with coverage, it is desirable to regenerate and reconstruct the "complete skin," that is, the skin and its appendages, especially sweat glands, sebaceous glands, and nerve innervation. Therefore, the relationship between hair follicle stem cells and sebaceous glands is worthy of further study.

### 4.2.5 Development and Regeneration of Skin Blood Vessels

At the 3rd week of the embryo, a part of mesenchymal cells of the dermis aggregate to form a blood island, and then there is a gap between the blood island cells. The surrounding cells gradually differentiate into endothelial cells, and the central hematopoietic stem cells form primitive blood cells which are free from the cavity. Endothelial cells are connected to each other in a tubular shape, producing blood vessels and lymphatic vessels. At the 5th month of the fetus, larger blood vessels are visible on the skin and naive smooth muscles appear on the wall.

The neonatal dermis lacks a papillary vascular plexus, which is compensated by a disorderly mutual traffic capillary network to complete its physiological function. One week after birth, the capillary plexus that communicated with each other began to degenerate and gradually formed a more ordered vascular network. At the 2nd week after birth, the papillary plexus begin to appear, and a clear and distinct structure is seen until the 4th to 5th week. By the 14th to 17th week, almost all newborns have complete papillary plexus structures. The formation and changes in blood vessels in the skin folds of newborns are very obvious. In summary, vascular development of the skin occurs mainly in the first 3 months of the embryo, and the developed blood vessels are significantly absent or devoid of the basement membrane compared to adults.

The development of blood vessels includes vasculogenesis (VG) and angiogenesis (AG). Vasculogenesis refers to the process of differentiation from primitive mesenchymal cells into endothelial progenitor cells (EPCs) or angioblasts (angioblasts) into endothelial cells during embryonic development, eventually forming a vascular network. Among them, vascular endothelial growth factor receptor 2 (VEGFR-2) plays a key role in the regulation of VG. Angiogenesis refers to the production of new blood vessels from existing blood vessels, the degradation of extravascular matrix, and the proliferation and migration of vascular endothelial cells to form a new progeny vascular network.

These two forms of blood vessel development exist during embryonic development, but in adults, blood vessels development is mainly achieved by angiogenesis.

Angiogenesis is an important biological phenomenon involved in wound healing, tissue repair, and regeneration.

Angiogenesis is a complex process that is regulated by many signaling molecules, such as vascular endothelial growth factor (VEGF), angiopoietin, fibroblast growth factor, transforming growth factor, platelet-derived growth factor (PDGF), etc., through direct or indirect effects to promote blood vessel growth and participate in vascular stabilization and formation. Angiogenesis is mainly caused by the induction of angiogenic factors, remodeling of intercellular connections, degeneration of the basement membrane, and changes in the polarity of some vascular endothelial cells to form apical cells. The apical cells have the ability to form an extended pseudopod, and mediate the development of vascular buds and the proliferative ability of adjacent stem cells, which promote the extension of vascular buds to form lumens, while recruiting pericytes. The choice of apical cells and stem cells is a dynamic competitive process in which endothelial cells dynamically compete to form apical cells. The final formation of functional blood vessels is a process in which the vascular buds generated by the apical cells fuse with each other and thereby conform to the vascular lumen. The newly generated blood vessels further perform basement membrane deposition and recruitment of parietal cells to form mature blood vessels, in which the upregulation of platelet-derived growth factor B (PDGF-B) and transforming growth factor-1 (TGF-1) plays an important role.

The development and regeneration of skin vascular are complex processes affected by a variety of factors, involving multiple signaling pathways. In-depth understanding of its developmental mechanism is important for the research and treatment of skin-related diseases.

## References

1. Liu HW, Cheng B, Li JF, et al. Characterization of angiotensin-converting enzyme expression during epidermis morphogenesis in humans: a potential marker for epidermal stem cells. Br J Dermatol. 2009;160:250–8.
2. Fu XB, Sun XQ, Sun TZ, et al. Epidermal growth factor induce the epithelial stem cell island formation in the regenerated epidermis. Nat Med J China. 2001;81(12):733–6.
3. Li JF, Fu XB, Shen ZY. Study on the relationship between epidermal stem cells and the developing process of sweat gland in human fetal skin. Chin J Burns. 2002;18:369.
4. Li JF, Fu XB, Sheng ZY. Immunohistochemical study on remodeling rule of extracellular matrix during sweat gland development in human fetal skin. Infect Inflamm Repair. 2001;

# Tissue Repair and Regeneration Disorders: Repair and Regeneration of Chronic Refractory Wounds

# 5

Yufeng Jiang, Xiaobing Fu, Shuliang Lu, Yiwen Niu, Qi Wang, Ting Xie, Wei Dong, Chiyu Jia, Rungong Yang, Yao Lu, and Jialiang Zhu

## 5.1 Epidemiological Characteristics of Chronic Refractory Wounds in Chinese Human Body

Chronic refractory wounds (commonly known as ulcers) can be formed by many reasons. The International Society for Wound Healing defines it as a wound that fails to achieve anatomical and functional integrity and secondary healing through a normal, orderly, and timely repair process. Clinically, it mostly refers to those who fail to heal and have no tendency to heal after more than one month of treatment. It depends on the wound size, the cause, the general health of the individual, and other factors. It mostly occurs in patients with severe chronic and acute injuries such as diabetes mellitus, trauma, varicose veins, angiosclerosis, paraplegia, and long-term bedridden. It has the characteristics of complicated pathogenesis, long course of disease, many disciplines involved, difficult treatment, and high treatment costs.

Y. Jiang
The Chinese People's Liberation Army Strategic Support Force Characteristic Medical Center, Beijing, China

X. Fu (✉) · R. Yang · Y. Lu · J. Zhu
The Chinese People's Liberation Army General Hospital, Beijing, China

S. Lu · Y. Niu
Ruijin Hospital, Shanghai Jiaotong University School of Medicine, Shanghai Burns Institute, Shanghai Wound Healing Institute, Shanghai, China

Q. Wang · T. Xie
The Ninth People's Hospital, Shanghai Jiaotong University School of Medicine, Shanghai, China

W. Dong
The First Affiliated Hospital of Jinan University, Guangzhou, China

C. Jia
Xiang'an Hospital Affiliated to Xiamen University, Xiamen, China

### 5.1.1 The Pathogenetic Characteristics of Chronic Refractory Wounds on the Body Surface

In 1998, Academician Xiaobing Fu completed the first epidemiological study on chronic refractory wounds on the body surface in China. Through the investigation of more than 30,000 inpatient surgical patients in 15 hospitals in different regions, it was found that patients with chronic refractory wounds on the surface accounted for 1.5–3%, mainly due to traumatic infection (67.5%), pressure ulcer (9.2%), venous ulcer (6.5%), diabetic ulcer (4.9%), and other factors (11.9%). In terms of the affected population, the chronic refractory wounds caused by trauma are mainly young and middle-aged people aged 20–50 years old, while those caused by diabetes, pressure ulcers, and venous ulcers are mainly elderly people over 60 years old [1].

A cross-sectional, retrospective epidemiological study completed in 2009 found that patients with chronic refractory wounds accounted for 1.7‰ of all hospitalized patients, and complications of age-related diseases such as diabetes mellitus and pressure ulcer have become the main causes of chronic refractory wounds on the body surface (Fig. 5.1) indicating that the characteristics of chronic refractory wounds in Chinese human body have been consistent with those in western developed countries. In this study, more than 1/3 of patients with chronic refractory wounds were caused by diabetes, especially in the 40–60 and 60–80 age groups, accounting for 29.4% and 49.0%, respectively. This is highly correlated with the rapid growth of diabetes in our country. Since 1980, China has conducted five surveys on the prevalence of diabetes in 1980, 1994, 2002, 2007, 2008, and 2010 and found that the prevalence of diabetes has experienced a catastrophic development from 0.67% → 2.28% → 2.60% → 9.70%, rising to 11.6% in 2010. In 2013, the top three countries with diabetes in the 20–79 age group were China, India, and the United States, with 98.4 million, 65.1 million, and 24.4 million, respectively. It is expected that the rankings of these three


X. Fu (ed.), *Regenerative Medicine in China*, https://doi.org/10.1007/978-981-16-1182-7_5

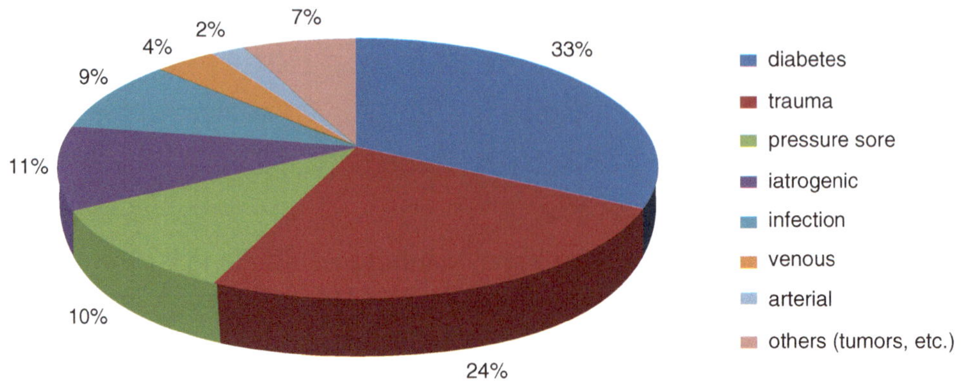


**Fig. 5.1** Causes of wound formation (2009)

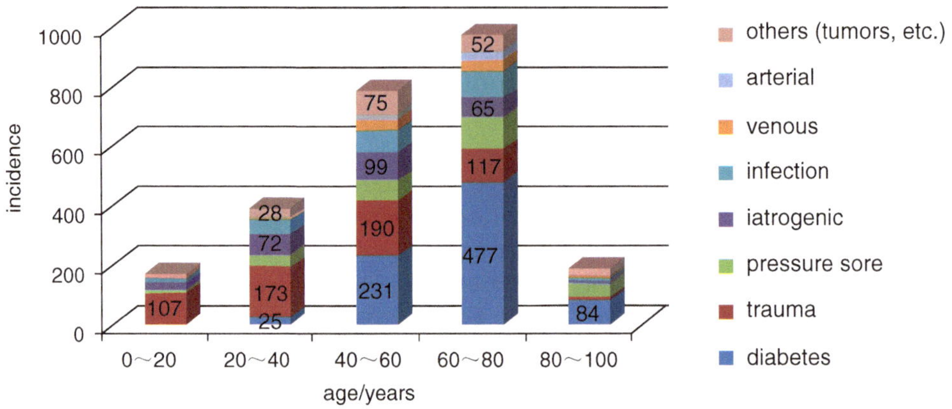


**Fig. 5.2** Age distribution of chronic refractory wounds on the surface (2009)

countries will remain unchanged in 2035, with the number of patients increasing to 142.7 million, 109 million, and 29.7 million, respectively [2]. According to the China Health Statistics Yearbook in the past 5 years, the incidence of trauma due to various reasons has not changed significantly in 10 years [3]. From this we can understand that diabetes has replaced trauma as the primary cause of chronic refractory wounds on the surface.

Our study also found a significant change in the age distribution of patients with chronic refractory wounds on the surface. The average age of patients 10 years ago was 36 years old, which is a whole difference of 22 years compared with the average age of 58 years old. Older patients now occupy a significantly larger proportion, with the highest age of onset being 40–60 years old and 60–80 years old (Fig. 5.2). Retired people become the main patient group. A US-wide survey of pressure ulcers found that 73% of these patients occurred in the elderly over 65 years old, and the characteristics of the disease in China are consistent with those reported in developed countries. The incidence of chronic refractory wounds on the surface shows an aging trend, and these changes are related to the recent aging of China's population.

Regarding diabetic foot, a multicenter prospective study in 2003 showed that the majority of patients with foot disease in China were elderly, with low education and low income, and many had complicated complications of macrovascular and microvascular disease. Neuropathic ulcers are more common in patients with foot ulcers. The foot disease patients in the northern region are young, have a long course of diabetes, and have a short course of foot disease. The common factor affecting the severity of diabetic foot in the north and south is ABI. Recent studies have found that the annual incidence of new-onset ulcers in diabetic patients in China is 8.1%, the annual incidence of new-onset ulcers in diabetic foot ulcers is 31.6%. Independent risk factors leading to the occurrence of foot ulcers include kidney disease, insulin levels, and a decrease in HDL levels [1, 4, 5].

The most serious consequences of diabetic foot disease, as well as the greatest psychological and life effects on patients, are the problem of amputation. The investigation of amputation rate in 39-grade 3A hospitals nationwide in 2009 found that diabetes amputation (toe) accounted for 28.2% of all amputations (toes), accounting for 39.5% of nontraumatic amputations; in 2010, we found that amputation (toe) of diabetic foot ulcers accounted for 19.03% of total amputation (toe), including 2.14% for large amputations and 16.88% for small amputations, and the annual incidence of amputation was 5.1%. The independent risk factors of large amputations in patients with diabetic foot ulcers included the increase of

WBC and the previous history of foot ulcers, independent risk factors of small amputations included prolonged course of diabetes, elevated WBC, foot ulcer infection, foot deformity, history of revascularization surgery, and decreased postprandial blood glucose levels [6–9].

Pressure sores, as another type of chronic refractory wounds that are highly correlated with the elderly, bring heavy burden on families and society. The occurrence of pressure sores will prolong the length of hospital stay and increase the mortality rate of the disease, so the nursing staff must strengthen the prevention knowledge of pressure sores. A survey of 39,951 patients in 12 hospitals nationwide completed in 2012 found that the prevalence of pressure sores was 1.577%, and the prevalence of hospital-acquired pressure sores was 0.628%. Excluding reversible stage I pressure sores, the prevalence rate was 1.121%. The prevalence rate of pressure sores was slightly higher in military hospitals (1.72%) than in local hospitals (1.498%), higher in tertiary hospitals (1.694%) than in secondary hospitals (1.114%), and higher in traditional Chinese medicine hospitals (1.684%) than in western hospitals (1.55%). The prevalence rate of pressure sores in different hospitals was 1.114–1.72%. Among them, only 46.517% of hospitalized patients with Braden score $\leq 16$ used decompression mattresses, 75.149% could turn over regularly, and nearly 1/3 of the patients did not use any decompression devices. In 76 patients with Braden score > 16 still occurred pressure sores, accounting for 12.063% of patients with pressure sores, and only 35.526% of these patients used decompression mattresses, and 56.579% could turn over regularly. It is believed that the cause of pressure sores may still be related to the lack of decompression mattresses and unscheduled turn over.

Iatrogenic injury refers to injury caused by the operation of medical personnel and not related to the primary disease during the medical procedure. The distribution of iatrogenic wounds involves all departments of the hospital, including surgery, internal medicine, and other specialties. Because both subcutaneous and deep artificial implants can cause wounds, so there are more surgical occurrences (including brain surgery using titanium mesh instead of skull implantation after exposure, brain pacemaker exposure, cardiovascular pacemaker exposure, artificial blood vessel exposure, oral and maxillofacial surgery/head and neck surgery implant exposure), especially in orthopedics and plastic surgery, due to the extensive use of biological materials (internal fixation equipment after limb fractures, prostheses after joint replacement, various plastic surgery materials), resulting in a higher incidence of iatrogenic wounds. This is mainly due to the continuous emergence of various biological materials, the expanding indications of surgery, and the increasing number of operations for elderly patients as their life expectancy increases.

### 5.1.2 The Pathogenic Microbiological Characteristics of Chronic Refractory Wounds on the Body Surface

Through a study of 1,488,201 cases, we screened 2513 patients with chronic refractory wounds that met the criteria and organized the contents of the bacterial culture in their medical records. It was found that 1853 cases were not cultured, 660 records could be analyzed, 144 records showed negative culture results, 4 records could not be classified, and up to 77.8% of patients in the records were treated with intravenous antibiotics. This suggests that in the clinic the bacterial culture rate of the wound and the use of antibiotics should be emphasized and strengthened. Analysis of 660 positive results showed that 36 species (347 strains) of Gram-negative bacilli, 17 species (265 strains) of Gram-positive cocci, 5 species (7 strains) of Gram-positive bacilli, and 1 specie (4 strains) of Gram-negative cocci, 7 species (42 strains) of fungi, a total of 66 sortable positive records (665 strains). *Staphylococcus aureus* (without methicillin-resistant *Staphylococcus aureus*) is the most common pathogen, followed by *Pseudomonas aeruginosa, Escherichia coli*, and coagulase-negative *Staphylococci*. Gram-positive bacilli and Gram-negative cocci are rare. *Candida albicans* is the most common fungus (Figs. 5.3 and 5.4). In this study, 473 cases with 1 pathogenic microorganism, 55 cases with 2 species, 12 cases with 3 species, 5 cases with 4 species, and 2 cases with 5 species were sequentially detected. Monopathogenic bacterial infection is the most common.

### 5.1.3 Health Economics Characteristics of Chronic Refractory Wounds on the Surface

Through comparative studies, it was found that although the proportion of self-pay was significantly reduced (58.9%, 42.3%) in 10 years, the individual treatment burden of patients was reduced, compared with 8.9 days (2007) and 8.6 days (2008) published in the National Statistical Bulletin on Health Development, the average hospital stay for chronic refractory wounds in the study was 21 days (P50; P25, P75: 12, 40), increasing the hospital stay for up to 13 days. Males with chronic refractory wounds due to diabetes had the longest hospital stay (P50 = 31 days; P25, P75: 19, 52.3) ($P < 0.01$). The average cost per patient was 12227.0 yuan ($1798.1) (P50; P25, P75: 6801.7, 26794.4) (Table 5.1), compared with the average medical expenses of 4123 yuan (P50 = 1600 yuan) for urban and rural residents, including 7606 yuan (P50 = 3375 yuan) in urban area and 2649 yuan (P50 = 1100 yuan) in rural area, the average indirect cost per hospitalization (mainly including transportation, escort, etc.) was 360 yuan (including 514 yuan in urban area and 294

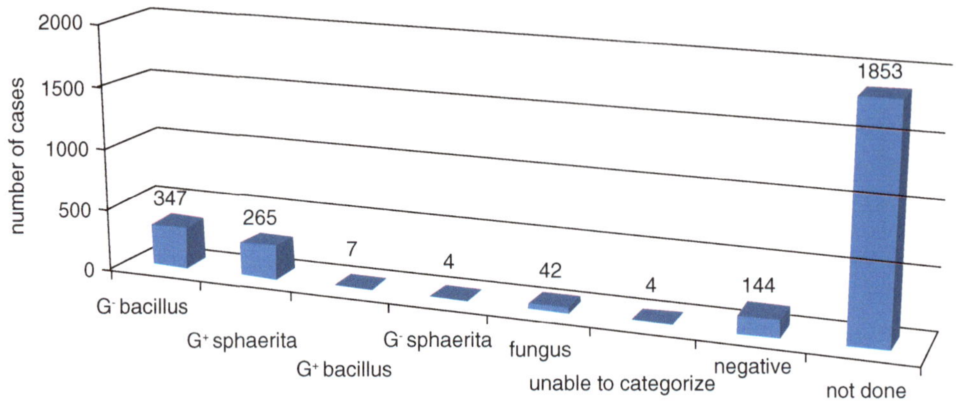


**Fig. 5.3** Classification of pathogenic microbiological examination results of chronic refractory wounds on the surface

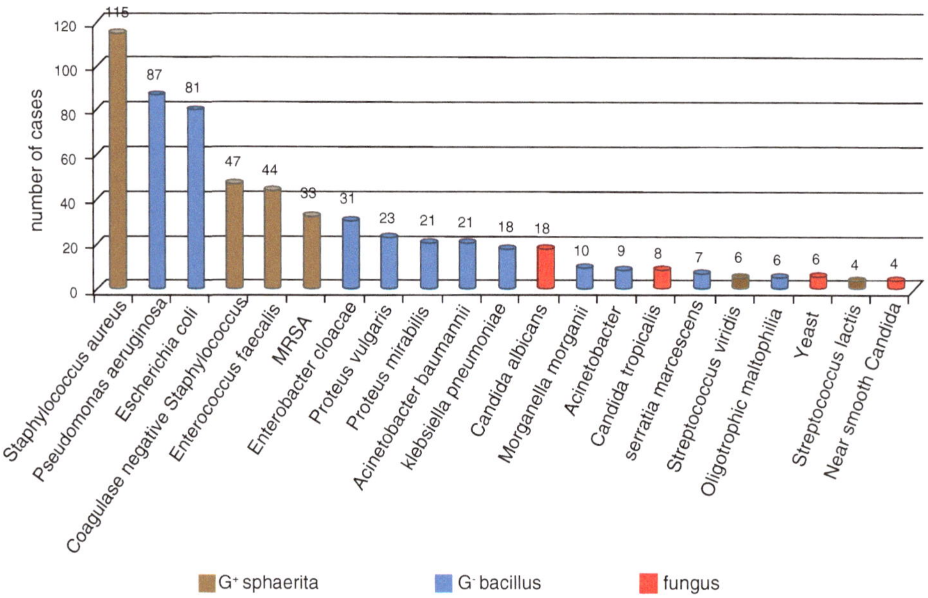


**Fig. 5.4** Top 20 pathogenic microorganisms in positive test results of chronic refractory wounds on the surface

yuan in rural area), as well as the national per capita health cost was 854.4 yuan/person (2007) and 984 yuan/person (2008), it can be seen that the chronic refractory wounds caused a heavy health economic burden. In addition, the analysis of the distribution of medical expenses found that the cost of nursing is only 4%, and the cost of medicines accounts for 38% of the total cost. Uneven and unreasonable distribution of medical expenses may be related to relevant national policies.

Through the above research, it can be found that with the rapid development of China's society and economy, the aggravation of population aging, changes in lifestyle patterns and the accompanying changes in disease spectrum, diabetes mellitus has become the primary cause of chronic refractory wounds in China. The treatment of these wounds is particularly difficult due to the advanced age, infectious factors and basic diseases such as diabetes. The country needs to develop an overall plan for early prevention, early detection and early treatment of chronic wounds, and further improve the universal health care system to effectively reduce the incidence of chronic refractory wounds on the surface.

## 5.2 Study on the Mechanism of Local Skin Damage on Refractory Diabetic Wounds

Skin tissue wound healing refers to a series of pathophysiological processes in which local tissues are repaired by proliferation or regeneration after traumatic or other disease processes because skin tissue defects to form wounds [10]. Wound healing is regulated by the body's genes, making wound healing events have their own laws. The regulatory capacity of organisms can withstand the adverse effects of systemic or local factors through related mechanisms. Once the systemic disease or local pathological changes exceed the body's ability to regulate, it may lead to delayed wound healing or nonhealing, thus forming "out of control" wound repair.

**Table 5.1** Health economics characteristics of different causes of chronic refractory wounds

| Pathogeny | Diabetes | Trauma | Oppression | Iatrogenic | Infectivity | Venous | Arterial | Other | Total |
|---|---|---|---|---|---|---|---|---|---|
| **Observed indicator** | **Male** | | | | **Median (P25,P75)** | | | | |
| Average length of stay (d) | 31 (19,52.3) | 30 (17,52) | 29.5 (19,55.5) | 21 (12,35) | 24 (15.5,41.5) | 15 (9,26) | 23 (11,33.5) | 19 (10.3,29.5) | 23 (13,42) |
| Average hospitalization fee (yuan) | 17181.67 (9064.8,34219.1) | 13689.1 (7671.4,33067.3) | 17755.1 (8892.7,41064.8) | 10444 (5234.4,18962.4) | 10139.2 (5517.2,16087.4) | 8694.1 (5391.3,11901.5) | 18052.1 (9830,41138.3) | 11837.9 (6374.3,22863.3) | 13308.2 (7136.4,29870.1) |
| Mean healing time (d) | 76 (45,163) | 80 (45,176) | 106 (53,383) | 113 (60,259) | 88.5 (47,234.8) | 112 (53,601.5) | 96 (62.5,156) | 80 (53.5,389) | 81 (46,208.8) |
| **Observed indicator** | **Female** | | | | **Median (P25,P75)** | | | | |
| Average length of stay (d) | 27.5 (17.8,50) | 27.5 (16,48.3) | 13 (9.8,30) | 19 (12,29) | 23 (12,44) | 18 (12,24) | 23 (11,37) | 17 (9,23) | 20 (12,35) |
| Average hospitalization fee (yuan) | 14068.6 (8391,26699) | 13870.6 (6757.3,25191.6) | 9839.7 (4975,20804.2) | 8575 (4931.3,17223.9) | 8411.1 (5330.9,13633.6) | 9938.9 (6912.8,13875.1) | 11602.9 (9168,20286.3) | 10987.2 (5395.2,23139.3) | 10942.6 (6052.4,22078.1) |
| Mean healing time (d) | 117 (69,195) | 71 (43,160) | 76 (40,186.5) | 132.5 (61.8,329.8) | 70 (44,111) | 205 (67,493.5) | 67 (52.5,79.3) | 220.5 (87.5,464.5) | 89 (46,208) |

Among all the related factors leading to the "out of control" wound repair, diabetes combined with refractory wounds is one of the most important areas for attention.

So far, it has been considered that the occurrence of diabetic foot is based on diabetic vascular neuropathological changes [11], which are generally manifested as delayed wound healing and ulcer formation with insufficient blood supply and infection. Related molecular biology studies show that:

(a) The migration of macrophages is inhibited, directly or indirectly impairing the chemotaxis of neutrophils and other tissue cells.
(b) Abnormal expression of a variety of growth factors, these growth factors are involved in cell proliferation, chemotaxis, synthesis, secretion, and other activities [12].
(c) Neuropeptide regulation pathway disorder, which inhibits cell proliferation, chemotaxis, and growth factor synthesis related to wound healing [13].
(d) The imbalance between matrix metalloproteinases (MMPs) and tissue inhibitor of metalloproteinases (TIMPs) leads to new extracellular matrix (ECM) deposition and neovascular reconstruction disorders, which may be due to abnormal expression of growth factors.
(e) Abnormal cell biological behaviors: the number and bactericidal ability of inflammatory cells decreased, the chemotactic ability of monocytes decreased; fibroblast proliferation ability, response to growth factors, and collagen synthesis decreased significantly.
(f) The formation of glycation end products (AGEs) leads to an increase in oxygen free radicals, triggering an imbalance of oxidative stress.
(g) Inhibition of capillary regeneration in wound.

Recent studies have noted that vascular lesions in diabetic lower extremity ulcers are characterized by stenosis caused by thickening of the vascular basement membrane. After ulceration, vascular repair penetrates from residual diseased capillaries to the ulcer, mainly due to insufficient blood supply leading to the regeneration of capillaries in the wounds. Vascular regeneration after exogenous trauma includes revascularization, in addition to the above mechanisms. The possible reason for this difference is that the occurrence of diabetic lower extremity ulcers is due to the numerous biological behavioral abnormalities already existing in the diabetic skin, which leads to the pathological process with peripheral neuropathy and vascular lesions as the main clinical features and gradually develops into spontaneous ulcers. Although the repair process after the ulcer contains all the elements of wound healing, it is essentially a continuation of the same pathological process, which is related to several characteristic differences associated with the initiation of wound healing after the integrity has not been damaged in the case of external trauma. It is based on such differences that they differ in many aspects related to healing. Therefore, the study of the "out of control" mechanism of diabetic wound healing includes not only the occurrence of lower extremity ulcers but also the difficulty of wound healing caused by exogenous trauma.

Whether it is a spontaneous ulcer of diabetes or a wound caused by exogenous trauma, it has the same clinical feature—difficult to heal. Although diabetic vasculoneuropathy is considered to be the mechanism for diabetes refractory to healing, this understanding does not explain many biological behavioral abnormalities in diabetic skin and wound healing, and the treatments based on this understanding has only achieved unsatisfactory results in a large number of human experiments and clinical practice. The reason is that diabetic vasculoneuropathy may be only the pathological outcome of diabetic complications. Therefore, it is necessary to understand whether the various biological behavioral abnormalities in the healing process of diabetic wounds have a common "switch" by understanding the characteristics of diabetic skin and its posttraumatic healing, so as to clarify the initiating factors of the occurrence of refractory in mechanism and provide a more effective starting point for clinical treatment.

### 5.2.1 The Characteristics of Diabetic Skin

Diabetic wound healing is a noninvasive—invasive—repairing biological process. Therefore, whether there are abnormal histological, cytological, and molecular biological behaviors of diabetic skin before trauma is obviously important for the "out of control" of the whole wound repair process.

Studies shown that the wound healing in diabetic rats is inextricably linked to the increase of blood glucose and the high concentration of sugar in local tissues. Diabetic wound healing is associated with metabolic changes in diabetes, and local high glucose and AGEs accumulation are important features of biochemical changes in diabetic skin [14].

AGE Reader (DiagnOptics, Groningen, Netherlands) can simply and noninvasively detect the skin of the forearm and automatically obtain the skin autofluorescence (SAF) value. In clinical practice, the SAF value is used to reflect the accumulation of AGEs in human tissues. Studies have shown that the accumulation of type I collagen AGEs in the skin of patients with diabetic foot ulcers is significantly increased, and the accumulation of AGEs is correlated with SAF. SAF test can be used as a simple, rapid, and noninvasive method to screen chronic vascular complications of diabetes. Compare to glycosylated hemoglobin test, SAF can more accurately reflect the actual time of diabetic patients with glucose metabolism disorders and oxidative stress. Therefore,

SAF test may be used as a simple method to assess local skin tissue and overall metabolic control status.

Diabetic skin usually has a thin appearance. At the histological level, the thickness of the epidermis and dermis are obviously thinned. In addition, in animal experiments, it was found that the layers of keratinocytes in diabetic skin were not clear, some epidermis lacks stratified arrangement, and the number of spinous cells was significantly reduced. The collagen in dermis of the diabetic is thin and disorderly arranged, and some collagens can be denatured and broken. The focal infiltration of chronic inflammatory cells can be seen in the collagen degeneration area [15].

In addition to histological changes, the content and properties of collagen in diabetic skin tissue also showed abnormal changes, and the hydroxyproline content and collagen solubility of skin tissue decreased significantly.

Tissue repair cells include epidermal keratinocytes, fibroblasts, and vascular endothelial cells. Immunohistochemical examination showed that the number of apoptotic cells in the skin of diabetic patients increased significantly.

A large number of reports have reported abnormal expression of growth factors in diabetic skin. It is generally believed that growth factors with healing-promoting effects in diabetic skin tend to be downregulated, but many experimental studies provide contradictory evidence. In the diabetic rat model, the expression of FGF-2 was also not decreased, and the expression of FGFR was higher than that of normal skin. However, the immunofluorescence double labeling technique showed that FGF-2 was coexpressed with AGEs at the same site [16, 17], thus it is reasonable to presume that there is a lack of growth factors with normal functional activity in diabetic skin.

Inflammatory cells usually play a role in entering the periphery of the wound after wound formation [18].

However, in the skin of noninvasive diabetes, focal infiltration of inflammatory cells in the region of collagen degeneration can be observed, and the increase in myeloperoxidase (MPO) content suggests the number of neutrophils in diabetic skin tissue increased significantly, and the content of malondialdehyde (MDA), which indirectly reflected the oxidative damage of cell membrane, was significantly higher than normal, aMMP-2 level and aMMP-2/TIMP-2 ratio were significantly higher than normal. Combined with the positive expression of Vimentin antigen, it reflects the excessive infiltration of inflammatory cells and a certain degree of tissue damage in the skin tissue under the pathological condition of diabetes.

The above characteristics of diabetic skin tissue indicate that there are histological and cellular biological changes without being subjected to exogenous trauma. This series of diabetic skin tissue behaviors involves various aspects related to wound healing, meaning that diabetic skin has a different starting point from normal wound and will inevitably affect the healing process after trauma.

### 5.2.2 The Characteristics of Wound Healing in Diabetes

Diabetic wounds showed pathological features of chronic prolonged inflammatory response and tissue repair delay [19].

Fibroblasts are one of the major repair cells [20]. The number of local fibroblasts in diabetic skin burn wounds was significantly reduced, and collagen deposition was also significantly reduced.

Vascular endothelial cells are involved in the initiation and development of inflammatory responses. The functions of chemotaxis, activation, migration, proliferation, and differentiation play an important role in the formation of new blood vessels. There is a neovascularization disorder in the healing process of diabetic wounds [21, 22], which is characterized by a decrease in the number of functional neovascularizations. The mechanism depends not only on the proliferation of vascular endothelial cells but also on the assembly of new blood vessels, which is an important link leading to the inhibition of vascular remodeling [14].

An important sign of wound healing is the reepithelialization of the wound. The proliferative activity of epidermal keratinocytes during re-epithelialization is one of the most important repairing actions in wound healing. Normal and orderly proliferation regulation is a necessary guarantee for the smooth healing of wounds. Studies shown that the decreased expression and activity of cell cycle regulators in epidermal keratinocytes is one of the mechanisms leading to delayed re-epithelialization and refractory wound healing under diabetic pathological conditions.

The expression of growth factors in diabetic wound healing showed different degrees of change. In the mechanism of diabetic wound healing, there is not only a change in the amount of growth factors, but also the deficiency of growth factors with normal functional activity caused by glycosylation of growth factors is an important condition of the growth factor. The local application of the exogenous growth factor FGF-2 can promote collagen neogenesis, improve repair cell function, and increase the expression of FGF-2 mRNA in diabetic wound tissue, which supports this inference.

The inflammatory response is an important stage in wound healing [23]. After the normal skin trauma, the acute inflammatory cells accumulate to the wound edge under the chemotaxis of inflammatory mediators to exercise their mission, forming a relatively clear inflammatory reaction zone in histology. After the diabetic skin trauma, a large number of inflammatory cells are diffusely infiltrated, and persist in the wound healing process. Furthermore, diabetic wounds often stagnate in abnormal inflammatory states, suggesting that there are not only abnormal inflammatory reactions in diabetic wounds but also obstacles in the transition from the inflammatory phase to the subsequent phase.

It was confirmed that the repair process of diabetic full-thickness injury showed delayed inflammatory phase, unsmooth transition in inflammatory phase-repair period and delayed repair period, that is, the wound showed an imbalance of inflammation/repair (Fig. 5.5) [24]. So what are the characteristics of macrophages that are closely related to them in this process?

Macrophage infiltration and polarization transformation were observed in the full-thickness skin defect repair model of diabetic rats. It was found that macrophage infiltration in diabetic wounds was "slow-in and slow-out." The number of macrophage infiltration in the diabetic group was less than that in the normal group on the first and third days after trauma (Figs. 5.6 and 5.7). On the third day after injury, the

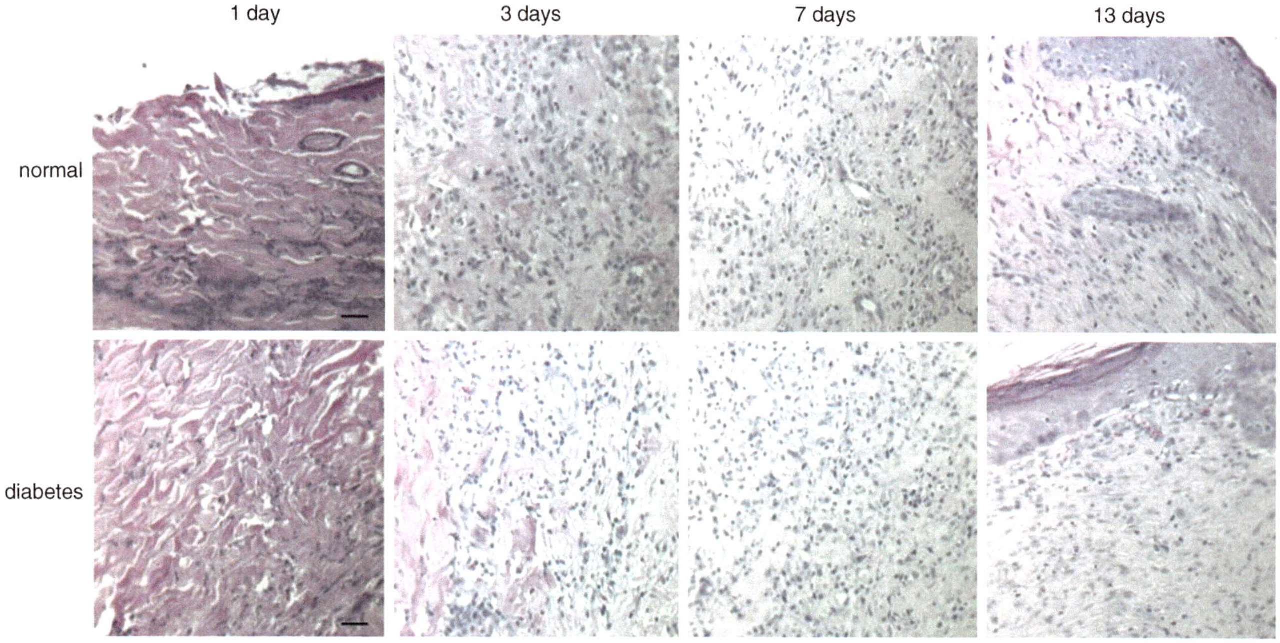


**Fig. 5.5** HE staining shows the histological morphology of the wounds at each time point in both groups. (Scale 20 μm)

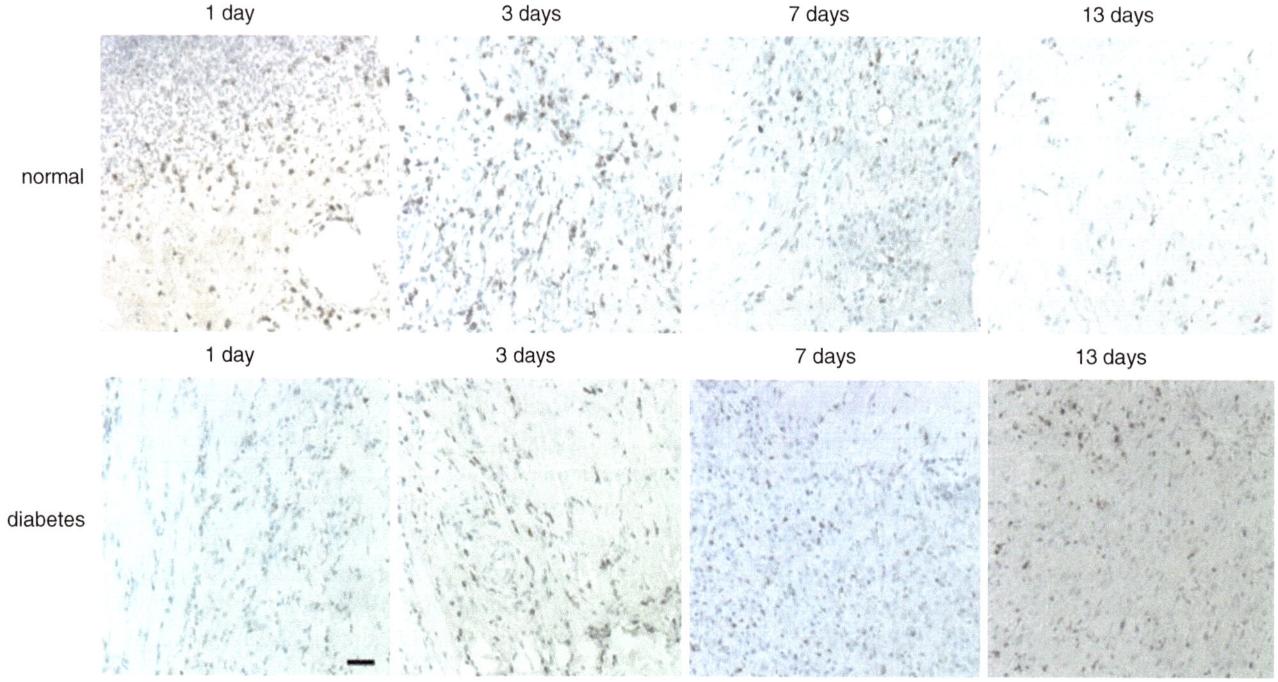


**Fig. 5.6** Immunohistochemistry showed a difference in macrophage infiltration and regression between the two groups (scale 20 μm)

number of macrophages in the diabetic group was not only insufficient, but no typical phagocytosis was seen (Fig. 5.8).

On the seventh day after injury, there were still more M1 macrophages infiltrated in the diabetic wound, and the number of M2 macrophages was far less than that of the normal group. It is suggested that the wounds of diabetic mice show an imbalance of inflammation/repair accompanied by abnormal macrophage infiltration and polarization.

The exploration of the tissue characteristics and healing characteristics of diabetes skin has revealed the regularity of the diabetic wound healing, that is, the healing factors such as tissue cells, extracellular matrix, and growth factors interact and influence each other at various stages of healing through their own behavioral abnormalities, forming a "out of control" network for diabetic wound healing. It is worth noting that the diabetic skin is always accompanied by the presence of a high-glucose environment, the accumulation of AGEs, or the associated glycosylation effects, whether in the noninvasive skin tissue or in the wound repair process. This raises the question of how the product of glucose metabolism play a role in the "out of control" network of diabetic wound healing.

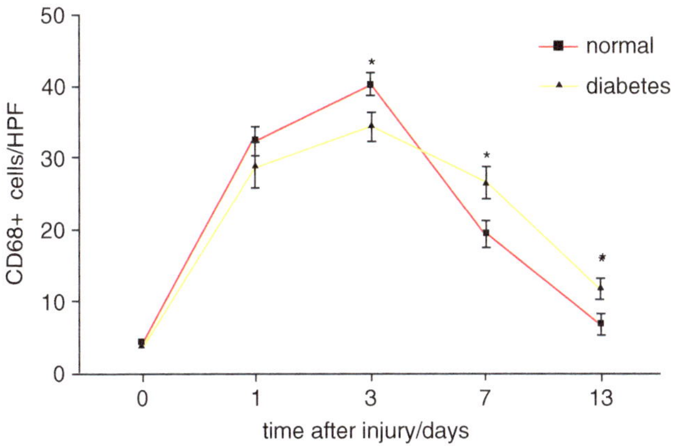


**Fig. 5.7** Macrophage infiltration in the dorsal wound of diabetic rats was "slow-in and slow-out"

### 5.2.3 The Relationship Between Metabolic Disorders and Healing Factors

Diabetes is characterized by persistent pathological hyperglycemia, which triggers the activation of abnormal metabolic pathways, leading to the disorder of the internal environment on which cells depend to survive, causing pathological changes in the function and structure of cells, tissues, and organs. It is an important factor causing the occurrence and development of diabetic complications. Among them, nonenzymatic glycosylation induced by long-term hyperglycemia is one of the main metabolic remodeling activities, and its biochemical outcome is local high glucose and AGEs accumulation. Numerous studies have confirmed that the characteristic of short-term diabetes is mainly increased sugar content in skin tissue, while the characteristics of long-term diabetes are increased sugar content in the skin tissue and a large accumulation of AGEs. AGEs have a wide range of biological activities. Diabetic skin tissue is a predisposing site for glycosylation due to the presence of a large number of long half-life tissue components. At the same time, long-term high glucose environment makes tis-

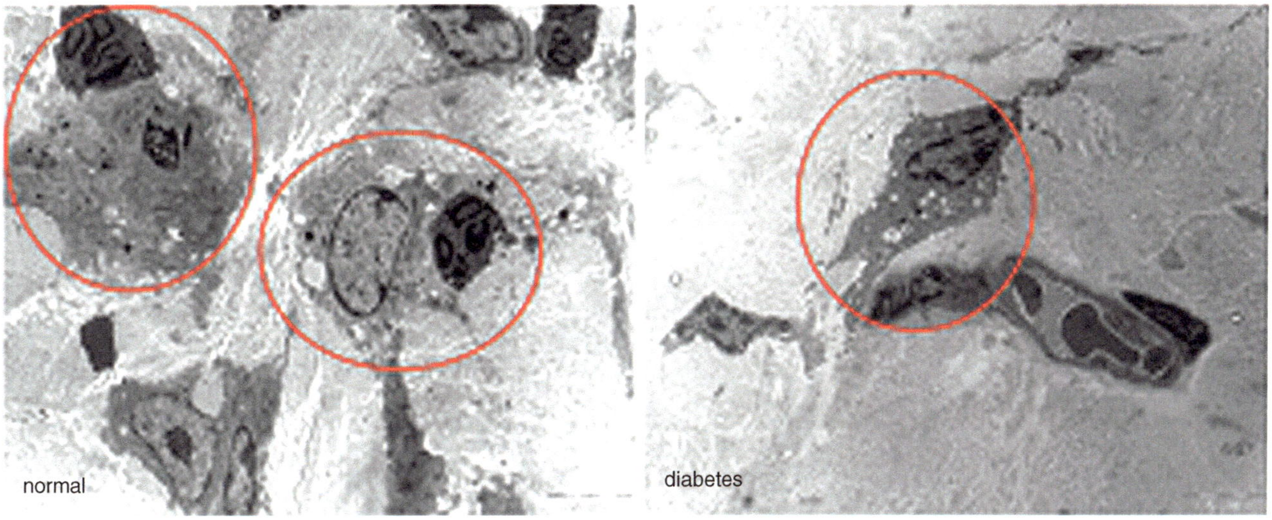


**Fig. 5.8** Phagocytosis of neutrophils by macrophages observed under electron microscopy on the third day after trauma (×3400)
In a mouse model of full-thickness skin defect repair, on the third day after trauma, typical phagocytosis of neutrophils neutrophils (segmented cells) by macrophages (including vesicle cells) was observed, while only a small number of macrophage infiltration was observed in the diabetic group, and no typical phagocytosis of neutrophils by macrophages was observed

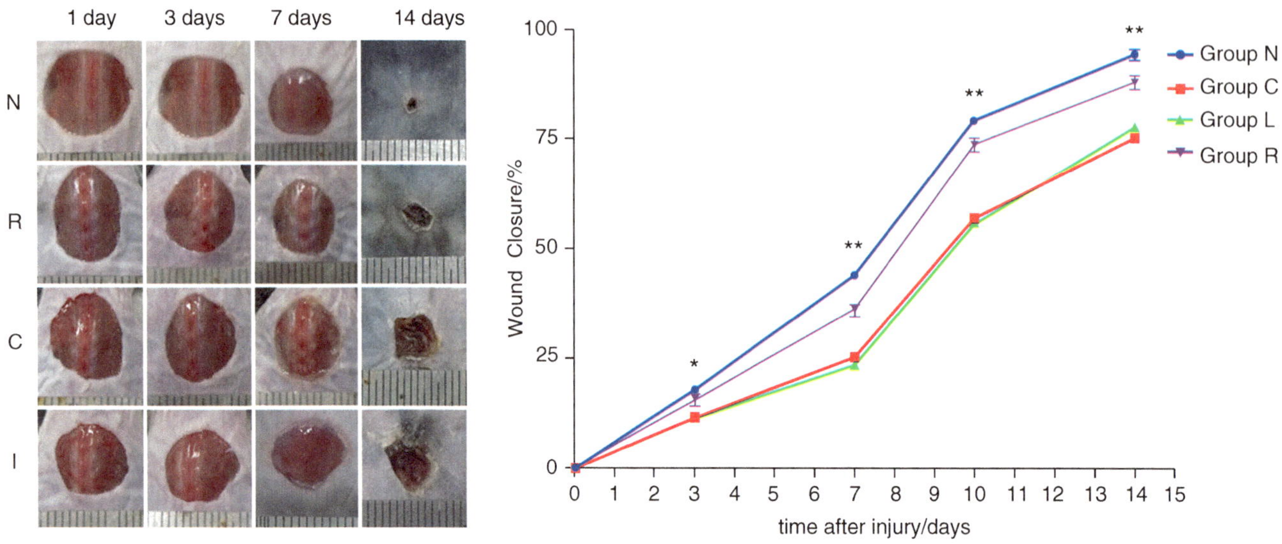


**Fig. 5.9** Diabetic rat model of full-thickness skin defect and trauma The healing speed of RAGE antibody intervention group (R Group) was faster than that of diabetic control group, but it was lower than that of normal mice (N Group). On the third day after injury, the percentage of wound healing in R Group was significantly higher than that in normal saline control group with diabetes (C Group). There was significant difference between the two groups ($P < 0.05$), which was more obvious on the seventh and tenth day after injury. There was no significant difference between the IgG control group (I Group) and the C Group. Comparison of wound healing rate in each group: $*P < 0.05$

sue cells involved in wound healing easily express glycosylation product receptor (RAGE), thereby constructing a structural pathway for the pathological effect of glycosylation products (Fig. 5.9).

In vitro experiments showed that cultured endothelial cells and fibroblasts have strong adherence ability and good cell viability. After high glucose intervention, the cell growth speed is accelerated, the cell volume is enlarged, and the metabolism is vigorous. After 48 h of AGE-BSA intervention, the number of endothelial cells decreased, parts of the cell membranes were intact, and cytoplasm appeared foaming. Under the intervention of AGE-BSA, the volume of endothelial cells and fibroblasts became smaller, the cell membrane shrunk, the division phase decreased, the cell adhesion ability decreased, the proliferation of fibroblasts and endothelial cells was inhibited, and apoptosis increased, angiogenesis of microvascular endothelial cells was inhibited (Fig.5.10).

By establishing a glycosylated extracellular matrix model to better mimic the environment of diabetes, it was further confirmed that glycosylation of extracellular matrix secreted by fibroblasts could inhibit fibroblast adhesion and proliferation and lead to increased apoptosis cells. The expression of RAGE, the receptor of AGEs, was increased in diabetic skin tissue. Glycosylated extracellular matrix upregulates p53 and p21 gene expression in human fibroblasts by RAGE mediation, affecting the orderly operation of cell cycle and promoting apoptosis by regulating the expression of Bcl-2 family proteins.

Study on the differences between high glucose and AGEs on the behavior of repair cells showed that AGEs could inhibit the proliferation of repair cells in 48 h. The adverse effects of high glucose and AGEs on the biological behavior of repair cells were time-effect relationship and dose-effect relationship, and the damage of AGEs was greater than that of high glucose. In addition, the study also found that fibroblasts were more tolerant to high glucose and AGEs damage than endothelial cells, and endothelial cells were more tolerant than keratinocytes, indicating that pathological damage of diabetes has different degrees of pathological effects on different tissue repair cells.

In vitro experiments also confirmed that with the increase of high glucose and AGEs concentration, the apoptotic rate of neutrophils decreased, and the release of neutrophil elastase and reactive oxygen species increased. While macrophages stimulated by high glucose, the expression of iNOS protein was enhanced and the expression of Arg-1 protein was inhibited, and the high glucose environment impaired the pro-vascularization ability of activated macrophages. At the same time, AGEs intervention inhibited the phagocytosis and inflammation-promoting ability of macrophages and enhanced their pro-inflammatory ability, all of which were dependent on RAGE pathway.

Pathological hyperglycemia persists in diabetic patients, and the formation of AGEs is accompanied by accumulation of various active intermediate metabolites. High glucose can spontaneously oxidize to form AGEs in an open aerobic environment, during which glyoxal (GO) and $H_2O_2$

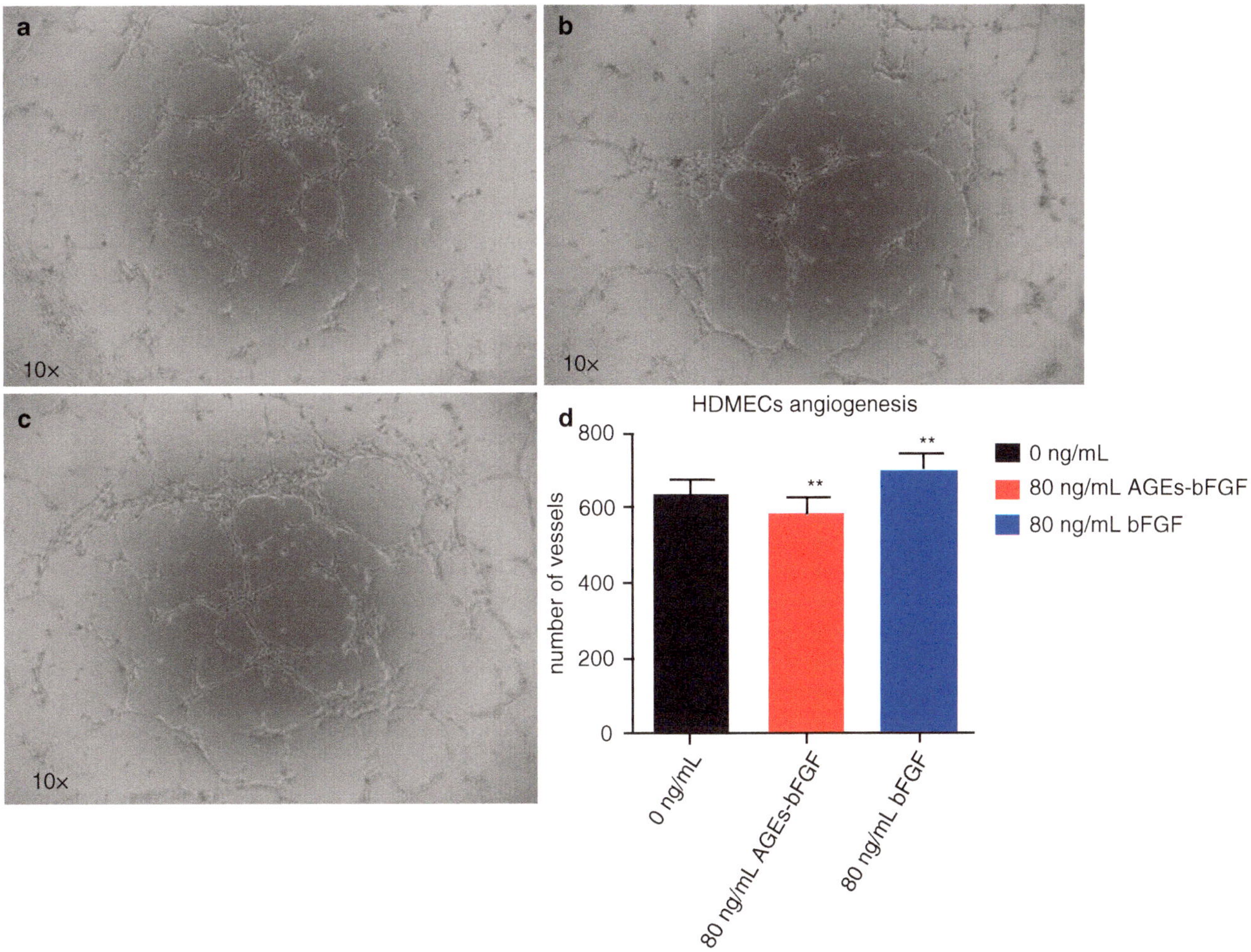


**Fig. 5.10** Angiogenesis ability of human dermal microvascular endothelial cells under different intervention conditions (inverted microscope ×10)
The results of angiogenesis experiments showed that 80 ng/mL bFGF significantly promoted HDMEC angiogenesis (637.25 ± 15.97 vs. 701.00 ± 14.73, $P < 0.01$, A, C, D), while 80 ng/mL AGEs-bFGF significantly inhibited angiogenesis of skin endothelial cells (637.25 ± 15.97 vs. 586.00 ± 10.82, $P < 0.01$, A, B, D). Compared with the 0 ng/mL group: $^{**}P < 0.01$. A—normal endothelial cell culture medium; B—80 ng/mL AGEs-bFGF; C—80 ng/mL bFGF; D—comparison of cell angiogenesis ability of human dermal microvascular endothelial cells under different intervention conditions.

can be produced. AGEs can increase the release of neutrophil reactive oxygen species (ROS) in a dose-dependent manner. GO can promote the glycosylation of proteins and has a toxic effect on repair cells. The production of reactive oxygen species accelerates the formation of AGEs, affects the viability of repair cells, and promotes the production of ROS and MDA, thus forming a vicious circle between oxidative stress and AGEs independent of the high-glucose environment, affecting each other, causing each other, resulting in a series of chain reactions and amplification effects.

The local accumulation of high glucose and AGEs as the direct products of metabolic remodeling in diabetes initially mediated the biological abnormalities in diabetic skin by altering the skin microenvironment. These phenotypically different biological abnormalities are an integral and interrelated group of syndromes due to the common initiating factors of metabolic abnormalities in nature, namely, "Underlying Disorder" of diabetic skin. At the same time, local metabolite accumulation is one of the important sources of environmental stimuli, acts as a "switch" for the "out of control" network of diabetic wound healing during the whole process of wound repair. The presentation and confirmation of this series of concepts provides a powerful basis for the ultimate understanding of the nature of "out of control" in the healing of diabetic wounds.

### 5.2.4 The Exploration of Intervention Methods for Diabetes Complicated with Refractory Wounds

#### 5.2.4.1 Overview of Mechanisms and Interventions for Diabetic Refractory Wounds at Home and Abroad

A lot of researches have been carried out on the related mechanisms of diabetic refractory wounds at home and abroad, especially the occurrence and development of diabetic foot, and some achievements have been made [25].

So far, it has been considered that diabetic vascular neuropathological changes are an important cause of diabetic refractory wound. With the deepening of research, people also noticed the relationship between biochemical changes of diabetes and diabetic complications. It is believed that in the mechanism of high glucose-mediated diabetes complications damage formation, four metabolic remodeling constitute the main pathways of metabolic abnormalities: polyol pathway, formation of AGEs, protein kinase C (PKC) pathway, and hexosamine pathway. These metabolic remodeling can affect the development of diabetic complications through the excessive production of peroxide.

On this basis, people have explored relevant interventions. These interventions can be broadly divided into two categories. One is for the main causes of vascular neuropathy, including antiinfective treatment, improving blood supply and neurotrophy, growth factors application, reducing local mechanical load, and diabetic foot care. The second type of means is to achieve the purpose of promoting healing by intervention of certain drugs on biochemical abnormalities of diabetes and subsequent pathways. Studies have shown that aminoguanidine can selectively inhibit the activity of nitric oxide synthase (iNOS) by blocking AGEs and advanced lipoxidation end products (ALE), and promote the healing of diabetic refractory wounds [26].

In summary, the research to date has greatly promoted the research progress of related mechanisms through the description of the pathophysiological and molecular biological abnormalities of diabetic wounds. However, it is worth noting that the exploration of interventions based on this is still unsatisfactory.

#### 5.2.4.2 Establishment of Intervention Means

In view of the experience and deficiencies in the previous researches on the mechanism of diabetic refractory wounds, we believe that the following factors must be considered in the establishment of interventions:

(a) The establishment of interventions must be based on systematic mechanism research.

Previous mechanism studies involved various factors including cells, extracellular matrix, growth factors, etc., in the process of wound repair, and many pathophysiological changes in diabetic skin were also observed. At the same time, the possible pathways of metabolic remodeling caused by abnormal glucose metabolism on the occurrence of diabetic complications were explored. However, an obvious drawback of the above studies is the lack of systematic organic correlation among the various elements.

Diabetic skin tissue already has histological and cellular biological changes in the absence of exogenous trauma. At the same time, local high glucose and AGEs accumulation, as the direct product of metabolic remodeling in diabetes, initially mediates the biological abnormalities of diabetic skin by changing the skin microenvironment. The different biological abnormalities on these appearances are a collective and interrelated group of syndromes, namely, "Underlying Disorder" of diabetic skin, due to the common initiating factors of metabolic abnormalities in nature. Based on this understanding, the interventions we have chosen can reverse or reduce the "Underlying Disorder" of diabetic skin, thus achieving the goal of improving the wound healing.

(b) Interventions should give priority to upstream events in the pathogenesis.

Although diabetic vascular neuropathy is considered to be a mechanism of diabetes refractory to healing, this understanding does not fully explain many biological behavioral abnormalities in diabetic skin and wound healing. The reason is that diabetic vascular neuropathy may be only the pathological outcome of diabetic complications. Through the analysis of the "Underlying Disorder" of diabetic skin and the characteristics of posttraumatic healing, we summarized the nature of the diabetic refractory wounds, that is, the diabetic refractory wound is a pathological evolution process based on diabetic metabolic disorders and mediated by subsequent events of metabolic abnormalities [27, 28]. Compared with diabetic skin blood vascular neuropathy, the accumulation of metabolites in local tissues is an upstream event in the development of this disease. The microenvironmental change caused by the increase of glucose content and accumulation of metabolites in skin tissue caused by diabetic metabolic disorders, namely, "cutaneous environmental disorders," is one of the initiating factors leading to the diabetic refractory wounds. Therefore, for the prevention and treatment of diabetes complicated with refractory wounds, it is undoubtedly the focus should be placed on the initial stage of "cutaneous environmental disorders," that is, through the intervention of the upstream link related to wound healing, to stop the occurrence or development of its follow-up effects, so as to provide means for effective and feasible prevention and treatment strategies, and achieve an ideal preventive and therapeutic effect on diabetes complicated with refractory wounds.

(c) Interventions should try to avoid strategies that are specific to a particular aspect of the wound healing process.

The exploration of the skin tissue characteristics and healing characteristics of diabetes has revealed the regularity of the diabetic refractory wound healing, that is, the healing elements such as tissue cells, extracellular matrix, and growth factors interact and influence each other through their respective behavioral abnormalities at various stages of healing, forming a network of "out of control" for diabetic wound healing. Therefore, a single intervention, or an intervention strategy for a single process, is often difficult to achieve a better healing effect.

Based on the above principles, we have selected arginine and aminoguanidine as interventions to improve and prevent "Underlying Disorder" and refractory wounds of diabetic skin tissue on the basis of a large number of experimental studies.

#### 5.2.4.3 The Main Role of Arginine and Aminoguanidine in the Mechanism of Diabetes Complicated with Refractory Wounds

##### The Effect of Arginine on the "Underlying Disorder" of Diabetic Skin Tissue

Arginine is a conditionally essential amino acid, which can be synthesized by the body to meet the metabolic needs under normal circumstances. Arginine not only has the effect of lowering blood glucose and promoting insulin secretion but also promotes the repair of diabetic refractory wounds by accelerating collagen synthesis and reconstituting the nitric oxide pathway to restore the normal proliferation of cells.

The content of glucose in the skin tissue was significantly decreased after the application of arginine, indicating that arginine can effectively correct the increase of local tissue glucose content caused by glucose metabolism disorder, which may reduce the pathophysiological changes of local tissues. Arginine can reduce hyperglycemia in diabetic rats through the polyamine formation pathway, and arginine can also lower blood glucose by stimulating insulin release or increasing tissue sensitivity to insulin.

Current studies have confirmed that arginine mainly affects cell physiology through the conversion of arginine to polyamines and nitric oxide (NO), while polyamines and NO regulate and stimulate cell proliferation. Arginine is a precursor for the synthesis of NO. NO can activate guanylate cyclase in cells and participate in a variety of intracellular metabolic processes [29]. Arginine is converted to putrescine and polyamine by ornithine. Polyamines are closely related to cell growth, which can stimulate DNA and RNA biosynthesis. Putrescine also promotes cell proliferation. In diabetic skin tissue, the NO content is insufficient due to the decrease of iNOS activity [30]. This lack of NO may be an important cause of tissue repair cell proliferation disorders. The supplement of exogenous arginine can significantly increase the activity of iNOS and increase the level of local NO, so as to achieve the purpose of reconstructing cell proliferation behavior [31, 32].

In view of the above pharmacodynamic effects of the arginine, prophylactic application of arginine to diabetic patients can improve the "Underlying Disorder" phenomenon of diabetic skin, thereby reducing the occurrence of diabetic skin tissue complications.

##### The Prevention and Treatment of Aminoguanidine on Refractory Wounds

Aminoguanidine is a hydrazine compound with a nucleophilic effect. It can competitively bind to the early glycosylation product to form inactive substitutes that cannot cause protein cross-linking, thereby inhibiting the formation of AGEs and ameliorating the biological behavioral abnormalities of healing factors such as tissue repair cells, extracellular matrix, and growth factors mediated by AGEs.

Our study shows that after prophylactic application of aminoguanidine, the content of AGEs in diabetic skin tissue is significantly reduced, the collagen solubility of skin is significantly increased, and the wound healing rate is significantly increased. In addition, aminoguanidine significantly inhibits the vicious circle between AGEs and oxidative stress, and improves the toxic effects of $H_2O_2$ on fibroblasts.

#### 5.2.4.4 Prospects for the Intervention of Diabetes Complicated with Wound Healing

Diabetes is one of the most common diseases in daily life. With the development of the economy and the improvement of living standards, the incidence is increasing year by year.

Diabetes combined with refractory wound healing is one of the important complications of diabetes.

In our country, in stark contrast to the increasing incidence of diabetes with refractory wound healing, there is a lack of awareness and means of prevention and treatment. Patients with diabetes complicated with refractory wounds and high-risk groups have neither specialist treatment nor effective health education. At the same time, some western developed countries attach great importance to the prevention and treatment of diabetic refractory wounds, and have begun to form the principles of diagnosis, treatment, prevention and care, and conducted a large number of researches on relevant interventions. In this field, China is clearly in a backward state.

Therefore, relying on systematic research accumulation of the mechanism of diabetes wound healing and interventions with independent intellectual property rights, in-depth study on the prevention and treatment mechanism and optimal application of arginine and aminoguanidine for diabetes combined with refractory wound, and finally complete the pre-clinical experiments of arginine and aminoguanidine, thus laying the foundation for the establishment of standardized and systematic diagnosis and treatment of diabetic refractory wounds, which not only has academic value but also has broad market prospects.

## 5.3 Establishment of Innovative Treatment Methods for Refractory Wounds

For a long time, people have been looking for ways or drugs to shorten the healing time of wounds while improving the quality of wound healing to make perfect healing. For representative diabetic foot and radiation ulcers, we have created four innovative key treatment technologies based on routine surgery, wound negative pressure therapy, modern moisturizing functional dressings, etc., which significantly improved the cure rate:

(a) Surgery plus photon therapy.
(b) Modified cytokine therapy.
(c) A new comprehensive treatment technology system based on scaffold materials and cell therapy.
(d) For the first time in the world, the "4G" system has been used to realize the same standard in different levels of medical institutions for the treatment of complex wounds, which has played an important role in improving the cure rate of refractory wounds.

### 5.3.1 Surgery Plus Photon Therapy

He-Ne laser can accelerate local blood flow velocity and increase capillary permeability, thereby improving inflammation local microcirculation, affecting enzyme activity, strengthening intracellular ribonucleic acid, protein and glycogen synthesis, enhancing the activity of phagocytes, enhancing their phagocytic ability, improving the immune function of tissue cells, improving the body's immunity and metabolic level, and improving the body's nutritional status. In addition, it also promotes fibroblasts proliferation, neovascularization, collagen synthesis and granulation tissue growth, and helps control infection. Semiconductor gallium, aluminum, and arsenic lasers can expand microvessels, promote blood circulation, increase oxygen carrying capacity of red blood cells, improve tissue utilization of oxygen, activate red blood cell surface enzyme system, increase ATP production and DNA and RNA synthesis, promote material metabolism and energy metabolism, and improve the immunity of the individual, thereby facilitating the repair and regeneration of the damaged tissue.

In addition, electrical stimulation can promote blood vessel formation and enhance the migration of epidermal cells. The mechanism is mainly magnetic field nonthermal biological effects. The electromagnetic effect generated by the applied magnetic field is transmitted to the target tissue through a rich neural network. As a result, the metabolic activity of the cell is strengthened, including the biological activity of macrophages, granulocytes, and lymphocytes, which plays a more active role in the antiinfective process. Increased red blood cell metabolic activity improves hemoglobin oxygen carrying capacity, increases oxygen supply, and improves internal respiratory function. The cell activity of the lesion tissue is enhanced, on the one hand; it can promote the absorption of inflammatory exudate, on the other hand; it can accelerate the repair of damaged tissue and inhibit the adhesion of scar. The generation of microcurrent can have a series of effects on the bioelectrical activity in the body, such as strengthening the activity of $Na^+$, $K^+$, $Cl^-$, changing the membrane potential, enhancing the permeability of cell membrane, and promoting the exchange of substances inside and outside the cell membrane. Therefore, the magnetic field has the effects of sedation, analgesia, and alleviation of inflammatory response, which may be associated with the increased activity of cholinesterase, monoamine oxidase, histamine, and kininase.

Short-wave has the function of promoting blood circulation and promoting the absorption of inflammatory substances, at the same time, it can increase the function of phagocytic cells, and the action site is deep, which has a good effect on the control of wound inflammation. At present, there is a kind of warm-up therapy (TM) on the foreign market. The device uses advanced medical foam dressing to retain the thermal temperature of the wound surface as the greenhouse effect, and the wound temperature rises to 38 °C. Because it is not directly contact with the wound, there are no adverse reactions, and good results have been achieved for the treatment of venous ulcers and pressure sores.

In response to radiation ulcers, we innovatively expand the debridement domain, excise more tissues outside the wound margin, reduce and optimize the ineffective necrosis-clearance-repair process based on the characteristics that the necrosis scope of this type of ulcers exceeds the naked eye observation domain. In addition, innovative photon therapy technology is used to accelerate the healing speed of chronic refractory wounds represented by diabetic foot, improve the quality of healing, and achieve remarkable results. Related studies have shown that high-power red photons can promote the synthesis of adenosine triphosphate (ATP); enhance the body's antioxidant capacity; promote the synthesis of DNA, RNA, and protein; promote the material exchange and metabolism of cells; increase glycogen utilization; increase cell respiration; improve blood circulation; reduce wound exudate and promote exudate recovery; promote cytokines production and accelerate cell division; accelerate the regeneration of damaged nerves; promote the growth of granulation tissue and skin, wound healing and ulcer healing; accelerate division of bone cells, promote the healing of callus; increase the phagocytosis of white blood cells and enhance the body's resistance; reduces the 5-hydroxytryptamine (5-HT) content in the inflammation site and acts as an analgesic effect. At present, relevant products in China have been applied in clinical practice and achieved good therapeutic effects.

### 5.3.2 Modified Cytokine Therapy

Growth factors not only directly participate in the inflammatory response of the wound but also affect a series of biological processes such as the transformation of tissue repair cell cycle. After exogenous application of growth factors such as platelet-derived growth factor (PDGF), fibroblast growth factor (FGF), and epidermal growth factor (EGF), the wounded "inactivated" macrophages are activated and release growth factors such as TGF, TNF and FGF. Exogenously applied growth factors plus endogenously released growth factors can act directly on tissue repair cells, thereby initiating the repair process. In the early 1990s, scholars abroad used the autologous platelet-derived growth factor to treat chronic wounds including diabetic ulcers, bedsores, ulcers caused by arteriovenous diseases of the lower extremities, and all of them achieved unexpected results.

The therapeutic effect of transgenic growth factor therapy on wound healing has received more and more attention in recent years. At the beginning of the twentieth century, a multicenter, large-sample clinical study completed in China showed that the recombinant bovine basic fibroblast growth factor (bFGF) had 2.5 days, 4 days, 5 days, and 3.5 days earlier healing promoting effect on shallow II degree, deep II degree burn, granulation wound and donor site than the control in the same period, and no adverse reactions occurred. So far, the domestic pharmaceutical administration has officially approved the recombinant bovine basic fibroblast growth factor, and recombinant human epidermal growth factor (EGF), which are widely used in clinical treatment of various acute and chronic wounds. Modified cytokines are currently widely used in ophthalmology, otolaryngology, gynecology, etc., due to their good repair effects and are also used to repair damaged myocardium and islet cells.

### 5.3.3 A New Comprehensive Treatment Technology System Based on Scaffold Materials and Cell Therapy

In the course of clinical practice, aiming at diabetic foot wounds, radioactive refractory wounds, and other causes, such as wound healing or refractory wounds caused mainly by repairing cell damage or dermal scaffold loss, we have established a "one-stop" approach to promote tissue repair by supplementing repair cells and providing scaffold materials, which plays an important role in promoting repair and reducing the amputation rate.

In the past half century, with the deepening of people's understanding of the mechanism of wound repair and tissue regeneration, especially Dr. Winter's research on the wet environment and wound healing effect and related mechanisms in the 1960s, people gradually realized that the dressing should also be endowed with functions such as promoting or accelerating wound healing and improving repair quality.

Tissue engineering is the comprehensive application of cell biology and engineering principles. In the laboratory, a part of human tissue cells are cultured and expanded in vitro, then these cultured cells are planted and adsorbed on a biomaterial scaffold, and then transplanted to the needed parts of the human body to repair tissue defects, replace part or all of the functions of the tissues and organs, or as an extracorporeal device, temporarily replace some of the functions of the organs to achieve the purpose of improving the quality of life and prolonging life. At present, the tissue engineering products that can be applied in the local treatment of trauma wounds mainly include tissue engineering artificial skin, tissue engineering cartilage (bone), tissue engineering tendon, and tissue engineering peripheral nerve. Now the most researched and most likely to be applied clinically are various types of stem cells. Stem cell application plays two main roles in wound repair and tissue regeneration. On the one hand, pluripotent stem cells transform into related tissue repair cells to promote repair and regeneration under the action of local microenvironment in the injury site. On the other hand, stem cells exert autocrine and paracrine effects on wounds, secrete a large number of growth factors related to tissue repair and regeneration, and participate in the process of repair and regeneration. At present, there have been reports that local application of mesenchymal stem cells has a positive effect on angiogenesis of diabetic foot and regeneration of skin sweat glands after severe burns.

Under the guidance of this idea, we combine a variety of derived stem cells (umbilical cord, bone marrow, etc.) with scaffold materials (chitosan, hydrocolloid, hydrogel, etc.), which have a good affinity with tissue cells, and then through 3D printing and other technologies form a three-dimensional structure with a variety of biologically active factors, which plays an important role in promoting repair and reducing amputation rate.

### 5.3.4 Utilizing the "4G" System to Improve the Cure Rate of Refractory Wounds

For the first time in the world, the "4G" system has been used to achieve the treatment of complex wounds with the same standard in different levels of medical institutions, which has played an important role in improving the overall cure rate of refractory wounds.

The community is the basic unit for the distribution of urban residents in China. By working with community health institutions, we extend the medical services for wound repair to the community, provide a convenient medical environment, and have better operability to meet the medical requirements of most patients with wound diseases. Taking the wound repair department as the core and the community medical care as the network, the layout of the wound repair medical service constructed is obviously adapted to the occurrence law of wound diseases and is represented as the overall pattern of "small wards and big outpatient service." In order to realize this pattern, we have realized the treatment of complex wounds with the same standard in the different levels of medical institutions for the first time in the world by using the "4G" system. This system enables the wound treatment experts of large hospitals to truly observe the wounds while away from the grassroots or community health institutions, thereby directly participating in the wound treatment process, which not only facilitates patients' medical treatment but also ensures the quality of medical care and plays an important role in improving the cure rate of refractory wounds. The specific operation of the wound repair department and the community medical linkage mechanism involves the coordination and interaction of the wound repair department, the health administrative department, and the community health institution. To this end, based on the experience accumulated in the initial operation phase of the linkage mechanism, through repeated communication with the health administrative departments and community health institutions, we have determined the policy direction of institutional guarantees and mechanism incentives, which laid a good foundation for mobilizing the subjective initiative of all parties. We have been specially commented by international peers and highly praised the topic of "Looking to the East." [33–38]

## 5.4 Theory and Practice of Wound Healing Center Construction

With the rapid development of the social economy, the human disease spectrum has undergone significant changes. In the past, some major infectious diseases that seriously endangered the physical and mental health of the people have been eliminated, but the wounds caused by trauma and various diseases have become one of the diseases with the highest incidence in society today. Wound formation involves a variety of factors including trauma, systemic (local) diseases, and aging population, involving a wide range of people. Wound treatment is not only the basis of all trauma treatments but also the key to preventing late complications and promoting the early recovery of trauma patients. Whether in Europe and the United States or in China, wound epidemiological studies have shown that due to socio-economic development, the main factors leading to wound formation have been transformed from traditional trauma-infective factors to complications caused by various chronic diseases and senile diseases, such as ulcers and bedsores caused by diabetic foot and varicose veins of the lower extremities. In the past 20 years, the increasing number of various wounds and the complexity of various causes of wound formation have led to an increasing demand for wound treatment [39]. Multicenter epidemiological survey of chronic refractory wounds shows that the age group with high incidence of chronic wounds in China is 40–59 years old (3 1%) and 60–80 years old (38%), which not only includes the young and middle-aged people but also covers the ageing population who requires a large amount of medical care. The changes in the spectrum of these diseases are closely related to economic development and harmonious development of society. The development of high technology has provided many new treatments and methods for wound healing and has made wound treatment more complicated and diversified. Establishing a scientific and rational diagnosis and treatment model is a guarantee to promote the development of new technologies for wound healing and to benefit trauma patients. In traditional treatment systems, it will be very difficult to continue to treat complex wounds by a single surgery (such as orthopedics, burns, or general surgery) or a subject in the internal medicine (such as diabetes and endocrinology). The establishment of a comprehensive wound center (specialist), which consists of personnel in surgery, anesthesia, internal medicine and nursing, makes it necessary to obtain systematic treatment of complex wounds caused by multiple factors, and is the key to improving the cure rate. This model, like the previous treatment of severe diseases, is based on the integration of multiple disciplines according to the critical illness treatment needs. Wound centers and intensive care units are innovative treatment models that follow the development of medical technology [40].

After Professor Xiaobing Fu and other experts systematically proposed the idea of constructing a standardized and exemplary wound center in 2005, China began to practice in related fields [41]. In the early stage, Professor Han Chunmao, from the Second Affiliated Hospital of Zhejiang University, started the practice of establishing a wound therapy specialty in a medical unit based on the burns department and using the academic and technical advantages of the burn department in treating wounds. Later, some medical units carried out the construction of wound treatment specialist for a single disease, such as Professor Xu Zhangrong from the 306 Hospital of the People's Liberation Army, using the technical advantages of diabetes specialists in the treatment of diabetes and introducing surgical personnel, established the Diabetes Foot Treatment Specialist in the 306 Hospital of the People's Liberation Army, which achieved remarkable results in the treatment of diabetic foot. In addition, the outpatient departments of some hospitals have formed a specialist dressing room for wound treatment through the strengthening of the dressing room technology and equipment. According to the survey, there are more than 200 wound centers (specialties). In 2014, we conducted a survey of the composition of wound healing centers or specialists named after Wound Healing Centers or Wound Care Units in 69 third grade A hospitals in China. Among the 69 wound centers, 46% developed from the expansion of the original burn surgery function, 32% developed from the strengthening of the original outpatient dressing room, and 12% were set up in the endocrinology department or diabetes center, the other 10% were branch departments established by departments such as vascular surgery, orthopedics, hand and foot surgery, and plastic surgery. The characteristics of these wound centers are as follows: the treatment team is under the doctor's guidance (leadership) and participated by the nurses, which has changed the situation in which there were only nurses but no doctors in the past; most of the doctors and nurses involved in the wound treatment have carried out wound treatment specialist training or participated in related study classes in the early stage, and systematically understand the basic theories and basic skills of wound treatment; because doctors and nurses participate in wound treatment together, the scope and disease types of wound treatment specialists are significantly expanded; because of the formation of specialty, many new treatment techniques and methods can be used centrally, improving the utilization rate of treatment equipment and treatment technology; the cure rate, average hospitalization days, bed occupancy rate, and drug proportion of chronic refractory wounds are greatly improved. Great results have been achieved in both health economic and social benefits.

In view of the characteristics of "small wards and big outpatient service" for chronic refractory wounds [1], we combined the current characteristics and operation modes of Chinese medical treatment, changed traditional treatment methods, and innovatively established a new mode of bidirectional linkage and referral between complex refractory wound treatment specialists and community medical institutions. The new model has initially solved the problem of patients with chronic refractory wounds that have difficulty in seeing a doctor, expensive medical treatment and long hospital stay, and are highly recognized by international colleagues. According to incomplete statistics, by the end of October 2014, we had advocated the establishment of more than 50 wound centers in China. The cure rate of these centers for refractory wounds increased from 54% before the establishment of the centers to 93%, and the average hospitalization days decreased from 47 days to 26 days, and the proportion of drugs decreased from 17% to 14%.

The specialized training of doctors and nurses and the development and rapid transformation of innovative treatment technology are the key to ensuring the connotation development of the construction of wound specialty centers and improving the success rate of treatment. In March 2010, led by Academician Xiaobing Fu of the Chinese Academy of Engineering, the China Organizational Rehabilitation Society applied to the World Diabetes Foundation (WDF) and the Access to Healthcare (AtH) for the project—"National Chronic Wound Care Training Program for Doctors and Nurses Dealing with Patients with Diabetic Mellitus" and received a total of $550,000 support from the two foundations [42]. The project is composed of well-known domestic professors and scholars in China, who are responsible for the preparation, development, implementation and management of educational courses, compiling teaching materials, and teaching as a main lecturer in the training course. In 2011, the People's Military Medical Publishing House officially published the book *Treatment of Diabetic Foot and Related Chronic Refractory Wounds*, which was widely welcomed and concerned by trainees as a project training textbook and a reference book for understanding the basic knowledge in this field [43]. In 2013, the book was further revised and updated on the basis of the first edition and the *Treatment of Diabetic Foot and Related Chronic Refractory Wounds* (second Edition) was reprinted, which further enriched and improved the textbook content. It has been expanded to 10 people based on the original 6-person project expert group. By the end of the project in 2015, more than 60 classes have been opened in more than 20 cities across the country, with more than 8600 participants, highly recognized by international counterparts. From the perspective of project development, the project has the following characteristics:

(a) The project is highly targeted.
(b) The training content keeps pace with the times.
(c) The teaching standard of the project is unified.
(d) The project has strong teaching staff.
(e) The project has good practicability.
(f) The training form is pragmatic. Recently, we have followed up the learning effects of some trainees, especially the theoretical knowledge and practical skills, which proved to be good.

Many modern advanced technologies and products can be well transformed and applied in the wound treatment specialty, so that the technical requirements of wound treatment can be met to the greatest extent [44]. The emergence of modern advanced dressings has developed the traditional dressings into a new function of actively promoting wound repair by isolating the wound and preventing re-contamination [45]. The research, development, and application of a class of new drug, genetic engineering growth factors, has made people take a solid step toward the dream of intervention and regulation of wound healing. The application of red light in American aerospace technology has shown significant effects on chronic wounds. Negative pressure therapy, hyperbaric oxygen therapy, traditional medicine, etc. have also played an important role in wound healing.

The innovative wound management model is the foundation for the orderly development of wound centers (specialties). Establishing a two-way linkage mechanism between wound treatment specialists (centers) in large hospitals and community health institutions is an important means to solve the problem of treating patients with wounds and reducing medical expenses. This single-disease two-way linkage mechanism is collaboration between the doctor in a community health institution after specialized training by wound therapists and the wound treatment specialist in a large hospital in the treatment of complex and refractory wounds. The usual technical guidance of community health institutions can be guaranteed through the established "Wi-Fi-networking+" technology. In 2011, we established the first professional wound treatment specialist in Shanghai Ninth People's Hospital. In the first year of operation, 125 patients were treated, and all of them had wounds that failed to heal using traditional conventional methods. Among them, 121 cases were cured, with a cure rate as high as 96.8%. Especially in 2015, the newly built wound treatment specialist of Shanghai Ninth People's Hospital successfully cured the chronic wounds caused by the Japanese artillery shrapnel 68 years ago and the wounds caused by electric shock 52 years ago, which caused good responses in the academic circles. The practice of the Shanghai Ninth People's Hospital shows that with this innovative model, the cure rate for patients who need wound treatment has increased from 60% in the past to around 94%, and the cost of each treatment has dropped from around 150 yuan to 30–40 yuan. Especially, the treatment of patients in community medical institutions at home has saved a lot of time and effort. For the hospital, the average hospitalization day has dropped from more than 20 days to 14 days, and the proportion of drugs is only 16%, which achieve significant social and economic benefits. The adoption of this innovative model has greatly promoted the orderly flow of patients, reduced the average hospitalization days, and significantly reduced medical expenses.

The Chinese Medical Association Trauma Surgeons Branch has started to promote the "1239" three-year action plan for the construction of China's wound center (wound repair specialist) to form the basic framework for the development of wound repair discipline, and standardize and enhance the professional level of wound repair in China. According to the plan, we will achieve corresponding results in the following aspects:

(a) Establish an expert platform representing the national level.
(b) Two wound repair training institutions with good teaching and clinical practice conditions have been built and incorporated into the training system of the Chinese Medical Association.
(c) Build three distinctive wound treatment specialists that can represent the national level and form a demonstration unit for the construction of wound repair specialists in China.
(d) According to the regional distribution, nine regional wound repair specialists will be established nationwide within three years.

At present, great achievements have been made at the academic and technical levels. In 2016, the first *Chinese Guideline for Diagnosis and Treatment of Skin Wounds* (2015 Edition) was published.

It is believed that under the joint efforts of medical workers at all levels of the country dedicated to the prevention and treatment of wounds, the wound center will surely usher in a leap forward.

## 5.5 Chronic Ulcer

### 5.5.1 Introduction

Chronic ulcer is a general term for wound associated with the wounded site and the host which does not be healed normally in the desired time or for a long time [46]. Its definition has not yet been uniformly given. Clinically, it is customary to treat wounds that have not been healed by regular treatment for one month and have no obvious healing tendency as chronic ulcers. Chronic ulcer on the surface is a difficult problem in surgical clinics. Due to the different reasons for its formation, the time of prolongation, the depth of ulceration, and the location of the disease, the treatment methods and prognosis are not the same [47].

#### 5.5.1.1 The Classification of Ulcers

There is no uniform classification standard for ulcers at present. The main classification criteria are as follows:

1. According to the concept of traditional wounds.
   Divided into surgery, burns, daily injuries, bedsores, infectious ulcers.
2. According to the time of ulcer prolongation and degree of contamination Divided into clean, contaminated, infected, and ulcer wounds.

3. Using skin continuity as a measure and according to anatomical depth.
   Divided into superficial, half-thickness, full-thickness, and deep tissue ulcers below the skin.
4. European RYB classification.
   The open wounds of stage 2 or delayed healing are divided into red, yellow, black, and mixed wounds according to the tissue morphology.
5. According to the cause of ulcer formation.
   (a) Traumatic ulcer: with a clear history of trauma, such as car accidents, gunshot wounds, crushing or thermal burns; it can form residual ulcer wound in the late stage, deep to the skin layers or even the muscles, tendons, joints and bone tissue; extensive unstable scars formed after a burn can be broken due to local tension or infection without healing persistently. Much longer duration, and it will cause cancer and form Marjolin's ulcer [48] (Fig. 5.11).
   (b) Autoimmune ulcer (drug induced ulcer): The patient is in a high immune state, which leads to the ulcer gradually expanding and deepening, lasting for several years or even decades.
   (c) Tuberculous ulcer: A special infection combined with sinus, which is caused by *Mycobacterium tuberculosis*.
   (d) Pressure ulcer: It is an ulcer formed by ischemic necrosis of the skin or subcutaneous tissue due to local compression. It occurs in the bony protrusion of elderly patients in bed (Fig. 5.12). Clinical manifestations are generally divided into the following three phases. The first phase: erythema phase. The second phase: vesicular phase. The third phase: ulcer phase. The prevention of bedsore generally has the following aspects. Avoid local compression for a long time. Skin care: keep the skin clean and dry. Strengthen functional exercise: relieve the pressure of local tissue constantly. Preventive cushions and devices. Behavioral and psychological education.
   (e) Cancerous ulcer (malignant ulcer): refers to the primary or secondary cancerous ulcer on the body surface (Fig. 5.13).
   (f) Radiation ulcers: it is often complicated in the treatment of radiotherapy accompanied by chronic inflammation and fibrotic changes in the deep and surrounding tissues of the ulcer. More frequently, it is also accompanied by intractable pain and other sequelae (Fig. 5.14).
   The clinical manifestations are as follows: varying ulcer size and depth; extensive fibroplasia; and degeneration around ulcer.
   (g) Vascular ulcer: lower extremity ulcers caused by varicose veins and vasculitis of lower limbs are much common in the distal leg and ankle [49] (Fig. 5.15), with dark base, rough skin around the wound obvious pigmentation.
   (h) Diabetic ulcer: one of the serious complications of diabetic patients (Fig. 5.16). Most diabetic patients with foot ulcers are associated with neurological diseases.

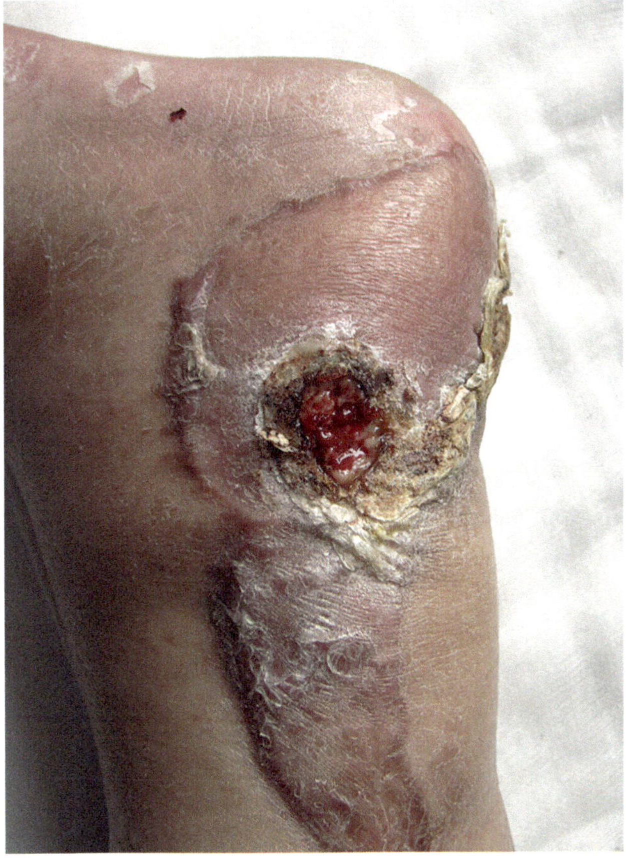

**Fig. 5.11** Marjolin's ulcer

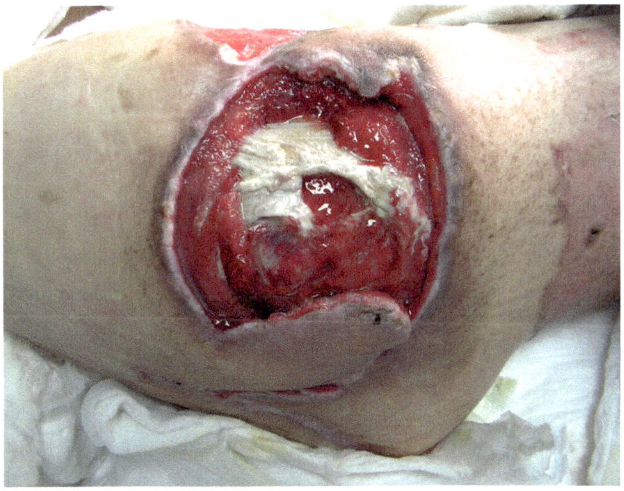

**Fig. 5.12** Pressure ulcer

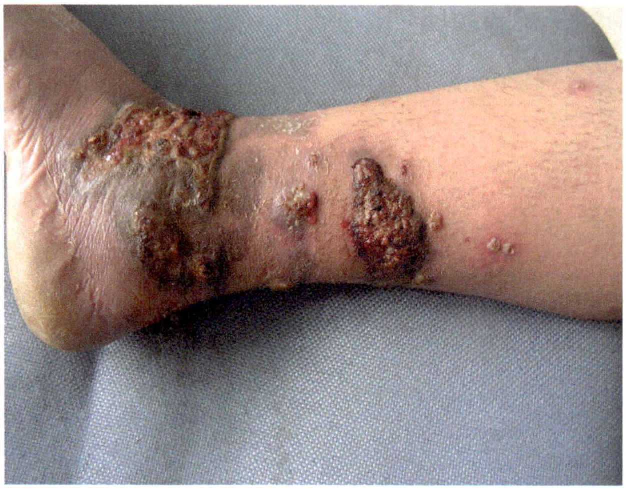

**Fig. 5.13** Cancerous ulcer

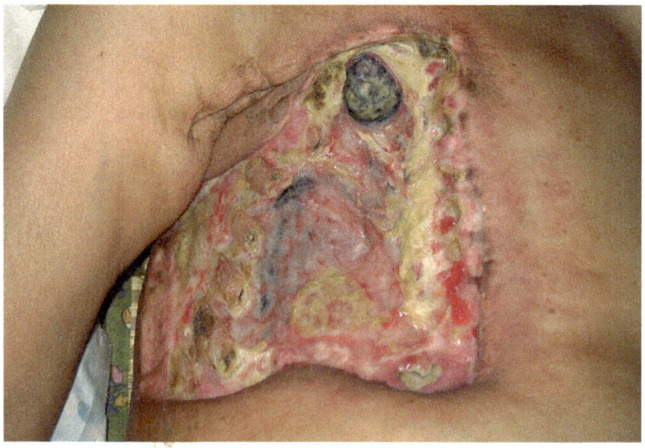

**Fig. 5.14** Radiation ulcer

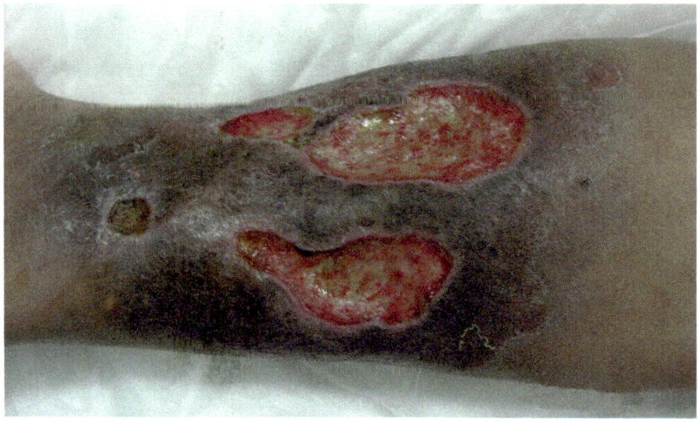

**Fig. 5.15** Vascular ulcer

(i) Infectious ulcer: ulcers that cannot heal due to repeated wound infections (Fig. 5.17).

The etiological classification can guide the treatment of the cause and highlight the individual characteristics of

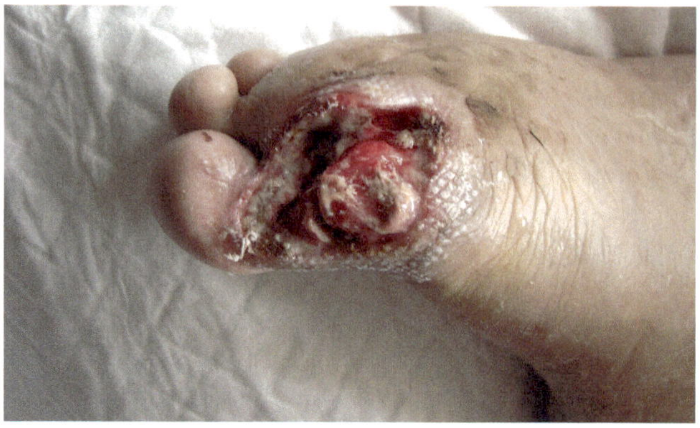

**Fig. 5.16** Diabetic foot

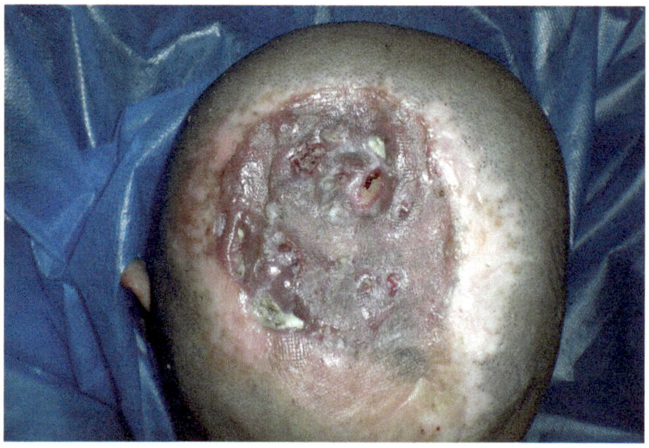

**Fig. 5.17** Infectious ulcer

different ulcers. However, although the causes of various ulcers are different, once the ulcers are formed, the local pathophysiology, and healing mechanism are roughly the same [50].

### 5.5.2 The Healing of Chronic Ulcers

The essence of chronic ulcer healing is the common result of the dynamic interactive response of the body to damage stimulation, orderly and controllable proliferation and differentiation of tissue cells. Due to the pathophysiological state of chronic ulcers, it is determined that microscopically involved complex interactions and responses among various cells, extracellular matrix, soluble mediators, and cytokines, and macroscopically experienced three different but overlapping stages:

(a) Inflammation stage.
(b) Proliferation stage.
(c) Maturation and reconstruction stage.

#### 5.5.2.1 Inflammation Stage

Monocytes in the blood circulation are concentrated by the chemokines at the wound and differentiate into macrophages. Macrophages migrate into the wound 48–96 h after trauma. The anti-infective effects of macrophages include phagocytosis and the production of active free radicals such as nitrous oxide, oxygen, and superoxide. Once the infiltration of macrophages is blocked, the wound healing process will be severely impaired.

#### 5.5.2.2 Proliferation Stage

Fibroblasts and endothelial cells are the main cells growing at this stage. The new collagen-rich matrix produced by fibroblasts replaces the original fibrin clot and plays an important role in the formation of granulation tissue.

Angiogenesis activated during healing and repair is a fundamental biological mechanism. This process is characterized by invasion, migration and proliferation of endothelial cells.

#### 5.5.2.3 Maturation and Reconstruction Stage

The main feature of the maturation stage is the deposition of collagen on the wound surface. The rate, quality, and total amount of matrix deposition determine the strength of the scar.

### 5.5.3 The Treatment of Chronic Ulcers

#### 5.5.3.1 Etiology Treatment

For chronic ulcers caused by diabetes, the first thing is to control blood glucose level. Fasting blood glucose is generally required to be stable below 10 mmol/L stablely. For vascular factors, local blood circulation and oxygen supply should be improved, including bed rest, elevation of the affected limb, and application of improved microcirculation drugs [51]. For pressure ulcers, relieve local pressure and pay attention to changing position. For radioactive ulcers, local radiation exposure should be stopped.

#### 5.5.3.2 Conservative Therapy

It is the basis and premise of surgical treatment. The focus is on symptomatic treatment, such as systemic nutritional metabolism support, preparation of a local wound bed [52]. Physiotherapy such as ultrashort wave, infrared irradiation is adopted to improve local blood circulation. Cleaning the wound local dressing, timely removing necrotic tissue and secretions, and carrying out bacterial culture of secretion and drug sensitivity test is also the part of conservative therapy.

#### 5.5.3.3 Debridement

Surgical intervention is used to treat ulcer wounds to achieve the transformation from contaminated (yellow, black, or a mixed) wounds to relatively clean (red) wounds, from unprepared healing to ready healing wounds [53].

#### 5.5.3.4 Application of Various Flaps and Myocutaneous Flaps

The principle is to completely remove the necrotic tissue, together with the scar tissue around and at the base. If the bone is damaged, the necrotic bone tissue should be removed together. The remaining cavity is preferably covered with an adjacent flap or myocutaneous flap [54]. It is easy to recur after skin grafting because of weak skin friction resistance, so it is not the first choice for repairing bedsores. Unless the condition is serious, in order to prevent the loss of protein and temporarily relieve pain, it can be considered to temporarily close the wound before the flap is transferred [55, 56].

At present, the use of various flaps and musculocutaneous flaps to repair wounds is still a very effective means [57, 58]. The flaps and myocutaneous flaps have rich blood supply and good anti-infective ability, as well as the advantages in pressure resistance and friction resistance. The repair of wounds generally uses island-shaped myocutaneous flaps, axial flaps, arbitrary flaps, or other tissue flaps with abundant blood supply and abundant tissue. These tissue flaps have rich blood supply, strong anti-infective ability, and can improve local blood circulation, improve the biological effects of growth factors, help to remove residual necrotic tissue, and promote wound healing.

It should be selected according to the cause, location, wound condition, patient occupation, and age [59, 60]:

(a) For the head wound, because the scalp is thick and the blood supply is rich, in the case of no bone exposure, as long as the tissue above the skull periosteum can be preserved, it can be treated with full thickness skin; if the skull is exposed, the wound can be repaired with a local flap or a trapezius myocutaneous flap.
(b) For face and neck wounds, the skin flaps can be selected include local flaps, thoracic triangle flaps, trapezius myocutaneous flaps, pectoralis major myocutaneous flaps, and sternocleidomastoid myocutaneous flaps.
(c) For the front chest wound, the selected flaps include the ipsilateral latissimus dorsi musculocutaneous flap, the contralateral pectoralis major myocutaneous flap, and the rectus abdominis myocutaneous flap.
(d) For abdominal, thoracodorsal wounds, local flap is generally used for repair. If the defect is large, two flaps can be used in parallel for repair (Fig. 5.18).

##### Wound Medication

Scientific and proper use of wound medication can greatly accelerate the healing of ulcers [61]. Cell aging, tissue ischemia, and bacterial colonization are the main factors for

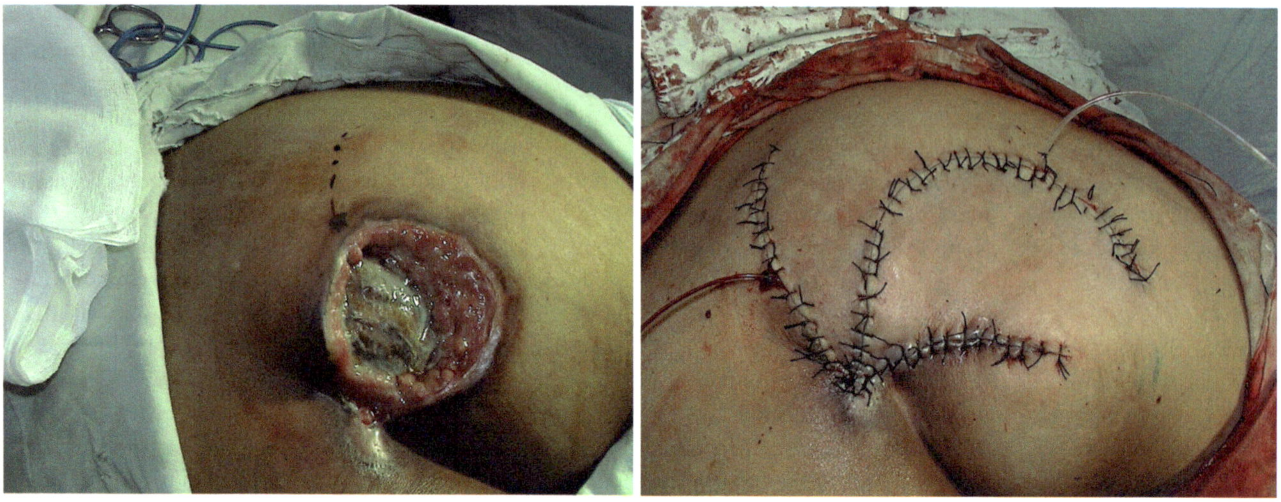

**Fig. 5.18** Repair of sacrococcygeal wound with local flap

ulcer formation and prolonged unhealing. The compatibility of local drugs should focus on the control of infection, promoting tissue regeneration and improving local ischemia, follow the stage law of ulcer repair, and make the overall consideration of many factors such as systemic and local conditions, effectiveness and adverse reactions, compatibility, and dosage forms [62].

### Vacuum Sealing Technology

It is a new therapeutic technology for repairing and covering soft tissue wounds by using medical polymer composite composed of polyvinyl alcohol-absorbent gelatin sponge. The principle is that this material acts as an intermediary between the drainage tube and the drainage surface, making the drainage from the point to the surface, changing the open wound into a relatively closed wound to prevent pollution and secondary infection; under the action of negative pressure, the blood flow of the wound increases, stimulating the growth of granulation tissue, and having the effect of compression hemostasis [63].

### Hyperbaric Oxygen Therapy

By increasing oxygen diffusion, the blood oxygen content and the oxygen partial pressure of the wound are increased, the oxygen supply of the lesion tissue is corrected, and the bactericidal ability of the white blood cells is enhanced. The hyperbaric oxygen can reduce the whole blood viscosity, plasma viscosity and platelet aggregation rate, can increase red blood cell deformability, and improve microcirculation. The hyperbaric oxygen can promote the establishment of collateral circulation, improve capillary permeability, effectively prevent extravasation of plasma water, and reduce wound edema, thereby improving the microenvironment of wound healing [64, 65].

### Bioengineered Skin Products

With the rapid development of materials science and life sciences, more and more bioengineered skin or skin substitutes have been used to treat acute and chronic wounds including burns [66–68].

Bioengineered skin may work by delivering living cells that are suitable for the environment. There is evidence that some viable "skins" release growth factors and cytokines, but fail to fully explain the mechanisms by which they work.

### Gene Therapy

This technology can now be used to introduce specific genes into wounds using a variety of physical or biological vectors, including viruses. To date, most of the research on wound healing gene therapy has been limited to laboratory and animal models, but some gene therapy that promotes human wound healing still makes us look forward to.

### Stem Cell Therapy

It is speculated that pluripotent hematopoietic stem cells are more effective than the introduction of specific genes. Because it can differentiate into various cell phenotypes, including fibroblasts, endothelial cells, keratinocytes, etc., which are the key cells in the healing process. There have been many reports of successful clinical applications [69–73]. However, stem cell research itself is still controversial. The main problem is that although the results in the laboratory are very encouraging, the results in clinical practice are not satisfactory.

### Platelet-Rich Plasma Therapy

Platelet-rich plasma (PRP) usually is defined as plasma with higher platelet concentration than healthy whole blood. It can also refer to plasma rich in platelets, high platelet concentrates, and autologous platelet gels [74]. After injecting it into the tissue defect, it can make up for the defect of too little growth factor in the wound, and start the repair mechanism faster, induce tissue regeneration.

#### Antioxidant Treatment

One way to correct abnormalities in wound healing in diabetic patients is to reduce the amount of free radical products. Raxofelast, an antiallergic drug, is a protective membrane antioxidant that improves wound healing in diabetic rats by stimulating angiogenesis.

## 5.5.4 Tuberculous Wounds

### 5.5.4.1 Overview

Tuberculosis (TB) is infected by *Mycobacterium tuberculosis* (MT). In recent years, tuberculosis has been classified as a major infectious disease by the World Health Organization. In China, the tuberculosis epidemic is equally serious as well [75]. The fifth national tuberculosis epidemiological sampling survey report shows that the annual incidence of tuberculosis in China is about 1.3 million, accounting for about 14% of the total number of tuberculosis cases worldwide, ranking second in the world. According to relevant study, about 100,000 patients in China suffer from subcutaneous and skin soft tissue damage caused by tuberculosis bacilli each year, and some tuberculous wounds are formed [76, 77]. In recent years, the incidence of TB in patients with diabetes mellitus (DM) ranks first in the world [78]. It is predicted that the incidence of tuberculous wounds will increase further.

Because tuberculous wounds have the characteristics of insidious onset, slow progress, and high rate of misdiagnosis and missed diagnosis, sinus-type wounds have been formed in most patients when they visit the hospital [79]. Most of the sinus-type tuberculous wounds are sporadic and scattered in clinics, which leads to low attention in the academic circles. There are few reports at home and abroad [80, 81]. At present, medical diagnosis and treatment of such diseases is mainly based on internal medicine in China, and there are few studies on tuberculous wounds.

### 5.5.4.2 Epidemiological Characteristics of Tuberculous Wounds

So far, the epidemiological data of tuberculous wounds in China have rarely been officially reported [82]. The epidemiological data has positive guiding significance for the government to formulate prevention and control policies and to specifically improve the level of clinical tuberculous wounds diagnosis and treatment. Recently, we reviewed the clinical data of hospitalized patients with extra-pulmonary tuberculous wounds in a hospital from January 2010 to December 2012, systematically analyzed the clinical epidemiological characteristics and rules, in order to fill the gap in this aspect of China, and broaden the theoretical and practical areas of wound healing field, so as to provide reliable epidemiological data for improving the quality of tuberculous wound healing and enhancing overall prevention and control measures for tuberculosis. Of the 5863 extra-pulmonary tuberculosis patients, 235 had tuberculous wounds, with an incidence of 4.01%. The age distribution of the patients ranged from 1 to 87 years (median 35 years), with an average age of 6.9 ± 17.9 years. Among them, 163 (69.4%) were rural patients and 72 (30.6%) were urban patients (Fig. 5.19). Among the causes, the peripheral lymph node tuberculosis was the first (112 cases, 47.7%), followed by bone and joint tuberculosis (95 cases, 40.4%). The main site of the disease was neck, 99 cases (88.4%). There were 173 patients (73.6%) without systemic symptoms. Patients with erythrocyte sedimentation rate greater than 20 mm/h accounted for 76.1%, and the positive rate of *Mycobacterium tuberculosis* culture was 43.8%. In the pathological examination, 129 cases (74.6%) were found to be tuberculosis, and 44 cases (25.4%) were negative samples. The average time from the onset of clinical symptoms to the diagnosis of tuberculosis was 4.4 months, which was much higher than that reported in the literature from 9 to 54 days. Among the patients with a diagnosis time of more than 6 months, rural residents accounted for 85.4%.The patient treated with dressing change was 54.9%, but the cure rate was only 4.7%; the cure rate of surgical treatment was 89.8%. To a certain extent, this reflects the epidemiological data and epidemic status of local areas in China during a certain period.

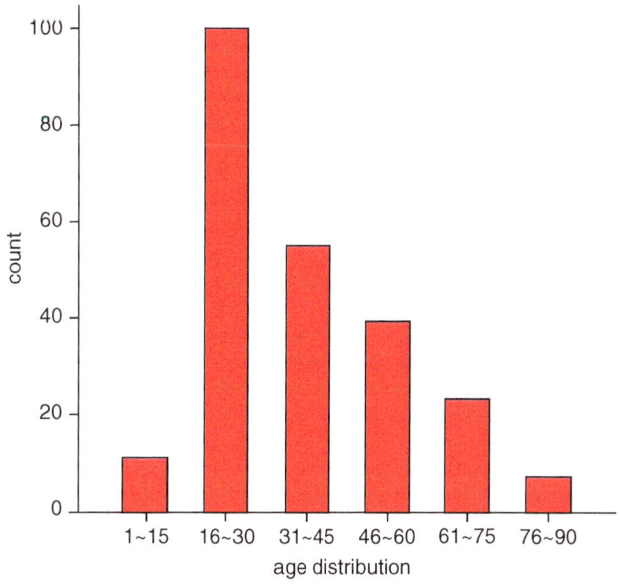


**Fig. 5.19** Age distribution of patients

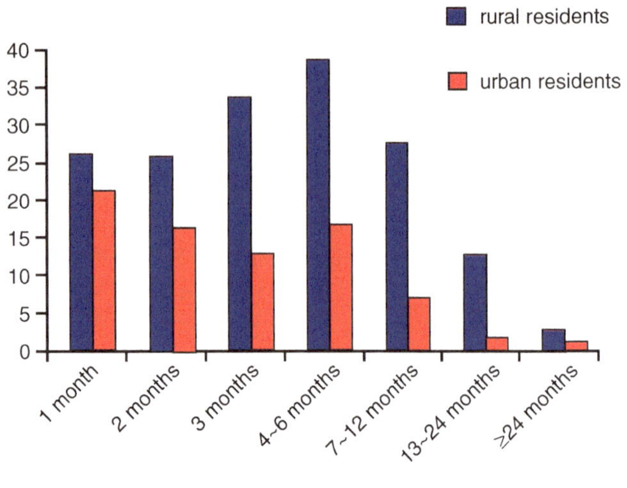


**Fig. 5.20** Time distribution of tuberculous wounds diagnosis

The average time from the onset of clinical symptoms to the diagnosis of tuberculosis was 4.4 months (median 3 months), and the time distribution ranged from 1 to 32 months. Among them, the majority of patients were diagnosed within the first 3 months (Fig. 5.20). Among patients with a diagnosis time of more than 6 months, the rural residents have a relatively high composition.

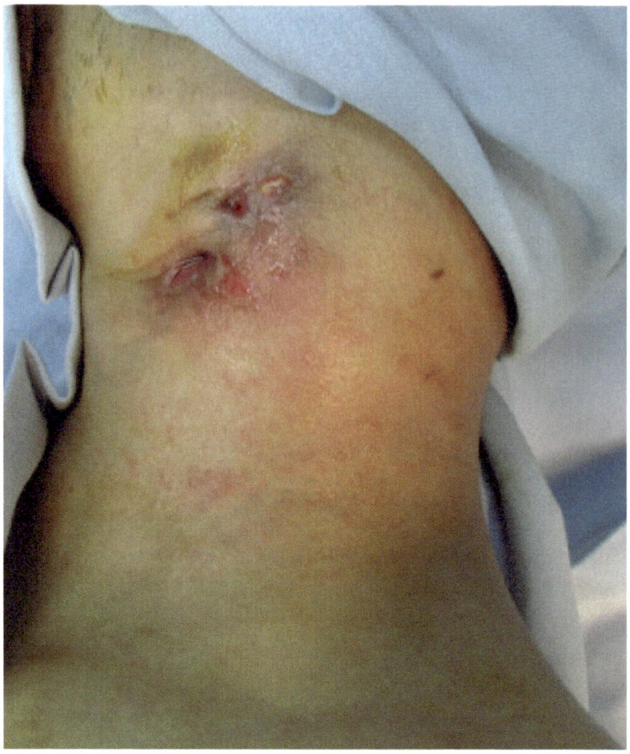

**Fig. 5.21** Neck tuberculosis wound

#### 5.5.4.3 The Concept of Tuberculous Wounds

At present, there is no standard concept for wounds caused by *Mycobacterium tuberculosis* in the international and domestic medical community. Based on the initial cause of wound formation, combined with the final clinical features, we proposed the concept of tuberculous wounds, which is caused by *Mycobacterium tuberculosis* invading the local tissues of the body, leading to necrosis of the affected site or adjacent skin and subcutaneous soft tissue, eventually leading to skin ulceration. Tuberculous wounds are a big concept, referring to the wounds caused by *M. tuberculosis*. The common clinical tuberculous wounds are caused by the spread of lymphoid tuberculosis and bone tuberculosis lesions to surrounding tissues and skin. Skin tuberculosis refers to the invasion of skin by *M. tuberculosis*. Once a wound is formed, it is also a category of tuberculous wounds.

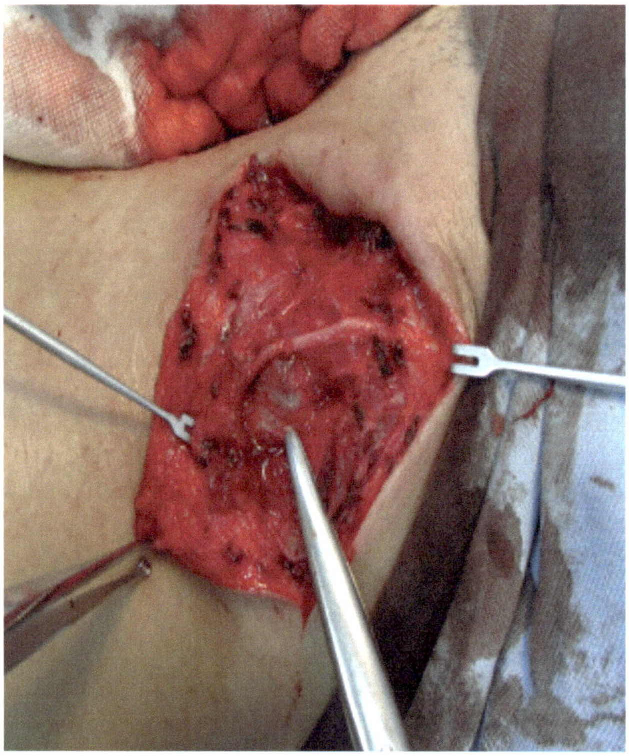

**Fig. 5.22** Seen during surgery

#### 5.5.4.4 Clinical Manifestations of Tuberculous Wounds

Because tuberculous wounds are caused by *Mycobacterium tuberculosis* infection, the wounds have their unique clinical manifestations:

(a) A small mouth and a large bottom, and the skin ulcers are generally small, but the invasion of subcutaneous tissue is large and the invaded level is deep (Figs. 5.21 and 5.22).
(b) Easy to invade bone. For example, the chest wall tuberculosis wounds often involve the sternum, and the wounds near the joints are often accompanied by bone and joint tuberculosis.

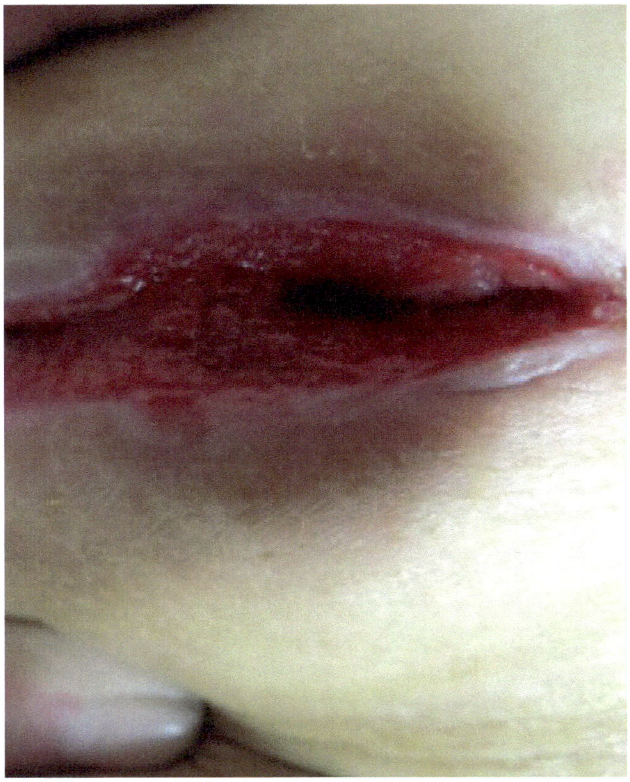

**Fig. 5.23** Waist wound

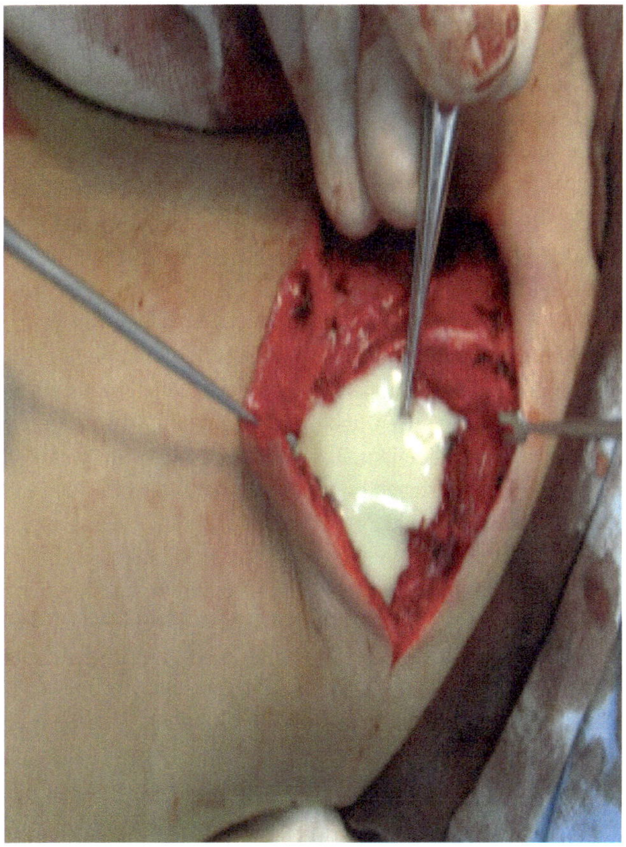

**Fig. 5.24** Yellow-green necrotic purulent secretions

(c) Often multiple sinuses are formed, the trajectory is tortuous into a mouse hole (Fig. 5.23), reaching deep into the muscles and even the bone surface.
(d) The affected tissue is necrotic to caseous necrosis, may be accompanied by yellow-green purulent secretions and no obvious foul odor (Fig. 5.24).
(e) Most of the patients have deep and clear primary lesions. Due to the positional factors, the wound site is often lower than the original lesion.

Most patients have no systemic symptoms, and clinical symptoms are different, which may lead to misdiagnosis and missed diagnosis. Most of the wounds are single, while the number of multiple wounds is relatively small. The skin around the sores is red and swollen, with tenderness.

#### 5.5.4.5 Diagnosis of Tuberculous Wounds

The diagnosis of tuberculous wounds needs to be combined with the clinical features of the wound (caseous necrosis, yellow-green purulent secretions, and mouse-hole-like sinus), imaging features, and ultrasound and laboratory tests. However, due to the atypical symptoms in the early stage of tuberculous wounds, it is easy to be confused with inflammatory granulomatosis, tumors, chronic inflammation, and other diseases, and it is difficult to specifically exclude other diseases in imaging, which brings certain difficulties to the diagnosis of tuberculous wounds, so the rate of early misdiagnosis is extremely high.

Tuberculous wounds are caused by *Mycobacterium tuberculosis* infection. Because of its unique strains and immune response, laboratory tests have a higher diagnostic value. Our small-scale epidemiological survey found that PPD test had the highest positive rate in laboratory tests, which was of great significance for diagnosing *M. tuberculosis* infection. However, the PPD test can also be positive after previous infection with *M. tuberculosis* or BCG vaccination. At present, there is no reliable standard to distinguish the natural tuberculosis infection and the reaction after BCG vaccination, so it cannot be used as a diagnosis standard. The diagnosis of tuberculous wounds requires the discovery of M. tuberculosis in wound secretions, but it has the disadvantages of long culture time, high price, high requirements for laboratory and inspectors, and low positive rate. Although the positive rate of biopsy histopathology is higher than that of tuberculosis cultivation, it can be the gold standard for the diagnosis of tuberculous wounds; many patients still have negative results. Therefore, even if the pathological examination is negative, the possibility of tuberculosis cannot be ruled out.

#### 5.5.4.6 Treatment of Tuberculous Wounds

**Preoperative Evaluation**

Ideal preoperative analysis of indicators for assessing wound conditions should include accurate positioning, assessment of wound area, depth, presence and shape of the subcutaneous sinus, nature of the wound contents, anatomical levels invaded by the wound tissue, and anatomical relationship with adjacent bones and soft tissue.

The sinus tract formed by tuberculous wounds has the remarkable characteristics of small mouth and large bottom, and mouse hole, the appearance and the actual situation in the deep are very different, so it is deceptive. Most patients think it is a superficial small wound, and the surgery should be simple. Inexperienced doctors also tend to think that the lesion is not large and ignore the preoperative assessment, which leads to surgery failure. Conventional methods are susceptible to uneven wound edges, patient position, wound site, and tissue swelling. It is not possible to accurately assess deep wounds with cystic segmentation and musculoskeletal involvement.

In recent years, the authors research team has attempted to use magnetic resonance imaging and 3D reconstruction software to achieve a 3D reconstruction of tuberculous wounds with sinus, attempting to achieve a panoramic and accurate display of its deep morphology and adjacent anatomical relationships, and initially achieved satisfactory results (Figs. 5.25, 5.26, and 5.27), which greatly facilitates the formulation of individualized surgical plans and the notification of the condition [83]. The technology is mainly divided into three parts: image acquisition, image segmentation reconstruction, and visualization. The acquired magnetic resonance images are imported into the medical 3D reconstruction software, and the signal recognition threshold selection tool is used to segment the inflamed tissue, sinus and normal muscle, then 3D reconstruction is performed, and the organization is displayed in different colors. The reconstructed 3D image can clearly show the deep stereoscopic shape of tuberculous wounds, including the anatomical adjacent relationship between inflammatory tissue and normal tissue, the sinus movement and depth, and can be

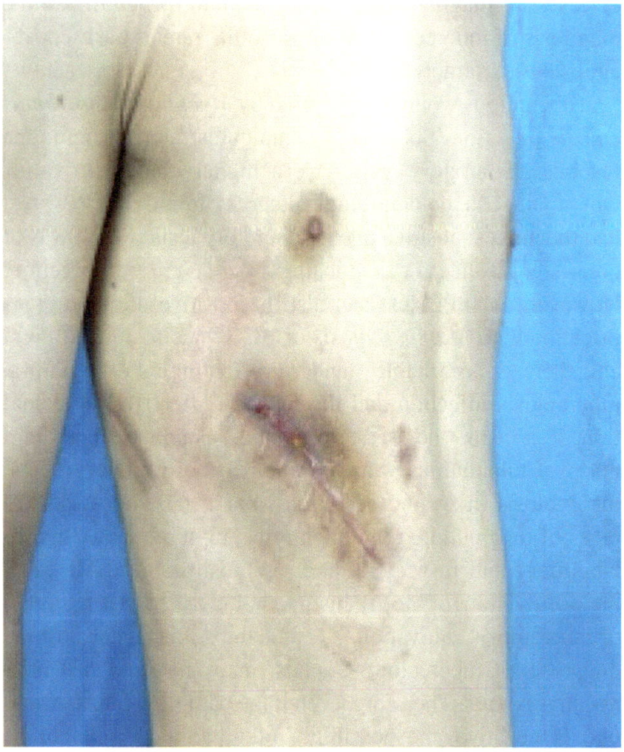

**Fig. 5.25** Chest wall tuberculosis wound

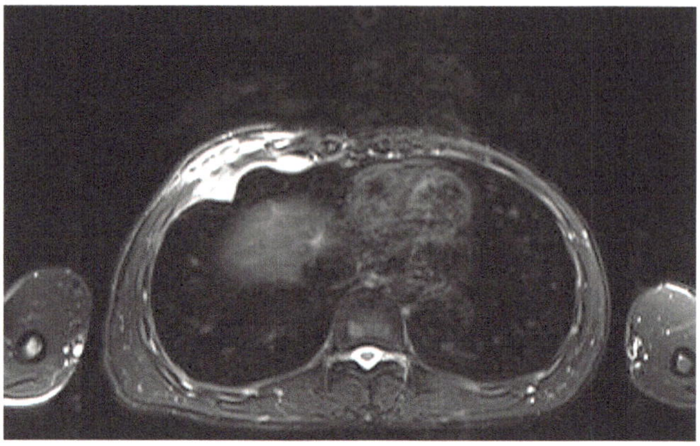

**Fig. 5.26** Nuclear magnetic resonance scanning

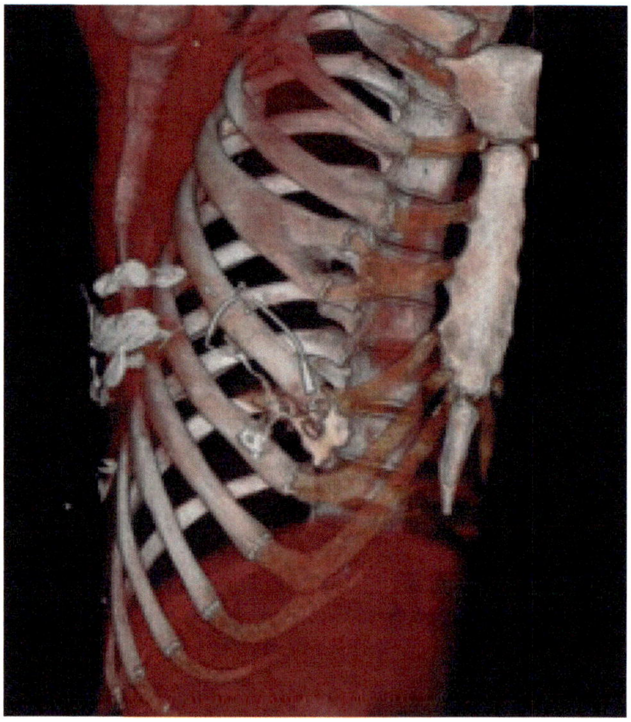

**Fig. 5.27** 3D reconstruction

rotated, translated, scaled to observe the internal morphology of the wound from different perspectives. The images obtained are detailed and intuitive, which facilitates the communication among the members of the surgical team and the formulation of surgical plans, so as to reduce the damage to the surrounding normal tissues and reduce the risk of surgery. At the same time, the 3D reconstruction image is intuitive and easy to understand, and also makes the communication between doctors and patients more concise and smooth.

### Treatment Plan and Efficacy

In the early stage of the disease, when the local tissue necrosis range is small, after a long period of time, the treatment has a certain effect. However, if the medical history is long, the primary lesion is large, the local necrotic tissue is wide, and the depth of involvement is deep, it is difficult to work by traditional treatments alone. Not only the course of the disease is prolonged but also the condition tends to gradually worsen. Surgical intervention (lesion clearance+wound coverage) is essential (Figs. 5.28, 5.29, 5.30, and 5.31).

Surgery is one of the important means of treating refractory wounds [84]. In surgical debridement, only the complete removal of necrotic tissue can achieve the final complete healing of the ulcer, otherwise the remaining lesions will become the cause of recurrent ulcer. The wounds covers generally require muscle flaps, musculocutaneous flaps, or free flaps. Of course, in order to achieve a complete wound healing, preoperative and postoperative standard anti-tuberculosis

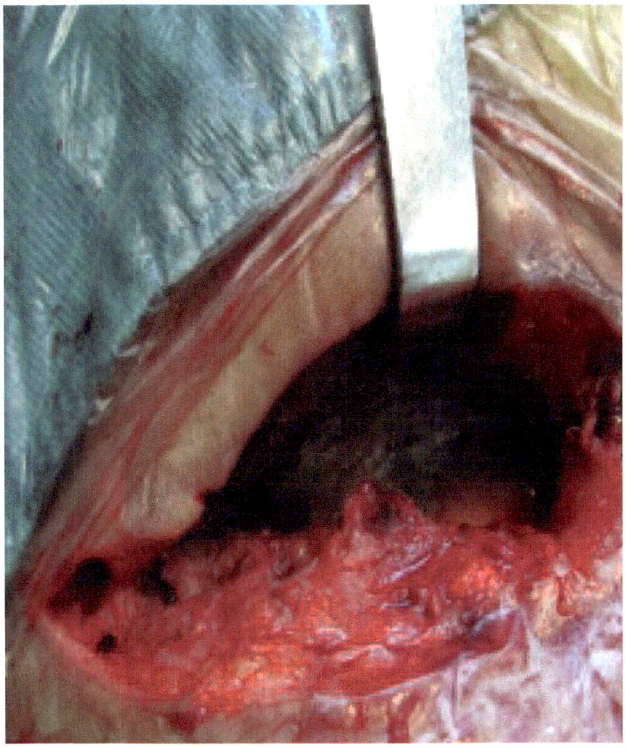

**Fig. 5.29** Postoperative debridement

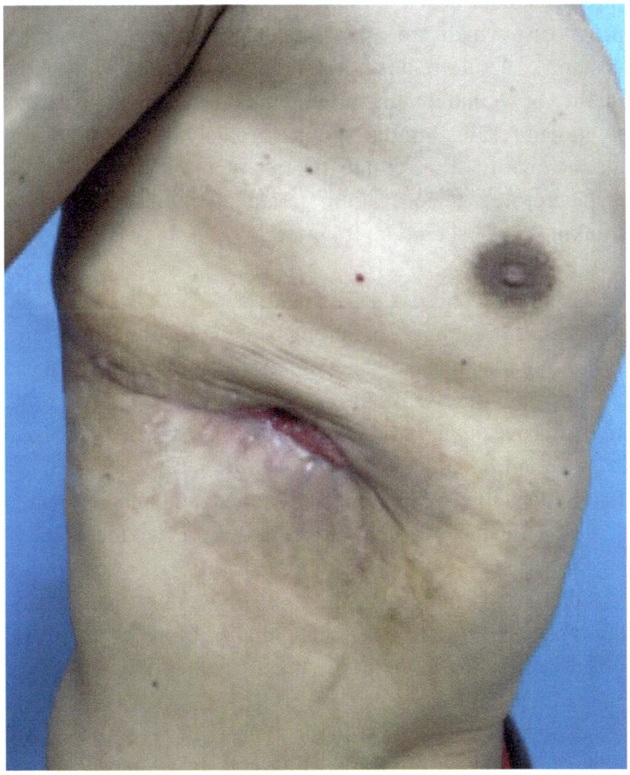

**Fig. 5.28** Chest wall tuberculosis wound

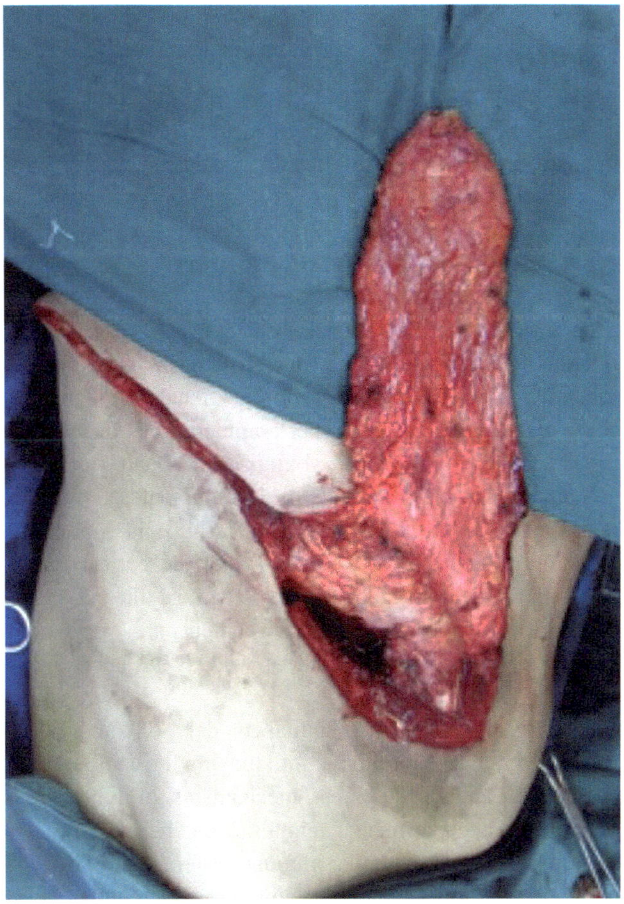

**Fig. 5.30** Flap transfer

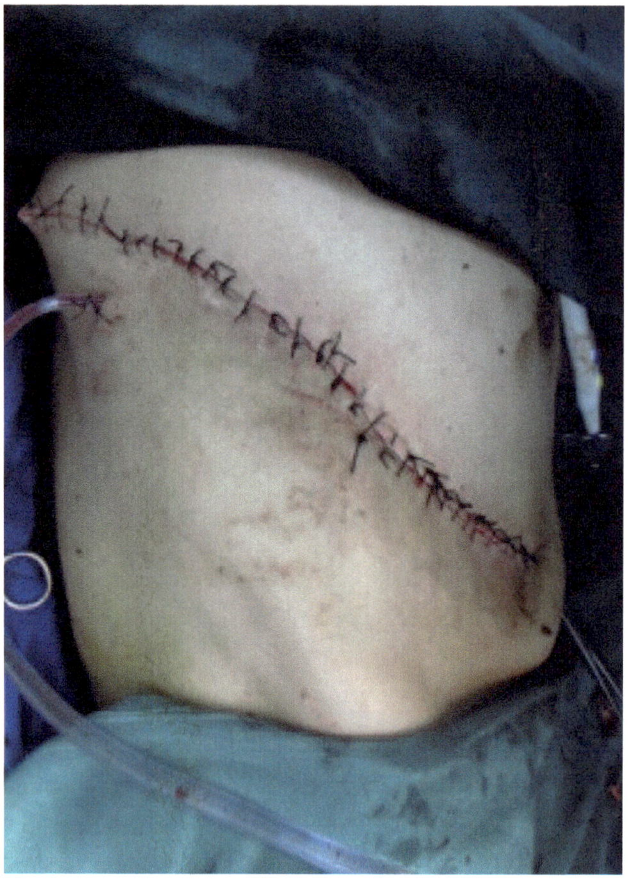

**Fig. 5.31** Wound healing

chemotherapy is also necessary. Recently, we have adopted a new treatment strategy of "lesion clearance+VSD + flap" and achieved good clinical results [85].

#### 5.5.4.7 Research Trends and Prospects of Tuberculous Wounds

Most of these diseases are mainly diagnosed and treated by internal medicine in China, and no systematic study on tuberculous wounds has been reported. Analysis of the reasons, first, compared with other common types of wounds, the incidence of tuberculous wounds is lower and people pay less attention to them; second, the development is slower, the diagnosis cannot be confirmed in time; third, the replication of animal models is very difficult, and the corresponding basic research is difficult to carry out; four, the protective conditions of the research environment are very high. Therefore, research on tuberculous wounds has been almost blank for many years.

The establishment of animal models of tuberculous wounds is the necessary basis for studying the causes, rules; occurrence and development mechanisms of tuberculous wounds. First, experimental animals should be susceptible to mycobacteria, have a similar immune system to humans, and can form pathological changes similar to human tuberculous wounds. Secondly, the choice of animal models of tuberculous wounds should also consider laboratory biosafety issues. Based on the above requirements, animals that meet the requirements are very limited.

At present, the research on tuberculous wounds is still in its infancy, and the animal model of tuberculous wounds is still not mature and stable enough, and there may still be a certain gap from the clinical practice. Although there are still some problems in the animal model of tuberculous wounds, as far as the actual situation is concerned, the research potential of the molecular mechanism related to tuberculosis wounds in the zebrafish model infected by *Mycobacterium marinum* is not to be underestimated. Genes and transcriptional expression pathways associated with tuberculous wounds can be found, and the target genes and target proteins associated with tuberculous wound treatment can be found, making biological target therapy for tuberculous wounds possible.

The future development trend should be the application of high-frequency ultrasound, CT scan, and magnetic resonance imaging without non-invasive real-time imaging (3D reconstruction accurately shows the location, size, shape, internal structure of the wound, and its relationship with surrounding structures), and in the basic research, the occurrence and development mechanism of tuberculous wounds should be systematically in-depth studied.

### 5.5.5 The Conclusion

Chronic ulcers are a class of diseases with high prevalence, high treatment costs, variable clinical conditions, and poor prognosis, which are often treated by disparate treatment systems. Therefore, it is not advisable to simply evaluate the quality of wound treatment without considering the patient's treatment results. Similarly, it is extremely difficult to evaluate the quality of the clinician's treatment.

Therefore, when making treatment strategies, such a thinking mode should be followed:

(a) Diagnosis and risk assessment.
(b) Active treatment, including stabilizing the ulcer, promoting healing early, and treating complications that can increase the risk of chronic ulcers.
(c) Improve quality of life and reduce pain when ulcers have unconditionally healed.
(d) Make a long-term targeted treatment and nursing plan to slow the development of ulcers and prevent recurrence.

Of course, China's research in the field of chronic ulcers, still exists a large gap between China and foreign countries. Mainly reflecting in the following aspects:

(a) Conceptual backwardness. Chronic ulcers are not deemed to be life-threatening and to belong to natural physiological processes.

(b) Insufficient capital investment. The deficiency of scientific research funds will inevitably lead to the shortage of human resources and the difficulty in forming a scale of the project, and it is unlikely to make a breakthrough at a certain point.
(c) Poor use of funds. Since there is no overall plan, the limited funds are scattered, resulting in low-level duplication.
(d) Academic institutions are not fully equipped.

Therefore, we should strive to do the following works.

(a) Conduct universal education on wound healing, making its importance recognized by most people, which is the basis of other kinds of works.
(b) Improve organizational structure and straighten out relationships. A strong organization is the core of the development of the discipline, which can grasp the development direction and overall planning of the discipline.
(c) Break the traditional concept and take a new road of "medical and commercial cooperation, common development." At present, China's economy is still underdeveloped, and science and technology funds are not sufficient. It is not enough to rely solely on the various research funds. We must find our own way and "medical and commercial cooperation, common development" is a practical way. It has been implemented in foreign countries for many years and proved to be beneficial to both medicine and business.
(d) Hold regular academic meetings on wound healing to learn from each other in order to strengthen academic exchanges. At the same time, top talents should be selected to participate in appropriate international conferences, so as to timely understand the international basic research trends and clinical treatment levels, and track the international advanced level.
(e) Grasp the relationship between basic research and clinical research. Basic research to a great extent reflects the level of science and technology in a country. Once it lags behind, it is difficult to catch up in a short period of time. Therefore, we must pay attention to basic research work. But only focusing on basic research is not enough, because our ultimate goal is to solve clinical practical problems, so it is critical to correctly grasp the relationship between the two. Contemporarily, the situation in China is that there is a serious disconnect between basic and clinical research results, many of which cannot be transformed into clinical services. Only by combining the two closely, accelerating the development and application of new products, can wound healing research really go on the track of healthy development.

## 5.6 Treatment of Chronic Refractory Wound with Osteomyelitis

### 5.6.1 Overview

#### 5.6.1.1 The Concept and Mechanism of Osteomyelitis

Osteomyelitis is an infectious inflammatory response of bone caused by microorganisms, which can be limited to a certain part of the bone and can also involve various areas of the bone, such as bone marrow, cortical bone, periosteum, and surrounding soft tissue. In clinical practice, it is often divided into acute osteomyelitis (several days to weeks) and chronic osteomyelitis (several weeks to months or even longer) according to the course of disease. The latter generally develop from the former to the formation of dead bones and become chronic.

The pathogenesis of osteomyelitis is mainly divided into two types: exogenous and hematogenous. Exogenous osteomyelitis is caused by open fractures, surgery or spread of infection in adjacent tissues. Hematogenous osteomyelitis is mainly caused by bacteria reaching a certain bone tissue through the blood circulation from other infection lesions in the body.

Chronic osteomyelitis is a biofilm infection, in which only a very small proportion of the microorganisms are free to swim (plankton), active (culturable), and sensitive to systemic medication. However, the vast majority of pathogens are colonized, elastically adherent (on dead bone, autologous or external grafts), and deeply implanted in microbial adhesion membranes (biofilms). Once the microorganism enters a colonized state, it cannot be cleared by the host's immunity, nor can high concentrations of antibiotics in the blood kill it. Over time, the toxins produced by microorganisms and the alkaloids produced by host cell-related immune side effects accumulate, causing severe local and systemic damage (sepsis, soft tissue loss, and chronic edema). At the body level, when the inflammation blocks the blood vessels, partial ischemic osteonecrosis is secondary. Bone tissue that lacks blood supply will gradually separate from normal bone tissue and gradually become the so-called dead bone. In the vicinity of the infected area, reactive hyperemia occurs with an increase in local osteoclast activity, which further aggravates bone loss. The hallmark of chronic osteomyelitis is that the diseased soft tissue is wrapped with infected dead bone. The infected area of the bone is surrounded by sclerotic and relatively ischemic bone, which is covered with thickened periosteum, scarred muscles, and subcutaneous tissue. Because of the ischemic scar tissue surrounding the lesion, systemic antibiotics are difficult to achieve.

#### 5.6.1.2 The Classification and Diagnosis of Osteomyelitis

**Classification**

In 1985, Cierny and Mader proposed the Cierny-Mader classification for adult patients with osteomyelitis, becoming the first osteomyelitis classification system that combines the course, classification and the treatment plan [86]. The Cierny-Mader classification classifies the main factors affecting treatment, that is, the extent of osteonecrosis, the overall health of the patient, and the impact of the disease on function, consisting of patient classification and anatomical classification.

Patients with osteomyelitis can be classified into three types according to the physiological indicators of the patient's response. Type A: The patient has a normal response to infection and surgical treatment. The patient has normal immune function and good local blood supply. Type B: The patient's body is damaged and the wound healing ability is reduced, and the B-Local (BL) and B-Systematic (BS) factors damage the immune function and healing ability of the patient. Type C: Patients with mild disability, other illnesses, and after treatment may be worse than untreated.

According to anatomical indexes, osteomyelitis can be classified into four types. Type I: Intramedullary osteomyelitis, characterized by endosteal lesions. Type II: Superficial osteomyelitis, lesions limited to the bone surface, secondary to surface defects. Type III: Localized osteomyelitis, the lesion is a stable and well-defined dead bone and cavity of full-thickness cortex, completely eliminating the lesion will not cause instability. Type IV: Diffuse osteomyelitis, which is mechanically unstable before or after treatment and requires complex reconstruction.

The combination of anatomical and physiological indexes can divide osteomyelitis into 12 clinical stages. For example, type B patients with systemic impairment factors have type III osteomyelitis, which is defined as stage III BS of osteomyelitis. This classification method is very helpful for the choice of treatment options, and it can decide whether to adopt simple method or complex method, radical surgery or palliative treatment, limb saving, or amputation.

**Diagnosis**

The diagnosis of osteomyelitis should be a combination of clinical manifestations, laboratory tests, and imaging examinations, but there is no non-invasive examination to completely diagnose or exclude osteomyelitis. The gold standard for diagnosis is histological and microbiological examination of dead bone by biopsy. During physical examination, attention should be paid to the integrity of the skin and soft tissue, determine the location of the tender point, check the stability of the bone, and judge the condition of the limb nerves and blood vessels. Laboratory tests are generally not specific and the severity of the infection cannot be determined. The vast majority of patients had elevated ESR and CRP, but only 35% of patients with elevated white blood cell counts.

It can be examined by a variety of imaging methods, but there is no way to clearly confirm or exclude osteomyelitis. The purpose of imaging examination is to help confirm the diagnosis and preoperative preparation.

The gold standard for diagnosing osteomyelitis is bacterial culture and susceptibility testing after biopsy. Biopsy not only confirms the diagnosis but also helps to select sensitive antibiotics. *Staphylococcus* is the most typical pathogen, especially in posttraumatic infections. Anaerobic and Gram-negative bacteria are generally rare, soft tissue, and bone specimens should be submitted for microbiological studies.

#### 5.6.1.3 Overview of the Treatment of Osteomyelitis

Chronic osteomyelitis with chronic refractory wounds must be treated surgically, with the goal of treating infection, reconstructing soft tissue and bone structures. The principles of surgery are as follows.

(a) Thorough debridement: remove all kinds of internal plants; completely remove dead bones, fistula, abscesses, necrosis and bad granulation tissue according to the preoperative evaluation range.
(b) Treatment of ineffective cavities: application of flap transfer or antibiotic bone cement bead filling.
(c) Maintain stability: external fixes, etc.
(d) Closed wounds: in order to prevent recurrence of infection, it must be covered with well-vascularized tissue. At the same time, the treatment of osteomyelitis requires a multifaceted approach, in addition to antibiotic application, surgical debridement and reconstruction, should also consider the patient's accompanying disease and appropriate treatment, such as smoking cessation, blood glucose control.

**Classification for Different Patients**

Type B patients are those who have underlying disease, and they are affected by the primary disease and respond to stress, trauma, or infection. There is a risk of failure in the treatment of type B patients, because there may be a higher probability of metabolic disorders, impaired immune function, bacterial infections, wound rot, and excessive bleeding. If the risk and/or complications of treatment exceed the benefits of the treatment itself, the patient is defined as a type C patient. Type C patients are not treated with surgery, but simply given palliative symptomatic treatment. During the treatment process, improving patients' basic health condition could bring benefits to type B patients which could eventually make the outcome similar to type A patients. Choosing a safe surgical procedure and avoiding the use of surgical grafts can also reduce the risk of treatment. However, if the treatment does need the application of internal plants, the entire treatment process is best staged, and reconstructed surgically after the application of antibiotics in order to reduce the tissue tension generated by the local inflammatory reaction, remove the remaining pathogenic strains, and protect soft tissue coverage to increase treatment success rate.

#### Classification for Different Anatomies

Classification for different anatomies (Fig. 5.32). Type I (intramedullary) osteomyelitis is not associated with skin and soft tissue wounds and is not described here.

Type II (superficial) osteomyelitis. This type of osteomyelitis is associated with skin and soft tissue defects, so normal soft tissue coverage must be restored when making a preoperative plan. Clinical physical examinations, vascular ultrasound, and angiography are often used to assess defect conditions and potential surgical procedures for repair surgery. Remove the diseased soft tissue to a vigorous, soft edge and bite off the diseased bone until the "red pepper sign" appears. Thereafter, it is necessary to synthesize vascular perfusion and local tissue conditions to develop a long-term and feasible surgical approach for soft tissue coverage. Reconstruction of type II osteomyelitis is often performed by closed vacuum suction with skin grafting, local transfer flap or free tissue flap transplantation.

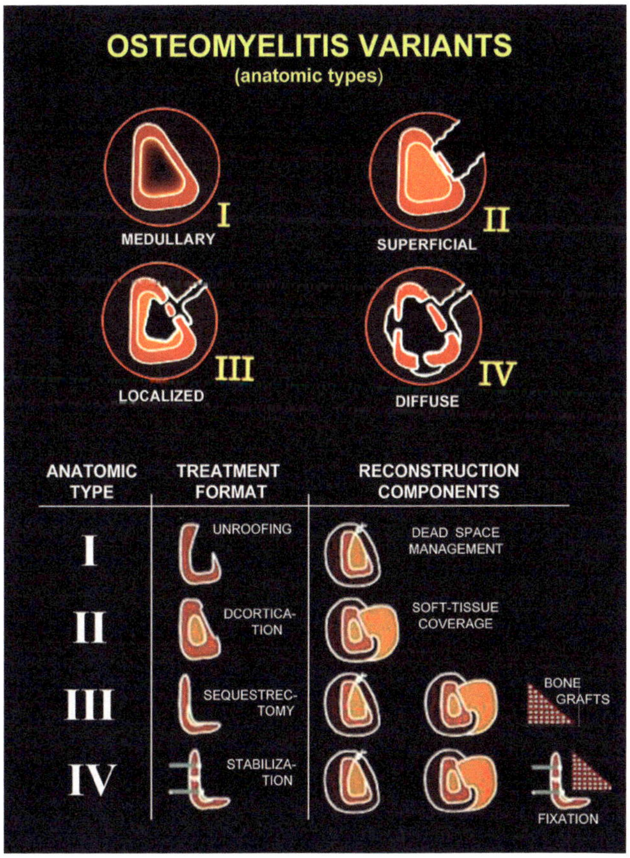


**Fig. 5.32** Cierny-Mader classification

(a) Type III (limited) osteomyelitis. Type III osteomyelitis is characterized by both type I and type II osteomyelitis, and there are often severe soft tissue defects after debridement surgery. If debridement removes bone tissue to a large extent that may affect the mechanical stability of the remaining bone, prophylactic stabilization of the affected limb is required to achieve stable results, including the use of bone metastasis, external fixators, or the implantation of antibiotic loads (antibiotic-coated plants or fillers, antibiotic rods, etc.) in situ after debridement surgery. The soft tissue defect is the same as the type II osteomyelitis that has been discussed. If it is necessary to treat the ineffective cavity or reconstruct the mechanical structure after debridement, local antibiotic treatment is often required for a period of time before the reconstruction surgery.
(b) Type IV (diffuse) osteomyelitis. Debridement surgery for type IV osteomyelitis lesions can cause bone instability. Mechanical instability, potential cavities, bone defects, and other serious underlying diseases (type B patients) make the treatment of type IV osteomyelitis most difficult. On the one hand, almost all treatments require staged reconstruction to make later reconstructions as clean and sterile as possible. On the other hand, it can also complete the soft tissue recovery and bone reconstruction in the form of free bone flap with vascular pedicle flap transformation, or open bone metastases, or different combinations of shortening and lengthening of bone, in order to replace the above-mentioned staged surgical plan.

### 5.6.1.4 The Main Differences and Difficulties Between the Refractory Wounds with Osteomyelitis and Common Conventional Refractory Wounds

(a) Refractory wounds with osteomyelitis are more difficult to accurately assess and diagnose than conventional refractory wounds, and are easily missed diagnose, misdiagnosed, or neglected. The main lesions of refractory wounds with osteomyelitis tend to be deep and may be multilacunar, the wounds that can be observed by the naked eye are often only the tip of the iceberg. Not only the patients often do not care at the beginning, but the inexperienced clinicians may also missed diagnose and misdiagnosed, making the disease unable to be effectively treated and controlled in the early stage.
(b) Refractory wounds with osteomyelitis differ from conventional ones in the presence of dead bone lesions. In addition, the lesions often involve the bone marrow cav-

ity and are often accompanied by the presence of orthopedic implants. Bacteria will form biofilms on the surface of dead bones and implants that cannot be removed by routine flushing and antibiotics. Even if extensive debridement is carried out, as long as the debridement of dead bone or intramedullary cavity is not complete and bacterial biofilm remains, it will soon return to the level before debridement. However, in clinical practice, it is often difficult to confirm the extent of dead bone and bone infection, and it is difficult to remove intramedullary lesions. Expanding debridement for complete removal will not only increase the size of invalid cavity but also further damage the mechanical stability. It is very difficult to give consideration to both "effective and thorough" and "minimally invasive and precise" and to further maintain clean and stable wound after debridement.

(c) Refractory wounds with osteomyelitis often involve the bones and joints stability, resulting in abnormal activities of the soft tissues around the wounds and making the wounds difficult to heal. The maintenance of local stability must be strengthened during the treatment.

### 5.6.2 The Osteomyelitis-Diagnose-Score (ODS) and Diagnosis and Treatment Process

#### 5.6.2.1 The Osteomyelitis-Diagnose-Score

In 2011, Professor Schmidt et al. [87] in Germany established the osteomyelitis-diagnose-score (ODS) to assign scores to five indicators of "clinical history and risk factors," "clinical manifestations and laboratory test results," "imaging examination results," "microbial culture," and "histopathology." Each index is scored from 0 to 6 points, and the total score is obtained by adding the five scores. When the total score is≥18 points, the diagnosis is grade A, that is, the diagnosis of osteomyelitis is "reliable"; when the total score is in the range of 8–17 points, the diagnosis is grade B, that is, the diagnosis of osteomyelitis is "possible"; when the total score is<8 points, the diagnosis is grade C, that is, the diagnosis of osteomyelitis is "less likely." Among the five indicators, each diagnostic factor can only be rated as 6 points at most. This means that even if a diagnosis score of one indicator is greater than 6 points, its weight in the total score will not be greater than the other 4 diagnostic indicators. The detailed scores of each indicator are shown in Table 5.2.

**Table 5.2** Diagnosis and treatment of osteomyelitis

| |
|---|
| I. Assess patients |
| II. Preoperative examination |
| 1. Laboratory tests: biochemistry, blood routine, coagulation, urine routine, erythrocyte sedimentation rate, C-reactive protein, calcitonin |
| 2. Diagnostic examination: vascularity index, ultrasound, transcutaneous oxygen partial pressure |
| 3. Imaging examination: X-ray, magnetic resonance, CT, radionuclide scanning |
| 4. Tissue biopsy: culture, histological section, PCR |
| III. Clinical classification |
| 1. Anatomical classification: medullary cavity, superficial, localized, diffuse |
| 2. Physiological classification: type A patient, type B patient (BL/BS), type C patient |
| IV. Treatment |
| 1. Limb salvage |
| 2. Amputation |
| 3. Palliative: type C patient, incurable patient |
| V. Improve the general condition of the patient: treatment of concomitant diseases |
| VI. First operation |
| A. One-time surgical reconstruction: |
| 1. Debridement, tissue biopsy, local and systemic antibiotics |
| 2. Dealing with invalid cavities: limb salvage or amputation |
| (a) Wound: self-healing in the second stage; directly closing or delaying the closure of the wound |
| (b) Bone: with vascularized bone flap; first stage shortening |
| (c) Fixation: orthopedic surgery, external fixator |
| (d) Drug sustained release: antibiotic beads |
| B. The first step in multi-stage surgery: |
| 1. Debridement, tissue biopsy, systemic antibiotics |
| 2. Replace: replace the instrument, re-rinse, lay the sheet and replace the gloves |
| 3. Temporary fixation: external fixator, antibiotic coated plants |
| 4. Dealing with invalid cavities |
| (a) Wound: self-healing in the second stage; directly closing or delaying the closure of the wound |
| (b) Bone: bone removal; with vascularized bone flap |
| (c) Fixation: orthopedic surgery, external fixator, antibiotic coated plants |
| (d) Drug sustained release: antibiotic beads, antibiotic filler |

**Table 5.2** (continued)

| |
|---|
| VII. Discharge, outpatient follow-up: monitoring wounds, rechecking indicators (erythrocyte sedimentation rate/C-reactive protein); rehabilitation exercise |
| VIII. Second surgery |
| A. One-time surgical reconstruction |
| 1. Prophylactic application of antibiotics, removal of internal plants, debridement, tissue biopsy (negative frozen section: no inflammation) |
| 2. Replace: replace the instrument, re-rinse, lay the sheet and replace the gloves |
| 3. Reconstruction |
| (a) Wound: direct closure |
| (b) Bone: bone graft; with vascularized bone flap; joint prosthesis |
| (c) Fixation: orthopedic surgery; external fixation or internal fixation; joint prosthesis |
| (d) Drug sustained release: antibiotic beads; permanent filler; antibiotic-coated plants |
| B. The second step of multi-stage surgery |
| 1. Prophylactic application of antibiotics, removal of internal plants, debridement, tissue biopsy (positive frozen section: acute inflammation) |
| 2. Same as VI B (above) or amputation |
| IX. Discharge and outpatient follow-up: monitoring wounds, rechecking indicators (erythrocyte sedimentation rate / C-reactive protein); rehabilitation exercise |
| X. Third surgery |
| A. One-time surgical reconstruction: (negative frozen section: no inflammation) same as VIII A (above) |
| B. The third step of multistage surgery: (positive frozen section: acute inflammation) same as VI B (above) or amputation |
| XI. Fourth surgery: biological reconstruction: callus healing, shortening of operation, bone removal, joint resection |
| XII. Discharge, outpatient follow-up: monitoring wounds, rechecking indicators (erythrocyte sedimentation rate/ C-reactive protein); rehabilitation exercise |

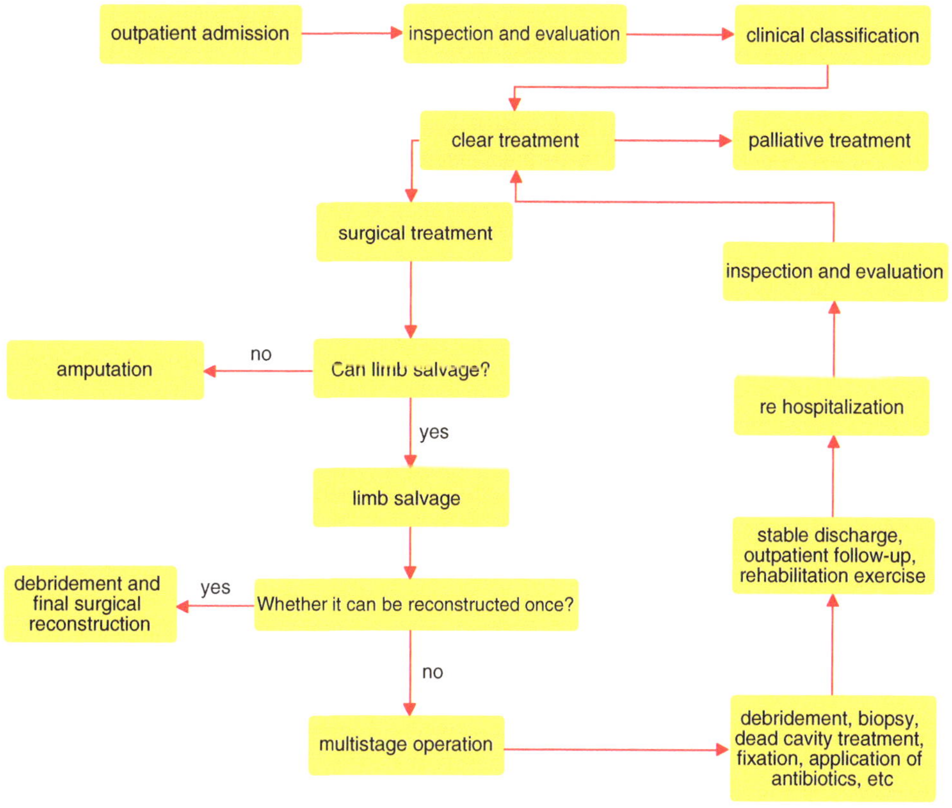


**Fig. 5.33** Flowchart of diagnosis and treatment of osteomyelitis

### 5.6.2.2 The Diagnosis and Treatment Process of Osteomyelitis

The diagnosis and treatment process of osteomyelitis is shown in Table 5.2.

Flowchart of diagnosis and treatment of osteomyelitis (Fig. 5.33).

### 5.6.3 The "6R Technology" for the Treatment of Chronic Refractory Wounds with Osteomyelitis

In the long-term treatment of various types of osteomyelitis, we have accumulated a lot of valuable clinical treatment experience and summarized them as "6R technology" for osteomyelitis treatment, namely, low temperature plasma radiofrequency debridement (radiofrequency), reaming, rinsing, monitoring reliable wounds (reliable), revascularization, reconstruction/regeneration.

#### 5.6.3.1 Low-Temperature Plasma Radiofrequency Debridement

For bacteria, biofilms and necrotic lesions that affect wound healing, debridement must be effective and thorough, while at the same time, local blood circulation and metabolic disorders in the lesion area require debridement to be minimally invasive and precise, with no or less damage to normal tissue structure. Therefore, the key to the treatment of chronic refractory wounds is debridement, and the difficulty of debridement lies in the consideration of the two principles of "effective and thorough" and "minimally invasive and precise." There are many debridement techniques in clinical application, including self- debridement, enzyme debridement, biological debridement, sharp surgical debridement, ultrasonic debridement, and water knife debridement, but these methods have their own distinct shortcomings in the treatment of chronic wounds. Even the sharp surgical debridement, which is considered to be the gold standard for wound debridement, cannot be tolerated by old, weak, and critically ill patients because of its large trauma and bleeding during operation, especially for patients with coagulopathy disorders or in the process of anticoagulant therapy.

Low-temperature plasma radiofrequency technology was developed in the 1990s and matured by ArthroCare. It uses the energy generated by the high-frequency plasma motion to excite the electrolyte between the bipolar electrode and the tissue into the ion-vapor layer of the plasma, and uses the high-speed plasma to open the intercellular bond and gradually decompose the cells into carbohydrates, so as to realize the ablation of soft tissue. When the temperature reaches 40–70 °C, the target tissue is ablated accurately and limited by the plasma between the electrodes, which makes the water evaporate, the protein degenerate and necrosis, and the blood vessels and tissues around the tissue shrink, close, and solidify. Plasma ablation technology has the advantages of low temperature during operation and precise ablation, which makes it less damage to surrounding tissues during work, thus reducing postoperative pain and healing time. Moreover, the plasma ablation system offers a variety of tool tip options, which can be used in open surgery or closed surgery such as arthroscopy. It has been widely used in the surgical treatment of departments such as otolaryngology, plastic surgery, joint, and spinal surgery.

At the beginning of the twenty-first century, Axel Kramer et al. [88] and other scholars first proposed the use of low-temperature plasma radiofrequency ablation technology for wound treatment. Since then, the research teams at home and abroad have verified the debridement effects of low-temperature plasma radio frequency through in vitro and in vitro experiments [89]. In 2012, the author's team verified the in vivo sterilization effect of low-temperature plasma radiofrequency technology through animal experiments, and compared plasma debridement with traditional surgical debridement and electric knife debridement, confirming the effect of low-temperature plasma radiofrequency debridement is significantly better than that of surgical debridement and electric knife debridement [90]. After the success of the animal experiment, the author's team applied the low-temperature plasma radiofrequency technology for debridement treatment of clinical chronic osteomyelitis wounds and obtained very satisfactory therapeutic results. It is fully verified that the low-temperature plasma radiofrequency technology can take into account the "effective and thorough" and "minimally invasive and precise" of debridement in the treatment of chronic refractory wounds with osteomyelitis, which is a new technology worthy of vigorously promotion.

#### 5.6.3.2 Reaming

Due to the infection in the medullary cavity of type I (intramedullary), type III (limited), and type IV (diffuse) osteomyelitis, and the medullary cavity in the lesion site of patients is often occluded by the infection lesions or abnormal hyperplasia of bone, so it is necessary to perform a debridement in the medullary cavity and open the closed medullary cavity during the operation. There are various potential risks in the conventional graded reaming, including injury of intramedullary blood supply, fat embolism, and osteonecrosis caused by the thermal effects of cortical bone. In order to reduce the various complications that may occur during the reaming process, Synthes in the United States produced a new "reamer-irrigator-aspirator" (RIA) reaming system in 2003. During the process of reaming, it can maintain continuous saline perfusion and continue suction to reduce the pressure in the medullary cavity. The materials in the medullary cavity are sucked away at the head of the reaming knife, and the continuous and stable infusion of normal saline driven by gravity can ensure the smooth suction channel. Compared with the traditional reaming method, the RIA reaming system has the following advantages:

(a) It can effectively reduce the pressure in the medullary cavity and prevent the fat particles from infecting the bacteria into the systemic circulation system.
(b) It can effectively reduce cortical osteonecrosis caused by high temperature of reaming.

(c) One-time reaming can significantly shorten the operation time and reduce trauma.
(d) The fragments produced by reaming can be collected for microbial bacterial culture, drug sensitivity test and histopathological examination.

#### 5.6.3.3 Rinsing

##### Flush

Pulsed flushing can spray the flushing liquid according to the set pressure and frequency, which is convenient for flushing the wound attachments away from the tissue. It is a safe and more effective method of wound cleaning than ordinary rinsing. The flushing fluid in the debridement surgery is aseptic isotonic saline, at least 9000 mL. Generally, no other drugs are added to the rinsing liquid, and hydrogen peroxide solution with a volume fraction of 3% can be used when it is identified or suspected to be contaminated or infected with anaerobic bacteria.

##### Lavage

In the First World War, Carrel and Dakin underwent continuous lavage treatment for the wounded soldiers, and they received amazing results. After continuous practice and improvement, now closed lavage drainage has the advantages of promoting the rapid discharge of necrotic tissues and infections, local high concentration of antibiotics that are conducive to local bactericidal, reducing the cavity of negative pressure suction promote healing, painless patients in the lavage process, and simultaneous lavage of multiple lesions. It has become one of the important means of osteomyelitis treatment.

#### 5.6.3.4 Monitoring Reliable Wounds

In the first stage of repair and reconstruction, the chronic osteomyelitis wounds that have been initially treated by surgery have a recent recurrence caused by poor infection control, which leads to surgical failure. This is often related to the fact that the wound bacterial level cannot be controlled within a certain range.

It is necessary to monitor the stable level of the osteomyelitis wounds. If debridement is doubtful or the level of debridement is not good or the condition is complex, it is necessary to closely monitor the wound and systemic inflammatory reaction in time to ensure the deep wound is stable recently. After no severe inflammatory reaction, the next step is to cover the wound and rebuild the continuity of the bone. Vacuum sealing drainage (VSD) can be used as a temporary cover for osteomyelitis wounds in this process.

In 1992, Dr. Fleischman was the first to use VSD in Germany. In 1994, Professor Juward introduced VSD technology to China, which was gradually widely used in surgical clinics. The mechanism of vacuum sealing drainage is to significantly increase the blood flow of the wound, promote the removal of necrotic tissue and bacteria, accelerate the growth of granulation tissue and cell proliferation and repair, promote capillary neogenesis, promote collagen synthesis in the proliferative phase and contractile fiber synthesis in repairing phase, rapidly enhance leukocyte activity, and phagocytic function reduces the number of bacteria, thus promoting accelerated healing of various wound including osteomyelitis.

In 1960, Canadian doctor L.J. Papineau [91] first proposed the Papineau method for the treatment of osteomyelitis, namely open cancellous bone grafting, which mainly includes:

(a) Complete lesion removal.
(b) Open cancellous bone transplantation.
(c) Continuous repeated washing.

Since then, Cierny has discussed it in more detail, that is, after thorough debridement, one-stage granular cancellous bone grafting is performed in the invalid cavity of the bone defect, after the operation, the dressing is continued until the surface of the grafted bone covered the granulation tissue, and then free skin grafting is performed to cover the wound. With the widespread application of VSD technology in orthopedics, if it is difficult to close the wound after the lesion is completely removed, VSD technology can be combined with the Papineau method to promote the growth of fresh granulation and accelerate wound healing.

The Papineau method combined with VSD technology has the following advantages over the ordinary Papineau method:

(a) The method is simple without changing dressings.
(b) Effective antibiotic flushing is possible.
(c) Granulation grows more quickly and evenly. However, it must also be noted that if ivory-like sclerotic bone or dead bone is found to be exposed without granulation when replacing the VSD, the sclerotic bone or dead bone must be removed again.

Infect necrotic tissues and exudates on chronic refractory wounds with osteomyelitis are often very viscous, making the effect of VSD greatly discounted and the tube easily blocked. Therefore, it is necessary to apply VSD on the basis of thorough debridement and to design each sponge and each tube during the operation. After the operation, saline should be continuously or intermittently applied to lavage multiple tubes of VSD. This not only ensures the patency of the VSD device but also further flushes the local tissue necrotic exudates and metabolites to accelerate wound healing.

#### 5.6.3.5 Revascularization

After extensive and thorough debridement of the lesion, soft tissue transfer techniques are used to fill the invalid cavity and reconstruct local blood supply. There are various methods for soft tissue flap transfer, including the local vascularized pedicled myocutaneous flap, and the free tissue flap with microsurgical anastomosis. For larger skin and soft tissue defects, the choice of flaps is a very challenging task, requiring clinicians to have very rich clinical experience, and should follow the principle of "from the near to the distant, simple, and not complex." First of all, it is necessary to make a comprehensive evaluation according to the specific conditions of the affected limbs. This includes the area of the skin defect, the surrounding tissue condition, the blood supply of the limb (angiography if necessary), and whether or not a bone defect is combined. The appropriate donor sites are selected according to the results of these evaluations. The commonly used flaps include local flaps, sural nerve flaps, medial and lateral head flaps of the gastrocnemius, medial and lateral flaps of the calf, dorsalis pedis flaps, cross leg flaps, thoracic umbilical flaps, and latissimus dorsal myocutaneous flaps. Secondly, larger defects such as upper leg preferred medial and lateral head flaps of the gastrocnemius; lower leg can choose sural nerve flaps, dorsalis pedis flaps, medial and lateral leg flasps, the middle leg has a larger choice, and the above flaps can be used. When the skin defect is very large or combined with tibia defect, the soft tissue condition of the lower leg is very poor, and there is no alternative flaps locally, the cross-leg flap, free thoracic umbilical flap, latissimus dorsi flap, or composite tissue flap of the contralateral fibula should be considered. In addition, when designing skin flaps, consideration should be given to the area of the skin defect to be repaired and the amount of soft tissue required for invalid cavity filling. The preferred flap is the myocutaneous flap or the flap with some fascial tissue. Finally, for the filling of ineffective cavities without skin defects, the muscle flap is preferred because the local muscle flap has complete blood supply and good antiinflammatory effects [92]. The flaps after removal of the epithelium can also be used to fill the invalid cavity with the tissue flaps that preserve the dermis, subcutaneous fat, and deep fascia [93]. It must be borne in mind that before the soft tissue is transplanted; the infected lesion should be thoroughly debrided so that the tissue flap can have a healthy recipient area, which helps to ensure the success of the operation.

#### 5.6.3.6 Structural Reconstruction and Tissue Regeneration

Postoperative infections in orthopedics often require complete removal of the implant at the expense of stability to control infection, while extensive and thorough debridement of osteomyelitis often affects the stability of the limbs, so the external fixation becomes the most commonly used fixation to stabilize and reconstruct the structure. The external fixation has many advantages, such as minimally invasive, easy to operate, and wide indications. It is the most commonly used fixation technique for the treatment of chronic osteomyelitis with severe bone and soft tissue defects.

In the 1950s, Dr. Ilizarov of the Soviet Union designed and applied a ring-shaped external fixator and minimally invasive technique (Ilizarov technique) for the treatment of chronic osteomyelitis with bone defects, nonunion, bone and joint deformity, and obtained good clinical results. And after years of animal experiments and clinical experiments, the stimulating effect of stretch stress on tissue growth and regeneration has been found, that is, the law of stretch regeneration, also known as the law of tension-stress (LTS). LTS believes that a certain tension generated by slow and continuous stretching of living tissue can secondary and maintain the regeneration and active growth of certain tissue structures, which are consistent with fetal tissues and are the same cell division. Based on the biological theory of LTS, Ilizarov has continuously developed and summarized a technology of traction bone regeneration, also known as distraction osteogenesis (DO) technology, that is, continuous distraction can stimulate bone growth and induce proliferative compensatory adaptation of muscles, fascia, nerve, and skin. After distraction, the new bone tissue is mineralized by the original intramembranous osteogenesis process, which can be transformed into normal bone structure under physiological stress stimulation. Both bone transport technology and bone reconstruction technology originate from the basic principles of tractive osteogenesis [94].

The mechanisms of DO technology in the treatment of chronic osteomyelitis are as follows: completely clearing the infected lesions, repairing the tissue defect by distraction osteogenesis, and reconstructing the blood supply and function of the affected limb. A large number of basic researches and clinical observations have demonstrated that sustained stretch stress stimulation within physiological limits can activate and maintain the ability of tissue regeneration. According to DO technology theory, after a suitable stretching stress is given to the bone, the bones and their attached muscles, fascia, blood vessels and nerves grow synchronously, which increases the extent of limb extension to some extent [95]. Slow and continuous stretching will stimulate cell proliferation and biosynthesis, and active tissue metabolism. A large number of histological studies of the Ilizarov method have confirmed that bone formation is intramembranous ossification in homogeneous region. Histology has shown that there is thin capillary growth between the bone columns, and vessels of uniform diameter extend from the surface of the original bone end. Microangiography confirms that the neovascularization is in the same direction as the longitudinal axis of the new bone. After the Ilizarov external fixation is firmly fixed, the osteotomy site is still elastically connected. The slow stretching makes the tissue metabolism abnormally active and stimulates cell proliferation and biosynthesis. A growing zone can be formed in the middle of the extended region, with fibroblast-like forming collagen fibers (aligned with the direction of distraction). Osteoblasts on collagen fibers produce bone-like tissue, which gradually forms bone trabecula bone and gradually ossifies after fixation. Active smooth muscle cells appear in the middle layer of blood vessel wall, and new capillaries have many communicating branches that anastomose with the blood vessels in the soft tissue surrounding the traction area, constituting the blood circulation in the extended area and its surroundings [96].

Ilizarov external fixation technology provides a solid and adjustable fixation system for the treatment of osteomyelitis, which maximizes the protection of soft tissue around the bone and promotes bone tissue to play its potential. The Ilizarov external fixator penetrates the limb and bone tissue through multi-planar fine Kirschner wires, connects ring-shaped fixator, and assembles into three-dimensional structure with 3–4 screws. This design is firmly fixed, which can not only eliminate shear and rotation stress but also play its role of simple stretching stress or compression, and at the same time, it can also exert its periodic axial micro-motion during weight-bearing walking to promote bone healing. It can be adjusted in many directions and has the functions of de-angulation, de-rotation, de-lateral displacement, and axial compression with biomechanical requirements. It has more advantageous than single-arm external fixator [97].

### 5.6.4 The Application of Antibiotics

#### 5.6.4.1 Systemic Application of Antibiotics

Effective antibiotic use is the basis for the treatment of chronic osteomyelitis [98]. Systemic application of antibiotics to control infection must meet two conditions: effective bactericidal concentration and maintenance for a sufficient period of time. Although there are many expert opinions and scientific evidences on the treatment of pediatric hematogenous osteomyelitis or endophyte-associated osteomyelitis, in the treatment of adult osteomyelitis without grafts, the optimal antibiotic medication is still unclear and there is a lack of treatment guide that are universally accepted worldwide [99].

In the past, experts often recommended intravenous antibiotics for 4–6 weeks before continuing oral antibiotics for 2 weeks to 2 months [100–103]. According to expert opinion, the purpose of prolonging the course of intravenous medication is to increase the blood drug level. But now, new opinions suggest intravenous administration only during the first 2 weeks [104]. Although intravenous antibiotics facilitate drug penetration into the bone, in 2009 a Cochrane Meta-analysis that included eight trials comparing the efficacy of oral versus intravenous administrations in adult chronic osteomyelitis found that there was no statistically significant difference between oral and intravenous administration in disease remission rate at 12-month follow-up, but the incidence of adverse reactions was significantly higher with intravenous administration than with oral administration [105]. In multivariate logistic regression analysis, the effectiveness of intravenous administration for 1 week did not differ from 2 to 3 weeks or more.

After surgical treatment, antibiotics can help treat residual infections and prevent further spread of chronic infections. The choice of antibiotics should be based on the results of bacterial culture at the site of infection. Because different pathogens have different sensitivities to antibiotic treatment, fine needle bone biopsy or bone biopsy must be performed. In addition, treatment-related drug resistance needs to be considered during long-term treatment, and multiple antibiotics should be used in combination. The antibacterial spectrum should cover every pathogen. In addition, the time of intravenous antibiotics should be as short as possible, and replaced with oral antibiotics until the symptoms disappear. Adjustments and decisions should be made based on a combination of cost and efficacy.

Overall, the duration of antibiotic treatment for osteomyelitis adjuvant to surgery is generally limited to 6 weeks [106]. Long-term (6 months or more) intravenous or oral antibiotics did not show any significant improvement in the condition compared to 6 weeks of treatment [107].

#### 5.6.4.2 Local Application of Antibiotics

Because scar formation or vascular damage often occur in the injured area, leading to blood circulation disorders, it is difficult for systemic application of antibiotics to achieve an effective drug concentration in the lesion. Therefore, the application of local antibiotics is very necessary. The local antibiotics should have the following characteristics:

(a) The antibacterial spectrum is broad.
(b) The local drug concentration of the antibacterial drugs is high, it is easily soluble in water, and it needs to have sufficient stability.
(c) The adverse reactions of the drugs are small.
(d) Thermal stability, suitable for manufacturing process. In addition to the above-mentioned application of antibiotics for lavage, antibiotic sustained release system, namely, polymethyl meth acrylate (PMMA) beads rich in antibiotics, are commonly used for local treatment. After debridement, the antibiotic beads are packed into the ineffective cavity can significantly increase the local drug concentration and is widely used in clinical practice.

However, PMMA itself has certain defects, mainly including:

(a) Cannot be absorbed, need second operation to remove.
(b) No osteogenesis.
(c) The heat generated by the polymerization leads to the inactivation of antibiotics. In order to make up for the shortcomings of PMMA, high-dose antibiotic mixtures

of calcium sulfate are now widely used in the treatment of osteomyelitis.

Although calcium sulfate beads can avoid secondary surgery removal compared with traditional antibiotic beads as potential foreign bodies, these biodegradable products also have a number of disadvantages, such as:

(a) Not strong enough to bear the role of load-bearing filler.
(b) The number and types of antibiotics that can be carried are limited.
(c) Side effects during the degradation process can release inflammatory stimuli, increasing the probability of spontaneous fistula formation in the wounds.

## References


1. Fu XB, Sheng ZY, Cherry GW, et al. Epidemiological study of chronic dermal ulcers in China. Wound Repair Reg. 1998;6:21–8.
2. Guariguata L, Whiting DR, Hambleton I, et al. Global estimates of diabetes prevalence for 2013 and projections for 2035. Diabetes Res Clin Pract. 2014;103(2):137–49.
3. National Bureau of Statistics of China. China health statistical yearbook 2008. Beijing: China Statistics Press; 2008. http://www.moh.gov.cn/publicfiles/business/htmlfiles/mohbgt/s8274/200809/37759.htm
4. Iang YF, Huang S, FU XB, et al. Epidemiology of chronic cutaneous wounds in China. Wound Repair Regen. 2011;19(2):181–8.
5. Jiang YF, Wang X, Xia L, et al. A cohort study of diabetic patients and diabetic foot ulceration patients in China. Wound Repair Regen. 2015;23(2):222–30.
6. Reiber GE. Epidemiology of foot ulcers and amputations in the diabetic foot//Bowker JH, MA Pfeifer. The Diabetic foot. St.Louis: Mosby; 2001. p. 13–32.
7. Frykberg RG, Habershaw GM, Chrzan JS. Epidemiology of the diabetic foot: ulcerations and amputations//Veves A. Contemporary endocrinology: clinical management of diabetic neuropathy. Totowa NJ: Humana Press; 1998. p. 273.
8. Li X, Xiao T, Wang Y, et al. Incidence, risk factors for amputation among patients with diabetic foot ulcer in a Chinese tertiary hospital. Diabetes Res Clin Pract. 2011;93(1):26–30.
9. Jiang YF, Ran X, Jia L, et al. Epidemiology of type 2 diabetic foot problems and predictive factors for amputation in China. Int J Low Extrem Wounds. 2015;14(1):19–27.
10. Zhengguo W. Wound healing and tissue repair. Jinan: Shandong Science Technology Publishing House; 1998. p. 350.
11. Jeffcoate WJ, Harding KG. Diabetic foot ulcers. Lancet. 2003;361:1545–51.
12. Brunner G, Blakytny R. Extracellular regulation of TGF-βactivity in wound repair: growth factor latency as a sensor mechanism for injury. Thromb Haemost. 2004;92:253–61.
13. Antezana MA, Sullivan SR, Usui ML, et al. Neutral endopeptidase activity is increased in the skin of subjects with diabetic ulcers. J Invest Dermatol. 2002;119:1400–4.
14. Lin WD, Lu SL, Qing C, et al. Proliferation-inhibiting effect of advanced glycation end products modified human serum albumin to vascular endothelial cell ECV304. Zhonghua yi xue za zhi. 2003;83(7):572–6.
15. Xie T, Lu SL, Niu YW, et al. Study on the proliferation of epidermal cells of wound edge in deep partial thickness scald injury in rat. Chin J Burns. 2005;21(2):128–31.
16. Lin WD, Lu SL, Qing C, et al. The expression pattern of VEGF and bFGF in the deep partial thickness scald wound of diabetic rats and its relationship with the microvessel density of the wound. Chin J Burns. 2003;83(19):1702–4.
17. Yang YM, Lu SL, Dong JY, et al. Expression of epidermal growth factor receptor on superficial second-degree scald wounds in rats. Chin J Burns. 2003;19(4):243.
18. Gibran NS, Jang YC, Isik FF, et al. Diminished neuropeptide levels contribute to impaired cutaneous healing response associated with diabetes mellitus. J Surg Res. 2002;108:122–8.
19. Niu YW, Lu SL, Qing C, et al. Effect of extracellular matrix glycation on dermal fibroblasts. J Shanghai Jiaotong Univers (Medical Science). 2004;24(9):697–700.
20. Wang MJ, Lu SL, Sheng ZY, et al. Effect of high concentrations of glucose on the biological behavior of dermal fibroblast in diabetic rat. Chin J Diabetes. 2006;14(2):137–41.
21. Teixeira AS, Andrade SP. Glucose-induced inhibition of angiogenesis in the rat sponge granuloma is prevented by aminoguanidine. Life Sci. 1999;64:655–62.
22. Griffioen AW, Molema G. Angiogenesis: potentials for pharmacologic intervention in the treatment of cancer, cardiovascular disease and chronic inflammation. Pharmacol Rev. 2000;52:237–68.
23. Singer AJ, Clark RAF. Cutaneous wound healing. N Engl J Med. 1999;341:738–46.
24. Dong J, Takami Y, Tanaka H, et al. Protective effects of a free radical scavenger, MCI-186, on high-glucose-induced dysfunction of human dermal microvascular endothelial cells. Wound Repair Regen. 2004;12(6):607–12.
25. Falanga V. Wound healing and its impairment in the diabetic foot. Lancet. 2005;366:1736–43.
26. Ge K, Lu SL, Qing C, et al. A study on aminoguanidine improving wound healing of diabetic burn. Chin J Burns. 2004;20(8):463–7.
27. Lu SL, Qing C, Xie T, et al. Research on olfactory mechanism of the cutaneous "underlying disorder" in diabetic rats. Chin J Trauma. 2004;20(8):468–73.
28. Niu YW, Xie T, Ge K, et al. Cell proliferation and apoptosis in diabetic dermal tissues. J Shanghai Jiaotong Univers (Medical Science). 2007;27(4):376–9.
29. Lee RH, Efron D, Tantry U, et al. Nitric oxide in the healing wound: a time-course study. J Surg Res. 2001;101:104–8.
30. Shi HP, Efron DT, Most D, et al. The role of iNOS in wound healing. Surgery. 2001;130:225–9.
31. Witte MB, Thornton FJ, Tantry U, et al. L-Arginine supplementation enhances diabetic wound healing: involvement of nitric oxide synthase and arginase pathways. Metabolism. 2002;51:1269.
32. Ge K, Lu SL, Qing C, et al. The influence of L-arginine on angiogenesis in burn wounds in diabetic rats. Chin J Burns. 2004;20:210–3.
33. Fu XB, Wang DW. Modern trauma repair. Beijing: People's Military Medical Press; 1999.
34. Fu XB. Growth factor and wound repair. Beijing: People's Military Medical Press; 1991.
35. Fu XB, Wang DW. Foundation of wound repair. Beijing: People's Military Medical Press; 1997.
36. Fu XB, Wang ZG. Modern high technology and wound repair. Beijing: People's Military Medical Press; 2002.
37. Fu XB, Wu ZG. Modern wound dressings: theory and practice. Beijing: Chemical Industry Press; 2007.
38. Fu XB, Wang ZG. Regenerative medicine: principle and practice. Shanghai: Shanghai Science and Technology Press; 2008.
39. Fu XB, Lu SL, Jiang JX, et al. The construction of wound treatment center is imperative. Chinese J Trauma. 2009;25(9):769–70.
40. Fu XB. Pay more attention to the role of new and old technology in the battle (create, burn) wound surface repair. J Trauma Surg. 2007;9(4):293–5.
41. Yu Y, Fu XB. Establishing an education program for chronic wound care in China. Intern J Lower Extrem Wounds. 2012;11(4):320–4.

42. Fu XB. The practice of wound healing center construction in China. Chin J Burns. 2011;27(1):8–9.
43. Jiang YF, Xu ZR, Fu XB. Healing diabetic foot ulcers step by step. Intern J Extrem Wounds. 2012;11(4):307–10.
44. Fu XB. Translational medicine in wound treatment: research and application and thinking of some achievements. Chinese J Burns. 2014;30(1):3–5.
45. Heyer K, Augustin M, Protz K, et al. Effectiveness of advanced versus conventional wound dressings on healing of chronic wounds: systematic review and meta-analysis. Dermatology. 2013;226(2):172–84.
46. David OP, Sierra-Sosa D, Zapirain BG. Pressure ulcer image segmentation technique through synthetic frequencies generation and contrast variation using toroidal geometry. Biomed Eng Online. 2017;16(1):4. https://doi.org/10.1186/s12938-016-0298-3.
47. Tanywe A, Fernandez RS. Effectiveness of rifampicin-streptomycin for treatment of Buruli ulcer: a systematic review. JBI Database System Rev Implement Rep. 2017;15(1):119–39. https://doi.org/10.11124/JBISRIR-2016-003235.
48. Alhysoni KA, Bukhari SM, Hajjaj MF. Acute Marjolin's ulcer in a postauricular scar after mastoidectomy. Case Rep Otolaryngol. 2016;2016:2046954. https://doi.org/10.1155/2016/2046954.
49. Hinojosa CA, Olivares-Cruz S, Laparra-Escareno H, et al. Impact of optimal anticoagulation therapy on chronic venous ulcer healing in thrombophilic patients with post-thrombotic syndrome. J Wound Care. 2016;25(12):756–9.
50. Zhao R, Liang H, Clarke E, et al. Inflammation in chronic wounds. Int J Mol Sci. 2016;17(12):pii: E2085. Review
51. Hinojosa CA, Olivares-Cruz S, Laparra-Escareno H, et al. Impact of optimal anticoagulation therapy on chronic venous ulcer healing in thrombophilic patients with post-thrombotic syndrome. J Wound Care. 2016;25(12):756–9.
52. Molnar JA, Vlad LG, Gumus T. Nutrition and chronic wounds: improving clinical outcomes. Plast Reconstr Surg. 2016;138(3 Suppl):71S–81S. https://doi.org/10.1097/PRS.0000000000002676.
53. Dawson C, Naranjo C, Sanchez-Maldonado B, et al. Immediate effects of diamond burr debridement in patients with spontaneous chronic corneal epithelial defects, light and electron microscopic evaluation. Vet Ophthalmol. 2017;20(1):11–5. https://doi.org/10.1111/vop.12337.
54. Foster JA, Shukla P, Azar O, et al. Marjolin's ulcer of the pleural surface within a long-standing Eloesser Flap. Ann Thorac Surg. 2016;102(5):e383–5. https://doi.org/10.1016/j.athoracsur.2016.04.004.
55. Fourgeaud C, Mouloise G, Michon-Pasturel U, et al. Interest of punch skin grafting for the treatment of painful ulcers. J Mal Vasc. 2016;41(5):329–34. https://doi.org/10.1016/j.jmv.2016.08.002.
56. Hulsey A, Linneman P, Litt J. Clinical usage and economic effectiveness of a recently developed epidermal autograft harvesting system in 13 chronic wound patients in a university-based wound center. Cureus. 2016;8(11):e878. https://doi.org/10.7759/cureus.878.
57. Al Maksoud AM, Barsoum AK, Moneer M. Squamous cell carcinoma of the heel with free latissimus dorsi myocutaneous flap reconstruction: case report and technical note. J Surg Case Rep. 2016;2016(5):pii: rjw067. https://doi.org/10.1093/jscr/rjw067.
58. Johnston BR, Ha AY, Kwan D. Surgical management of chronic wounds. R I Med J (2013). 2016;99(2):30–3. Review
59. Grandjean A, Romana C, Fitoussi F. Distally based sural flap for ankle and foot coverage in children. Orthop Traumatol Surg Res. 2016;102(1):111–6. https://doi.org/10.1016/j.otsr.2015.10.010.
60. Lee BL, Ma H, Perng CK, et al. Clinical manifestation, diagnosis, and surgical treatment of chronic radiation ulcers related to percutaneous coronary intervention. Ann Plast Surg. 2016;76(Suppl 1):S68–73. https://doi.org/10.1097/SAP.0000000000000688.
61. Raposio E, Libondi G, Bertozzi N, et al. Effects of topic simvastatin for the treatment of chronic vascular cutaneous ulcers: a pilot study. J Am Coll Clin Wound Spec. 2016;7(1-3):13–8. https://doi.org/10.1016/j.jccw.2016.06.001.
62. Avijgan M, Kamran A, Abedini A. Effectiveness of aloe vera gel in chronic ulcers in comparison with conventional treatments. Iran J Med Sci. 2016;41(3 Suppl):S30.
63. Leclercq A, Labeille B, Perrot JL, et al. Skin graft secured by VAC (vacuum-assisted closure) therapy in chronic leg ulcers: a controlled randomized study. Ann Dermatol Venereol. 2016;143(1):3–8. https://doi.org/10.1016/j.annder.2015.06.022.
64. Enomoto M, Yagishita K, Okuma K, et al. Hyperbaric oxygen therapy for a refractory skin ulcer after radical mastectomy and radiation therapy: a case report. J Med Case Rep. 2017;11(1):5. https://doi.org/10.1186/s13256-016-1168-0.
65. Yu J, Lu S, McLaren AM, et al. Topical oxygen therapy results in complete wound healing in diabetic foot ulcers. Wound Repair Regen. 2016;24(6):1066–72. https://doi.org/10.1111/wrr.12490.
66. Stone R5C, Stojadinovic O, Rosa AM, et al. A bioengineered living cell construct activates an acute wound healing response in venous leg ulcers. Sci Transl Med, 2017. 9(371):pii: eaaf8611. https://doi.org/10.1126/scitranslmed.aaf8611.
67. Liu YC, Chhabra N, Houser SM. Novel treatment of a septal ulceration using an extracellular matrix scaffold (septal ulceration treatment using ECM). Am J Otolaryngol. 2016;37(3):195–8. https://doi.org/10.1016/j.amjoto.2016.01.013.
68. Capobianco CM, Zgonis T. Soft tissue reconstruction pyramid for the diabetic charcot foot. Clin Podiatr Med Surg. 2017;34(1):69–76. https://doi.org/10.1016/j.cpm.2016.07.008. Review
69. Julianto I, Rindastuti Y. Topical delivery of mesenchymal stem cells "secretomes" in wound repair. Acta Med Indones. 2016;48(3):217–20.
70. Hu J, Zhao G, Zhang L, et al. Safety and therapeutic effect of mesenchymal stem cell infusion on moderate to severe ulcerative colitis. Exp Ther Med. 2016;12(5):2983–9.
71. Meneses JV, Fortuna V, de Souza ES, et al. Autologous stem cell-based therapy for sickle cell leg ulcer: a pilot study. Br J Haematol. 2016;175(5):949–55. https://doi.org/10.1111/bjh.14326.
72. Gerami-Naini B, Smith A, Maione AG, et al. Generation of induced pluripotent stem cells from diabetic foot ulcer fibroblasts using a nonintegrative Sendai virus. Cell Reprogram. 2016;18(4):214–23. https://doi.org/10.1089/cell.2015.0087.
73. Raposio E, Bertozzi N, Bonomini S, et al. Adipose-derived stem cells added to platelet-rich plasma for chronic skin ulcer therapy. Wounds. 2016;28(4):126–31.
74. Afradi H, Saghaei Y, Kachoei ZA. Treatment of 100 chronic thalassemic leg wounds by plasma-rich platelets. Int J Dermatol. 2017;56(2):171–5. https://doi.org/10.1111/ijd.13443.
75. Zumla A, George A, Sharma V, et al. The WHO 2014 global tuberculosis report—further to go. Lancet Glob Health. 2015;3(1):10–2. https://doi.org/10.1016/S2214-109X(14)70361-4.
76. Unnetcioglu A, Sunnetcioglu M, Binici L, et al. Comparative analysis of pulmonary and extrapulmonary tuberculosis of 411 cases. Ann Clin Microbiol Antimicrob. 2015;14:34. https://doi.org/10.1186/s12941-015-0092-2.
77. Wang LX, Cheng SM, Chen MT, et al. Report of the fifth Chinese tuberculosis epidemiological sampling survey in 2012. Chin J Antituberc. 2012;34(8):485–508.
78. Wang HT, Zhang J, Ji LC, et al. Frequency of tuberculosis among diabetic patients in the People's Republic of China. Ther Clin Risk Manag. 2014;10:45–9.
79. Jia CY. Tuberculous wound - a neglected clinical problem worthy of attention. Chin J Inj Repair Wound Heal (Electronic

Edition). 2014;9(4):9–11. https://doi.org/10.3877/cma.j.issn.1673-9450.2014.04.003.
80. Li PC, Zheng ML, Qiu YB, et al. 8 cases with tuberculous ulcer wound on chest wall were repaired with skin flap combined with true skin flap. Chin J Burns. 2012;28(1):55–6. https://doi.org/10.3760/cma.j.issn.1009-2587.2012.01.014.
81. Moon MS, Kim SS, Moon YW, et al. Surgery-related complications and sequelae in management of tuberculosis of spine. Asian Spine J. 2014;8(4):435–45.
82. Chang N, Jia CY, Liu Z, et al. Epidemiological survey of 235 patients with extrapulmonary tuberculous wound. Chin J Burns. 2015;31(2):122–5.
83. Cheng L, Wang RC, Jia CY, et al. Clinical exploration of three-dimensional reconstruction of tuberculous wound. Chin J Burns. 2015;31(6):434–5. https://doi.org/10.3760/cma.j.issn.1009-2587.2015.06.011.
84. Slaninka I, Klein L, Čáp R, et al. Optimizing the treatment procedure in crural ulcers - a pilot study of the surgical method. Rozhl Chir. 2015;94(2):69–73.
85. Jia CY, Li PC, Cheng L, et al. Clinical application of surgical intervention in tuberculous wound of sinus tract. Chin J Burns. 2016;32(6):326–30.
86. George Cierny MD III, Mader JT, Penninck JJ. A clinical staging system for adult Osteomyelitis. Contemp Orthop. 1985;10:17–37.
87. Schmidt HG, Tiemann AH, Braunschweig R, et al. Definition of the diagnosis osteomyelitis diagnosis score (ODS). Z Orthop Unfall. 2011;149(4):449–60.
88. Kramer A, Hübner N-O, Weltmann K-D, Lademann J. Polypragmasia in the therapy of infected wounds conclusions drawn from the perspectives of low temperature plasma technology for plasma wound therapy. GMS Krankenhaushygiene Interdisziplinär. 2008;3(1)
89. Sönnergren HH, Strömbeck L, Faergemann J. The antimicrobial effects of plasma mediated bipolar radiofrequency ablation on bacteria and fungi relevant for wound infections. Acta Derm Venereol. 2012;92:29–33.
90. Yang R, Tantan Z, Zhu J, et al. Effect of radiofrequency ablation on healing of infected full-thickness wounds in minipigs. Int J Lower Extrem Wounds. 2013;12(4):265–70.
91. Cierny GD. Chronic osteomyelitis: results of treatment. In: Greene WB(ed). Instructional course lectures, vol. 39. Park Ridge, IL: AAOS; 1990. p. 495–508.
92. Santiago Restrepo C, Gimenez CR, McCarthy K. Imaging of osteomyelitis and musculoskeletal soft tissue infections. Rheum Dis Clin N Am. 2003;29:89–109.
93. Serkan Y, Kaan G, Tayfun A. The simple and effective choice for treatment of chronic calcaneal osteomyelitis. Plast Reconstr Surg. 2003;111:753–60.
94. Aronson J. Limb-lengthening, skeletal reconstruction, and bone transport with the Ilizarov method. J Bone Joint Surg Am. 1997:1243–58.
95. Barker KL, Lamb SE, Simpson AH. Functional recovery in patients with nonunion treated with the Ilizarov technique. J Bone Joint Surg Br. 2004;86(1):81–5.
96. Yang L, Nayagam S, Saleh M. Stiffness characteristics and interfragmentary displacements with different hybrid extemal fixators. Clin Biomech(Bristol, Avon). 2003;18(2):166–72.
97. Madhusudhan TR, Ramesh B, Manjunath K, et al. Outcomes of Ilizarov ring fixation in recalcitrant infected tibial nonunions — a prospective study. J Trauma Manag Outcomes. 2008;2(1):6.
98. Stange LD, Bauwens K, Sehouli J, et al. Systematic review and metaanalysis of antibiotic for bone and joint infection. Lancet Infect Dis. 2001;1(3):175–81.
99. Lazzarini L, Lipsky BA, Mader JT. Antibiotic treatment of osteomyelitis: what have we learned from 30 years of clinical trials ? Int J Infect Dis. 2005;9:127–38.
100. Lew DP, Waldvogel FA. Osteomyelitis. Lancet. 2004;364:369–79.
101. Haidar R, Der Boghossian A, Atiyeh B. Duration of post-surgical antibiotics in chronic osteomyelitis. Int J Infect Dis. 2010;14:752–8.
102. Parsons B, Strauss E. Surgical management of chronic osteomyelitis. Am J Surg. 2004;188:57–66.
103. Mader JT, Shirtliff ME, Bergquist SC, Calhoun J. Antimicrobial treatment of chronic osteomyelitis. Clin Orthop Relat Res. 1999;360:47–65.
104. Uçkay I, Lew DP. Infections in skeletal prostheses. In: Lippincott JW, editor. Bennet & Brachman's hospital infections. Philadelphia: Williams & Wilkins; 2007. p. 665–72.
105. Conterno LO, da Silva Filho CR. Antibiotics for treating chronic osteomyelitis in adults. Cochrane Database Syst Rev. 2009;3:CD004439.
106. Spellberg B, Lipsky BA. Systemic antibiotic therapy for chronic osteomyelitis in adults. Clin Infect Dis. 2012;54:393–407.
107. Calhoun JH, Manring MM. Adult osteomyelitis. Infect Dis Clin North Am. 2005;19:765–86.

# Tissue Repair and Over-regeneration: Prevention and Treatment of Scars During Tissue Repair and Regeneration

6

Xiao Wang, Lei Liu, Duyin Jiang, Shuliang Lu, Yingkai Liu, Wei Dong, Yongjun Qi, Jixun Zhang, Ya Jiao, Hongmin Gong, Wei Wang, and Xiaochuan Wang

## 6.1 Genomics and Genetics of Scar Formation

Wound healing is an extremely complex process, including the remodeling of parenchymal cells and surrounding cell matrix, angiogenesis and neurogenesis, immune system reconstruction, and other processes [1]. If the healing process is abnormal, the tissue around the wound continues to proliferate, causing excessive repair and regeneration of the tissue, eventually leading to the formation of abnormal scars [2].

In recent years, researches on scars are not limited to histology, biochemistry, cell biology, and other fields, using more advanced techniques to make more in-depth exploration of scar genomics and genetics from the molecular gene level. However, no specific cause of scar formation has been found so far. The production of scars is not caused by a single gene or a single factor, but by the interaction of multiple gene pathways and the combined effects of environmental factors. The research on the genomics and genetics of scar formation is of great significance for the prevention and treatment of scars.

Pathological scars mainly refer to hypertrophic scars and keloids. The pathogenesis and the treatment of these two are different.

X. Wang · L. Liu · D. Jiang (✉) · Y. Qi · J. Zhang
Y. Jiao · H. Gong · W. Wang · X. Wang
The Second Hospital of Shandong University, Jinan, China
e-mail: jdybs2@vip.163.com

S. Lu · Y. Liu
Ruijin Hospital, Shanghai Jiaotong University School of Medicine, Shanghai Burns Institute, Shanghai Wound Healing Institute, Shanghai, China

W. Dong
The First Affiliated Hospital of Jinan University, Guangzhou, China

### 6.1.1 Hypertrophic Scars

Hypertrophic scars are usually secondary to burns, trauma, and surgery. The prolongation of proliferative phase during healing leads to the continuous expression of collagen, elastin, α-smooth muscle actin (α-SMA), and fibronectin, forming non-functional tissues that protrude from the surface of the wound, which has a great negative impact on the local appearance and function of the patients.

High-risk factors for hypertrophic scar formation include severe burns, women, young age, dark skin, location (neck or upper limb), multiple operations, delayed healing, etc., especially after burns, and the incidence is as high as 30–72% [2, 3].

The study of genetic factors in the pathogenesis of hypertrophic scars is in its infancy, and the current research has not found specific genetic loci that lead to the onset of hypertrophic scars. DNA genotyping suggests that genetic variation may be related to the severity of hypertrophic scars [3].

Abnormal miRNA expression promotes pathological processes such as fibrosis, inflammation, cell proliferation, and ECM metabolism in hypertrophic scars. Mu et al. applied miRNA microarray technology to analyze miRNAs in hypertrophic scars, and found that compared with normal skin, 21 miRNAs showed significant differential expression, and MiR-143-3p inhibited the formation of hypertrophic scars. According to Zhou Renpeng et al., 24 miRNAs showed significant differential expression, including miR-21 and miR-200b, which are closely related to the TGF-β pathway and fibrosis process. In addition, miR-181c, miR-10a, and miR-199a-5p have all been shown altered expression levels in hypertrophic scars [4–6].

Abnormalities in mRNA expression profiles are also associated with the onset of hypertrophic scars. Differential genes are mainly involved in cell cycle, cell proliferation, immune response, and cell adhesion, and are mainly involved in focal adhesion formation, TGF-β signaling pathway, cell cycle signaling pathway, p53 signaling pathway,



X. Fu (ed.), *Regenerative Medicine in China*, https://doi.org/10.1007/978-981-16-1182-7_6

and tumor-associated signaling pathway, which further illustrates that hypertrophic scars are regulated by multiple pathways. These differentially expressed mRNAs and their involved signaling pathways may become new targets for gene intervention therapy of hypertrophic scars with potential clinical significance.

### 6.1.2 Keloids

Keloid is a benign dermal proliferative tumor, which is a pathological reaction secondary to abnormal repair of skin lesions. It is characterized by excessive ECM deposition, mainly excessive proliferation of fibroblasts and accumulation of collagen, showing a tumor-like growth pattern [7]. The high-risk factors of keloids include ethnic factors, the site of injury, tissue tension around the wound, infection, hormone levels, and the presence of foreign bodies.

Keloids have obvious genetic susceptibility, which is mainly manifested in the family hereditary, and the high incidence of specific races. Data have shown that people with dark skin are more susceptible to keloids. The incidence of African-American, Hispanic, and Asian-born people is as high as 15–20%, which is much higher than that of Caucasians, while albino patients have on incidence [7, 8].

Keloid is a disease caused by multi-gene involvement and mutation of many genes, and its genetic pattern and pathogenic genes are not clear [9]. In cases of familial hereditary keloids, single or multiple genetic loci are mutated, but these susceptibility loci are heterogeneous, racially specific and lack universality. Some scientists have found that 15q21.2–22.3, 2q23, 7p11, and other loci are associated with the occurrence of keloid in different families. In a study of two keloid families, Marneros et al. found that the genetic susceptibility locus of African-American black pedigrees is located in the 7p11 region, and the susceptibility locus of Japanese pedigrees is located in the 2q23 region. Liu Xiaojun et al. excluded the effects of chromosome 7p11 and 2q23 regions on the disease in the study of family genetic patients of Chinese Han population, demonstrating the heterogeneity and race susceptibility of susceptibility loci [10, 11].

Bian Xi et al. compared differentially expressed genes between keloid and normal skin, performed bioinformatics analysis of keloid-related genes, and screened 94 keloid-related genes (71 upregulated, 23 downregulated). Among them, key genes such as TGF-β1, FN1, COL1A1, MMP9, VEGFA, TP53, IL-6, and MMP2 may play important roles in TGF-β1 signal transduction, cell proliferation and apoptosis, tumor formation, and other related pathways, leading to the occurrence and development of keloids [12, 13].

## 6.2 Scar Formation Mechanism: Dermis "Template Defect" Theory

The wound healing process is completed by cells, cytokines, extracellular matrix, etc. Therefore, previous researches on the mechanism of scar formation have started from cells, cytokines, and extracellular matrix. With the deepening of research and the further expansion of the research scope, it is gradually realized that in the process of wound healing, cells, cytokines, and extracellular matrix play the role of "participants" or "executors." Their changes and the interactions are the follow-up "chain" or "waterfall" effects on scar formation, which is an "intermediate process" of repair, rather than the initiating factors leading to excessive hyperplasia of scar. So what are the initiating factors that affect scar formation? Some clinical and experimental phenomena have given us great inspiration.

Clinical practice found that:

(a) There is a great difference in outcomes after natural healing of burn wounds of different degrees. Shallow burn wounds do not leave or only leave slight scars after healing, and deep burn wounds often form obvious scars after healing [14].
(b) The healing results of autologous skin grafts with different thicknesses are also different. The degree of scar hypertrophy after deep wound skin grafting is inversely proportional to the thickness of the skin graft. Full-thickness skin grafts leave no scar.
(c) In frostbite wounds, although the blood vessels and cellular components in the skin tissue have lost their activity, if the dermal tissues other than blood vessels and cells are retained, there will be almost no hypertrophic scar after healing. These phenomena suggest that hyperplasia of scars may be related to the degree of dermal tissue loss. The use of skin substitutes (such as Integra, DermagraftTC, AlloDerm) can alleviate the excessive formation of scars to a certain extent [15, 16]. Further studies have found that such dermal analogs mimicking the structure of dermal tissue can support the infiltration of host FB, the formation of new blood vessels, and epithelialization [17]. Some researchers have referred to this role of dermal analogs as "template-like action," further suggesting that the reconstruction of the structure and function of the skin tissue at the injury site requires the involvement of certain layers and/or components of the dermal tissue in order to be completed smoothly. Such skin layers or components may mimic certain properties of the dermal tissue that are necessary for the outcome of cell function in wound healing and serve as a "template" to guide the trend of cell function. Defects in dermal tissue result in the absence of a "template" leading to excessive scar formation. So how does dermal

tissue play a "template" role? What mechanisms affect the changes in cells, cytokines, and extracellular matrix to produce a series of effects? Is it through the structure or components of the dermal tissue? Therefore, the study of its mechanism is helpful to understand the biological mechanisms of scar formation, for which we have conducted a series of studies.

### 6.2.1 The Effect of Skin Dermis Defect and Its Defect Degree on Scar Formation

In order to understand the relationship between the degree of skin dermis defect and scar formation, we observed the degree of scar hyperplasia under different degrees of skin dermal tissue defects and the formation of scars after autologous skin replantation with different thicknesses of tissue defects in the same degree.

In this study, 45 donor sites of 24 burn patients' limbs were selected as the study wounds, which were divided into the split-thickness skin donor sites (group A) and the intermediate split-thickness skin donor sites (group B). According to whether or not to transplant autologous skin with a certain thickness, group A is divided into the following subgroups, respectively, group A1 (without autograft) and group A2 (split-thickness autograft) and group B into group B1 (without autograft), group B2 (split-thickness autograft) and group B3 (intermediate split-thickness autograft). Skin graft specimens are retained, and the thickness of the dermis is measured by microscopic imaging system and image analysis system after tissue sectioning. The degree of scar hypertrophy in the above donor sites was scored in Vancouver Score 6 months after surgery. The results showed that the thickness of defective dermal tissue in group A was 0.146–0.163 mm, and in group B was 0.456–0.656 mm (Table 6.1) [18]. After healing, the Vancouver Score increased with the degree of dermal tissue defect, and there was a positive correlation between the two ($r = 0.597$, $P < 0.01$). After autologous skin grafting, the scar score was reduced correspondingly and the thickness of the grafted skin was negatively correlated ($r = -0.569$, $P < 0.01$) (Table 6.2) [19]. It can be seen that the degree of scar hyperplasia increases with the degree of dermal tissue defect, and the degree of scar hyperplasia relieved by skin graft replantation is directly proportional to the thickness of the replanted dermal tissue. For the first time, it is demonstrated theoretically that the degree of dermal tissue defect during wound healing process is closely related to the degree of scar hypertrophy.

The above experimental results suggest that the degree of scar hyperplasia increases with the degree of dermal tissue defect, the replantation of dermal tissue can alleviate scar hyperplasia, and the degree of scar hyperplasia reduction is

**Table 6.1** Measurement of dermal tissue thickness of wound defects and thickness of replanted dermal tissue in each group (mm, $\bar{x} \pm s$)

| Group | Number of wounds | Thickness of defect dermis | Thickness of replanted dermis |
|---|---|---|---|
| A1 | 9 | 0.146 ± 0.022 | 0 |
| A2 | 9 | 0.163 ± 0.035 | 0.138 ± 0.084 |
| B1 | 9 | 0.456 ± 0.150* | 0 |
| B2 | 9 | 0.656 ± 0.277* | 0.152 ± 0.071 |
| B3 | 9 | 0.603 ± 0.122* | 0.558 ± 0.095# |

Note: Compared with group A, $^*P < 0.05$; comparison of the thickness of replanted dermal tissue between group B3 and groups A2, B2, $^*P < 0.05$

**Table 6.2** Comparison of wounds Vancouver scores 6 months after skin replantation with different thicknesses ($\bar{x} \pm s$)

| Group | Number of wounds | Vancouver score of scar |
|---|---|---|
| A1 | 9 | 0.182 ± 0.050 |
| A2 | 9 | 0.111 ± 0.033 |
| B1 | 9 | 3.714 ± 0.498* |
| B2 | 9 | 1.050 ± 0.057# |
| B3 | 9 | 0.636 ± 0.055△ |

Note: Compared with each group, #compared with group A2, $^*P < 0.05$; △ compared with groups B2, A2, $^*P < 0.05$

related to the thickness of replanted dermal tissue. This led to another level of thinking, that is, why does the degree of dermal tissue defect affect the formation of scars? What is the effect of different degrees of dermal tissue defect on wound healing process?

### 6.2.2 The Effect of Skin Dermis Defect Degree on Wound Healing Process

In order to study the effects of different degrees of skin tissue defects on wound healing process, we carried out clinical experiments within the scope of ethics, and further verified and improved the results of clinical experiments through animal experiments.

In clinical trials, 94 cases of deep burn wounds after escharectomy were selected. The experimental group was acellular dermal matrix + autologous split-thickness skin graft, and the control group was autologous split-thickness skin graft. The wound healing process was dynamically observed from histomorphology and cell biology. In the animal experiment, 120 male Sprague-Dawley rats were used to create a 2.5 cm × 2.5 cm full-thickness skin tissue defect in the middle of the back. They were divided into four groups: natural healing group (control group), split-thickness skin graft group, full-thickness skin graft group, and composite graft group (acellular dermal matrix + autologous split-thickness skin graft). The changes in wound histomorphology, tissue biomechanical compliance, and repair of cell function were observed dynamically for 20 weeks.

Clinical trials confirmed that the granulation tissue was less in the composite graft group, fibroblasts (FB) and blood vessels could grow through the collagen gap of the acellular dermal matrix, and the structure after tissue repair (12 months after surgery) was closer to the structure of normal dermal tissue than that after simple split-thickness skin graft. Compared with the composite graft group, there was a large amount of new collagen deposition in the wound of the split-thickness skin graft group, and the ratio of FB differentiation into myofibroblast (MFB) was high and lasted for a long time, which was manifested by the sustained high expression of α-smooth muscle actin (α-SMA) in FB; high expression of endothelial cell marker CD34 suggested that vascular endothelial cells were active in function, proliferated vigorously, and had obvious capillary proliferation; TGF-β1 and its receptor TGF-βRI, II and its downstream signal transduction protein Smad3 were highly expressed, while the level of apoptosis was significantly lower than that of the composite graft group (Tables 6.3, 6.4, 6.5, 6.6, and 6.7). It can be seen that the reduction of tissue defect by composite transplantation not only decreased the proliferation, secretion, and synthesis functions of the repairing cells but also promoted the upregulation of apoptosis level. Its effect on repairing cell function is beneficial to reduce scar formation [20–24].

In view of the ethical limitations of clinical trials, we have further refined relevant research through animal experiments.

The histological observation in animal experiments showed that in the early stage of wound healing, FB morphology in the new wounds of the control group and each experimental group was spindle-shaped with obvious polarity, the long axis of the cells and the new collagen were arranged parallel to the skin surface, and the collagen fibers were thin and densely arranged; the collagen in the dermal tissue part of the graft (including the autologous dermis and the acellular dermal matrix) was thick, loose, and woven, the proliferating FB was arranged along the interstitial space of the collagen, and the cells were star-shaped with no obvious polarity. In the late stage of wound healing, compared with the control group, the new collagen in the wounds of each experimental group gradually became thick, loose, and woven, and the arrangement structure of the new collagen was close to that of normal skin tissue, the number of FB decreased significantly, and the cell morphology tend to be star-shaped from the bipolar shape in the early stage of wound healing. The proximity of collagen arrangement and cell morphology changes to normal skin tissue was most obvious in the full-thickness skin graft group, while the effect of autologous thin skin graft alone is poor, and the effect of composite graft group was close to that of full-thickness skin graft group. The above results indicate that the replantation of the dermal tissue accelerates the process of tissue remodeling in the state of natural healing.

In the first week after surgery, the collagen in the new granulation tissue of wound is thin and arranged parallel to the skin surface. In the 20th week after surgery, the procollagen gradually becomes thicker and arranged in a woven pattern, which tend to be characteristic of collagen arrangement in normal skin tissue. Among them, the full-thickness

**Table 6.3** Image analysis data of positive expression of mRNA in type III collagen and type III procollagen in each group ($\bar{x} \pm s$, $n = 9$)

| | Postoperative time (weeks) | | | |
|---|---|---|---|---|
| Test index group | 1 | 2 | 3 | 4 |
| Type III collagen composite transplantation group | 65.89 ± 5.25 | 58.27 ± 8.36 | 52.02 ± 4.85 | 51.83 ± 5.49 |
| Thick skin group | 66.35 ± 3.24 | 68.23 ± 5.60* | 68.28 ± 4.49* | 65.64 ± 6.92* |
| Composite transplantation group | 13.63 ± 3.40 | 17.34 ± 4.89 | 14.16 ± 3.32 | 5.29 ± 1.07 |
| Thick blade skin transplantation group | 24.40 ± 3.02 | 24.74 ± 1.87* | 22.54 ± 1.65* | 19.71 ± 4.16* |

Note: Compared with composite graft group, *$P < 0.05$

**Table 6.4** Comparison of CD34 expression in wound tissue of each group

| | Postoperative time (weeks) | | | |
|---|---|---|---|---|
| Group | 1 | 2 | 3 | 4 |
| Composite transplantation group | 4.0 ± 0.7 | 4.3 ± 0.9* | 3.5 ± 0.5* | 3.1 ± 1.13* |
| Thick blade skin transplantation group | 5.3 ± 2.0 | 5.4 ± 0.8 | 4.9 ± 1.72 | 5.6 ± 2.3 |

Note: Compared with split-thickness skin graft group, *$P < 0.05$

**Table 6.5** Comparison of p53 expression in wound tissue of each group ($\bar{x} \pm s$, $n = 9$)

| | Postoperative time (weeks) | | | |
|---|---|---|---|---|
| Group | 1 | 2 | 3 | 4 |
| Composite transplantation group | 19.87 ± 3.67 | 30.57 ± 10.90* | 27.08 ± 7.12* | 22.85 ± 5.19* |
| Thick blade skin transplantation group | 16.04 ± 3.67 | 18.60 ± 2.74 | 19.30 ± 3.02 | 18.16 ± 1.51 |

Note: Compared with split-thickness skin graft group, *$P < 0.05$

**Table 6.6** Comparison of positive expression rates of TGF-β1, TβRI, II, and Smad3 proteins in each group ( $\bar{x} \pm s$ , $n = 10$)

| Test index group | Group | Time after transplantation (weeks) | | | |
|---|---|---|---|---|---|
| | | 1 | 2 | 3 | 4 |
| TGF-β1 | Composite transplantation group | 13.08 ± 4.65 | 12.36 ± 1.51 | 11.18 ± 1.88 | 9.03 ± 1.89 |
| | Thick skin group | 19.24 ± 4.59* | 14.91 ± 4.17* | 13.66 ± 1.58* | 11.46 ± 2.37* |
| TβRI | Composite transplantation group | 6.87 ± 2.60 | 4.30 ± 2.19 | 2.92 ± 1.21 | 2.22 ± 0.68 |
| | Thick skin group | 10.62 ± 3.95* | 6.21 ± 2.09* | 4.22 ± 0.86* | 3.51 ± 0.74* |
| TβRII | Composite transplantation group | 4.34 ± 1.95 | 3.51 ± 0.88 | 2.76 ± 1.04 | 2.32 ± 0.49 |
| | Thick skin group | 6.81 ± 1.20* | 5.23 ± 0.86* | 3.99 ± 0.58* | 2.93 ± 0.64* |
| Smad3 | Composite transplantation group | 14.59 ± 4.22 | 11.36 ± 4.06 | 10.12 ± 2.02 | 6.32 ± 1.56 |
| | Thick skin group | 23.38 ± 4.00* | 16.54 ± 1.99* | 13.39 ± 2.03* | 9.60 ± 3.07* |

Note: Compared with composite graft group, $^{*}P < 0.05$

**Table 6.7** Comparison of apoptosis rate in wound tissues of each group ( $\bar{x} \pm s$ , $n = 9$)

| Group | Postoperative time (weeks) | | | |
|---|---|---|---|---|
| | 1 | 2 | 3 | 4 |
| Composite transplantation group | 15.90 ± 6.88 | 15.40 ± 2.61 | 23.54 ± 2.48* | 34.02 ± 7.20* |
| Thick blade skin transplantation group | 10.98 ± 2.34 | 13.36 ± 2.52 | 19.12 ± 3.44 | 4.61 ± 2.29 |

Note: Compared with split-thickness skin graft group, $^{*}P < 0.05$

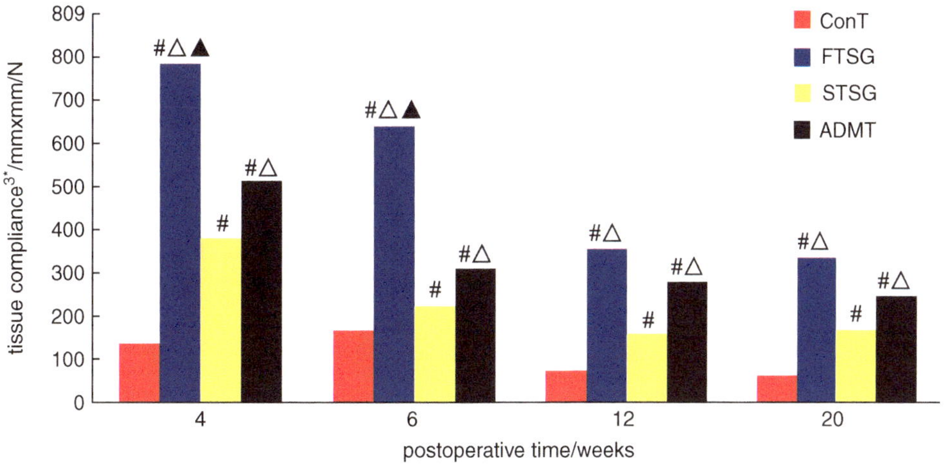


**Fig. 6.1** Comparison of biomechanical compliance of wound tissue in each group
Note: Comparison of biomechanical compliance of wound tissue in each group during wound healing
ConT is the natural healing group; FTSG is the full-thickness skin graft group; STSG is the autologous split-thickness skin graft group; and ADMT is the composite graft group
#Compared with the control group, $P < 0.05$; △ FTSG, ADMT compared with STSG, $P < 0.05$; ▲FTSG compared with ADMT, $P < 0.05$

skin graft group is the most obvious, while the effect of autologous split-thickness skin graft alone is worse, and the effect of composite graft group is close to that of full-thickness skin graft group.

Comparison of tissue mechanics compliance and FB function found: in naturally healed full-thickness skin tissue defect wounds, the mechanical compliance of wound skin tissue is poor, the proportion of FB to MFB differentiation is high and lasts for a long time, and cytokines and extracellular matrix components promoting scar formation such as TGF-β1, FN, and integrin α2β1 are highly expressed. If the tissue defect is compensated by dermal tissue replantation, the mechanical compliance of the wound skin tissue is significantly improved, and the functional status of FB including cell differentiation, expression of various extracellular matrix, and expression of matrix and the expression of cytokines promoting scar formation are significantly downregulated. Moreover, this effect is closely related to the thickness of the replanted dermal tissue. Full-thickness skin graft has the best effect and is superior to split-thickness skin graft. If the acellular dermal matrix is applied simultaneously with the transplantation of split-thickness skin (i.e., composite graft), the effect of simple split-thickness skin graft can be significantly improved (Fig. 6.1, Tables 6.8, 6.9, 6.10, 6.11,

**Table 6.8** Comparison of α-SMA-positive expression rates in wound tissue of each group ( $\bar{x} \pm s$ , $n = 6$)

| Group | Postoperative time (weeks) 1 | 2 | 4 | 6 | 12 |
|---|---|---|---|---|---|
| Natural healing group | $28.02 \pm 2.73$ | $33.53 \pm 1.62$ | $26.99 \pm 2.90$ | $8.60 \pm 0.74$ | $4.85 \pm 0.58$ |
| Full-thickness skin transplantation group | $8.32 \pm 1.44^{\#,*}$ | $15.71 \pm 1.82^{\#,*,\blacktriangle}$ | $6.29 \pm 0.77^{\#,*}$ | $5.39 \pm 0.44^{\#,*}$ | $1.71 \pm 0.32^{\#,*,\blacktriangle}$ |
| Thick blade skin transplantation group | $20.42 \pm 2.20^{\#}$ | $22.91 \pm 2.22^{\#}$ | $12.18 \pm 2.79^{\#}$ | $6.87 \pm 0.41^{\#}$ | $2.50 \pm 0.26^{\#}$ |
| Composite transplantation group | $10.28 \pm 3.99^{\#,*}$ | $21.78 \pm 1.66^{\#}$ | $7.53 \pm 0.98^{\#,*}$ | $5.70 \pm 0.46^{\#,*}$ | $2.20 \pm 0.28^{\#}$ |

Note: Other groups compared with the control group, $^{\#}P < 0.01$; comparison of FTSG, ADMT and STSG, $*P < 0.01$; comparison of FTSG and ADMT, $\blacktriangle P < 0.01$

**Table 6.9** Comparison of FN-positive expression rates in wound tissue of each group ( $\bar{x} \pm s$ , $n = 6$)

| Group | Postoperative time (weeks) 1 | 2 | 4 | 6 | 12 |
|---|---|---|---|---|---|
| Natural healing group | $33.23 \pm 0.88^{\#}$ | $33.00 \pm 2.38^{\#}$ | $36.76 \pm 2.88^{\#}$ | $31.43 \pm 2.06^{\#}$ | $17.93 \pm 1.66^{\#}$ |
| Full-thickness skin transplantation group | $19.48 \pm 2.00^{*,\blacktriangle}$ | $20.86 \pm 1.34^{*,\blacktriangle}$ | $18.65 \pm 2.24^{*,\blacktriangle}$ | $18.03 \pm 0.77^{*,\blacktriangle}$ | $5.86 \pm 0.66^{*,\blacktriangle}$ |
| Thick blade skin transplantation group | $25.66 \pm 1.71$ | $29.18 \pm 1.28$ | $26.59 \pm 2.61$ | $24.55 \pm 1.72$ | $8.59 \pm 1.09$ |
| Composite transplantation group | $22.06 \pm 1.43$ | $23.70 \pm 1.41^{\blacktriangle}$ | $21.94 \pm 2.24^{\blacktriangle}$ | $19.27 \pm 1.28^{\blacktriangle}$ | $6.10 \pm 0.41$ |

Note: Other groups compared with the control group, $^{\#}P < 0.01$; comparison of FTSG, ADMT, and STSG, $*P < 0.01$; comparison of FTSG and ADMT, $\blacktriangle P < 0.01$

**Table 6.10** Comparison of integrin α2-positive expression rates in wound tissue of each group ( $\bar{x} \pm s$ , $n = 6$)

| Group | Postoperative time (weeks) 1 | 2 | 4 | 6 | 12 |
|---|---|---|---|---|---|
| Natural healing group | $22.15 \pm 2.04$ | $26.96 \pm 3.18$ | $16.69 \pm 3.26$ | $7.94 \pm 1.26$ | $4.89 \pm 0.69$ |
| Full-thickness skin transplantation group | $14.40 \pm 1.62^{\#,*,\blacktriangle}$ | $16.78 \pm 3.08^{\#,*,\blacktriangle}$ | $7.76 \pm 1.06^{\#,*}$ | $5.11 \pm 0.43^{\#,*}$ | $3.49 \pm 0.99$ |
| Thick blade skin transplantation group | $19.45 \pm 1.22^{\#}$ | $23.12 \pm 1.51^{\#}$ | $11.72 \pm 1.56^{\#}$ | $6.48 \pm 0.56^{\#}$ | $4.35 \pm 0.63$ |
| Composite transplantation group | $17.26 \pm 1.38^{\#,*}$ | $19.97 \pm 2.04^{\#,*}$ | $8.18 \pm 1.07^{\#,*}$ | $5.69 \pm 0.66^{\#}$ | $3.95 \pm 0.68$ |

Note: Other groups compared with the control group, $^{\#}P < 0.01$; comparison of FTSG, ADMT, and STSG, $*P < 0.01$; comparison of FTSG and ADMT, $\blacktriangle P < 0.01$

**Table 6.11** Comparison of integrin β1-positive expression rates in wound tissue of each group ( $\bar{x} \pm s$ , $n = 6$)

| Group | Postoperative time (weeks) 1 | 2 | 4 | 6 | 12 |
|---|---|---|---|---|---|
| Natural healing group | $25.25 \pm 1.13^{\#}$ | $34.35 \pm 2.96^{\#}$ | $40.68 \pm 3.23^{\#}$ | $10.56 \pm 1.08^{\#}$ | $8.12 \pm 1.35^{\#}$ |
| Full-thickness skin transplantation group | $17.61 \pm 1.59^{*,\blacktriangle}$ | $18.71 \pm 1.07^{*,\blacktriangle}$ | $13.16 \pm 1.44^{*,\blacktriangle}$ | $5.89 \pm 0.44^{*,\blacktriangle}$ | $4.31 \pm 0.36^{*,\blacktriangle}$ |
| Thick blade skin transplantation group | $20.57 \pm 2.17$ | $26.51 \pm 2.61$ | $20.28 \pm 1.94$ | $9.04 \pm 0.98$ | $6.46 \pm 0.36$ |
| Composite transplantation group | $21.72 \pm 1.17$ | $21.64 \pm 1.46^{*}$ | $17.96 \pm 1.15^{*}$ | $7.05 \pm 0.79^{*}$ | $5.20 \pm 0.98$ |

Note: Other groups compared with the control group, $^{\#}P < 0.01$; comparison of FTSG, ADMT, and STSG, $*P < 0.01$; comparison of FTSG and ADMT, $\blacktriangle P < 0.01$

and 6.12). The results suggest that tissue compliance and functional status of FB are closely related to the degree of dermal tissue defect. The smaller the defect, the better the tissue compliance and the regulation of FB function, thus promoting the process of tissue repair to reduce scar formation [25, 26].

The mechanical compliance of wound tissue healed naturally is poor. Skin transplantation can improve the mechanical compliance of wound tissue, among which, the full-thickness skin graft group has the best effect, while the split-thickness skin graft group has the worst effect, and the effect of the composite graft group is between the full-thickness skin graft group and the split-thickness skin graft group.

The results of animal experiments are basically consistent with the trend of clinical experiments, indicating that the degree of skin dermis defect can regulate multiple aspects in wound healing process and is a key factor affecting scar formation.

Then, why does the defect of dermal tissue affect the mechanical compliance of skin tissue and the function of FB? What mechanism does dermal tissue play its regulation during wound healing? Is it through the structure or composition of dermal tissue? For this, we have carried out further research.

**Table 6.12** Comparison of TGF-β1-positive expression rates in wound tissue of each group ( $\bar{x} \pm s$ , $n = 6$)

| Group | Postoperative time (weeks) | | | | |
|---|---|---|---|---|---|
| | 1 | 2 | 4 | 6 | 12 |
| Natural healing group | 24.09 ± 0.96# | 36.83 ± 2.63# | 28.24 ± 1.62# | 24.23 ± 2.43# | 23.29 ± 2.11# |
| Full-thickness skin transplantation group | 18.27 ± 1.18 | 15.79 ± 0.80* | 16.74 ± 1.13*,▲ | 13.22 ± 1.89*,▲ | 10.67 ± 0.93*,▲ |
| Thick blade skin transplantation group | 18.88 ± 2.13 | 19.12 ± 1.93 | 22.66 ± 1.33 | 19.72 ± 1.44 | 16.79 ± 0.85 |
| Composite transplantation group | 18.31 ± 1.62 | 16.41 ± 1.88* | 18.66 ± 0.79* | 14.94 ± 1.11* | 14.39 ± 0.99* |

Note: Other groups compared with the control group, #$P < 0.01$; comparison of FTSG, ADMT, and STSG, *$P < 0.01$; comparison of FTSG and ADMT, ▲$P < 0.01$

### 6.2.3 The Role of Three-Dimensional Structure and Composition of Dermal Tissue in Regulating Biological Behavior of FB

The dermal tissue consists of two parts: the tissue structure and the composition. In vitro studies have shown that various extracellular matrix components can have different effects (inhibition or promotion) on cell function, and the relevant results are often obtained without involving their three-dimensional structure. Tissue structure can also have an important impact on cell function. So is the effect of dermal tissue on the wound healing process achieved through its structure or its composition? What is the relationship between the structure and composition of the tissue? For this reason, we have carried out further research.

#### 6.2.3.1 The "Permissive Effect" of the Dermal Tissue Structure on the Composition

We studied the effects of three-dimensional structures and three-dimensional structures of different materials on FB. The decalcified cancellous collagen and the biological sponge (porous material) were implanted into the subcutaneous of SD rats, and the samples were taken at the first week and the second week, respectively. The histological observation revealed that the collagen arrangement of the fibrous wrapping part (i.e., the part without the three-dimensional scaffolds) outside the decalcified cancellous collagen and the biological sponge was single and uniformly parallel, and the FB morphology was spindle-shaped with obvious polarity, which was similar to the FB morphology and collagen arrangement in the granulation tissue of the wound. While the morphology of FB migrating into the pores of decalcified cancellous collagen and biological sponge (i.e., the part with three-dimensional scaffolds) was diverse, and the collagen was arranged along the scaffold in a multidirectional manner, which was similar to the cell morphology and collagen arrangement of the autologous dermal part or acellular dermal matrix part of the wound graft. It is worth noting that:

(a) FB showed distinct cell morphology in different parts of the same wound (with three-dimensional structure part and no three-dimensional structure part).
(b) There were no significant differences in the effects on cell morphology and collagen arrangement between two different materials, decalcified cancellous collagen and biological sponge. Does this suggest that the three-dimensional structure of the tissue may play a dominant role in the effect of repairing cell function, and that the effect of dermal tissue on the wound healing process is mainly through its physiological structure? In order to further clarify the relationship between structure and composition, we carried out in-depth studies.

We used an in vitro culture model to study the relationship between structure and composition. The in vitro culture system of adherent cells is basically divided into two-dimensional culture and three-dimensional culture. Inoculation of cells directly on the culture dish or coating the culture dish with a certain extracellular matrix component and then inoculating the cells on it all belong to two-dimensional culture. Traditional three-dimensional culture coats the suspension of collagen and cells on the culture dish. If the collagen gel adheres to the culture dish base, it forms an anchoring matrix; if the collagen gel is separated from the culture dish base, it is a floating matrix. The anchoring matrix is in a high tension state due to adhesion to the culture dish base, similar to the two-dimensional culture, and the situation is similar to the hypertrophic scar. And the floating matrix has low tension, similar to normal skin, and is relatively close to the physiological state. A new three-dimensional culture model is currently established, which utilizes repeated passages of cells in situ and accumulates extracellular matrix secreted by cells during growth. This three-dimensional culture model has been proven to be more in line with the physiological situation in terms of composition, structure, and mechanical properties, and can more mimic the physiological state, known as the new three-dimensional matrix. On this basis, the new three-dimensional matrix is compressed by external pressure, which is called the new three-dimensional culture compressed matrix; or the new three-dimensional matrix is dissolved by enzymatic digestion and coated on the Petri dish, which is called the new three-dimensional culture dissolved matrix. The latter two methods aim to destroy their three-dimensional structure and essentially belong to two-dimensional culture.

The experiments were grouped as follows: FN, LN, collagen-coated culture matrix and new three-dimensional culture matrix, new three-dimensional culture compression matrix, and new three-dimensional culture dissolution matrix were used to observe the effects of different substrates on MFB induction. The results showed that FN, LN, collagen-coated culture matrix, and new three-dimensional culture dissolution matrix could induce MFB, especially the FN-coated culture matrix; the new three-dimensional culture compression matrix with structural damage can also induce the production of MFB compared with the new three-dimensional culture dissolution matrix, but the new three-dimensional matrix is difficult to induce MFB.

Why can different matrix components induce MFB under two-dimensional culture conditions? Why does the dissolved matrix or the compressed matrix with damaged three-dimensional structure can induce MFB, whereas the more physiological three-dimensional matrix does not induce MFB? Studies have shown that the mechanical properties of the two-dimensional culture system are similar to those of tissues in the early stage of wound healing, and can make the cell function in the culture system more active. The new three-dimensional matrix has been proven to be more physiological in terms of composition, structure, and mechanical properties. It can be seen that although the components of the extracellular matrix may have an effect on the function of FB, the effect is conditional and closely related to the structure of the extracellular matrix and its corresponding mechanical properties. Under non-physiological conditions, extracellular matrix components can promote the development of FB function toward over proliferation; when the structural and mechanical properties of the extracellular matrix return to the physiological state, the abnormal effects of the extracellular matrix components on cell function will disappear. Therefore, the three-dimensional structure of the extracellular matrix plays a "permissive role" in regulating cell function and affecting the outcome of tissue repair.

#### 6.2.3.2 Tissue Structure Is the "Template" that Guides the Trend of Cell Function

We observed that the morphology and collagen arrangement of FB in the larger pore size of decalcified cancellous collagen were closer to the granulation tissue wound, while those of FB in the smaller pore size were closer to the autologous dermis. This phenomenon suggests that the size of tissue spatial structure may have an effect on the function of the cells, and we have studied this phenomenon.

In the experiment, collagen membranes with three-dimensional spatial structure and pore sizes of 200 μm, 500 μm, and 1000 μm were implanted subcutaneously in SD rats, and the samples were taken for three consecutive weeks to observe the effect on FB function. It was found that the cell proliferation level of the 500 μm collagen membranes reached its peak at the second week, which was higher than that of the 200 μm and 1000 μm, and began to decline rapidly at the third week, which was lower than the latter two materials. The apoptotic level was opposite: The apoptotic level of 500 μm collagen membrane was lower than that of the 200 μm and 1000 μm collagen membranes in the first 2 weeks, and higher than the latter two materials in the third week.

The results suggest that there is a degree of regulation of cell function by tissue spatial structure. The appropriate three-dimensional structure can promote the completion of the cell cycle as soon as possible, and the inappropriate tissue structure is not conducive to the recovery of cell function.

This result was further confirmed in vitro experiments. The new three-dimensional matrix cannot induce MFB, and the cell morphology recovered quickly. Five hours after cell inoculation, the FB morphology was short fusiform and spread, basically normal FB morphology, indicating that the physiological cycle of cells on the physiological matrix was shortened. The cell adherent rate on the new three-dimensional matrix was about six times that of the two-dimensional culture (Fig. 6.2), and there was no significant difference in cell adherent rate between different two-dimensional culture matrices.

The above results indicate that the structure of the extracellular matrix is a "template" to guide the functional trend of cells, and the closer its structure is to the physiological state, the more favorable it is for the recovery of cell biological behavior [27–30].

#### 6.2.3.3 The Integrity and Continuity of the Tissue Structure Is the Key for Dermal Tissue to Play a "Template Role"

In vivo experiment, we observed that the acellular dermal matrix was filled with more granulation tissue in the void portion caused by dermatome in the composite graft, and the function of FB in this part was also active. Does this suggest

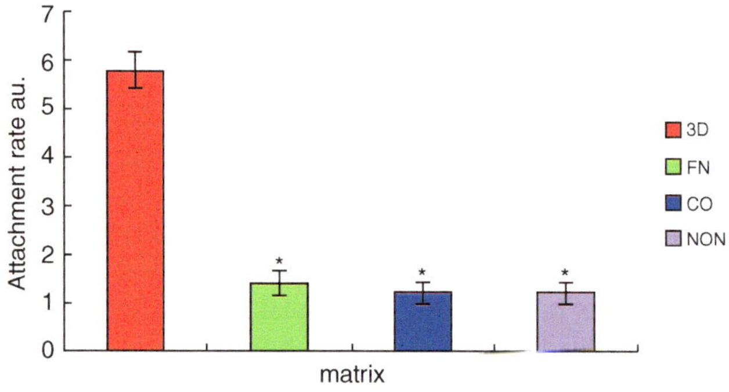


**Fig. 6.2** Comparison of FB adherent rate on different matrices in 10 min
Note: Compared with the 3D group, $*P < 0.01$

that the tissue integrity or continuity has a great impact on tissue repair? To verify this hypothesis, we designed experiments in which collagen membranes cut into pieces and structurally intact collagen membranes (with three-dimensional structure) were implanted subcutaneously into the back of SD rats, respectively, and sampled 1–3 weeks after the operation. Histological observation of sections showed that the granulation tissue with incomplete collagen membrane structure proliferated obviously, while the granulation tissue with intact structure was less. It can be seen that the integrity or continuity of the tissue structure is also crucial to the full play of its "template role."

In summary, the defect of the dermal tissue and its degree are the fundamental causes of scar hypertrophy. The mechanism is that the degree of dermal tissue defect affects the wound healing process. The three-dimensional structure of dermal tissue has a "template" guiding effect on the function of repairing cells, which can not only induce the growth of repairing cells but also improve the mechanical state of wound skin tissue, regulate the biological behavior of repairing cells, and promote tissue remodeling. The structure of the dermal tissue has a "permissive" effect on the composition. Under the non-physiological conditions, the extracellular matrix components can have an abnormal effect on the function of the repairing cells. Once the structural and mechanical properties of the extracellular matrix return to the physiological state, the abnormal effect of the extracellular matrix components on cell function will disappear. The appropriate three-dimensional structure can promote the completion of the cell physiological cycle, and the closer the structure is to the physiological state, the more favorable to the recovery of cell biological behavior. The integrity and continuity of the dermal tissue is the necessary prerequisite for tissue structure to fully play the role of "template." The damage of integrity and continuity of dermal tissue caused by trauma, which leads to the loss of "template effect" of dermis, may be one of the important mechanisms affecting the function of repairing cells and leading to scar formation. Therefore, the "template defect theory" of scar formation is proposed.

### 6.2.4 The Microscopic Discussion of "Template Defect Theory"

#### 6.2.4.1 The Influence of the "Bridge Piers" Like Structure of the Dermal Template Unit on FB

What is a suitable three-dimensional structure? What characteristics should a suitable three-dimensional structure have? To understand the role of the dermal template, it is necessary to be explored at the microscopic level.

We conclude that the template-like function of the dermis, as a functional manifestation of the dermal tissue structure, must have its basic composition. It has the necessary information of the dermal template, including the basic structure and composition of the dermal template. We call this basic composition the "dermal template unit." The dermal tissue can regulate normal biological behavior and phenotype of the cells through dermal template unit at the microscopic level.

So, how can we understand the regulation of dermal template unit on cells at the microscopic level? Firstly, fibroblasts in dermal tissue have adhesion characteristics. Secondly, the adhesive components are widely distributed in the extracellular matrix of the dermal tissue, and the cells can only function by forming adhesion points (focal adhesion) in combination with the adhesive components. Therefore, these adhesion components, which form focal adhesion with adherent cells, are arranged in the extracellular matrix like "bridge piers" to guide cell proliferation, migration, and expansion. In the local wound, the appropriate arrangement of "bridge piers" can effectively guide the cells to play normal functions, participate in the wound repair process, and maintain the original mechanical properties of the wound.

In this study, type I collagen was selected as the cell adhesion point material. A "bridge piers" like structure array consisting of type I collagen was fabricated on a planar matrix using micro printing technology. Meanwhile, molecular self-assembly technology was applied to cover cell non-adhesive material poly-lysine-grafted polyethylene glycol (PLL-g-PEG) molecules around the "bridge piers" to ensure that cells only adhere to the "bridge piers" (Fig. 6.3). This allows us to explore the regulatory effect of micropier grid used for cell culture (MPGCC) on cell function by adjusting the size and spacing of the piers within the micro scale of cells. After culturing with different parameters of MPGCC, FB morphology showed diversity, α-SMA expression increased, cell viability decreased, and hydroxyproline level increased, suggesting that MPGCC with cell adhesion characteristics can regulate cell biological behavior. However, the impact of the "bridge piers" like array design on cell biological behavior is far from the expected [31]. Therefore, how to understand the rational layout of cell adhesion points in the dermal matrix, that is, how to set the arrangement and effective spacing between the "bridge pier" and the "bridge pier," in order to achieve the desired purpose of tissue repair by regulating cell function, is worth our deep exploration.

#### 6.2.4.2 Mathematical Derivation of the Spatial Relationship of the "Bridge Piers" Structure Array of the Dermal Template Unit in the Three-Dimensional Structure

In order to clarify the relationship between the "bridge piers" like structure and the dermal template and the template unit, and to explore the rational layout of the "bridge piers" like structure in depth, we synthesized the previous research

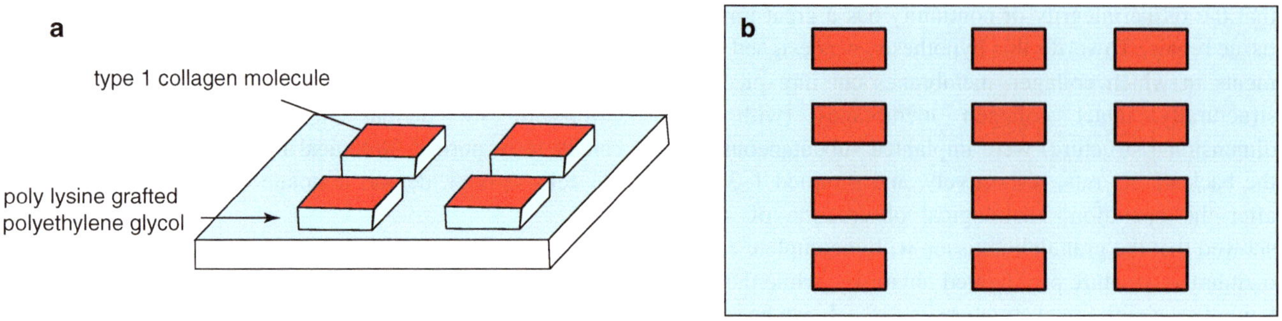


**Fig. 6.3** Schematic diagram of "bridge piers" like structure array for cell adhesion

Note: **a**—stereogram; **b**—plan. Red is slightly convex, coated with cell adhesion material; blue is base, coated with non-adhesive material

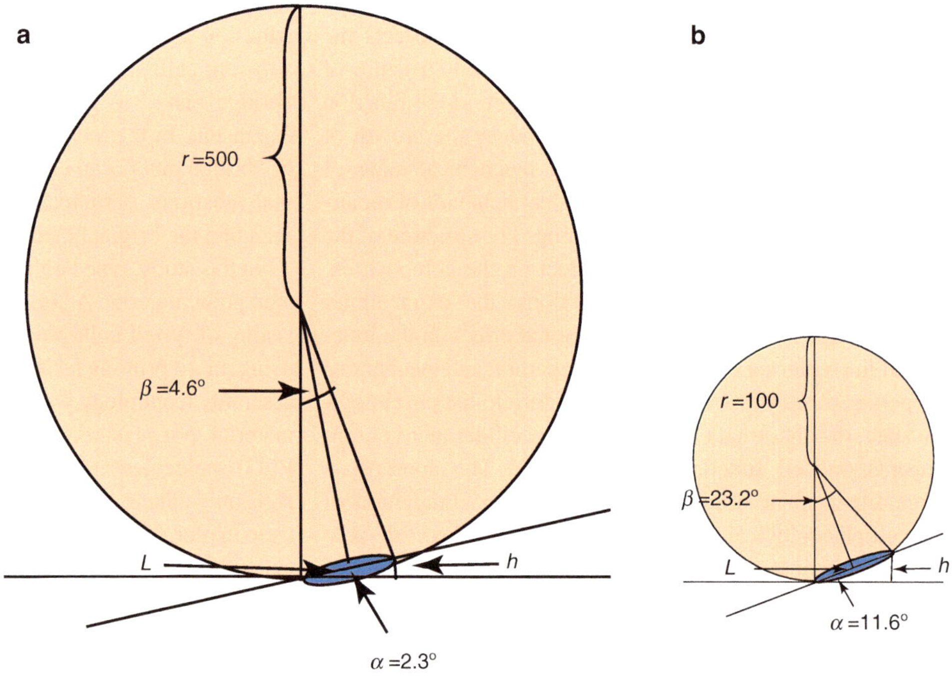


**Fig. 6.4** Mathematical schematic of cell adhesion in different pore sizes
**Note: *h* represents the height difference between the two ends of cells' long axis after cell adhesion. *L* represents the long axis of the cell. *r* represents the pore size. α represents the adhesion angle, and β represents the arc angle occupied by cells after adherence to the pore. ∠ $\beta = 360°/(2\pi r/L)$, $\sin\alpha = h/L$, $\sin(\beta/2) = (L/2)/r$, $\sin\alpha = \sin(\beta/2)$, therefore, $h/L = (L/2)/r$, $h = L^2/2r$**

results and used mathematical methods such as trigonometric function and plane geometry for analysis and verification.

Previous studies have suggested that the geometry in three-dimensional structures of tissues can alter the biological function of cells. The change of geometric shape in three-dimensional structure can be summarized as a combination of various curvatures. So, how to find the intrinsic relationship related to cell regulation in such a complex and variable curvature combination? We select circles with a single curvature for analysis. Assuming that the diameters of the circles are 100 μm and 1000 μm, and assuming that the length of the adherent cells is the same (40 μm), a mathematical derivation is used to illustrate the effect of curvature on cells. It is found (Fig. 6.4) that different curvatures have different deviation angles ($\angle\gamma$).

The larger the curvature, the smaller the aperture and the larger the deviation angle. Since dermal fibroblasts have the properties of contact adhesion with the material surface, the proliferation, migration, and extension of the cells are inseparable from the presence of adhesion points on the material surface. Therefore, the adhesion points on the material surface play a key role in the influence of curvature on the bending of the cell. When the cells adhere to the curved surface, the two ends of the cells' long diameter have different heights ($h$) from the cross-sectional observation. The smaller the aperture, the larger the deviation angle, the larger the height difference between the two ends of the cells' long diameter, and the greater the bending degree of cell adhesion on the curved surface. Ingber's study also suggests that the bending of the cell body will cause the cytoskeleton to bend, which in turn causes changes in cell function. It indicates that curved surfaces with different deviation angles can cause different degrees of cell body bending, which may be one of the reasons for the difference of cell function [32].

#### 6.2.4.3 Study on the Effect of Spatial Angle Arrangement of "Bridge Piers" Like Structure of Dermal Template Unit on Fibroblasts

Studies have shown that the movement of adherent cells in the extracellular matrix is fan-shaped, and this special shape is related to the distribution of focal adhesion on the cells. According to our view that the cells are regulated by the angle formed by the adhesion points, this sector shape seems to be simulated with different triangles. In order to verify this hypothesis, this study used CAD to design a "bridge piers" like structure array with different angles to observe their effects on cell biological behavior.

The horizontal and vertical lines are arranged on a 2 × 2 cm plane, and the spacing between the horizontal lines and vertical lines is 40 μm, forming a square grid with a side length of 40 μm. In each square, make a circle with a diameter of 40 μm. A vertical line from the center of the circle intersects with the circle as the first line, intersects with the circle through the center of the circle, and forms a $\theta$ angle with the first line as the second line, forming a sector area. Take the three vertices of the sector area as the center to make a circle with a diameter of 5 μm as the pier. The "bridge piers" like structure arrays with different angles are prepared by changing the angles of $\theta$ (20°, 40°, 60°, and 80°). The array consists of isosceles triangles with different apex angles. Define the two same sides (pier spacing) of the isosceles triangle as $L$ and the apex angle as $\theta$.

Then, the area of the triangle ($S$) = (bottom × height)/2 = $[L \times (L \times \sin\theta)]/2 = (L^2 \times \sin\theta)/2$.

That is to say, the area formed by the triangular "bridge-piers" like array is related to the angle change. The larger the angle is, the larger the area is. Fibroblast function test showed that with the increase of the regulation angle, the cell proliferation increased, the expression of α-SMA was downregulated, and the level of hydroxyproline secreted by the cells decreased, showing a trend of benign cell growth. It can be seen that the triangular structures with different angles composed of three cell adhesion points can regulate the cell functions differently.

Donald's research found that with the increasing of cell adhesion area, the extent of cytoskeleton stretching increased, and the cells could expand effectively, which was beneficial to cell survival. In this study, by changing the angle, the triangle area in the array increases with the angle, and the line between the three vertices of the triangle determines the area of the triangle. Therefore, through the variation of the spatial position of the three apexes with adhesion, the degree of stretch of the cells exerts an influence. Mathematical analysis found that this effect was related to the cell effect caused by the increase of adhesion area.

By adjusting the different triangular structures formed by cell adhesion points and their relationship with the degree of cell stretching, this study further demonstrates the view that cell biological behavior is regulated by the environmental structure. It is speculated that the triangle formed by the three cell adhesion points may be the basic framework for cells to manifest their functions in the matrix environment or the basic unit of the dermal template—"dermal template unit."

This study not only further enriches and supports the "dermal template defect" theory of scar formation mechanism but also provides a research platform for further studying the relationship between extracellular matrix material, three-dimensional structure, and cell biological behavior at the microscopic level by establishing a cell culture system of "bridge piers" array.

## 6.3 Scar Prevention

The formation of scars not only affects the appearance but also the severe scar deformity affects the function of the body [33]. The prevention and treatment of scars caused by different reasons are also different.

### 6.3.1 The Prevention of Therapeutic Scars

The therapeutic scars mainly refer to scars caused by iatrogenic injuries such as surgery, injection, and laser treatment.

(a) Prevention during operation: Superb suture technique is the key to scar prevention. Appropriate choice of operation timing and mode, aseptic technique during operation, elimination of invalid cavity, no foreign body residue, adequate reduction of wounds, and layered suture are all crucial [34]. The knot should be buried under the skin in subcutaneous suture, and the skin edge should be slightly everted [35] using the noninvasive suture needle thread and the knot strength to prevent the formation of "centipede-like scar" in the future [36].
(b) Prevention after operation: firstly, prevent wound infection. Antibiotic treatment is used prophylactically for contaminated or susceptible wounds [37]. After wound healing, early application of drugs and appropriate pressure therapy, at least 3–6 months [38]. Recent studies have confirmed that regular and quantitative injection of botulinum toxin type A around wounds can effectively inhibit the formation of postoperative scars [39].

### 6.3.2 The Prevention of Non-therapeutic Scars

Non-therapeutic scars mainly refer to scars caused by trauma and burns. These injuries are often severe and have different degrees of pollution. Therefore, the prevention of such scars focuses on prevention and control of infection, reduction of inflammatory reaction in wound healing, promotion of wound healing, and early closure of wounds.

(a) For large wounds that are difficult to heal with autologous skin, the transfer of adjacent flaps or autologous skin grafting can be considered to promote wound healing [40].
(b) Intervention in wound healing process. Physiotherapy can be used in the healing process, such as hyperbaric oxygen therapy, wax therapy, infrared therapy, and He-Ne laser treatment after the injury, to promote the early healing of wounds [41].
(c) Intervention after wound healing. The wound is healed, continuous compression therapy is applied for half a year. Early application of anti-scar hyperplasia drugs to prevent scar hyperplasia [42].

The prevention of scars is very complicated. A single method is sometimes difficult to work, and comprehensive intervention in a variety of methods can achieve better results.

## 6.4 Keloid Treatment

### 6.4.1 Surgical Resection

Surgical treatment is the main method for mature scars or keloids, which has the characteristics of direct operation and the most significant effect of reducing scar area in the near future. In view of the high recurrence rate after surgery, no single surgical treatment is used, but the combination of radiotherapy, drug injection therapy, and surgery is advocated. It should be emphasized that it is impossible to remove the scar completely by any surgical method, but to minimize or correct the damage caused by the scar; and after the healing of the surgical knife edge, it is faced with the occurrence of new scars, and the evaluation of the therapeutic effect needs to be observed for more than 1 year [43].

### 6.4.2 Physical Therapy

Commonly used are compression therapy, cryotherapy, laser therapy, radiation therapy, silicone gel sheeting, and adhesive tape therapy.

#### 6.4.2.1 Compression Therapy

Commonly used compression methods include binding elastic bandages, wearing stretch fabrics, wearing pressure earrings (for keloids on the earlobe), and wearing compression clothing. The effect of compression therapy on keloids is slow, the treatment time is long, and some body parts are inconvenient to operate.

#### 6.4.2.2 Cryotherapy

Cryotherapy uses cryogens such as liquid nitrogen to destroy cells and micro vessels in scars at low temperatures, resulting in hypoxic necrosis and exfoliation of tissues, so as to eliminate scars. The main adverse reactions are blister formation, delayed wound healing, depigmentation, or pigmentation.

#### 6.4.2.3 Laser Therapy

Laser therapy is currently the most promising and constantly updated treatment model for keloids. However, the main problems are insufficient penetration, insufficient treatment depth, unsatisfactory efficacy, and inevitable recurrence, which need further improvement [44].

#### 6.4.2.4 Radiation Therapy

Radiation therapy can be used as a single treatment or an adjuvant treatment after surgery. Side effects of radiation therapy include erythema, skin atrophy, ulceration, telangiectasia, pigmentation, and delayed wound healing. For younger people, potentially carcinogenic sites (breast and thyroid) and large area, multi-site lesions should be prohibited [45].

#### 6.4.2.5 Silicone Gel Sheeting

The application of silicone gel sheeting is easy to use, no pain and fewer side effects, which has been gradually promoted. It can avoid spinal growth and development deformity caused by chest bandage compression therapy in children, and is suitable for patients who cannot tolerate other methods.

#### 6.4.2.6 Adhesive Tape Therapy

Adhesive tape is used to prevent and treat keloids. It is characterized by low sensitization, suitable viscosity, multi-microporous, and some elasticity.

### 6.4.3 Drug Treatment

These drugs mainly include steroid hormones, retinoic acid, antitumor drugs, cytokine-related treatments, drugs regulating collagen metabolism, antihistamines, and traditional Chinese medicine, as well as calcium antagonists and tacrolimus (FK506), bleomycin and newly emerged drugs botulinum toxin type A (BTX-A), and other drugs [46].

#### 6.4.3.1 Apoptosis-Related Drug Therapy

(a) Steroid hormones: Corticosteroids for the treatment of keloids are mostly topical, and can be used alone or in combination with other methods. Postoperative steroid hormone therapy has become one of the most popular treatments for keloids. Common adverse reactions of corticosteroid therapy include skin atrophy, pigmentation or depigmentation, necrosis, ulceration, Cushing's syndrome, and physiological dysfunction, which can be reversed in a small part after withdrawal.
(b) Retinoic acid: Retinoic acid is a vitamin A-related drug that interferes with the synthesis of DNA in fibroblasts, inhibits proliferation, prevents collagen synthesis, and thus inhibits the growth of keloids [47].
(c) Fluorouracil: 5-Fluorouracil is a tumor chemotherapy drug, which can inhibit the proliferation of fibroblasts and the ability to synthesize collagen, and at the same time degrade the total amount of collagen, thereby achieving the purpose of treating keloids.

#### 6.4.3.2 Cytokine-Related Therapy

Anti-positive growth factors and negative growth factors such as interferon-γ can inhibit the secretion of recombinant basic fibroblast growth factor by fibroblasts, thereby inhibiting collagen synthesis, reducing wound inflammation, and inhibiting scar hypertrophy [48].

#### 6.4.3.3 Traditional Chinese Medicine Treatment

Traditional Chinese medicine believes that keloid is qi and blood stagnant in the meridians, is a sputum disease, is a meridian sputum, sinister poison and body turbidity, blood stasis caused by the disease. Traditional Chinese medicine has provided new ideas for the treatment of keloids with its advantages of syndrome differentiation and treatment, natural, non-toxicity, and various kinds [49].

Although there are many treatments for scars at present, there is a lack of recognized and universally effective standard methods. At present, it is generally advocated that a variety of methods should be used in combination at home and abroad, such as surgery, drugs, radiotherapy, cryotherapy, laser, and other therapies should be combined with two, three, or even four to achieve better results [50]. In general, surgical treatment is the main treatment for various mature scars, while compression therapy, radiation therapy, and drug injection therapy have a poor effect on mature scars, which are often used as auxiliary measures for surgical treatment. For keloids, surgery and drug injection therapy or surgery and radiation therapy should be used in combination, or drug injection therapy or radiation therapy alone can be used, but surgery should not be used alone. The research on the treatment of keloids has progressed rapidly and has now reached the level of gene and cell molecular biology. The recent development of gene therapy, stem cell therapy, and bioengineering technology will undoubtedly bring new hope for keloid treatment [51].

## References


1. Wells A, Nuschke A, Yates CC. Skin tissue repair: matrix microenvironmental influences. Matrix Biol. 2016;49:25–36.
2. Hompson CM, Hocking AM, Honari S, et al. Genetic risk factors for hypertrophic scar development. J Burn Care Res. 2013;34(5):477–82.
3. Finnerty CC, Jeschke MG, Branski LK, et al. Hypertrophic scarring: the greatest unmet challenge after burn injury. Lancet. 2016;388(10052):1427–36.
4. Sand M, Gambichler T, Sand D, et al. MicroRNAs and the skin: tiny players in the body's largest organ. J Derm Sci. 2009;53:169–75.
5. Mu S, Kang B, Zeng W, et al. MicroRNA-143-3p inhibits hyperplastic scar formation by targeting connective tissue growth factor CTGF/CCN2 via the Akt/mTOR pathway. Mol Cell Biochem. 2016;416(1–2):99–108.
6. Li C, Zhu HY, Bai WD, et al. Aberrant miR-21 and miR-200b expression and its pro-fibrotic potential in hypertrophic scars MiR-10a and miR-181c regulate collagen type I generation in hypertrophic scars by targeting PAI-1 and uPA. FEBS Lett. 2015;589(3):380–9.
7. Andrews JP, Marttala J, Macarak E, et al. Keloids: the paradigm of skin fibrosispatho- mechanisms and treatment. Matrix Biol. 2016;51:37–46.
8. Marneros AG, Norris JE, Olsen BR, et al. Clinical genetics of familial keloids. Arch Dermatol. 2001;137:1429–34.
9. Xiaojun L, Gao J, Song MEI, et al. Location analysis of susceptibility loci in Chinese Han keloid family. China J Cosmetic Plastic Surg. 2008;19:179–82.
10. Heitzer E, Seidl H, Bambach I, et al. Infrequent p53 gene mutation but UV gradient-like p53 protein positivity in keloids. Exp Dermatol. 2012;21:277–80.
11. Brown JJ, Bayat A. Genetic susceptibility to raised dermal scarring. Br J Dermatol. 2009;161(1):8–18.
12. Teng GD, Liu C, Chen ML, et al. Differential susceptible loci expression in keloid and hypertrophic scars in Chinese Han population. Annals of plastic surgery. Ann Plastic Surg. 2015;74(1):26–9.
13. Bian B, Wei H, Bolun L, et al. Bioinformatics analysis of keloid related genes. Chinese J Minim Invasive Surg. 2012;12:444–9.
14. Wainwright D, Madden M, Luterman A, et al. Clinical evaluation of an acellular allograft dermal matrix in full-thickness burns. J Burn Care Rehabil. 1996;17(2):124–36.
15. Jia SX, Liao ZJ, Huang BG, et al. The clinical application of composite transplantation of acelluar dermal matrix with autograft. Chin J Plast Srug. 2001;17:227–9.
16. Livesey SA, Herndon DN, Hollyoak MA, et al. Transplanted acellular allograft dermal matrix: potential as a template for the reconstruction of viable dermis. Transplantation. 1995;60(1):1–9.
17. Yannas IV. Studies on the biological activity of the dermal regeneration template. Wound Repair Regen. 1998;6(6):518–23.
18. Su HT, Li ZY, Lu SL, et al. The clinical study of the relationship between the defect of different thickness dermal tissues and the proliferative scar formation. Chin J Traumatol. 2005;21(7):517–9.
19. Xiang J, Hu QS, Qing C, et al. The dynamic histological observations of grafting dermal regeneration template with thin autogenic skin in burn patients. Acta Universitatis Medicinalis Secondae Shanghai. 2003;23(6):492–4.
20. Zhang J, Xiang J, Wang ZY, et al. The effect of dermal regeneration template on wound collagen synthesis. Acta Universitatis Medicinalis Secondae Shanghai. 2003;23(5):393–5.

21. Xiang J, Qing C, Liao ZJ, et al. Effect of dermal regeneration template on myofibroblasts and cell apoptosis during wound healing. Chin J Traumatol. 2004;20(2):85–8.
22. Wang XQ, Xiang J, Hu QS, et al. The angiogenesis effect after application of dermal template on wound. Chin J Clin Rehab. 2003;7(23):3194–5.
23. Xiang J, Wang XQ, Qing C, et al. The influence of dermal template on the expressions of signal transduction protein Smad 3 and transforming growth factorβ1 and its receptor during wound healing process in patients with deep burns. Chin J Burns. 2005;21(1):52–4.
24. Wang XQ, Su HT, Xiang J, et al. The influence of dermal template on the p53 gene expression and apoptosis during wound repairing in burn patients. Chin J Burns. 2004;20(6):351–3.
25. Liu YK, Lu SL, Qing C. The effects of tissue mechanical compliance on the biological behaviors of fibroblasts during wound healing. Shanghai: Shanghai Second Medical University; 2003.
26. Liu YK, Lu SL, Qing C, et al. Influence of dermal template on the biomechanical compliance of wound tissue. Chin J Burns. 2005;21(2):122–4.
27. Liu YK, Lu SL, Qing C, et al. Effects of dermal template on the biological behaviors of fibroblasts during wound healing. Chin J Reparative Reconstruct Surg. 2005;19(1):10–4.
28. Mao ZG, Lu SL, Qing C. The effect of three-dimensional structure on the biological behaviors of fibroblasts. Shanghai: Shanghai Second Medical University; 2005.
29. Liu YK, Lu SL. Effect of mechanical stimulation on the outcome of myofibroblasts. Chin J Traumatol. 2002;18(11):703–4.
30. Cukierman E, Pankov R, Stevens DR, et al. Taking cell-matrix adhesions to the third dimension. Science. 2001;23(294):1710.
31. Zhang FS, Lu SL, Qing C. Study on the mechanism of scar formation-the induction of myofibroblasts and their signal transduction. Shanghai: Shanghai Jiao Tong University School of Medicine; 2006.
32. Jiang YZ, Ding GP, Lu SL, et al. Exploratory study on the microremodeling of dermal tissue. Chin J Burns. 2009;25(5):343–51.
33. Borovikova AA, King K, et al. Current concepts related to hypertrophic scarring in burn injuries. Wound Repair Regen. 2016;24(3):466–77.
34. Lim JY, Song WK, Whang KK. Scar-saving flap during serial excision by borrowing from the opposite side. Ann Dermatol. 2008;20(3):120–5.
35. Zhang X, Diao JS, Guo SZ, et al. Wedge-shaped excision and modified vertical mattress suture fully buried in a multilayered and tensioned wound closure. Aesthet Plast Surg. 2009;33(3):457–60.
36. Saleh F, Palmieri B, Lodi D, et al. An innovative method to evaluate the suture compliance in sealing the surgical wound lips. Int J Med Sci. 2008;5(6):354–60.
37. Fijan S, Frauwallner A, Langerholc T, et al. Efficacy of using probiotics with antagonistic activity against pathogens of wound infections: an integrative review of literature. Biomed Res Int. 2019;2019:7585486.
38. Atiyeh BS, Chahine F. Local injection of botulinum toxin type a to prevent postoperative scar: comment. J Craniofac Surg 2020.
39. Appropriate timing of early postoperative botulinum toxin type a injection for thyroidectomy scar management: a split-scar study: correction. Plast Reconstr Surg. 2020;145(1):289.
40. Olbrisch RR. Continuous Y-V-plasty. Handchir Mikrochir Plast Chir. 1984;16(4):246–50.
41. Writing group of consensus on treatment of skin traumatic scars with photoelectric therapy and radio-frequency technology (0 8 version); [Consensus on treatment of skin traumatic scars with photoelectric therapy and radio-frequency technology (2018 version)]. Zhonghua Shao Shang Za Zhi. 2018;34(9):593–7.
42. Caviggioli F, Vinci V, Vappiani M, et al. Evidence-based scar management: how to improve results with technique and technology. Plast Reconstr Surg. 2017;139(6):1371e–3e.
43. Longowal MS, Humphreys RN B, Remington TK. Multidisciplinary treatment of a massive head and neck keloid scar: a case report. SAGE Open Med Case Rep. 2020;8 https://doi.org/10.1177/2050313X20936033.
44. Fuenmayor P, Quiñonez H, Salas R, et al. Experience treating earlobe keloids with laser diode 980?nm excision followed by triamcinolone infiltration. Lasers Surg Med. 2020.
45. Anderson EM, David J, Phillips T, et al. Interstitial high-dose-rate brachytherapy in the treatment of keloids: moving toward a volumetric approach. Brachytherapy. 2020.
46. Limmer EE, Glass DA. A review of current keloid management: mainstay monotherapies and emerging approaches. Dermatol Ther (Heidelb). 2020.
47. Mirza FN, Mirza HN, Khatri KA. Concomitant use of isotretinoin and lasers with implications for future guidelines: an updated systematic review. Dermatol Ther. 2020:e14022.
48. Sohrabi C, Goutos I. The use of botulinum toxin in keloid scar management: a literature review. Scars Burn Heal. 2020;6:2059513120926628.
49. Si L, Zhang M, Guan E, et al. Resveratrol inhibits proliferation and promotes apoptosis of keloid fibroblasts by targeting HIF-1α. J Plast Surg Hand Surg. 2020:1–7.
50. Ojeh N, Bharatha A, Gaur U, et al. Keloids: current and emerging therapies. Scars Burn Heal. 2020;6:2059513120940499.
51. Yang D, Li M, Du N. Effects of the circ_101238/miR-138-5p/CDK6 axis on proliferation and apoptosis keloid fibroblasts. Exp Ther Med. 2020;20(3):1995–2002.

# Repair and Regeneration After Important Visceral Injury

# 7

Biao Cheng, Xiaobing Fu, Jianxin Jiang, Ce Yang, Haisheng Li, Shuyong Wang, Yunfang Wang, Yuesheng Huang, Xiaoguang Li, Zhaoyang Yang, Hongmei Duan, Wen Zhao, Yudan Gao, and Peng Hao

## 7.1 Overview of Visceral Injury Repair and Regeneration

### 7.1.1 Recognition of Visceral Injury and Repair

Visceral organs are the participants and maintainers of various life activities of the body. Various injuries such as trauma, surgery, organ transplantation, inflammatory bowel disease, and other serious diseases will cause damage to internal organs. The main reason is the double impact of ischemia and reperfusion, which in turn causes the activation of complement-phagocytic-lymphocyte in the body, causing local and systemic inflammatory reactions, dysfunction of coagulation system, hypermetabolic status, etc., eventually leading to multiple organ dysfunction syndrome (MODS), and even multiple systemic organ failure (MSOF) also called multiple organ failure (MOF). Visceral organ damage, especially multiple organ function damage, is an important feature of the aggravation of traumatic injury and the occurrence of complications. For open wounds, damaged organs can be repaired and reconstructed by surgery. However, for closed injury such as ischemia-reperfusion injury to intestine, liver, kidney, and lung; ischemic injury of donors during organ transplantation; and multiple organ damage after traumatic (burn) injury, especially the occult shock of the intestinal tract, etc., the organ itself has ischemic damage that is difficult to distinguish with the naked eye; the pathogenesis of such damage is complex, wide, and concealed; there is a lack of effective prosthetic measures; and the repair after injury is often not easy to attract people's attention, thus leading to the death of patients. According to experts' statistics, more than half of all deaths are caused by visceral complications after severe burns; two-thirds of the injured in serious traffic accidents are accompanied by visceral injury, which is the primary cause of disability and death. MODS is also ranked first in the cause of death in the intensive care unit. In general, the death of the visceral injury after severe trauma is mainly divided into two stages: early death, which is closely related to shock or severe brain injury; and late death, which is mainly caused by MODS or multiple system organ failure (MSOF), and its occurrence is associated with systemic inflammatory response syndrome (SIRS), ischemia-reperfusion injury, and endotoxemia. Among them, organ ischemia-reperfusion injury and microcirculatory dysfunction (the second hit) are one of the central links of visceral complications after severe trauma. For visceral injury, previous studies focused on the pathogenesis of visceral injury and initially clarified the role of infection, uncontrolled inflammatory response, and oxygen-free radical activation in the occurrence of severe visceral injury. However, it is worth noting that previous studies have focused too much on the pathogenesis of organ damage, while there is a lack of in-depth discussion on the outcome of damaged organs. Therefore, it is essential to strengthen the prevention and treatment of vis-

B. Cheng
General Hospital of Southern Theater Command of Chinese People's Liberation Army, Guangzhou, China

X. Fu (✉) · S. Wang
The Chinese People's Liberation Army General Hospital, Beijing, China

J. Jiang · H. Li · C. Yang
State Key Laboratory of Trauma, Burns and Combined Injury, Research Institute of Surgery, Daping Hospital, Army Medical University, Chongqing, China

Y. Wang
Academy of Military Medical Sciences, Military Medical Research Institute, Beijing, China

Y. Huang
Shenzhen People's Hospital, The First Affiliated Hospital of Southern University of Science and Technology, The Second Clinical Medical College of Jinan University, Shenzhen, China

X. Li · Z. Yang · H. Duan · W. Zhao · Y. Gao · P. Hao
Department of Neurobiology, School of Basic Medical Sciences, Capital Medical University, Beijing, China


X. Fu (ed.), *Regenerative Medicine in China*, https://doi.org/10.1007/978-981-16-1182-7_7

ceral injuries and promote the early repair and reconstruction of damaged organs to guarantee life safety. How to accelerate and promote the repair of damaged internal organs has become the key to determine the success of serious trauma treatment, especially to prevent MODS and MSOF.

It has been thought that higher animals contain many cell types, mainly postmitotic cells and mitotic cells. The former include mature neurons, muscle cells, and adipocytes, while the latter include epithelial cells, etc. Due to their differences in proliferative capacity, the repair of the organism has two forms: physiological and nonphysiological. Even tissues or organs composed of dividing cells, there are two extreme pathological repair outcomes beyond the physiological range: insufficient repair and excessive repair. Traditionally, the repair processes of tissue injuries are divided into three main stages: inflammation and exudation, granulation tissue hyperplasia, and scar formation and remodeling. Regenerative repair is the ideal ending for tissue repair, which is composed of signals of biological development and prosthodontics. The repair of visceral ischemic injury after severe trauma, as well as other basic problems after trauma, such as shock prevention and infection treatment, is an important and unresolved issue in this field. They are not only related to the recovery of damaged visceral anatomy and function under severe trauma and critical illness conditions but also important for the prevention and treatment of late complications, such as multiple organ dysfunction syndrome (MODS). With the increasing harm of trauma to modern society and the deepening of people's understanding of the concept and connotation of tissue repair, especially the successful application of techniques and methods in the field of molecular biology to surface wound repair makes it possible to repair the visceral ischemic injury after severe trauma, especially the active repair. It has not only attracted the attention of scholars but also gradually become a hot spot in this field.

### 7.1.2 The Repair and Regeneration of Visceral Injuries

#### 7.1.2.1 Heart Damage and Repair

Cardiomyocytes lack the ability to proliferate and differentiate. Myocardial cells cannot regenerate after myocardial infarction, and eventually become the scar tissue, which is the main cause of refractory heart failure and death in patients with myocardial infarction. Current treatments are difficult to fundamentally restore the number of cardiomyocytes and improve myocardial contractile and relaxant function. In 1999, Makino et al. first discovered that mouse mesenchymal stem cells (MSCs) can induce spontaneous beating cells with morphology and electromechanical characteristics of cardiomyocytes after 5-azacytidine treatment in vitro. Wang et al. further demonstrated that MSCs can induce and differentiate into cardiomyocyte-like cells in the local microenvironment of the heart in vivo, which provided a theoretical basis for MSC transplantation for myocardial ischemia-reperfusion injury. Silva et al. injected MSCs into an animal model of acute myocardial infarction and found that MSCs can differentiate into vascular endothelial cells, enhance angiogenic ability, and enhance blood flow recovery in ischemic areas. Yoon et al. also found that transplanted MSCs not only promoted the formation of new blood vessels but also had the ability to differentiate into cardiomyocytes. Subsequently, the clinical application of MSC transplantation for ischemic heart disease has also been fully developed. Recent animal experiments and early clinical studies have shown that stem cell transplantation can replace necrotic cardiomyocytes, increase the number of functional cardiomyocytes, and improve cardiac function. In 2004, the team of Planat-Bénard identified a very small subset of cardiomyocyte-like cells (0.02–0.07%) in murine stromal vascular fraction (SVF), showing contractile behavior in 24 days of primary culture. These cells are positive for several cardiac-specific genes, including GATA-4 and Nkx2.5. In 2007, Song et al. demonstrated a similar small subset of human SVF cells that spontaneously beat (0.005–0.07%). The combination of ADSCs and bFGF-β in the mouse hindlimb ischemia model and control the release of bFGF can lead to angiogenesis and maturation. This is partly due to the secretion of hepatocyte growth factor, vascular endothelial growth factor, and transforming growth factor β1. In 2011, Friis et al. published a study on the safety and feasibility of intramyocardial injection of cultured bone marrow mesenchymal stem cells in patients with stable coronary artery disease (CAD). They treated a total of 31 patients and concluded that the treatment was safe and could significantly improve left ventricular function and exercise tolerance. Young et al. pointed out that ADSCs can improve cardiac function through cell differentiation and paracrine pathways. It is expected that clinical trials will be carried out in the near future to open up a new way for the treatment of heart injury, which has become the focus of cardiovascular disease researchers in recent years.

Embryonic stem cells (ESCs) are pluripotent stem cells that can differentiate into functional cardiomyocytes and improve left ventricular function. The problems with the use of ESCs are mainly immune rejection and tumorigenicity. At the same time, ethical issues are fundamental problems that constrain its widespread application. Takahashi et al. found that induced pluripotent stem cells (iPSCs) are cells with similar immunophenotype to ESCs, which solve the rejection problem of allogeneic ESC transplantation, but cannot avoid tumorigenicity. Inducing somatic cell reprogramming into iPSCs is inefficient, complicated, and cumbersome, which is not suitable for large-scale clinical application.

Since the clinical trials of stem cell transplantation are still in the exploratory stage, the stem cell transplantation techniques used include direct thoracotomy injection, catheter intervention, and transvenous transplantation, so there is controversy. The evaluation of the therapeutic effect of stem cell transplantation includes the survival of reinfused stem cells, the proportion of stem cells into normal cardiomyocytes, and whether the neonatal cardiomyocytes have the physiological characteristics of normal cardiomyocytes. However, there is still a lack of authoritative conclusions on the appropriate evaluation index of clinical effect. In short, stem cell transplantation is a new method for treating heart damage, and it has great application prospects with its unique advantages.

#### 7.1.2.2 Pancreatic Injury and Repair

Islet transplantation is a hot spot for the treatment of diabetes, but the lack of donors and the existence of immune rejection limit its application. Pancreatic stem cells can be differentiated into islet cells, which provides a new source of material for islet transplantation. Pancreatic stem cells can be directionally induced to the exocrine gland tissue, which plays an important role in the study of the occurrence, development, and treatment of acute and chronic pancreatitis, and can repair pancreatic insufficiency caused by pancreatic trauma. Studies have shown that pancreatic stem cells have important research value for the occurrence, development, regulation, and treatment of pancreatic cancer. The mechanism of bone marrow mesenchymal stem cells in the treatment of chronic pancreatitis may be related to the following points: (a) Bone marrow mesenchymal stem cells as "seed" cells can colonize the damaged pancreas in chronic pancreatitis and transform into pancreatic "target tissue cells," such as pancreatic stem cells, ductal cells, acinar cells, and islet (like) cells, to play a tissue repair role. (b) Bone marrow mesenchymal stem cells can directly transform into "target tissue cells" to repair tissue, and also secrete a variety of bioactive molecules (such as stem cell-specific growth factors) in a paracrine/autocrine secretion manner, antagonize the release of inflammatory factors and pathological effects, and inhibit the activation of pancreatic stellate cells to promote tissue repair and improve the function of tissues and organs. (c) Bone marrow mesenchymal stem cells can play a therapeutic role in reducing immune inflammatory response in the diseased pancreatic tissue by exerting their immunomodulatory effect (by paracrine/autocrine means), inhibiting T lymphocytes, cytotoxic T lymphocytes, and natural killer cells.

#### 7.1.2.3 Liver Damage and Repair

In recent years, research on liver stem cells has gradually deepened, and more and more studies have shown that liver stem cell transplantation has extremely attractive clinical application value. Firstly, in vitro culture of liver stem cells provides a new cell source for biological artificial liver, and its strong proliferative capacity provides a new idea to solve the difficulty of hepatocyte proliferation and the lack of donors for transplantation. Secondly, liver stem cell transplantation can not only replace necrotic tissue but also stimulate the regeneration of recipient tissue to treat liver damage caused by various reasons. In addition, liver stem cells are genetically modified in vitro and then transplanted to the recipient liver with corresponding gene deficient to differentiate into normal-function liver cells, which served as a good carrier for in vitro gene therapy to improve liver metabolic diseases.

Although the research on liver stem cells has made great progress, it is still in its infancy, and there are still many problems to be solved. How to obtain a large number of high-purity liver stem cells in vitro, how to establish a stable culture system of liver stem cells in vitro, what is the specific mechanism of liver stem cells repairing liver damage, how to apply animal liver stem cell transplantation to the clinic, and how to maintain its safety, need further research.

#### 7.1.2.4 Intestinal Damage and Repair

The results of recent years suggest that MSCs may migrate to the small intestine and play a role in protecting the intestinal epithelial barrier. Studies have shown that MSCs can promote the repair of intestinal epithelium in mice with radiation-induced intestinal injury, promote the closure of fistula in patients with Crohn's disease, colonize intestinal epithelium of rats with ulcerative colitis, reduce the permeability of small intestine in ischemia-reperfusion (I/R) rats, and reduce the damage of intestinal villi. The protection of MSCs against intestinal I/R injury may play a role through the following aspects: controlling the inflammatory response at a lower level, which not only reduces the inflammatory damage of tissues but also has no effect on the immune protection of the body. MSCs may reduce the effects of TNF-α and IL-1 by secreting anti-inflammatory cytokines, or directly inhibit the secretion of TNF-α and IL-1 by immune cells, reduce intestinal inflammatory response, reduce oxidative stress in the body, and maintain the stability of the plasma membrane. Ulcerative colitis (UC) is often associated with accelerated apoptosis of colonic epithelial cells, while a large number of inflammatory cytokines and mediators produced in the intestine exacerbate the damage of intestinal mucosal barrier function. Therefore, inhibiting intestinal inflammatory response, repairing epithelial cells, and improving intestinal epithelial barrier function are new ideas for the treatment of UC. According to the role in inflammatory response, cytokines can be divided into pro-inflammatory factors such as TNF-α, IL-6, and anti-inflammatory factors such as IL-10 and IL-4. The imbalance of these two cytokines is closely related to the pathogenesis of UC. IL-6 plays an important role in the pathogenesis of UC, and its increase is one of the main features of UC. Its plasma concentration is positively correlated with the extent of ulcerative colitis and the severity of the lesion. IL-10 is an important factor in maintaining normal intestinal mucosal immune regulation and stabilizing the intestinal mucosal environment, and it plays an important role in the development and healing of colitis. MSCs have strong immunomodulatory ability, which can inhibit T-cell proliferation, affect the maturation and function of dendritic cells, inhibit the proliferation and differentiation of B cells, and have immunomodulatory effects on other immune cells such as NK cells and macrophages. The expression of IL-6 decreased and IL-10 increased in colon tissue after MSC transplantation, indicating that MSCs can treat UC rats by regulating the imbalance of pro-inflammatory cytokines and anti-inflammatory cytokines. In addition, the decreased level of inflammation in MSC group may be related to the recovery of hemodynamics after MSC treatment, thus promoting the absorption of inflammation.

#### 7.1.2.5 Lung Damage and Repair

Studies have shown that bone marrow mesenchymal stem cells (MSCs) have a repairing effect on lung injury induced by silica dust. After silica dust enters the lungs through the respiratory tract, alveolar macrophages engulf silica dust particles, and the cells activate and produce a large number of inflammatory factors and fibrogenic factors, causing pulmonary inflammation and fibrosis. At the same time, after the change of macrophage function, the immune response is initiated and antigen-antibody complexes are formed and precipitated on the reticular fibers, forming silicon nodules. The antagonism effect of exogenous MSC on pulmonary fibrosis in rats has a dose-effect relationship. Therefore, the number, frequency, and time of MSC infusion for the treatment of silicosis should be further studied.

#### 7.1.2.6 Others

For the repair of visceral injuries such as kidney, ovary, and even cranial nerves, active repair is currently a research hot spot and focus. MSCs can be induced to differentiate into neuron-like cells and glial-like cells under in vitro culture conditions. In 2000, Woodbury and Sanchez et al. demonstrated that MSCs from rats and human can express neural cell precursor marker nest in mRNA and protein, in the culture medium of epidermal growth factor (EGF) or brain-derived neurotrophic factor (BDNF), and have the morphology of nerve cells. These cells also express glial fibrillary acidic protein (GFAP) and neuron-specific nuclear antigen (NeuN). In 2002, Zhao et al. transplanted MSCs into the brain of ischemia-reperfusion rats and found that the sensory function of injured rats was significantly improved, and some transplanted cells expressed markers of astrocytes, oligodendrocytes, and neurons. It indicated that MSCs can survive and migrate in ischemic brain tissue, and differentiate into parenchymal cells to reduce neurological dysfunction caused by cerebral ischemia.

### 7.1.3 Growth Factors and Visceral Repair and Regeneration

In recent years, with the continuous improvement of the regeneration theory, especially the rapid development of molecular biology, the concept of posttraumatic healing and regeneration process has been gradually standardized. It is currently believed that tissue repair and regeneration are the results of the coordinated action of various repairing cell activities, such as proliferation, differentiation, migration, autophagy, and apoptosis under neuroendocrine-immune regulation, which involves the interaction of a series of different types of cells, structural proteins, growth factors, and protein kinases.

After cells enter the cell cycle, a series of morphological changes and molecular events related to proliferation occur in different phases of the cycle. The G1 phase is the stage of cell growth and development. According to the time sequence and the characteristics of molecular events, the G1 phase can be divided into early G1 and late G1. There is a restriction point (R point) between the two phases. Animal cells operate mainly by extracellular growth factors in the cell cycle. Under the stimulation of appropriate growth factors, the cells can pass the G1 phase restriction point. Once the restriction point is passed, even if the stimulation of the growth factor is removed, the cells can complete a cell cycle through the S phase. If there is no proper growth factor stimulation, the cells stop at the G1 phase restriction point and cells that stop at the early G1 phase for a long time are called G0 phase cells. If cells do not pass the restriction point and do not enter the late G1, they will not be able to enter the S phase. Late G1 phase is the key point for cells to enter the S phase. The main activity of cells in the late G1 phase is to prepare for DNA synthesis, such as various deoxyribonucleic acid, thymidine kinase, DNA polymerase, DNA helicase, and other substances required for DNA replication. In addition, there are also a number of proteins closely related to cell cycle operation, such as cyclin, calmodulin, and trigger proteins, which are also synthesized in large amounts. It can be seen that growth factors play an important role in the proliferation of epithelial cells. Growth factors also play an important role in the gene regulation of the mammalian cell cycle. After cells are stimulated by growth factors in G0 phase, cyclin D and cyclin E begin to transcribe, produce corresponding proteins, and bind to DCK2, CDK4, and CDKs, respectively; reach the peak at the junction of G1 phase and S phase, that is, the G1 restriction point; and degrade quickly in the S phase. The growth factors directly bind to the corresponding receptors on the target cells to generate second messenger substances in the cell, which along all levels of the intracellular signaling system cause a series of cascade reactions until they cause changes in the expression of cell cycle regulatory proteins in the nucleus. In conclusion, growth factors play an important role in the proliferation of epithelial cells.

In the mid and late 1980s, it was found that the natural process of wound repair was actually controlled by a variety of growth factors. It is envisaged that the regulation of tissue repair and regeneration could be achieved at the molecular and genetic levels by the application of growth factors.

In view of the characteristics and pathogenesis of visceral ischemic injury after severe trauma, the main measures to promote and accelerate the repair of visceral injury include modern and traditional aspects. In the 1990s, scholars proposed that the active repair and regeneration of visceral injury are mainly based on the new concept of active repair of visceral damage based on growth factors and transgenes, which breaks through the constraints and limitations of traditional concepts. Modern repair, that is, active repair, is based on the principles of molecular biology, using the close relationship between growth factors, receptors, and internal organs in embryonic development and growth maintenance, to actively promote and accelerate the repair of damaged organs from the cellular and molecular levels by regulating the activity or gene expression of endogenous growth factor in vitro, or by exogenous administration of growth factors, or by gene transduction. Studies in the basic field have shown that embryonic development of important viscera such as brain, heart, liver, kidney, and gastrointestinal tract is participated and regulated by growth factors including nerve growth factor (NGF), transforming growth factor (TGF), and fibroblast growth factor (FGF); at the same time, their repair process after maturation is also finely regulated by the above growth factors. In China, the team led by Academician Xiaobing Fu has completed animal experiments and hopes to apply it to the clinic for the benefit of mankind in the future. It breaks through the traditional symptomatic therapy, mainly aiming at the pathogenesis of severe posttraumatic visceral injury and taking corresponding treatment measures. It not only blocks a link in the mechanism of the organ damage to avoid further damage but also provides a suitable internal and external environment for organ repair, so that the active repair of the damaged organ itself can be initiated and restored, and directly promotes tissue regeneration.

Academician Xiaobing Fu led the team to complete the "Basic and Applied Research on Active Repair of Important Visceral Ischemic Injury Caused by Severe Trauma" and won the second prize of National Science and Technology Progress Award in 2005. The study lasted for 18 years and was the first to propose the concept of using growth factors to promote the active repair of important visceral injuries, systematically elucidated the relevant mechanisms of growth factors in regulating active repair of important visceral injuries, proposed and confirmed that the metabolic disorders of the amino acid system in the body lead to delayed repair of important visceral environmental factors after severe trauma, systematically established a series of indicators and methods to determine organ damage and repair, and actively developed new drugs to promote active repair of visceral injuries.

In addition, in order to further study the factors affecting the active repair of important visceral injuries, the team led by Academician Xiaobing Fu dynamically observed the changes of free amino acid content in the body fluids and organs of 28 trauma patients and 170 burn patients, and found that in the course of trauma and burn developing into sepsis, multidigestive tract dysfunction syndrome, and multiple organ failure, the metabolic disorders of amino acids were progressively aggravated. The above results were also confirmed in different trauma animal model experiments. According to this, they clearly state that the disturbance of amino acid metabolism destroys the vital visceral to actively repair the internal environment, and they successfully developed a new drug to improve the environment of viscera repair and promote the active repair of internal organs, which treats nearly 10,000 patients.

### 7.1.4 The Outlook

In the past, most of the treatments for organ dysfunction have been passively waiting for their own repairs, and the results have been unsatisfactory due to the gap in their respective repair capabilities. In recent years, with the rapid development of regenerative medicine, tissue engineering, stem cells, gene therapy, and growth factors have been applied to the active repair of damaged internal organs with certain means and approaches. Regenerative medicine using stem cells and growth factors has allowed stem cells to differentiate into a variety of functional tissues. EGF has not only achieved gratifying research results in intestinal epithelial cells with ischemia-reperfusion injury but also made great progress in the proliferation of damaged alveolar type II epithelium, lung fluid transport, reduction of pulmonary edema, and acceleration of lung repair in acute lung injury (such as inhalation injury).

Researchers at home and abroad used stem cells to treat ischemia-reperfusion injury of vital organs, such as heart, brain, and kidney, which reduced organ damage and cell apoptosis rate, shortened organ repair time, controlled organ reinjury, and also increased the survival rate of organs. The application of stem cells has shown a broad prospect in the treatment of clinical diseases.

Cell protection in ischemia-reperfusion injury is important, which is of great significance to reduce SIRS and prevent MODS. This protection has both physical (low temperature) and chemical drugs. Find and develop drugs with comprehensive effects of protecting vascular endothelial cells, anti-inflammation, and antioxidant-free radicals and reducing parenchymal cell metabolism.

Liver transplantation is currently the gold standard for the treatment of patients with end-stage liver disease and liver tumor with liver dysfunction. Ischemia-reperfusion injury is inevitable during liver transplantation and is an important factor affecting the function of postoperative liver and the occurrence of acute and chronic rejection after liver transplantation. Its related cell therapy research has been very popular in recent years. Bone marrow mesenchymal stem cells (BMSCs) have anti-inflammatory and immunosuppressive effects, can express various cytokines, promote liver cell regeneration, or differentiate into cells with a hepatocyte-like phenotype, play the role of hepatocytes, and promote the repair of damaged liver.

Although the existing research results show diversity, the overall trend shows that adult stem cells (ASCs) have different degrees of repair effects on damaged internal organs. Regardless of the type of ASCs, the repair effects are mainly as follows. (a) Cell mechanism: structural repair, that is, transplanted ASCs proliferate and differentiate into corresponding tissue cells (such as cardiomyocytes, alveolar epithelial cells, and vascular endothelial cells) under the local microenvironment after entering the corresponding target organs to repair the damaged tissue cells, so that the damaged organs can be structurally repaired. The differentiation of such stem cells into various mature tissue cells is stem cell engraftment. Some scholars believe that cell engraftment may be cell fusion, not cell differentiation. In addition, the mechanism of transdifferentiation of stem cells is highly praised by the academia. Transplanted MSCs can be reprogrammed in a local microenvironment and differentiate into cells with similar biological properties to their surrounding cells. (b) Paracrine mechanism: Stem cells improve local microcirculation and antiapoptosis or promote local tissue repair by secreting some cytokines and growth factors (VEGF, bFGF, HGF, IGF-1). Using their characteristics, some important genes are transfected into stem cells to become drug-release carriers. (c) Immunomodulatory effect: For example, mesenchymal stem cells (MSCs) can inhibit the proliferation and function of a variety of immune cells, including T cells, B cells, NK cells, and dendritic cells, and the mechanism may be related to cell-cell direct contact and secretion of soluble factors. In addition, MSC does not express HLA-n molecules, as well as costimulatory molecules CD40, CD80, and CD86, so MSCs are not immunogenic. Studies have treated Crohn's disease with allogeneic MSCs and found no significant side effects. (d) Initiating endogenous repair: In the process of MSC transplantation promoting the repair of damaged tissues, endogenous cell repair still dominates, while transplanted MSCs can be used as a strong signal to promote the homing of other endogenous stem cells to the damaged site. Therefore, tissue regeneration is mainly attributed to the proliferation and differentiation of endogenous stem cells, and transplanted MSCs only play a role in stimulating host cell regeneration. In addition, MSCs may have the potential to increase localized damage signals, attract more endogenous stem cells and other precursor cells to the damaged area, and promote tissue repair.

Transplantation of MSCs can alleviate tissue damage caused by organ ischemia-reperfusion, especially for ischemia-reperfusion injury of heart, brain, kidney, gastrointestinal, and other organs. But the exact mechanism is still unclear. Cell transdifferentiation, paracrine mechanism, and initiation of endogenous repair are major roles, but standardized clinical observations and studies are still few. In the future, we should focus on how to apply it in clinic and carry out more clinical researches on the relationship between active molecules such as growth factors and the repair and regeneration of internal organ damage, in order to further evaluate its clinical application value. With the in-depth study and promotion of active repair and perfect regeneration of visceral injury by various new means, it is expected to make a major breakthrough in clinical treatment.

## 7.2 Repair and Regeneration After Lung Injury

### 7.2.1 Lung Development and Molecular Regulation Mechanisms

#### 7.2.1.1 Lung Development

Lung development is generally divided into three periods: embryonic period, fetal period, and postnatal period (Fig. 7.1). The embryonic period (third to seventh week) is the initial stage of lung development, marked by the formation of the main respiratory tract and lung buds. Except that the nasal epithelium is derived from the ectoderm, the epithelium of other parts of the respiratory system is differentiated from the endoderm of the primitive digestive tract. At the fourth week of the embryo, a longitudinal shallow groove (laryngotracheal groove) appears in the middle of the caudal basal wall of the original pharynx. The groove gradually deepens and begins to heal from its tail end. The healing process moves toward the head and finally forms a long-shaped cecum, the tracheal diverticulum, which is the primordia of the larynx, trachea, bronchus, and lung. The end of the

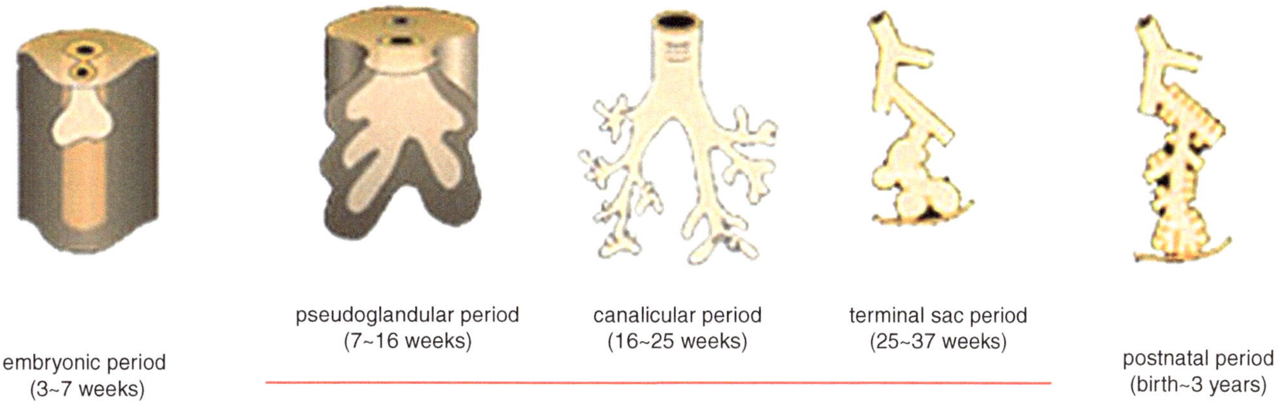


**Fig. 7.1** Basic process of lung development

diverticulum is enlarged and divided into left and right branches, the lung buds, which are the primordia of the bronchus and lung. The groove between the lung buds and the esophagus is deepened, and the lung buds extend and branch between the mesenchymal tissues to form the future main bronchus. Lobar bronchus, segmental bronchus, and subsegmental bronchus formed on about 37th day, 42nd day, and 48th day, respectively.

The fetal period is divided into three periods: pseudoglandular period, canalicular period, and terminal vesicle period. The pseudoglandular period (7th to 16th week of the embryo) is mainly from the development of the main respiratory tract to the formation of the terminal bronchus. It is characterized by the formation of fetal lung (including 15–20 respiratory branches), which then branches to form future alveolar ducts. The developing respiratory tract is covered with a single layer of cubic cells containing large amounts of glycogen. At the 13th week, epithelial differentiation occurs in the proximal respiratory tract with the appearance of ciliated cells, goblet cells, and basal cells. Epithelial differentiation is centrifugal. Undifferentiated cells are distributed in the terminal tubules, and differentiated cells are distributed in the proximal tubules. The upper lobes develop earlier than the lower lobes. The early respiratory tract is surrounded by loose mesenchymal tissues, and loose capillaries are free to extend in these mesenchymal tissues. The pulmonary artery grows with the respiratory tract, and the main arterial ducts appear at the 14th week. The pulmonary veins also develop at the same time, but the pattern is different. The pulmonary veins divide the lung into segments and subsegments. At the end of the pseudoglandular period, the developmental patterns of the respiratory tract, arteries, and veins correspond to those of adults. The canalicular period (16th to 25th week of embryo) is mainly acinar development and angiogenesis. During this period, lung tissue has changed from no gas exchange function to potential exchange function, including acinar appearance, potential blood-gas barrier formation, and differentiation of type I and type II epithelial cells, and gradually began to secrete surfactant after 20 weeks. The acini consist of a cluster of respiratory tracts and alveoli, originating from the terminal bronchioles, including 2–4 respiratory bronchioles, with 6–7 branch buds at the end. Its initial occurrence is a crucial first step for the development of the gas exchange interface of the lung tissue in the future. The mesenchymal tissue, initially less vascularized around the respiratory tract, is further vascularized and closer to the respiratory epithelium. The capillaries initially form a bi-capillary network between the future respiratory tracts, and then fuse into a single capillary. With the fusion of capillaries and epithelial basement membranes, the blood-air barrier structure gradually forms. During the canalicular period, the area of the blood-air barrier increases exponentially, thereby reducing the average thickness of the wall and increasing the gas exchange potential. Epithelial differentiation is characterized by thinning of the epithelium from the proximal to the distal end, transformation from cubic cells to thin cell layers, the latter are distributed in wider ducts. Therefore, as the interstitial becomes thinner, the length and width of the tubules increase, and blood supply gradually increases. Many cells in the canalicular period are called intermediate cells because they are neither mature type I epithelial cells nor type II epithelial cells. About 20 weeks of human embryos, more lamellar bodies begin to appear in the cytoplasm of glycogen-rich cubic cells, usually accompanied by smaller multivesicles, the latter being the initial form of lamellar bodies. The level of glycogen in type II epithelial cells decreases as the level of glycogen in the lamellar body increases, and glycogen provides the matrix for the synthesis of surfactants. The terminal vesicle period (from the 25th week to the full term of the embryo) is mainly the re-differentiation of the vesicle duct caused by the second cristae. This period is important for the formation of the final respiratory tract. The terminal vesicles are prolonged, branched, and widened until alveolarization is completed. With the appearance of alveolar septum, capillaries, elastic fibers, and collagen fibers, the terminal vesicles further develop into primitive alveoli. The inner surface of the primitive alveoli is covered with epithelial cells derived from endoderm, which are considered to be stem cells of the alveolar epithelium. Initially, the cells are cuboidal and called type II alveolar epithelial cells. Later, some type II cells become thin monolayer squamous epithelium and develop into type I alveolar epithelial cells. By birth, alveoli and capillaries have developed quite well. Therefore, the fetus has a respiratory function that can survive independently as soon as it is born.

Postnatal period, also known as the alveolar period, is the period of alveolar development and maturation, and it is also the last link of lung development. Most gas exchange surfaces are formed at this stage. Lung development at birth is basically mature, and further developed and perfection is required to reach the age of 3 years. Differentiation of alveolar surface epithelial cells to form the thin blood-air barrier is a morphological marker of lung development and maturation. Alveolarization progresses rapidly from late fetus to early neonatal period, accompanied by the development and maturation of lung tissue structure, and the functional development is also becoming mature.

#### 7.2.1.2 The Regulation Mechanism of Lung Development

The lungs are derived from two different tissues, the endoderm and the mesoderm. The lung develops from a lung bud into a complete organ with respiratory function, undergoing extremely complex developmental biology processes such as the appearance of the lung primordia, tracheal formation and separation from the esophagus, morphogenesis of tracheal branches, differentiation of specific epithelial cells along the proximal-distal axis to form the lung basic structure, alveolar development, and differentiation of distal epithelial cells. These changes occur in an interlaced and orderly manner. Therefore, there are fine and strict regulation mechanisms in lung development. Studies have shown that lung morphogenesis is closely related to the effects of growth factors and morphogens in the local microenvironment (Fig. 7.2). In the lung, growth factors that promote lung morphogenesis include fibroblast growth factor (FGF), epidermal growth factor (EGF), transforming growth factor (TGF), bone morphogenetic protein 4 (BMP-4), and platelet-derived growth factor (PDGF). The morphogens associated with lung development are Sonic hedgehog (SHH) and retinoic acid. The spatiotemporal regulation of transcription factors on the expression of serial effector genes is an important part of the fine regulation mechanism of embryonic development. The morphogenetic signal in the microenvironment regulates the target genes through transcription factors, thereby achieving orderly embryonic development. The transcription factors associated with lung development include hepatocyte nuclear factor-3 (HNF-3), thyroid transcription factor-1 (TTF-1) or NKX2.1, GATA6, glial nuclear protein (Gli), Hox cluster transcription factor, Myc, etc. At different stages of the lung development, there are different biologically active substances, forming a strict and orderly law of temporal and spatial changes, jointly regulating the morphogenesis of bronchial trees, the differentiation and evolution of alveolar epithelial cells, and the establishment of a blood-air barrier.

The lung primordium is the basis of lung formation, which originates from the ventral side of the foregut. Although there is not much direct information on the mechanism of lung primordia formation, more and more studies have shown that a series of transcription factors are involved in the spatial and temporal regulation of lung primordia pattern formation. HNF-3 is an early and well-defined transcription factor with a high degree of similarity to members of the forkhead (fkh) gene family in Drosophila. The formation of lung primordia is limited to the boundaries of HNF-3β and HNF-3α expression. HNF-3α and HNF-3β are expressed as early as the differentiation of the esophagus and laryngotracheal groove. Expression of HNF-3α and HNF-3β is also retained in the fully differentiated adult bronchial epithelium. Studies have shown that they regulate the expression of lung-specific genes, such as surfactant protein B. HNF-3γ, another member of the HNF-3 family, appears in the differentiation of the hindgut and is involved in the morphogenesis of the liver and

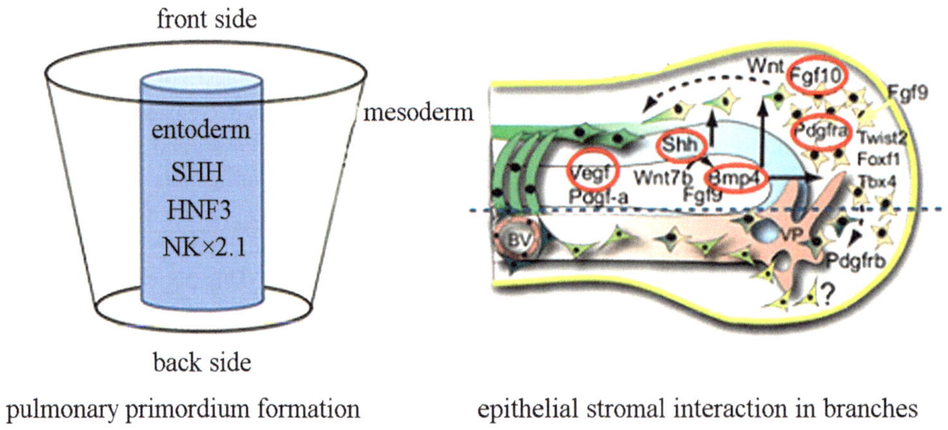


**Fig. 7.2** Regulation mechanism of lung development

stomach. Thus, the region-specifically expressed HNF-3 gene family may form molecular axial signals that specifically mediate cellular changes within the tissue structure derived from the intestinal endoderm. With the knockout of HNF-3β, the embryo dies before lung formation. There is no direct evidence as to whether HNF-3 gene family activation is required for lung primordium formation. Recent studies have shown that glial nuclear protein (Gli) may also play an important role in the development of lung primordia. Gli transcription factors are expressed in the pulmonary interstitium in different temporal and spatial patterns. Combined knockout of Gli2 and Gli3 significantly blocked lung development. The morphogen SHH is involved in the phylogeny of hedgehog in Drosophila, and the hedgehog in Drosophila participates in the formation of multiple parts of Drosophila. SHH is expressed in the lung epithelium and interacts with cellular receptors on interstitial cells. SHH signaling plays a role in promoting lung morphogenesis through the activation of Gli family transcription factors. Studies have shown that although the pulmonary interstitial of SHH knockout mice is abnormal, there is a formation of pulmonary interstitial structure, suggesting that SHH signaling plays only a partial role in the formation of pulmonary interstitium.

The homologous domain transcription factor Nkx2.1/TTF-1 is expressed in the dorsoventral margin of the foregut during the formation of lung buds, clearly distinguishing the lung primordium and esophageal primordium. At present, little is known about the mechanism by which the lung primordium develops into trachea. Studies have shown that by knocking out the Nkx2.1 gene, the trachea of newborn mice is significantly shorter and fuses with the esophagus. The tracheal-esophageal phenotype also occurs in $SHH^{-/-}$, $Gli2^{-/-}$, $Gli3^{+/-}$, and retinoic acid receptors RAR-$\alpha 1^{-/-}$ and RAR-$\beta 2^{-/-}$ mice. There is SHH expression in the lungs of $Nhx2.1^{-/-}$ mice, as well as Nhx2.1 expression in the lungs of $Shh^{-/-}$ mice, suggesting that the roles of the two in lung morphogenesis may be independent of each other, but there may be a functional and parallel relationship. In vertebrates, the trachea includes a series of different phenotypic cells, such as ciliated and nonciliated columnar epithelial cells, and secretory cells (serous cells). The specific signaling and transcription factors required for cell differentiation and spatial composition along the trachea are not fully understood.

HNF-3/forkhead homolog-4 (HFH-4) is expressed in the bronchial epithelium and appears to be required for differentiation of ciliated epithelial cells in the lung. HFH-4 is not lung specific and is also expressed in fetal kidneys, fallopian tubes, and other embryonic organs. Embryos of HFH-$4^{-/-}$ lack the entire ciliogenesis process. Ectopic expression of HFH-4 can lead to columnar cells in the distal lung, an area rich in alveolar epithelial cells, suggesting that HFH-4 seems to be required for the differentiation of ciliated columnar epithelial cells.

Branching is an important part of lung morphogenesis. Branch morphogenesis depends on the epithelial-mesenchymal interaction, which is mediated through a complex molecular network, including growth factors, transcription factors, extracellular matrix proteins, and their receptors. The nature of the epithelial-interstitial interaction depends on the developmental signals, which establish location information at the individual cell level. Based on developmental signals, cells undergo behavioral changes. Cell proliferation, migration, or differentiation is based on the location information of morphogenesis. The developmental signals required for morphogenesis and cell differentiation pass through the location information of cell-cell interactions, and cell-cell interactions initiate specific effector gene expression by activating transcription factors. Key components of the epithelial-mesenchymal interactions include signaling molecules and transcription factors. In the lung epithelium, well-defined key signaling molecules include BMP-4, SHH, and PDGF. Within the pulmonary interstitium, the most important mediator of branching morphogenesis is the FGF pathway, especially FGF-10. In addition to the Gli family, Hox cluster transcription factors are also expressed in the pulmonary interstitium. The transcription factors HNF-3, HFH-4, GATA6, N-Myc, and Nkx2.1 are expressed in the lung epithelium. Studies have shown that HNF-3 and GATA6 are key regulators of epithelial-mesenchymal interactions.

Tissue recombination experiments have shown that two different functional stroma may guide morphogenesis of tracheal (nonbranched) and parenchymal (branched) lung epithelium. It is believed that the signals produced and transcription factors expressed in these two interstitials may be different. The transcription factor encoded by the Hox family is expressed in the pulmonary interstitium. Hoxa-5 gene targeting experiments have shown that this family plays a key role in guiding lung epithelial morphogenesis. Hoxa-$5^{-/-}$ mice die rapidly after birth due to abnormal tracheal morphogenesis and decreased production of surfactant in the lungs. Another key interstitial medium for lung development is the FGF signaling pathway. Disruption of this pathway can result in significant impairment of lung morphogenesis. FGF is produced by the interstitium and acts by homologous receptors on epithelial cells. Targeted knockout of FGF-10 can result in loss of lung structure at the distal end of the main bronchus. The role of FGF in guiding epithelial morphogenesis may be related to its direct induction of epithelial cell proliferation and differentiation. When FGF induces cell proliferation, the intracellular transcription factors c-Fos and c-Myc are activated. They may play a similar role in the proliferation of lung epithelial cells and stromal cells. In limb morphogenesis, ectopic application of FGF results in activation of the zinc finger transcription factor SnR and Tbx family transcription factors. Tbx family transcription factors are also expressed in the lung epithelium. However, the relationship between these transcription factors and FGF signaling-induced lung morphogenesis is unclear.

Cell-cell interactions between epithelium and mesenchyme are key to normal morphogenesis throughout lung development. Transcription factors mediate guiding signals produced by cell-cell interactions. In lung branching morphogenesis, the ability of epithelial cells to receive mesenchymal signals is dependent on the normal activity of N-Myc. N-Myc is expressed in the lung epithelium. Targeted knockout of N-Myc results in significant abnormalities in lung development in mice. In FGF-$10^{-/-}$ embryos, significant impairment to lung growth and differentiation along the proximal-distal axis. Blocking Nkx2.1 also results in severe defects in the proximal-distal morphogenesis. In Nkx2.$1^{-/-}$ embryos, there is no formation of lung structure after secondary or tertiary bronchus. Blocking SHH signaling also affects proximal-distal lung morphogenesis, but limited lung development and cell differentiation can be observed. Therefore, proximal lung morphogenesis is independent of the regulation of Nkx2.1, FGF-10, and SHH, while distal lung morphogenesis is significantly dependent on the regulation of Nkx2.1 and FGF-10, and to a certain extent also dependent on the role of SHH.

Alveolar formation refers to the process by which the lung compartment is divided into different alveoli. Physiologically, alveolar formation is a critical step in the maturation of the respiratory system and the establishment of effective gas exchange. FGF and PDGF signaling pathways are involved in alveolar formation, but transcription factors downstream of these pathways are unclear. There are few reports on the signaling mechanisms and transcription factors involved in alveolar formation. Some factors involved in early lung morphogenesis and present in mature lungs may also be involved in alveolar formation. These factors include HNF-3, GATA6, and Nkx2.1, but direct evidence is lacking. Retinoic acid and glucocorticoids affect alveolar formation. Studies have shown that retinoic acid can alter the expression pattern of transcription factor of Hox gene cluster in the developing pulmonary interstitium. This change has the potential to alter the interstitial induction or initial action, thereby affecting the morphogenesis of the epithelium. However, except for Hoxa-5, neither ectopic expression nor loss-of-function mutations in the Hox gene caused significant abnormalities in the lung phenotype. The glucocorticoid receptors are transcription factors belonging to the same superfamily as the retinoic acid receptors. Loss of glucocorticoid receptor function results in postnatal death from respiratory dysfunction. Glucocorticoid-binding functional sites are present on the pulmonary surfactant protein genes. However, lung development is normal in embryos with mutations in the glucocorticoid receptor DNA-binding domain (blocking their dimerization and gene activation), suggesting that the effects of glucocorticoids on lung development may be independent of DNA binding and transactivation of downstream target genes.

### 7.2.2 Lung Stem/Progenitor Cells

Lung is an important and complex organ in the body. Different anatomical parts have different cell types, and there are 40–60 kinds of cells in the adult lung. Under physiological conditions, the renewal of adult lungs is very slow. For example, it takes 4 months for normal adult rat lung cells to renew once. Because the lung communicates with the outside world and requires frequent exposure to harmful particles and microorganisms, the repair ability of the lung tissue itself is the basis for maintaining homeostasis. In recent years, different types of stem cells have been found in different parts of the lung (Fig. 7.3, Table 7.1), which may play a key role in lung tissue repair. Because they are located in the lung tissue and have the characteristics of stem cells, they are also referred to as endogenous lung stem/progenitor cells.

#### 7.2.2.1 Common Lung Tissue Stem Cells

**Basal Cells**

Basal cells (BCs) are mainly located in the basement membrane of the proximal airway epithelium of the trachea and bronchus. BCs are triangular, mainly expressing K5, K14, and p63. BCs cultured in vitro have strong clonality and can differentiate into various tracheal epithelial cells such as ciliated cells and goblet cells under certain conditions. BCs cultured in vitro were transplanted onto the damaged tracheal basement membrane and implanted under the skin of immunodeficient mice. After a period of time, BCs differentiated into goblet cells and ciliated cells and regenerated epithelial tissue similar to normal trachea. Therefore, BCs have the potential to self-renew and differentiate into a variety of tracheal epithelial cells. Hong et al. observed changes in various types of tracheal epithelial cells after naphthalene injury. It was found that Clara cells were almost completely shed 3 days after injury, and BCs rapidly increased to 4.5 times normal and were the main proliferating cells; the number of Clara cells began to increase 6 days after injury, while the number of BCs began to decrease; the number of Clara cells and BCs returned to normal levels 9 days after injury. Dynamic changes in BCs and Clara cells suggest that basal cells are the main repairing cells of tracheal epithelium after naphthalene injury and may differentiate into Clara cells. This pedigree was confirmed by subsequent pedigree tracking experiments. The researchers used gene-conditional knockout technology to selectively label $K14^{+}$BCs and their progeny cells. It was found that the cells genetically labeled at 4 days after naphthalene injury were few but all were BCs,

Fig. 7.3 Common lung stem/progenitor cells

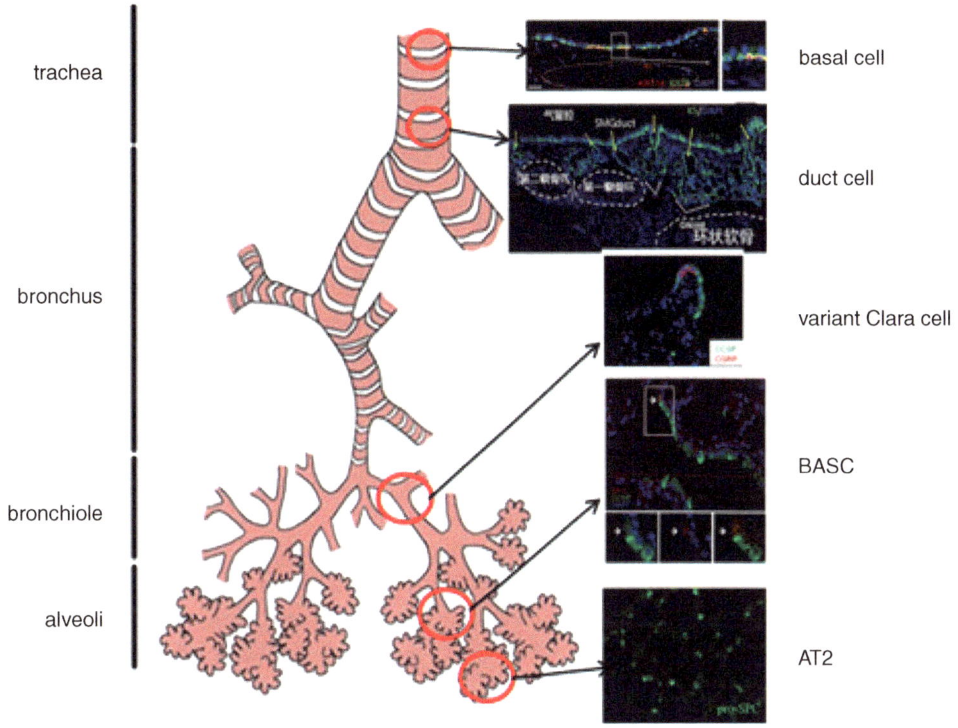


**Table 7.1** Common lung stem/progenitor cells

| Cell type | Cell marker | Distribution | Stem cell level | Daughter cell |
|---|---|---|---|---|
| Basal cell | K5, K14, p63 | Trachea, bronchus | Unipotent stem cell | Goblet cell, ciliated cell, mucilage cell, serous cell |
| Duct cell | K5, K14 | Submucous gland of trachea | Unipotent stem cell | Goblet cell, ciliated cell, mucilage cell, serous cell, myoepithelial cell |
| Clara cell | $CCSP^+CYP450^-2F2^+$ | Bronchiole epithelium | Transient expansion cell | Ciliated cell |
| Variant Clara cell | $CCSP^+CYP450^-2F2^-$ | NEB, BADJ | Unipotent stem cell | Clara cell, ciliated cell, PNEC |
| BASC | $CCSP^+pro^-SPC^+$ | BADJ | Unipotent stem cell | Clara cell, AT2, AT1 |
| AT2 | $Pro^-SPC^+$ | Alveolar epithelium | Ancestral cell | AT2, AT1 |
| Human lung stem cells | C-kit, OCT4, Nanog, Klf4, SOX2 | Bronchioles, alveolar epithelium | Multipotential stem cell | Clara cell, AT2, AT1, vascular endothelial cell, smooth muscle cell |
| SP cell | Sca1, CD31, Hoechst33342 | Not yet positioned | Not clear | Not clear |
| Smooth muscle progenitor cells | FGF-10 | Muscularis of airway at all levels | Ancestral cell | Smooth muscle cell |
| Angioblasts | Flk1 | Blood vessels at all levels | Ancestral cell | Capillary endothelial cell |

and the number of labeled cells increased significantly at the 12th day and the 20th day after injury, and most cells have the morphology of ciliated cells or express Clara cell secretory protein (CCSP), demonstrating that BCs can differentiate into ciliated cells and Clara cells.

### Duct Cells

The duct cells are located in the ductal portion of the tracheal submucosal gland. The duct cells are cuboidal and express K5 and K14. Tracheal submucosal glands (SMGs) are located between the tracheal rings and the epithelial layer of trachea. Human SMGs are distributed in the airways from the larynx to the main bronchus, while mouse SMGs are confined between the cricoid cartilage and the first tracheal ring. The SMGs consist of serous/mucous tubules, collecting ducts and ciliary ducts, and finally open to the tracheal epithelial layer. The serous/mucous tubules are covered with polygonal serous cells and mucous cells surrounded by flat myoepithelial cells. Mucous cells secrete mucus which can be stained by AB/PAS and labeled with DMBT1; serous cells secrete serum, mainly expressing lactoferrin and pIgR; myoepithelial cells express K5, K14, and α14. Mucous tubules and serous tubules are connected to each other and gradually merge to form collecting ducts, which turn into ciliary ducts before opening to the epithelium. Due to their concealed anatomical site, SMGs are less susceptible to damage than epithelial cells and are suitable for stem cell survival.

After BrdU or H3-TdR labeling, cells that are still labeled for some time are called label-retaining cells (LRCs), which may contain stem cells. Liu et al. found that LRCs are mainly located in SMG duct of the trachea and proximal bronchus using BrdU marker. Tracheal epithelial tissue can be regenerated by implanting duct cells on the epithelial-depleted tracheal basement membrane and transplanting them together under the skin of immunodeficient mice. Hegab et al. obtained TROP-2-positive duct cells by differential digestion and flow sorting, and double-positive BCs by TROP-2 method and flow sorting, and compared the characteristics of the two stem cells in vivo and in vitro. TROP-2 is a hallmark of prostate basal cells and is expressed in all epithelial cells and duct cells, but not in myoepithelial cells and mucous/serous cells. In vitro culture showed that the cloning ability of BCs was higher than that of duct cells, and both cells could differentiate into mucous cells, serous cells, ciliated cells, and myoepithelial cells. The researchers inoculated $RFP^+$ duct cells cultured in vitro into the fat pad of the scapula of mice without any labeling and found that about 50% of the mice could form submucosal gland tubule-like structures, and 20% of the tubule-like structures were surrounded by duct-like structures, and even wrapped with myoepithelial cells. The submucosal glands formed have the function of secreting mucous and serous, and all cells express RFP. The results indicate that transplanted $RFP^+$ duct cells can form functionally and structurally intact submucosal glands, further validating the multi-differentiation potential of duct cells. In vivo studies have found that only $K5^+K14^+$ duct cells and a small amount of $K5^+K14^-$BCs remain in the trachea after ischemia-hypoxia injury in mice. Lineage tracking of $K14^+$ duct cells revealed that duct cells were involved in repairing epithelial cells in submucosal glands, submucosal gland ducts, and near the opening after ischemia-anoxia injury, but BCs could only differentiate into epithelial cells. It should be noted that only 1% of human BCs and 10% of mouse BCs express K14, and most of the $K14^+$ cells are duct cells, so the $K14^+$ cells tracked by Hong et al. may be duct cells instead of BCs. In conclusion, duct cells are more stem than BCs and belong to pluripotent stem cells.

#### Clara Cells

Clara cells are mainly distributed in the bronchiolus epithelium, but their distribution and number are slightly different among different species. In terms of distribution, human Clara cells are only distributed in the bronchioles, neither in trachea nor bronchi, while mouse Clara cells are distributed in all tracheal branches below the trachea, including bronchi and bronchioles. In terms of number, human Clara cells account for 11% and 22% of the terminal bronchioles and respiratory bronchioles, respectively, and the distal airways of mice are almost Clara cells. Clara cells are cubic or columnar, and specifically express Clara cell secretory protein (CCSP) and CYP450-2F2. CYP450-2F2 can convert naphthalene in cigarettes into cytotoxic substances and cause cell death. Therefore, naphthalene can cause specific damage to Clara cells.

It is currently believed that Clara cells are the main transit-amplifying cells (TACs) at the bronchioles, that is, they have the function of terminal cells in quiescent state, but can rapidly proliferate and differentiate into ciliated cells after injury. Under physiological conditions, only 0.2–0.5% of Clara cells proliferate in rat and mouse bronchioles with a cell cycle of 30 h, but 15% and 44% of the proliferating cells in the human terminal bronchioles and respiratory bronchioles are Clara cells, respectively. The protein CCSP secreted by Clara cells, also known as CC10, CC16, Clara cell antigen, secretory globulin, and uteroglobin, is the main component of the airway surface fluid. CCSP is a 10–16 ku protein that is resistant to proteases and is stable in high heat and strong acid environments. The gene encoding this protein in humans is about 4.1 kb in size and contains 3 exons and 2 introns, which can be regulated by leucine zipper factor basic region CCAAT, enhancer binding protein α, Nkx2.1, and thyroid transcription factor 1. The main functions of CCSP are as follows: (a) Main components of the liquid substances on the airway surface. (b) Immunomodulation: It can enhance the release of anti-inflammatory mediators. (c) Inhibition of tumor formation. (d) Regulation of the niches of stem cells in the airway. (e) Enhanced lung ability to cope with oxidative stress. (f) Elevated serum levels may serve as an early marker of lung injury.

#### Variant Clara Cells

Also known as variant CCSP-expressing cells (vCEs), they are mainly located in the bronchiolar bifurcation and bronchoalveolar duct junction (BADJ). As mentioned earlier, Clara cells can be specifically damaged by naphthalene due to the action of CYP450-2F2. However, after naphthalene injury, a group of cells expressing CCSP remain in the neuroepithelial body (NEB) at the bronchiolar bifurcation and BADJ, which lack CYP450-2F2 and are resistant to naphthalene, so they are known as variant Clara cells.

Hong et al. found LRCs in NEB and adjacent tissues after naphthalene injury by H3-TdR labeling residue method, suggesting that there may be stem cells in this area. Further studies found that LRCs include vCE expressing CCSP, PNECs expressing calcitonin gene-related peptide (CGRP), and vCE expressing CCSP and CGRP. After conditional knockout of CCSP-expressing cells in mice, it was found that PNECs could not completely repair the airway epithelium, suggesting that the variant Clara cells at NEB may be the main cells for bronchiolar repair. The possible stem cell levels are as follows: vCE self-renews and differentiates into Clara cells, Clara cells self-renew and differentiate into ciliated cells, while PNECs can only self-renew, in addition, vCE may also differentiate into PNECs, while PNECs can regulate the proliferation and differentiate of vCE and maintain its characteristics. Therefore, vCE at NEB is a stem cell in the bronchiolar epithelium.

Giangreco et al. found that the vCE at the BADJ after naphthalene injury was the earliest and most important proliferating cell in the terminal bronchioles after injury, accounting for about 90% of all proliferating cells in this area. But are vCEs at BADJ and NEB the same group of cells? Morphological quantitative analysis found that about 57% of the vCEs at BADJ were located within 40 μm from BADJ, and about 75% of the proliferative vCEs were located within 80 μm from BADJ, so the two are not a group of cells from the anatomical site. CGRP immunostaining showed that vCE at BADJ did not express CGRP, and the distribution was completely unrelated to NEB, while vCE at NEB partially expressed CGRP and distributed in NEB and its surrounding tissues. Therefore, the vCE at BADJ is not the same group of cells as the vCE at NEB. In the early stage of naphthalene injury, the majority of Clara cells in the terminal bronchioles were necrotic and exfoliated, while vCE at BADJ rapidly proliferated and gradually migrated to the proximal end. In the late stage of naphthalene injury, the density of Clara cells returned to normal, and some vCEs entered the resting phase. Therefore, vCE at BADJ is primarily involved in homeostasis maintenance and repair of the terminal bronchiolar epithelium.

### Bronchioloalveolar Stem Cells

Bronchioalveolar stem cells (BASCs), located at BADJ, are stem cells expressing Clara cell marker CCSP and type II alveolar epithelial cell marker pro-SPC, which were first discovered and named by Kim in 2005. BADJ is the boundary between the conductive airway and the alveoli. Since tissue-specific stem/progenitor cells have been found in the migration regions of different cells in tissues such as the esophagus and cornea, BADJ is also a potential stem cell nest, and searching for common regulatory mechanism within the migration regions of different tissues helps to discover stem cell regulatory factors. In fact, $CCSP^{+}SPC^{+}$BASC only exists at BADJ, while Giangreco et al. also found variant Clara cells at BADJ. Under physiological conditions, the number of BASCs is very small, accounting for about 0.34% of total lung cells. Since cytoplasmic markers cannot be used for the isolation and functional analysis of living cells, the surface markers Sca-1, CD34, CD45, and CD31 were selected as sorting markers, and the flow-sorted $CD45^{-}CD31^{-}Sca1^{+}CD34^{+}$ lung epithelial cells were almost all $CCSP^{+}pro^{-}SPC^{+}$BASC. It was inoculated into the trophoblast culture of mouse embryonic fibroblasts after irradiation, and it was found that a single BASC could form clones with a significantly higher clone formation than AT2. At the ninth passage, it still expressed both CCSP and pro-SPC and maintained strong colony formation ability, indicating that BASC has strong self-renewal and colony formation ability. Matrix gel is a basement membrane component extracted from mouse sarcoma cells, such as extracellular matrix proteins and growth factors, and is often used as a medium for stem cell induction and differentiation. BASC can differentiate into $CCSP^{+}$ Clara cells, pro-$SPC^{+}$ type II alveolar epithelial cells, and $AQP5^{+}$ type I alveolar epithelial cells after culture in matrix gel, but cannot differentiate into ciliated cells, indicating that BASC has multidirectional differentiation potential. After naphthalene injury, bleomycin injury, and left lung resection in mice, the number of BASCs increased significantly, the proliferative capacity increased significantly and began to migrate to alveoli, and finally the tracheal epithelium and alveolar epithelium were effectively repaired. However, Rawlins et al. found that BASC was not involved in the repair of bronchioles and alveolar epithelium by pedigree tracking of $CCSP^{+}$ cells. Although this study has problems such as a small sample size and inadequate morphological quantitative analysis, the results still suggest that the completion of lung repair requires the participation of multiple stem cells, and a large number of stem cells play a major role. Since BASC is also resistant to naphthalene and expresses CCSP, BASC is very similar to vCE at BADJ. So what is the relationship between them? Kim et al. found that only a part of $CCSP^{+}$ cells remaining in BADJ after naphthalene injury expressed pro-SPC at the same time, while others only express CCSP, so BASC may be a subgroup of vCE at BADJ, but no studies have confirmed it. It was found that there was a kind of epithelial cells expressing CCSP, CGRP, and SPC in mouse fetal lung, suggesting that Clara cells, neuroendocrine cells, and AT2 may all develop from a common precursor cell, and BASC may be this precursor cell.

The isolation and culture of BASC is the premise and basis for studying its biological characteristics and important regulatory molecules. At present, the isolation of BASC mainly refers to the method of Kim laboratory. That is, the epithelial cells of the distal airway are digested into a single-cell suspension by intrapulmonary infusion of dispase, collagenase, and other digestive enzymes, and then the $CD45^{-}CD31^{-}$ $Sca1^{+}CD34^{+}$ cells are sorted out as BASCs by flow sorting, which are then inoculated into the mouse embryonic fibroblast trophoblasts and cultured in DMEM medium. Further analysis of BASC flow sorting markers revealed that $CD34^{+}$ cells were not present in the airway epithelium. Immunofluorescence staining revealed that Sca1 was mainly expressed in cells outside the airway epithelium, especially in vascular endothelial cells (95% of $CD31^+$ cells expressed Sca1). In the airway epithelium, Sca1 is only expressed on the basal and lateral membrane of the proximal airway epithelial cells in the lung, while the distal airway epithelial cells do not express Sca1. Therefore, Sca1 is a widely expressed marker in lung tissue, and the expression levels of different cells are different: endothelial cells are the highest, proximal airway epithelial cells are the second, and distal airway epithelial cells are the weakest. The results indicate that Sca1 could not distinguish between stem cells (BASC) and transit-amplifying cells (Clara cells) in the bronchioles. However, Clara cells were found to have higher autofluorescence (AF), while BASC has lower autofluorescence, thus proposing a new sorting marker $CD45^-CD31^-CD34\ Sca1^{low}A^{Flow}$. The reason for the different results may be the different methods of cell separation. Kim uses dispase, collagenase digestion, and isolation of AT2, while the latter uses elastase to isolate all epithelial cells from the conducting airway to the alveoli, which contain Clara cells at BADJ and NEB. In addition to flow sorting, the BASC purification methods include whole-cell adherence screening. The main reason is that AT2 cells have completely differentiated after 1 week of culture, and then enter the apoptotic stage, while BASC culture for 1 week before forming clonal colonies, so the majority of AT2 can be removed after 2 weeks of whole-cell suspension culture; the addition of FIBROOUT in the culture system can remove fibroblasts. However, regardless of the sorting and purification methods, it is necessary to use CCSP and pro-SPC co-staining to analyze the purity.

### Type II Alveolar Epithelial Cells

The alveolar epithelium is mainly composed of alveolar type 1 cells (AT1) and alveolar type 2 cells (AT2). AT2 is cubic, accounting for about 16% of total lung cells, but covers only 5% of the alveolar surface area, mainly distributed at the junction of adjacent alveolar walls. The AT2 cytoplasm is rich in lamellar bodies, and there are a large number of surfactant proteins (SPs) in the lamellar bodies, including SP-A, SP-B, SP-C, and SP-D, which can maintain the alveolar surface tension and clear dust or pathogens entering the alveolar space. AT1 is the squamous epithelial cell, accounting for 8% of the total lung cells, but covering 95% of the alveolar surface. AT1 mainly constitutes the blood-air barrier to complete gas exchange and clears the fluid in the alveoli to maintain the dry state of the lung. According to stem cell theory, in continuously renewed tissues, the stem cell populations can proliferate, differentiate, and produce excessive daughter cells, some of which replace senescent or lost cells, and the remaining daughter cells eventually apoptosis. Therefore, in order to maintain tissue homeostasis and normal repair, the proliferation, differentiation, and apoptosis of stem cells must be in balance.

The H3-TDR labeling of adult mice revealed that a complete cell cycle of AT2 is about 22 h, which is identical to that of AT2 in rats after $NO_2$ injury. The entire cell cycle and the time of each phase of AT2 are related to the developmental stage of the organism and toxic damage, and the culture in vitro is different from that in vivo. In general, the S phase of AT2 is 7–9 h in different species, different developmental stages, toxic damage, cell culture, etc., while the G2 and M phases lasted 1–12 h. In primary culture, only a portion of AT2 can continuously proliferate and form clones, suggesting that AT2 may consist of different subpopulations. Recent studies have confirmed this view. Reddy et al. found that the response of AT2 to E-cadherin was inconsistent after hyperoxia injury, and accordingly divides AT2 into two subtypes: one subtype does not express cadherin, and this group has high telomerase activity, has high proliferative activity, and is more tolerant to injury; another subtype expresses cadherin, which has low telomerase activity, has no proliferative activity, and is susceptible to damage. Liu et al. found that the ratio of AT2-expressing stem cell antigen (Sca-1) was significantly increased after *S. aureus* pneumonia, and $Sca\text{-}1^+AT2$ has stronger potential for differentiation into AT1 than Sca-1-AT2 in vitro, suggesting that $Sca\text{-}1^+AT2$ may be the major subpopulation of AT2 exerting progenitor cell function.

Evans et al. used H3-TdR to label $NO_2$ lung injury rats and found that 88% of the labeled cells in alveolar epithelium were AT2 and only 1% were AT1 at 1 h after labeling; cells between AT1 and AT2 appeared in the alveolar epithelium at 24 h after labeling, accounting for 40% of labeled cells, while AT2 decreased to 60%; AT1 increased significantly 3 days after labeling, and the number of cells in the intermediate state decreased significantly. The results suggest that after alveolar epithelial injury, AT2 can proliferate and differentiate into AT1, and finally repair the alveolar epithelium. Adamson et al. also used H3-TdR marker technology to confirm that AT2 can also differentiate into AT1 during lung development. Since then, AT2 has been considered to be the progenitor cell of AT1. However, when AT2 was cultured in DMEM containing 10% FBS, it began to differentiate into AT1 on the fourth day, and completely differentiated into the flat AT1 from paving stone-like cells on the seventh day, and differentiated immediately after AT2 passage. Therefore, AT2 is also considered to be a transit-amplifying cell. At present, the differentiation of AT2 to AT1 mainly depends on the judgment of various cells. The gold standard for identifying AT2 is still that its ultrastructure under electron microscope meets the following conditions: there are lamellar bodies, apical microvilli, cell-cell junctions, and cuboid shape in the cytoplasm, through which AT2 and AT1 can be clearly distinguished. In addition, AT2 has other identification methods such as modified Papanicolaou staining, cell-specific lectin, and immunohistochemical markers. However, the expression of immunohistochemical markers depends on the developmental stage of the body and is affected by pathological changes. For example, after lung injury, there will be AT2-to-AT1 differentiated intermediate cells, while expressing AT2 and AT1 markers.

An important mechanism for the body to clear cells is apoptosis. Although there are many basic studies on apoptosis inducers, apoptotic pathways, and effectors, there are few studies on the apoptosis of lung tissue cells. The AT2 cell membrane expresses the Fas receptor, and the binding of the Fas receptor to the Fas ligand or Fas antibody can initiate apoptosis. Apoptosis of AT2 is an integral part of pulmonary septal remodeling during lung morphogenesis and epithelial repair after lung repair. In the remission period of adult acute lung injury, a large number of apoptotic cells appeared in the epithelial recovery period after AT2 hyperplasia induced by intratracheal injection of KGF in rats, which was eventually cleared by macrophages or adjacent cells in the lung.

It is currently believed that AT2 may be a key stem cell for alveolar epithelial repair. Mollar et al. transplanted male rat alveolar type II epithelial cells cultured in vitro into the lungs of female rats with bleomycin-induced lung injury, and found that transplanted alveolar type II epithelial cells not only are directly involved in the repair of alveolar tissue but may also prevent/reduce pulmonary fibrosis and improve lung function through endocrine effects. Nolen-Walston et al. found that the number of AT2 in the residual lung of the left lung resected mice began to increase on the 7th day after surgery, with the highest proliferative activity, reaching the peak on the 14th day. The cell dynamics model found that AT2 contributed more than 75% of alveolar epithelium.

### Smooth Muscle Progenitor Cells

The smooth muscle progenitor cells are distributed in the muscular layers of all levels of the airway wall and express fibroblast growth factor-10 (FGF-10), belonging to a kind of peripheral mesenchymal cells. Lineage tracing of FGF-10 genetically labeled lacZ mice revealed that airway smooth muscle cells were derived from FGF-10-positive cells. As the airway continues to sprout and elongate, the FGF-$10^+$ cells gradually wrap around the airway along the long axis of the airway, as if a person is wearing a sock while stretching his legs. It was found that Shh and BMP4 can regulate the differentiation of FGF-$10^+$ smooth muscle progenitor cells into α-$SMA^+$ smooth muscle cells, while Shh and BMP4 were distributed throughout the airway from proximal to distal.

### Hemangioblasts

Hemangioblasts are distributed in all levels of blood vessels in the lung and express Flk1. At 9–10 days in mice and 4–5 weeks in humans, a longitudinal shallow groove appears in the middle of the bottom wall of the primitive pharynx, which is called laryngotracheal groove. Capillary plexus appears simultaneously in the laryngotracheal groove, and mice labeled with Flk1 marker can specifically visualize all capillary plexus at this time, so Flk1 is the earliest marker of hemangioblasts. Under the stimulation of VEGF secreted by the primitive epithelial layer, hemangioblasts proliferate and differentiate, eventually forming a complex capillary network in the lung. The correct formation of the capillary network is important for airway branching and tissue perfusion, and the correct matching of capillary endothelium and alveolar epithelium determines the ultimate maximum gas diffusion capacity of the lung. Among them, mesothelial-mesenchymal-epithelial-endothelial cross talk is essential in the whole process of lung development: mesothelial-expressed FGF-9 can activate and regulate FGF-10 through intraepithelial molecules, such as FGFR2b, SHP2, Grb2, Sos, and Ras, and Sprouty2 is an important inducer.

### Other Types of Lung Stem/Progenitor Cells

Kajstura, a scientist at Harvard Medical School in the United States, first discovered a true stem cell in human lungs in 2011, which has three characteristics: self-renew, clone formation, and multidirectional differentiation, and named it human lung stem cells (HLSCs). The cell membrane of HLSC specifically expresses c-Kit, and the nucleus expresses four stemness transcription factors: NANOG, OCT3/4, SOX2, and KLF4. c-Kit, namely CD133, is a stem cell antigen. c-$Kit^+$ cells colonize the yolk sac, liver, and other organs during embryogenesis and are mainly expressed in hematopoietic stem cells in adulthood, and the colonized organs express c-Kit ligand stem cell factor. Fibroblasts can dedifferentiate into pluripotent stem cells, namely induced pluripotent stem cells (iPS), after being transfected into four stem transcription factors: NANOG, OCT3/4, SOX2, and KLF4. Therefore, it is speculated from the stem cell phenotype that the stem capacity of HLSC is quite high. Using c-Kit surface markers, the researchers sorted HLSCs from adult and fetal lung tissues, and then single cells were inoculated into Terasaki plates. It was found that cell colonies appeared in the culture holes after 8 days, the colonies increased significantly after 20 days of culture, all of them were c-Kit-positive cells, and the total colony-forming efficiency was about 1%, indicating that HLSC had strong clone formation ability. It has also been observed in the experiment that HLSC has two modes of division, symmetry and asymmetry, which can produce daughter cells identical to themselves, so HLSC has self-renewal ability. After adding dexamethasone to the culture medium, HLSC can differentiate into lung epithelial cells such as AT2 and BCs, vascular endothelial cells, and smooth muscle cells, so HLSC has multidirectional differentiation potential. In vitro experiments show that HLSC has three major characteristics of stem cells and belongs to a pluripotent stem cell.

To further examine the stem cell characteristics of HLSC, the researchers prepared a mouse model of local lung cryo-damage and injected the EFP-labeled HLSC in vitro into the lung tissue surrounding the injured area. It was found that regardless of whether the injected cells were monoclonal or polyclonal, HLSC began to undergo symmetric and asymmetric division 12–48 h after transplantation, and HLSC completely settled in the injured area and surrounding lung tissues after 10–14 days, and differentiated into Clara cells (CC10), type I/II alveolar epithelium (AQP5/SPC), vascular endothelial cells (VWF), and smooth muscle cells (ACTA2), which confirms the multidirectional differentiation potential of HLSC. The integrity of the alveolar epithelium and vascular endothelium was examined by two-photon imaging with tracheal and pulmonary artery perfusion of rhodamine, respectively. The results showed that the newly formed alveolar epithelium and vascular endothelium were tightly connected without rhodamine leakage, indicating that the new lung tissue had the structural basis for normal alveolar ventilation. The researchers verified the self-renewal and clone formation ability of HLSC through continuous transplantation experiments commonly used in hematopoietic stem cells. They isolated EGFP$^+$ c-Kit$^+$ cells from the lung tissue of mice that had received EGFP$^+$HLSC transplantation for 14 days and injected them directly into another frozen-injured lung without culture. After 10 days, the second one was found to still have the same effect as the first one.

The HLSC content in human lungs is extremely rare. Morphological quantitative analyses reveal that HLSCs are mainly distributed in the noncartilage-supported trachea (below terminal bronchioles) with diameters of 25–1200 μm and in the distal airway such as alveoli. Seventy-nine percent were distributed in bronchioles and 21% in alveoli. The proportion in the whole lung, trachea, and alveoli of adults is 1/24000, 1/6000, and 1/30000, respectively. Although the discovery of HLSC has been questioned, it still brings hope for stem cell treatment for lung diseases.

Side population (SP) cells, also known as marginal group cells, bypass cells. The cell expresses an ATP-binding-dependent transporter protein, Bcrp1, which actively effluxes Hoechst 33342 and PI that have entered the cell against dye concentration gradients, thereby separating it from Hoechst 33342-positive or PI-positive host cells during flow sorting. SP cells were first isolated and extracted from bone marrow and were therefore thought to have hematopoietic stem cell activity. In recent years, it has been found that SP cells are nonhematopoietic stem cells, and specific SP cells have been successively extracted from tissues such as heart, liver, pancreas, and breast and have the potential for stem cell differentiation. SP cells in the lung accounted for 0.03–0.07% of the total number of cells. Nonbone marrow-derived CD45$^-$SP cells expressed Sca1, mesenchymal cell marker vimentin, and Clara epithelial cell marker CCSP, but did not express CYP450-2F2. However, the tissue localization of SP cells, the specific role, and molecular mechanism involved in lung injury have not been clearly defined.

#### 7.2.2.2 The Role of Lung Tissue Stem Cells in Lung Disease

Because the lungs communicate with the external environment, the proliferation and differentiation ability of respiratory epithelial cells is continuously affected by factors such as pathogens, dust, and toxicants. The functional changes of airway epithelial cells, especially stem cells, directly affect the development of acute and chronic lung injury. For example, inadequate repair capacity of airway epithelial is the earliest event of chronic lung injury, and defects in lung tissue stem cells to terminal cells differentiation can lead to changes in the proportion of epithelial cells, and eventually worsen the condition. In addition, the conversion of part-time progenitor cells to specialized progenitor cells may make airway epithelial cells more susceptible to damage, thereby promoting the occurrence and permanent existence of chronic lung diseases. Take Clara cells that have an acute response after airway injury as an example: once Clara cells begin to proliferate, they lose cell functions, such as secreting CCSP; if Clara cells proliferate continuously, their differentiation function will be limited, but differentiation will also make them lose their proliferative potential; the apoptosis and senescence of Clara cells will cause defects in epithelial function.

##### Acute Lung Injury

The clearance of pulmonary edema and the repair of alveolar epithelium after acute lung injury (ALI)/acute respiratory distress syndrome (ARDS) are the key links in the repair of lung injury. Diffuse alveolar damage is a major marker of ALI/ARDS, whether caused by direct or indirect factors. Pathological biopsy of patients who died of ALI/ARDS found that the earliest injury was interstitial edema, followed by severe alveolar epithelial damage, characterized by extensive necrosis of AT1, residual bare basement covered with hyaline membranes, and loss of epithelial integrity leading to the infiltration of protein-rich edema fluid into the alveolar space. After intratracheal injection of 5 mg/kg O111: B4 lipopolysaccharide (LPS) in male Wistar rats, focal infiltration of neutrophils and monocytes appeared 24 h later, and gradually increased. After 48 h eosinophils and amorphous substances appeared in the alveolar cavity, AT1 did not change significantly, AT2 was more numerous and contained lamellar bodies, and some AT2 showed immature expressions such as ribosomes and rough endoplasmic reticulum. AT2 is more resistant to damage than AT1, and AT2 remaining after ALI is a repairing cell for alveolar epithelium. The normal alveolar epithelial repair process is: AT2 first undergoes rapid adhesion and migration after ALI, and the whole process takes 8–16 h, which is the earliest repair event; then AT2 begins to rapidly proliferate along the pulmonary septum, covering the bare basement membrane and reconstructing the continuity of the epithelium, which is most obvious after 1–2 days after ALI, is the main manifestation of the proliferative phase of ALI/ARDS, and is also the most obvious and most easily observed repair reaction; finally, AT2 differentiates into AT1 and completes the repair 10–14 days after injury. If the adhesion, migration, and proliferation are insufficient and the apoptosis is too strong, it will cause the alveolar epithelium to fall off, eventually leading to the repair of pulmonary fibrosis. Studies have found that loss of cell adhesion sites can slow cell migration and induce apoptosis. Therefore, integrin-associated cell adhesion plays a key role in alveolar epithelial repair after ALI. However, due to the lack of specific, effective, real-time in vivo monitoring techniques, there is no in vivo evidence of migration and adhesion. In addition, residual epithelial cells at the wound edge can also release a variety of pro-inflammatory factors and growth factors, attract proteins and cells needed to restore the extracellular matrix, and promote re-epithelialization.

### Chronic Obstructive Pulmonary Disease

Chronic obstructive pulmonary disease (COPD) is a chronic lung disease caused by chronic inflammation and characterized by progressive irreversible airflow limitation. Due to the progressive decline in lung function, it seriously affects the workforce and quality of life of patients, resulting in a huge social and economic burden. WHO expects COPD to become the third largest disease in the world by 2030. The main pathological changes in COPD are epithelial hyperplasia and metaplasia. Studies have found that basal cells and AT2 may be involved in the development of COPD. There is a clear boundary between the proliferative zone of mucinous cells and the associated flat metaplastic zone, and there is a continuous layer of $P63^+$ basal cells on the basal surface of the proliferative zone and the metaplastic zone. The stratified $P63^+K14^+$ or $K5^+K14^+$ basal cells also appeared in the flat metaplasia zone of epithelium. AT2 in emphysema patients expressed higher cyclin-dependent kinase (CDK) inhibitors p16INK4a and p21Waf1/CIP1, which leads to increased apoptotic AT2. In addition, AT2 has shorter telomeres, suggesting AT2 is senescent in emphysema patients.

### Cystic Fibrosis

Cystic fibrosis (CF) is a lung disease characterized by epithelial remodeling and induced by recurrent infection and inflammation. It is currently believed that the pathogenesis of CF is that the mutation of cystic fibrosis transmembrane conductance regulator (CFTR) gene in columnar epithelial cells causes disorder of ion transport, which ultimately leads to limited mucus clearance, chronic bacterial infection, release of pro-inflammatory factors, severe and persistent leukocyte exudation, and epithelial damage and repair. The main pathological changes of CF are bronchiectasis caused by goblet cell and basal cell proliferation, wall tissue destruction, and the like. $K5^+K14^+$ basal cells in the airway epithelium of CF patients proliferate excessively and express epidermal growth factor receptor (EGFR). Hajj et al. isolated epithelial cells from CF patients and healthy individuals, inoculated them into tracheal grafts with epithelial removal, and implanted under the skin of nude mice. It was found that the regeneration ability of epithelial cells from CF patients was weakened, and only an epithelial layer with abnormal tissue structure was formed.

### Asthma

Asthma is a chronic inflammatory disease of the airway characterized by reversible airflow limitation caused by airway hyperresponsiveness. Data from five major cities in China show that the prevalence of asthma in children aged 13–14 years is 3–5%, which is the main disease causing students' absence from school. The main pathological changes of asthma are goblet cell hyperplasia and mucus hypersecretion, and others include repeated ciliated cell shedding, basement membrane thickening, subepithelial fibrosis, smooth muscle cell hypertrophy, angiogenesis, and submucosal gland hyperplasia. Basal cells appear in the area of goblet cell hyperplasia, suggesting that epithelial cell shedding and goblet cell hyperplasia may be caused by incorrect fate selection during basal cell differentiation. Kicic et al. isolated epithelial cells from asthmatic patients and found that the intrinsic "asthmatic epithelial cell phenotype" was maintained after several passages in vitro, suggesting that the epithelial cell types of asthma patients may have been transformed.

### Bronchiolitis Obliterans

Bronchiolitis obliterans is a major chronic rejection phenomenon after lung transplantation, resulting in a 5-year survival rate (less than 50%) that is much lower than other organ transplants. The main pathogenesis is that epithelial cell shedding causes mucosal lamina propria cells such as fibroblasts to invade the epithelial layer, eventually leading to blockage of bronchioles. Epithelial shedding in small airways is earlier than metaplasia and hyperplasia, suggesting that the loss of epithelial cells in bronchiolitis obliterans may be caused by defects in stem cell function. The balance between basal cell self-renewal and the production of suitable ratio of goblet cells and ciliated cells is an important basis for maintaining normal airway epithelial function. This balance requires regulation by stem cells and potential intermediate progenitor cells. Changes in basal cells and their daughter cells can lead to airway remodeling: excessive self-renewal without differentiation can lead to the proliferation of basal cells; the wrong choice of cell differentiation fate leads to the proliferation of goblet cells and the metaplasia of ciliated cells; phenobarbital cells produce stratified upper basal cells that may lead to flat metaplasia, and dysplasia of basal cell proliferation with increased apoptosis or incorrect differentiation leads to hypoplasia. Abnormal changes in basal cell proliferation and differentiation are caused by intrinsic transcriptional and regulatory mechanisms.

#### 7.2.2.3 Important Molecules that Regulate the Biological Characteristics of Lung Tissue Stem Cells

**CARM1**

Coactivator-associated arginine methyltransferase 1 (CARM1), also known as protein arginine methyltransferase 4 (PRMT4), is one of the nine members of the arginine protein methyltransferase family. CARM1 is a regulatory factor that regulates gene transcription, mRNA processing stability, and translation. CARM1 is also a transcriptional co-activator that increases transcription and translation of steroid receptors via methylated steroid receptor co-activators SRC3 (NCOA3) and CBP/p300 (CREBBP). In addition, CARM1 can increase the transcriptional activity of other factors such as cFOS, p53 (TRP53), NF-κB, and LEF1/TCF4. Under normal conditions, CARM1 is expressed in AT2, Clara cells, BASC, and vascular endothelial cells, with the highest expression of AT2. After knocking out CARM1 in mice, the number of alveoli was reduced, the pulmonary septum was thickened, and the lungs could not be filled, so effective gas exchange could not be performed, resulting in death from respiratory distress soon after birth. Further studies found that the AT2 proliferation ability of CARM1 knockout mice was enhanced, but they could not differentiate into AT1, thus failing to form an effective blood-air barrier. The expression of the cell cycle suppressor Gadd45g and the pro-apoptotic gene Scn3b was downregulated after knockout of CARM1 in mice. In vitro studies have found that CARM1 can form a complex with glucocorticoid receptor and p53, bind to the promoter region of the Scn3b gene, and initiate transcription of Scn3b. Therefore, CARM1 can improve cell responsiveness to glucocorticoids, and glucocorticoids can promote the differentiation of lung tissue stem cells such as AT2. In conclusion, CARM1 can inhibit the proliferation of lung tissue stem cells and promote apoptosis and differentiation.

**HNF-3α (Foxa1)**

It is a subtype of the hepatocyte nuclear factor-3 family. The HNF-3 family has three types: HNF-3α, HNF-3β, and HNF-3γ. Its structural features are as follows: the HNF-3 family shares an N-terminal conserved transcriptional activation region, which mainly regulates the interaction of HNF-3 proteins with other proteins; the 100 amino acid residues at the C terminus are essential transcriptional activation regions of HNF-3, including two important conserved regions II and III; there is a homologous wing-loop DNA-binding region between the N-terminus and the C-terminus. HNF-3α and HNF-3β proteins share 93% homology in the wing-loop DNA-binding region, can bind to the same DNA sequence, and are strong transcriptional activators. Under normal circumstances, multiple specific transcription factors act synergistically to activate the promoter of lung-related genes. HNF-3α and HNF-3β proteins can jointly regulate the expression of Clara cell-specific protein CCSP and AT2-specific protein SP. HNF-3α and HNF-3β are interlaced in lung development, but HNF-3γ is not involved in lung development. HNF-3 is mainly expressed in AT2 in adult lungs, and HNF-3α expression is increased in lung tissue 24 h after ALI. It can inhibit the expression of antiapoptotic genes by binding to the promoter regions of antiapoptotic genes BCL2 and UCP2, thereby promoting AT2 apoptosis after ALI and slowing down repair.

**HNF-3β (Foxa2)**

HNF-3β exhibits a decreasing expression pattern from the proximal to the distal airway: high expression in bronchiolar epithelial cells and low expression in AT2. HNF-3β can regulate the expression of Clara cell marker CCSP and pulmonary surfactant SP alone or in combination with other factors, and participate in the maintenance of normal lung development and repair. Xu et al. found that HNF-3β/SREBP/CEBPA together maintained the stability of SP by gene chip, promoter analysis, and protein interaction studies. Using immunohistochemical techniques, Porter et al. found that GATA-6 and HNF-3β co-regulate the expression of the nicotinic acetylcholine receptor (nAChR) alpha subunit in AT1, AT2, Clara cells, and ciliated cells. IFNγ released after ALI promotes the binding of IFNγ regulatory factor 1 to the HNF-3β promoter, which stimulates the expression of HNF-3β. IFNγ also promotes the co-binding of HNF-3β and STAT to the CCSP promoter and induces the expression of CCSP. The lack of SP and increased secretion of CCSP in the acute phase after ALI suggest that the recovery of HNF-3β activity after ALI may improve the repair efficiency of ALI. HNF-3β$^{-/-}$ knockout mice died at E9.5 and were found that they could not form pulmonary nodules, lung ridges, foregut endoderm, visceral endoderm, and neural tube, suggesting that HNF-3β is indispensable in lung development. Transgenic mice with HNF-3β sequence inserted after SPC promoter expressed high expression of HNF-3β in alveolar epithelial cells, and disrupted the decreasing expression pattern of HNF-3β from the proximal airway to the distal airway. The fetal lung of this transgenic mouse mainly contains a large number of primitive tubules, which cover the cubic epithelial cells with high expression of HNF-3β, but the branching and angiogenesis are inhibited, and the expression of E-cadherin and VEGF disappears, suggesting that normal concentration gradient of HNF-3β promotes alveolar formation.

#### TTF-1 (Nkx2.1)

Thyroid-specific enhancer-binding protein (T/EBP) is expressed in endodermal-derived epithelial cells of organs such as lung, thyroid, and diencephalon. In the early stage of lung development, TTF-1 is expressed in all airway epithelial cells and is mainly expressed in alveolar epithelium and bronchiolar epithelium in the late stage, which is involved in the regulation of SP, T1α, and CCSP expression, while TTF-1 expression is co-regulated by HNF-3β and GATA6. TTF-1 plays a key role in lung development. $TTF\text{-}1^{-/-}$ knockout mice have developmental defects in the lung, thyroid, and pituitary gland, with only the stem bronchus in the lungs and no alveolar structure, suggesting that TTF-1 may promote the formation of lung branches during the pseudoglandular phase. $TTF\text{-}1^{-/-}$ mouse alveolar epithelial cells do not express SPB, SPC, and CCSP, and low expression of BMP4, suggesting that TTF-1 promotes the differentiation of lung stem cells into alveolar epithelial cells and Clara cells. Lungs of premature infants with bronchopulmonary dysplasia are rich in TGF-β, which activates the downstream transcription factors SMAD3, and the combination of SMAD3 and TTF-1 inhibits SPB expression. Therefore, TTF-1 promotes maturation and differentiation of lung tissue stem cells.

#### HFH-4 (FOXJ1)

It is a potent transcriptional activator in the FOX family. During embryogenesis, FOXJ1 is mainly expressed in ciliated epithelial cells of trachea, bronchi, and bronchioles, and it is also expressed in cells of esophageal ciliated epithelium, paranasal sinus, ovary, testis, kidney, and ependyma. In adult mice, it is mainly expressed in ciliated epithelial cells of the lung, choroid plexus cells, and sperm cells at specific stages. Loss of ciliated cells in the bronchioles and ventricles of $FOXJ1^{-/-}$ knockout mice causes pulmonary dysfunction and hydrocephalus, leading to stillbirth. In addition, $FOXJ1^{-/-}$ mice have random translocation of internal organs, so FOXJ1 can regulate the differentiation of ciliated cells and the left-right asymmetric distribution of internal organs. Using transgenic technology to express FOXJ1 in the distal airway of mice, it was found that the distal airway of fetal mice contained atypical cubic or columnar epithelial cells and highly expressed FOXJ1 and β-tubulin IV. Although these cells can still express TTF-1 and HNF-3β, they no longer express SPB/SPC/CCSP. Therefore, ectopic expression of FOXJ1 can promote differentiation into ciliated cells and inhibit expression of genes in nonciliated cells.

#### GATA6

The GATA family was initially found to regulate the gene expression of hematopoietic stem cells, including GATA4, GATA5, and GATA6. GATA4 is mainly expressed in the heart, intestinal endoderm, mesenchymal epithelium, liver, testis, and ovary, and $GATA4^{-/-}$ mice die early due to developmental disorders of foregut endoderm and visceral endoderm. GATA5 and GATA6 exhibit nonoverlapping expression patterns during lung development. GATA5 is mainly expressed in smooth muscle cells of the trachea and bronchus, and GATA6 is expressed only in bronchial epithelial cells. $GATA5^{-/-}$ mice have normal lung development, whereas $GATA6^{-/-}$ mice have stillbirth due to defects in extraembryonic tissues. Zhang et al. found that after knocking out GATA6 in mouse $SPC^{+}$ cells, the mice could not survive, the number of BASCs in the lungs increased, and the proliferative capacity increased, but they could not differentiate into AT2, AT1, and Clara cells. Further studies found that the downregulation of the nonclassical Wnt pathway receptor FZD2 in knockout mice, artificially elevating FZD2 or downregulating the classical receptor β-catenin, can reverse the effects after knockout of GATA6. Mice that specifically knock out GATA6 of $CCSP^{+}$ cells can survive, and 14 days after naphthalene injury, the proliferative capacity of BASC is significantly stronger than that of wild-type mice. Therefore, GATA6 can inhibit the proliferation of BASC and promote its differentiation into AT2, AT1, and Clara cells.

#### Bmi1

Bmi1 is an epigenetic chromatin modifier in the Polycomb group family, inhibits gene transcription, and is an important component of the PRC1 complex. It was discovered that Bmi1 cooperated with c-Myc to promote the development of B-cell lymphoma and was therefore considered to be an oncogene. Bmi1 mainly inhibits the expression of p16INK4a and p19ARF proteins, thereby promoting cell proliferation and inhibiting apoptosis. Bim1 is important for maintaining self-renewal of hematopoietic stem cells and neural stem cells. The lungs of mice that knocked out Bmi1 developed normally, but the proliferative capacity of BASC was lost. Knockout of Bmi1 in a K-ras knockout mouse model of lung adenocarcinoma slowed down the number and progression of lung cancer cells, which may be related to defects in BASC proliferation. And the expression of p19ARF was decreased in both knockout mice. This indicates that Bmi1 promotes the proliferation of BASC.

#### C-Myc

Myc is a family of widely used transcription factors that bind to the E-box element of 10–15% genomic DNA with ligand Max to regulate the transcription of thousands of genes. c-Myc is highly expressed in many proliferating cells and tumors, regulating cell growth, proliferation, dedifferentiation, and apoptosis. c-Myc regulates gene expression in two ways: one is to regulate gene expression at the transcriptional level by binding E-Box elements in the promoter region of target genes via the c-Myc/Max complex; another is the regulation of gene expression at the posttranscriptional level by Myc-induced miRNAs. The ability of embryonic stem cells and adult tissue stem cells to self-renew and multidirectionally differentiate is called "stemness." It is currently believed that the transcription factors and genes required for stem cells to maintain stemness are consistent. Among the 34 genes that maintain the stemness of embryonic stem cells and the 19 genes that maintain the stemness of IPS cells, c-Myc is the most significantly upregulated transcription factor in BASC. The expression of c-Myc in BASC is increased in the early stage of lung development, and gradually decrease with the maturation of lung development. BASC proliferative capacity decreases after knocking out c-Myc. Further studies reveal that c-Myc may regulate the biological properties of BASC through miRNA and E-Box elements.

#### 7.2.2.4 Important Signaling Pathways that Regulate the Biological Characteristics of Lung Tissue Stem Cells

##### Wnt/β-Catenin Pathway

There are three pathways of Wnt pathway: classical Wnt/β--catenin cell biology pathway, Wnt-$Ca_2^+$ pathway, and PCP signaling pathway. Among them, Wnt/β-catenin cell biological signaling pathway has been the most extensively studied on the regulation of various tissue stem cells. The genetic destruction of the β-catenin degradation complex leads to an increase in the level of β-catenin in the cells, leading to uncontrolled proliferation of small intestinal stem cells/transition cells and loss of differentiation and migration capacity. The enhancement or inhibition of uncontrolled signal of β-catenin cells leads to enhanced or inhibited proliferation of small intestinal crypt cells and loss of differentiation into intestinal epithelial cells. The enhancement of β-catenin or the enhancement of inhibitory signal may also lead to enhanced proliferation and decreased differentiation of other types of stem cells such as hematopoietic stem cells and epidermal stem cells. E16.5 mice were at the peak of lung endoderm development, and β-catenin mice were at the peak of lung endoderm expression. Enhanced β-catenin reached its peak, airway epithelial development defects after enhancement, and the number of BASCs increased in adulthood. After naphthalene injury, the proliferative capacity of the increased BASC was approximately equal to that of normal BASC, and the increased BASC returned to a resting state after epithelial repair. Therefore, β-catenin is at rest. It is necessary to maintain the activity of BASC, and enhancing its expression can enhance its proliferative ability and reduce the differentiation ability.

##### Rho GTPase Pathway

The Rho GTPase family includes Rho, Rac, Cdc42, Rnd, and other types, which are involved in cytoskeleton remodeling and cell contraction by regulating actin remodeling, adhesion site formation and renewal, and actomyosin contraction. As a member of the Rho family, RhoA is involved in actin aggregation into muscle fibers, formation of stress fibers, local adhesion macromolecules, and the stretching of actomyosin. Rac1 stimulates the formation of local complexes and actin aggregation in lamellipodia, while Cdc42 performs similar functions in filopodia. Inactivation of RhoA by the bacterial toxin ExoT can inhibit wound healing in the AT2 cell line A549, while protein kinase A (PKA) can enhance RhoA activity and promote bronchial epithelial migration. After high-flux ventilation injury in rats, RhoA activity in AT2 is increased and adhesion ability is increased, while KGF could inhibit RhoA with increased activity and decrease the adhesion ability of AT2. Studies have shown that overexpression of both constitutively active (CA) and dominant negative (DN) of RhoA and Rac1 can inhibit wound healing in human bronchial epithelial cell line 16HBE14, indicating that the balance of activity of CA and DN is essential for normal epithelial repair. In addition, Rho GTPase activity is different in different parts of the cell. The activity of Rac1 on the margin of the migrating cells is increased, while the center of the cells has a higher activity of RhoA to produce the adhesion site and tension of cell contraction. Therefore, Rho GTPase mainly regulates the migration and adhesion of lung tissue stem cells.

#### 7.2.2.5 MAPK Pathway

Mitogen-activated protein kinases (MAPKs) are a class of serine/threonine protein kinases that widely exist in mammalian cells, which are involved in cell proliferation, differentiation, and migration. The MAPK pathway transmits signals in a highly conserved kinase cascade, that involves the sequential phosphorylation of three kinases termed as MAPK kinase kinase (MAPKKK), MAPK kinase (MAPKK), and MAPK. The MAPK family includes 8 subfamilies: p38 MAPK, extracellular signal-regulated protein kinase (ERK), c-Jun N-terminal kinase (JNK), big MAP kinase-1 (ERKS/BMK1), ERK3, ERK7, NLK, and ERK8. These subfamilies can form multiple pathways, among which ERK1/2 pathway, JNK/SAPK pathway, and p38 pathway are the most important. p38 and JNK are rapidly activated in wound margin cells, and inhibiting the activity of p38 MAPK, JNK, ERK1/2 can slow down the migration of primary cultured human airway epithelial cells. Elevated levels of inflammatory factors nitrogen oxides can reduce the activity of ERK1/2 and inhibit the migration of bronchial epithelial cells. Ventura et al. found that after knocking out p38α (also known as MAPK14), the number of BASCs increased and the proliferative capacity increased, but the differentiate ability lost. In vitro culture of BASC from p38α knockout mice found that BASCs could not differentiate into AT2 and Clara cells, and BASCs from wild-type mice could not differentiate into AT2 and Clara cells after adding p38α inhibitor SB203580. Therefore, although the main role of the MAPK pathway is to promote cell proliferation and migration, the biological effects of different tissues and different stimulating factors on the MAPK pathway are also different.

#### 7.2.2.6 PI3K/PTEN Pathway

PI3K and PTEN are a pair of signal pathways that can inhibit each other. PI3K activation induces the synthesis of PIP3, which in turn activates AKT and PKB, exerting antiapoptotic, proliferative and cancer-promoting effects. PTEN is a phosphatase that degrades PI3K and inhibits the action of PI3K. Inhibition of PTEN activity, overexpression of inactivated form PTEN, or introduction of PTEN-specific siRNA can accelerate wound healing in primary cultured human airway epithelial cells, whereas inhibition of PI3K activity and expression of inactivated form PI3K can slow cell migration after lung injury. Yang et al. found that in the K-ras knockout mouse lung adenocarcinoma model, an increased number of BASCs expressed a subunit P110 of PI3K and a downstream target AKT. The number of BASCs decreased after treatment with the PI3K inhibitor PX-866, and the number of BASCs in K-ras$^{-/-}$ mice increased after knockout CCSP$^{+}$ intracellular PTEN. PX-866 can inhibit the colony formation rate of BASC. The above results indicate that the activation of PI3K or the inhibition of PTEN can promote the proliferation of BASC. Shigehisa et al. specifically knocked out PTEN gene in SPC$^{+}$ cells and revealed that the alveolar space of PTEN knockout neonatal rats could not expand, the pulmonary septum was thickened, and the survival rate was significantly decreased. Flow cytometry found that the proportion of BASC and SP cells was significantly increased, but the differentiation into AT2 and AT1 was defective. It indicates that the inactivation of PTEN promotes the proliferation of BASC and SP cells and inhibits their differentiation.

#### 7.2.2.7 TGF Pathway

TGF-β is the most important morphogen in mammals. According to its biological functions, the TGF-β family can be divided into the following categories: activins, inhibins, bone morphogenetic proteins (BMPs), and Mullerian-inhibiting substances (MISs). After binding to class I and class II receptors, various TGFs act through Smad molecules. TGF-β is an immunosuppressive factor and pro-inflammatory factor that induces the expression of many genes, including connective tissue growth factor (CTGF), α-smooth muscle actin (α-SMA), type II collagen, and type II plasmin activator inhibitors. TGF enzyme can promote the migration of A549 cells and primary AT2 cells in rats and mice through Smad3 and transgelin-dependent pathways, but inhibits the migration of fetal bovine bronchial epithelial cells. Manoj et al. found that rat SPC$^{+}$AT2 expressed TGF-β and Smad4. During the in vitro culture of AT2, the expression of TGF-β, Smad2, Samd3, and cell cycle inhibitors p15Ink4b and p21Cip1 decreased during the proliferative phase, and the expression of the above molecules increased at the peak of AT2 differentiation to AT1, and the medium contained more TGF-β. When TGF-β antibody or Smad4 siRNA was added to the medium during the differentiation phase, the differentiation of AT2 into AT1 was inhibited. Therefore, the TGF-β pathway can promote the migration and differentiation of lung tissue stem cells.

### 7.2.3 Lung Tissue Repair and Regeneration

#### 7.2.3.1 Extrapulmonary Stem/Progenitor Cells Participate in Repairing Lung Tissue Damage

##### Bone Marrow Stem/Progenitor Cells Are Involved in Repairing Damaged Lung Tissue

The bone marrow is the largest stem cell bank in the body, and the main source of extrapulmonary stem/progenitor cells is the bone marrow pool. The cells involved in the repair of lung injury mainly include bone marrow-derived mesenchymal cells (BDMCs), epithelial progenitor cells (EPCs), and hematopoietic progenitor/stem cells. Under the action of pulmonary infection, acute lung injury, or bone marrow mobilization agent (such as G-CSF, HGF, or adrenomedullin), the above cells flow out of the bone marrow pool and migrate directionally, and participate in the repair of damaged lung tissue in a specific differentiation form. Previous studies have demonstrated that bone marrow mobilizers G-CSF, HGF, or adrenal medullary proteins can induce an increase in bone marrow-derived endothelial progenitor cells in the pulmonary capillary lumen during alveolar regeneration in a mouse emphysema model. However, whether bone marrow-derived cells differentiate into alveolar cells or merge with colonized cells remains to be confirmed. In patients with bacterial pneumonia and acute lung injury, the number of circulating endothelial progenitor cells is significantly increased, and the increased number is associated with disease prognosis, suggesting that bone marrow-derived progenitor cells are released into the circulation under inflammatory stimuli, and these cells promote the regression of inflammatory processes and repair of damaged lung tissue. The promotion of alveolar regeneration by bone marrow-derived mesenchymal cells has been well demonstrated in the elastase-induced emphysema model.

**Repair Effect of Bone Marrow Stem/Progenitor Cell Transplantation on Lung Tissue Injury**

In the current clinical stem cell therapy, mesenchymal stem cells (MSCs) are important candidate cells for cell therapy. MSCs are easily isolated from bone marrow and tissues. Allogeneic MSCs are susceptible to receptor tolerance due to their low expression of major histocompatibility complex (MHC) type I and II proteins and lack of co-stimulatory molecules of T cells. Therefore, the use of allogeneic MSCs is theoretically feasible, and MSCs can be stored for therapeutic use without ethical controversy. In recent years, more than 100 clinical MSCs have been registered and conducted in the United States. As mentioned above, MSCs are able to alleviate lung tissue damage and promote the repair process. These beneficial effects are based on the ability of MSCs to modulate the immune system and produce growth factors and cytokines (such as epidermal growth factor, HGF, and prostaglandin E2). In view of the above anti-inflammatory effects, the potential of MSCs for the treatment of severe lung disease (acute lung injury, COPD, pulmonary hypertension, asthma, and pulmonary fibrosis) has been extensively studied. At the same time, in the experimental model, MSCs were injected intravenously or tracheally into the injured lung. Intravenous or intratracheal injection of bone marrow cells or bone marrow-derived MSCs attenuated LPS-induced lung injury in mice, and bleomycin-induced inflammation, collagen deposition, and fibrosis were also attenuated after intratracheal or intravenous infusion of MSCs. The mechanism of action mainly involves the immunomodulatory effect directed at increasing anti-inflammatory mediators and reducing the secretion of pro-inflammatory mediators, the repair effect of the blood-air barrier directed by secretory growth factors, the clearance effect of alveolar edema, and the inhibition of alveolar epithelial cells apoptosis. Therefore, MSCs have important clinical value in the repair and regeneration of acute lung injury.

In the model of acute lung injury caused by endotoxin, lung tissue damage includes apoptosis and necrosis. This requires normal repairing cell replacement and maintenance of the organ homeostasis. Previous studies have confirmed that bone marrow MSCs have strong plasticity in the microenvironment of lung injury and can differentiate into various types of lung tissue cells such as alveolar type I and type II epithelial cells, fibroblasts, endothelial cells, and bronchial epithelial cells. Green fluorescent protein (GFP) chimeric mice with bone marrow reconstitution showed flat GFP-positive BDMCs in the alveolar wall 7 days after LPS injection. These cells are positively stained for molecular markers keratin (epithelial cell marker) or CD34 (endothelial cell marker). This suggests that bone marrow BDMCs can differentiate or fuse with alveolar epithelium and vascular endothelial cells, indicating that transplanted BDMCs may be involved in the repair process of lung injury. However, as the observation time prolonged, BMDCs gradually and significantly decreased. In addition, bone marrow-derived mononuclear cell (BMDMC) treatment can improve inflammatory damage and fibrosis in acute lung injury. Although there are many controversies about the number residence time, and paracrine regulation of bone marrow-derived cells colonized in the lungs, the above results suggest that BMDCs initially migrate to damaged organs and differentiate or fuse with organ parenchymal cells; as BMDCs colonize damaged organs, they are difficult or unable to differentiate or develop into new cells. At this time, the main role should be to regulate the local microenvironment of the injury and stimulate the endogenous repair reaction.

Recent studies suggest that intravenous infusion of mesenchymal stem cells (MSCs) can significantly ameliorate lung injury induced by hyperoxia in neonatal mice, reverse the pathological reduction of alveolar surface area, and reduce respiratory function. Further studies have found that MSC medium also have similar therapeutic effects. Regarding its mechanism, the study further confirmed that during this process, bronchoalveolar stem cells (BASCs) in the bronchoalveolar junctions, a group of Clara cells with secretory function, were increased significantly. Moreover, in vitro clone formation experiments found that the proliferation of BASCs may not be caused by growth factors, and lineage tracking techniques found that BASCs contribute to the reconstruction of epithelial structures after lung injury. Therefore, the repair effect of MSCs on acute lung injury may be caused by stimulating the proliferation of BASCs.

#### 7.2.3.2 Involvement of Intrapulmonary Stem/Progenitor Cells in the Repair of Lung Tissue Damage

Recent studies on stem cell therapy for various lung diseases have shown that both stem cells from the lung tissue and the stem cells derived from the extrapulmonary tissue can participate in the repair of lung injury tissue. Based on the extremely low growth rate and limited regenerative capacity of the airway epithelium itself, exogenous stem cells have been used for a long time and some therapeutic effects have been achieved, but the repair and regeneration of exogenous stem cells in lung tissue is limited and it is difficult to produce sufficient tracheal epithelial cells or alveolar epithelial cells. Therefore, it is currently difficult to treat lung diseases by promoting the repair and regeneration of damaged lung tissue. In fact, a small number of endogenous adult stem/progenitor cells exist in many organs and tissues in mammals, and they are distributed in specific microenvironments: niches, which may be an important cell source for maintaining normal organ tissue stability and repairing damaged tissue. Studies of lung endogenous stem cells in the lungs showed that stem/progenitor cells with certain differentiation ability were distributed in the trachea, bronchus, bronchioles, and alveoli of adult mice. Similar distribution of stem/progenitor cells was also found in lung tissues of mammals such as humans, rats, rabbits, and the like. Although there is still lack of strict endogenous markers for lung stem/progenitor cells, isolation and culture are still difficult, and the classification of stem/progenitor cells is still controversial, their role in maintaining lung structural stability and lung tissue repair has been widely recognized.

### Alveolar Stem/Progenitor Cells Participate in the Regeneration of Damaged Lung Tissue

During lung injury repair, intrapulmonary stem/progenitor cells (such as tracheal stem cells, bronchial stem cells, bronchiolar stem cells, bronchioloalveolar stem cells, alveolar stem cells, and alveolar type II epithelial cells) play an important role in restoring the stability of the lung environment and participating in the repair of damaged tissues. Alveolar type I and type II epithelial cells cover most of the alveolar space in the constituent cells of the alveolar wall, the main area of gas exchange. In the occurrence of lung injury, type I alveolar epithelial cells with large surface area are damaged and necrotic, and the number of type II alveolar epithelial cells with absolute dominance can differentiate and replace type I alveolar epithelium. Studies have shown that under intrapulmonary inflammatory stimuli (LPS and bleomycin), type I alveolar epithelial damage and type II alveolar epithelium may differentiate and replace the damaged type I alveolar epithelium, and a portion of the type II alveolar epithelial group may become hypertrophic in morphology. These phenomena are often seen in a variety of damaged lungs. At present, studies have further suggested that there are subpopulations of stem cells with different morphological structures in the type II alveolar epithelium, which are distributed in the terminal bronchioles, alveolar duct junctions, and alveolar walls. Therefore, in the process of structural remodeling of lung injury, how to effectively mobilize the repair potential of type II epithelial cells from the quantitative, distribution, and cell transformation pathways analysis undoubtedly has absolute weight advantage.

Experiments in GFP chimeric mice found that alveolar regenerated after lung injury consisted of bone marrow-derived (GFP-positive) and nonbone marrow-derived (GFP-negative) cells. This suggests that colonized lung cells, including endogenous stem cells, contribute to alveolar development. It has been demonstrated that type II alveolar epithelial cells are capable of repairing damaged alveolar epithelium. However, the potential of lung endogenous stem cells to replace injured type II alveolar epithelium is unclear. It has recently been suggested that mouse stem cell antigen (Sca)-1-positive cells may be lung endogenous stem cells. Hegab et al. reported that elastase-induced lung injury increased the number of cells with stem cell markers (such as Sca-1, CD34, and c-Kit), and the number of Sca-$1^+$/SPC$^+$ cells increased significantly under the action of HGF or elastase, and the combination effect is the strongest. Most Sca-$1^+$ cells are endogenous stem cells of the lung; however, most c-Kit$^+$ cells are bone marrow-derived. Therefore, how to effectively increase the number of endogenous stem cells in the lung may be one of the key links to effectively repair damaged lung tissue. Fortunately, in recent years, American scholar Edward Morrisey et al. found that the activation of Wnt signaling pathway can significantly increase the number of BASCs, and pharmacological regulators such as lithium can enforce the expansion and differentiation of key stem cell populations in lung tissue. Undoubtedly, this will provide new possibilities for the idea of repairing damaged lungs with lung stem cells as the starting point.

At the same time, Nolen-Walston et al. observed the response of lung endogenous stem cells (Sca-$1^+$/SP-C$^+$/CCSP$^+$/CD45$^-$) and type II alveolar epithelial cells during compensatory lung growth in mice after pneumonectomy. It was found that the number of Sca-$1^+$ cells and type II alveolar epithelial cells increased in compensatory lung growth and reached 220% and 124% of the basic value, respectively. The role of Sca-$1^-$ cells accounts for 0–25% of compensatory lung growth. However, according to the cell dynamics model, type II alveolar epithelial cells, which have the absolute advantage in number, are still essential for lung tissue regeneration.

At present, compared with reports on the increase of endogenous stem cells in mouse lungs, although *New England Journal of Medicine* reported evidence of human lung stem cells in 2011, our understanding of human lung stem cells is still very limited. There are two main reasons for this: (a) lack of specific markers of human lung endogenous stem cells and (b) limited access to lung specimens. Nevertheless, this study on lung stem cells has demonstrated the characteristics of c-Kit-positive cells in vitro and in vivo and provided some experimental preparations for the future clinical application of lung stem cells. However, stem cell transplantation from the discovery of lung stem cells to the final application to the clinic requires a lot of follow-up experiments. First, how effective is lung stem cell transplantation? Does the new lung tissue differentiated from lung stem cells have the physiological function of normal lung tissue? Second, what is the feasibility of lung stem cell transplantation? For patients with lung disease, will their lung stem cells lose their ability to self-proliferate and multipotent to differentiate due to the poor microenvironment of the lungs? Again, can the transplantation of allogeneic lung stem cells have similar efficacy as autologous transplantation? Finally, how to solve the technical problems in a series of processes from isolation, culture to final transplantation of lung stem cells?

In view of this, StemSurvive stock solutions for tissue stem cells have been developed in recent years. With this solution, human lung tissue can be stored for 7 days, and tissue stem cells and niche cells are not affected. Subsequently, alveolar progenitor cells (AEPCs) were isolated from human lungs stored in StemSurvive solution. AEPCs are endothelial cell phenotypes characterized by mesenchymal stem cells. By microarray analysis, AEPCs share many genes with mesenchymal stem cells and type II alveolar epithelial cells, suggesting a phenotypic overlap between alveolar epithelium and its interstitial cells. In fact, studies have found an increase in the number of AEPCs in fibrotic lungs and some types of adenocarcinoma. AEPCs undergo transformation of mesenchymal and epithelial phenotypes, suggesting that these cells play a role as lung tissue stem cells in tissue repair and cancer development. For alveolar repair, mesenchymal properties such as antiapoptotic activity and activity may be beneficial for functional epithelial progenitor cells. Further experimental exploration is needed to elucidate the pathophysiological role of AEPCs in lung diseases.

#### Lung Mesenchymal Stem Cells Participate in Regeneration of Injured Lung Tissue

Lung MSCs, a subset of endogenous stem cells, have the ability to self-renew and differentiate into mesenchymal cell lines. Given the inconsistent characteristics of MSCs from different organs, and the absence of specific cell surface markers, the current basic criteria for MSCs are: ability to adhere to plastic culture dishes; potential for differentiation of osteoblasts, adipocytes, and mesenchymal cells in vitro; and positive molecular markers usually selecting CD73/CD90/CD105 and negative molecular markers usually choosing CD34/CD45/CD14 or CD11b/CD79a or CD19/HLA-DR.

Lung MSCs can be isolated from newborn lungs and bronchoalveolar lavage fluid. Karoubi et al. isolated MSCs from surgical human lung tissue and successfully differentiated them into type II alveolar epithelial cells expressing aquaporin 5 and CCSP. Although the role of MSCs in lung regeneration is unknown, the beneficial effects of MSCs on lung injury have been extensively studied. MSCs can produce a variety of cytokines and growth factors. In addition, co-culture of LPS-stimulated lung cells with MSCs resulted in decreased secretion of pro-inflammatory cytokines, suggesting that soluble factors secreted by MSCs inhibit inflammatory responses, and/or direct effects of lung cells and MSCs produce anti-inflammatory effects. MSCs have immunomodulatory effects on immune cells (T cells, B cells, and NK cells). In addition, recent studies have found that endogenous lung stem cells with MSC phenotype can be used in mice lungs after elastase injury, and intratracheal administration of stem cells can reduce elastase-induced lung injury and improve survival rate. Transplanted stem cells can reach the alveolar space, and only some cells remain in the alveolar wall. The above results do not support the differentiation of cells, but suggest the immunomodulatory effects of stem cells in lung injury. In addition, Spees et al. reported that mitochondrial DNA can be transferred from MSCs to other cells, which regulate the mitochondrial function of recipient cells. Therefore, we speculate that the inhibitory effect of MSCs on lung injury may be due to the anti-inflammatory effect of MSCs rather than the differentiation into lung cells.

### 7.2.3.3 Effects of Drugs on the Repair and Regeneration of Damaged Lung Tissue

#### Retinoic Acid

Retinoic acid (RA) is an active metabolite of vitamin A, and airway epithelial cells are specific target cells for vitamin A action. RA is involved in lung development, especially the occurrence of alveoli and the process of lung repair after injury. RA regulates the morphological branching of the embryonic lungs and promotes alveolar septation. Knockout of mouse RA receptors leads to alveolar dysfunction, that is, abnormal formation of normal alveolar and alveolar elastic fibers. Elastin synthesis is increased in lung fibroblasts after RA treatment and is related to lipofibroblasts (retinoid reserve cells). These results suggest that RA plays an important role in the development of lung morphology. Since Massaro et al. found that all-trans retinoic acid (ATRA) can reverse the anatomy and functional lesions of rat emphysema models, a series of studies have been carried out in this field. In particular, RA can induce the proliferation of type II alveolar epithelial cells. The mechanism of action is to interfere with the activity of cyclin-dependent complex in late G1 phase and inhibit the expression of Cdk inhibitory protein CKI p21Cip1, which regulates cell cycle in cell mitosis, leading to the weakening of cell division cycle inhibitory factors, promoting cells into the proliferative cycle, thus promoting the growth of residual lung after lung resection, and playing a role in promoting lung tissue repair. Massaro found that the use of RA after birth can increase the number of alveoli. In addition, RA can inhibit the inhibitory effect of dexamethasone on alveolar formation. It is currently believed that the promotion of alveolar regeneration by RA may be an important component in the treatment of lung diseases such as reduced gas exchange surface area. To date, a total of 14 studies have used RA to prevent and treat emphysema models. Interestingly, 8 of them showed that RA promoted lung tissue regeneration, while the other 6 showed negative results. The possible causes of this inconsistency include (a) species differences in animal models and (b) RA dose domain value difference. During compensatory lung growth, small animals such as rodents show a good regeneration process because their somatic cells have proliferative potential throughout their life, which can affect the therapeutic outcome of RA. Another factor is the RA dose that promotes lung regeneration. Stinchcombe and Maden have evaluated the effects of RA on lung regeneration in three strains of mice (TO, ICR, NIHS) and found that the RA dose domain values are different for different strains of mice. In comparison, the effect of RA on improving the function of injured lung in rats was weaker than that in mice.

In addition to exogenous RA, the lipid interstitial cells in the lung tissue store retinol, the substrate of endogenous retinoic acid; the lipid interstitial cells accumulate in the alveolar germinal site; and the retinol plays a key role in the formation of alveolar tissue, suggesting that retinol in these cells forms endogenous retinoic acid in alveolar tissue. The study found that rat lipid interstitial cells can synthesize and secrete ATRA, which can increase the expression of CRBP-1 mRNA in type I epithelial cells. Retinol-binding protein-retinol complex is a substrate for the synthesis of retinoic acid in vivo. All-trans retinoic acid mediates the expression of related genes via nuclear receptor RARs and RXRs. Exogenous all-trans retinoic acid can increase the amount of retinol storage particles and thereby increase the secretion of endogenous retinoic acid, thereby inducing or increasing the formation of alveolar tissue. Therefore, endogenous retinoic acid is also involved in the repair of injured lung tissue promoted by exogenous RA.

The pharmacokinetic results of exogenous RA by intraperitoneal injection showed that after RA (2.0 mg/kg) injection into mice, it rapidly entered the peripheral blood and was present in the lungs at 5 min; reached a peak of 4178 pg/mg at 15 min, then decreased, and could not be detected in the plasma at 4 h; however, retinoic acid in the lung remained during the observation period and existed in the form of all-trans retinoic acid. Previous studies have demonstrated that RA can cause rapid expression of related genes in the lung: expression of RA response elements such as RA receptors, RA-binding proteins, and tropoelastin. Therefore, exogenous RA has a good targeting in the lung tissue and is one of the effective components for repairing damaged lung tissue.

### Hepatocyte Growth Factor

Hepatocyte growth factor (HGF) was initially used as a mitogen for primary culture of hepatocytes.

HGF is a pluripotent growth factor secreted by mesenchymal cells, which promotes cell division, proliferation, migration, and differentiation. After lung injury or during lung development, it plays a mitogenic role through the tyrosine phosphorylation of its receptor c-Met and also has a certain role in the development of lung morphogenesis. In particular, HGF is a mitogen for the alveolar type II epithelium. In lung compensatory growth after lung resection in mice, HGF stimulates proliferation of airway epithelial cells. In addition, HGF can also activate the migration and proliferation of endothelial cells and induce angiogenesis. In the formation of alveolar septum, HGF promotes proliferation, migration, and microtubule formation of lung epithelial cells and endothelial cells through four kinds of cells (fibroblasts, macrophages, smooth muscle cells, and activated epithelial cells) in three common secretory ways. In view of the above effects, the role of HGF in lung regeneration has been extensively studied. Intraperitoneal injection of HGF significantly increased the proportion of Sca-$1^+$/Flk-$1^+$ in peripheral blood mononuclear cells of mice. HGF can also induce the proliferation of bone marrow-derived and alveolar wall-resident endothelial cells, reverse elastase-induced emphysema in mice, reduce collagen deposition in mice with lung fibrosis, and induce lung compensatory growth. In the rat emphysema model, transfection of cDNA encoding human HGF promotes efficient expression of human HGF in the alveolar endothelium and epithelium, resulting in more extensive pulmonary vascularization and inhibition of alveolar wall cell apoptosis. Intravenous injection of adipose-derived interstitial cells secreting HGF can improve emphysema in rats. Hegab et al. reported that inhalation of HGF twice a week for two consecutive weeks significantly reduced elastase-induced alveolar cavity expansion and alveolar wall destruction, increased static lung compliance, and returned to normal levels. HGF promotes chemotaxis of epithelial cell line A549. After HGF receptor blockade, A549 chemotaxis was inhibited, but the same concentration of KGF did not have this effect. Under specific culture conditions, HGF induces differentiation of nonadherent lung stem cells into alveolar-like cells.

### Granulocyte Colony-Stimulating Factor

Granulocyte colony-stimulating factor (G-CSF) relieves the pathological process of acute lung injury by mobilizing bone marrow stem cells into peripheral blood. In the mouse emphysema model, G-CSF can reduce emphysema lesions. For mice treated with G-CSF, the mean linear intercept (Lm) of alveoli is significantly shorter than that in the injured group. This phenomenon is consistent with the extent of reduction of RA-induced emphysema lesions in mice. G-CSF can increase the number of bone marrow-derived endothelial progenitor cells in the blood circulation. G-CSF combined with RA treatment has a significant additive effect, manifested by further shortening of Lm. Bone marrow-derived cells play an important role in G-CSF-induced lung regeneration. These results suggest that the lack of circulating stem cells in elderly patients with COPD may be a limiting factor affecting the efficacy.

### Keratinocyte Growth Factor

Keratinocyte growth factor (KGF), that is, fibroblast growth factor-7, belongs to the FGF family and is mainly produced by mesenchymal cells. It acts on alveolar type II epithelial cells expressing KGF receptors and plays an important role during lung development. KGF receptor is expressed in alveolar type II epithelial cells. KGF promotes the survival, proliferation, and migration of alveolar type II epithelial cells and cell adhesion to extracellular matrices. Intratracheal injection of KGF induces proliferation of alveolar type II epithelial cells. For pulmonary resected rats, KGF induces compensatory formation of new alveoli in mature lungs. In addition, in vitro experiments confirmed that KGF has a significant reversal effect during the transformation of AT2 to AT1 phenotype, which may be an important regulatory molecule to maintain the AT2 phenotype or AT1 dedifferentiation. Although KGF pretreatment prevented elastase-induced emphysema, KGF treatment (3 weeks after elastase action) did not reverse the pathological expansion of alveolar. rhKGF pretreatment may not alleviate alveolar inflammatory exudation and may not alleviate epithelial cell damage. Studies suggest that KGF may not be directly involved in alveolar epithelial repair and restoration of its integrity. The results of blood gas and lung compliance tests suggest that the improvement of gas exchange function by KGF may be mainly due to the increase of surfactant protein secreted by AT2 proliferation. KGF gene therapy (attenuated *Salmonella typhimurium* vaccine + recombinant human KGF gene therapy) can alleviate pneumococcal injury in radiation-induced rats. These results suggest that KGF may play an important role in anti-inflammatory effects and does not effectively promote alveolar repair.

#### Adrenomedullin

Adrenomedullin is a multifunctional regulatory polypeptide isolated from human adrenal pheochromocytoma. Adrenomedullin can induce cAMP production, and cell growth regulation; inhibit apoptosis and angiogenesis; and antagonize microbial activity. Adrenomedullin receptors are highly expressed in airway epithelial cells and alveolar type II epithelial cells, while both cells are involved in lung epithelial regeneration. In a mouse emphysema model, continuous infusion of adrenomedullin by subcutaneous osmotic pump increases the number of Sca-$1^+$ cells in peripheral blood and promotes alveolar regeneration and pulmonary vascularization.

#### Simvastatin

In addition to the effect of lowering cholesterol, simvastatin, one of the HMG-CoA reductase inhibitors (statins), has other pharmacological effects, such as anti-inflammatory effects (regulation of nuclear factors, anti-inflammation, and reduction of leukocyte infiltration), improvement of endothelial cell function, inhibition of the apoptosis of alveolar type II cells, and promotion of the proliferation of alveolar type II cells by upregulating the expression level of phosphorylated Akt. Studies on tissue regeneration effects of statins confirmed that intraperitoneal injection of simvastatin shortens elastase-induced emphysema Lm and increases the number of alveolar PCNA$^+$ cells. Inhalation of a 50 μg endotoxin model in healthy adults revealed that simvastatin antagonized excessive inflammatory responses including (a) reduction of neutrophil aggregation by reducing the production of local cytokines and chemokines (such as TNF-α, MMP-7); (b) direct increase of neutrophil apoptosis, decrease of recruitment and other mechanisms, and decrease of the number and activation of neutrophils; (c) inhibition of MMP-7 and MMP-9 release from macrophages and reduction of macrophage activation; and (d) reduction of CRP concentration in plasma. In addition, for radiation-induced lung injury (RILI) mice, simvastatin can act as an anti-inflammatory molecule and protective component of lung barrier; reduce vascular leakage, leukocyte infiltration, and oxidative stress; reverse the dysregulation of RILI-related gene expression such as p53, nuclear factor-erythrocyte 2-related factor, and protective component of lung barrier; and reverse sphingolipid metabolic pathway genes. To confirm that simvastatin protects key effector regulatory molecules, the whole lung gene expression data were obtained by single-network analysis of proteins in simvastatin-treated injured mice, and topological analysis of gene product interactions confirmed that eight priority genes (Ccna2a, Cdc2, fcer1g, Syk, Vav3, Mmp9, Itgam, Cd44) were key nodes affecting the RILI network. This further confirms the protective mechanism of statins against acute lung injury from the perspective of signaling pathways. At present, it is suggested that in clinical practice, 5 mg/(kg·d) simvastatin starting 3–7 days before surgery may be beneficial to relieve lung ischemia-reperfusion injury, which is beneficial to the recovery of pulmonary function after surgery.

### 7.2.3.4 Factors Affecting the Repair of Damaged Lung Tissue by Stem/Progenitor Cells

#### The Etiology of Acute Lung Injury

Previous studies on lung injury cell treatment found that the injury factors (endotoxin, live bacteria, oleic acid, and bleomycin) are different and stem/progenitor cells have different effects on structural remodeling and functional recovery of damaged lung tissue, suggesting that the effect of clinical stem/progenitor cells on acute lung injury may be closely related to the etiology of injury. It is necessary to make informed choices and prudent judgment about the relationship between primary lung injury, secondary lung injury, pathogen species (bacteria, virus, and fungi), and the effect of cell therapy.

#### Neuroendocrine-Immune Network Coordination

There is a serious damage stress response in lung injury, and a large amount of neuroendocrine hormone released by the body has an important influence on the repair of stem/progenitor cells from various sources.

Glucocorticoids, epinephrine, norepinephrine, and acetylcholine released from the hypothalamus-pituitary-adrenal axis, sympathetic adrenal medullary system, cholinergic system, and local neuroendocrine cells in the lung can affect the mobilization response and chemotactic activity of stem/progenitor cells. In recent years, it has been found that melatonin secreted by the pineal gland also contributes significantly to the repair of lung injury by mesenchymal stem cells. At the same time, it was found that human MSC reduced immune tolerance rather than immunocompetent lung injury in mice, suggesting that the immune status of the body determines the effect of MSC treatment. The above results suggest that the coordination of neuroendocrine-immune network is directly involved in the regulation of lung injury repair and affects the therapeutic effect of stem/progenitor cells.

#### Differences Between Endogenous and Exogenous Stem/Progenitor Cells

At present, among stem/progenitor cells that have positive effects on lung injury, the greatest advantage of exogenous stem/progenitor cells is the controllable number, but they need to be obtained through in vitro procedures such as isolation, purification, and amplification, and the potential safety risks such as in vitro contamination and differentiation cannot be excluded. After the completion of transplantation, the outcome of the cells in the body still needs to be further reduced to prevent potential risks of transplant rejection, teratogenicity, and tumor formation. In contrast, the greatest advantage of endogenous stem/progenitor cells is the safety, which requires only mobilization agents or regulators to fully mobilize the redistribution of stem/progenitor cells against lung injury in vivo and does not require in vitro cell manipulation steps, but the quantitative limitations (such as the responsiveness of the body to mobilization agents) will affect the therapeutic effect.

#### Stem/Progenitor Cell Species, Age, and Transplantation Path

First, in the treatment of lung injury, the stem/progenitor cells of the same species have better therapeutic effects than the stem/progenitor cells of different species. Second, studies found that senescent stem cells are at a disadvantage in the treatment of lung injury due to their decline in migration capacity, anti-inflammatory activity, and immunomodulatory capacity. Therefore, the selection of stem cells derived from young individuals is better than stem cells derived from elderly individuals. Finally, there are some differences in the effect of intravenous, tracheal, intrapulmonary, and intraperitoneal injection of target cells. Studies have confirmed that intravenous injection is better than intraperitoneal injection. Therefore, the selection of the same species, younger age, and direct pathway injection method in the treatment of lung injury will have better therapeutic effect.

### 7.2.3.5 Bioartificial Lung Replacement Therapy to Repair Lung Function

So far, lung transplantation still has many bottlenecks due to limited lung donors. Therefore, the idea of transplanting stem/progenitor cells or fetal lung cells to repair damaged lungs or constructing artificial lungs replacement for decompensated lungs has been a concern of the scientific community. Since the lung is a complex organ with a three-dimensional structure composed of more than 40 cells, it is difficult to construct the lung artificially at present. Recently, several artificial lung models have been reported. Mainstream studies use acellular lung scaffold materials with better biocompatibility, supplemented by new endothelial and epithelial cells transplanted to scaffold. In addition, the source of artificial lung cells also involves fetal lung cells, human umbilical endothelial cells, etc.

Researchers at Harvard Medical School in the United States have eluted mouse lung parenchymal cells by SDS solution, leaving only the extracellular matrix as a scaffold for new lung growth. The scaffold still retains basic morphological structures such as blood vessels, airways, and alveoli. Subsequently, vascular endothelial cells and alveolar epithelial cells were implanted in the scaffold and cultured in containers mimicking the biological environment. The results showed that stem cells rapidly grew and differentiated on the residual lung scaffolds and began oxygen exchange after 7 days, simulating normal lung respiratory function, and lung regeneration can be completed in about 2 weeks. After implanting it in mice, the artificial lungs continued to work and the mice survived for 6 h. It is believed that with the progress of research and improvement of technology, complications such as pulmonary edema will be gradually overcome, and the survival time of regenerative lung will gradually prolong. With the deepening of stem cell research, it is possible to obtain sufficient adult stem cells (such as bone marrow mesenchymal stem cells), embryonic stem cells, and even induced pluripotent stem cells (iPS cells). Under the action of regulatory factors in specific differentiation stages, cell types (alveolar epithelial cells, vascular endothelial cells, etc.) can be generated to promote lung regeneration, thereby achieving lung regeneration and functional recovery based on the basic scaffold structure of the lung. In addition, artificial lung researchers combined human alveolar cells with vacuum chips to create chip lungs that breathe freely. The micro-device simulates the most active alveolar part of the lung, combines the two layers of the lung blood-air barrier (the inner layer is the alveolar layer and the outer layer is the blood circulation layer), and makes use of vacuum principle to enable air to operate in a highly reductive manner through the whole system, which can effectively realize the process of oxygen mixing into the blood. Although these cells are not yet suitable for clinical applications, and the pulmonary interstitium has not been scientifically configured and integrated in structural remodeling, the concept of bioartificial lungs, with its low rejection and controllable source of lung organs, may be potential candidates for the treatment of lung disease in the future and may bring new hope to about 50 million patients with advanced lung disease worldwide.

#### 7.2.3.6 Consideration of Stem/Progenitor Cells in Lung Tissue Repair

At present, in the repair, remodeling, and regeneration of lung structural as a central link in the treatment of refractory lung diseases, there are still some aspects worthy of attention: First, most acute lung injury treatment researches are based on the results in rodent model, in which the lung maintains a vigorous proliferative potential throughout its life cycle, while the human lung has a very limited self-regeneration potential. Therefore, species differences should be further considered for many effective stem/progenitor cell treatments, and because human lung stem/progenitor cells are limited in number and poorly understood, there are still many uncertainties in transplanting it to the mature lung. In comparison, the use of secondary endogenous lung stem/progenitor cell repair strategy can effectively improve the self-renewal, proliferation, migration, and differentiation potential of lung stem/progenitor cells, and it has positive significance in overcoming the bottleneck of cell transplantation therapy and improving the biological safety of injury treatment. Second, in view of the biosafety of endogenous stem/progenitor cells and the controllability of the number of exogenous stem/progenitor cells, the combination of two source cells to repair lung injury is expected to enhance treatment. Third, in view of the complexity of lung injury repair, it is necessary to consider the number of stem/progenitor cells and repair efficiency and to fully understand the local microenvironment of the lungs. We need to improve the repair microenvironment of lung damage from the perspective of neuroendocrine-immune network to provide a suitable environment for stem/progenitor cell repair. Fourth, lung injury repair involves a variety of cellular responses, and the regulation and integration of inflammation-related factors and pro-repairing factor clusters (such as the synergistic effects of statins and retinoic acid, statins, and growth factors) will help grasp the timing of repair and promote the functional repair of damaged lungs. Fifth, for the method of obtaining stem/progenitor cells to promote lung repair through bone marrow mobilization, synergistic treatment with different stem/progenitor cell groups will have more advantages than single-cell population, which has been supported by evidence in previous studies of bone marrow mononuclear cell therapy. Sixth, in view of the strong endocrine and paracrine effects of stem/progenitor cells, the transmitters and microbubbles released by them will be the active components for lung injury repair, and the development of stem/progenitor cell repair solutions based on such components will also have beneficial effects on lung injury repair. Seventh, in view of the previous unsuccessful experience in the bio-artificial lung research, the role of extracellular matrix components in the repair of lung injury should be emphasized on the basis of fully considering the number, and the important contribution of pulmonary extracellular matrix to the restoration of alveolar structural integrity in structural remodeling should be highlighted. At the same time, more attention should be paid to the lineage of intrapulmonary stem/progenitor cells, the changes and outcomes of extrapulmonary stem/progenitor cells before and after lung tissue repair, and the functional integration of extrapulmonary and intrapulmonary stem/progenitor cells in lung tissue repair.

### 7.2.4 Summary

The lungs are developed from the mesoderm and endoderm of the embryo. The lung primordia are the basis of lung formation, and the lung development undergoes three stages: embryonic period, fetal period, and postnatal period. Mature lung tissue consists of more than 40 cells. Under physiological conditions, the renewal of adult lungs is very slow. Because the lung communicates with the outside world and its structure is very fragile, it is extremely vulnerable. Therefore, the repair ability of lung tissue itself is important for maintaining its structural integrity and exerting its normal function. In recent years, a variety of tissue cells with certain self-renewal and differentiation potential have been found in lung tissues, collectively known as endogenous lung stem/progenitor cells, such as basal cells and duct cells located in the trachea, Clara cells and variant Clara cells located in the epithelium of bronchi and bronchioles, and bronchioloalveolar stem cells and type II alveolar epithelial cells located at the bronchioloalveolar junction. In addition, smooth muscle progenitor cells, angioblasts, and marginal cells in lung tissue also have certain stemness. Studies have shown that these endogenous stem cells may play a role in the repair and regeneration of chronic obstructive pulmonary disease, cystic fibrosis, acute lung injury, and other diseases.

## 7.3 Liver Regeneration and Liver Stem Cells

### 7.3.1 Liver Regeneration

In Greek mythology, Prometheus stole fire from the gods for human use. His punishment was that a giant eagle ate his liver every day, after which his liver regenerated every night. In concurrence with Greek mythos, science has proven that mammals possess livers with strong regenerative capabilities. A healthy liver can rapidly initiate consecutive synergistic changes and restore itself to its initial volume and structure after resection or injury [1]. In 1931, Higgins and Anderson established the classic model of liver regeneration in rats, in which after a 70% partial hepatectomy (2/3 liver) the liver was able to completely regenerate in just 20 days. The resected portion exhibited no new growth, while the remaining hepatic lobe demonstrated compensatory hyperplasia and discontinued growth when returned to its original volume [2]. This model revealed key mechanisms of liver regeneration, including the roles of different cell types such as hepatic stellate cells, macrophages, sinusoidal endothelial cells, and cytokines such as HGF, IL-6, EGF, TNF, 5-HT, norepinephrine, and bile [3]. Because stem cell and tissue engineering technology are some of the most rapidly developing fields used in life science research, they have great potential for further use in clinical use such as liver cell therapy, tissue and organ repair, developmental biology, and pharmacology.

### 7.3.2 Liver Stem Cells

The liver possesses stem cells which can differentiate into hepatocytes and cholangiocytes, which can aid the repair of liver injury. These are known as oval cells or atypical epithelial cells which are found in the Hering canal located at the end of the hepatobiliary duct [4]. Small bile duct hyperplasia, the primary biliary response, triggers oval cell differentiation [5]. An excellent model of induced oval cell response is the 2-AAF/PHx rat model, where rats are treated with 2-acetylaminofluorene (2-AAF) to inhibit the proliferation of hepatocytes and then subjected to partial hepatectomy, resulting in a large amount of oval cells during regeneration. Mouse models were found to be incompatible with this method so a different approach was developed [6, 7] using common markers such as EPCAM, CK19, CD133, and SOX9, and cells were isolated from fetal or adult livers, proliferated in vitro, differentiated into hepatocytes and biliary cells, and allowed to repopulate the liver when transplanted into liver injury models [8]. In recent years, lineage-specific tracing technology based on genetic markers has made great progress, which can faithfully display the fate of cells in vivo and provide a powerful tool for studying the fate of specific groups of cells. Therefore, scientists use this technology to further study the regeneration mechanism of livers.

### 7.3.3 The Regulation of Liver Regeneration In Vivo

Krt19 (CK19) is a cell marker specific to the bile duct epithelium, a source of oval cells or atypical bile duct epithelial cells. Yanger et al. used Krt19 to label hepatic stem/progenitor cells and lineage tracing to observe the fate of their derived cells [9]. They observed virtually no Krt19-positive oval cell-derived hepatocytes in any of the models of liver injury or in stable liver, only observing generation of new biliary cells. Lineage traced cells revealed that new hepatocytes were not derived from nonhepatocytes, but from existing hepatocytes. Nucleoside analogue labeling of rapidly proliferating cell populations revealed that nonhepatic parenchymal cells also did not differentiate to hepatocytes. Similarly, Tarlow et al. used Sox9, another well-recognized marker of liver stem/progenitor cells [10]. The Sox9-positive cells did not differentiate to hepatocytes, instead becoming part of the bile duct epithelium. Conversely, the overexpression of cell cycle suppressor gene p21 and knockout of integrin β1 both inhibited proliferation and resulted in bile duct stem cell-derived hepatocyte regeneration.

Lgr5, of the Wnt-signaling pathway and a stem cell marker, was used by Huch et al. to observe stem cell populations in the liver. Lgr5-positive cells were not present in homeostatic liver, nor in $CCl_4$-induced acute liver injury; however, it did appear near the portal vein, expressing the marker Sox9 of cholangiocytes, making them closer to cholangiocytes rather than hepatocytes in their gene expression profile. $CCl_4$-induced acute liver parenchymal injury model tracing revealed that bile-duct-derived cells can gradually differentiate into mature liver cells, while CDE-induced and DDC-induced injury can differentiate into both liver cells and cholangiocytes [11]. Regardless of the type of damage, the Lgr5-positive cell population has a weak effect on the overall regeneration of the liver parenchyma. These cells can be expanded through organoids culture in vitro and can also differentiate into hepatocytes and cholangiocytes, acting as stem cells in Fah−/− mouse liver (Fah gene deficiency will lead to hypertyrosinemia, which will lead to severe liver injury. NTBC drugs can block tyrosine metabolism and terminate the downstream pathway. It is a better model to study liver reproduction) [12].

Axin2, another target gene of the Wnt signaling pathway, was found to be expressed in a population of hepatocytes of the central vein. Wang et al. used Axin2 to label these cells, diploid cells that express glutamine synthetase (GS), the hepatic progenitor cell marker Tbx3, but not carbamoyl phosphate synthase (CPS-1) of mature cells. Fate tracing indicates that while Axin2-positive cells are found near the central vein, their derivatives gradually migrate to the portal area and become new mature liver cells that express CPS-1 instead of GS or Tbx3 [13].

Wnt2 and Wnt9b, ligands of the Wnt signaling pathway secreted by central venous endothelial cells, constitute the microenvironment of Axin2-positive hepatocytes. Knocking out the Wnt signaling pathway in endothelial cells of the central vein caused significant downregulation in the expression of Axin2 and GS in cells of the central vein and inhibited proliferative ability, confirming that the Wnt signaling pathway is necessary for the normal functioning of Axin2-positive cells.

Font-Burgada et al. found bile duct cells of the portal region in Sox9-GFP transgenic mouse model [14], which have low expression of Sox9 but also express hepatocyte genes, appropriately called hybrid hepatocytes (HybHP) [15]. These cells exist in the homeostatic liver, adjacent to the terminal branches of the portal vein and bile duct. The chronic hepatic parenchymal injury model, induced by CCl4 or through overexpression of MUP-uPA, has cells that exhibit strong proliferative ability; however, Sox9-positive or CK19-positive biliary epithelial cells are not involved in the generation of new liver cells. HybHP regeneration is damage-dependent, playing a major role in liver regeneration during mild chronic injury, but not in severe chronic injury. In severe injury models that illicit oval cell response, mature hepatocytes can transdifferentiate into Sox9-positive hepatic stem/progenitor cells, which then undergo expansion and re-differentiate into both hepatocytes and cholangiocytes [16].

Pu et al. discovered a class of molecules, Mfsd2a, expressed specifically in hepatocytes of the portal vein of adult mice. Fate tracing showed that Mfsd2a-positive hepatocytes gradually decreased in homeostatic environments and expanded after major hepatectomy or CCl4-induced acute liver injury [17]. During chronic bile duct injury, Mfsd2a-positive cells are also reduced, while in CCl4-induced chronic liver injury, most intact hepatic lobes completely regenerate. A small population of hepatocytes with high expression of telomerase (TERThigh) also exist in the liver. Lineage tracing of these cells has shown self-renewal ability and participation in the generation of a large number of hepatocytes in a steady state of liver, and regeneration of hepatocytes in the case of injury.

Lineage tracing strategies using different models for liver regeneration revealed that hepatocytes have significant heterogeneity. Axin2-positive hepatocytes of the central vein, hybrid hepatocytes with low expression of Sox9, the Mfsd2a-positive hepatocytes of the portal vein, and the TERThigh hepatocytes also have a large population of common hepatocytes with no specific markers. Under normal homeostasis, Axin2-positive hepatocytes of the central vein and TERThigh hepatocytes of other types of hepatocytes throughout the hepatic lobules facilitate the renewal of hepatocytes; under acute liver injury or partial hepatectomy, liver regeneration mainly depends on preexisting hepatocytes, and Lgr5-positive stem cells are very limited in regeneration of hepatocytes. Under mild chronic liver parenchymal injury, hybrid hepatocytes with low expression of Sox9 or Mfsd2a-positive hepatocytes are responsible generating new hepatocytes. Studying the underlying mechanisms and factors of hepatocyte regeneration and identifying its key players will better help us develop interventions such as using genes or compounds to directly target the target cells and enhance or activate the repair and regeneration of endogenous cells. It is imperative for donors and recipients of living donor liver transplantation to adopt routine measures to promote rapid regeneration of endogenous hepatocytes. In addition to making significant advances in vivo studies of liver regeneration, there have been many breakthroughs in the studies of obtaining hepatocytes in vitro for liver regeneration using stem cells and lineage tracing-related technologies.

### 7.3.4 Strategies for Obtaining Hepatocytes In Vitro

Currently, orthotopic liver transplantation is the only effective treatment for end-stage liver disease; however, shortages in suitable organ donors impede new developments in liver transplantation technology. Although hepatocyte transplantation is an alternative option, primary hepatocytes cannot achieve the culture and expansion efficiency needed of large-scale production. Because pluripotent stem cells (PSCs) have an almost limitless self-renewal capacity, a multistep differentiation strategy to recapitulate the liver development pathway was established in vitro. Ethical issues, along with the possibility of immune rejection and tumorigenic risk associated with ESCs, prevent it from being considered as treatment. Although iPSCs are able to circumvent the issues of ethicality and immune rejection, there is still a risk that long-term culture will cause gene mutations that lead to tumorigenesis.

In 2011, the scientists Hui Lijian and Suzuki used lineage reprogramming techniques to convert mouse fibroblasts into hepatocytes through two combinations of liver development-specific transcription factors, GATA4 + HNF1a + FOXA3 and HNF4a + FOXA1 + FOXA2/FOXA3, respectively. In both methods, cells expressed hepatocyte-specific genes such as Alb, HNF4a, and Afp [18, 19] and performed functions of primary hepatocytes, including glycogen synthesis, albumin secretion, urea synthesis, low-density lipoprotein uptake, P450 enzyme metabolism, etc. The cells were also able to alleviate liver damage in Fah−/− mice. Nevertheless, the hepatocytes obtained cannot be considered mature because they still express genes markers of early development, and their regeneration and function of liver recovery in injured mice are inferior to that of primary hepatocytes.

In 2014, Hui Lijian et al. used overexpression of the transcription factors FOXA3, HNF-1A, and HNF-4A [20], and Deng Hongkui et al. used the transcription factors HNF-1A, HNF-4A, HN6, ATF5, PROX1, CEBPA, c-Myc, and p53 shRNA to transform human fibroblasts into functionally mature liver cells [21]. Both sets of reprogrammed cells had a P450 enzyme metabolism comparable to those of primary hepatocytes and allowed recovery in liver injury model mice.

However, because the overexpression of these transcription factors depends on viral methods, it cannot be used for clinical use.

Many scientists began to consider using a small molecule mediated reprogramming strategy as an alternative. The Wang Yunfang led team successfully reprogrammed human primary gastric epithelial cells into endodermal progenitor cells (hiEndoPCs) using four small molecule compounds: A8301, BIX01294, BayK8644, and RG108 [22]. Quantitative amplification and specifically induced differentiation resulted in hepatocytes that express a variety of functional genes related to liver maturation, and also perform various functions of liver maturation such as albumin synthesis, urea secretion, glycogen synthesis, HCV susceptibility, and P450 enzyme metabolism [23]. Transplantation of the cells into a Fah−/− mouse model also resulted in liver recovery. These techniques can be used to treat multiple liver diseases and provide a novel cell source for drug metabolism, toxicological research, and anti-HCV drug development. Because hepatocytes produced by reprogramming methods have non-hepatic lineages, characteristics of the original cells are retained and thus differ from primary hepatocytes. Huch et al. established an in vitro expansion and culture system of hepatic stem/progenitor cells obtained from the bile duct through human liver surgeries or biopsies [24]. After being expanded in vitro for over 1 year, using three-dimensional organoid culture methods, it was re-differentiated into functional hepatocytes and integrated into the livers of liver injured mouse models. The chromosomal structure of the cells remained stable even after long-term expansion, making it ideal for individualized disease models, drug development, and cell therapy.

Katsuda et al. used small molecules Y27632, A8301, and CHIR99021 to reprogram rodent primary hepatocytes (mainly diploid hepatocytes) into hepatic stem/progenitor cells which can differentiate into both hepatocytes and cholangiocytes in vitro, almost completely regenerate, and repopulate injured liver with high efficiency (75%–90%) when transplanted into liver injury model mice [25]. The high efficiency and safety of these small molecule applications have made it a highly sought-after method for obtaining hepatocytes. Recently, Hui Lijian et al. and Yan Hexin et al. reprogrammed human primary hepatocytes into expandable hepatic stem/progenitor cells using different small molecule combinations, which can be differentiated into functional hepatocytes. Based on previous in vitro hepatocyte reprogramming, scientists have recently developed in vivo hepatocyte reprogramming. Myofibroblast development is crucial for understanding liver fibrosis and cirrhosis, as well as formation of scar tissue. Song et al. used a p75 neurotrophic receptor peptide (p75NTRp)-labeled adenovirus to target four liver-specific transcription factors FOXA3, GATA4, HNF1a, and HNF4a of hepatic myofibroblasts [26]. Rezvani et al. specifically targeted hepatic myofibroblasts using hepadnavirus-adenovirus vector (AAV6) carrying transcription factors FOXA1, FOXA2, FOXA3, GATA4, and HNF1a/HNF4a [27]. While this method is relatively effective in transporting transcription factors to target cells and can be used to treat chronic liver fibrosis and cirrhosis by converting some hepatic myofibroblasts into hepatocytes (efficiency <1%), the efficiency is still too low and the method for overexpressing transcription factors is too complex. Although the maturity of hepatocyte cellular functions, safety, and effectiveness still have room for further improvements, these technologies have made great improvements in the cell therapy development for liver diseases.

### 7.3.5 Establishment of Tissue-Engineered Liver

Direct transplantation of healthy cells into damaged livers for the treatment of liver diseases is very effective, particularly where the function of the liver cells is destroyed, while liver structure is intact. Having a suitable extracellular matrix in combination with specific cells is still a challenge as well as the question of whether or not tissues and organs constructed in vitro can perform the complete functions of specific organs. Due to the complicated structure of the liver, and the importance of its many functions, there is currently no adequate product available, despite its promising progress in basic and tissue engineering research.

Previously, Bhatia et al. of MIT used a microfabrication method to try to simulate the natural structure of the liver, fabricating micron-scale network channels of microvascular structures such as hepatic sinusoids and capillary bile ducts on solid substrates, then implanting hepatocytes, sinusoidal endothelial cells, and cholangiocytes into the network to establish an artificially perfused, functional hepatocyte units. This engineered liver is small in size and simple in structure, making it more suited for in vitro studies, including drug metabolism, toxicity detection, and viral infection rather than transplantation [28].

Three-dimensional organoid culture technology has provided ways to solve the problems associated with 2D cell culture. Organoid culture places cells in suitable extracellular matrix microenvironments for self-driven three-dimensional organization, forming miniature organs with complex layered intercellular interactions and functions, that is able to more accurately represent the occurrence and development of certain diseases.

Organoid culture technique was first developed by Hans Clevers to recapitulate the 3D structures of the intestinal wall, such as the villi and crypts. In 2013, Takabe et al. used induced pluripotent stem cell (iPSC)-derived hepatic endoderm cells (iPSC-HEs) as a source of hepatocytes, umbilical vein endothelial cells (HUVECs) as hepatic sinusoidal endothelial cells, and human umbilical cord mesenchymal stem cells as hepatic stellate cells in co-culture, in order to obtain what is known as a liver bud [29]. A liver buds hepatocyte function is significantly higher than those induced by traditional iPS, later even forming complex structures, including hepatic sinusoids and hepatic cord, and connections with the blood vessels of the host animal. Transplantation of liver buds improved survival in acute liver injury mouse models. Liver buds are an important clinical breakthrough because before there were very few limited cell types that have been used to produce three-dimensional, vascularized primary liver in vitro that can improve the prognosis of acute liver failure models. However, liver buds have neither the lobular structure of the normal livers nor do they have an extrahepatic biliary system, potentially leading to toxic levels of accumulated bile. Liver buds also cannot be transplanted orthotopically and are only viable for temporary heterotopic mesenteric transplantation in patients with hereditary metabolic liver disease, or improving the survival period of patients on the waiting list for liver transplantation.

Development of an acellular-recellular technique has brought hope to creating a complete tissue engineered liver, using physical or chemical (detergent or enzymes) methods to first remove the parenchymal and interstitial cells, while retaining the three-dimensional structural scaffold, original extracellular matrix components, and the perfusion vasculature. The decellularized organ is recellularized by circulating perfusion of parenchymal and interstitial cells. Because it maintains and maximizes the original structure and components, it is a favorable regenerative environment for the growth and function of perfused cells. The lack of immunogenicity and good histocompatibility also means that xenogeneic organs can be used, thus solving the problem of insufficient sources. It is clear that it will have broad application prospects in future organ replacement therapy.

Currently, the decellularization technology of intact organs has been realized in organs such as heart [30], liver [31, 32], and lung [33], and preliminarily in the kidney and pancreas [34]. Wang Yunfang's team had independently established an early-stage rapid and mild liver decellularization technique, removing cells within a few hours and preserving the various extracellular matrixes and complete structure of the liver [35]. This technology has obtained international patents and is currently undergoing research related to recellularization. After allotransplantation, recellularized livers can survive for 8 h in recipient mice [31]. After transplantation, rat lungs can only participate in gas exchange for 45–120 min [33], and the longest survival time is 3 days [36]. Due to incomplete recellularization of the vascular system leading to subendothelial collagen exposure, activation of the coagulation system leading to coagulation, and organ blockages, improvements can still be made. There may be more problems that need to be examined and solved in future clinical application, such as the choice of source of decellularized organs, which organs of the species are more suitable for reconstruction after decellularization and transplantation in vivo, and how to rebuild the biliary system to avoid bile leakage.

The development of 3D printing technology has also provided new options for the construction of tissue engineered liver. 3D printing can accumulate material layer by layer to form a three-dimensional structure similar to the original object. By printing the liver frame and various types of cells layer by layer, it is expected that the printed liver will possess a structure and function close to the real liver. There are some challenges from 3D printing the liver, including choosing printing materials and the use of biocompatible natural or artificial materials with mechanical properties of the liver that will facilitate transplantation applications. Due to the highly complex structure of the liver, printing will be a time-consuming and laborious process, requiring continuous development and improvements of the printing process.

The bioartificial liver support system (BAL) also provides a new way to treat liver disease, the purpose of which is to eliminate toxic wastes such as ammonia and various inflammatory factors in liver failure, synthesize albumin and blood coagulation factors, correct metabolic disorders, promote endogenous liver regeneration, or enable liver transplantation. Constructing bioartificial liver requires a large number of functional hepatocytes, usually in the hundreds of millions. The most commonly used cell sources are hepatoma cell lines HepG2/C3A, HepaRG, or porcine hepatocytes, all of which have corresponding problems. The use of porcine hepatocytes presents a risk of spreading heterologous genes or viruses, and the function and survival of the cells rapidly downregulate over time. The emergence of stem cells use in recent years has provided a new path to the cellular source of the bioartificial liver.

In 2016, Chinese scientist Hui Lijian tried to use reprogrammed hepatocytes to construct bioartificial liver by reprogramming human fibroblasts into hepatocyte-like cells (hiHeps) using overexpression of transcription factors and introducing SV40 large T antigen into hepatocyte-like cells to enable hepatocytes to be expanded in large quantities in a multilayer radial flow bioreactor to the quantity of three billion [37]. There are two main strategies of cellular expansion that show great potential: firstly, improving the efficiency and function of hepatic differentiation of pluripotent stem cells and improving the metabolic function of hepatocytes derived from reprogramming and secondly, the establishment of immunodeficient FAH-deficient genetically engineered large-animal models such as pigs as bioreactors to amplify hepatocytes in vivo in order to obtain a large number of mature hepatocytes will be an important direction of effort.

### 7.3.6 Summary and Outlook

Liver regeneration is a fundamental issue commonly studied in both basic research and clinical settings. This review focuses on the scientific breakthroughs accumulated in the last 5 years and attempts to clarify various mechanisms and multiple theories, with the ultimate goal of sorting out the challenges faced in the field and the direction of future development. Some basic concepts and knowledge will be provided for readers interested in beginning studying in this field. Currently, liver regeneration requires a more credible lineage tracing system to further clarify the mechanisms of in vivo, identify the major cell types responsible in different disease types, and then develop drugs or methods that directly regulate the function of major cell types, thereby promoting the regeneration of endogenous hepatocytes. Large numbers of functional liver cells are required to be obtained in vitro for direct transplantation, such as the development of safe and efficient reprogramming technology to convert fibroblasts into mature hepatocytes or the development of long-term large-scale culture of primary hepatocytes or liver stem cells to obtain large numbers of hepatocytes. In short, both in vitro and in vivo approaches are aimed at liver regeneration and the treatment of liver diseases, which show great potential for application.

## 7.4 Repair and Regeneration of Digestive Tract Injury

Gastrointestinal injury often manifests as ulcers and gastrointestinal ischemia-reperfusion. The renewal rate of gastrointestinal epithelial cells is very fast; apoptosis is important to maintain the number, morphology, and function of cells; and various pathogenic factors can cause apoptosis in gastrointestinal cells. The absorptive cells of the small intestinal mucosa are derived from the lacuna, and the progeny cells produced by the proliferation of the lacuna stem cells continue to migrate upward, divide at the same time of migration, and have differentiated and matured when reaching the villi. In this dynamic system, the excess stem cells produced by symmetric division under normal conditions are also cleared by apoptosis or rapid differentiation, and the cell proliferation and death are balanced. If apoptosis is blocked, the damaged cells cannot reactively die, which may promote the development of the disease and make other traditional therapeutic drugs insensitive, which further indicates the importance of apoptosis for the digestive tract.

### 7.4.1 Classification of Digestive Tract Injuries

#### 7.4.1.1 Peptic Ulcer

Peptic ulcer (PU) refers to the inflammation and necrotic lesions of the mucosa under the action of various pathogenic factors. The lesions reach the muscularis mucosae and often occur in the gastric acid-related digestive tract mucosa, among which the stomach and duodenum are the most common. There is also a more refractory ulcerative colitis (UC), first described by Willks and Moxon in 1875, named ulcerative colitis by Willks and Boas in 1903, and officially named chronic nonspecific ulcerative colitis by the World Health Organization (WHO) in 1973. Epidemiological data show that the incidence of ulcerative colitis has increased year by year both at home and abroad. Ulcerative colitis is a chronic, nonspecific inflammation that primarily affects the rectum and colonic mucosa. The pathogenesis of UC is still unclear and may be related to the interaction of multiple factors such as heredity, infection, psychology, and immunity. It is currently believed that environmental factors act on genetically susceptible individuals and initiate intestinal immune responses and inflammatory processes in the presence of intestinal flora (or microorganisms that are not yet clear), possibly due to persistent stimulation of antigens or immune regulation disorders, making the inflammatory immunity difficult to self-limit.

The healing of peptic ulcers is extremely complex, including the elimination of necrotic substances, the formation of fibrous tissue and scar tissue in the basal granulation tissue, the growth and remodeling of blood vessels and epithelial cells, and a series of cells are involved in the process. Through histological and ultrastructural analysis of experimental ulcer healing, Tarnawski found that although the epithelium of the newly healed ulcer was intact, there were obvious histological and ultrastructural abnormalities. Therefore, the concept of quality of ulcer healing (QOUH) was first proposed. It is believed that the healing of ulcers is not only the repair of mucosal defects but also the repair and reconstruction of submucosal tissue structure and the improvement of mucosal defense function. In addition, Tarnawski also observed in the experiment that in QOUH, sucralfate was more effective than omeprazole treatment through the nutrition effect of gastric mucosa and the expression of growth factors and their receptors. Therefore, the evaluation of QOUH should not only observe the regenerative mucosa under endoscopy or direct vision but also include the structural maturity and functional maturity of the regenerative mucosa, so as to determine its effect on ulcer recurrence and the efficacy of drugs on PU.

#### 7.4.1.2 Ischemia-Reperfusion

Tissue damage caused by ischemia-reperfusion injury (I/R) is particularly pronounced. The small intestine is highly sensitive to ischemia-reperfusion, mitochondrial damage caused by short-term ischemia is reversible, and long-term ischemia or reperfusion after ischemia can cause irreversible damage to the mitochondria of cells. The role of growth factors EGF and bFGF in the repair of intestinal injury has been confirmed by many experiments. Intestinal I/R causes complement-phagocytic-lymphocyte activation in the body, which not only causes local inflammation in the intestine but may also cause distal organ damage through activation of granulocytes, in which the activation of the terminal complement component C5 is a critical step in the process of damage to local and distant organ damage after intestinal I/R. Upon activation of C5, C5a and C5b-9 produced can mediate the activation of polymorphonuclear leukocytes (PMNs), which aggregate in intestinal tissues and distant organs and induce tissue damage. Treatment of superior mesenteric artery I/R with C5 monoclonal antibody not only significantly alleviated the loss of microvascular tension and release of lactate dehydrogenase from intestinal cells but also inhibited the significant increase of myeloperoxidase activity in lung and intestine, and the expression of inter cellular adhesion molecule (ICAM), thereby blocking activation of the complement system and activation of granulocytes. Therefore, anti-C5 monoclonal antibody significantly improved intestinal I/R tissue damage and lung injury, and it is expected to provide new ideas and means for studying measures to prevent and treat MSOF.

Intestinal ischemia-reperfusion can not only cause damage to its structure and function but also cause damage to a variety of organs such as kidney and lung. It is one of the causes of various complications after burns and trauma. Therefore, it is clinically important to promote and accelerate the repair of viscera after injury. Two important regulators in the process of wound repair, represented by basic fibroblast growth factor and transforming growth factor, can promote wound healing on the body surface by promoting the formation and remodeling of capillaries, effective chemotaxis to various repair cells, and increasing the deposition of extracellular matrix. The research by Xiaobing Fu team initially confirmed that the expression of endogenous bFGF and TGF-β induced by intestinal ischemia-reperfusion injury may be a protective mechanism of the body after severe trauma [38]. At the same time, it was found that the administration of exogenous growth factors has obvious promoting effects on damaged internal organs, but there is still no deep understanding of its molecular mechanism. We will introduce in detail in later chapters.

### 7.4.2 The Determination of Digestive Tract Injury

In 1990, at the Hawaii International Conference, Tarnawski et al. first proposed the concept quality of ulcer healing (QOUH). It is pointed out that ulcer healing requires not only the repair of mucosa but also the repair and reconstruction of submucosal tissue structure. QOUH pays more attention to its functional maturity while evaluating the structural maturity of the localized regenerated mucosa and connects the quality of QOUH with future ulcer recurrence.

#### 7.4.2.1 Evaluation Method of QOUH

##### Endoscopic Evaluation

Takemoto et al. performed a new endoscopic staging of duodenal ulcer, with the presence of white fur as the regeneration phase (R phase) and the disappearance of white fur as the scar phase (S phase). Stage R0: There is no regenerated villi on the edge of the ulcer. Stage R1: A small amount of regenerated villi can be seen on the edge of the ulcer. Stage R2: Coarse granular regenerated villi can be seen on the edge of the ulcer. Stage Sa: Depression in the central part of the ulcer scar. Stage Sb: The depression disappears in the central part of the ulcer scar, and the regenerative mucosa is coarse and granular. Stage Sc: The depression disappears in the central part of the ulcer scar, the regenerated villi are fine grained, and the mucosa of the scar is flat, close to the normal mucosal morphology.

##### Evaluation Method of Histological Maturity of Regenerated Mucosa

(a) Epithelial tissue: the thickness of the regenerated mucosa; the number of epithelial cells; the ratio of the number of epithelial cells to the number of connective tissue cells; the ratio of epithelial cells to the number of glandular cavities; the height, number, and arrangement of glands; the degree of glandular cystic expansion; and the morphology and differentiation of gland cells are measured.
(b) Granulation tissue: the number of fibroblasts and neovascularization, differentiation conformation, innervation status, regeneration of collagen fibers and muscularis mucosae, and degree of inflammatory cell infiltration are measured.

##### Evaluation Method of Functional Maturity of Regenerated Mucosa

The function of the regenerated mucosa is evaluated by biopsy:

(a) Microcirculation status: gastric mucosal blood flow (GMBF) is measured.
(b) Glycoprotein content determination and glycoprotein composition analysis.
(c) Prostaglandin (PGs), epidermal growth factor (EGF) level determination, and adenosine triphosphate (ATP), adenosine diphosphate (ADP), adenosine monophosphate (AMP) quantitative analysis.
(d) Detection of mucus production by regenerated mucosa and epithelial cells.
(e) Receptor expression (EGF, dopamine receptor).

#### 7.4.2.2 Factors Affecting QOUH

##### *Helicobacter pylori* (Hp)

Most patients with gastric ulcer and duodenal ulcer have Hp infection. Eradication of Hp can not only accelerate ulcer healing but also greatly reduce the recurrence rate. If Hp is permanently removed, peptic ulcer can be cured. Furata studied the effect of lansoprazole with or without amoxicillin on QOUH. The results suggest that the eradication of Hp by high-dose amoxicillin is helpful for improving QOUH, and indirectly explains the adverse effects of Hp on QOUH.

##### Blood Circulation

Studies have shown that NSAIDs inhibit microvascular formation in granulation tissue, resulting in delayed ulcer healing. During the healing of human ulcers, it is observed that the blood flow at the edge of the ulcer increases first, and then the ulcer heals. The increase of peripheral blood flow is more significant in fully healed ulcers than in unhealed ulcers. All of the above suggest that the microcirculation of the regenerated mucosa is closely related to QOUH.

##### Growth Factor

It is known that the gastric mucosa contains EGF, bFGF, etc. These factors play a role in protecting gastric mucosa, promoting mitosis and angiogenesis, and promoting the proliferation and injury of normal mucosa or the repair and healing of ulcer epithelium.

##### Arachidonic Acid (AA) Metabolites

Prostaglandins (PGs) and leukotrienes (LTs), the major metabolites of AA, play an important role in the injury and repair of gastric mucosal cells. PGs can reverse the inhibition of NSAIDs on the DNA synthesis of ulcer marginal epithelial cells, and can accelerate ulcer healing, improve QOUH, and reduce ulcer recurrence through cytoprotection and stimulation of cell proliferation, angiogenesis, extracellular matrix reconstruction, and anti-inflammatory effects.

##### Oxygen-Free Radical

When the gastric mucosa is inflamed or ulcerated, the production of free radicals exceeds the clearance of free radicals, thus accumulating locally in the mucosa, which has pathogenic effects on chronic gastric ulcer and duodenal ulcer.

##### Heat-Shock Proteins

Heat-shock proteins (HSPs) are ancient and highly conserved proteins. It can protect cells, resist external damage, and participate in the transmission of cellular information and gene regulation, which is thought to be of positive significance to promote ulcer tissue repair and improve QOUH. Studies have suggested that promoting the expression of HSPs can reduce the damage of gastric mucosa and promote ulcer healing.

##### Aging

Tsukimi et al. induced chronic gastric ulcer in young rats and old rats by intracavity injection of acetic acid. It was found that the regeneration of ulcer mucosa in old rats was significantly worse than that in young rats, and tissue contraction response was also observed. This indicates that aging may result in a decrease in QOUH due to various gastric dysfunctions that affect ulcer healing.

##### Other

Various endogenous or exogenous damage factors such as NSAID drugs, smoking, drinking and other bad habits, irregular life, bad mental stimulation, depression, or anxiety can damage the mucosal barrier function, disrupt the metabolism of cytoprotective factors, and affect neurohumoral regulation, resulting in a low QOUH and ulcer recurrence.

#### 7.4.2.3 Antiulcer Drugs and QOUH

##### Drugs that Reduce Mucosal Invasiveness

(a) High gastric acid can delay ulcer healing. Ito et al. studied the influencing factors of QOUH in lansoprazole treatment of ulcers and found that low gastric acid and low ratio of pepsinogen I to II can result in poor healing quality of PU, and on the contrary high healing quality.
(b) Hp clearance can accelerate the healing of ulcers and improve QOUH. Animal experiments and clinical observations confirm that amoxicillin can not only kill Hp but also prevent the formation of duodenal ulcer and gastric ulcer induced by mercamine hydrochloride and acetic acid in rats.

##### Gastric Mucosal Protective Agent

(a) Sucralfate: Sucralfate enhances the expression of EGF, bFGF, and their receptors through the trophic effects on gastric mucosa and activation of EGF, bFGF, and their receptor genes. Some of them are directly combined with ulcer marginal cells or indirectly through the action of PGs and somatostatin, which can increase the protective effect on regenerated mucosa and glands and stimulate the formation of microvessels in granulation tissue, thereby increasing QOUH.

(b) Bismuth: Bismuth can improve QOUH through the following three aspects. In acidic environment, it can chelate with proteins to form a protective barrier against the invasion of acid and protease and form a complex with mucous membranes, thus forming an effective barrier to prevent hydrogen ion diffusion. It also reduces pepsin excretion and its activity, and promoting the synthesis of prostaglandins as well. It has an anti-Hp effect.

(c) Prostaglandins: Prostaglandins achieve this by inhibiting gastric acid secretion, increasing mucosal blood flow, promoting mucosal epithelial regeneration, and stimulating mucus and bicarbonate secretion. Arakawa et al. treated acetic acid ulcer in rats with rebamipide, a new prostaglandin inducer, and found that the cumulative recurrence rate of ulcers treated with rebamipide was significantly lower than that of cimetidine, suggesting that rebamipide is beneficial for improving the quality of healing.

(d) Growth factor: The experimental ulcer was treated with recombinant human basic fibroblast growth factor (rh2b-FGF), and it was found that the width of the regenerated gland epithelium, the capillary density in the granulation tissue, and the collagen content in the scar tissue were increased, and the maturation of regenerated gland and RNA synthesis in ulcer margin tissues were promoted.

#### The Influence of Traditional Chinese Medicine on QOUH

Traditional Chinese medicine can repair local pathological changes through the overall regulation, maximally adjust the ability of the body to resist disease, effectively regulate the imbalance between attack factors and protective factors of peptic ulcer, and adjust the disordered digestive function, so to improve QOUH. The treatment of experimental gastric ulcer in rats with Jianpi Liqi Granules found that the particles can improve QOUH and prevent ulcer recurrence. This effect may be related to the fact that granule can strengthen the spleen and replenish qi, improve autoimmunity, protect gastric mucosa from damage, enhance defensive factors, and restore overall function.

#### The Relationship Between QOUH with Ulcer Recurrence

In recent years, a large number of studies have shown that the recurrence rate of completely cured ulcers is very low, and the level of QOUH is one of the important factors affecting recurrence. The more abnormal structures that exist after healing, the greater the possibility of recurrence. Arakawa also confirmed that the histological maturity, PAS-positive substance, and PGE activity of the flat, fine-grained regenerated mucosa were better than those of the coarse-grained regenerated mucosa, and the recurrence of ulcer in the former was significantly less than that in the latter, suggesting that QOUH was closely related to ulcer recurrence. Therefore, a more detailed and accurate evaluation of scar tissue after ulcer healing will be of great significance for the selection of drugs, combination therapy, and search for methods to control the recurrence of ulcer disease.

## 7.4.3 The Role of Growth Factors in the Repair and Regeneration of the Digestive Tract Injury

Peptic ulcer healing is regulated by growth factors and their receptors throughout the process. Among them, transforming growth factor-α (TGF-α) and epidermal growth factor (EGF) are activated by receptors, regulate cell proliferation, and reconstruct epithelial tissue. Fibroblast growth factor, platelet-derived growth factor (PDGF), transforming growth factor-β (TGF-β), and vascular endothelial growth factor (VEGF) promote the regeneration of connective tissue and microvessel. When the chronic ulcer heals, the neonatal epithelium secretes EGF and other growth peptides and promotes overexpression of local EGF receptors. Others such as insulin-like growth factor-1 (IGF-1), keratinocyte growth factor (KGF), hepatocyte growth factor (HGF), and trefoil peptide play a role in the regeneration of injured mucosa. Therefore, the role of growth factors in the intestines should not be underestimated. Studying its relationship with the intestines and the mechanism of action will provide new targets for the treatment of gastrointestinal diseases.

### 7.4.3.1 Growth Factors and Intestinal Development

In the process of intestinal development, a variety of growth factors are expressed simultaneously, and exogenous regulation of intestinal growth factors can promote or inhibit the development of the intestine, of which EGF is more typical. The effect of EGF on the division of the lacuna is most obvious in the colon, which can strongly stimulate the lacunar division in the short term, and reduces the division of the lacuna in the resting state. Previous studies have suggested that the increase in the number of stem cells is a factor that causes the division of the lacuna. When the intestinal mucosa is intact, EGF cannot be absorbed, but can be absorbed after mucosal injury, which plays a role in promoting local division. Administration of growth factors via the gastrointestinal tract may be one of the clinical treatment methods.

#### Epidermal Growth Factor

EGF is a single-chain polypeptide with 53 amino acids, which is abundant in the submandibular gland and can hardly be expressed in normal gastric mucosa. EGF stimulates the proliferation of epithelial cells and peripheral cells. Therefore, EGF has a proliferative effect in combination with receptors on gastral epithelium and gastric mucous cell membranes. Epidermal growth factor receptor (EGFR) is a glycoprotein with molecular weight of 170 ku, which exists in gastric epithelial cells and parietal cells. EGFR has high affinity to EGF. The EGFR tyrosine kinase receptor family plays an important role in the repair of gastric mucosal injury. The activation of EGF-EGFR pathway can upregulate gastric mucosal cell proliferation, increase gastric mucosal blood flow, and promote the healing of acute and chronic injury.

EGF can promote the differentiation and proliferation of gastrointestinal mucosal epithelium and can stimulate the synthesis of DNA and RNA in various cells in vitro and in vivo. The gastric mucosa also has the ability to produce EGF, and the EGF in the gastric juice is likely to be a balanced response of the human body to ulcer.

EGFR is expressed in gastrointestinal epithelial tissues and has the function of regulating cell proliferation, differentiation, and apoptosis. Previous studies have shown that EGFR tyrosine kinase receptor family plays an important role in the repair of gastric mucosal injury. The activation of EGFR pathway can upregulate gastric mucosal cell proliferation, increase gastric mucosal blood flow, and promote the healing of acute and chronic injury. It was found that the expression of EGFR did not increase in the early stage of ulceration, but increased continuously for 25 days in the healing period and scar period. The upregulation of EGFR can promote the proliferation and differentiation of epidermal cells on the edge of ulcer to migrate to the granulation tissue, cover the ulcer surface, and extend into granulation tissue to reconstruct gastric mucosal glands in ulcer scars. It was observed that EGFR was weakly positive in normal gastric mucosa of rats, and the expression of EGFR was higher in the tissue adjacent to the ulcer than in normal tissues during ulcer healing. It is suggested that EGFR may play an important role in cell proliferation, differentiation, migration, and inhibition of gastric acid during ulcer healing.

It is currently believed that the mechanism by which EGF participates in the repair of peptic ulcer may include the following:

(a) It can activate ornithine decarboxylase (ODC).
(b) It can promote the differentiation and proliferation of gastrointestinal mucosal epithelium. It can stimulate the synthesis of DNA, RNA, collagen fiber, and hyaluronic acid in vivo and in vitro.
(c) It can inhibit gastric acid secretion and promote the synthesis and secretion of mucus glycoprotein in gastric mucosa.
(d) It can increase gastric mucosal blood flow. Smoking can delay ulcer healing and may be associated with inhibition of EGF release from salivary glands and duodenal. In addition, it has been suggested that gastric ulcer in any part of the gastrointestinal tract can induce stem cells to form a new EGF secretory cell system and secrete a large amount of EGF, thereby stimulating cell proliferation, regeneration, and ulcer healing.

The team led by Academician Xiaobing Fu observed the effects of exogenous epidermal growth factor on intestinal mucosal permeability and intestinal, hepatic, and renal function changes after intestinal ischemia-reperfusion in rats [39]. Eighty grade 3 male Wistar rats were randomly divided into sham-operated group (C), intestinal ischemia group (I), intestinal ischemia-reperfusion group (I/R), and EGF treatment group. In the I/R group and the EGF treatment group, the root of superior mesenteric artery was clamped with microvascular clamp for 45 min, and then the vessel clamp was released to form reperfusion. Normal saline or EGF (100 μg/kg) was injected through the jugular vein immediately after reperfusion, and the animals were sacrificed at 2 h, 6 h, 12 h, and 24 h after injury. In group C, the root of superior mesenteric artery was isolated without clamping. Group I was killed immediately after 45-min ischemia. The liver function, renal function, plasma diamine oxidase (DAO) activity, and D-lactic acid concentration were taken, and the morphology of small intestine, liver, and kidney was observed. The results showed that: a. Compared with group C, plasma alanine aminotransferase (ALT) and urea nitrogen (BUN) were significantly increased in each group, but the increase in EGF treatment group was significantly lower than that in I/R group ($P < 0.05$). b. The increase of plasma D-lactate concentration and DAO activity in the EGF treatment group were significantly lower than those in the I/R group ($P < 0.01$). The degree of mucosal congestion, edema, inflammatory cell infiltration, and focal necrosis of liver, kidney, and small intestine in the EGF treatment group were significantly less than that in the I/R group. Studies have shown that exogenous EGF can significantly reduce the intestinal, liver, and kidney injury caused by ischemia-reperfusion, and its main role is to promote the signal transduction pathway after EGF binding with receptor.

#### Acidic Fibroblast Growth Factor

Acid fibroblast growth factor (aFGF) can promote connective tissue formation, induce epithelial cell migration and proliferation, stimulate angiogenesis, and play a role in multiple aspects of wound healing, such as proliferation, differentiation, and migration. However, the specific mechanism of acidic fibroblast growth factor after visceral injury is still unclear. Acidic fibroblast growth factor binds to its receptor to form dimer, which can transfer a variety of extracellular stimuli to the cytoplasm; the tyrosine protein kinases in the cytoplasm are phosphorylated and activated, and then the signals are transmitted to the nucleus to activate the nuclear transcription factors (c-Fos, c-Jun, etc.); transcription factors promote transcription and translation and can form growth factors, receptors, etc., forming a cascading effect. Mitogen-activated tyrosine kinases, as intracellular tyrosine protein kinases, are activated during tissue regeneration and wound healing that can cause cell proliferation and differentiation, and they are closely related to the quality and outcome of tissue repair. Extracellular regulated protein kinase is one of the four signal transduction pathways of mitogen-activated tyrosine kinase, which can participate in many physiological processes such as cell growth, development, division, and synchronization of intercellular functions. In addition, the role of extracellular regulated protein kinase and acidic fibroblast growth factor receptor-2 in the repair of intestinal ischemia-reperfusion injury has not been reported. Sun Hong et al. found that acidic fibroblast growth factor intervention can upregulate the expression of acidic fibroblast growth factor receptor-2 and extracellular regulated protein kinase after ischemia-reperfusion injury. It is suggested that exogenous acidic fibroblast growth factor promotes the generation of endogenous acidic fibroblast growth factor receptor-2, and extracellular regulated protein kinase may be one of the mechanisms in the repair of visceral injury.

Since the mitogenic activity of wild-type aFGF may be related to cell proliferation, differentiation, and tumorigenesis, it is limited in large-scale applications. Therefore, it is hoped that the wild-type aFGF will be modified by genetic engineering technology, and the nuclear translocation region will delete, and the ability of aFGF to induce DNA synthesis and cell proliferation is lost, but still retain binding to aFGF receptor and induce receptor-mediated tyrosine phosphorylation and c-Fos expression, resulting in a mutant aFGF, called modified acidic fibroblast growth factor (maFGF). The team led by Academician Xiaobing Fu constructed maFGF, which lost its mitogenic effect but retained nonmitogenic hormone-like activity [40]. At the same time, their study found that exogenous maFGF had an effect on intestinal cell apoptosis after ischemia-reperfusion. They randomly divided 54 rats into a sham-operated group, a saline control group, and a maFGF treatment group. Rats in the sham-operated group exposed superior mesenteric artery without clamping. Rats in the saline control group and maFGF treatment group were subjected to intestinal ischemia by SMA clamping for 45 min, and the loosening clamp formed ischemia-reperfusion. At the moment of reperfusion, 0.1 mL saline and 4 μg maFGF were intravenously injected. At 2 h, 6 h, 12 h, and 24 h of ischemia-reperfusion, small intestinal tissues were taken to observe the histological changes, and the apoptosis rate of intestinal cells was detected by terminal deoxynucleotidyl transferase-mediated dUTP-biotin nick end labeling assay (TUNEL). Histological examination showed that the intestinal injury was severe in the saline control group after 2–24 h of ischemia-reperfusion, and the intestinal damage in the maFGF treatment group was less than that in the saline control group. The results of apoptosis test showed that the apoptosis rate of intestinal cells in the sham-operated group was lower, and the apoptosis rate of the saline control group and the maFGF treatment group was significantly higher than that of the sham-operated group. After 12 h of ischemia-reperfusion, the apoptosis rate of the saline control group was as high as 62.8 ± 1.7%, and that of the maFGF treatment group was 42.5 ± 2.6%. The difference between the two groups was statistically significant ($P < 0.05$). Studies have shown that maFGF can help reduce intestinal cell apoptosis induced by intestinal ischemia-reperfusion in rats.

### Basic Fibroblast Growth Factor

Basic fibroblast growth factor (bFGF) is a single-chain polypeptide with a molecular weight of 5–20 ku, which is present in normal gastric mucosa. bFGF, as an important mitogen, can directly act on the cycle of tissue repair cells (such as fibroblasts), reducing the proportion of cells in G1 phase, increasing the proportion of S phase and G2 phase + M phase, shortening the cell cycle transition time, and accelerating cell division and proliferation. bFGF not only has a growth-stimulating effect on fibroblasts but also is a strong angiogenic agent, which has a strong angiogenic effect and plays an important role in the repair of peptic ulcer. Satoh et al. found that there was an increase in endogenous bFGF during the healing of gastric ulcer in mice. Exogenous bFGF can promote the healing of experimental gastric and duodenal ulcers. Szabo et al. used bFGF to promote angiogenesis and accelerate healing of chronic wounds. bFGF (bFGF-CS23) with acid stability was used to treat duodenal ulcer in mice. The results showed that bFGF did not affect the secretion of gastric acid and pepsin, but it was more effective than cimetidine to promote the formation of blood vessels on ulcer surface and accelerate ulcer healing. Wang et al. found that the width of regenerated epithelium at ulcer margin, the density of capillaries in granulation tissue, and the content of collagen in scar tissue increased and promoted the maturation of regenerated glands and RNA synthesis in ulcer margin tissue. Topical application of bFGF accelerates healing of chronic gastric ulcer in rats, while anti-bFGF antibodies delay healing. Intragastric administration of bFGF can reverse epithelial migration due to gastric acid inhibition. Ulcer healing was accelerated after rh-bFGF administration in patients with NSAID-associated gastric ulcer. Immunohistochemical studies showed that bFGF expression was higher in ulcer margin tissues of peptic ulcer than in normal gastric mucosa.

In an article published in 1999 by the team led by Academician Xiaobing Fu, the effects of bFGF on the expression of endogenous bFGF and TGF-β in the intestine after ischemia-reperfusion were observed in animals [41]. Sixty-four healthy male Wistar rats (provided by the Animal Center of the Academy of Military Medical Sciences) weighing 200–250 g were randomly divided into the sham-operated group (group A), the ischemia-reperfusion group (group B), and the bFGF treatment group (group C). Group B was divided into four groups according to the time of ischemia 45 min, and reperfusion 6 h, 24 h, and 48 h. Group C was divided into three groups according to the time of reperfusion 45 min after ischemia: reperfusion 6 h, 24 h, and 48 h, with eight animals in each group. The rats were anesthetized by intraperitoneal injection of 20 g/L sodium pentobarbital, and superior mesenteric artery (SMA) was isolated under sterile conditions. The SMA roots were clamped with noninvasive vascular clamps, and the blood flow was completely blocked for 45 min; then the vascular clamp was relaxed to restore the intestinal blood flow and form reperfusion. The sham-operated group only separated the SMA, but did not clamp it, and closed the abdomen after 45 min. Group C animals were clamped with SMA according to the method of group B. At the time of reperfusion, 0.15 mL bFGF heparin saline (bFGF 4 μg/mouse) was injected from the right jugular vein, the abdominal cavity was closed, and 3 mL normal saline was injected subcutaneously to prevent shock. All animals were killed at different time points, and small intestine tissues were taken and fixed in 100 ml/L formalin. Animal small intestine tissues were taken at different time points and embedded in paraffin. The expression of bFGF and TGF-β was observed by light microscopy using HE staining and immunohistochemistry. The results showed that at 6 h of reperfusion after 45 min of ischemia, the intestinal structure was most severely damaged, with obvious tissue edema, mucosal shedding, and a large number of neutrophil infiltration, and some mucosal cells degenerated and were necrotic and homogeneous. The intestinal mucosal structure recovered partially at 24 h of reperfusion, and basically restored at 48 h. In the bFGF treatment group, intestinal damage was alleviated, and only a small amount of mucosal cells showed focal degeneration and shedding after 6 h of reperfusion. Endogenous bFGF is mainly distributed in neutrophils, lymphocytes in the lamina propria of intestinal villi, and vascular endothelial cells in the submucosa. TGF-β is mainly distributed in lymphocytes, plasma cells, and macrophages in the lamina propria of the intestinal villi, as well as in the connective tissue of the submucosa. After 6-h reperfusion, it was abundantly distributed in detached mucosal cells and neutrophils released into the lumen. The main effects of exogenous bFGF on the changes of bFGF and TGF-β expression in the intestine were as follows: in the small intestinal tissue (sham-operated group), there was only a small amount of bFGF and TGF-β expression; immediately after 45 min of ischemia, the expression of bFGF and TGF-β began to increase, and the increase of TGF-β was more obvious, with statistical significance ($P < 0.01$); at 6 h, 24 h, and 48 h after reperfusion, the expression levels of bFGF and TGF-β increased significantly ($P < 0.01$), and the difference was extremely significant compared with the sham-operated group and peaked at 24 h and 6 h after reperfusion, which was about 3.4 times and 3.3 times of that in the sham-operated group; the expression level began to decrease at 48 h after reperfusion, but the difference of bFGF was still significant compared with sham-operated group ($P < 0.05$). The possible mechanism of bFGF secretion was preliminarily elucidated, that is, inactive bFGF was secreted into the surrounding tissues in an active form through the destruction of the protoplasm membrane after injury. In addition, the inflammatory response during the injury period concentrates a large number of inflammatory cells such as monocytes and lymphocytes and secretes a large amount of TGF-β, and local high concentration of TGF-β may positively regulate the expression of bFGF, thereby promoting the repair. Therefore, as a protective mechanism of the body itself, the expression of endogenous bFGF and TGF-β is upregulated after injury to promote the repair of the organ itself, which may be one of the mechanisms for promoting the repair of visceral damage by bFGF. They hypothesized that the mechanisms by which bFGF reduces intestinal ischemia-reperfusion include the following: bFGF's vasodilating effect is beneficial to the opening of microvessels, further reducing intestinal mucosal damage caused by local embolism under intestinal ischemia; FGF is involved in the regulation of extracellular calcium concentration, which is beneficial to alleviate the cytotoxicity caused by intracellular calcium overload under ischemia-reperfusion conditions; the intestinal tract as a visceral organ has FGF-like growth factor receptors on its mucosa, and its biological effect is beneficial to the repair of damaged organs. The team's follow-up studies further confirmed that after exogenous administration of bFGF, bFGF and TGF-β expression levels were increased at 6 h and 24 h after reperfusion, but only bFGF reached significant levels at 6 h after reperfusion compared with group B ($P < 0.05$). It is suggested that part of the effect of exogenous bFGF on the repair of intestinal damage may be achieved by upregulating the expression level of bFGF in the intestine itself. At the same time, their study found that exogenous basic fibroblast growth factor (bFGF) had an effect on liver function and intestinal substance P (SP) content after intestinal ischemia-reperfusion in rats, thereby interfering with tissue damage repair. Fifty-four Wistar rats were randomly divided into three groups: sham-operated group, saline control group, and bFGF treatment group. Each rat was perfused with 4 μg bFGF. Animals in saline control group and bFGF treatment group were sacrificed at 2 h, 6 h, 24 h, and 48 h after reperfusion, and specimens were collected to detect the SP content in small intestine tissue and plasma D-lactate, diamine oxidase (DAO), and alanine aminotransferase (ALT) levels. The experimental results showed that plasma ALT was significantly lower in the bFGF treatment group than in the saline control group. The plasma DAO in the two groups increased significantly from 2 h to 6 h after reperfusion, and in the bFGF treatment group, the plasma DAO increased more significantly after 6 h, but returned to normal after 24 h. In the saline control group, the SP content in the small intestine increased significantly 6 h to 48 h after injury, and the plasma D-lactate and SP increased in parallel, while the SP and plasma D-lactate in the bFGF treatment group did not change significantly. Studies have confirmed that early application of bFGF after ischemia-reperfusion injury can alleviate liver function damage and may aggravate intestinal epithelial damage, but late inhibition of small intestinal SP excessive release may be beneficial to the repair of intestinal injury. Inhibition or antagonism of endogenous basic fibroblast growth factor (bFGF) also has the same effect on intestinal, hepatic, and renal functions induced by intestinal ischemia-reperfusion. Ninety-six rats were divided into three groups: bFGF antibody pretreatment group, serine threonine protein kinase inhibitor H7 pretreatment group, and normal saline control group. The superior mesenteric artery roots were clamped with microvascular clamps for 45 min and then relaxed to form reperfusion. The other six were used as normal controls (sham-operated group). The animals were killed immediately, 2 h, 6 h, 24 h, and 48 h after perfusion, and blood was taken to detect the changes of liver and kidney functions and diamine oxidase (DAO), and samples of intestine, liver, and kidney were taken for morphological observation. The results showed that compared with the sham-operated group, the indexes of liver, kidney, and intestinal injury were significantly increased in the three groups. At 2 h and 6 h after injury, the plasma alanine aminotransferase (ALT) of animals in the bFGF antibody group and the H7 group increased by 2.5–3.5 on average compared with control group ($P < 0.05$, $P < 0.01$). The changes of plasma DAO and pathological results indicated that the intestinal barrier function of the three groups was significantly destroyed at 2 h and 6 h after injury. It is confirmed that inhibiting or antagonizing endogenous bFGF activity will further aggravate intestinal, liver, and kidney damage caused by ischemia-reperfusion, and its main role is to affect the binding of bFGF to receptors and the consequent signaling pathways.

## Transforming Growth Factor-α

Transforming growth factor-alpha (TGF-α) is another major regulatory peptide involved in the repair of gastric mucosal injury in the EGF family. EGF family members include epidermal growth factor (EGF), transforming growth factor-α (TGF-α), amphiregulin, heparin-binding epidermal growth factor (HB-EGF), vaccinia virus growth factor (VVGF), myxoma virus growth factor (MVGF), growth factors of Shope fibroma virus (SFGF), and the like. The complete TGF-α molecule is a straight-chain polypeptide consisting of 50 amino acid residues, which is obtained by two cleavages of transmembrane transforming growth factor-α (TM-TGF-α) containing 160 amino acids, known as secreted transforming growth factor-alpha (S-TGF-α), commonly referred to as TGF-α. Mucosal injury is an important factor in stimulating the secretion and synthesis of TGF-α, and its increase plays an important role in the repair of local tissues. In addition to injury regulation, TGF-α also has a role in self-enhancing regulation. TGF-α is expressed not only in tumor tissues but also in many normal tissues, such as skin keratinocytes, activated macrophages, mammary epithelium, placenta, anterior pituitary, liver, pancreas, and gastrointestinal tract.

In humans and a variety of mammals, TGF-α can be synthesized in all segments of the gastrointestinal tract. It is produced in the entire gastrointestinal tract, especially in the antral mucosa, which is three times higher than the gastric body mucosa. Immunoelectron microscopy revealed that TGF-α is present on the tubular capsule in parietal cells and is also expressed in chief cells and mucous cells. The distribution of EGF receptor (EGFR) is similar to that of TGF-α, but strongly expressed on the basolateral membrane of cells. The results of radioimmunoassay showed that the concentration of TGF-α in gastric mucosa was significantly higher than that of EGF. This suggests that TGF-α may be the major physiological ligand for EGF receptors under normal conditions. Early studies have shown that reactive expression of TGF-α can be rapidly induced after gastric mucosal injury; during the healing process of gastric and duodenal ulcers, the expression of TGF-α in the mucosa also gradually increases, with the most significant increase in the ulcer healing and scarring stages. In the gastrointestinal tract, TGF-α is involved in the regulating the renewal of mucosal epithelium and the repair of mucosal damage, and is an important mediator for maintaining mucosal integrity, known as "mucosal intact peptide." During the repair of gastric mucosa damaged by acetic acid, especially 6 h after injury, the expression of TGF-α was significantly increased. *Helicobacter pylori* may affect the repair of gastric mucosa by investigating the expression of its receptor by affecting the repair of ulcerative colitis by transplantation of EGF and TGF-α bone marrow mesenchymal stem cells. Immunohistochemistry also showed that adaptive stimulation can significantly increase the expression levels of TGF-α, EGF, and EGFR. Preadministered exogenous TGF-α in rats by intraperitoneal or intravenous injection has obvious anti-injury effect on mucosa. Japanese scholars have found through animal experiments that the mucosal protective effect of TGF-α is related to the increased $Na^+/H^+$ exchange and has nothing to do with the increase of DNA synthesis. The study found that TGF-α reduces the area of gastric mucosal damage in a dose-dependent manner and also promotes capsaicin-sensitive nerve to release calcitonin-related peptide (CGRP), thereby increasing gastric mucosal blood flow and reducing gastric mucosal damage. In addition, Akiba et al. found that TGF-α also plays a protective role in gastric mucosa by promoting the synthesis of prostaglandin E2 (PGE2) through arachidonic acid metabolic pathway.

TGF-α is involved in the regulation of gastrointestinal mucosal epithelial renewal and mucosal injury repair. During the healing process of ulcers, two autocrine systems, EGF/EGFR and TGF-α/EGFR, play an important role in cell proliferation, differentiation, migration, and inhibition of gastric acid secretion. However, TGF-α plays a decisive role in regulating the reconstruction of local gastric structure.

#### Transforming Growth Factor-β

Transforming growth factor-beta (TGF-β) is a growth factor consisting of 390 amino acid residues. It is active due to the presence of two peptide chains, of which TGF-β1 is particularly attractive. TGF-β1 is a high-molecular-weight complex with a molecular weight of about 235 ku. In the healing process of peptic ulcer, TGF-β1 is of great significance for the formation of granulation tissue and scar in ulcers. First, TGF-β1 is an important inflammatory cell chemokine in the early stages of trauma. The specific effects of TGF-β1 are as follows:

(a) TGF-β1 can promote fibroblasts to synthesize collagen type I, collagen type III, collagen type VIII, elastic fibers, and fibronectin in large quantities. These components are interconnected in the wound, providing temporary ECM for capillary ingrowth and migration of basal cells.
(b) The synthesis of ECM molecules and cell adhesion are the main contents of tissue repair. TGF-β1 completes its regulation of tissue repair by inhibiting the production of collagenase, increasing the production of tissue inhibitors of collagenase inhibitor matrix metalloproteinase inhibitor (TIMP) and α2-macroglobulin, reducing protein breakdown around cells, and adjusting cell surface adhesion receptors.
(c) In the angiogenesis of granulation tissue, TGF-β1 can promote the proliferation and division of endothelial cells in the small blood vessels at the bottom of the wound and grow into granulation tissue in the form of buds, and gradually form cavities, interconnected into loops, and finally form blood vessels.
(d) TGF-β1 can also stimulate the transformation of fibroblasts into myofibroblasts, which have the ability to synthesize and secrete α-smooth muscle actin filaments. And α-smooth muscle actin filaments can pull the basal cells of wound margins to migrate to the center of the wound, which manifests as wound contraction. Some researchers have found that TGF-β directly stimulates vascular proliferation in vivo. Scholars have found that recombinant transforming growth factor-β3 (rHTGF-β3) treatment can accelerate the healing of gastric ulcer in mice.

Studies have shown that transforming growth factor-β (TGF-β) plays an irreplaceable role in intestinal immune balance and can inhibit the occurrence and development of inflammation by downregulating excessive immune response. Smads family members are signaling protein molecules downstream of TGF-β, and Smad3 is its key initiator. It is suggested that TGF-β is not only related to mucosal damage but also involved in the process of repair after injury. However, the expression of its downstream Smad3 phosphorylated protein was significantly inhibited during the injury phase, which may be mainly due to the inhibition of anti-inflammatory Smad3 activation by the overexpression of the pro-inflammatory protein Smad7 during the injury phase. During the repair phase, Smad3 was significantly activated, consistent with the trend of crypt cell proliferation, and at the same time, epithelial cell apoptosis decreased, suggesting that TGF-β is involved in UC mucosal repair by activating Smad3 phosphorylation.

In normal connective tissue, CTGF produced by fibroblasts is directly regulated by TGF-β1 and mediates part of the biological effects of TGF-β1, including stimulation of fibroblast proliferation and extracellular matrix production, and involvement in the process of wound repair and organ fibrosis formation of body tissues. The weak positive expression of CTGF between the gastric mucosa and epithelial cells of normal rats indicates that a small amount of CTGF can ensure the physiological renewal of connective tissue in the gastric wall, and keep the related components in connective tissue in a dynamic balance. However, the mechanism by which CTGF plays a role in the healing of gastrointestinal ulcers through signaling pathways such as TGF-β/SMADs and Ras/Raf/ERK and signaling molecules is still unclear.

#### Platelet-Derived Growth Factor

Platelet-derived growth factor (PDGF) is a glycoprotein with a molecular weight of 30 ku and a polypeptide composed of two chains A and B. Both platelets and activated macrophages produce PDGF. PDGF has three isomers: PDGF-AA, PDGF-AB, and PDGF-BB. The molecular weight of PDGF receptor is 164–185 ku and consists of two subunits, α and β. The structure of PDGF receptor correlates with the expression products of proto-oncogene c-Fms, c-Kit. PDGF is a mitogen of fibroblasts, endothelial cells, vascular smooth muscle cells, osteoblasts, and glial cells. In the process of cell proliferation, it promotes the transition from M1 phase to G2 phase and completes the regulation of cell proliferation by synergizing with somatostatin.

#### Vascular Endothelial Growth Factor

Vascular endothelial growth factor (VEGF) is also called vascular permeability factor (VPF) or angiopoietin. It is a glycoprotein isolated and purified by Ferrara from bovine pituitary follicular stellate cells in vitro for the first time in 1989, which specifically acts on vascular endothelial cells and promotes their mitosis. It is a homodimer formed by two identical subunits with molecular weights of 17–22 ku through a disulfide chain. The receptors for VEGF include the kinase insert domain receptor (KDR) and Fms-like tyrosine kinase-1 (KLT-1), which are only found in vascular endothelial cells and are membrane receptors. VEGF and its family members are indispensable inducers in physiological or pathological angiogenesis. VEGF is expressed in many normal human and animal tissues, but its expression is generally low. In some metabolic and blood-rich tissues, the expression of VEGF tends to be higher due to growth and angiogenesis. VEGF specifically acts on vascular endothelial cells and has the functions of maintaining normal state and integrity of blood vessels, improving vascular permeability, and promoting angiogenesis. Therefore, great attention has been paid to tissue repair and angiogenesis. VEGF also stimulates endothelial cells to produce nitric oxide and increase its concentration in a dose-dependent manner, thereby maintaining vascular function. VEGF plays a dual role in the protection of gastric mucosa and the healing of chronic ulcers. It not only protects the gastric mucosa by diluting harmful substances in the stomach by increasing microvascular permeability but also promotes the healing of ulcers by stimulating glands and angiogenesis. The expression of VEGF mRNA increased 3 h after ethanol-induced gastric mucosal injury. RT-PCR confirmed that VEGF mRNA in ulcer tissue of patients with gastric ulcer was significantly higher than that in normal gastric mucosa.

#### Hepatocyte Growth Factor

Hepatocyte growth factor (HGF) was discovered in mouse serum as a factor-promoting hepatocyte proliferation in 1984. HGF can significantly promote the proliferation of gastric mucosal epithelial cells, and this effect is much stronger than EGF. HGF not only promotes proliferation but also promotes chemotaxis and migration of gastric mucosal epithelial cells, which is far stronger than other growth factors. In the early stages of epithelial cell regeneration, chemotactic migration plays a leading role, and HGF plays an important role in this early chemotactic migration. Hori et al. suggest that HGF is the most important endogenous stimulator that affects the migration and proliferation of gastric and intestinal epithelial cells. Studies have shown that during gastric ulcer healing, the expression of HGF and its receptors is increased, and HGF is produced in gastric fibroblasts. After gastric mucosal defects, they are first replaced by granulation tissue and then covered by epithelial cells. Therefore, HGF is thought to be involved in the information transmission between mesenchymal cells and gastric mucosal epithelial cells. It transmits information such as granulation formation or fibrosis to epithelial cells, thereby promoting the chemotaxis, migration, and proliferation of gastric mucosal epithelial cells, and finally accelerating the repair of gastric mucosa.

### 7.4.4 The Role of Traditional Chinese Medicine in Repair and Regeneration After Digestive Tract Injury

Peptic ulcer is one of the most common chronic gastrointestinal dysfunction diseases in the world. Its main causes are imbalance of gastric mucosal defensive factor and aggressive factor, *Helicobacter pylori* infection, and the use of NSAIDs. The treatment of gastrointestinal ulcer is mainly based on drug treatment, mainly including H2 receptor blockers, proton pump inhibitors (PPIs), alkaline acid inhibitors, gastric mucosal protective agents, antibiotics, etc., which are combined in inhibiting gastric acid secretion, protecting gastric mucosa, and eradicating Hp. At the same time, remove the damage factors and the primary causes; try to avoid overwork, drinking, smoking, mental tension, and stimulating food; improve living habits; and maintain a good mentality. However, there are still some problems in the current treatment of peptic ulcer, such as adverse drug reactions and easy recurrence of ulcers. In recent years, related studies show that the effective ingredients of traditional Chinese medicine in the treatment of ulcers have better effects in ulcer prevention, acceleration of mucosal healing, improvement of quality of ulcer healing (QOUH), and reduction of the related adverse reactions and ulcer recurrence rate. Ancient Chinese medicine literature does not record the name of gastric ulcer disease, but it can be attributed to the category of TCM diseases such as "stomachache," "acid regurgitation," and "distention and fullness" according to its symptoms, accompanied by acid regurgitation, epigastric upset, belching, and other symptoms, with a long course of disease, repeated and difficult to heal. In long-term clinical practice, traditional Chinese medicine plays an important role in the treatment of gastric ulcer, and the efficacy is increasingly recognized.

Traditional Chinese medicine believes that the cause of this disease is closely related to the "three major injuries" (emotions, diet, fatigue). Among them, the emotional injury, liver qi attacking stomach, and prolonged unhealing can be transformed into heat accumulation of liver and stomach, weakness of spleen and stomach, gastric collateral fatigue, and so on. Combining with modern scientific methods, traditional Chinese medicine medical workers study the pathological essence of digestive tract injury in TCM. They agree that liver qi attacking stomach is mainly affected by autonomic nervous dysfunction; heat accumulation of liver and stomach is mainly affected by *Helicobacter pylori* infection; weakness of spleen and stomach is due to the destruction of gastric mucosal barrier and low regeneration function; and blood stasis syndrome is mainly caused by local microcirculation disorder, resulting in insufficient blood supply. Once the patient is ill, there will be two points: one is "virtual," that is, the spleen and stomach yang deficiency, the deficiency due to imaginary cold, and the other is "stagnation," referring to spleen and stomach qi stagnation, liver qi stagnation, and stasis, and dampness pathological products such as stagnation, food stagnation, heat lag, and blood stasis. The former is the pathological essence, and the latter is the pathological appearance. The combination of various factors causes the disease to occur and has the possibility of recurrence. The disease is in the stomach and intestine, but it is closely related to the spleen, liver, gallbladder, and other viscera.

In gastrointestinal injury, traditional Chinese medicine treatment still surrounds:

(a) Attenuating the aggressive factors of gastric ulcer (mainly referring to inhibiting gastric acid, pepsin, etc.).
(b) Antifree radical damage.
(c) Enhancing the gastric mucosal defense factor (improve gastric mucosal blood flow, protect gastric mucosal integrity, and promote mucosal repair).
(d) Anti-*Helicobacter pylori*.
(e) Regulating immune and anti-inflammatory responses: Domestic and foreign scholars have studied the antiulcer of traditional Chinese medicine. It can be found that single or combined application of Anwei Decoction, Compound Danshen Dripping Pills, Cuyu Granules, and other compound preparations can improve the QOUH of ulcers. The possible mechanisms include increasing mucosal blood flow, inhibiting Hp, inhibiting pepsin, and stimulating mucosal protective functions of bioactive substances.

In terms of active repair, epidermal growth factor (EGF), as an important mucosal protective factor, can maintain mucosal integrity, inhibit parietal cell secretion of gastric acid, promote DNA/RNA and protein synthesis of mucosal cells, and regulate mucosal cell apoptosis. The role of traditional Chinese medicine in promoting the healing of gastric ulcer by affecting the expression of EGF is still receiving attention, and studies have shown that this effect is determined. At present, there has been a more in-depth discussion on experimental research and great progress has been made. The administration of a certain dose of Cangzhu Lizhong Pill (Decoction) to the experimental animals can increase the EGF in the serum or stomach tissue of the animal, suggesting that related drugs may play an antiulcer role by stimulating the secretion of EGF. The effect of Cuyu Granule on the healing quality of acetic acid-induced gastric ulcer in rats was also reported [42]. Immunohistochemical image analysis of EGF expression in gastric mucosa of rats in each group showed that compared with the expression of EGF in gastric mucosa of rats in the blank model group, there was significant differences in EGF expression between the Cuyu Granule group and the ranitidine group ($P < 0.01$, $P < 0.05$), and the effect of the Cuyu Granule group was better than that of the ranitidine group ($P < 0.05$). This suggests that the Cuyu Granule may increase the expression of EGF in tissues around the ulcer, improve the functional maturity of regenerative mucosa, and then improve the quality of ulcer healing. It has also been reported that the use of ulcer cream can affect the expression of EGF and EGFR mRNA in gastric mucosa of rats with gastric ulcer. The ulcer cream has a good healing effect on gastric ulcer. The mechanism may be through improving the healing quality of ulcer and enhancing the expression of EGF and EGFR mRNA in epithelial cells at the edge of gastric ulcer, thus promoting the proliferation of epithelial cells in gastric mucosa and tissue repair and preventing ulcer recurrence. Astragalus can also promote the expression of EGF, which is significantly higher than that of omeprazole in the control group, so that the gastric mucosal epithelial tissue and gland structure can be better repaired and reconstructed, promote ulcer healing, and improve QOUH. In the study of the effect and mechanism of Danshen Decoction on promoting the healing of gastric ulcer, it was found that compared with the model group, Danshen Decoction can significantly promote ulcer healing in rats ($P < 0.01$), promote the expression of EGFR, and infer that promoting ulcer healing through gastric mucosal defense factors and inhibiting apoptotic pathways may be one of the mechanisms of Danshen Decoction in the treatment of gastric ulcer. Some scholars have observed the protective effects of Weitongning (dutchmanspipe root, potentilla, draconis resin, dandelion, debark peony root, costusroot, licorice, etc.) on gastric mucosa of rats with acetic acid-induced gastric ulcer. It was found that the content of EGF and NO in the high-dose group of Weitongning increased significantly, which was better than that in cimetidine group, but there was no significant difference. The Weitongning group and cimetidine group had obvious effects on the growth of regenerative mucosa, and the effect of the two groups was similar, $P < 0.01$ compared with the model group. It shows that Weitongning can increase the thickness of regenerative mucosa in gastric ulcer, increase the content of EGF and NO, and promote ulcer healing [43]. Other studies have shown that Western medicine and traditional Chinese medicine have their own advantages in improving and promoting the quality of ulcer healing. Compared with omeprazole, traditional Chinese medicine has more obvious effects on granulation tissue repair, capillary proliferation, and EGF secretion. Some studies have shown that different combinations of traditional Chinese medicines have different effects on increasing the content of EGF and the most prominent increase in the sugar supplement group.

Some Chinese medicines have effects on the expression of epidermal growth factor receptor (EGFR) in gastric tissue of rats with gastric ulcer. EGF needs to bind to its receptor (EGFR) to work. There is a close relationship between EGFR and gastric mucosal protection and gastric ulcer repair. Studies have shown that the expression of EGFR in gastric tissue of rats with gastric ulcer is higher than that in normal group, while the expression of EGFR in Jianwei Yuyang treatment group is higher, which is significantly different from that in the control group. When rats with gastric ulcer were treated with *Salviae miltiorrhizae*, the content of nitric oxide (no) in serum and expression of EGFR in gastric mucosa are significantly increased ($P < 0.05$). Many traditional Chinese medicines can induce and promote the synthesis of NO, reduce the content of plasma endothelin, increase the expression of EGFR around the ulcer, and finally promote the healing of ulcers.

As a natural preparation, Rehabilitation New Liquid is rich in amino acids, growth factors, and active substances; has good anti-inflammation, detumescence, regeneration, and repair effects; and also has obvious effects in enhancing the immunity of the body, as well as safe drug use and small adverse reactions. By searching the full-text database of CNKI journals from 1999 to 2014, the relevant literatures on Rehabilitation New Liquid were collected, and their effects on blood stasis blockage, stomach pain and bleeding, gastrointestinal ulcers, and adjutant treatment of tuberculosis were summarized.

In addition to its role in growth factors and their receptors, other mechanisms of antiulcer traditional Chinese medicines, such as H2 receptor blockers and proton pump inhibitors (PPIs), have also been discovered. The related studies on the active ingredients of antiulcer traditional Chinese medicine provide us with new ideas for the treatment of peptic ulcer. The combination of various antiulcer traditional Chinese medicine compound preparations and Western medicine can effectively shorten the healing time of ulcers, improve QOUH, and reduce the recurrence of ulcers.

Because the active ingredients of traditional Chinese medicine have the above advantages in the treatment of ulcers, the research on antiulcer traditional Chinese medicine has become a hot topic. However, there are still many shortcomings in the current studies and related literatures, and most of the current studies are experimental studies and few clinical studies. Due to different experimental subjects, the guidance of clinical research on clinical medication is irreplaceable, and relevant clinical research should be strengthened in the future as a basis for guiding clinical medication. There are fewer clinical cases for more than 2 years in relevant clinical studies, and most studies lack long-term follow-up and lack corresponding observation on the long-term effect of drugs. Current studies mainly focus on single-agent or compound preparations of traditional Chinese medicine, and the research level is relatively low. There are few studies on molecular pharmacology of active ingredients of traditional Chinese medicine. Traditional Chinese medicine has a history of thousands of years and has accumulated rich experience in the treatment of ulcers. On the basis of this, through in-depth research, making full use of the advantages of the overall multitarget regulation of traditional Chinese medicine, combined with the current treatment methods, the treatment of gastrointestinal ulcers will surely achieve greater breakthroughs. In the future, the focus of clinical research and observation should be on which types of traditional Chinese medicines (such as invigorating or activating blood circulation to dissipate blood stasis), or what compatibility can promote the production of EGF, and even the study of some single drugs. It is necessary to further observe the relationship between different periods of the ulcer surface and EGF content and strengthen the correlation study between TCM syndrome differentiation in traditional Chinese medicine and EGF for peptic ulcer. At the same time, light microscopy, electron microscopy, histochemistry, and immunohistochemistry can be used to evaluate the results of traditional Chinese medicine on promoting EGF production. It is believed that with the deepening of research, traditional Chinese medicine will make greater breakthroughs in this area.

Some people have used bone marrow-derived mesenchymal stem cells (BMSCs) with self-renewal ability and multidirectional differentiation potential to repair damaged gastric mucosa, which not only accelerates the healing of gastric ulcer but also greatly improves the healing quality of gastric mucosa. The poor quality of ulcer healing is an important factor causing ulcer recurrence.

Some scholars use bone marrow mesenchymal stem cell transplantation to treat ulcerative colitis [44]. Eighty patients with ulcerative colitis were divided into study group and control group. Patients in the control group were treated with conventional methods, while patients in the study group were given bone marrow mesenchymal stem cell transplantation for repair. The results showed that the clinical symptoms and signs of the study group were significantly less than those of the control group, and the intestinal mucosal inflammation was greatly improved without adverse reactions. It has been initially confirmed that bone marrow mesenchymal stem cell transplantation for ulcerative colitis can greatly improve symptoms.

## 7.5 Repair and Regeneration of Cardiac Damage in the Early Stage of Burn Injury

As early as the 1960s, cardiac dysfunction during severe burn shock has been found. Until the early 1980s, the main cause of postburn cardiac dysfunction was attributed to reduced blood volume (i.e., the result of shock) caused by increased capillary permeability after burn, or the role of myocardial inhibitors. At that time, it was thought that under stress conditions such as burns, the body can ensure the blood perfusion of the main organs such as the heart through blood flow redistribution, so that the myocardial blood flow will not be significantly reduced in the early stage of burns (especially in the early stage of shock), and there are no obvious structural damage and organic dysfunction. Therefore, it is believed that burn shock is mainly caused by increased vascular permeability, and the heart does not participate in the occurrence of burn shock in the early stage. The treatment of shock is mainly to "capacity replenishment" for blood volume reduction, and a series of fluid replenishment formula for burn shock is proposed. However, through a large number of clinical practice, it is found that even if the injury is treated immediately according to the fluid replenishment formula, some severely burned shocks are not only difficult to avoid but also difficult to correct, resulting in long-term ischemia and hypoxia of tissues and organs, organ dysfunction, and even failure, which has become one of the important bottlenecks for the further improvement of the cure rate of severe extensive burns.

### 7.5.1 Myocardial Damage Can Occur in the Early Stage of Severe Burns

In the past, it was thought that under stress conditions such as shock, the blood perfusion of the main organs such as heart could be guaranteed in the early stage by redistribution of blood flow. Therefore, it has long been believed that there is no ischemia and hypoxia damage to the myocardium during burn shock (especially in the early stage of shock), while the reduction of cardiac function after severe burns is mostly due to effective circulating blood loss and/or the role of myocardial inhibitors. Through a series of animal and clinical experiments, it was confirmed that myocardial damage can occur in the early stage of severe burns. The main findings are as follows [45–47].

#### 7.5.1.1 Myocardial Specific Structural Protein Leakage

CM-LC1 and TnT play important roles in myocardial contraction. Myosin light chain 1 (CM-LC1), troponin T (TnT), and troponin I (TnI) are specific indicators reflecting myocardial cell damage. Under normal conditions, they cannot enter the blood circulation through cells. When cells are degenerated and necrotic, TnT and others diffuse through the damaged cell membrane and enter the blood. At 1 h after the 30% TBSA III degree burn in rats, CM-LC1, TnT, and TnI significantly increased in the blood.

#### 7.5.1.2 Impairment of Cardiomyocyte Cytoskeleton

At 1 h after 30% TBSA burn in rats, some myocardial microtubule was broken, the fluorescence intensity of the skeleton protein was significantly reduced; in vitro experiments also found microtubule destruction in cardiomyocytes.

#### 7.5.1.3 Impairment of Cardiomyocyte Stress (Biomechanics)

The burn serum was added to the cultured cardiomyocytes, and the cell stress was detected by the cell microtubule suction technique. It was found that after the burn serum was added, the myocardial cells were deformed quickly and not easy to recover. Three hours after the addition of burn serum, the elastic coefficient and viscosity coefficient of myocardial cells decreased significantly. The stiffness of elastic component and viscous component of myocardial tissue are two factors that determine myocardial compliance. The elastic stiffness affects the degree of tissue deformation, while the viscous stiffness affects the rate of myocardial tissue deformation. The viscoelasticity of myocardial cells is reduced after burn, resulting in decreased myocardial compliance.

#### 7.5.1.4 Cardiomyocyte Apoptosis

TUNEL-positive cardiomyocytes were observed at 6 h after severe burns in rats, and apoptosis was further increased at 12 h after burn. Myocardial apoptosis was consistent with changes of cardiac function.

#### 7.5.1.5 Pathological Changes

One hour after burn, the myocardial muscle transverse disorder was observed, and then myocardial interstitial edema was seen, some muscle fibers were broken, and some muscle fibers were dissolved in sheet. Under the electron microscope, the myofilament was disordered or broken, focally dissolution, swelling and cavitation of mitochondrial, expansion and disintegration of sarcoplasmic reticulum, and partial nuclear dissolution.

#### 7.5.1.6 Decreased Cardiac Function and Myocardial Mechanics

Cardiac function indexes such as stroke volume (SV), stroke volume index (SVI), cardiac output (CO), and cardiac output index (CI) are decreased after burn; myocardial mechanical indexes such as left ventricular systolic peak pressure (LVSP), left ventricular end-diastolic pressure (LVEDP), and maximal rate of rise (decrease) of left ventricular pressure (±d*p*/d*t* max) begin to decrease at 1 h after injury, progressively decrease within 12 h, and remain below normal level at 24 h after injury. Among the indexes of myocardial mechanics, AOSP, AODP, and MAP mainly reflect the state of cardiac afterload and peripheral vascular resistance. LVSP reflects the maximum isometric tension. +d*p*/d*t* max is the maximum rate of increase of ventricular pressure, which reflects the contractile performance of the myocardium to a certain extent. -d*p*/d*t* max is the maximum rate of decrease of ventricular pressure in isovolumic diastolic period, which reflects the maximum rate of myocardial contraction component prolongation during myocardial relaxation, and is a good index to reflect the state of myocardial relaxation. LVEDP mainly reflects the left ventricular preload state and the degree of ventricular wall tension. It is not difficult to see that in the early stage of severe burns, the myocardial mechanics of rats is at a low level. Further analysis shows that LVSP and + d*p*/d*t* max decrease before LVEDP; that is, before the blood volume decreases, the myocardial contractility has begun to decrease, suggesting that in the early stage of serve burn, myocardial contraction and myocardial mechanical indexes have been damaged, resulting in the decrease of cardiac pump function and the cardiac output.

### 7.5.2 The Mechanism of Immediate Myocardial Damage in the Early Stage of Severe Burns

Why is myocardial damage and cardiac function reduced immediately after severe burns? Stress is an important factor. The cellular molecular mechanisms of early myocardial damage in burns include the following aspects.

#### 7.5.2.1 Mechanism of Immediate Reduction of Myocardial Blood Flow and Cardiac Function After Burns

(a) Activation of RAS system in the myocardium itself is an important initiating factor for early myocardial ischemia and hypoxia [48]: in early stage of severe burn, the local renin-angiotensin system (RAS) is activated and the local Ang II production is increased. Ang II has a direct toxic effect on cardiomyocytes. The pathophysiological level of Ang II can cause strong vasoconstriction and increase peripheral resistance, thus causing obvious damage to myocardial cells due to factors such as ischemia and hypoxia, changes in sarcolemmal permeability, and myocardial cell necrosis, leading to the reduction of myocardial perfusion. It is an important initiating factor for the immediate reduction of myocardial blood flow and early myocardial ischemia and hypoxia damage after burn. It was found that the Ang II content in myocardial tissue homogenate was significantly higher than normal value at 1 h after 30% TBSA III scald in rats, peaked at 6 h, decreased gradually, and remained significantly higher than normal at 24 h. At 1 h after injury, the cTnI in the burn group was significantly higher than the normal value, and gradually decreased after reaching the peak at 6 h, and was still significantly higher than the normal value at 24 h. The CK-MB was significantly higher than the normal value at each time point after burn, and reached the peak at 3 h. At 1 h after burn, myocardial tissue began to show lesions. At 3 h after burn, myocardial cells were swollen, myofilament was arranged disordered, cell boundaries were unclear and disappeared, interstitial blood vessels were dilated, and congestion, edema, bleeding, inflammatory cell infiltration, and the above lesions were further aggravated 12 h after burn. Some muscle fibers were wavy and sarcoplasmic condensation and red staining. The change trend of Ang II in myocardial tissue was consistent with the content of cTnI and CK-MB in plasma and pathological changes of myocardial tissue.

Further studies have found that the RAS system is also closely related to changes of cardiac function in the early stage of burn. At 1 h after burn, LVSP, +LVd*p*/d*t* max, and -LVd*p*/d*t* max were significantly lower than those in the control group; LVEDP was significantly increased and reached the peak at 6 h; Ang II, ACE in serum, and myocardial tissue also significantly increased, reaching the peak at 6 h; and ACE2 in myocardial tissue did not change significantly before and after burn. It is suggested that the change trend of ACE-Ang II axis is consistent with the changes of myocardial mechanical indexes and serum cTnI. ACE-Ang II axis in RAS plays an important role in the changes of cardiac function and myocardial damage in the early stage of burn. The main substrate of ACE2 is Ang II and produces Ang (1–7) which is antagonistic to Ang II. The rapid activation of ACE leads to the mass production of Ang II in the early stage of burn, while ACE2 has no obvious change in the early stage of burn, which is one of the important reasons for the decrease of Ang II degradation and overactivation of the ACE-Ang II axis. Active regulation of the ACE2-Ang (1–7) axis and the ACE-Ang II axis may reduce myocardial damage in the early stages of burns.

(b) Membrane receptor (β-AR)-mediated signal transduction system and "molecular switch Gsα/Giα" changes are important molecular mechanisms of early cardiac function inhibition. Previous studies have found that increasing cardiac preload and coronary blood flow velocity in scalded guinea pigs does not improve myocardial contractility, but the mechanism is still unclear. Adrenergic receptors are important receptors that affect myocardial systolic and diastolic function, and severe scald stress can cause significant changes in catecholamine neurotransmitters; the signal transduction system mediated by β-adrenoceptor and "molecular switch" Gsα/Giα is systematically studied. The results showed that: the signal transduction system of β-adrenoceptor in myocardial tissue changed significantly after severe burns. At 3–48 h after scald, the left ventricular pressure, maximal rate of left ventricular pressure rise, and maximum rate of left ventricular pressure decline significantly reduced, and the maximum decrease rate was at 6 h after burn and remained low until 48 h. The ventricular β receptors were significantly lower than those in the control group after scald, with the lowest level at 6 h after injury, but there was no significant change in Kd. The activities of cAMP and its metabolic key enzymes, adenylate cyclase (AC)/phosphodiesterase (PDE), in myocardium changed significantly. After 30% III degree scald in rats, the content of cAMP and the basal activity of adenylate cyclase (AC) in myocardium significantly decreased, and the decrease of cAMP content was positively correlated with the decrease of AC activity. There was no significant change in the activity of phosphodiesterase in myocardium. It is suggested that the main reason for the decrease of cAMP content is production obstacle. Further studies found that AC basal activity and isoproterenol (Iso)-stimulating activity of myocardial membrane significantly decreased after scald, while there were no significant changes in the stimulating activity of sodium fluoride (NaF) and forskolin (FSK), suggesting that the decrease of AC activity was mainly caused by the downregulation of β-AR. At 12 h, 24 h, and 48 h after scald, AC basal activity and Iso-stimulating activity decreased more significantly, and NaF-stimulating activity also significantly decreased, but FSK-stimulating activity had no significant change, suggesting that the decrease of AC activity was related to the dysfunction of G-protein-coupled AC catalytic subunit. One of the important advances in AC research in recent years is that myocardial AC is mainly distributed in V/VI type. Gsα can upregulate myocardial V/VI AC activity by activating almost all subtypes of AC and promote cAMP production, thus amplifying cardiac systolic and diastolic index; Giα mainly inhibits the AC of V/VI subtype, so it is an important factor in the negative regulation of myocardial V/VI AC. Therefore, Gsα/Giα subunit is considered a key molecular component (also known as a signal transducer) that regulates myocardial AC activity in the receptor's posterior phase and regulates myocardial function. The results showed that the expression of Gsα and its mRNA in myocardial tissue was significantly decreased after burn and reached the valley point at 3 h and 9 h, respectively, while Giα and its mRNA increased significantly, reaching peak at 3 h and 12 h, respectively. These results indicate that the downregulation of β-AR in the early postinjury and the consequent inversion of Gsα/Giα molecular ratio are important molecular mechanisms of early systolic and diastolic dysfunction.

#### 7.5.2.2 Mitochondrial Damage Is the Core of Myocardial Damage in Early Stage of Burns

1. Myocardial mitochondrial DNA deletion and downregulation of NRF1, mtTFA, and CPT-III mRNA expression are important factors in energy metabolism disorders. The study found that after 30% TBSA III degree burn in rats, 4.8 kb large fragment deletion occurred in myocardial mtDNA, ATP content of myocardial mitochondrial decreased, ADP and AMP levels increased, and TnI content in serum increased significantly. The 4.8 kb large fragment of myocardial mtDNA deletion contains the key enzymes of oxidative phosphorylation F0, F1-ATPase subunit 6 (ATPase6), cytochrome C oxidase subunit III (COX III), NADH reductase 3, 4 L, 4, and so on. The deletion of these genes severely affects the activities of related enzymes and further causes mitochondrial energy metabolism disorders, resulting in decreased ATP production in myocardial tissue of burned rats. We focused on the effects of F0, F1-ATPase activity encoded by myocardial mitochondrial DNA on energy metabolism. It was found that the content of ADP increased after 30% TBSA III degree burn, suggesting that mitochondrial F0,F1-ATPase activity is an important factor in ATP synthesis and maintenance of mitochondria membrane potential; mitochondrial energy metabolism disorder caused by the deletion of 4.8 kb mtDNA fragment after burn may be an important mechanism of myocardial damage in the early stage of burn and the formation of "shock heart" after burn. The content of MDA in myocardial tissue homogenate was significantly increased and the activity of SOD continued to decrease after burn, suggesting that oxidative damage is an important factor in the deletion of 4.8 kb mtDNA [49]. Results also demonstrate the mitochondrial responses to severe burn and indicate a pathway by which decreased EF-Tumt expression mediates oxidative damage in postburn myocardium.

   Hypoxia can downregulate the expression of NRF1, mtTFA, and CPT-II mRNA and reduce the level of cellular energy metabolism. Pretreatment of myocardial cells with L-carnitine and transfection of carnitine acyltransferase (CAT) gene can antagonize hypoxia/reoxygenation injury of cardiomyocytes. The results show that: (a) the contents of ATP and ADP in cardiomyocytes decrease significantly after hypoxia/reoxygenation. The expression of NRF1 and mtTFA, which regulate mitochondrial energy metabolism, decreases significantly after hypoxia/reoxygenation, and further decreases at 2–8 h after reoxygenation. This indicates that hypoxia/reoxygenation can cause a significant decrease in mitochondrial ATP synthesis and energy metabolism, which is related to the inhibition of the expression of NRF1 and mtTFA, which are important factors regulating the expression of mitochondrial respiratory chain subunits. After hypoxia/reoxygenation, the expression of CPT-II mRNA in cardiomyocytes is significantly reduced, suggesting that the transport of long-chain fatty acids to peroxisomes in mitochondrial for fatty acid β oxidation is significantly inhibited, leading to energy synthesis disorders. (b) After pretreatment with L-carnitine, cardiomyocytes were exposed to hypoxia/reoxygenation. The results show that ATP content is significantly increased; DNA fragmentation rate and apoptotic cell percentage are significantly decreased; and the expression of NRF1, mtTFA, and CPT-II mRNA is significantly increased, showing the protective effect of L-carnitine pretreatment on hypoxia/reoxygenation injury in cultured cardiomyocytes. (c) The recombinant retroviral pcDNA4/TO vector carrying CAT gene is transfected into cardiomyocytes to detect the expression of CAT gene in cardiomyocytes after transfection, and to detect changes in mitochondrial energy metabolism and whether it could antagonize hypoxia-induced cardiomyocyte apoptosis. The results show that the expression of CAT gene in primary cultured cardiomyocytes is significantly expressed after transfection with recombinant retrovirus pcDNA4/TO carrying CAT gene; the ATP production rate of CAT gene transfected group is upregulated by 37%, which significantly improved the inhibition of energy metabolism induced by hypoxia; the percentage of cardiomyocyte apoptosis in CAT gene transfected group decreases to 7%, indicating that transfection of CAT gene can significantly antagonize hypoxia/reoxygenation-induced cardiomyocyte apoptosis. The above results comprehensively show that CAT gene is one of the important functional genes regulating cardiomyocyte energy metabolism. It is confirmed that transfection of CAT gene is an important measure to antagonize myocardial ischemia/anoxia damage and has potential clinical application value.

2. Hypoxia activates the mitochondria-dependent apoptotic pathway and induces apoptosis. The study has found that hypoxia can activate mitochondria-dependent caspase-3-mediated cardiomyocyte apoptosis:
   (a) The main way of hypoxia-induced cardiomyocyte injury is to induce apoptosis. The survival rate of cardiomyocytes is significantly reduced at 6 h after hypoxia. By 24 h, the cell survival rate decreases by about 42%. At the same time, the increase of apoptotic cell rate, the typical morphological features of apoptosis, and the characteristic fragmentation of chromosomal DNA show that apoptosis is the main death mode of cardiomyocyte injury induced by hypoxia. (b) Hypoxia can cause a large amount of mitochondrial cytochrome c (Cyt c) release into the cytoplasm, and the Cyt c content in mitochondria and cytoplasm is a typical growth and decline relationship. The results indicate that hypoxia can induce activation of the endogenous apoptotic pathway (mitochondrial pathway), and mitochondria release a large amount of Cyt c, further activating downstream signal transduction molecules related to apoptosis. (c) Hypoxia can upregulate the expression of caspase-3 and caspase-9 genes in cardiomyocytes, and the expression trends of both are consistent. The quantitative analysis of enzyme activity indicates that the activation of caspase-3 is consistent with the upregulation of gene expression, indicating that hypoxia can activate downstream apoptosis-related signaling caspase-9, caspase-3 by inducing the release of Cyt c from mitochondria. (d) Calcium overload of cardiomyocytes induced by hypoxia appeared earlier than mitochondrial Cyt c release and caspase-3 activation, suggesting that hypoxia can cause a significant increase in the concentration of free calcium in cardiomyocytes, and it is earlier than the decline of cell survival rate and the occurrence of apoptosis. Therefore, calcium overload is an early important molecular event to initiate mitochondrial Cyt c release and caspase-3 activation. The direct evidence is that chelated intracellular calcium blocks hypoxia-induced caspase-3 activation and antagonizes the occurrence of cardiomyocyte apoptosis. (e) Pretreatment of cardiomyocytes with specific inhibitors of caspase-3 and intracellular calcium chelating agents can antagonize hypoxia-induced cardiomyocyte apoptosis. The combination of BAPTA/AM and caspase-3 inhibitor has better protection effect. On one hand, this result confirms the important role of caspase-3 activation in hypoxia-induced cardiomyocyte apoptosis; on the other hand, it provides new clues for clinical prevention and treatment of ischemic/hypoxic myocardial damage.
3. The activation of mtPLA2 and the opening of mPTP by $Ca^{2+}$ overload are important mechanisms of mitochondrial damage and cardiomyocytes apoptosis. Based on the following two characteristics of DOG, [$^3$H]DOG was

used to directly detect the opening and closing characteristics of mitochondrial PTP in burned cardiomyocytes. (a) DOG can enter the cytoplasm through the myocardial cell membrane, but it cannot penetrate the normal mitochondrial membrane and only enters the mitochondria when PTP is open. (b) The cells have no metabolic effects on DOG. Three hours after 30% TBSA III degree burn in rats, the contents of [$^3$H]DOG, MDA and $Ca^{2+}$ in myocardial mitochondria were significantly increased and the content of Cyt c was significantly decreased. The content of [$^3$H]DOG in mitochondria was positively correlated with $Ca^{2+}$ and MDA ($r = 0.8547, 0.9117, P < 0.01$), and the apoptosis of cardiomyocytes was increased and the activity of caspase-3 was enhanced, indicating that the opening of myocardial mitochondrial PTP increased significantly after burn. The opening of mitochondrial PTP in burned myocardium causes the disorder of mitochondrial oxidative phosphorylation and the release of Cyt c, thus activating caspase-3, which is an important mechanism of cardiomyocyte apoptosis. The overload of mitochondrial $Ca^{2+}$ and the increase of free radicals may be the important reasons for opening of myocardial mitochondrial PTP after burn. Myocardial mitochondrial $Ca^{2+}$ overload after burn may induce PTP opening by promoting structural changes of mitochondrial matrix cyclophilin D(CyP2D) and binding to ANT.

After burn, mtPLA2 activity increased, RCR decreased, and RCR was significantly negatively correlated with mtPLA2 activity ($r = -0.6835, P < 0.01$). It is suggested that the increase of $Ca^{2+}$ can activate mtPLA2, which can degrade mitochondrial membrane phospholipids, reduce the activities of certain respiratory enzymes and F0F1-ATPase, and decrease RCR.

#### 7.5.2.3 The Expression of Pro-Inflammatory Factors in Cardiomyocytes Is Upregulated

Ischemia and hypoxia are associated with uncontrolled inflammatory response, which are involved in the occurrence of myocardial damage in early stage of burn [46].

Studies have shown that the essential of organ function damage after burn is ischemia and hypoxia damage, the uncontrolled inflammatory response is its basic pathophysiological change, and vascular endothelial cells play a key role in it. After burn, stimulating factors such as ischemia-reperfusion activate neutrophils, endothelial cells, monocytes/macrophages, and other effector cells to release a variety of pro-inflammatory cytokines, such as tumor necrosis factor, and then activate effector cells of the body to produce secondary cytokines or inflammatory mediators, and form a cascade reaction of cytokines or inflammatory mediators, resulting in uncontrolled release of cytokines or inflammatory mediators, ultimately leading to organ damage. Therefore, pro-inflammatory cytokines are key factors in triggering "cascade amplification" inflammatory responses and leading to the development of SIRS. The process of cytokine release by effector cells includes primary signaling-kinase cascade pathway-nuclear transcription factor-mRNA transcription-translation-protein precursor processing-secretion-cell utilization. In this process, the most "bottleneck" is the nuclear transcription factor, and NF-κB is the most common nuclear transcription factor. NF-κB is a pleiotropic transcriptional regulator and a member of the Rel family. It is a class of proteins that can specifically bind to the κB site of various gene promoters or enhancers and promote their transcriptional expression. NF-κB is involved in regulating the transcription of many cytokines, inflammatory mediators, and adhesion molecules that are closely related to inflammation, immune response, growth, and differentiation. At rest, NF-κB (P50/P65) binds to its inhibitory protein IκB (including IκB, INBβ, IκBr, IκBδ, and IκBε) to form inactive trimers in the cytoplasm. When the cells are stimulated, IκB phosphorylates and degrades, and detaches from NF-κB, which activates NF-κB and shifts from cytoplasm to nucleus, thereby initiating the transcription of corresponding genes.

After 35% TBSA III degree burn in rats, TNF-α in plasma increased rapidly and reached the peak at 6 h after injury, and maintained a high level to 24 h after injury; the level of IL-8 in plasma gradually increased, and the level of IL-8 reached three times of normal value at 6 h after injury, and continued to increase to 24 h after injury. Administration of PDTC immediately after burn in rats can effectively reduce the contents of TNF-α and IL-8 in plasma.

After burn, the content of TNF-α in rat myocardium did not increase significantly within 6 h after injury, but increased rapidly from 12 h after injury to 24 h after injury. PDTC can significantly reduce the level of TNF-α in myocardial tissue at 12 h and 24 h after injury.

After burn, the expression of TNF-α mRNA in myocardium increased significantly, reached the peak at 6 h after injury, and maintained a high level within 24 h after injury. The results of in situ hybridization were consistent with the results of RT-PCR. PDTC can significantly inhibit the expression of TNF-α mRNA in myocardial tissue at 6 h and 12 h after injury.

The expression of ICAM-1 in myocardial tissue increased gradually, peaked at 12 h, and maintained at a high level until 24 h after injury. PDTC can significantly reduce the level of TNF-α level in myocardial tissue at 12 h and 24 h after injury.

MDA in the myocardial tissue homogenate of burned rats increased rapidly after injury, and the difference was significantly higher than that of the control group at 3 h after injury, and maintained at a high level within 24 h after injury. PDTC can effectively reduce the content of MDA in myocardial tissue.

After severe burns, MPO activity in myocardial tissue increased significantly at 3 h after injury, and reached the peak at 12 h after injury and maintained a high level within 24 h after injury. PDTC can significantly reduce MPO activity in myocardial tissue after injury.

After burns in rats, LVSP and ± dp/dt max decreased significantly, while LVEDP increased, indicating that both systolic and diastolic functions decreased. PDTC can effectively improve left ventricular systolic and diastolic function.

These results showed that after 35% TBSA III degree burn in rats, NF-κB in myocardial tissue was rapidly activated and continued for 24 h after injury, and the peak was at 3 h after injury. After injury, the content of MDA and the expression of TNF-α, IL-8, ICAM-1, mRNA, and protein were increased in the myocardium, the neutrophil aggregation increased, and the myocardial contractile and diastolic function decreased. Immediate application of NF-κB inhibitor (PDTC) in rats can effectively inhibit NF-κB activation, decrease the expression of TNF-α, IL-8, and ICAM-1, and reduce PMN aggregation and myocardial contractile function damage. It is suggested that NF-κB activation in myocardium is involved in the regulation of some cytokine expression in early severe burns and the accumulation of PMN in burn organs, which plays an important role in early organ damage.

In summary, activation of NF-κB in cardiopulmonary tissues in early stage of severe burns results in increased expression of TNF-α, IL-8, and ICAM-1 in cardiopulmonary tissues, increases aggregation of PMN in cardiopulmonary tissues, and decreases myocardial contractile function. NF-κB inhibitor (PDTC) can reduce ROS production or inhibit its activity through its antioxidant properties, inhibit NF-κB activation, downregulate cytokine expression, and reduce PMN aggregation and myocardial contractile function damage caused by increased cytokines in cardiopulmonary tissues of rats in the early stage of severe burn, which can prevent and treat cardiopulmonary damage after severe burns.

Thus, ischemia and hypoxia are associated with uncontrolled inflammatory responses. In ischemia and hypoxia, inflammatory cells, especially PMN and endothelial cells in myocardial tissue, are activated, so that PMN adheres to and accumulates in the microvessels of myocardial tissue, which can obstruct microvascular blood flow and exacerbate microcirculation disorder of myocardial tissue and ischemia and hypoxia. MPO is present in the cytoplasm of PMN, and MPO is significantly increased in myocardial tissue after burn, indicating that PMN aggregated more in myocardial tissue after burn. Activated PMN produces a large amount of MPO, elastase, oxygen free radicals, and cytokines such as TNF-α, causing damage to tissue cells. Therefore, there is a certain intrinsic relationship between ischemia-hypoxia and uncontrolled inflammatory response (Fig. 7.4). At 1 h after burn injury, the activity of nuclear transcription factor NF-κB in myocardium is significantly increased and maintained at a high level within 24 h. The expression of TNF-α, IL-8, and ICAM-1 in myocardial tissue and the level of tissue homogenate are all increased, suggesting that NF-κB activation upregulates the expression of the above cytokines. Increased MDA content and MPO activity in myocardial tissue reflect the decrease of LVSP, +d*p*/d*t* max and -d*p*/d*t* max, suggesting that NF-κB activation leads to the release of pro-inflammatory cytokines, which is an important mechanism of myocardial damage and the occurrence of "shock heart."

#### 7.5.2.4 p38 Kinase Is an Important Signaling Pathway Mediating Myocardial Damage in the Early Stage of Burns [50]

Signal transduction is a key intermediate link in the induction of cellular effects by most stimuli. Intervention of key signaling pathways can eliminate or reduce the cellular effects induced by stimuli. The MAPKs pathway is an important intracellular signal transduction pathway, including three family members, ERK, p38 kinase, and JNK. Among them, p38 kinase and JNK pathways are mainly activated by a variety of stress stimuli, such as ischemia and hypoxia, inflammatory factors, free radicals, and endotoxin, which play an important role in mediating stress cell damage.

(a) The overall animal level studies found that MAPK activation in myocardial tissue is associated with myocardial damage in the early stage of burn. The activation of p38 kinase, ERK, and JNK is detected by immunoblot chemiluminescence assay. The results showed that p38 kinase and ERK were activated after 40% III degree scald in rats, and no activation was observed in JNK. The p38 kinase is weakly activated in normal rat myocardial tissue. The activation of p38 kinase increased rapidly at 1 h after scald and peaked at 1 h, 3 h, and 6 h. The activa-

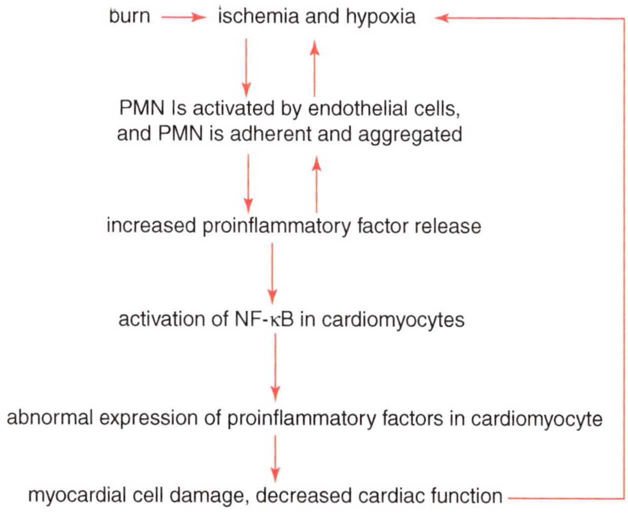


**Fig. 7.4** Relationship between ischemia-hypoxia and uncontrolled inflammatory response

tion degree of p38 kinase was 8.79, 9.05, and 8.26 times higher in the control group, decreased at 12 h, and was the lowest at 24 h, but the activation degree was still 374% of that in the control group. There are two subtypes of ERK, which are less activated in normal rats. The activated ERK1 and ERK2 increased rapidly at 1 h after scald, reached the peak at 3 h after injury (ERK1 and ERK2 were 7.44 and 7.67 times higher in the normal group), and decreased significantly after 12 h. The activation laws of ERK1 and ERK2 are basically the same.

The activation and intracellular distribution of p38 kinase, ERK, and JNK in myocardial tissue cells are detected by immunohistochemistry, showing that no activated JNK-positive cells were detected in normal and burned rat myocardial cells. Phosphorylated p38 kinase and ERK were not observed in normal rat myocardial tissue cells, and no nuclear translocation occurred. At 1 h after burn, p38 kinase and ERK showed significant activation characteristics with nuclear translocation, showing that brown-positive granules were diffusely distributed in the cytoplasm of the cardiomyocytes and concentrated in the nucleus. The positive characteristics, especially the nuclear translocation, were most obvious at 3 h after injury, remained strong at 6 h after injury, and weakened significantly at 12 h and 24 h after injury, and only a few positive myocardial tissue cells could be seen. The positive characteristics of p38 kinase are stronger than ERK.

P38 kinase was significantly activated in the myocardium after burn, whereas JNK failed to activate significantly, indicating that the p38 kinase pathway (non-JNK) is the major stress stimulatory signal transduction pathway in this experimental model. At 1 h after burn, the activation of p38 kinase in myocardial tissue increased by 8.8-fold and reached the peak at 1 h, 3 h, and 6 h, and was 3.7-fold higher than that in the control group at 24 h after injury. The rapid activation of p38 kinase suggests that not only ischemia-hypoxia and a large number of inflammatory cytokines can lead to p38 kinase activation after burn but also the immediate postburn stress response may be a stimulator of activation of this pathway. After burns, the body releases a lot of substances such as catecholamines, which causes stress reactions. Studies have confirmed that norepinephrine activates the p38 kinase pathway and plays an important role in norepinephrine-mediated cell damage. The sustained activation of p38 kinase reflects the persistence of damaging stimuli such as stress, hypoxia, and inflammatory factors after burn, suggesting that the sustained activation of p38 kinase pathway may play a very important role in mediating myocardial damage in the early stage of burns. Nuclear translocation accompanies the whole process of p38 kinase activation. Activated p38 kinase can regulate the transcriptional activity of multinuclear transcription factors by translocating into the nucleus, and then participate in the regulation of multigene expression, suggesting that rapidly activated p38 kinase in myocardial cells after burn may play an important role in mediating early myocardial damage by regulating gene expression. The study found that the peak of p38 kinase activation appeared earlier than the peak of myocardial damage, and p38 kinase was continuously activated within 24 h of observation, suggesting that p38 kinase pathway may play an important role in early myocardial damage after burns. At the same time, it was found that the activation of ERK1 and ERK2 in myocardial tissue was significantly enhanced with nuclear translocation after burn, peaked at 3 h and 6 h after injury, and decreased after 12 h without significant difference from normal. What role of ERK pathway activation plays in myocardial tissue after burn is unclear. Previous studies have suggested that the stress-activated ERK pathway can protect cell survival, and it is speculated that the activation of ERK pathway in myocardial tissue in the early stage of severe burn may be the self-anti-injury mechanism initiated by cells when stimulated by damaging stress.

It can be seen that the p38 kinase and ERK are activated in the MAPK pathway of myocardial tissue cells in the early stage of severe burns, and postburn stress, ischemia, hypoxia, and inflammatory factors are the main factors for their activation. The activation rule of p38 kinase and ERK suggests that not only the signaling pathway mediating tissue damage is activated after burns but also the signaling pathway that promotes cell survival is also activated, which initiates the body's own anti-injury mechanism to protect cardiomyocytes from ischemia, hypoxia, and inflammatory factors. The imbalance between these two factors may be an important intracellular mechanism that determines early myocardial cell damage.

(b) In vitro cell studies have found that the p38 kinase pathway plays an important role in myocardial cell damage induced by hypoxia and burn serum. Hypoxia and burn serum can rapidly and continuously activate the p38 kinase pathway in cardiomyocytes. At rest, the pathway is almost inactivated in cells. Activation of p38 kinase was not detected in cardiomyocytes without experimental stimuli. However, the activation of p38 kinase was significantly increased at 0.5 h after hypoxia and burn serum stimulation of cardiomyocytes, and reached a peak at 1 h, indicating that this pathway can be rapidly activated by injurious stimulus signals such as hypoxia and burn serum. Significant nuclear translocation occurred at 1 h after injury, suggesting that rapidly activated p38 kinase may play its biological role in the nucleus of cardiomyocytes. Nuclear transcription factors are the major downstream substrates of p38 kinase. It is speculated that p38 kinase may mediate myocardial cell effect induced by burn serum by regulating the activity of nuclear transcription factors and thus participating in a large number of gene expression. During the 12 h of experimental observation, the p38 kinase in cardiomyocytes was continuously activated, and the second activation peak appeared at 6 h after hypoxia and burn serum stimulation. It is suggested that hypoxia combined with burn serum can prolong the activation of p38 kinase in cardiomyocytes, which may be due to the fact that burn serum contains a lot of inflammatory factors, toxins, and other substances, and these stimulating factors are superimposed with hypoxia, resulting in sustained and long-term activation of p38 kinase. The rapid and sustained activation of p38 kinase suggests that this pathway may play an important role in hypoxia and burn serum-mediated cardiomyocyte damage.

Sustained activation of the p38 kinase pathway mediates cardiomyocyte damage in vitro. Previous studies have confirmed that hypoxia combined with burn serum can aggravate cardiomyocyte damage compared with single hypoxia. After hypoxia combined with burn serum for 6 h, the viability of cardiomyocytes decreased slightly; after 12 h, the viability of cardiomyocytes decreased significantly ($P < 0.05$). Further analysis showed that the content of LDH in the culture supernatant increased after stimulation of cardiomyocytes by hypoxia and burn serum for 3 h and increased significantly after 6 h. LDH is present in the cytoplasm of cardiomyocytes and leaks out of the cytoplasm only when cell membrane permeability increases or integrity is disrupted. It can be seen that hypoxia and burn serum stimulated cardiomyocytes for 3 h, which led to a certain degree of cardiomyocyte membrane damage; while the LDH content in the culture supernatant was significantly increased at 12 h after hypoxia and burn serum acted on cardiomyocytes, reflecting cardiomyocytes injury was significantly aggravated at this point, and the cell viability also decreased significantly at this point.

It was found that cardiomyocyte apoptosis increased significantly after hypoxia and burn serum stimulation of cardiomyocytes for 12 h, and the apoptosis rate of cardiomyocytes increased further after 18 h, indicating that cardiomyocyte apoptosis is one of the reasons for the decline in cardiomyocyte vitality under hypoxia and burn serum stimulation. To clarify the relationship between the sustained activation of the p38 kinase pathway and cardiomyocyte damage induced by hypoxia and burn serum, the p38 kinase selective inhibitor SB203580 was added to the culture medium to a final concentration of 10 μmol/L to inhibit the activation of p38 kinase and further demonstrate the role of p38 kinase pathway in cardiomyocyte injury induced by hypoxia and burn serum. The results showed that 10 μmol/L SB203580 could effectively inhibit the activation of p38 kinase in cardiomyocytes induced by hypoxia and burn serum. At the same time, the leakage of LDH in cardiomyocytes was decreased at 3 h after SB203580 administration, and the apoptosis of cardiomyocytes decreased and the viability of cardiomyocytes was improved after 12 h, demonstrating that the sustained activation of p38 kinase pathway plays an important role in mediating cardiomyocyte damage induced by hypoxia and burn serum.

#### 7.5.2.5 Damage to the Myocardial Cytoskeleton

(a) Ischemia and hypoxia induce increased expression of c-Fos and c-Jun, which can cause myocardial cytoskeleton damage by affecting the expression of cardiac troponin and β-Tubulin. When cardiomyocytes were treated with hypoxic combined burn serum, the expression of nuclear transcription factors c-Fos and c-Jun in cardiomyocytes increased significantly, and they bound to AP-1-binding sites of downstream genes troponin and β-Tubulin, which decreased the expression of cardiac troponin and β-tubulin significantly, and damaged myocardial cytoskeleton. Under electron microscope, the reticular structure of cardiomyocyte cytoskeleton is disordered. Some of the cytoskeletons are broken in granular shape and scattered around the nucleus, resulting in the damage to cardiomyocyte morphology, necrosis, and apoptosis. It is indicated that c-Fos and c-Jun are the main factors causing cardiomyocyte damage in hypoxia combined with burn serum. Using self-constructed antisense c-Fos gene recombinant and antisense c-Jun gene recombinant to transfect cardiomyocytes, it was found that the expression of c-Fos and c-Jun was inhibited and the expression of troponin and β-tubulin was upregulated, and the morphological structure, functional protein expression, protein composition, and protein ratio of cardiomyocytes tended to be normal in the cardiomyocytes treated with hypoxia-combined burn serum, which alleviated the damage of cardiomyocytes and protected cardiomyocytes.
(b) To explore the effect and mechanism of mechanical load on ischemia-anoxia cardiomyocytes by simulating mechanical load with mechanical stretch and to prove that the cardiac high load caused by excessive and rapid fluid replacement in the early stage of burn can aggravate myocardial damage in vitro cell level. The study found that the positive rate of LDH and PI staining in culture supernatant was not significantly different from

normal after static stretch stimulation with physiological stimulus intensity of 10%, suggesting that 10% stretch has no obvious damage to cell (membrane). After 10% stretching, the cardiomyocytes spread further, the cell body is wide, and the pseudopod is increased, suggesting that the cells are active. Ten percent static stretch stimulation is not only an acute injury factor for normal cardiomyocytes cultured in vitro but may also upregulate the function of cardiomyocytes.

However, under ischemic and hypoxic conditions, the resistance of cardiomyocytes to mechanical stretch is reduced. After static stretch stimulation with 10% of the same physiological stimulation intensity was applied, the morphological damage of ischemia-anoxia cardiomyocytes aggravated, cell spreading area and length increased, pseudopod increased, and cell membrane was damaged. Compared with the ischemia-hypoxia group alone, the number of PI-positive cells increased significantly and the LDH in the culture medium increased sharply after mechanical stretch + ischemia-hypoxia stimulation. Mechanical stretch also aggravated the upregulation of inflammation-related genes in ischemia-hypoxia cardiomyocytes. The 10% stretching group + ischemia-hypoxia group significantly upregulated the expression of TNF-α mRNA, decreased the expression of contractile protein gene β-MHC mRNA in cardiomyocytes, and further decreased myocardial contractile function. Because mechanical stretch can aggravate the damage of ischemic-hypoxic cardiomyocytes, in clinical work, for patients with severe cardiac insufficiency who have experienced delayed resuscitation, a large number of rapid fluid replacement needs to be combined with effective cardiac function monitoring and carried out according to the heart's endurance capacity, so as to avoid excessive rapid fluid replacement to cause excessive cardiac preload, excessive myocardial stretch, and aggravate myocardial damage.

Mechanical stretching under normoxia revealed that the expression of microfilaments and tubulin in cardiomyocytes is enhanced and the morphology is intact. Mechanical stretching under hypoxic-ischemic conditions revealed that microfilaments and microtubules were severely damaged, and the content of β-tubulin protein in microtubules was reduced. Laser confocal microscopy showed that nonsarcomeric microfilaments were damaged obviously, no obvious microtubules in the polymerization state existed, the cell morphology was irregular, the periphery was rough, the membrane integrity was destroyed, and the cell morphology was seriously damaged, indicating that mechanical stretch aggravates the myocardial cytoskeletal damage caused by ischemia and hypoxia is an important mechanism leading to myocardial damage.

The results of the whole animal experiment showed that the tolerance of rats to a large amount of rapid fluid replacement was significantly decreased after burn, which showed that the cardiac function indexes (LVSP, +d*p*/d*t* max, -d*p*/d*t* max) decreased after fluid replacement, and the amount of fluid needed to reach the same level of LVEDP (10–15 mmHg) in rats in burn group was less than that in normal rats. The above results indicate that under the condition of ischemia and hypoxia, mechanical stretch of physiological strength leads to severe damage of myocardial cells, cell structure destruction, and cytoskeleton changes, which is one of the mechanisms of myocardial damage in early burns. This suggests that the appropriate volume and speed should be given during clinical antishock fluid replacement to prevent excessive and rapid fluid replacement from overloading the heart, resulting in excessive stretch of the myocardium, aggravating myocardial damage, and leading to the occurrence of "shock heart."

(c) The molecular mechanism of cardiomyocyte damage caused by burn serum combined ischemia and mechanical stretch is multifaceted, mainly including the following aspects: (a) Increase the release of pro-inflammatory cytokines from cardiomyocytes and cause myocardial damage. The contents of IL-1 and TNF-α in cardiomyocytes were significantly increased, indicating that mechanical stretch can promote the secretion of inflammatory factors by cardiomyocytes. (b) p38 kinase is an important signaling pathway mediating cardiomyocyte damage induced by burn serum combined ischemia and mechanical stretch. Under hypoxic combined burn serum + mechanical stretch, p38 expression increased, nuclear translocation occurred within 1 h, but JNK was not expressed. (c) Enhanced activation of NF-κB is one of the important factors that mechanical stretch aggravates cardiomyocyte damage. Under the stimulation of hypoxia and burn serum, when combined with 10% axial static stretch, the expression of NF-κB and nuclear translocation were more significant, and the expression level of IκB-α decreased with the prolongation of stimulation time. NF-κB is a nuclear transcription factor with multidirectional regulation, which regulates genes related to immune response, stress response, and inflammatory response, and its enhanced activation is one of the important factors that mechanical stretch aggravates cardiomyocyte damage.

(d) Stabilizing the cytoskeleton can alleviate the damage of ischemia-hypoxia cardiomyocyte caused by high mechanical load. On the basis of elucidating the effects of mechanical stretch on the damage (mainly cytoskeletal damage) of cardiomyocytes induced by ischemia-hypoxia, the protective effects of actin cytoskeletal stabilizer phalloidin and taxol on cardiomyocyte ischemia-hypoxia combined with stretch injury were studied. It was found that cytoskeletal microfilament or (and) microtubule stabilizer can significantly reduce the release of LDH from cultured cardiomyocytes, upregulate the expression of MHC mRNA in cardiomyocytes in the 10% stretch + ischemia-hypoxia group, inhibit the transformation of MHC mRNA from α type to β type in cardiomyocytes, downregulate the expression of TNF-α mRNA, and significantly reduce the number of PI-positive cells, and the combination of taxol and phalloidin is more effective.

(e) Disruption of microtubule stability may be one of the factors leading to mitochondrial structure and function damage. Hypoxia is one of the most common pathophysiological phenomena in severe burns, trauma, and other various diseases. Energy metabolism disorder is the fundamental cause of cell and tissue damage caused by hypoxia. Cellular energy metabolism disorders during hypoxia manifest as inhibition of aerobic metabolism (mitochondrial pathway) and initiation of compensatory glycolysis. In the past, studies on energy metabolism disorders under hypoxia or ischemia and hypoxia mostly started from mitochondria in terms of aerobic metabolism. Despite a lot of work, the exact mechanism of energy metabolism disorders, especially mitochondrial damage, under hypoxic conditions is still unclear, and there is a lack of effective conditioning measures in the clinic.

The results showed that the beaded structure disappeared at 10 min after hypoxia; the microtubules were distorted and fractured at 20 min of hypoxia, with disruption of continuity and integrity, disordered distribution, and loss of microtubules away from the nucleus; the structural damage of microtubules was aggravated at 30 min and 1 h of hypoxia until the distribution regularity was lost. Fluorescence intensity of tubulin and Western blot also showed that microtubule damage and depolymerization occurred at 10 min of hypoxia and aggravated with the prolongation of hypoxia time. It shows that under hypoxia, microtubules depolymerize very early and disrupt their distribution and structure; the respiratory function and energy synthesis of cardiomyocytes began to decrease at 30 min of hypoxia; within 1 h of hypoxia, mitochondria only showed changes in distribution and structural damage, while the overall structure and staining activity of mitochondria did not change significantly, indicating that the hypoxia damage of microtubules occurred earlier than mitochondrial damage. Regarding the causes of microtubule damage, it has been thought that mitochondrial damage leads to energy starvation and depletion. Skeletal protein phosphorylation can inhibit aggregation and assembly of skeleton proteins, leading to depolymerization of the skeleton, thereby causing damage to the cytoskeleton including microtubules. However, a large number of studies in recent years have begun to cast doubt on the traditional understanding. Studies have shown that cardiomyocyte ischemia and hypoxia can directly lead to myocardial cytoskeletal damage. As an important skeleton to maintain the integrity of muscle fibers and organelles, microtubules show significant damage before irreversible damage occurs in severe ischemia. Myocardial cytoskeletal changes precede the ultrastructural changes in myocardial ischemia.

To demonstrate whether the early microtubule damage is involved in subsequent mitochondrial damage, microtubule depolymerizers were used to further explore this. It was found that the use of microtubule depolymerizer under normoxia significantly reduced the mitochondrial function indexes such as RCR and ATP, although the morphological and structural changes of mitochondria were not obvious. Further studies also found that the damage changes of mitochondrial arrangement, distribution, and morphology after depolymerization of microtubules and hypoxia treatment for 30 min and 1 h were aggravated compared with the corresponding hypoxia group, and the RCR and ATP content in the hypoxia depolymerization group were also decreased compared with hypoxia group at the corresponding time points. These results suggest that microtubules are involved in the intracellular localization of mitochondria and the regulation of mitochondrial respiratory function and energy metabolism in early hypoxia.

(f) The effect and mechanism of microtubule destruction on MPT in hypoxia cardiomyocytes: Hypoxia can cause the obvious destruction of the polymeric microtubule structure and the obvious reduction of the content of polymeric microtubule in cardiomyocytes, and the hypoxic damage is gradually aggravated with the prolongation of treatment time. The important role of mitochondrial permeability transition pore (mPTP) in cell damage, apoptosis, and necrosis is receiving more and more attention. mPTP is a multiprotein complex that forms a large, nonselective permeable pore on the mitochondrial inner membrane. Its irreversible opening leads to the occurrence of mitochondrial permeability transition (MPT), which leads to a decrease in mitochondrial inner membrane potential, the released of mitochondrial cytochrome C into the cytoplasm, causing cell necrosis and apoptosis. Studies have shown that the opening of mitochondrial permeability transition pore is a key link in myocardial ischemia and hypoxia damage, and calcium overload and ROS increase are the two main factors leading to mPTP opening in hypoxic cardiomyocytes. Our study demonstrates that microtubule destruction can lead to mPTP opening and plays an important role in hypoxia damage of cardiomyocytes.

Mitochondrial immunofluorescence of cardiomyocytes in normal group was strong and granular. After 0.5-h treatment, obvious mPTP opening occurred in the hypoxia group and the normoxia + microtubule depolymerization group, which showed that the mitochondrial fluorescence intensity was weaker than that in the control group. The immunofluorescence of mitochondria in the hypoxia + stabilizer group was not significantly different from that in the control group. With the prolongation of treatment time, the degree of mPTP opening in the hypoxic group and the normoxia + microtubule depolymerization group was increasing, showing that the ratio of the immunofluorescence intensity in the ROI region to that in the control group was smaller and smaller; the degree of mPTP opening in the hypoxia + stabilizer group was significantly reduced compared with the hypoxic group.

In normal group, the mitochondrial inner membrane potential of cardiomyocytes is higher, and the mitochondrial fluorescence intensity is stronger. After 0.5-h treatment, the mitochondrial inner membrane potential in the hypoxia group and the normoxia + microtubule depolymerization group decreased significantly, showing that the mitochondrial fluorescence intensity was weakened. The immunofluorescence of mitochondria in the hypoxia + stabilizer group was not significantly different from that in the control group. With the prolongation of treatment time, the degree of membrane potential loss in the hypoxia group and the normoxia + microtubule depolymerization group increased continuously, while the loss of the membrane potential in the hypoxia + stabilizer group was significantly improved compared with the hypoxia group.

Cytochrome C was almost undetectable in the cytoplasm of cardiomyocytes in normal group. After 0.5-h treatment, cytochrome C in mitochondria of the hypoxia group and the normoxia + microtubule depolymerization group leaked into the cytoplasm, and cytochrome C in cytoplasm increased significantly. No significant increase in cytochrome C was detected in the cytoplasm of the hypoxia + stabilizer group. With the prolongation of treatment time, the cytochrome C leaking into the cytoplasm increased in the hypoxia group and the normoxia + microtubule depolymerization group, while the cytochrome C leakage from mitochondria was significantly less in the hypoxia + stabilizer group than in the hypoxia group. After 0.5-h treatment, the cell viability of hypoxia group and normoxia + depolymerization group was significantly decreased, and with the prolongation of treatment time, the cell activity decreased continuously; the cell activity of hypoxia + stabilizer group was significantly improved than that of hypoxia group.

At 0.5 h after hypoxia, the concentration of free calcium in cardiomyocytes increased significantly. With the prolongation of hypoxia, the concentration of free calcium increased gradually, reaching a peak at 6 h after hypoxia, and slightly decreased at 12 h. After 0.5 h cardiomyocyte treatment in the normoxia + depolymerization group, the concentration of free calcium was also significantly increased, and the change trend was consistent with that in the hypoxic group. The increase of intracellular calcium concentration in hypoxia + microtubule stabilizer group was significantly lower than that in the hypoxia group at the same time points. Although the calcium concentration in the hypoxia group and the normoxia + microtubule depolymerization group was significantly higher than that in the control group, the calcium concentration in the normoxia + microtubule depolymerization group was significantly lower than that in the hypoxia group.

After 0.5-h hypoxia, the content of ROS in cardiomyocytes increased significantly, and with the prolongation of hypoxia, the ROS content in cardiomyocytes increased gradually. After 0.5 h of treatment in the normoxia + depolymerization group, the ROS content in cardiomyocytes also increased significantly, and the trend was consistent with that in the hypoxic group. While the ROS levels in the hypoxia + microtubule stabilizer group were significantly lower than those in the hypoxia group at the same time points. Although the ROS levels in the hypoxia group and the normoxia + microtubule depolymerization group were significantly higher than those in the control group, the increase of ROS level in the normoxia + microtubule depolymerization group was significantly lower than that in the hypoxia group.

The above results indicate that after the disruption of microtubules in normal cardiomyocytes by colchicine, a microtubule depolymerization agent, the cell mPTP is opened, resulting in MPT in the cells, causing a corresponding decrease in the mitochondrial inner membrane potential, a significant increase in cytochrome C released from the mitochondria, and a significant decrease in cell activity. When paclitaxel, a microtubule stabilizer, was used to alleviate the hypoxic injury of microtubules, the opening of mPTP in cardiomyocytes was effectively prevented, indicating that microtubule destruction in hypoxic cardiomyocytes is an important factor leading to MPT. The mechanism of microtubule destruction in hypoxic cardiomyocytes leading to MPT is not fully understood. $Ca^{2+}$, inorganic phosphate, and ROS are the key factors leading to MPT in hypoxic cardiomyocytes.

Ischemia, hypoxia, and other factors act on the cells, causing abnormal $Ca^{2+}$ transport in the cells leading to intracellular $Ca^{2+}$ overload and increase of free radicals. High concentrations of $Ca^{2+}$ can cause the binding of recombinant CyP-D to ANT, while ROS acts on the thiol of ANT to oxidize it, which causes the opening of mPTP, leading to the occurrence of MPT.

(g) Microtubule destruction in hypoxic cardiomyocytes has an important influence on key enzymes and energy production of glycolytic pathway. Cardiomyocytes provide energy primarily through oxidative phosphorylation of mitochondria in the presence of sufficient oxygen supply. However, after extensive and severe burns, the main energy supply of cardiomyocytes is converted to anaerobic glycolysis pathway due to ischemia and hypoxia in the myocardium. Three key enzymes in the glycolytic pathway: phosphofructokinase (PFK), hexokinase (HK), and pyruvate kinase (PK) are critical in providing ATP required for myocardial metabolism. Among the three enzymes that catalyze three irreversible reactions during glycolytic process, PFK is considered the most important, catalyzing the conversion of fructose 6-phosphate to fructose 1,6-diphosphate; HK phosphorylates glucose to glucose-6-phosphate; PK converts phosphoenolpyruvate to pyruvate and releases ATP. LDH reduces pyruvic acid to lactic acid.

The study found that the PK activity in the cardiomyocytes of group B and group D increased slightly at first and then decreased, reaching a peak at 1 h and then gradually decreased. Compared with group A at each time point, group B and group D were significantly lower than group A at 0.5 h after hypoxia; group B and group D were significantly lower than group A after 1 h of hypoxia, and reached a peak at 1 h; while group A gradually decreased after reaching the peak at about 3 h. The trend of group C was similar to that of group A; it increased immediately after 0.5 h, reached the peak around 6 h, and then decreased rapidly, but was significantly lower than that of group A at 3 h and 6 h; group D was significantly lower than group C at each time point.

With the prolongation of treatment time, the HK activity of cardiomyocytes in group B and D gradually decreased to half of that in group A at 3 h, and the change trended to be stable after 6 h, but the activity is maintained at a very low level, and there was no significant difference between the two groups. Compared with group A, the activity of enzymes in the two groups was significantly lower than that in group A at all-time points from 0.5 h after hypoxia; the change trend of group A and group C was similar, and there was no significant difference. It gradually increased from 0.5 h, peaked at about 3 h, and then decreased rapidly, but it was still significantly higher than that of group B and group D at 12 h. At this time, the HK activity of group C was significantly higher than that of group A.

The PFK activity of cardiomyocytes in group A increased first, reached the peak after 6 h, and then decreased rapidly. After 0.5 h of hypoxia, the activity of PFK in group B and group D was significantly lower than that in group A, and then decreased slowly. After 6 h, PFK activity tended to ease and decreased to the lowest level at 12 h. PFK activity in group B and group D was lower than that in group A at all-time points, and there was no significant difference between the two groups. PFK activity in group C began to rise rapidly at 0.5 h after hypoxia, slowly decreased after reaching the peak at 3 h, decreased rapidly after 6 h, and decreased to 0.5 h level after 12 h; this trend was similar to that in group A, but the PFK activity at each time point was significantly higher than that in group B and group D.

The LDH activity of cardiomyocytes in group A showed a gradually increasing trend, and the activity of LDH at 12 h was twice as high as that at 0.5 h. The trend of LDH activity in group C also increased gradually. Although it was lower than that in group A at 0.5 h, it increased significantly from 1 h and was higher than the activity of LDH in group A at each time point. The LDH activity at 12 h was four times of that at 0.5 h. Compared with group A, the LDH activity in group B increased significantly from 0.5 h, peaked at 3 h, and was significantly higher than that in group A, but then decreased rapidly and was significantly lower than that in group A at 12 h. The change of LDH activity in group D was similar to that in group C within 3 h, and was still significantly higher than that in group A at 3 h, but it decreased sharply thereafter, and was lower than 0.5 h at 12 h, and significantly lower than the other groups from 6 h.

After 0.5-h hypoxia, the LC content of cardiomyocytes in group B and group D was significantly higher than that in group A, and then the LC content increased slowly, reached stable at 1–3 h, and increased slowly after 3 h, but then it was significantly lower than that in group A at all-time points, and the trend of the two groups was gentle and similar. The LC content in group A increased gradually, increased rapidly at 1–3 h, and was higher than that in group B, group C, and group D at 3 h, 6 h, and 12 h. Compared with group A, the LC content in group C also showed an upward trend. The LC content in group C was not significantly different from that in group A from 0.5 h to 1 h, and increased sharply after 1 h, but was still significantly lower than that in group A.

Detection of cardiomyocyte activity showed that after treatment with different factors, the mortality rate of cardiomyocytes increased gradually. The mortality rate of cardiomyocytes in group A after 12 h was about 10 times higher than that in group after 1 h, and more than half of the cells died after 24 h. Compared with group A, the cell death rate of group B and group D at each time point was significantly increased, more than half of the cells died at 12 h, and 80% of the cells died after 24 h, and there was no significant difference between the two groups. There was no significant difference between group C and group A within 1 h after hypoxia, but then the dead cells gradually increased, but the number of dead cells in group C at each time point was significantly lower than that in group A, and the survival rate was about 65% after 24 h.

After 0.5- to 6-h treatment, the CK activity in group B and group D increased rapidly and the increase slowed after 6 h. After 1 h, the activity of group B was significantly higher than that in group A at each time point, but it was lower than that in group D at each time point. The CK activity in group D was significantly higher than that in group A at each time point, while CK activity in group C was lower than that in group A at each time point.

The ATP content in group A showed a steady decreasing trend, and after 12 h, the ATP content decreased to about 1/4 of 0.5 h. Compared with group A, the ATP content in group C was significantly higher than that in group A in the early period after hypoxia, then gradually decreased, and the decrease of ATP was more obvious at 1–6 h, but the ATP content at each time point was significantly higher than that in group A during the 6-h period, and there was no significant difference between the two groups after 12 h. The ATP content in group B was significantly lower than that in group A in the early stage of hypoxia (0.5 h), then gradually decreased and was significantly lower than that in group A at all-time pints, among which the decrease of 0.5–3 h was most obvious. The ATP content in group D decreased from hypoxia and was significantly lower than group A and group C at all-time points. Contrary to the change of ATP content, the ADP content in each group showed a gradual increase trend.

The above results showed that under hypoxia alone, the key enzyme activities of glycolysis in cardiomyocytes increased significantly at first and then decreased, suggesting that cardiomyocytes glycolysis activity is significantly enhanced under hypoxia. Hypoxia is one of the important factors to initiate glycolysis. However, with the prolongation of hypoxia, the hypoxia condition is further aggravated, and the key enzyme activities of glycolysis are further enhanced, while LDH maintains high activity for a certain period of time with the prolongation of time, resulting in the accumulation of LC, a glycolysis metabolite. Under hypoxia, the microtubule depolymerization (colchicine) keeps the microtubules in a state of over-depolymerization, and the activities of key enzymes of glycolysis decrease with time. Using large doses of microtubule stabilizers transformed the dynamic depolymerization process of microtubules into an overstable state, and the key enzyme activities of glycolysis in cardiomyocytes still showed a significant decrease trend, but the appropriate concentration of microtubule stabilizers can reverse the depolymerization state of microtubules in the early stage of hypoxia. Fluorescence microscopy revealed that there was no significant difference between the microtubule morphology under appropriate concentration of microtubule stabilizer and the normal microtubule morphology under normoxia for a period of hypoxia, but this effect only occurred in the early stage of hypoxia, and the microtubule stabilizer had little effect on the microtubule depolymerization process after 12 h. Under the action of appropriate concentration of microtubule stabilizer, the key enzymes activities of glycolysis in cardiomyocytes increased significantly, and the metabolite LC also increased rapidly. After 12-h hypoxia, cell microtubules were gradually not affected by the low concentration of microtubule stabilizers, and at the same time, the rapid decrease of glycolytic energy was also observed.

Over-depolymerization or over-stabilization of microtubules in hypoxic cardiomyocytes induced by microtubule depolymerization can accelerate cardiomyocytes damage and even death, while energy production activity is significantly weakened. Proper microtubule stabilization during hypoxia can significantly slow down cell damage and death in an early stage, thereby promoting cell energy production, but this protection is only effective in a short period of time. Once the hypoxia is aggravated and the cell structure is irreversibly damaged, the protective effect of stable microtubules is lost.

The use of microtubule depolymerization and high-dose microtubule stabilizers can accelerate cell damage and even death by altering the structure of microtubules. Small doses of microtubule stabilizers can significantly alleviate cell damage and death. After moderately stabilizing the microtubules of cardiomyocytes, the ATP content increased significantly and was significantly higher than that in group A at all-time points within 12 h. However, with the prolongation of hypoxia, the oxidative energy supply of mitochondria is significantly weakened, the cytoskeleton is irreversibly damaged, and the mitochondria detach from the microtubules and the structure is irreversibly changed. At this time, stabilizing the microtubules cannot change the energy production of the cells.

It can be seen that the activity and energy production of cardiomyocytes under hypoxia are closely related to the structure of cytoskeletal microtubules. Stabilizing microtubules can significantly reduce cell damage and delay cell death, but this effect is time-dependent, that is, occurs in the early period after hypoxia.

Microtubule-associated protein 4 (MAP4), which belongs to type II microtubule-associated protein, is a fibrillar protein with thermal stability and sensitivity to proteases, and is one of the major microtubule-associated proteins constituting the nonneuronal cytoskeleton. When MAP4 is coated outside the microtubules, the tubulin subunits cannot be separated from the end of the microtubules and are important substances for stabilizing microtubules under physiological conditions. Studies have shown that in normal cardiomyocytes, MAP4 is located in a bundle of polymeric microtubules formed by α-tubulin and β-tubulin proteins. Hypoxia can destroy microtubules in cardiomyocytes, and MAP4 is significantly reduced. With the prolongation of hypoxia time, the content of α-Tubulin protein and MAP4 in cardiomyocytes decreased gradually. Transfection of the replication-deficient recombinant adenoviral vector containing the rat MAP4 gene can upregulate the expression of MAP4, help maintain the stability of microtubules in hypoxic cardiomyocytes, and maintain the energy metabolism and physiological activity of cardiomyocytes in the early stage of hypoxia, but does not affect the activity and physiological function of cardiomyocytes in normal culture. Upregulation of MAP4 expression can significantly improve ATP and energy charge levels of cardiomyocytes in the early stage of hypoxia (0.5–3 h) and maintain cell viability. However, with the prolongation of hypoxia time, cardiomyocytes eventually still suffer inevitable energy metabolism disorders and the relative viability of cells declines.

### 7.5.3 The "Shock Heart" Hypothesis of Ischemia and Hypoxia Damage in the Early Stage of Burn

The above results indicate that after severe burns, the activation of RAS system in myocardium leads to early myocardial ischemia and hypoxia; changes of blood components after burns cause changes of erythrocyte membrane viscoelasticity, which leads to the decrease of myocardial local blood flow; changes of the signal transduction system mediated by myocardial cell membrane receptors (β-AR) and "molecular switch Gsα/Giα" cause the rapid inhibition of cardiac function, and so on, which make the myocardial ischemia and hypoxia damage cardiac dysfunction occur before the blood volume drops significantly due to the increase of capillary permeability. This early myocardial damage and weakened blood pumping function can not only cause cardiac dysfunction but also induce or aggravate shock, which is one of the important initiating factors for early ischemia and hypoxia. Based on the above findings, the "shock heart" hypothesis of early ischemia and hypoxia injury was proposed (Fig. 7.5). This theory corrects the previous understanding that the there is no obvious decrease of myocardial blood flow, no obvious structural damage and organic dysfunction of myocardium in the early stage of burn, that the burn shock is mainly hypovolemic shock due to increased vascular permeability, and the heart does not participate in the occurrence of early burn shock. It provides a new direction for the prevention and treatment of early ischemia and hypoxia damage. Later, with the further reduction of blood volume, if the timely and effective treatment is not available, the myocardium may severe more ischemia and hypoxia damage.

In order to clarify the effect of early myocardial damage on the ischemia and hypoxia injury of other tissues and organs and the "initiating" effect, the "shock heart" hypothesis of early ischemia and hypoxia injury was proved by experiments, and the effects of "shock heart" on liver, kidney, and intestinal damage in severely burned rats were studied. In the experiment, rats were burned with 30% TBSA III degree and were intraperitoneally injected with Ringer lactate solution according to the Parkland formula (4 mL·kg$^{-1}$·1% TBSA-1). The rats were divided into burn group and drug intervention group. The drug intervention group was further divided into propranolol group (β-blockers inhibit myocardial contraction, 0.75 mg/kg, intravenous drip), lanatoside C group (enhancing myocardial contraction, 0.2 mg/kg, intravenous drip), enalaprilat (improving myocardial blood flow, 1 mg/kg, intravenous drip), and combined treatment group of lanatoside C and enalaprilat (respective doses constant). The results showed that serum CtnI (myocardial damage index) was significantly increased at 0.5 h after burn, while serum TBA, β2-MG, and DAO (sensitive indicators reflecting liver, kidney, intestinal damage) increased significantly at 1–3 h after injury; the cardiac function of rats began to decrease significantly at 1 h after injury and gradually decreased within 12 h. After adequate fluid replacement, the cardiac function recovered after 24 h, but it was still significantly lower than that of the control group. At 6 h after injury, the β-blocker propranolol was used to inhibit myocardial contraction. It was found that myocardial damage was significantly aggravated; cardiac function was further reduced; at this time, the blood flow of liver, kidney, and intestine was also reduced; and the damage was aggravated. In the angiotensin-converting enzyme inhibitor enalaprilat group, the cardiotonic lanatoside C group, and the combined treatment group of lanatoside C and enalaprilat, myocardial damage was significantly reduced, myocardial mechanical indexes were improved, the blood flow of liver, kidney, and intestine was increased, and the damage was alleviated (Fig. 7.6) [51]. There was a significant negative correlation between myocardial damage index and cardiac function, and the cardiac function was positively correlated with the blood flow of liver, kidney, and intestine and negatively correlated with the changes of damage indexes. These results suggest that the occurrence time of myocardial damage after severe burns is not only significantly earlier than those of other organs but also significantly correlated with other organ

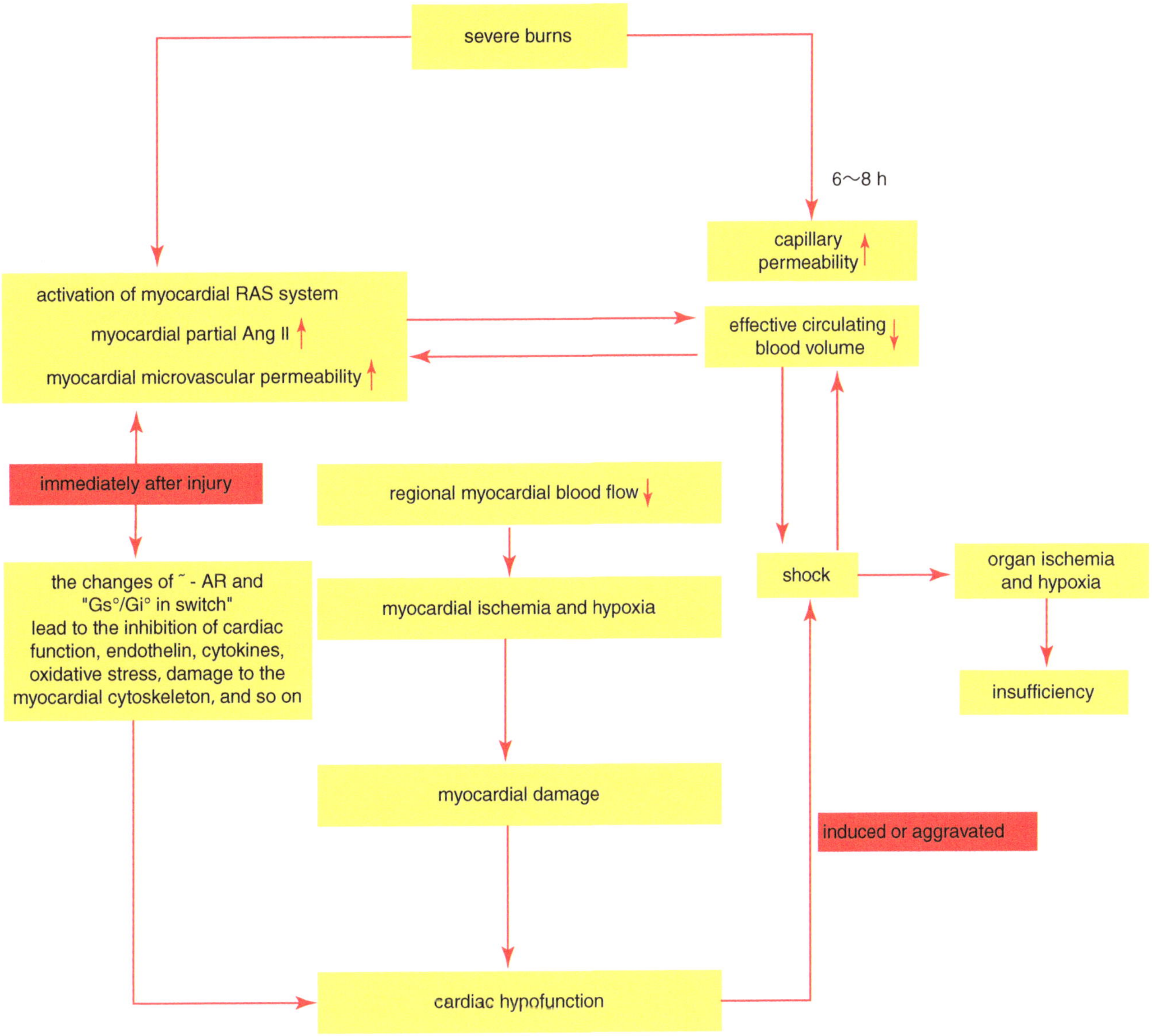


**Fig. 7.5** The "shock heart" hypothesis of early ischemia and hypoxia injury

damage indexes and blood flow, suggesting that "shock heart" is one of the important triggers for blood flow reduction and organ damage in liver, kidney, and intestine in the early stage of severe burn.

Of course, with the further reduction of blood volume, myocardial ischemia and hypoxia will be further aggravated. In addition to the reduction of aerobic metabolism, oxygen free radicals, cytokines, and other mediated damage may also occur. The core of early myocardial damage in burns is mitochondrial damage, which can cause energy metabolism disorders and initiate mitochondrial pathway apoptosis. The opening of MPTP caused by mitochondrial $Ca^{2+}$ overload and increased free radicals not only inhibits aerobic metabolism but also releases cytochrome C and activates cytoplasmic caspase-3, leading to mitochondrial pathway apoptosis. In addition, the endogenous protective mechanism is relatively weakened or damaged, which is also an important mechanism of myocardial damage.

### 7.5.4 Prevention and Treatment of Myocardial Damage in the Early Stage of Severe Burns

According to the mechanism of myocardial damage and "shock heart" in the early stage of burns, the prevention and treatment measures and strategies were proposed from various aspects.

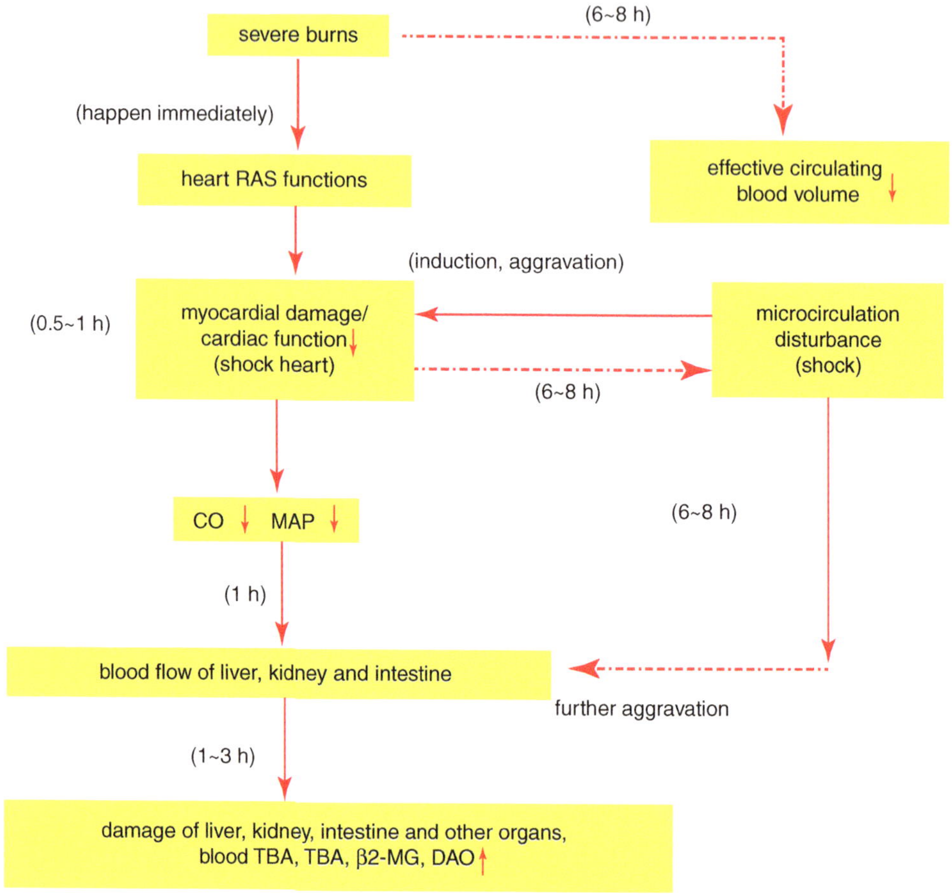


**Fig. 7.6** Schematic diagram of "shock heart" inducing and aggravating shock and liver, kidney, and intestinal damage in early stage of burn

#### 7.5.4.1 Angiotensin-Converting Enzyme Inhibitor

In the early stage of severe burns, the activation of renin-angiotensin system (RAS) increases the production of Ang II in myocardium, leading to the decrease of regional myocardial perfusion, which is an important initiating factor for early myocardial ischemia and hypoxia damage. Studies have shown that the low dose (1 mg/kg) of angiotensin-converting enzyme inhibitor (ACEI) can significantly improve myocardial ischemia and hypoxia injury in the early stage of severe burns and has no significant effect on blood pressure.

After 30% body surface area (TBSA) III degree burn, the enalaprilat injection, an angiotensin-converting enzyme inhibitor, can significantly reduce plasma Ang II. In the three enalaprilat injection groups, plasma Ang II levels were significantly negatively correlated with the dose of enalaprilat injection: although the plasma Ang II level in the low-dose (1 mg/kg) enalaprilat injection group was significantly lower than that in the control group, it was still higher than the normal level; the plasma Ang II levels in the middle-dose (2 mg/kg) group and high-dose (4 mg/kg) group were lower than that in the low-dose group, especially in the high-dose group.

The study found that the low dose of enalaprilat injection had no significant effect on circulating blood pressure during shock fluid replacement. After scald, the systolic and diastolic blood pressures of the scald control group and the high- and medium-dose enalaprilat injection treatment group were significantly lower than the normal values. At 6 h after scald, the systolic and diastolic blood pressure of the low-dose group was not significantly decreased, slightly higher than that of the scald control group; the diastolic blood pressure of the low-dose group was lower than normal at 12 h after injury, but significantly higher than that of the scald control group and the high- and medium-dose enalaprilat injection group. After scald, the mean arterial pressure of the scald control group and the three enalaprilat injection groups were significantly lower than the normal level, and the change of mean arterial pressure was negatively correlated with the dosage of enalaprilat injection. The mean arterial pressure of high-dose group was lower than that of the medium- and low-dose groups. The mean arterial pressure of the low dose group was not significantly different from that of the scald control group at 6 h after the burn; the mean arterial pressure of the low-dose group was higher than that of the scald control group at 12 h after scald, suggesting that the application of low-dose enalaprilat injection has no significant effect on circulating blood pressure at the same time of fluid replacement.

Application of low-dose enalaprilat injection can significantly reduce myocardial damage [48]. After scald, serum CK content of scald group was significantly higher than normal level; serum CK content of the three treatment groups was significantly lower than that of the scald control group at 6 h after scald; at 12 h after scald, serum CK content of the medium- and low-dose treatment group was still significantly lower than that of the scald control group. In the three treatment groups, the serum CK levels of the middle- and high-dose groups were higher than that of the low-dose group, and the high-dose group was the most obvious. The serum CK content of the low-dose group was not significantly different from the normal value at 12 h after injury. The CK-MB was significantly higher than the normal value at all time points after burn, reaching a peak at 3 h. At 1 h and 3 h after injury, the CK-MB of the treatment groups was also significantly higher than the normal value, but there was no significant difference from the normal value at 6 h after injury, but they were significantly lower than that of the scald group at each time point. At 1 h after injury, the cTnI of the scald group was significantly higher than the normal value ($P < 0.01$), gradually decreased after reaching the peak at 6 h, and was still significantly higher than the normal value at 24 h ($P < 0.01$). There was no significant difference in cTnl between the treatment groups and the normal value at each time point, but they were significantly lower than that of the scald group.

Application of the low-dose enalaprilat injection can significantly improve myocardial mechanical indexes. LVSP reflects left ventricular contractility. After scald, LVSP was significantly lower than normal, showing a downward trend. It fell to the lowest level around 12 h after injury, and rebounded at 24 h after injury, but it was still significantly lower than normal. At 3 h, 6 h, 12 h, and 24 h after injury, LVSP of the low-dose enalaprilat injection group was higher than that of the scald control group in varying degrees, suggesting that the early application of enalaprilat injection after severe burns can reduce the damage of left ventricular systolic function and protect cardiac function. At 6 h and 12 h after scald, the LVSP of each group was significantly lower than the normal value, but the LVSP of the low-dose treatment group was higher than that of the scald group and the medium- and high-dose groups; at 12 h after scald, the LVSP of the low-dose treatment group was significantly different from that of the medium- and high-dose treatment groups, suggesting that the medium and low dose of enalaprilat injection can improve left ventricular contractility after severe burns, but the effect of low dose is the most obvious. +d*p*/d*t* max reflects the changes of left ventricular systolic function. After burns, +d*p*/d*t* max showed a downward trend, fell to the lowest level around 12 h after injury, and rebounded at 24 h after injury, but still significantly lower than normal. At 1 h, 3 h, 6 h, 12 h, and 24 h after injury, the +d*p*/d*t* max of the low-dose treatment group had different degrees of elevation than that of the burn control group. At 6 h and 12 h after severe burns, the +d*p*/d*t* max of each group was significantly lower than the normal value. The +d*p*/d*t* max of the low-dose treatment group was significantly higher than that of the scald group, the medium-dose group, and the high-dose group; at 6 h after scald, the +d*p*/d*t* max of the medium-dose treatment group was also significantly higher than that of the high-dose treatment group, suggesting that the medium and low doses of enalaprilat injection can improve the left ventricular systolic function after severe burns, but the effect of low dose is the most obvious. -d*p*/d*t* max showed a downward trend, fell to the lowest level around 12 h after injury, and rebounded at 24 h after injury, but still significantly lower than normal. At 1 h, 3 h, 6 h, 12 h, and 24 h after injury, the -d*p*/d*t* max of the low-dose treatment group was increased to different extents than the scald control group. At 6 h and 12 h after scald, the -dp/dt max of each group was significantly lower than the normal value, and the -d*p*/d*t* max of the low-dose treatment group was higher than that of the scald group and the medium- and high-dose groups; at 6 h after scald, the difference of -dp/dt max between the middle-dose group and the high-dose group was significant, suggesting that the medium and low doses of enalaprilat injection can alleviate the left ventricular diastolic function after severe burns, but the effect of low dose is better. LVEDP, an index reflecting left ventricular diastolic performance after burns, also showed a downward trend, fell to the lowest level around 12 h after injury, and rebounded at 24 h after injury, but it was still significantly lower than normal. At 3 h, 6 h, 12 h, and 24 h after injury, the LVEDP of the low-dose treatment group was increased to different extents than the scald control group. At 6 h and 12 h, the LVEDP in each group was significantly lower than the normal value, and the LVEDP of the low-dose group was higher than that of the scald group and the medium- and high-dose groups. At 6 h and 12 h, the LVEDP of the low-dose group was significantly different from that of the medium- and high-dose treatment groups; the LVEDP of the middle-dose treatment group was significantly different from that of the high-dose treatment group at 6 h, suggesting that the medium and low doses of enalaprilat injection can improve the LVEDP after severe burns, but the effect of low dose is better.

These results indicate that in the early stage of severe burns, the use of low-dose enalaprilat to improve myocardial function during effective fluid replacement will not only significantly affect circulating blood pressure but also be beneficial to the prevention and treatment of myocardial damage in the early stage of burns.

There are two mutually antagonistic systems in RAS: ACE-Ang II axis and ACE2-Ang (1–7) axis. Under normal circumstances, the two are in a state of balance and maintain the normal function of the cardiovascular system. Ang II, the main bioactive substance of RAS, plays an important role in regulating the physiological and pathological processes of the heart. In addition to directly regulating vascular blood flow, Ang II can also increase oxidative free radicals, promote the expression of adhesion molecules, induce the inflammatory process, and cause endothelial dysfunction through its receptor ATR. ACE2, as an analog of ACE, has a limited distribution, mainly in the endothelial system of the heart and kidney, as well as the smooth muscle cells in the coronary artery. Its main function is to degrade Ang II into bioactive peptide Ang (1–7) and antagonize the various biological effects of Ang II, which has positive significance for the protection of early heart damage in burns. The authors found that the rapid activation of ACE in the early stage of burn resulted in the mass production of Ang II, while the change of ACE2 was not significant, which makes the balance between the positive and negative regulation of ACE-Ang II axis and ACE2-Ang (1–7) axis in RAS system is broken. Rats were given Ang (1–7) in the early stage of burns in an attempt to negatively regulate the RAS system. The experiments found that after 30% TBSA III degree burn in rats, the administration of 1 μg/kg Ang (1–7) could not significantly reduce the serum Ang II level in burned rats, but LVSP, LVEDP, +d*p*/d*t* max, and -d*p*/d*t* max significantly improved, SBP and SDP of arterial blood pressure significantly increased, and serum cTnI decreased significantly, indicating that it has protective effect on early heart damage in burns. It is further proved that early heart damage in burns is closely related to ACE-Ang II axis activation in RAS. Adjusting the balance of ACE-Ang II axis and ACE2-Ang (1–7) axis has protective effect on myocardial damage.

#### 7.5.4.2 Regulation of β-AR-Mediated Signal Transduction and "Molecular Switch Gsα/Giα" Ratio

The results showed that clonidine could improve cardiac function in the early stage of burns by upregulating the β-AR signaling system of myocardium, prevent the decrease of LVSP, ±d*p*/d*t* max, and Bmax in a dose-dependent manner, increase the Bmax of β-AR after burns, increase the expression of Gsα and its mRNA, inhibit the expression of Giα, significantly increase the basic activity of AC and increase the Gpp(NH)P stimulating activity, and increase cAMP content after burns. The study found that *Panax notoginseng* saponins (PNSs) can also upregulate the β-AR signaling system after scald, significantly increase the expression of Gsα mRNA, reduce the expression of Gi2α mRNA, increase the content of cAMP, and enhance the basic activity of AC. Within 12 h after burn, AOSP, AODP, MAP, LVSP, LVEDP, and ±d*p*/d*t* max continuously decreased. The myocardial morphological damage was alleviated in the rats treated with PNS, and the myocardial mechanical indexes were gradually improved, suggesting that PNS can effectively improve myocardial mechanical indexes of severely burned rats and reduce the cardiac damage caused by severe burns. The results of the study have guiding significance for clinical prevention and treatment of cardiac dysfunction immediately after burns.

#### 7.5.4.3 Early and Timely Fluid Replacement

For rats with 30% TBSA III degree burn, the regional myocardial blood flow decreased significantly at 1 h after burn, reached the lowest point at 6 h, and then increased gradually, reaching a normal value at 48 h. At 3 h after injury, the erythrocyte membrane viscoelasticity increased significantly, peaked at 6 h, and then gradually decreased to the normal value at 24 h. There was a significant negative correlation between regional myocardial blood flow and erythrocyte membrane viscoelasticity and viscosity coefficient. The stiffness of erythrocyte membrane is mainly determined by the structure of cell membrane. Its lipid bilayer structure is the structural basis to ensure the fluidity and strong deformability of erythrocyte membrane, and the membrane skeletal protein network has an important regulatory role. The lipid fluidity of erythrocyte membrane decreased and the content of macromolecular cross-linked protein increased after severe burns. The mechanism may be related to the direct damage of heat to erythrocyte membrane and the saponification of erythrocyte membrane lipid, sulfhydryl, and membrane skeleton proteins by increasing the content of oxygen free radicals in blood. The deformability of red blood cells after burns decreases, leading to a decrease in myocardial blood flow, which is one of the important causes of myocardial damage after burns.

Early and timely fluid replacement can significantly improve hemorheology indexes, including low shear rate blood viscosity, medium shear rate blood viscosity, high shear rate blood viscosity, plasma viscosity, erythrocyte aggregation index, hematocrit, and erythrocyte electrophoresis rate. The results showed that the elastic modulus and viscosity coefficient of erythrocyte membrane in the early fluid replacement group were significantly lower than those in the delayed fluid replacement group; regional myocardial blood flow significantly increased; and myocardial microvascular permeability, endothelin-1 content, NO-2 content, ACE activity, Ang II content, and plasma myosin light chain-1 (MLC1) content were significantly lower than those in the delayed fluid replacement group. The mortality rate of animals at 24 h after injury was significantly lower than that in the uniform fluid replacement group (14.66% vs 46.66%). It suggests that rapid fluid replacement can effectively prevent myocardial ischemia and hypoxia damage caused by delayed resuscitation of burns and reduce the degree of myocardial damage. The contents of ACE and Ang II in myocardial tissue of the rapid fluid replacement group were significantly lower than those in the delayed fluid replacement group, and the levels of ACE and Ang II were significantly positively correlated with plasma CM-LC1 level; regional myocardial blood flow (hydrogen clearance method) was significantly increased in the rapid fluid replacement group, and pathological changes were significantly reduced. It suggests that rapid fluid replacement can improve the activity of myocardial RAS system, reduce the production of local Ang II and endothelin-1 in myocardium, increase myocardial regional blood perfusion, improve the mechanical properties of erythrocyte membrane, reduce myocardial microvascular permeability, and play a protective role in myocardial damage.

#### 7.5.4.4 Drugs to Support Cardiac Function and Improve Myocardial Nutrition

In addition to fluid replacement and antishock for burn patients, nondigitalis drugs, such as dobutamine, should be timely given to patients with weak myocardial contraction and low heart rate on the basis of supplementing blood volume; for patients with weak myocardial contraction and fast heart rate, give lanatoside C in time to support the heart. In addition, GIK solution, fructose sodium diphosphate, energy mixture, and other drugs are routinely administered to improve myocardial nutrition to reduce myocardial damage in the early stage of burn.

The special nutrients rhITF and glycylglutamine dipeptide have protective effects on cardiomyocytes in burned rats. The rhITF recombinant expression system was successfully constructed, and the high-purity and bioactive human ITF was obtained. Its physical and chemical properties were consistent with the theoretical values and had an extremely high stability, which laid a foundation for further research on the role and mechanism of ITF in protecting cardiomyocytes. The synthesis process of glycylglutamine was established, and the protective effect and mechanism of glycylglutamine on myocardial injury in burned rats were discussed. The results showed that myocardial interstitial edema and myocardial fiber disorders were observed at 12 h after burn injury in rats; at 24 h after injury, the edema was aggravated; some myofibers were broken or arranged in a wavy pattern, focally dissolved in the cytoplasm; and myocardial fibrinolysis and necrosis, fiber rupture, and nucleus disappearance could be observed at 48–72 h. The damage of the glycylglutamine group was significantly less compared with the burn control group; the AST, CK, and LDH of the glycylglutamine group were significantly reduced, suggesting that the administration of glycylglutamine can reduce the degree of myocardial cell damage after burn. Compared with the normal control group, the myocardial dynamic indexes, such as LVSP, LVEDP, AOSP, AODP, MAP, and ±d*p*/d*t* max of rats in each group, are decreased after burn and decreased to the lowest value at 48 h. Comparing the treatment group with the burn control group, there was no significant difference between the two groups within 24 h, and each index decreased to a lesser extent at 48 h, suggesting that the administration of glycylglutamine could significantly improve the myocardial dynamic indexes in burned rats. The content of ATP in each group decreased with the change of time phase and decreased to the lowest level at 72 h, and the degree of decrease was lower in the administration group than in the burn group. The content of ADP and AMP was increased with the change of time and reached the highest at 48 h, and the level of ADP and AMP in the administration group was lower than that in the burn group. The content of adenylate pool increased after injury and reached the highest at 48 h. There was no significant difference between the administration group and the burn group within 12 h, and the degree of increase was higher in the administered group after 24 h. It is suggested that the administration of glycylglutamine can improve the energy metabolism of myocardial tissue after burn. The expression of HSP70 protein in the glycylglutamine group was higher than that in the burn group, suggesting that the protective mechanism of glycylglutamine in attenuating the degree of myocardial damage in burned rats is related to improving myocardial blood supply, maintaining myocardial energy metabolism, alleviating peroxidative damage, and promoting HSP70 and MT synthesis.

#### 7.5.4.5 Antagonize or Reduce Inflammatory Mediators

(a) A large-scale escharectomy is performed in the early stage of burn. Wound is one of the main sources of inflammatory mediators in burns. Subeschar tissue and edema fluid contain a large amount of inflammatory mediators, and burn eschar may also contain "burn toxins." Therefore, timely and effective removal of wounds can not only accelerate the repair of wounds but also effectively block the source of inflammatory mediators and reduce organ damage caused by inflammatory mediators, which has an important impact on the cure rate and treatment quality of severe burns. In the absence of effective treatment for inflammatory mediators, we have proposed the idea of accelerating burn wound repair, reducing systemic inflammatory response, and preventing early organ damage by performing an early large-scale escharectomy. That is, for patients with large-area deep burns, after the hemodynamic indexes are basically stable, the large-area III degree and its surrounding deep II degree wounds should be resected as soon as possible, and covered with allogeneic skin and autologous skin to make infected or necrotic burn wound a relatively healthy closed wound to improve the nutritional status of the body, accelerate wound healing, reduce SIRS, and prevent early organ damage. Animal experiments found that all eschars were removed immediately after burn, the levels of TnT and MLC1 in blood were reduced immediately, the indexes of myocardial mechanics were improved compared with those in the control group, the myocardial mechanical indexes such as LVSP, LVEDP, ±d*p*/d*t* max, AOSP, AODP, and MAP decreased slightly, and the vascular permeability decreased significantly. Clinically, a large area of escharectomy can significantly shorten the healing time of wounds. After escharectomy, serum TNF and endotoxin levels are significantly decreased, and the SIRS performances are reduced or disappeared. Postoperatively, the damage effect of patients' serum on cultured vascular endothelial cells was alleviated, the visceral dysfunction and systemic infection rates of patients were reduced, and the cure rate was increased.

The mechanism by which early large-area escharectomy reduces myocardial damage is multifaceted. Reducing damage caused by inflammatory mediators is an important mechanism. Immediate escharectomy in the early stage of burn can significantly inhibit the activation of NF-κB in cardiomyocytes, downregulate the expression of TNF-α and IL-8 mRNA in cardiomyocytes, and reduce the levels of TNF in myocardial tissue and plasma, and plasma TNF is positively correlated with TnT ($r = 0.9409$, $P < 0.001$), suggesting that a escharectomy in the early stage of burn can inhibit the activation of NF-κB in effector cells of the body, thereby inhibiting the release of cytokines or inflammatory mediators, enzymes, etc., which is beneficial to block or reduce myocardial damage after burns.

A large area of escharectomy in the early stage of burn can inhibit the activation of NF-κB in myocardial tissue. A large area of escharectomy in the early stage of severe burns in rats can effectively inhibit the increase of NF-κB activity in cardiomyocytes.

A large area of escharectomy in the early stage of burn can reduce the expression of TNF-α and IL-8 in myocardium. In the early stage of burn, escharectomy can reduce the increase of TNF-α and IL-8 in myocardial tissue homogenate after severe burns in rats. In situ hybridization of TNF-α and IL-8 also confirmed that early escharectomy could inhibit the expression of TNF-α and IL-8 mRNA in myocardium.

A large area of escharectomy in the early stage of burn can improve aortic systolic pressure, aortic diastolic blood pressure, and mean arterial pressure; reduce plasma troponin T, myosin light chain I, and creatine kinase isoenzyme MB; and significantly improve left ventricular systolic and diastolic function in rats after burn.

(b) Early application of ulinastatin (UTI) [52]: Clinical and animal studies have shown that ulinastatin has preventive and therapeutic effects on early myocardial damage in burns. A clinical study was conducted on 34 patients with severe burns whose burn area was more than 50%. The results showed that after treatment with ulinastatin (group U), plasma cTnI and CK-MB levels were significantly reduced, and plasma PMN elastase content was significantly lower than that of burn control group (group B) at all time points.

Animal experiments showed that after 30% TBSA III degree burn in rats, the levels of plasma cTnI and CK-MB in the ulinastatin treatment group were significantly lower than those in the burn control group; the TNF-α content significantly decreased and basically decreased to normal at 24 h. At 1 h, 3 h, 6 h, 12 h, and 24 h after burn, IL-10 content in myocardium of rats increased significantly, and the IL-10 content in the ulinastatin treatment group was significantly higher than that in the burn control group at 3 h, 6 h, 12 h, and 24 h after burn. Application of ulinastatin can also significantly reduce MDA content, caspase-3 activity, and myocardial apoptosis index in myocardial tissue and alleviate myocardial tissue pathological changes.

Ulinastatin is a urinary trypsin inhibitor that is isolated and purified from male urine and has two active functional regions. Both active functional regions have a wide spectrum of inhibitory enzymes and do not completely overlap, and they can simultaneously competitively or noncompetitively inhibit the activities of various hydrolases such as trypsin, phospholipase A2, hyaluronidase, and elastase, as well as the release of inflammatory mediators. The results showed that ulinastatin can effectively inhibit the expression of TNF-α, which proves that the myocardial protective effect of ulinastatin is related to the reduction of uncontrolled inflammatory response after burn. Ulinastatin can significantly increase the expression of IL-10 in myocardial tissue, thereby enhancing the inhibition of inflammatory mediator TNF-α, further reducing the myocardial damage caused by uncontrolled inflammatory response, suggesting that the protective effect of ulinastatin on myocardial injury after severe burns is related to the balance of pro-inflammatory/anti-inflammatory mediators. Severe lipid peroxidation injury occurred in myocardial tissue in the early stage of burn. The MDA content in the ulinastatin treatment group (group U) was significantly reduced, indicating that ulinastatin can reduce the degree of lipid peroxidation in myocardial tissue, and its myocardial protective effect is also related to the reduction of lipid peroxidation damage in myocardial tissue. Combined use of caspase-3 activity and TUNEL in situ apoptosis dual-index detection can reduce the false positive/negative caused by a single index and improve the specificity and reliability of apoptosis detection. The results show that ulinastatin may also affect the signaling pathway of apoptosis in a certain way, thereby reducing the apoptosis rate of cardiocytes and reducing myocardial damage in scalded rats.

(c) Application of antioxidants—early application of Shengmai injection: Clinical and animal studies have found that the application of Shengmai injection in the early stage of severe burn can effectively reduce myocardial damage, improve myocardial function, reduce complications, and improve the success rate of large-area burn treatment. After early application of Shengmai injection in clinical burn patients, cTnI, CK-MB, and LDH were significantly lower than those of the control group.

In animal experiments, after 30% TBSA III degree scald rats were treated with Shengmai injection, myocardial mechanical indexes such as LVSP, LVEDP, +d*p*/d*t* max, and -d*p*/d*t* max significantly improved, and myocardial tissue pathological changes were alleviated, suggesting that early application of Shengmai injection after severe burn can improve left ventricular function to varying degrees and reduce left ventricular function damage.

In situ labeling (TUNEL) of apoptosis in left ventricular myocardium of rats after severe burn showed that there were no apoptosis-positive cells in the myocardium of rats in both groups before scald, a small amount of apoptotic cells were detected in the myocardium at 3 h after injury, and the number of apoptotic cells increased significantly at 6 h and 12 h after injury and remained significant until 24 h. At 3 h, 6 h, 12 h, and 24 h after injury, the number of apoptosis-positive cells in the Shengmai injection group was reduced compared with the scalded control group, and was significantly reduced after 6 h compared with the scald control group.

After severe burns, the activity of caspase-3 in the left ventricular myocardium of rats in the Shengmai injection group was significantly lower than that in the control group, and the content of MDA in the Shengmai injection group was also significantly lower than that of the control group.

Shengmai injection is a compound preparation of traditional Chinese medicine, and its main components are red ginseng, *Ophiopogon japonicus*, and Schisandra. Among its active ingredients, ginsenosides have the effects of strengthening heart, regulating blood pressure, improving circulation, and promoting substance metabolism and protein synthesis. Ophiopogonin has the effects of improving myocardial contractility and cardiac pump function, antiarrhythmia, and hypoxia tolerance. Clinical studies have shown that when Shengmai injection was used early on the basis of conventional treatment, serum cTnI, CK-MB, and LDH were significantly lower than those of conventional resuscitation and fluid replacement therapy. It is suggested that the early application of Shengmai injection can reduce myocardial damage, improve myocardial intrinsic contractility, improve myocardial contractile function, reduce the decrease of myocardial diastolic function caused by severe burns, and improve myocardial diastolic function. The mechanism may be related to the reduction of cardiomyocyte apoptosis and the reduction of lipid peroxidation damage in myocardial tissue.

(d) Astragaloside reduces oxidative damage in hypoxic cardiomyocytes [53]. Astragaloside is a saponin compound extracted from *Astragalus membranaceus*, which is used in the Chinese Pharmacopoeia to judge the quality standard of Astragalus and its products, such as Astragalus Oral Liquid. The study found that after application of astragaloside (AST), myocardial cell viability from high to low was in the order of normoxia group, hypoxia group, hypoxia + AST 50 mg/L group, hypoxia + AST 25 mg/L group, and hypoxia + AST 12.5 mg/L group, while the LDH value reflecting cell damage from low to high was in the order of normoxia group, hypoxia + AST 50 mg/L group, hypoxia + AST 25 mg/L group, hypoxia + AST 12.5 mg/L group, and hypoxia group. MDA value reflecting cellular oxidative damage decreased and SOD value increased, indicating that astragalosides have the effects of scavenging reactive oxygen species and alleviating oxidative damage in hypoxic myocardium

Fluorescence inverted microscope and laser confocal microscope were used to observe the intracellular distribution of AST markers. It was found that there was diffuse green fluorescence in the cytoplasm of cardiomyocytes, uneven distribution, and no fluorescence distribution in the nucleus. It is indicated that AST-BSA-FITC has entered cells, mainly distributed in the cytoplasm, and there are relatively concentrated areas in the cytoplasm. Under the transmission electron microscope, it was found that the ultrastructure of the cells was intact, the dark brown large particles with high electron density were distributed on the mitochondria, and the particle diameter was slightly larger than the mitochondrial crista gap diameter, but the mitochondrial crista structure was intact, without distortion and degeneration. Therefore, it was judged that it did not enter the mitochondrial cavity, but attached to the mitochondrial membrane, and no distribution of the particles was observed in other organelles. No high electron density particle distribution was observed in the negative control cells.

The ability of AST to scavenge $OH^-$, $O2^-$ in vitro found that AST had a significant clearance of $OH^-$ in the concentration range of 12.5–100 mg/L, and enhanced with increasing dose, and AST had no significant clearance of $O^{2-}$ in the concentration range of 12.5–100 mg/L.

The ability of AST to scavenge reactive oxygen species in cells was tested, and it showed that the green fluorescence intensity in the picture was proportional to the ROS concentration after 12 h hypoxia, and the fluorescence intensity in the hypoxia group was significantly higher than that in the normal group; and the fluorescence intensity was significantly decreased after adding astragaloside (AST, 25 mg/L) compared with that in the hypoxia group. After the action of SOD blocker sodium diethyldithiocarbamate (DDC, 25 μM), the fluorescence intensity increased compared with the simple hypoxia group. After treatment with astragaloside, the fluorescence intensity did not change significantly, and the effect of scavenging intracellular ROS basically disappeared.

Detection of SOD mRNA and protein expression in cardiomyocytes showed that compared with the normal group, the expression of SOD mRNA was significantly increased after hypoxia; the expression of SOD mRNA was increased after AST treatment under normoxia and hypoxia. The change trend of hypoxia 12 h and hypoxia 3 h was consistent. Compared with the normal group, the expression of SOD protein was significantly increased after 12 h hypoxia. The expression of SOD protein was higher after AST treatment under normoxia and hypoxia than before.

These results suggest that after entering the cells, astragaloside may increase SOD mRNA expression and SOD protein expression through mitochondrial membrane-related receptors, increase SOD activity, and accelerate intracellular $O^{2-}$ disproportionation into $OH^-$. At the same time, astragaloside molecules entering the cytoplasm can react with the generated $OH^-$ to scavenge part of $OH^-$, thereby reducing the accumulation of intracellular ROS; reducing the oxidative damage of cell membranes, proteins, nucleic acids, etc.; stabilizing and improving the activities of endogenous antioxidant enzyme such as SOD; enhancing the ability of cells to scavenge oxygen free radicals; strengthening endogenous protective effect; and decreasing cell damage and apoptosis.

Antioxidant PDTC: Animal experiments have shown that the antioxidant PDTC can reduce the aggregation of PMN in myocardial tissue, inhibit the increase of NF-κB activity in myocardial cells in the early stage of burn, inhibit the expression of TNF-α mRNA and IL-8 mRNA in myocardial tissue of burned rats, reduce the content of TNF-α and IL-8 in myocardial tissue and plasma, and reduce MDA content and MPO activity in myocardial tissue after burn, significantly improving left ventricular systolic and diastolic function.

#### 7.5.4.6 Mitochondrial Damage Reduction or Regulation of Ion Channels

(a) $K^+$-ATP opener and $Ca^{2+}$ transport blocker: It was found that in 30% TBSA III burned rats, the mitochondrial $K^+$ influx rate was significantly accelerated, the mitochondrial respiratory control rate (RCR) and III state respiratory rate (ST3) significantly improved. Furthermore, $[Ca^{2+}]$m, MDA content and serum CK, LDH levels were significantly reduced in the treatment group of mitochondrial $K^+$-ATP opener diazoxide (dose 10 mg/kg), suggesting that $K^+$-ATP channel opener diazoxide can alleviate cardiomyocyte damage in the early stage of severe burns, and its mechanism is related to the opening of mitochondrial $K^+$ channels, inhibiting mitochondrial $Ca^{2+}$ overload and reducing free radical production. Ruthenium red, a $Ca^{2+}$ transport blocker, also reduces cardiomyocyte and mitochondrial damage in the early stage of severe burns. The mechanism of these change is related to the opening of mitochondrial $K^+$ channels, leading to mitochondrial $Ca^{2+}$ overload and free radical production. The results showed that for 30% TBSA III degree burned rats, ruthenium red treatment group had a significant decrease in the myocardial $[Ca^{2+}]$ m, a significant increase in mitochondrial RCR, ST3, and ATP, and a significant decrease in serum CK, LDH. This result indicates that ruthenium red can effectively inhibit the uptake of $Ca^{2+}$, reduce mitochondrial $Ca^{2+}$ overload, improve myocardial mitochondrial respiratory function, and alleviate myocardial damage after severe burns.

(b) Regulation of adenosine A1 receptor agonists [54]: The opening of mitochondrial permeability transition pore (MPTP) is a key link leading to necrosis and apoptosis of hypoxic cardiomyocytes. Immunofluorescence staining showed that in normal cardiomyocytes, protein kinase C (PKC) was distributed in the cytoplasm, with weak fluorescence intensity and low expression, and no expression was observed in the nucleus and cell membrane. There was no significant change in the fluorescence intensity and distribution of PKC in hypoxic cardiomyocytes. The fluorescence intensity of PKC in the hypoxia + CCPA (adenosine A1 receptor agonist) group and the hypoxia + CCPA +5-HD (mitoKATP blocker) group was significantly increased, but no significant fluorescence intensity changes were observed in the nucleus and cell membrane.

Western blot showed that the expression of PKC in normal cardiomyocytes was low, mainly distributed in the cytoplasm, and a small amount was expressed on the membrane. The expression of total protein and PKC in cytoplasm and membrane protein of hypoxia cardiomyocytes did not change significantly, which showed that the absorbance values of corresponding protein bands were not significantly different from that of normal group.

However, in hypoxia + CCPA group and hypoxia + CCPA + 5-HD group, the total protein and PKC content in membrane protein increased significantly, but the PKC content in the cytoplasmic protein did not change.

Using the co-incubation method of calcein-AM and cobalt chloride ($CoCl_2$) to observe the changes of mitochondrial permeability transition pore (MPTP) under different treatment factors by laser confocal microscopy, it was found that the fluorescence of mitochondria in normal cardiomyocytes was strong and granular. In the hypoxia group, hypoxia + CCPA + 5-HD group, and hypoxia + CCPA + CHE group, there was obvious MPTP opening, which showed that the mitochondrial fluorescence intensity was significantly weakened compared with normal group. The mitochondrial fluorescence intensity in hypoxia + CCPA group was not significantly different from that in normal group. After hypoxia for 6 h, the mitochondrial membrane potential of hypoxia group, hypoxia + CCPA + 5-HD group, and hypoxia + CCPA + CHE group was significantly lower than that of the normal group, showing a decrease in red fluorescence intensity, while the fluorescence intensity of mitochondria in the hypoxia + CCPA group was not significantly different from that of the normal group.

Normal cardiomyocytes have less reactive oxygen species and show weak green fluorescence. After 6-h hypoxia, the green fluorescence and reactive oxygen species increased significantly in hypoxia group, hypoxia + CCPA + 5-HD group, and hypoxia + CCPA + CHE group, while the reactive oxygen species did not change significantly in hypoxia + CCPA group compared with the normal group. After 6-h hypoxia, the viability of cardiomyocytes in hypoxia group, hypoxia + CCPA + 5-HD group, and hypoxia + CCPA + CHE group was significantly lower than that in the normal group, while the cell viability in hypoxia + CCPA group was not significantly decreased compared with the normal group.

These findings suggest that the adenosine A1 receptor agonist CCPA can significantly reduce the opening of MPTP in hypoxic cardiomyocytes and maintain cell viability; both PKC and mitoKATP-specific blockers can block the effect of CCPA on reducing the opening of MPTP in hypoxic cardiomyocytes, suggesting that CCPA can regulate the opening of MPTP through the PKC and mitoKATP pathways. PKC plays an important role in cell signaling, apoptosis regulation, and myocardial protection. The adenosine A1 receptor activates PKC by coupling with the G protein receptor on the membrane, causing a series of intracellular signaling, reducing cell apoptosis and necrosis. Studies have shown that in hypoxic cardiomyocytes, the use of the adenosine A1 receptor agonist CCPA not only increased the total amount of PKC but also increased the expression of PKC in the membrane protein, but the expression of PKC on the cell membrane was not found to be increased. Therefore, under hypoxic conditions, the effect of CCPA on PKC may be to increase the expression of PKC in certain organelles (such as mitochondria) rather than the cell membrane, thereby activating it and exerting cytoprotective effects. mitoKATP, a channel complex composed of various proteins, is present in mitochondria and is considered the key link and terminal effector of IPC to play a protective effect. The mitoKATP blocker 5-HD did not block the effect of CCPA on PKC expression in hypoxic cardiomyocytes, suggesting that PKC is upstream of mitoKATP in the CCPA signaling pathway of hypoxic cardiomyocytes. The use of CCPA inhibits hypoxia-induced mitochondrial membrane potential reduction and increases in reactive oxygen species concentration, while mitoKATP blockers counteract this effect of CCPA. Therefore, CCPA may maintain mitochondrial membrane potential and reduce reactive oxygen species production by promoting mitoKATP opening, thereby reducing MPTP opening in hypoxic cardiomyocytes.

(c) Glycine receptor pathway: Our results indicate that glycine has significant protective effects on cultured ischemic-hypoxic cardiomyocytes and burned rat myocardial tissues, which can reduce the release of CK and LDH from ischemic-hypoxic cardiomyocytes, significantly improve the viability of ischemic-hypoxic cardiomyocytes (CCK-8), decrease the positive rate of PI staining in cardiomyocytes, and increase the ATP content. The glycine receptor (G1yR) is a ligand-gated ion channel, and we are the first to discover the presence of the $\alpha 1$ subunit of the glycine receptor in cardiomyocytes. L-type calcium channel exists on the cell membrane, and the change of membrane potential can affect the opening and closing of L-type calcium channel. When the cell membrane potential is depolarized, the opening of L-type calcium channel increases. Glycine can significantly reduce the calcium overload of cardiomyocytes after hypoxia for 6 h. After adding anti-GlyR$\alpha 1$ to block the $\alpha 1$ subunit of glycine receptor, the calcium overload of hypoxic cardiomyocytes is obviously aggravated; after adding the glycine receptor agonist taurine, the calcium overload is obviously alleviated. It is proved from different sides that glycine exerts its protective effect through its receptor $\alpha 1$ subunit. These results suggest that after hypoxia, depolarization of myocardial cell membrane leads to an increase in cell membrane voltage-dependent calcium channel opening, increasing calcium influx and myocardial cell damage; while after glycine binds to its receptor, the cardiomyocyte membrane depolarization is significantly alleviated, thereby reducing the opening of voltage-dependent calcium channels in the cell membrane, and significantly reducing the calcium ion influx, thus exerting its protective effect.

#### 7.5.4.7 Regulate Endogenous Protection Mechanisms

After severe burns, the body also initiates an anti-injury, that is, cell protection mechanism while producing damage effects. Cytoprotection refers to the ability of certain substances secreted by cells or some of their structures to prevent or reduce the harmful substances from damaging cells and leading to necrosis. The current research believes that all the ability to prevent or significantly reduce the damage and lethality of harmful substances to the body cells belongs to cytoprotection, and the substances with cytoprotective effects are collectively referred to as cytoprotective factors. The studies have found that endogenous protective substances play an important role in the body's resistance to severe traumatic secondary damage, which can mobilize the intrinsic protective mechanisms of cells, regulate the homeostasis balance of cells, and become a new strategy to prevent or reduce cell damage.

Hypoxia-inducible factor-1 (HIF-1), heat-shock protein (HSP), and some protective signaling pathways are the endogenous protection mechanisms that have been studied more. Studies suggest that upregulation of endogenous protective molecules is an important mechanism for the body to resist myocardial damage in the early stage of burns. Animal experiments showed that after 40% III degree burn in rats, myocardial HIF-1α mRNA levels and protein increased, left ventricle was significantly higher than the right ventricle, and HIF-1α was mainly expressed in the nucleus. In vitro studies have shown that after cultured cardiomyocytes are hypoxic, HIF-1α undergoes nuclear translocation and its protein expression increases, and glycolytic enzyme activity increases. Within 12 h of hypoxia, ATP and energy of cardiomyocytes can still be maintained at a certain level, so that cells have a basic energy supply without irreversible damage. In order to clarify the endogenous protective effect of HIF-1α on myocardial damage after burn, the expression structure of hypoxia-inducible factor-1α siRNA U6 promoter was constructed, and the expression of HIF-1α was downregulated by iRNA interference technique to observe the effect of HIF-1α expression on myocardial energy metabolism and myocardial damage after inhibition of HIF-1α expression. It was found that the RNAi group can effectively inhibit the expression of HIF-1α, reduce the activity of glycolytic enzyme, and make the cell ATP and energy level sustained, rapid decline, and cause irreversible damage to cells in advance, indicating that the protective effect of HIF-1α on hypoxic cardiomyocytes is to delay the time that cells enter irreversible damage.

The study also found that the expression of HSP70 protein in myocardial tissue increased significantly at 3 h after 30% TBSA III scald in rats and decreased slightly at 6 h and 12 h after injury, and then the expression increased gradually, reaching a peak again 48 h after burn. Pretreatment with sodium arsenite (SA) could induce a significant increase in HSP70 protein expression and a significant decrease in serum cTnI levels in rat myocardium after burn injury. These results suggest that preinduced high expression of HSP70 can effectively alleviate myocardial damage in the early stage of severe burns, and the increased expression of HSP70 in the myocardium after burn is an important mechanism of anti-injury.

The protective effect of PI3K/Akt signaling pathway on cardiomyocytes in the early stage of burns is mainly to inhibit cardiomyocyte apoptosis [55]. PI3K is an important signal transduction molecule in the cell. It can be divided into three types according to the structural characteristics of the P110 subunit of PI3K and the substrate molecules. The most widely studied type I PI3K can be activated by cell surface receptors.

In mammalian cells, type I PI3K is further divided into two subtypes, IA and IB, which transmit signals from tyrosine kinase-linked receptors and G-protein-linked receptors, respectively. Type IA PI3K is a dimeric protein composed of catalytic subunit P110 and regulatory subunit P85. PI3K is activated in two ways, one by interacting with growth factor receptors or a connexins with phosphorylated tyrosine residues, causing dimeric conformational changes and thus activated; the other by direct binding of Ras and P110 leading to the activation of PI3K. The result of PI3K activation is the production of the second messenger PIP3 on the plasma membrane. PIP3 binds to Akt, a signaling protein that contains a PH domain, which promotes phosphorylation of Akt protein kinase. Activated Akt further activates or inhibits its downstream target protein through phosphorylation, thereby regulating cell proliferation, differentiation, glucose metabolism, and migration. Whether the PI3K/Akt signaling pathway is activated in myocardium after burn, whether PI3K/Akt signaling can affect the sensitivity of cardiomyocytes to ischemia-hypoxia injury, and the effect and mechanism of PI3K/Akt signaling pathway on cardiomyocyte apoptosis in the early stage of burn are unclear. It is speculated that the PI3K/Akt signaling pathway is activated at the same time as cardiomyocytes undergo ischemia-hypoxia injury in the early stage of burn and may play an antiapoptotic role by regulating calcium concentration, mitochondrial membrane stability, and apoptosis gene expression. PI3K/Akt/HIF-1α may be an important molecular mechanism of this antiapoptotic effect.

The results showed that the expression of PI3K protein increased significantly at 1 h after 30% TBSA III scald in rats, reached a peak at 3 h, and did not decrease to normal level until 24 h after injury. As a direct target protein downstream of PI3K, Akt kinase phosphorylation is a hallmark of

PI3K/Akt pathway activation. The phosphorylation level of Akt increased significantly at 1 h after burn, reached a peak at 3 h, and returned to normal at 24 h after burn, and the change trend was basically consistent with PI3K. The results of RT-PCR showed that there was no significant change in PI3K mRNA in the early stage of severe burns, and the mRNA increased significantly at 6 h after injury, which was later than the activation of PI3K/Akt pathway protein, suggesting that the PI3K gene transcriptional activity is increased by the activation of PI3K/Akt pathway, which may be a feedback regulation for the level of protein activation.

Activation of the PI3K/Akt signaling pathway after burns can inhibit ischemia-hypoxia cardiomyocyte apoptosis. The study found that after the myocardial cells were stimulated by ischemia and hypoxia in the early stage of severe burns, the cell viability decreased gradually. The viability of cardiomyocytes decreased to 87% after 6 h of ischemia and hypoxia and to 22% of normal after 24 h. The activity of LDH in cardiomyocyte culture medium also increased gradually. It indicates that ischemia and hypoxia can cause destruction of cardiomyocyte membrane and decrease cardiomyocyte viability. After inhibiting the activation of PI3K/Akt with the specific inhibitor LY294002 (50 μM), the cell viability of cardiomyocytes treated with ischemia-hypoxia decreased more significantly than that of the ischemia-hypoxia group alone at each time point, and the LDH activity in the cell culture medium was significantly higher than that in the ischemia-hypoxia group at the same time point. This suggests that PI3K/Akt can alleviate cardiomyocyte membrane damage caused by ischemia and hypoxia, maintain cardiomyocyte activity, and have a protective effect on ischemia-hypoxia cardiomyocytes. Blocking this pathway will aggravate myocardial ischemia-hypoxia damage. LDH is present in the cytoplasm of cardiomyocytes and only leaks out of the cytoplasm when cell membrane permeability increases or integrity is disrupted. Therefore, the content of LDH in the culture supernatant can reflect the degree of cell membrane damage. Previous studies have shown that only when cells undergo significant apoptosis or necrosis, the permeability of cell membrane will increase or even disintegrate, and apoptosis itself is an important factor that reduces cell viability. This suggests that the PI3K/Akt signaling pathway may play an antiapoptotic role in maintaining cell membrane stability and cell viability.

To verify whether PI3K/Akt has antiapoptotic effects, PI3K/Akt inhibitor LY294002 and activator IGF-1 were further used to positively and negatively regulate the activation of this pathway, in order to confirm the effects of PI3K/Akt on apoptosis of hypoxic and ischemic cardiomyocytes. The results of TUNEL semiquantitative analysis showed that the apoptotic rate increased significantly after 6 h of ischemia-hypoxia treatment. When LY294002 (50 μM) was used to specifically block the PI3K/Akt pathway, the apoptotic rate of cardiomyocytes increased significantly after 6 h of ischemia-hypoxia treatment compared with the control group. However, after pretreatment with IGF-1 (200 ng/mL) and 6 h of ischemia-hypoxia, the apoptotic rate of cardiomyocytes was significantly lower than that of ischemia-hypoxia group. Quantitative analysis of apoptosis by ELISA also showed that the number of apoptotic cells was significantly increased at 1 h, 3 h, 6 h, and 12 h after myocardial ischemia and hypoxia compared with that before stimulation. After treatment with LY294002 and ischemia and hypoxia, the number of cardiomyocyte apoptosis at each time point was significantly higher than that of the hypoxic group. However, after IGF-1 treatment and the ischemic and hypoxic treatment, the number of cardiomyocyte apoptosis was significantly decreased at each time point. These results fully demonstrate that PI3K/Akt has a clear antiapoptotic effect on ischemia-hypoxia cardiomyocytes. Blocking or activating this pathway can aggravate or attenuate cardiomyocyte apoptosis induced by ischemia-hypoxia stimulation. It is indicated that the activation of PI3K/Akt in the early stage of burn is an important molecular basis for endogenous protective responses of cardiomyocytes. At the same time, the application of IGF-1, a selective activator of PI3K/Akt, may become a new means to prevent myocardial apoptosis induced by ischemia and hypoxia in the early stage of burns.

Caspase-3 is an important apoptotic caspase that can be activated by multiple apoptotic pathways, such as the caspase pathway and the mitochondrial pathway, which plays an important role in the apoptosis of many cells. The main substrate for caspase-3 is poly (ADP-ribose) polymerase (PARP), which is involved in DNA repair and gene integrity monitoring. At the initiation of apoptosis, PARP of 116 ku was cleaved into 31 ku and 85 ku two fragments by caspase-3 between Asp216-Gly217, which separated the two zinc finger structures bound to DNA in PARP from the catalytic region at the carboxyl end and could not function properly. As a result, the activity of $Ca^{2+}/Mg^{2+}$-dependent endonuclease affected by the negative regulation of PARP was increased, and DNA between nucleosomes was cleaved, causing apoptosis. This cleavage process can be inhibited by the specific inhibitor of caspase-3, Ac-DEVD-CHO, but not by CrmA. Caspase-3 also cleaves U1-70K, DNA-PK, PKCd, and PKCq. Both PKCd and PKCq belong to the novel PKC (nPKC). When cleaved by caspase-3, the regulatory region can be excised and become active forms of PKC. In addition, experiments have shown that overexpression of PKCd and PKCq can cause cell apoptosis, indicating that they are involved in the induction of apoptosis. It can be seen that once caspase-3 is activated, apoptosis will be inevitable, so caspase-3 activation is also known as a landmark biochemical event of apoptosis. The results of this experiment showed that the activity of caspase-3 in cardiomyocytes was low before ischemia-hypoxia stimulation. After 1-h ischemia and hypoxia, the caspase-3 activity of cardiomyocytes was not significantly different from that of the normal group, and then increased gradually; the activity of caspase-3 in cardiomyocytes increased significantly after 3 h; and at 12 h after hypoxia, the caspase-3 activity of cardiomyocytes increased to 2.6 times of the normal group. After treatment with LY294002, a PI3K/Akt-specific inhibitor, and ischemia and hypoxia for 3 h, it was found that caspase-3 was further increased in cardiomyocytes and was significantly higher than that in the hypoxia group. At preapplication of IGF-1 and ischemia and hypoxia for 1 h and 3 h, caspase-3 activity was not significantly different from that in the normal group; at 6 h and 12 h, the caspase-3 activity of cardiomyocytes increased gradually, but was significantly lower than that in the hypoxia group at the same time point. The results suggest that PI3K/Akt may play an antiapoptotic role by inhibiting the activation of caspase-3, blocking the activation of PI3K/Akt, thereby increasing the activation of caspase-3, and further activating subsequent apoptosis.

It is well known that mitochondria play a pivotal role in the process of apoptosis. A variety of apoptotic stimulating factors can induce apoptosis in different cells. The decrease of mitochondrial transmembrane potential $\Delta\Psi$mt is considered the earliest event in the process of apoptosis cascade, which often occurs before the appearance of nuclear apoptotic features (chromatin condensation, DNA fragmentation) and is a characteristic manifestation of mitochondrial permeability transition pores (MPTP) opening. The latter directly leads to the release of cytochrome C from the mitochondria into the cytoplasm, triggering downstream cascades and causing apoptosis. This experiment further clarified the upstream mechanism of PI3K/Akt regulating caspase-3 activity by observing changes of mitochondrial transmembrane potential $\Delta\Psi$mt. TMRE is a cationic lipophilic fluorescent dye with reduced fluorescence intensity, reflecting a decrease in the number of mitochondria and/or a decrease or loss of $\Delta\Psi$mt. The change of $\Delta\Psi$mt can be used as an early feature of apoptosis and a marker of irreversible apoptosis. The results of this experiment showed that after 6-h ischemia and hypoxia treatment, the intracellular fluorescence intensity decreased to 63% of the control group; after 12 h, the intracellular fluorescence intensity decreased more significantly, only 36% of the normal group. After intervention with LY294002, a PI3K-specific inhibitor, and ischemia and hypoxia for 6 h and 12 h, cardiomyocyte fluorescence intensity was significantly lower than that in the ischemia-hypoxia group at the same time. After intervention with IGF-1, a PI3K-specific activator, and ischemia and hypoxia for 6 h, the fluorescence intensity of cardiomyocytes was higher than that in the hypoxia group. It is suggested that PI3K/Akt can stabilize the mitochondrial membrane stability of ischemic and hypoxic cardiomyocytes, prevent the increase of membrane permeability caused by MPTP opening, lead to the release of cytochrome C to the cytoplasm, and initiate the downstream caspase apoptosis reaction.

Calcium overload is a common factor of myocardial ischemia and hypoxia injury, and also an important factor leading to cell apoptosis. Under normal conditions, the maintenance of intracellular $Ca^{2+}$ concentration depends on ATPase-dependent calcium pump, $Na^+/Ca^{2+}$ exchange and regulation of normal $Ca^{2+}$ channels. Hypoxia leads to inhibition of cellular oxidative phosphorylation, rapid decrease of intracellular ATP content, and dysfunction of sodium-potassium pump, and elevated intracellular $Na^+$ also causes cell membrane depolarization to cause transient voltage-dependent $Ca^{2+}$ channel opening, $Ca^{2+}$ influx, and mitochondrial dysfunction causes $Ca^{2+}$ release from mitochondrial storage, resulting in intracellular $Ca^{2+}$ overload. Increased intracellular $Ca^{2+}$ activates $Ca^{2+}$-dependent proteases, endonucleases, and phospholipases to initiate apoptosis-related pathways. Studies have also shown that calcium overload is a predisposing factor for mitochondrial dysfunction and activates phospholipases to cause membrane structural damage. In this study, the $Ca^{2+}$-specific fluorescent dye Fluo-3 was used to measure the change of $[Ca^{2+}]$i content in cells, and the effect of PI3K/Akt on intracellular calcium overload was observed. The results showed that the intracellular fluorescence intensity increased significantly after ischemia-hypoxia treatment for 6 h. After intervention with PI3K-specific inhibitor LY294002, the fluorescence intensity of cardiomyocytes increased more significantly after 6-h ischemia and hypoxia. After intervention with IGF-1, the fluorescence intensity of cardiomyocytes was significantly lower than that of the hypoxic group after 6 h of ischemia and hypoxia. This indicates that activation of PI3K/Akt can attenuate $Ca^{2+}$ overload in cardiomyocytes under ischemia-hypoxia conditions, thereby inhibiting the activation of phospholipase and aggravating membrane damage. This is consistent with the results of the LDH activity test mentioned earlier. At the same time, the reduction of calcium overload can also reduce the burden of mitochondria, maintain mitochondrial membrane stability, and inhibit apoptosis. Previous studies have found that the PI3K P110$\gamma$ subunit promotes the opening of voltage-dependent calcium channels on the cell membrane of myocytes or neurons, leading to the influx of calcium ions, causing excitation-contraction coupling. Under the stimulation of ischemia and hypoxia, intracellular ATP production is insufficient, and ion pump function is lost, causing calcium ion aggregation, and mitochondria and sarcoplasmic reticulum also have dysfunction due to ATP deficiency, resulting in reduced calcium uptake and even membrane structure damage, increased calcium permeability, and aggravated intracellular calcium overload. In this experiment, the intracellular calcium concentration was measured after 6 h of ischemia and hypoxia in cardiomyocytes. At this time, the action of calcium ion influx mediated by PI3K was not obvious, and calcium overload caused by damage of mitochondria and sarcoplasmic reticulum may dominate.

These above results suggest that under ischemia and hypoxia, the PI3K/Akt signaling pathway may play an endogenous protective role in antagonizing apoptosis and maintaining cell viability by attenuating intracellular calcium overload, maintaining membrane and mitochondrial membrane stability, and inhibiting caspase apoptotic cascade represented by caspase-3 activation.

Regarding the mechanism of PI3K/Akt signaling pathway inhibiting apoptosis of myocardial cells in hypoxia-ischemia, it is speculated that under ischemic and hypoxic conditions, PI3K/Akt may further regulate the transcriptional activity of apoptosis-related genes and inhibit apoptosis of myocardial cells in ischemia and hypoxia by regulating the expression of "hypoxia core regulatory molecule" HIF-1α. The results showed that the expression of HIF-1α mRNA in cardiomyocytes was significantly lower than that in the normal group after preapplication of LY294002 and ischemia and hypoxia for 3 h. At the protein level, the expression of HIF-1α was significantly increased after 3 h of ischemia and hypoxia. After pretreatment with PI3K-specific inhibitor LY294002 or mTOR inhibitor rapamycin, HIF-1α protein level was significantly lower than that of ischemia and hypoxia group after 3 h of ischemia and hypoxia (Table 7–82). It is suggested that the activation of PI3K/Akt signaling pathway in ischemic and hypoxic cardiomyocytes can upregulate the transcriptional activity of HIF-1α mRNA, and phosphorylation of PI3K/Akt and mTOR can upregulate the expression of HIF-1α at the protein level. It has also been suggested that the regulation of HIF-1α in hypoxia occurs mainly at the protein level rather than at the transcription level, presumably related to cell species and stimulating conditions. It is worth noting that the ischemia-hypoxia stimulation in the experiment cannot change the transcriptional activity of HIF-1α mRNA in cardiomyocytes, and the activation of PI3K/Akt promotes the enhanced transcriptional activity of HIF-1α mRNA, which may be associated with certain nuclear transcription factor pathways that are not affected by ischemia and hypoxia, and this need further in-depth study. In order to explore the intermediate pathway of PI3K/Akt regulating HIF-1α protein expression in ischemia-anoxia cardiomyocytes, PI3K/Akt-specific inhibitor LY294002 and mTOR inhibitor rapamycin were used to observe the expression changes of p70S6K, p-mTOR, and p-Akt in cardiomyocytes after 3 h of ischemia and hypoxia. The results suggest that ischemia-hypoxia stimulation may regulate the protein expression of HIF-1α through the PI3K/Akt/mTOR/p70S6K pathway. Upregulation of HIF-1α protein expression can indirectly regulate the expression of apoptotic genes p53, Bcl-2, and Bax, and further reduce intracellular calcium overload and mitochondrial damage, thus playing an endogenous protective role against apoptosis.

The results showed that Bcl-2 mRNA increased gradually, while Bax mRNA decreased, p53 mRNA expression increased gradually, and c-Myc mRNA gradually increased after 1 h and 3 h of ischemia and hypoxia in cardiomyocytes. After preapplication of LY294002, the expression of Bcl-2 mRNA was significantly lower than that of ischemia-hypoxia group, the expression of Bax mRNA was significantly higher than that of ischemia-hypoxia group, the expression of p53 mRNA was more significantly increased than that of ischemia-hypoxia group, and the expression of c-Myc mRNA was significantly lower than that of the normal group after 1 h and 3 h of ischemia and hypoxia. The results suggest that under ischemia and hypoxia in cardiomyocytes, the activated PI3K/Akt signaling pathway can increase the ratio of Bcl-2/Bax and downregulate the expression of wild-type proapoptotic gene p53 by regulating the expression of Bcl-2 and Bax in order to reduce apoptosis and increase cell survival. In addition, upregulation of c-Myc expression after PI3K/Akt activation may not be related to its antiapoptotic mechanism. Since PI3K/Akt promotes cell proliferation and growth, it is considered that upregulation of c-Myc expression by this pathway may be related to alteration of cell cycle.

#### 7.5.4.8 NO Donor

We added three different concentrations of NO donor S-nitrosoglutathione (GSNO) into the cardiomyocyte culture medium to provide the cells with three stable concentrations of NO at low, medium, and high levels for a certain period of time. The results showed that the medium concentration of NO (7.5 μM) could enhance the anti-injury ability of hypoxic cardiomyocytes, and its mechanism may be to strengthen the endogenous protective mechanism of cardiomyocytes against hypoxia by increasing the level of HIF-1α protein in cardiomyocytes; high and low concentration of NO can promote the damage effect of hypoxic cardiomyocytes. The increase of HIF-1α protein level in hypoxic cardiomyocytes induced by moderate NO may be mainly due to the activation of PI3K signaling pathway. The mitochondrial respiratory chain may not be the main pathway for the increase of HIF-1α protein level. NO also has a protective effect on myocardial tissue in severely scalded rats. The mechanism may be that NO production promotes the increased expression of HIF-1α in the myocardial cells of scalded rats, thereby increasing the hypoxia tolerance of tissues. Inhibition of NO production can aggravate myocardial cell damage, and administration of L-arginine, a precursor of NO synthesis, can significantly improve cardiac function after burns.

#### 7.5.4.9 "Volume Replacement Plus Cardiac Dynamic Support" Resuscitation Regimen [56]

Rapid myocardial damage and weakened cardiac function after severe burns can not only cause cardiac insufficiency but also induce or aggravate shock, which is one of the important causes of shock/ischemia and hypoxia in the early stage of burns, so an effective shock recovery plan should not only consider the role of blood volume reduction caused by increased capillary permeability in shock development but also consider the role of impaired cardiac motility in burn shock. Based on the theory of "shock heart," we have established a new program of "Volume replacement plus cardiac dynamic support" shock recovery, namely, appropriate fluid replacement (volume replacement) combined with the prevention of cardiac damage (cardiac dynamic support), which not only contributes to effective recovery of severe burn shock but can also reduce visceral complications caused by insufficient or excessive fluid replacement. Applying the fluid replacement formula (immediate or delayed resuscitation formula) of the Army Military Medical University can meet the needs of "Volume replacement." "Cardiac dynamic support" is mainly aimed at the mechanism of early myocardial damage, such as using small doses of ACEI to reduce myocardial ischemia and using L-carnitine, fructose sodium diphosphate, and alprostadil injection to improve energy metabolism (fatty acids, glucose), cardiomyocyte protection, and antioxidant damage. The specific methods are as follows: while rapidly replenishing the fluid, give 5% glucose injection 100 mL + enalaprilat injection 1.25 mg, intravenous input once/day; 5% glucose injection 100 mL + fructose sodium diphosphate injection 10 g, intravenous input 2 times/day; and 5% glucose injection 100 mL + alprostadil injection 10 μg, intravenous input 2 times/day, 3 consecutive days. Under the major special support of the National Health Commission of the People's Republic of China, 11 famous burn treatment institutions nationwide were organized to conduct multicenter clinical research.

From the analysis of general clinical conditions, there were no significant differences in age, gender, injury factors, total burn area and III degree area, admission time after injury, vital signs, and composite moderate and severe inhalation injuries of burn patients among the three groups. The balance between the groups was good, and the results were comparable.

#### 7.5.4.10 Circulating Capacity and Blood Oxygenation-Related Indicators

(a) Fluid replacement volume and urine volume: The analysis found that on the basis that there was no difference in the volume of fluid replacement at the first 24 h and the second 24 h, the urine volume in group B and group C was significantly more than that in group A at 24 h and 48 h, and there was a statistically significant difference ($P$ values were 0.048 and 0.022, respectively), but there was no significant difference in urine volume between group B and group C.
(b) Changes of Hb and Hct: At 24 h after injury, the Hb level in group A was significantly higher than that in group B and group C ($P < 0.05$), and there was no significant difference between group B and group C. At 48 h after injury, group A was still higher than group C ($P < 0.05$). However, there was no significant difference between group A and group B, and group B and group C. At 24 h after injury, the Hct level in group A was significantly higher than that in group B and group C ($P < 0.05$), but there was no significant difference between group B and group C. At 48 h after injury, group A was still significantly higher than group C ($P < 0.05$), but there was no significant difference between group A and group B, and group B and group C.
(c) Changes of blood lactate: There were no significant differences in blood lactate between groups A, B, and C at admission; at 24 h and 48 h after injury, blood lactate in group A was significantly higher than that in group B and group C, but there was no significant difference between group B and group C. At 24 h after injury, Hb and Hct in group C were significantly lower than those in group A ($P = 0.029$), suggesting that blood concentration was reduced. However, there was no significant difference between group B and group C. The above results suggest that the circulating capacity of group B and group C is better than that of group A, blood concentration is reduced, tissue perfusion and oxygenation are significantly improved, and blood lactate is significantly reduced. However, there was no significant difference between group B and group C.

#### 7.5.4.11 Organ Damage Indexes

(a) Changes of serum troponin I (cTnI) and CK-MB, indexes of myocardial damage: Analysis of organ damage indexes of burn patients in three groups showed that serum troponin I (cTnI) increased at admission in all three groups, but there was no significant differences: at 12 h, 24 h, 36 h, 48 h, and 72 h after injury, cTnI in group A was significantly higher than that in group B and group C ($P < 0.01$), but there was no significant difference between group B and group C. Serum CK-MB increased in all three groups at admission, but there was no significant difference among the three groups. At 12 h, 24 h, 36 h, 48 h, and 72 h after injury, CK-MB in group A was significantly higher than that in group B and group C ($P < 0.01$), but there was no significant difference between group B and group C.

(b) Relationship between burn area and myocardial damage: This project also found the relationship between burn area and myocardial damage; when the burn area reached 51.5% or more, CK-MB had high specificity and sensitivity; and when the burn area reached 52.5%, cTnI had high specificity and sensitivity. This suggests that the incidence of myocardial damage is greatly increased when the burn area reaches 50%, and more positive measures should be taken to actively prevent myocardial damage.
(c) Changes of serum β2-MG, an index of kidney injury: The levels of serum β2-MG in the three groups were increased at admission, but there was no significant difference; at 12 h, 24 h, 48 h, 72 h after injury, serum β2-MG in group B and group C was significantly higher than that in group A ($P < 0.01$), but there was no significant difference between group B and group C. There were no significant differences in TBA and DAO among the three groups within 72 h after injury.
(d) Analysis of the mortality rate, an index of the ultimate efficacy: The mortality rate of patients in the three groups was analyzed. The mortality rate of the simple volume supplement group was as high as 25%; the mortality rate of the "Volume replacement plus cardiac dynamic support" group was only 10.3%. It can be seen that the cardiac dynamic support can improve the cure rate by 11–14.7%, and the clinical treatment effect is very obvious.

The above results suggest that patients admitted early after severe burns can improve myocardial ischemia by using enalaprilat for mobility support while applying the "volume replacement" formula of Military Medical University, or the combined application of enalaprilat, L-carnitine, fructose sodium diphosphate, and alprostadil can improve tissue and organ ischemia and hypoxia and improve tissue oxygenation and aerobic metabolism, thereby reducing visceral complications and improving the cure rate.

## 7.6 Repair and Regeneration After Brain, Spinal Cord, and Peripheral Nerve Injury

### 7.6.1 Repair and Regeneration After Brain Injury in Adult Mammals

#### 7.6.1.1 Response of Endogenous Neural Stem Cells in Adult Mammalian Brain After Traumatic Injury

In the neurogenic regions of the hippocampus in adult mammals, the subventricular zone (SVZ) and the dentate gyrus (DG) can produce new neurons throughout life [45–47, 57]. Over the past 20 years, scientists have conducted extensive studies on the extent of adult neurogenesis in the SVZ and DG regions, the role of newborn neurons in the normal brain, and the mechanisms of adult neurogenesis. At the same time, the degree and function of adult neurogenesis under pathological conditions were also studied in detail in different experimental animal disease models. Increasing evidence suggests that these endogenous neural stem/progenitor cells play an important role in the regeneration and repair of central nervous system damage or disease [48–51]. This section describes the potential functions of adult neurogenesis in injured brains, and future research strategies aimed at refilling and repairing brain damage with endogenous regenerative capacity.

Traumatic brain injury (TBI) can lead to death and disability, and there is currently no effective treatment in clinical practice. It has long been believed that mature brains cannot be repaired after injury. Recent studies have shown that during the entire life cycle of adult mammals, pluripotent neural stem/progenitor cells (NSC/NPC) are present in specific regions of the brain, producing new neurons and glial cells [48, 52]. Over the past 25 years, a large number of studies have shown that adult hippocampal dentate gyrus (DG) can produce mature neurons and play an important role in hippocampal-dependent learning and memory [53–55]; the subventricular zone (SVZ) can produce new olfactory ensheathing interneurons, which are essential for maintaining the normal operation of the olfactory bulb network and specific olfactory behavior [56, 58]. After TBI, there is increasing evidence that these endogenous NSC/NPC may play a role in regeneration and repair in central nervous system injury, and studies of different types of experimental animal TBI models and human TBI have found that injury improves the response of neurogenesis. In addition, hippocampal neurogenesis caused by TBI is associated with cognitive function recovery after initiation of TBI. These studies show that mature brains have intrinsic potential to restore damaged or destroyed neuronal populations. This suggests the possibility of establishing a therapeutic strategy that exploit this endogenous neurogenesis to regenerate and repair the injured brain.

**Neurogenesis of Normal Mammalian Brain**

In the brains of adult mammals, the endogenous neurogenesis regions are mainly confined to the SVZ region around the ventricles and the DG region of the hippocampus [45, 52]. The neural stem/progenitor cells (NSC/NPC) in the SVZ region produce new neurons and oligodendrocytes [59]. Most of the newborn neurons from the SVZ region migrate along the rostral migratory stream to the olfactory bulb, becoming olfactory bulb interneurons [60], and a small number of newborn neurons migrate to the cortical region. The relevant causes have not been determined, but may be related to repair or cell renewal mechanisms [61]. Similarly, newly generated cells in the DG region migrate laterally to the granule cell layer of the dentate gyrus and exhibit characteristics integrated with dentate gyrus neurons [62]. Most importantly, newly generated granule neurons in the DG region can form synapses and can extend axons to their normal target region, the CA3 region [63].

So far, a number of quantitative studies have been conducted on the degree of cytogenesis in these regions. The results suggest that a large number of new cells are continuously produced in the above regions [52], specifically, approximately 9000 new cells are produced in the dentate gyrus of rat hippocampus per day [64]. Considering that the total number of rat granular cells is 10,000 to two million, the addition of new cells is sufficient to affect the function of the neural network [65]. A recent study found that almost all of the deep granular cells and more than half of the upper cells of the olfactory bulb were replaced by newborn neurons within 12 months [65]. The same study reported that granule cells in the dentate gyrus accounted for 10% of adult newborn neurons in the hippocampus [65]. However, studies also found that in the brains of normal adult rodents, approximately half of the new neurons generated in the DG region and olfactory-related neurons generated in the SVZ region can only exist for 2 weeks or less. This time period is long enough to support the action of glial cells, the formation of neurons, and integration into existing networks, a process that typically takes 10–14 days [66]. However, it must be noted that most of the surviving neurons are mature neurons and can survive for months to years. Scholars strongly support the theory of neural network integration. In addition, the severe loss of new neurons may be a repetition of the network pruning process in early mammalian development. Whether the transient limited life cycle of newborn neurons originates from network pruning or specific cellular roles has not been determined.

With the discovery of persistent neuroneogenesis in the adult mammalian brain, the physiological role and importance of this adult neurogenesis, particularly the relationship between adult hippocampal neurogenesis and learning and memory functions, has been extensively studied. Studies have shown that growing in a rich environment, physical exercise or growth factor therapy can improve hippocampal neurogenesis and improve cognitive ability [67]. In addition, studies using different types of methods to inhibit adult neurogenesis have further confirmed the causal relationship between neurogenesis and hippocampal function. For example, when studying the effects of brain irradiation on adult rodent neurogenesis, the results of studies of systemic or local administration of antimitotic agents or hereditary elimination of progenitor cells to eliminate adult neurogenesis suggest that the generation of adult hippocampal dentate gyrus neurons plays an important role in hippocampal-dependent learning and memory tasks. These studies include tracking blinking and conditional fear [68], formation of contextual fear memory [65], long-term retention of spatial memory in water maze tasks [69], target recognition tasks [69], and active position avoidance tasks [67]. In addition, targeted deletion of adult newborn dentate gyrus neurons in the mature stage can induce retrograde memory impairment in experiments such as contextual fear memory, water maze, and visual memory discrimination. Although there are some inconsistencies and even some contradictions in the results of the study due to differences in methods of gene knockout neurogenesis or behavioral detection methods among the above research methods, more and more data provide convincing evidence that adult hippocampal neurogenesis is directly related to many aspects of hippocampal-dependent learning and memory function.

The role of neurogenesis in the SVZ region of the normal brain is unclear, compared with hippocampal neurogenesis. Newborn neurons from the SVZ region migrate to the olfactory bulb and differentiate into interneurons, with about 5% becoming peribulbar cells of the olfactory bulb [70]. The newly generated olfactory ensheathing inhibitory interneurons integrate into the olfactory loop and participate in some but not all olfactory functions. Using a research method similar to inhibiting hippocampal neurogenesis to inhibit olfactory neurogenesis, it turns out that adult newborn neurons in the olfactory bulb participate in olfactory discrimination, acquisition of olfactory perceptual learning and new odor-related behaviors, unique olfactory responses, short-term olfactory memory function, and flexible olfactory association learning and memory functions [71].

In the SVZ and DG regions, the fate of cell proliferation and maturation is regulated by multiple physical and chemical signals. For example, biochemical factors such as serotonin, glucocorticoids, ovarian steroids, and growth factors rigorously regulate cell proliferative responses, suggesting that cell proliferation in these regions is of physiological importance [72]. In addition, physical stimuli such as exercise, a rich environment, or stress can alter the proliferative capacity of cells. For example, physical exercise or abundant environmental stimuli can increase cell proliferation and neurogenesis in the SVZ and DG regions, whereas stress reduces this cellular response. However, the function of these new cells is manifested by the number of new cells, survival, differentiation, and integration with existing neural circuits [50].

### TBI-Induced Neurogenesis

Scientists have shown that TBI including fluid percussion injury (FPI) [73], controllable cortical crush injury (CCI) [74], closed head weight drop injury [75], and accelerated percussion injury [76] can significantly increase cell proliferation in the SVZ and DG regions of rats or mice. The most prominent feature of all reported common TBI models is the upregulation of endogenous cell proliferation responses in the DG and SVZ regions after TBI. Whether in the FPI model of the rats or the CCI model of the mice, the cell proliferation peaked in the DG region on the second day after the injury. The number of cell proliferation in the SVZ region in the FPI model also peaked on the second day after injury [77], and this proliferative response can last for 1 year [75]. As for the degree of neural differentiation, scientists have reported different results. In diffuse injury models such as closed head weight drop injury and FPI models, injury can increase the number of new neurons in the subgranular zone and granule cell layer of the dentate gyrus. In localized injury models such as CCI, the number of new neurons produced after injury did not increase significantly compared with the sham-operated group, although the number of proliferating cells increased [78]. The reason for this difference may be differences in the injury models, severity of the injury, time point of tissue assessment after injury, changes in the cell markers used, and/or quantitative methods. The difference in the injury model has a significant effect on the cellular response. For example, in the CCI model, TBI can trigger massive death of immature neurons in the DG region in the early stage of injury [79], while in the closed diffuse head injury model, hippocampal neurogenesis, that is, cell proliferation and new neuron production, can be increased simultaneously only when the injury is severe [75]. Despite differences, TBI can activate endogenous neural stem cells activation within the neurogenic region of the adult rodent brain.

The neurogenic ability of the neurogenic regions in normal brain tissue decreases with age. After TBI, the brains of adolescents have stronger neurogenesis than adults and older ones [77]. For higher animals with gyrencephalic brain, the endogenous cellular response induced by injury has a certain relationship with age. In 2015, Costine and colleagues found that in a piglet model of cortical crush injury, injury can lead to a significant increase in the proliferation rate of cells in the SVZ region at 7 days postpartum, but after 4 months postpartum, the injury does not cause a change in cell proliferation rate [80]. In addition, other scientists have demonstrated that injury-induced newborn granule cells integrate into the existing hippocampal network. This endogenous neurogenesis is directly linked to the congenital cognitive recovery observed after injury [81, 82]. TBI enhances cell proliferation and produces new neurons. In the stroke model, new neurons are observed to migrate from the SVZ region and migrate to the ischemic injury site [61]. In the TBI model, the phenomenon that newly generated neurons migrate to the injured site is not significant, but migration of new neurons along the white matter fiber bundle is observed [80]. These studies strongly suggest that repair and regenerate are attempted through endogenous neurogenic responses after mature brain injury. This concept is supported by evidence that the degree of injury that enhances hippocampal neurogenesis is associated with increased expression of the activity-dependent early gene c-Fos [75].

**Neurogenesis of the Human Brain**

The extent and function of adult neurogenesis in the human brain is unclear compared with rodent brains. Similar to rodent brains, the SVZ and hippocampus of the human brain are neurogenic regions [57, 83]. Proliferating NSC/NPC has been found in the above regions of autopsy brain specimens. Under culture conditions, cells isolated from the adult brain are capable of producing neurons and glia [84–86]. Using breakthrough labeling methods: by measuring the carbon 14 concentration ($^{14}C$) produced in the nuclear bomb test, the $^{14}C$ can persistently incorporate into the DNA of the dividing cell. Researchers at the Karolinska Institute in Sweden have published a series of studies on human brain neurogenesis, and they report that a large number of hippocampal neurogenesis in the human brain shows a mild decline during aging [87]. The degree of neurogenesis in the SVZ region and the subsequent migration of newly generated neurons from the SVZ region to the neocortex and olfactory bulb are quite limited and can be observed only in early childhood [88]. Surprisingly, unlike other species, a large number of new neurons are produced in corpus striatum, and the new interneurons of the striatum in adult brains are significantly reduced in the brains of patients with Huntington disease [89].

Due to the technical limitations of acquired brain tissue specimens and labeling NSC/NPC, few studies have reported on endogenous neurogenesis after human TBI. Using doublecortin (DCX), a marker for neural progenitor cells and migrating neuroblasts, Taylor and his colleagues found that the number of DCX-positive cells in SVZ, hippocampus, and periventricular white matter is closely related to age. Compared with older children, younger children have more DCX-positive cells in the above-mentioned areas. Brain injury had no effect on the number of DCX-positive cells in the brain, but abundant DCX-positive cells were observed around focal infarcts in nonbrain-injured patient. In contrast, Zheng and colleagues found that the number of DCX-positive cells in the brain of patients with cortical trauma is increased [90]. The differences between the two studies may be due to the source of the tissue, the markers used, or the timing of sampling. Studies of endogenous neurogenesis after human brain TBI are limited, and there is a lack of evidence that TBI induces new neurons in the human brain. However, this does not completely exclude the possibility of the existence of small-scale new neurons generated by injury in the human brain. This is because of evidence that neurogenic region exists in the human brain, ectopic production of new striatum neurons in the adult brain, and new neurons are observed around focal infarction and subarachnoid hemorrhage [87, 89, 91].

### Regulate TBI-Induced Neurogenesis

The basic regulatory mechanisms of adult neurogenesis have not been fully elucidated. Many important transcriptional, gene regulatory, and signal transduction pathways involved in neurogenesis during development are also involved in neurogenesis in adult brain [55]. In addition to these physiological regulatory mechanisms, brain trauma triggers additional pathways to regulate/affect the response of brain neurogenesis. For example, studies have shown that after brain injury, vascular endothelial growth factor expression is elevated, and vascular endothelial growth factor signaling pathway is involved in mediating the survival of newborn granular cell neurons rather than the proliferation of neuroblasts after LFPI [92]. Studies in transgenic animals have found that the neurotrophic factor p75 receptor [p75(NTR)] can affect endogenous neurogenesis at various stages. After brain injury, p75 (NTR) expression can regulate cell survival. Intranasal administration of LM11A-3, a small molecule receptor (NTR) ligand, can enhance hippocampal neurogenesis and reverse spatial memory disorders over a long period of time [93]. Studies in transgenic animals have also shown that Ephrins and Eph receptor B3 (ephrinB3–EphB3) signaling pathways are involved in the regulation of cell proliferation and survival in the SVZ region of the adult brain by negatively regulating cell cycle progression and apoptosis [94]. After TBI, the expression of EphB3 in the SVZ region was transiently decreased, and the EphB3 signal was downregulated, but the expansion and survival of endogenous adult stem cells in the SVZ region were observed [95]. Other growth factors such as bFGF, EGF, IGF-1, and BDNF are involved in promoting neurogenesis, production, and survival of new neurons after TBI [74, 96].

### Potential Strategies to Enhance Endogenous Neurogenesis for Traumatic Brain Injury

Both scientists and clinicians are interested in activating adult endogenous neurogenesis to improve regenerative capacity and repair adult TBI. Neurons produced from adult SVZ and DG are functional, and the use of this endogenous cell population to repair and regenerate damaged brains is an attractive strategy. Since the spontaneous congenital recovery of the brain is rather limited, it is necessary to enhance this endogenous process through exogenous means. So far, many factors have been identified to promote neurogenesis, particularly the improvement of cognitive function associated with hippocampal neurogenesis. Among these factors, many types of growth factors are effective in enhancing neurogenesis and functional recovery after brain injury. Scientists have shown that intraventricular injection of growth factor bFGF or EGF can significantly enhance cell proliferation and improve cognitive function in SVZ and hippocampus after adult TBI [97]. Intraventricular perfusion of S100β can increase hippocampal cell proliferation, produce new neurons, and improve the functional recovery in traumatic brain animals [98]. It has also been reported that the administration of recombinant VEGF after TBI can promote cell proliferation and functional recovery in the SVZ region [99] and increase the survival of new neurons in the DG region [92].

In addition to the growth factors mentioned above, drugs currently in clinical trials to treat brain trauma or other nervous systems such as statins [100], erythropoietin [101], and antidepressant imipramine [102] can also enhance neurogenesis and improve cognitive function in TBI animals. In the rat CCI model, daily administration of statins (simvastatin and atorvastatin) 1–14 days after injury significantly increased the number of BrdU-positive cells and BrdU-positive/NeuN-positive cells in the DG region and improved spatial learning function [100]. Similar results were obtained in the CCI animal model treated with erythropoietin [101]. In the mouse CCI model, treatment with imipramine, a commonly used tricyclic antidepressant, for 2 or 4 weeks significantly improved cognitive function and increased cell proliferation and total number of new neurons in the DG region [102]. Other agents or treatment strategies such as hypothermia, abundant environment, low-intensity laser therapy, CNTF-like peptide, and P7C3-aminocarbazole can affect the response of endogenous neural stem cells in injured animals [103–107]. For example, mild hypothermia treatment after TBI increases the neonatal neuronal survival [103]. Intravenous infusion of angiotensin receptor blocker (CGP42112A) into the brain of a closed-cranial brain injury for 3 days promoted cell proliferation in the DG and SVZ regions and promoted the increase in the number of new neurons in a dose-dependent manner [108]. After LFPI, treatment with aminocarbazole treatment agent P7C3 (P7C3-A20) for 30 min for 7 consecutive days promoted the proliferation of cells in SGZ and the survival of newly generated neurons [106]. In the CCI model, laser treatment significantly increased cell proliferation and the number of new neurons in the SVZ and DG regions [105]. Overall, these strategies can improve the cognitive function of injured animals by mobilizing increased endogenous stem cell pools. These therapeutic strategies can exert neuroprotective and/or neuroplastic effects to further promote functional recovery, for example, treatment with epidermal growth factor, statins, or erythropoietin can reduce the loss of mature neuronal cells caused by TBI [97, 100, 101], and treatment with VEGF, LM11A-3, P7C3-A20, or transcranial laser can reduce the volume of lesions and the number of degenerated neurons [93, 99, 105, 106]. These studies strongly support the link between enhanced endogenous neurogenesis and improved cognitive function, suggesting that activation of adult endogenous neurogenesis is an attractive research strategy for repairing TBI.

Although a large number of studies have shown that improving endogenous neurogenesis after adult brain injury is beneficial for functional recovery, any long-term adverse consequences of these cellular responses are unclear. It is well known that epilepsy or epileptic seizures are associated with abnormal hippocampal neurogenesis [83]. Elimination of abnormal hippocampal neurogenesis can reduce the frequency of chronic seizures and regulate cognitive dysfunction caused by epilepsy [109]. It is speculated that neurogenesis after traumatic brain injury can cause epileptic seizures [110]. If so, further enhancement of TBI-induced hippocampal neurogenesis may exacerbate this symptom. Another long-term concern is that the number of neural stem cell populations in adult brain is limited. In the neurogenesis region, neural stem cells self-renew by asymmetric division and produce specific progenitor cells [111]. When exogenous stimuli are unable to properly maintain the balance between self-renewal and generation of offspring, the endogenous neural stem cell pool is exhausted and neurogenesis is suspended. Although there is no direct evidence to prove that the relationship between epilepsy and neurogenesis after traumatic brain injury or the treatment after TBI will deplete the endogenous neural stem cell pool, it is necessary to be vigilant in achieving targeted induction of endogenous neurogenesis.

#### 7.6.1.2 Conclusion

Endogenous neurogenesis continues throughout the life of the adult mammalian brain, that is, the newly born neurons in the adult brain are functional and can be integrated into functional neural networks. After traumatic brain injury, the level of adult neurogenesis increases, accompanied by spontaneous cognitive recovery. For researchers, increasing or manipulating the response of endogenous cells may be a promising means of treating brain injury. To date, published studies have mostly been limited to increasing cell proliferation and survival of neonatal neurons in the neurogenesis area. Neural stem cells and their progeny have specific regions, and they are generated in specific regions and migrate to specific regions. For the repair of brain injury, it is imperative that these damage-activated neural stem cells can migrate to the injured site, survive, and become functional neurons to replace the injured or dead cells. Future research should focus on the targeted regulation of endogenous neural stem cell activation, migration, differentiation, and integration with the host and related mechanisms.

### 7.6.2 The Repair and Regeneration After Spinal Cord Injury in Adult Mammals

Spinal cord injury in adult mammals not only destroys the initial spinal anatomy, leading to cell death, but also triggers secondary damage by inflammation, demyelination, and gliosis, all of which ultimately lead to loss of function below the damage plane [112]. Spinal cord injuries are caused by car accidents, falls, sports, and work-related accidents. In Western Europe, there are 280–316 new cases per million people per year; in the United States, there are approximately 54 spinal cord injuries per million people or 17,000 new spinal cord injury cases per year. Spinal cord injury usually occurs in young adulthood, leading to impairment of motor and sensory function, neuropathic pain, and stiffness. The economical consumption of spinal cord injury is also striking: in 2016, depending on the age and anatomical segment of the injury, each patient with spinal cord injury (SCI), including his or her first year, spent an average of $340,000 to $one million [113]. Until now, the medical community has no effective intervention/repair methods for spinal cord injury in adult mammals.

Stem cell therapy for spinal cord repair is an attractive research strategy. Stem cells may play an important role in replacing damaged neurons and glial cells; promoting axonal regeneration and remyelination; restoring neuronal circuits; secreting neurotrophic factors, anti-inflammatory cytokines, and other molecules; and promoting tissue repair and neovascularization.

This section describes the role of transplantation of various exogenous stem cells such as human embryonic stem cells (hESCs), induced pluripotent stem cells (iPSCs), mesenchymal stem cells (MSCs), neural stem cells (NSCs), and olfactory ensheathing cells (OECs) in the treatment of SCI and a number of clinical trials aimed at transforming the results of laboratory stem cell research into the clinic. At the same time, in the past few decades, endogenous pluripotent stem cells have been discovered in specialized areas of the adult central nervous system, and some progress has been made in the application of endogenous neural stem cells in the treatment of central nervous system damage and neurodegenerative disease progress. These endogenous stem cells can continuously differentiate into neurons, which can participate in the formation of new loops and promote the recovery of some functions after nerve damage. However, these studies are limited to the activation and recruitment of endogenous neural stem cells in the brain, and there is almost no report on the activation of endogenous neural stem cells in the spinal cord to repair defects or diseases and promote functional recovery. Confirming the identity of endogenous neural stem cells in adult spinal cord and understanding their response to trauma will help to promote the development of new therapeutic pathways, such as the regulation of the behavior of these cells in situ after injury will become an operable and attractive idea. Although scientists have not been clear about the molecular mechanism of neurogenesis in recent years, with the help of genetic fate map, it has been confirmed that the ependymal cells in the central canal of the adult spinal cord are pluripotent and act as endogenous neural stem cells. This section will also address the concept of endogenous neurogenesis in adulthood, the response of ependymal cells after spinal cord injury, the heterogeneity and markers of ependymal cells, the factors that regulate ependymal cells, and the niches that affect the activation or differentiation of ependymal cells.

#### 7.6.2.1 Transplantation of Exogenous Stem Cells to Repair Adult Spinal Cord Injury

##### Human Embryonic Stem Cell

Embryonic stem cells originate from the inner cell mass of human blastocysts. They are proliferative, pluripotent, and can differentiate into almost all cell types, including neurons and glial cells. Modified experimental methods can differentiate hESCs into motor neuron progenitor cells (MPs) and oligodendrocyte progenitor cells (OPCs) [114]. Transplantation of MPs and OPCs derived from hESCs can effectively restore the motor function in laceration and traumatic transection in the SCI models. The regenerative mechanism of hESCs in the treatment of spinal cord injury depends on the differentiation potential of OPCs and MPs derived from hESCs into neurons and glial cells and the immunomodulatory properties of hESC-derived OPCs [114]. Based on the experimental data on transplantation of human embryonic stem cell-derived OPC for the treatment of spinal cord injury in rodents, the Food and Drug Administration (FDA) approved the first clinical trial of human embryonic stem cells in 2009. Geron Corporation of the United States has directly transplanted two million human embryonic stem cell-derived OPCs (GRNOPC1) into patients with acute ASIA grade A thoracic SCI in an attempt to test the safety and efficacy of clinical application of human embryonic stem cell-derived OPCs. In 2011, Geron discontinued this clinical trial for financial reasons. Preliminary results indicate that GRNOPC1s does not cause any harm to humans, but the controversy on the effectiveness of these cells continues.

The research of human embryonic stem cell-derived neural cell transplantation for spinal cord injury has the following problems: ethical issues related to cell source, immune rejection of transplanted cells, various media, growth factors, and animal-derived additives are involved in the differentiation process, incomplete or abnormal differentiation can lead to the formation of teratomas or nonneural cells, and these problems limit the clinical application of hESCs [115, 116].

##### Induced Pluripotent Stem Cells (iPSCs)

The iPSCs were originally produced in 2006 by Japanese scholars Takahashi and Yamanaka with the help of ectopic expression of four transcription factors, Oct4, Sox2, Klf4, and c-Myc, in fibroblasts. iPSCs are similar to embryonic stem cells in morphology, transcription, epigenetics, and phenotype and can differentiate into neurons, glial cells, neural progenitor cells (NPCs), and motor neurons [117].

Patient-specific iPSCs are produced by ectopic expression of a specific set of factors in somatic cells, with no ethical and immunological rejection problems [117]. Clinical trials using iPSCs involve reprogramming techniques including carrying viral vectors and their tumorigenicity [118]. Scientists have solved the risk of reprogramming iPSCs by means of nonviral methods such as mRNA or some chemical small molecules [119]. The regenerative potential of iPSCs cells has been demonstrated in rodent SCI models. However, it is necessary to optimize the growth and differentiation of iPSCs and complete reliability and safety testing before carrying out clinical application of iPSCs for SCI [120].

##### Mesenchymal Stem Cells

Mesenchymal stem cells (MSCs) are adult stem cells with self-replication ability and multidirectional differentiation potential, which can develop into osteoblasts, chondrocytes, adipocytes, and other types of cells [121]. In addition to their stem/progenitor properties, they have been shown to have extensive immune regulatory capabilities. The therapeutic effects of MSCs on SCI intervention are mainly reflected in the secretion of neurotrophic factors, angiogenesis, and anti-inflammatory effects, rather than direct trans-lineage transformation into functional oligodendrocytes or neurons [122–126]. Transplanted MSCs act as neuroprotectors and secrete brain-derived neurotrophic factor (BDNF), glial cell-derived neurotrophic factor (GDNF), nerve growth factor (NGF), vascular endothelial growth factor (VEGF), and hepatocyte growth factor (HGF) [127].

There are more and more clinical trials for the treatment of SCI with MSCs. Although there are still some problems to be solved before the clinic, MSCs are still considered candidate cells with transplant benefits [128]. Pathological changes in the injured area after SCI have temporal and spatial characteristics, ranging from acute to subacute to chronic, so transplantation of MSCs at different times after SCI may have different results [129]. Sykova et al. suggest that the optimal time window for transplantation of MSC for SCI is 3–4 weeks after SCI, which is related to the success of transplantation therapy [130]. Yoon et al. combined autologous bone marrow MSCs with granulocyte and macrophage colony-stimulating factor to treat 35 patients with acute, subacute, and chronic complete spinal cord injury. It was found that there were no serious complications in all patients, and 30.4% of patients in the acute and subacute phase had significant improvement in the ASIA score [131]. In the chronic phase of SCI, if glial scars have developed, there is little neurological improvement in the treatment of SCI by transplantation of MSC (via intradural and/or intravascular injection) [132, 133]. Although the results of MSC-based clinical studies are promising, there are still some important issues that need to be addressed, namely, cell-derived consistency, culture conditions, ideal cell number, and optimal administration method [128].

#### Olfactory Ensheathing Cells

Olfactory ensheathing cells (OECs) are unique astrocytes located in the lamina propria of the olfactory mucosa and distributed in the outer layers of the olfactory nerve bundle and the olfactory bulb. OECs have the dual properties of astrocytes and neuromembrane cells [134]. Transplanted OECs promote axonal extension, remyelination, and neuroprotection [135]. OECs that migrate to the injured area secrete large amounts of factors that promote growth, development, and differentiation and accelerate the maturation of different types of neurons and reduce the activity of astrocytes and the formation of scars. Spinal cord regeneration and functional recovery depend on the nature, source, injury model, preparation of transplanted cell, time window of transplantation, and transplantation procedures of transplanted OECs [129]. Mackay et al. performed a phase I clinical trial of single-blind autologous OECs transplantation in three patients with chronic SCI. Feasibility and safety were confirmed, but there was no evidence of clinical effectiveness [136]. Lima et al. reported that crushed olfactory mucosa was transplanted to patients with chronic SCI, but the paraplegic patients did not receive significant improvement [137].

#### Neural Stem Cells

Neural stem cells (NSCs) are pluripotent cells that differentiate into neurons, oligodendrocytes, and astrocytes, which are efficiently amplified in vitro [138]. The NSCs are located in the subventricular zone, the subgranular layer of the dentate gyrus, and the ependymal layer of the central canal [139]. After SCI, the stem cells located in the ependyma are activated, but not enough to repair SCI. Because the stem cells of the ependyma under the injured condition are mainly differentiated into a large number of astrocytes and a very small number oligodendrocytes, almost no neurons are generated [140]. Some preclinical studies have demonstrated that transplantation of NSCs promotes partial improvement of paraplegic limb function in experimental animals after SCI. Transplantation of OPCs differentiated from ependymal stem cells can effectively restore the motor function of SCI animals [139]. The source of NSCs, the method of cell isolation and preparation, the time window of transplantation, the selected immunosuppressive agents, and the injury model (laceration vs. transection) all affect the therapeutic efficacy of transplanted NSCs on SCI [140].

A large number of preclinical studies have shown that stem cells can improve the recovery of morphology and/or function after SCI. Ideal stem cell sources must be effective and safe. Cell transplantation-based treatments remain a challenging problem that requires further investigation, research, and sustained collaboration between clinicians and researchers.

### 7.6.2.2 Activation of Endogenous Neurogenesis in Adult Mammalian Spinal Cord to Repair Spinal Cord Injury

#### What Is Endogenous Neurogenesis in Adulthood? Which Are the Endogenous Stem Cells of the Adult Mammalian Spinal Cord?

The term adult endogenous neurogenesis was first used to refer to cells that produce the nervous system, and subsequently, it was thought to be activation of endogenous neural stem cells until it was restricted to the production of new neurons [113]. The Li Xiaoguang team re-added this concept in 2015. Adult endogenous neurogenesis means that endogenous neural stem cells in the adult central nervous system can be activated and recruited to migrate to the lesion site and differentiate into mature neurons, and new neurons can form functional neural circuits with host cells, ultimately leading to functional recovery [141, 142]. The main body of endogenous neurogenesis is neural stem cells, which are self-renewable and pluripotent, meaning that they can replicate themselves and produce different mature cell types. Neural stem cells exist in many areas of the central nervous system, such as the subventricular zone, the granule layer of dentate gyrus, and the ependyma of the central canal. These neural stem cells can be activated, proliferated, and differentiated under normal, injury, or stress conditions. But in the above cases, the activation degree of endogenous neural stem cells is low, the number is limited, and the direction of differentiation is uncontrollable, so the adult central nervous system injury or disease cannot recover spontaneously. In the intact adult mammalian spinal cord, there are three major dividing cell types, of which oligodendrocyte precursor cells (NG21/olig21) account for 80% of proliferating cells, astrocytes (GFAP1/Cx301/Sox91) account for less than 5% of proliferating cells, and ependymal cells (FoxJ11) account for less than 5% of proliferating cells. Oligodendrocyte precursor cells are the major dividing cell population in the adult intact spinal cord and can produce mature oligodendrocytes. After spinal cord injury, they increase the division ratio and produce a large number of remyelinated oligodendrocytes. In the intact spinal cord, astrocytes divide sporadically to maintain their population. After spinal cord injury, they reactively proliferate and divide, forming the boundary of glial scar. Astrocytes and oligodendrocyte precursor cells can self-renew but are not pluripotent, that is, they cannot differentiate into multiple types of terminal cells, proving that they are not stem cells in the adult spinal cord. Ependymal cells are ciliated cells arranged in the central lumen of the brain and spinal cord, responsible for the advancement of cerebrospinal fluid and as a barrier to the brain and spinal cord parenchyma. In the intact spinal cord, ependymal cells rarely divide, and during cell culture in vitro, it violently divides and can produce astrocytes, oligodendrocytes, and neurons, thus proving pluripotency. After spinal cord injury, ependymal cells initiate rapid division and self-renewal and produce a large number of astrocytes to participate in the formation of scars, while also producing a small fraction of oligodendrocytes that can myelinate axons. Thus, in the adult spinal cord, ependymal cells represent a potential population of neural stem cells [113].

### Response of Ependymal Cells after Adult Spinal Cord Injury

Spinal cord injury has the characteristics of triggering ependymal cell proliferation and multipotential differentiation potential. In a variety of spinal cord injury models including contusion, crush injury, and partial incision injury with intact central canal, injury in different ways and degrees can lead to extensive proliferation of ependymal cells. This result is similar in the mouse and rat models of spinal cord injury, suggesting that extensive proliferation of ependymal cells is a fundamental conserved response to injury. Proliferation of ependymal cells after spinal cord injury results in a significant increase in the number of neural stem cells. A few weeks after the low-thoracic spinal cord contusion injury in mice, an active proliferative response can still be observed in the cervical spinal cord far from the injury site, suggesting that the injury leads to a long-term, long-distance proliferative response. It is worth noting that scientists recently used cell lineage tracing technology to prelabel oligodendrocyte progenitors, astrocytes, and ependymal cells to track their fate after spinal cord injury. The results suggest that at the population level, ependymal cells are the only pluripotent cell population after spinal cord injury, that is, after spinal cord injury, Foxj1-positive ependymal cells produce a large number of astrocytes that form the core region of glial scar and oligodendrocytes scattered in the white matter. There is still a lack of evidence suggesting whether ependymal-derived astrocytes and oligodendrocytes have the same clonal origin or originate from different subpopulations of ependymal cells [113].

### The Ependymal Cells Are Morphologically Heterogeneous

The first subpopulation of ependymal cells, derived from radial glial progenitor cells during embryonic development, is produced at 14–16 days of embryonic development; during the first week after birth, these cells differentiate with a cilia appearance. The second subpopulation is formed 8–15 days after birth and may be associated with two thin bundles of radial glial cells that appear in the roof and floor of the spinal cord. These results suggest a potential heterogeneity of ependymal cells located in the central canal of the adult spinal cord [113].

### Markers of Ependymal Cells in Adult Spinal Cord

Nestin is a marker of undifferentiated stem and progenitor cells throughout the subventricular zone and also a marker of cells in the central canal of the adult spinal cord. In the central canal, nestin is expressed mainly by subpopulations of cells in the dorsal pole of the ependymal region. These dorsal nestin-positive cells have long filaments extending along the dorsal midline, as well as similar fibers extending from the ventral pole or occasionally from the lateral ependyma. Glial fibrillary acidic protein (GFAP) is a marker of forebrain neural stem cells and astrocytes and is detectable in the dorsal pole of the ependymal layer of the central canal and in the subependymal astrocytes adjacent to the ependymal layer of the spinal cord. The transcription factor Sox2 is a marker of the neural stem/progenitor cells in the subventricular zone and also a marker of ependymal cells in the central canal and some cells in the subependymal layers. Musashi1 and CD133/prominin are markers of forebrain progenitor cells and also markers of ependymal cells of the central canal of the adult spinal cord. Vimentin and S100b are markers of forebrain ependymal cells and also markers of ependymal cells of the central canal of the adult spinal cord. However, NG2, a marker of forebrain progenitor cells, and Olig2, an oligodendrocyte transcription factor, are not expressed in ependymal layer cells of the spinal cord, but are often expressed in areas adjacent to the ependymal layer. Mammalian achaete scute homolog 1(Mash1) is associated with neural progenitor cells in the subventricular zone, but is undetectable in the spinal cord [113].

### Possible Factors Regulating Ependymal Cells and Neurogenesis in Adult Spinal Cord

There are few findings on the mechanisms of activation and subsequent neurodifferentiation of adult spinal ependymal cell, and detailed description of this mechanism will help to optimize neurogenesis after spinal cord injury. Signals exposed to short distances such as Wnt, Notch, and/or myelin basic protein (MBP) ligands from niches can distinguish stem cells from progenitor cells that have begun to differentiate. Stem cells can also be regulated by external remote signals to reflect nutritional status, energy metabolism, oxygen levels, hormonal status, and other physiological changes. The ependymal cells in the central canal of the adult spinal cord can be regulated by intracellular and extracellular factors and have the characteristics of neural stem cells [113].

The main challenge in developing new therapeutic strategies with endogenous neural stem cells is to maintain the self-renewal ability of neural stem cells and control their ability to differentiate into specific neural cell types. Recent studies have shown that in addition to the intrinsic properties of stem cells, local microenvironments or niches such as adjacent cells, growth factors, cytokines, and circulating signals all synergistically regulate the survival, proliferation, and differentiation of stem cells. For example, in the niches of adult neurogenesis, astrocyte-derived Wnts affect the fate of adult neural stem cells to differentiate into neurons in vitro, and Wnts signaling enhances neurogenesis in the adult dentate gyrus in vivo. BMPs promote hippocampal-derived neural stem cells in adult ventricular-subventricular zone and differentiate into glial cells in vitro, while two BMP antagonists, Noggin expressed by ependymal cells and neurogenesin-1 expressed by dentate gyrus granule cells and astrocytes, prevent their differentiation into glial cells and redirect their differentiation into neurons. The Notch and Shh signaling pathways from microhabitats also play an important role in controlling adult neurogenesis. Shh signaling activation of resting adult neural stem cells facilitates the establishment and maintenance of a correct neural stem cell pool in the adult subventricular zone and the subgranular layer of the dentate gyrus. There are few studies on the niches of the spinal ependymal cell. Studies have shown that there is no clear definition of the subventricular zone of the adult spinal cord, but several types of cells are located at specific locations, express specific markers, and have different morphologies and functions. Hugnot et al. found that the microhabitat of the human and rodent spinal cord contains a subset of $Dcx^+$, Nkx $6.1^+$ neural cells that protrude into the central lumen; another subpopulation of $GFAP^+$ cells, which extend radial protrusions into the spinal cord parenchyma. These $GFAP^+$ cells are frequently observed either dorsally or ventrally in the ependymal cell subpopulations of the central canal or in the ependymal or subependymal regions [113].

The scientists found that $GFAP^+$ cells in the central canal of the spinal cord express the following genes: Notch (Jagged, Hes1), Wnt (Wnt7a, Fzd3), BMP (DAN, BMP6), and Shh pathways. In addition, these $GFAP^+$ cells highly express the transcription factors of the Zeb1-zinc finger homology domain and are considered important regulators of epithelial-mesenchymal transition. Zeb1 and Zeb2 are required for the formation and expansion of neurospheres and are also expressed in adult spinal cord neural stem cells. A deep understanding of the interaction mechanisms between neural stem cells and their niches is critical for accurately describing why stem cells are highly neurogenic in certain regions while remaining static in others [113].

Li Xiaoguang's team used biomaterial scaffold, chitosan composite collagen catheter, transplantation to repair the semi-transverse injury of thoracic spinal cord in adult rats, which not only promoted the regeneration of axons including corticospinal tract but also observed neuron-like cells in the injured area, and the behavioral and electrophysiological [somatosensory-evoked potentials (SEP) and motor-evoked potentials (MEP)] of paraplegic rats have a certain degree of recovery. Their results suggest that chitosan composite collagen catheter has the function of inhibiting scar infiltration into the damaged area, improving the inflammatory microenvironment of the damaged area, promoting axon regeneration, and prolonging the re-entry of the host spinal cord across the injured area into the caudal end. In 2015, the team transplanted NT-3 chitosan catheters capable of controlled release NT-3 for up to 14 weeks into a 5-mm defect of thoracic cord complete resection in adult rats. The results suggest that NT-3 chitosan can improve the microenvironment of the spinal cord injury zone and activate endogenous neurogenesis, that is, activate and recruit endogenous neural stem cells in the spinal cord, induce their migration to the injured area, differentiate into functional neurons, and establish functional synaptic connections with the host spinal cord, which eventually leads to a certain degree of recovery of motor and sensory functions of the paraplegic hind limbs. In addition, transcript analysis using the Weighted Gene Expression Network (WGCNA) suggests that NT-3 chitosan catheters have a role in promoting neurogenesis and angiogenesis and reducing inflammatory responses after spinal cord injury [113, 141, 142]. Although the origin, markers, and molecular mechanisms of neuronal differentiation of endogenous neural stem cells are not well understood, the next step is to use genetic fate mapping techniques and lineage tracking techniques to determine the source/identity, morphological characteristics, functions, and a series of molecular events after activation of endogenous stem cells, in order to reveal the mechanism of improving the local microenvironment in the injured area to promote adult spinal cord neurogenesis.

#### 7.6.2.3 Outlook

Stem cell transplantation has been reported to provide a new therapeutic strategy for the repair of adult spinal cord injury. The transplanted cells mainly involve neural stem cells, mesenchymal stem cells, embryonic stem cells, olfactory ensheathing cells, neurolemmal cells, activated macrophages, and recently induced pluripotent stem cells. Extensive research has been carried out in various animal models of spinal cord injury, and great progress has been made. However, each method has some limitations; for example, after transplantation of neural stem cells into normal or injured adult rat spinal cord, they remain either undifferentiated or differentiated along the glial lineage. Endogenous neural stem cell in the adult spinal cord, repairing spinal cord injury and promoting functional recovery by regulating endogenous neural stem cells in the spinal cord in situ, is the most promising therapeutic strategy. In lower vertebrates, activation of spinal ependymal cells promotes regeneration and functional recovery of the spinal cord. However, in adult mammals, the regenerative ability of ependymal cells is essentially limited. After adult spinal cord injury in adult mammals, most of the ependymal cells differentiate into glial cells that form the core of scar tissue, and a small amount of ependymal cells differentiate into oligodendrocytes and hardly differentiate into neurons. The main obstacles to nerve regeneration after spinal cord injury are the loss of neurons and demyelination of axons, so the main challenge of activating endogenous stem cells to repair spinal cord injury is to promote the generation of new neurons to supplement lost neurons and the generation of oligodendrocytes to demyelinate axons. Therefore, reprogramming ependymal cells to differentiate into oligodendrocyte and neuronal cell lines will result in reduced scar formation, complementation of neurons, and promotion of myelination. Given the safety and stability considerations of in vivo gene manipulation, the application of this method to clinical practice requires repeated validation of the effectiveness and safety in nonhuman primates.

After the central nervous system injury, many unfavorable factors for nerve repair make it difficult for a single nerve regeneration strategy to achieve significant results. In order to solve the key problem of nerve regeneration, Li Xiaoguang's team proposed the incubation theory of adult endogenous neural stem cells, that is, the microenvironment of the injured part of the central nervous system is like soil and endogenous neural stem cells are seeds, improving the damage or disease local microenvironment (soil) can activate endogenous neural stem cells (seeds), induce their differentiation into neurons, and functionally integrate into the host neural network. In their research, modified and characterized biomaterial scaffolds not only serve as a bridge supporting role but also continuously deliver neurotrophic factors to the injured area, aiming to create a microenvironment conducive to regeneration. The results demonstrate that endogenous neurogenesis is activated in the microenvironment created by NT-3 chitosan scaffold, challenging the traditional view that adult mammalian neurons cannot regenerate. This also indicates how to activate adult endogenous neurogenesis through the regenerative microenvironment provided by the composite treatment strategy of biomaterial scaffolds may be the key to treating central nervous system damage [113, 141, 142].

### 7.6.3 The Strategies and Prospects of Peripheral Nerve Injury Repair

Currently, the treatment of peripheral nerve injury is inadequate and unsatisfactory in clinic. This section summarizes the changes of cell bodies, lesions, and target organs after peripheral nerve injury. Various experimental intervention strategies include drugs and cell therapies aimed at increasing neuronal survival, axon regeneration, and target site reinnervation. In view of the complexity of nerve regeneration, further research is needed to address the biological characteristics of nerve damage, improve interaction with implanted scaffolds, and achieve cell therapy in neural tissue engineering.

The peripheral nervous system (PNS) has intrinsic repair and regeneration capabilities. Direct mechanical trauma is the most common cause of peripheral nerve injury, followed by damage during tumor resection. The ability of nerve regeneration is related to the age of the patient, the mechanism of injury, and especially the cell body of the nerve cells in the proximal end of the injury. Distal fingertip nerve damage can cause loss of sensation, but it can be regenerated very well. While proximal arm plexus tear is devastating to hand function, manifested by reduced motor performance, frequent pain, and cold intolerance [143]. Such injuries have a profound and permanent impact on the patient's living and working abilities.

Currently, fine and tension-free epithelial suture is clinical treatment option for microsurgery. When the nerve defects are too long to be sutured end-to-end, autologous nerve transplantation is still the gold standard [144]. However, this treatment not only causes further damage to the patient but also has problems such as limited supply of donor nerves. Nerve damage should be repaired as soon as possible, and delayed repair is obviously not conducive to the recovery of sensory and motor function [145]. These principles have not changed in clinical treatment of neurological deficits over the past 30 years. Although much progress has been made in the study of neuropathophysiological changes after peripheral nerve injury, the corresponding clinical outcomes are still poor [146].

Clearly, pure microsurgical methods cannot resolve the cellular and molecular events of complex peripheral nerve injury repair. Axonal damage has an effect on the entire neuron and brain function. A variety of factors have led to the failure of peripheral nerve regeneration, such as slow, inadequate, and misdirected axon growth, and rapid and prolonged cortical reorganization in the corresponding parts of the brain [143]. Perhaps the most important reason is the large number of normal cell deaths in the innervation pool, because the most basic neurobiological premise for regeneration is the survival of neurons [147].

#### 7.6.3.1 Neurobiology of Peripheral Nerve Injury

Because glial cells respond differently to injury, peripheral nerves are easier to regenerate than the central nervous system. The glial cells of the peripheral nervous system, Schwann cells (SCs), can be converted into a regenerative phenotype that promotes the formation of substrates, provides abundant signaling molecules, and promotes regenerative response of neurons [148]. After peripheral nerve injury, some molecular and cellular changes, as well as changes in the injury site (proximal and distal stumps) and target organs, can be observed at the cell level (spinal dorsal horn and anterior horn), which we will discuss in the section.

#### Cell Body

After axonal injury, the first signal received by neuronal cell body may be retrograde electrical activity, high-frequency burst action potential, which opens the calcium channel and initiates the Jun-kinase cascade, affecting transcription; however, withdrawal of target organ-derived neurotrophic support is the biggest determinant of neuronal survival [149]. This will result in a profound response to gene and protein expression, and these balances determine neuronal survival and regeneration or death leading to apoptosis. Compared with motor neurons in the spinal cord, primary sensory neurons are more susceptible to injury and apoptosis, and 40% of dorsal root ganglion (DRG) neurons die after peripheral nerve injury [147]. The time course of neuronal death determines the time window for clinical neuroprotection. In certain areas of urology, the large pelvic ganglion and its associated peripheral nerves are particularly vulnerable during pelvic surgery. Although the time course and extent of neuronal death in the large pelvic ganglion are not well understood, it is expected to be similar to the above results. After cavernous nerve injury, the molecular map of the changes in the large pelvic ganglion has been studied, and some genes related to apoptosis, neuroprotection, and regeneration are upregulated [150]. The expression characteristics of these genes and their effects on the fate of injured neurons will depend on the balance of apoptosis/neuroprotection.

#### Damage Site

The distal nerves at the peripheral nerve injury site undergo a series of molecular and cellular changes called Wallerian degeneration [151]. Within a few hours of injury, the axons and myelin sheaths at the distal end of the stump are degraded and macrophages migrate to the site of injury to engulf debris. In the first 24 h after injury, neurolemmal cells proliferate, transition from myelin to a regenerative phenotype, and exhibit some upregulated molecules to assist in the balance of degradation and regeneration process. In particular, the expression of inhibitory structural proteins, such as protein zero, myelin-associated protein, cell adhesion molecule (CAM), neuronal cell adhesion molecule (NCAM), and glial fibrillar acidic protein, and growth factors such as neural growth factor, brain-derived neurotrophic factor (BDNF), glial cell-derived neurotrophic factor (GDNF), basic fiber growth factor (bFGF), and neurotrophin 3 (NT-3) in denervated neurolemmal cells. When the neurolemmal cells and macrophages together remove debris, the neurolemmal cells form aligned column, forming a Büngner band, and constructing a free environment rich in trophic factors to guide axon regeneration [152].

#### Target Organ

At the distal end of the injury site, there are some obstacles before the regenerative axons reinnervate the target organ. Even with a certain amount of good axon regeneration, mismatching with the target can lead to loss of function; growth cones that fail to reach the correct target or lose nerve support are often "trimmed off." Loss of nerve contact at the distal end of the injured stump causes long-term denervated neurolemmal cells to downregulate the expression of growth factors and enter a dormant state, unable to support axon advancement [145]. Similarly, denervated target organs deplete trophic factors, leading to muscle fibers atrophy and progressive apoptosis of satellite cells. These reactions have a major impact on the functional recovery of the proximal end of the injured nerve [153].

### 7.6.3.2 Research Strategy and Tissue Engineering

#### Solving Neuronal Survival

Surgery repair of peripheral nerve injury plays at most a partial neuroprotective role and relies on early 24 h of repair [153]. When the diagnosis is delayed, the feasibility of clinical surgery is reduced, especially for those with closed brachial plexus injury, and the prognosis is usually not satisfactory. Therefore, another method of neuroprotection is needed. Exogenous growth factor replacement can reduce the loss of experimental neurons. However, adverse effects in clinical applications, unpredictability of interactions of various growth factors, heterogeneity, and adverse reactions of growth factors, have all affected clinical applications [154]. Recently, two agents, N-acetylcysteine (NAC) and acetyl-L-carnitine (ALCAR), have been shown to have sufficient neuroprotective effects in the clinic, while determining their safety for clinical use [155].

#### Treatment for Injury Sites

(a) Nerve-guiding stent: Autologous nerve graft is the current clinical gold standard when tension-free suture for peripheral nerve defects is not applicable. It provides support structure to guide axon regeneration and prevent neuroma formation and fibrous tissue invasion, but it will cause surgical trauma, feeling missing and structural mismatch at the donor site [156]. These problems motivate scholars to find nerve-guided stents to promote nerve regeneration, limit the infiltration of myofibroblasts, reduce scar formation, and locally accumulate high concentrations of neurotrophic factors. However, commercial stents (primarily biodegradable polymers or collagen-based hollow tubes) fail to achieve the effects of autologous nerve grafts, which can only bridge a limited short defect (≤2 cm) and have poor functional recovery [157].

Advances in tissue engineering in recent years have changed the concept that passive scaffolds, which provide only a simple protective space for nerve regeneration, are transformed to create an active environment that improves nerve sprouting and accelerates axon regeneration, and the surface topography in the lumen of the stent can be modified to accommodate and support cell adhesion, alignment, and morphological development [158]. Scholars have studied the effects of different topographical features such as grooves, electrospun fibers, gels, and membranes on the growth and migration of neurolemmal cells and neuronal cells [159]. In addition, the chemical characteristics of biological materials can help optimize cell behavior, such as grafting short peptide sequences (such as RGD) can promote cell adhesion to the polymer surface [160]; hydrolysis and aminolysis of polycaprolactone (PCL) membrane polymers can cause the neurolemmal cells to elongate and proliferate, and the ECM molecules can support the adhesion of neurolemmal cells to the wall and secrete stimulating neurite-promoting factors [161, 162].

(b) Drug treatment: There are currently no clinically available drugs to treat nerve damage. However, some small molecule peptides, such as hormones and growth factors, are considered potential candidates to increase nerve regeneration, reduce neuronal death, and promote regenerative axon growth after injury. Nerve growth factor promotes axon growth, whether locally or systemically. In a similar manner, BDNF and ciliary neurotrophic factor (CTNF) increase peripheral nerve regeneration distance and accelerate remyelination and functional recovery [163]. Topical administration of insulin growth factor-1 (IGF-1), FGF, or GDNF can improve axonal regeneration rate and functional recovery [164].

(c) Cell therapy: Given the complexity of events occurring after nerve injury and nerve regeneration, specific molecules or single methods to promote nerve repair have proven to be extremely challenging. There is a great hope in the field of regenerative medicine for nerve repair: developing the regenerative potential of cell therapy. When the peripheral nerve defect is relatively long, the successful regeneration cannot be achieved with the aid of nerve conduit alone. In view of the importance of Schwann cells in development and after nerve damage, transplantation of Schwann cells for nerve repair can significantly improve the regeneration effect [165]. Similarly, olfactory ensheathing cells, another source of specialized glial cells, can provide nutrients to the regenerative nerves and contribute to remyelination [166]. However, allogeneic or homologous neurolemmal cells need to sacrifice a segment of functional nerves, while the ability of olfactory ensheathing cells and SCs to expand is limited, which hinders their application in the field of neural tissue engineering. For this reason, scholars have conducted extensive research on other candidate cells, using stem cells as the most promising candidate for cell therapy in nerve repair. Embryonic stem cells (ESCs), neural stem cells (NSCs), induced pluripotent stem cells (iPSCs), and adult mesenchymal stem cells (MSCs) were studied in vitro and in vivo to investigate whether they are suitable for nerve repair.

#### Treatment of Target Organs

Even after many years of injury, if the survival of sensory neurons can be preserved, the skin receptors can be effectively reinnervated by the nerves, possibly restoring sensory function. In contrast, denervated muscles gradually lose the ability to reinnervate. Therefore, in addition to nerve regeneration, it is also necessary to prevent or reduce muscle atrophy caused by denervation. Experimental studies suggest that intramuscular injection of various growth factors or stem cells can be a useful means of assisting nerve repair. In addition, when the muscles are severely atrophied, the muscles can no longer receive effective innervation of the regenerative nerves.

(a) Growth factors and cell therapy: IGF-1, a potent myogenic molecule, can be efficiently delivered to damaged muscles by means of specific muscle nonviral vectors. Shiotani et al. injected IGF-1 into laryngeal paralyzed mice, resulting in increased muscle fiber diameter, reduced motor endplate length, and increased proportion of endplate innervation [167]. The same research team later found that the IGF-1 vector had the same effective effect when treating chronic nerve damage. Recent studies have shown that intramuscular infusion of IGF-1 works by upregulating the myogenic regulators myoD and myogenin [168].

In a variety of experimental models including muscle atrophy and age-related atrophy, intramuscular injection of adeno-associated virus (AAV) vectors can improve the conditions. In the rat model of median nerve injury, overexpression of vascular endothelial growth factor (VEGF) in the muscle with AAV-VEGF vector significantly reduced the progression of muscle atrophy [169]. Another study investigated the synergistic effect of intramuscular injection of a mixture of growth factors (NGF, CNTF, GDNF) to promote functional recovery after sciatic nerve injury in rats. Combined use of these three factors can increase muscle mass and promote functional recovery [170].

Various growth factors may contribute to the functional reinnervation of neurons by general systemic effects or reverse transport to the neuronal cell bodies of the spinal cord. Muscle satellite cells are intrinsic stem cells that rebuild the function of the denervated muscle after injury to the neuromuscular system. Denervated muscle function can be improved by injection of exogenous satellite cells expanded in vitro. Bacau and his colleagues injected high-density adult myoblasts or ASC into the tibialis anterior muscle of denervated rats, and after 4 months, there was no significant beneficial change in muscle and function of the experimental animals. In contrast, Halum et al. injected autologous myoblasts into the denervated laryngeal muscle of rats and found that the cells survived and fused into larger fibers, with fiber diameters and volumes higher than those of control animals. Some of these animals showed functional improvements, although there was no significant improvement in muscle nerve reinnervation [171, 172].

(b) Tissue engineering new muscles: In the cases where the intrinsic regenerative capacity of the muscle is exhausted, it may be necessary to replace the damaged muscle tissue. Any muscle tissue engineering should have the proper structural and mechanical properties to promote rapid muscle recovery. The basic requirements for construction are a suitable source of cells and easy to culture, expand, and differentiate into muscle cell lines. Satellite cells or myoblasts are obvious choices, but their optimal growth performance parameters have not been established. Many other types of cells, including embryonic stem cells, induced pluripotent stem cells, pericytes, and MSCs, have been tested. Various types of scaffolds have been developed that mimic the natural ECM function of muscles, which are typically reshaped by degradation of degradable substrates [173].

#### 7.6.3.3 Prospects for the Future

**Clinical Application Prospects**

The current peripheral nerve repair practice is similar to the detailed description of Gabriele Ferrara (1543–1627) more than 400 years ago, including disinfection, proper identification of nerve stumps, gentle suture technique, and limb fixation. The new technical concept was established for the treatment of injuries during the World War II, including the use of autologous nerve grafts and primary and secondary repairs. In the 1960s, combined with surgical microscopes and nerve repair techniques, it was recognized that the adverse effects of tension sutures improved the technique of nerve repair. Recently, in order to bypass complex and inhibitory factors, prolonged regenerative nerves through the denervated stump to the target organ, new surgical techniques such as free muscle transplantation and nerve transplantation have been established. These new methods can provide some functional alternatives, but for patients with nerve damage, there will be no substantial results. An in-depth understanding of the neurobiological characteristics of peripheral nerve injury and the above experimental strategies are possible for the next clinical advancement. Many studies are approaching clinical applications [174–177].

**Future Scientific Perspectives**

In view of the multifaceted peripheral nerve injury and various clinical conditions, it is necessary to combine drugs, molecular therapy, and new surgical methods, with new neural scaffolds and molecular targeting strategies, such as the construction of scaffold materials that can deliver drug and silent RNAs, to strengthen the intrinsic regeneration mechanisms. We should focus not only on how to improve axon regeneration but also on the neurolemmal cells of the distal stump and the molecular response of the denervated muscle. It should be recognized that many of the experimental advances made to date are still limited to short-distance peripheral nerve regeneration. New tissue-engineered nerve constructs should be able to achieve long-distance axon growth, and matching the effects of autologous nerve grafts is the ultimate goal. A deeper understanding of the structural anatomy of the peripheral nerves and the extracellular matrix can contribute to the design of the tissue engineered nerve. For example, simulating the Büngner band structure will more accurately replicate the architecture of the autologous nerve. In order to repair long-distance nerve defects, adequate blood supply is provided to ensure the survival of transplanted cells. Computer and mathematical modeling can be useful tools for the design of new scaffolds. Downstream advanced 3D in vitro models can more accurately mimic the anatomical and physiological properties of peripheral nerves. Repair of long-distance peripheral nerve injury still needs to be verified in large animals, and it remains a huge challenge for clinical application.

## References

1. Michalopoulos GK, DeFrances MC. Liver Regeneration. Science. 1997;276:60.
2. Forbes SJ, Rosenthal N. Preparing the ground for tissue regeneration: from mechanism to therapy. Nat Med. 2014;20:857–69.
3. Michalopoulos GK. Liver Regeneration. J Cell Physiol. 2007;213:286–300.
4. Kordes C, Häussinger D. Hepatic stem cell niches. J Clin Invest. 2013;123:1874–80.
5. Hu M, Kurobe M, Jeong YJ, et al. Wnt/β-catenin signaling in murine hepatic transit amplifying progenitor cells. Gastroenterology. 2007;133(5):1579–91.
6. Preisegger KH, Factor VM, Fuchsbichler A, et al. Atypical ductular proliferation and its inhibition by transforming growth factor beta1 in the 3,5-diethoxycarbonyl-1,4-dihydrocollidine mouse model for chronic alcoholic liver disease. Lab Investig. 1999;79:103–9.
7. Akhurst B, Croager EJ, Farley-Roche CA, et al. A modified choline-deficient, ethionine-supplemented diet protocol effectively induces oval cells in mouse liver. Hepatology. 2001;34:519–22.

8. Miyajima A, Tanaka M, Itoh T. Stem/progenitor cells in liver development, homeostasis, regeneration, and reprogramming. Cell Stem Cell. 2014;14(5):561–74.
9. Yanger K, Knigin D, Zong Y, et al. Adult hepatocytes are generated by self-duplication rather than stem cell differentiation. Cell Stem Cell. 2014;15:340–9.
10. Tarlow BD, Finegold MJ, Grompe M. Clonal tracing of Sox9+ liver progenitors in mouse oval cell injury. Hepatology. 2014;60:278–89.
11. Huch M, Dorrell C, Boj SF, et al. In vitro expansion of single Lgr5+ liver stem cells induced by Wnt-driven regeneration. Nature. 2013;494:247–50.
12. Azuma H, Paulk N, Ranade A, et al. Robust expansion of human hepatocytes in Fah(−/−)/Rag2(−/−)/Il2rg (−/−) mice. Nat Biotechnol. 2007;25:903–10.
13. Wang B, Zhao L, Fish M, et al. Self-renewing diploid Axin2(+) cells fuel homeostatic renewal of the liver. Nature. 2015;524:180–5.
14. Font-Burgada J, Shalapour S, Ramaswamy S, et al. Hybrid periportal hepatocytes regenerate the injured liver without giving rise to cancer. Cell. 2015;162:766–79.
15. Tarlow BD, Finegold MJ, Grompe M. Clonal tracing of Sox9+ liver progenitors in oval cell injury. Hepatology (Baltimore, Md.). 2014;60:278–89.
16. Tarlow BD, Pelz C, Naugler WE, et al. Bipotential adult liver progenitors are derived from chronically injured mature hepatocytes. Cell Stem Cell. 2014;15:605–18.
17. Pu W, Zhang H, Huang X, et al. Mfsd2a+ hepatocytes repopulate the liver during injury and regeneration. Nat Commun. 2016;7:13369.
18. Sekiya S, Suzuki A. Direct conversion of mouse fibroblasts to hepatocyte-like cells by defined factors. Nature. 2011;475:390–3.
19. Huang P, He Z, Ji S, et al. Induction of functional hepatocyte-like cells from mouse fibroblasts by defined factors. Nature. 2011;475:386–9.
20. Huang P, Zhang L, Gao Y, et al. Direct reprogramming of human fibroblasts to functional and expandable hepatocytes. Cell Stem Cell. 2014;14:370–84.
21. Du Y, Wang J, Jia J, et al. Human hepatocytes with drug metabolic function induced from fibroblasts by lineage reprogramming. Cell Stem Cell. 2014;14:394–403.
22. Wang Y, Qin J, Wang S, et al. Conversion of human gastric epithelial cells to multipotent endodermal progenitors using defined small molecules. Cell Stem Cell. 2016;19:449–61.
23. Levy G, Bomze D, Heinz S, et al. Long-term culture and expansion of primary human hepatocytes. Nat Biotechnol. 2015;33:1264–71.
24. Huch M, Gehart H, van Boxtel R, et al. Long-term culture of genome-stable bipotent stem cells from adult human liver. Cell. 2015;160:299–312.
25. Katsuda T, Kawamata M, Hagiwara K, et al. Conversion of terminally committed hepatocytes to culturable bipotent progenitor cells with regenerative capacity. Cell Stem Cell. 2017;20(1):41–55.
26. Song G, Pacher M, Balakrishnan A, et al. Direct reprogramming of hepatic myofibroblasts into hepatocytes in vivo attenuates liver fibrosis. Cell Stem Cell. 2016;18:797–808.
27. Rezvani M, Espanol-Suner R, Malato Y, et al. In vivo hepatic reprogramming of myofibroblasts with AAV vectors as a therapeutic strategy for liver fibrosis. Cell Stem Cell. 2016;18:809–16.
28. Bhatia SN, Underhill GH, Zaret KS, et al. Cell and tissue engineering for liver disease. Sci Transl Med. 2014;6(245):245sr2.
29. Takebe T, Sekine K, Enomura M, et al. Vascularized and functional human liver from an iPSC-derived organ bud transplant. Nature. 2013;499:481–4.
30. Ott HC, Matthiesen TS, Goh S-K, et al. Perfusion-decellularized matrix: using nature's platform to engineer a bioartificial heart. Nat Med. 2008;14:213–21.
31. Uygun BE, Soto-Gutierrez A, Yagi H, et al. Organ reengineering through development of a transplantable recellularized liver graft using decellularized liver matrix. Nature Med. 2010;16:814–20.
32. Baptista PM, Siddiqui MM, Lozier G, et al. The use of whole organ decellularization for the generation of a vascularized liver organoid. Hepatology. 2011;53:604–17.
33. Petersen TH, Calle EA, Zhao L, et al. Tissue-engineered lungs for in vivo implantation. Science (New York, N.Y.). 2010;329:538–41.
34. Song JJ, Ott HC. Organ engineering based on decellularized matrix scaffolds. Trends Mol Med. 2011;17(8):424–32.
35. Wang Y, Cui CB, Yamauchi M, et al. Lineage restriction of human hepatic stem cells to mature fates is made efficient by tissue-specific biomatrix scaffolds. Hepatology. 2011;53:293–305.
36. Ren X, Moser PT, Gilpin SE, et al. Engineering pulmonary vasculature in decellularized rat and human lungs. Nat Biotechnol. 2015;33:1097–102.
37. Shi XL, Gao Y, Yan Y, et al. Improved survival of porcine acute liver failure by a bioartificial liver device implanted with induced human functional hepatocytes. Cell Res. 2016;26:206–16.
38. Yang YH, Fu XB, Sun TZ. Effects of bFGF on the expression of endogenous bFGF and TGF in the intestinal tract after ischemia reperfusion. World Chin J Digestol. 1999;7(9):793–4.
39. Xing F, Guo BC, Li JY, et al. Effect of epidermal growth factor on gut function and mucosal permeability in rats after gut ischemia-reperfusion injury. Chin Crit Care Med. 2002;14(11):650–3.
40. Zhao JY, Fu XB, Chen W. Effects of modified acidic fibroblast growth factor on apoptosis in intestinal tissue after ischemia and perfusion in rats. J Traum Surg. 2005;6:441–3.
41. Fu XB, Yang YH, Sun TZ, et al. Effects of inhibition or antiendogenous basic fibroblast growth factor on functional changes in intestine, liver and kidneys in rats after gut ischemia reperfusion injury. Chin Crit Care Med. 2000.
42. Zhou HF, Shi SH, Zhang JM, et al. Influence of Cuyu granule on the healing quality of rat gastric ulcer due to acetic acid. Hubei J Trad Chin Med. 2006;28(3):1–13.
43. Zheng XG, Zhang GA, Yang XG, et al. Study of the mechanism of Weitongning protecting action on stomach membrane of rats with acetic acid gastric ulcer. Hubei J Trad Chin Med. 2003;25(6):7–8.
44. Wang GZ, Li CJ, Fang XC, et al. Effect of bone marrow mesenchymal stem cells on gastric ulcer repairing. Chin J Rep Reconstr Surg. 2015;29(7):889–92.
45. Altman J, Das GD. Autoradiographic and histological evidence of postnatal hippocampal neurogenesis in rats. J Comp Neurol. 1965;124(3):319–35.
46. Kempermann G, Kuhn HG, Gage FH. More hippocampal neurons in adult mice living in an enriched environment. Nature. 1997;386(6624):493–5.
47. Kempermann G, Kuhn HG, Gage FH. Experience-induced neurogenesis in the senescent dentate gyrus. J Neurosci. 1998;18(9):3206–12.
48. Gage FH, Kempermann G, Palmer TD, et al. Multipotent progenitor cells in the adult dentate gyrus. J Neurobiol. 1998;36(2):249–66.
49. Gould E, Tanapat P. Stress and hippocampal neurogenesis. Biol Psychiatry. 1999;46(11):1472–9.
50. Gould E, Tanapat P, Cameron HA. Adrenal steroids suppress granule cell death in the developing dentate gyrus through an NMDA receptor-dependent mechanism. Brain Res Dev Brain Res. 1997;103(103):91–3.
51. Gould E, Tanapat P, Hastings NB, et al. Neurogenesis in adulthood: a possible role in learning. Trends Cogn Sci. 1999;3(3):186–92.

52. Lois C, Alvarez-Buylla A. Proliferating subventricular zone cells in the adult mammalian forebrain can differentiate into neurons and glia. Proc Natl Acad Sci U S A. 1993;90(5):2074–7.
53. Deng W, Saxe MD, Gallina IS, et al. Adult-born hippocampal dentate granule cells undergoing maturation modulate learning and memory in the brain. J Neurosci. 2009;29(43):13532–42.
54. Clelland CD, Choi M, Romberg C, et al. A functional role for adult hippocampal neurogenesis in spatial pattern separation. Science. 2009;325(5937):210–3.
55. Aimone JB, Li Y, Lee SW, et al. Regulation and function of adult neurogenesis: from genes to cognition. Physiol Rev. 2014;94(4):991–1026.
56. Moreno MM, Linster C, Escanilla O, et al. Olfactory perceptual learning requires adult neurogenesis. Proc Natl Acad Sci U S A. 2009;106(42):17980–5.
57. Eriksson PS, Perfilieva E, Bjork-Eriksson T, et al. Neurogenesis in the adult human hippocampus. Nat Med. 1998;4(11):1313–7.
58. Breton-Provencher V, Lemasson M, Peralta MR III, et al. Inter neurons produced in adulthood are required for the normal functioning of the olfactory bulb network and for the execution of selected olfactory behaviors. J Neurosci. 2009;29(48):15245–57.
59. Ortega F, Gascon S, Masserdotti G, et al. Oligodendrogliogenic and neurogenic adult subependymal zone neural stem cells constitute distinct lineages and exhibit differential responsiveness to Wnt signalling. Nat Cell Biol. 2013;15(6):602–13.
60. Gritti A, Bonfanti L, Doetsch F, et al. Multipotent neural stem cells reside into the rostral extension and olfactory bulb of adult rodents. J Neurosci. 2002;22(2):437–45.
61. Parent JM, Vexler ZS, Gong C, et al. Rat forebrain neurogenesis and striatal neuron replacement after focal stroke. Ann Neurol. 2002;52(6):802–13.
62. Van Praag H, Schinder AF, Christie BR, et al. Functional neurogenesis in the adult hippocampus. Nature. 2002;415(6875):1030–4.
63. Hastings NB, Gould E. Rapid extension of axons into the CA3 region by adult-generated granule cells 56. J Comp Neurol. 1999;413:146–54.
64. Cameron HA, McKay RD. Adult neurogenesis produces a large pool of new granule cells in the dentate gyrus. J Comp Neurol. 2001;435:406–17.
65. Imayoshi I, Sakamoto M, Ohtsuka T, Takao K, Miyakawa T, Yamaguchi M, Mori K, Ikeda T, Itohara S, Kageyama R. Roles of continuous neurogenesis in the structural and functional integrity of the adult forebrain. Nat Neurosci. 2008;11:1153–61.
66. Kirn JR, Fishman Y, Sasportas K, et al. Fate of new neurons in adult canary high vocal center during the first 30 days after their formation. J Comp Neurol. 1999;411(3):487–94.
67. Burghardt NS, Park EH, Hen R, et al. Adult-born hippocampal neurons promote cognitive flexibility in mice. Hippocampus. 2012;22(9):1795–808.
68. Shors TJ, Townsend DA, Zhao M, Kozorovitskiy Y, Gould E. Neurogenesis may relate to some but not all types of hippocampal-dependent learning. Hippocampus. 2002;12:578–84.
69. Jessberger S, Clark RE, Broadbent NJ, Clemenson GD Jr, Consiglio A, Lie DC, Squire LR, Gage FH. Dentate gyrus-specific knockdown of adult neurogenesis impairs spatial and object recognition memory in adult rats. Learn Mem. 2009;16:147–54.
70. Lemasson M, Saghatelyan A, Olivo-Marin JC, et al. Neonatal and adult neurogenesis provide two distinct populations of newborn neurons to the mouse olfactory bulb. J Neurosci. 2005;25(29):6816–25.
71. Sakamoto M, Ieki N, Miyoshi G, et al. Continuous postnatal neurogenesis contributes to formation of the olfactory bulb neural circuits and flexible olfactory associative learning. J Neurosci. 2014a;34(17):5788–99.
72. Banasr M, Hery M, Brezun JM, et al. Serotonin mediates oestrogen stimulation of cell proliferation in the adult dentate gyrus 12. Eur J Neurosci. 2001;14(9):1417–24.
73. Rice AC, Khaldi A, Harvey HB, et al. Proliferation and neuronal differentiation of mitotically active cells following traumatic brain injury. Exp Neurol. 2003;183(2):406–17.
74. Gao X, Chen J. Conditional knockout of brain-derived neurotrophic factor in the hippocampus increases death of adult-born immature neurons following traumatic brain injury. J Neurotrauma. 2009;26(8):1325–35.
75. Villasana LE, Westbrook GL, Schnell E. Neurologic impairment following closed head injury predicts post-traumatic neurogenesis. Exp Neurol. 2014;261:156–62.
76. Bye N, Carron S, Han X, et al. Neurogenesis and glial proliferation are stimulated following diffuse traumatic brain injury in adult rats. J Neurosci Res. 2011;89(7):986–1000.
77. Sun D, Colello RJ, Daugherty WP, et al. Cell proliferation and neuronal differentiation in the dentate gyrus in juvenile and adult rats following traumatic brain injury. J Neurotrauma. 2005;22(1):95–105.
78. Gao X, Chen J. Moderate traumatic brain injury promotes neural precursor proliferation without increasing neurogenesis in the adult hippocampus. Exp Neurol. 2013;239:38–48.
79. Gao X, Deng-Bryant Y, Cho W, et al. Selective death of newborn neurons in hippocampal dentate gyrus following moderate experimental traumatic brain injury. J Neurosci Res. 2008;86(10):2258–70.
80. Costine BA, Missios S, Taylor SR, et al. The subventricular zone in the immature piglet brain: anatomy and exodus of neuroblasts into white matter after traumatic brain injury. Dev Neurosci. 2015;37(2):115–30.
81. Sun D, McGinn MJ, Zhou Z, et al. Anatomical integration of newly generated dentate granule neurons following traumatic brain injury in adult rats and its association to cognitive recovery. Exp Neurol. 2007;204(1):264–72.
82. Sun D, Daniels TE, Rolfe A, et al. Inhibition of injury-induced cell proliferation in the dentate gyrus of the hippocampus impairs spontaneous cognitive recovery after traumatic brain injury. J Neurotrauma. 2014;32(7):495–505.
83. Sanai N, Tramontin AD, Quinones-Hinojosa A, et al. Unique astrocyte ribbon in adult human brain contains neural stem cells but lacks chain migration. Nature. 2004;427(6976):740–4.
84. Kukekov VG, Laywell ED, Suslov O, et al. Multipotent stem/progenitor cells with similar properties arise from two neurogenic regions of adult human brain. Exp Neurol. 1999;156(2):333–44.
85. Nunes MC, Roy NS, Keyoung HM, et al. Identification and isolation of multipotential neural progenitor cells from the subcortical white matter of the adult human brain. Nat Med. 2003;9(9):439–47.
86. Murrell W, Palmero E, Bianco J, et al. Expansion of multipotent stem cells from the adult human brain. PLoS One. 2013;8(8):e71334.
87. Spalding KL, Bergmann O, Alkass K, et al. Dynamics of hippocampal neurogenesis in adult humans. Cell. 2013;153(6):1219–27.
88. Bergmann O, Liebl J, Bernard S, et al. The age of olfactory bulb neurons in humans. Neuron. 2012;74(4):634–9.
89. Ernst A, Alkass K, Bernard S, et al. Neurogenesis in the striatum of the adult human brain. Cell. 2014;156(5):1072–83.
90. Zheng W, Zhuge Q, Zhong M, et al. Neurogenesis in adult human brain after traumatic brain injury. J Neurotrauma. 2013;30(22):1872–80.
91. Taylor SR, Smith C, Harris BT, et al. Maturation dependent response of neurogenesis after traumatic brain injury in children. J Neurosurg Pediatr. 2013;12(6):545–54.

92. Lee C, Agoston DV. Vascular endothelial growth factor is involved in mediating increased de novo hippocampal neurogenesis in response to traumatic brain injury. J Neurotrauma. 2010;27:541–53.
93. Shi J, Longo FM, Massa SM. A small molecule p75(NTR) ligand protects neurogenesis after traumatic brain injury. Stem Cells. 2013;31(11):2561–74.
94. Ricard J, Salinas J, Garcia L, et al. EphrinB3 regulates cell proliferation and survival in adult neurogenesis. Mol Cell Neurosci. 2006;31(4):713–22.
95. Theus MH, Ricard J, Bethea JR, et al. EphB3 limits the expansion of neural progenitor cells in the subventricular zone by regulating p53 during homeostasis and following traumatic brain injury. Stem Cells. 2010;28(7):1231–42.
96. Carlson SW, Madathil SK, Sama DM, et al. Conditional overexpression of insulin-like growth factor-1 enhances hippocampal neurogenesis and restores immature neuron dendritic processes after traumatic brain injury. J Neuropathol Exp Neurol. 2014;73(8):734–46.
97. Sun D, Bullock MR, Altememi N, et al. The effect of epidermal growth factor in the injured brain after trauma in rats. J Neurotrauma. 2010;27(5):923–38.
98. Kleindienst A, McGinn MJ, Harvey HB, et al. Enhanced hippocampal neurogenesis by intraventricular S100B infusion is associated with improved cognitive recovery after traumatic brain injury. J Neurotrauma. 2005;22(6):645–55.
99. Thau-Zuchman O, Shohami E, Alexandrovich AG, et al. Vascular endothelial growth factor increases neurogenesis after traumatic brain injury. J Cereb Blood Flow Metab. 2010;30(5):1008–16.
100. Lu D, Qu C, Goussev A, et al. Statins increase neurogenesis in the dentate gyrus, reduce delayed neuronal death in the hippocampal CA3 region, and improve spatial learning in rat after traumatic brain injury. J Neurotrauma. 2007;24(7):1132–46.
101. Xiong Y, Mahmood A, Meng Y, et al. Delayed administration of erythropoietin reducing hippocampal cell loss, enhancing angiogenesis and neurogenesis, and improving functional outcome following traumatic brain injury in rats: comparison of treatment with single and triple dose. J Neurosurg. 2010;113(3):598–608.
102. Han X, Tong J, Zhang J, et al. Imipramine treatment improves cognitive outcome associated with enhanced hippocampal neurogenesis after traumatic brain injury in mice. J. Neurotrauma. 2011;28(6):995–1007.
103. Bregy A, Nixon R, Lotocki G, et al. Posttraumatic hypothermia increases double cortin expressing neurons in the dentate gyrus after traumatic brain injury in the rat. Exp Neurol. 2012;233(2):821–8.
104. Kovesdi E, Gyorgy AB, Kwon SK, et al. The effect of enriched environment on the outcome of traumatic brain injury; a behavioral, proteomics, and histological study. Front Neurosci. 2011;5:42.
105. Xuan W, Vatansever F, Huang L, et al. Transcranial low-level laser therapy enhances learning, memory, and neuroprogenitor cells after traumatic brain injury in mice. J Biomed Opt. 2014;19(10):108003.
106. Blaya MO, Bramlett HM, Naidoo J, et al. Neuroprotective efficacy of a proneurogenic compound after traumatic brain injury. J Neurotrauma. 2014;31(5):476–86.
107. Chohan MO, Bragina O, Kazim SF, et al. Enhancement of neurogenesis and memory by a neurotrophic peptide in mild to moderate traumatic brain injury. Neurosurgery. 2015;76(2):201–14.
108. Umschweif G, Liraz-Zaltsman S, Shabashov D, et al. Angiotensin receptor type 2 activation induces neuroprotection and neurogenesis after traumatic brain injury. Neurotherapeutics. 2014;11(3):665–78.
109. Cho KO, Lybrand ZR, Ito N, et al. Aberrant hippocampal neurogenesis contributes to epilepsy and associated cognitive decline. Nat Commun. 2015;6:6606.
110. Pitkanen A, Kemppainen S, Ndode-Ekane XE, et al. Posttraumatic epilepsy — disease or comorbidity[J]? Epilepsy Behav. 2014;38:19–24.
111. Kempermann G, Jessberger S, Steiner B, et al. Milestones of neuronal development in the adult hippocampus. Trends Neurosci. 2004;27(8):447–52.
112. Volarevic V, Erceg S, Bhattacharya SS, et al. Stem cell-based therapy for spinal cord injury. Cell Transplant. 2013;22(8):1309–23.
113. Duan H, Wei S, Wen Z, et al. Endogenous neurogenesis in adult mammals after spinal cord injury. Sci China Life Sci. 2016;59(12):1313.
114. Erceg S, Ronaghi M, Oria M, et al. Transplanted oligodendrocytes and motoneuron progenitors generated from human embryonic stem cells promote locomotor recovery after spinal cord transection. Stem Cells. 2010;28(9):1541–9.
115. Erceg S, Ronaghi M, Stojković M. Human embryonic stem cell differentiation toward regional specific neural precursors. Stem Cells. 2009;27(1):78–87.
116. Mothe AJ, Tator CH. Advances in stem cell therapy for spinal cord injury. J Clin Invest. 2012;122(11):3824–34.
117. Lukovic D, Moreno-Manzano V, Klabusay M, et al. Non-coding RNAs in pluripotency and neural differentiation of human pluripotent stem cells. Front Genet. 2014;14(5):132.
118. Lukovic D, Moreno Manzano V, Stojkovic M, et al. Concise review: human pluripotent stem cells in the treatment of spinal cord injury. Stem Cells. 2012;30(9):1787–92.
119. Warren L, Manos PD, Ahfeldt T, et al. Highly efficient reprogramming to pluripotency and directed differentiation of human cells with synthetic modified mRNA. Cell Stem Cell. 2010;7(5):618–30.
120. Nori S, Okada Y, Yasuda A, et al. Grafted human-induced pluripotent stem-cell-derived neurospheres promote motor functional recovery after spinal cord injury in mice. Proc Natl Acad Sci U S A. 2011;108(40):16825–30.
121. Volarevic V, Al-Qahtani A, Arsenijevic N, et al. Interleukin-1 receptor antagonist (IL-1Ra) and IL-1Ra producing mesenchymal stem cells as modulators of diabetogenesis. Autoimmunity. 2010;43(4):255–63.
122. Hawryluk GW, Mothe AJ, Chamankhah M, et al. In vitro characterization of trophic factor expression in neural precursor cells. Stem Cells Dev. 2012;21(3):432–47.
123. Himes BT, Neuhuber B, Coleman C, et al. Recovery of function following grafting of human bone marrow-derived stromal cells into the injured spinal cord. Neurorehabil Neural Repair. 2006;20(2):278–96.
124. Hawryluk GW, Mothe A, Wang J, et al. An in vivo characterization of trophic factor production following neural precursor cell or bone marrow stromal cell transplantation for spinal cord injury. Stem Cells Dev. 2012;21(12):2222–38.
125. Caplan AI, Dennis JE. Mesenchymal stem cells as trophic mediators. J Cell Biochem. 2006;98(5):1076–84.
126. Ruff CA, Wilcox JT, Fehlings MG. Cell-based transplantation strategies to promote plasticity following spinal cord injury. Exp Neurol. 2012;235(1):78–90.
127. Sasaki M, Radtke C, Tan AM, et al. BDNF hypersecreting human mesenchymal stem cells promote functional recovery, axonal sprouting, and protection of corticospinal neurons after spinal cord injury. J Neurosci. 2011;29(47):14932–41.
128. Martinez AM, Goulart CO, Ramalho Bdos S, et al. Neurotrauma and mesenchymal stem cells treatment: from experimental studies to clinical trials. World J Stem Cells. 2014;6(2):179–94.

129. Li J, Lepski G. Cell transplantation for spinal cord injury: a systematic review. Biomed Res Int. 2013;78(2):64–75.
130. Sykova E, Homola A, Mazanec R, et al. Autologous bone marrow transplantation in patients with subacute and chronic spinal cord injury. Cell Transplant. 2006;15(8–9):675–87.
131. Yoon SH, Shim YS, Park YH, et al. Complete spinal cord injury treatment using autologous bone marrow cell transplantation and bone marrow stimulation with granulocyte macrophage-colony stimulating factor: phase I/II clinical trial. Stem Cells. 2007;25(8):2066–73.
132. Kumar A, Kumar S, Narayanan R, et al. Autologous bone marrow derived mononuclear cell therapy for spinal cord injury: a phase I/II clinical safety and primary efficacy data. Exp Clin Transplant. 2009;7(4):241–8.
133. Cristante AF, Barros-Filho TE, Tatsui N, et al. Stem cells in the treatment of chronic spinal cord injury: evaluation of somatosensitive evoked potentials in 39 patients. Spinal Cord. 2009;47(10):733–8.
134. Rao YJ, Zhu WX, Du ZQ, et al. Effectiveness of olfactory ensheathing cell transplantation for treatment of spinal cord injury. Genet Mol Res. 2014;13(2):4124–9.
135. Munoz-Quiles C, Santos-Benito FF, Llamusi MB, et al. Chronic spinal injury repair by olfactory bulb ensheathing glia and feasibility for autologous therapy. J Neuropathol Exp Neurol. 2009;68(12):1294–308.
136. Mackay-Sim A, Feron F, Cochrane J, et al. Autologous olfactory ensheathing cell transplantation in human paraplegia: a 3-year clinical trial. Brain. 2008;131(9):2376–86.
137. Lima C, Pratas-Vital J, Escada P, et al. Olfactory mucosa autografts in human spinal cord injury: a pilot clinical study. J Spinal Cord Med. 2006;29(3):191–203.
138. Hsu YC, Lee DC, Chiu IM. Neural stem cells, neural progenitors, and neurotrophic factors. Cell Transplant. 2007;16(2):133–50.
139. Moreno-Manzano V, Rodriguez-Jimenez FJ, Garcia-Rosello M, et al. Activated spinal cord ependymal stem cells rescue neurological function. Stem Cells. 2009;27(3):733–43.
140. Ronaghi M, Erceg S, Moreno-Manzano V, et al. Challenges of stem cell therapy for spinal cord injury: human embryonic stem cells, endogenous neural stem cells, or induced pluripotent stem cells? Stem Cells. 2010;28(1):93–9.
141. Yang Z, Zhang A, Duan H, et al. NT3-chitosan elicits robust endogenous neurogenesis to enable functional recovery after spinal cord injury. Proc Natl Acad Sci U S A (PNAS). 2015;112(43):13354–9.
142. Duan H, Ge W, Zhang A, et al. Transcriptome analyses reveal molecular mechanisms underlying functional recovery after spinal cord injury. Proc Natl Acad Sci U S A (PNAS). 2015;112(43):13360–5.
143. Dahlin LB. The biology of nerve injury and repair. J Am Soc Surg Hand. 2004;4(3):143–55.
144. Millesi H. Bridging defects: autologous nerve grafts. Acta Neurochir. 2007;100:37–8.
145. Gordon T, Tyreman N, Raji MA. The basis for diminished functional recovery after delayed peripheral nerve repair. J Neurosci. 2011;31(14):5325–34.
146. Lundborg G. A 25-year perspective of peripheral nerve surgery: evolving neuroscientific concepts and clinical significance. J Hand Ther. 2000;25(3):391–414.
147. Hart MK, Brannstrom T, Wiberg M, et al. Primary sensory neurons and satellite cells after peripheral axotomy in the adult rat: time course of cell death and elimination. Exp Brain Res. 2002;142(3):308–18.
148. Geuna S, Raimondo S, Ronchi G, et al. Chapter 3: histology of the peripheral nerve and changes occurring during nerve regeneration. Int Rev Neurobiol. 2009;87(Chapter 3):27–46.
149. Makwana M, Raivich G. Molecular mechanisms in successful peripheral regeneration. FEBS J. 2005;272(11):2628–38.
150. Calenda G, Strong TD, Pavlovich CP, et al. Whole genome microarray of the major pelvic ganglion after cavernous nerve injury: new insights into molecular profile changes after nerve injury. BJU Int. 2012;109(10):1552–64.
151. Burnett MG, Zager EL. Pathophysiology of peripheral nerve injury: a brief review. Neurosurg Focus. 2004;16(5):1–7.
152. Scheib J, Hoke A. Advances in peripheral nerve regeneration. Nat Rev Neurol. 2013;9(12):668–76.
153. Allodi I, Udina E, Navarro X. Specificity of peripheral nerve regeneration: interactions at the axon level. Prog Neurobiol. 2012;98(1):16–37.
154. McArthur JC, Yiannoutsos C, Simpson DM, et al. A phase II trial of nerve growth factor for sensory neuropathy associated with HIV infection. AIDS Clinical Trials Group team 291. Neurology. 2000;54(5):1080–8.
155. Zhang CG, Welin D, Novikov L, et al. Motorneuron protection by N-acetyl-cysteine after ventral root avulsion and ventral rhizotomy. Br J Plast Surg. 2005;58(6):765–73.
156. Schlosshauer B, Dreesmann L, Schaller HE, et al. Synthetic nerve guide implants in humans: a comprehensive survey. Neurosurgery. 2006;59(4):740–7.
157. Pabari A, Lloyd-Hughes H, Seifalian AM, et al. Nerve conduits for peripheral nerve surgery. Plast Reconstr Surg. 2014;133(6):1420–30.
158. Gu X, Ding F, Williams DF. Neural tissue engineering options for peripheral nerve regeneration. Biomaterials. 2014;35(24):6143–56.
159. Mobasseri SA, Terenghi G, Downes S. Micro-structural geometry of thin films intended for the inner lumen of nerve conduits affects nerve repair. J Mater Sci Mater Med. 2013;24(7):1639–47.
160. Hersel U, Dahmen C. Kessler H.RGD modified polymers: biomaterials for stimulated cell adhesion and beyond. Biomaterials. 2003;24(24):4385–415.
161. de Luca AC, Terenghi G, Downes S. Chemical surface modification of poly-epsilon-caprolactone improves Schwann cell proliferation for peripheral nerve repair. J Tissue Eng Regen Med. 2014;8(2):153–63.
162. Armstrong SJ, Wiberg M, Terenghi G, Kingham PJ. ECM molecules mediate both Schwann cell proliferation and activation to enhance neurite outgrowth. Tissue Eng. 2007;13(12):2863–70.
163. Lewin SL, Utley DS, Cheng ET, et al. Simultaneous treatment with BDNF and CNTF after peripheral nerve transection and repair enhances rate of functional recovery compared with BDNF treatment alone. Laryngoscope. 1997;107(7):992–9.
164. Fine EG, Decosterd I, Papaloizos M, et al. GDNF and NGF released by synthetic guidance channels support sciatic nerve regeneration across a long gap. Eur J NeuroSci. 2002;15(4):589–601.
165. Kalbermatten DF, Erba P, Mahay D, et al. Schwann cell strip for peripheral nerve repair. J Hand Surg Eur Vol. 2008;33(5):587–94.
166. Radtke C, Vogt PM. Peripheral nerve regeneration: a current perspective. Eplasty. 2009;9:e47.
167. Shiotani A, O'Malley BW Jr, Coleman ME, et al. Reinnervation of motor endplates and increased muscle fiber size after human insulin-like growth factor I gene transfer into the paralyzed larynx. Hum Gene Ther. 1998;9(14):2039–47.
168. Nagata K, Itaka K, Baba M, et al. Muscle-targeted hydrodynamic gene introduction of insulin-like growth factor-1 using polyplex nanomicelle to treat peripheral nerve injury. J Control Release. 2014;183(1):27–34.
169. Moimas S, Novati F, Ronchi G, et al. Effect of vascular endothelial growth factor gene therapy on post-traumatic peripheral nerve regeneration and denervation-related muscle atrophy. Gene Ther. 2013;20(10):1014–21.

170. Chen J, Chu YF, Chen JM, et al. Synergistic effects of NGF, CNTF and GDNF on functional recovery following sciatic nerve injury in rats. Adv Med Sci. 2010;55(1):32–42.
171. Cesar M, Roussanne-Domergue S, Coulet B, et al. Transplantation of adult myoblasts or adipose tissue precursor cells by high-density injection failed to improve reinnervated skeletal muscles. Muscle Nerve. 2008;37(2):219–30.
172. Halum SL, Naidu M, Delo DM, et al. Injection of autologous muscle stem cells (myoblasts) for the treatment of vocal fold paralysis: a pilot study. Laryngoscope. 2007;117(5):917–22.
173. Fishman JM, Tyraskis A, Maghsoudlou P, et al. Skeletal muscle tissue engineering: which cell to use? Tissue Eng B Rev. 2013;19(6):503–15.
174. Artico M, Cervoni L, Nucci F, et al. Birthday of peripheral nervous system surgery: the contribution of Gabriele Ferrara(1543-1627). Neurosurgery. 1996;39(2):380–2.
175. Seddon HJ. Nerve grafting and other unusual forms of nerve repair. Spec Rep Ser. 1954;282:389–417.
176. Millesi H, Meissl G, Berger A. The interfascicular nerve-grafting of the median and ulnar nerves. J Bone Joint Surg Am. 1972;54(4):727–50.
177. Moore AM. Nerve transfers to restore upper extremity function: a paradigm shift. Front Neurol. 2014;5(5):40.

# Tissue Repair and Regeneration Process Regulation

# 8

Biao Cheng, Min Xuan, Xiaobing Fu, Hongwei Liu, and Chunmeng Shi

## 8.1 Systemic Factors Affecting Tissue Repair and Regeneration

As the bio-psycho-social medical model concept is widely accepted, the impact of these factors on various diseases is increasingly being valued by clinicians. Trauma itself is a process in which external harmful stimuli affect the overall function through local effects. Wound healing, especially in the repair of large wounds, requires the mobilization of a whole body of psycho-neuro-immuno-endocrine-based regulatory mechanisms to respond to injury stimuli. As far as systemic factors are concerned, the health of the overall function plays an important role in wound healing, and factors such as the surrounding environment can also interfere with the outcome of the repair, which should be the focus of attention.

### 8.1.1 Psychological Factors

Trauma itself is a serious psychological and physiological stress. In addition, patients lack reasonable understanding of treatment and prognosis. Therefore, traumatic patients generally have negative psychological states such as anxiety, fear, and depression, while anxiety has a signal function; it sends a dangerous signal to the individual. When anxiety occurs, the human autonomic nervous system is activated, the cardiovascular system is strengthened, and the secretion of the adrenal glands is increased. It is characterized by rapid heartbeat, feeling cold or fever, shortness of breath, accompanied by experiences of nervousness, worry, fear, etc. Negative psychological state can impair the body's immune system function, which indirectly affects wound healing. On the contrary, a positive state of mind can promote the normal immune response of the human body. The neuro-endocrine axis of the body maintains a virtuous cycle.

The effects of psychology on wound healing include stress, as well as coping style, rich emotions, complex environment, and social support. British medical researchers found that patient's immune system function will be rapidly enhanced after the patient's depressed emotional vent; this method is economical and effective. British medical researchers asked 18 of the 36 patients to be clinically tested to write down their most unpleasant experiences, and 18 others wrote daily chores. It was found that the group of patients who wrote their inner feelings healed faster. It is confirmed that the venting and adjustment of emotions have a direct impact on wound healing.

The rapid development of cell molecular biology has enabled people to have an unprecedented understanding of life phenomenon and a certain understanding of the biological basis of psychological stress. Psychological stressors regulate the function and fate of various target cells through a neuro-immuno- endocrine network, affecting many physiological and pathological processes including wound healing. In short, under psychological stress, changes in all organs of the body (including plasticity changes in central nervous system function) are guided and based on changes in neuro-endocrine system [1].

#### 8.1.1.1 Psychological Stress and Nerve: the Role of the Endocrine System in Skin Healing

Under stress, intricate neuroendocrine changes include those in the renin angiotensin system (RAS) and hypothalamic-pituitary-adrenal (HPA) axis activation, commonly known as the stress system. Adrenal catecholamines act on the HPA axis to maintain energy balance, RAS redistributes blood

B. Cheng · M. Xuan
General Hospital of Southern Theater Command of Chinese People's Liberation Army, Guangzhou, China

X. Fu (✉)
The Chinese People's Liberation Army General Hospital, Beijing, China

H. Liu
The First Affiliated Hospital of Jinan University, Guangzhou, China

C. Shi
Army Medical University, Chongqing, China


X. Fu (ed.), *Regenerative Medicine in China*, https://doi.org/10.1007/978-981-16-1182-7_8

flow to ensure blood supply to vital organs, nerve stimulation and fear, sadness, anxiety, contradiction, nervous changes from the high-level cortex, visual, taste and body, and the humoral signals such as hormones and cytokines activate the stress system and induce a series of behavioral and physiological responses. In the process of stress regulation, there are multiple levels of action sites in the central and peripheral stress systems. In addition to the HPA axis and the blue nucleus/norepinephrine-parasympathetic sympathetic system, there are other stress sites and mechanisms in the body, such as central dopaminergic neurons and hippocampus, and peripheral reproductive hormone axis, growth hormone axis, thyroid axis, and metabolic reactions. They play an important role in cognitive integration and neurohormonal and neurochemical effects in stress response. In order to adapt to psychological stress, neutrophils release substance P (SP) and activate mast cells or other inflammatory cells together with other inflammatory mediators from the sensory nerve to participate in the inflammatory response. The corticosteroid-releasing factor (CRF) and SP initiate a systemic stress response by activating neuroendocrine pathways such as the sympathetic nervous system, hypothalamic–pituitary axis, and the renin–angiotensin system. They release stress hormones (such as catecholamine, cortisol, growth hormones, glucagon, and renin). The skin and its attachments are important target organs for major stress mediators (such as corticotropic releasing hormone, ACTH, cortisol, catecholamine, prolactin, substance P, and nerve growth factor) and potential stress response immunoregulators. More skin exposure to a variety of exogenous and endogenous stressors than other organs provides an ideal clinical model for studying peripheral and systemic responses to stress, including psychological stress.

Brain–skin contact and local neuroimmune endocrine loops are both the pathophysiological basis of skin function and related changes, and the triggering factor for stress triggering and aggravation. To study the effects of psychological stress on wound healing, Detillion et al. performed adrenalectomy to remove endogenous cortisol to observe changes in psychological stress in solitary wound healing. It was found that positive social interaction participated in the activity change of HPA axis in rodents, which can promote wound healing. Ebrecht surveyed 24 non-smokers to determine the patient's sensory anxiety, healthy behaviors, and personal factors, as well as salivary cortisol levels at 2 weeks before and after biopsy. The results showed that the healing rate was negatively correlated with the perceived stress scale (PSS) and the general health questionnaire (GHQ).

Activation of the stress system leads to adaptive behavioral changes and physical changes. In addition to being closely related to the nervous and endocrine systems, the most basic stress hormones (glucocorticoids and catecholamine) can affect major immune functions and T helper (Th1) response to Th2 selectivity. To a certain extent, they may enhance the production of pro-inflammatory cytokines and activate the adrenocorticotropic hormone–mast cell–histamine axis, thereby feeding back the stress system and enhancing or reducing the immune response.

#### 8.1.1.2 The Role of Psychological Stress and the Immune System in Skin Wound Healing

Psychoneuroimmunology (PNI) is a discipline that has studied immune and endocrine, central, and peripheral nervous systems for nearly 40 years. Neurotransmitters, hormones, and neuropeptides have been shown to regulate immune cells and communicate with neural tissue by secreting large amounts of cytokines. A key role of the central and peripheral nerves is to maintain cell-mediated (Th1) and humoral (Th2) immune responses, and psycho-neuroimmunology becomes the pathophysiological basis for understanding the link between the immune systems. Stress-induced immune disorders are sufficient to cause health-related consequences. PNI is the basis for a close correlation between the spirit/brain and the immune system.

The relationship between the central nervous system and the immune system is mainly accomplished by chemical messengers secreted by nerve cells, endocrine cells, and immune cells. Psychological stressors can damage this network. Early investigations have found that mental stress affects the body's immune function, and stress plays a non-negligible role in the immune system. Emotional anger is associated with corticosteroid secretion, immune function, and non-adaptive changes in surgical recovery. Assuming the relationship between extroverted and introverted emotional anger or non-anger control and delayed healing, the results do show that human emotional anger is closely related to wound healing. In acute stress, endogenous stress hormones enhance the skin's immunity by increasing lymphocyte trafficking and cytokine gene expression at the site of antigenic invasion. In acute wounds, when women are in high stress, there are two key cytokines IL-1 and IL-8 in the wound area, indicating that the production of pro-inflammatory factors in the local microenvironment of wound healing is affected by psychological stress.

The regulation of the immune system by psychological stress is complex, so the effect on wound healing also shows different outcomes. As Weinman's research suggests, the openness of traumatic experience can lead to upregulation of the immune function, which is the key to promoting wound healing. In order to confirm that stress increases wound infection, Rojas found that the skin wounds had viable bacteria through quantitative observation. It was found that inhibition stress (RST) delayed the healing ability by 30%, and the conditional pathogen increased compared with the control group, and was statistically significant ($P < 0.05$). Further studies have found that RST-induced glucocorticoids play an important role in the mechanism of bacterial clearance. If treated with the glucocorticoid receptor antagonist RU486, pathogenic bacteria will be reduced ($P < 0.05$). Therefore, stress-damaged bacterial clearance during wound healing leads to a marked increase in the incidence of conditioned pathogen infections; psychological stress delays wound healing, reduces immune/inflammatory responses, and also influences bacterial clearance. In short, the complex effects of psychological stress on the immune response present a variety of patterns of response to wound healing.

The skin's nerve and the central nervous system (including psychology), the endocrine axis, and the immune system are a complete stress system. To fully understand the various physiological and pathological functions of the skin, including cell growth, immunity, inflammation, and healing, it is necessary to have a deeper understanding of the dense sensory neural network, the complex central nervous system (including psychology), the release of the multi-layered surface, as well as active specific receptors expressed on the target cells of a large number of skin.

#### 8.1.1.3 Related Signal Pathways Involved in Psychological Stress and Cytokines in Wound Healing

Psychological stress changes the cytokines around and in the brain, but physiological evidence is still lacking. At present, it is necessary to study the role of acute and chronic psychological stress factors in the cytokine network in humans, explore the pathophysiological significance of cytokines in the process of psychological stress, and investigate whether cytokines play a synergistic or antagonistic role in complex networks. The balance between pro-inflammatory cytokines (such as IL-1b, IL-6, TNF-α) and anti-inflammatory cytokines (such as IL-1 receptor antagonists, IL-4, IL-10, TGF-β) reflects neurological and mental strength, neuroimmunity, and neuroinflammatory reactions. Maes suggested that psychological stress as an immobilization can lead to activation of the inflammatory response system. Moreover, stress-induced cytokine secretion can induce and maintain depressive symptoms. Psychological stress (such as sleep deprivation) will reduce skin function recovery and increase the activity of IL-1β, TNF-α, and NK cells. Therefore, the effects of psychological stress on cytokines also affect skin function and wound healing. Wound healing is an orderly, complex physiological process involving inflammation, proliferation, and shaping, which are effected by different cells, cytokines, and matrix metalloproteinases. Cytokines are involved in inflammation and immune responses, as well as cell differentiation and proliferation. Therefore, changes in wound healing caused by the effects of psychological stress on cytokines have also become the focus of research. It has been shown that in animals, sustained stress induces changes in the kinetics of epidermal proinflammatory cytokines, such as IL-1α and IL-1β, as well as the expression of growth factors in the early stages of wound healing. The inflammatory response mediated is often considered to be a predisposing factor for scar formation. It is currently one of the strategies for the treatment and prevention of keloids by inhibiting the IL-6 receptor and its downstream effectors or molecules.

Environmental stress-induced biological and psychological changes are often accomplished by a number of signaling proteins, particularly in the HPA axis. This system also potentially acts on reactive oxygen species (ROS) and acts on cytokines, and finally controls DNA regulation to methylate the promoter regions of these genes. This also suggests that environmental stressors have mechanisms that induce long- term biological changes. In addition, two pathways for stress signaling, the JNK/SAPK and p38 pathways, were studied. The core molecules of these two pathways are c-Jun N-terminal kinase (JNK) and p38 kinase, which are also called stress-activated protein kinase 1/2 (SAPK1/2) and p38, both belonging to mitogen-activated protein kinase (MAPK). The amygdala is thought to be the key to mediating stress-induced changes in hippocampal function. Yang demonstrated that stress immediately causes phosphorylation of extracellular signal-regulated kinase (ERK) in the CA1 region of the hippocampus and central amygdala (CEA) and basolateral amygdala (BLA), indicating that the signal path is activated.

The team of Academician Xiaobing Fu has made some explorations in this regard. First, the animal model of psychological stress was observed for wound healing. C57BL/6 mice aged 6–8 weeks were used (provided by SPF Animal Laboratory, Institute of Neuroscience, Fourth Military Medical University). They were taken into lab 1 week before the experiment to adapt to the new breeding environment. The stress mice model was prepared according to the restraint stress model produced by Padgett et al. in 1998. After establishing this stress model, the serum cortisol level in mice was four times higher than that in the control group. At 20:00 h every night, the mice were introduced into a well-ventilated 50 mL centrifugal tube (four rows of appropriate holes were placed on the wall of the centrifuge tube, a hole was made at the tip of the centrifuge tube, and a hole in the middle of the centrifugal tube cover so that the mouse's tail reached out). Activities restriction,fasting and water cessation was done during period. After the mouse enters the 50 mL centrifuge tube, it cannot be turned over and turned around, it is not movable. After 12 h of restraint, the mice were taken out at 8:00 h the next morning. After three times of restraint, the model of full-thickness skin defect in the back of the mouse was made. (A special puncher was used on both sides of the back spine of the mouse, 0.8 mm in diameter, 0.64 $mm^2$ in area, and two round full-thickness skin wounds were cut), and continue to bind five times after the wound was made. At the same time, the control group and the stress group were fasted, water-free, and wounded in the same period of time, so that the experimental group and the control group had the same conditions except for the constraint factor. In a certain period after trauma, the re-epithelialization rate of the wound in the stress group was higher than that in the unstressed group. Reverse transcription PCR was used to detect the expression of ACE, AT1, and AT2 mRNA in skin tissue around the wound (Figs. 8.1, 8.2, and 8.3).

Compared with normal controls, the expression levels of ACE, AT1, and AT2 mRNA increased after infection, and the expression levels of ACE and AT1 were down-regulated and then increased in the stress group, while AT2 was not down-regulated and raised immediately after wounding. The peaks of the three mRNA expressions in the stress group and the unstressed group differed at time points. From the relative expression level, the expression level of AT2 was lower than that of ACE and AT1 in normal control tissues, but the up-regulation of AT2 expression was highest after trauma.

Images acquired with the Olympus Model FV-1000 laser scanning confocal microscope and image acquisition system (Figs. 8.4, 8.5, and 8.6).

It can be seen from the figure that in the skin of the normal control group, ACE is slightly expressed in the basal layer of the epidermis and the connective tissue of the dermis. At2 is expressed in the basal layer of the epidermis and in the hair follicles and sweat glands. At1 is not expressed.

In Figs. 8.4, 8.5, and 8.6, C represents the unstressed group, S represents the stress group, d represents the post-traumatic days, and M is the abbreviation of merge. Red is ACE, blue is AT1, and green is AT2. Compared with normal tissues, the expression of ACE, AT1, and AT2 was enhanced after trauma, both in the stress group and in the unstressed group. ACE is mainly expressed in dermal connective tissue. The expression of AT1 is the weakest and is relatively strong outside the hair follicle. AT2 is expressed in the epidermal base and hair follicles and sweat glands. There is almost no overlap in the expression of ACE and AT2. This study showed that the wound healing rate of mice under moderate stress was significantly higher than that of the unstressed group.

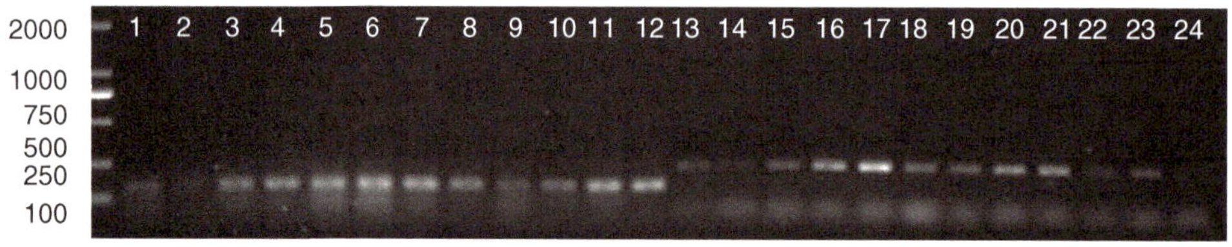


**Fig. 8.1** ACE mRNA expression

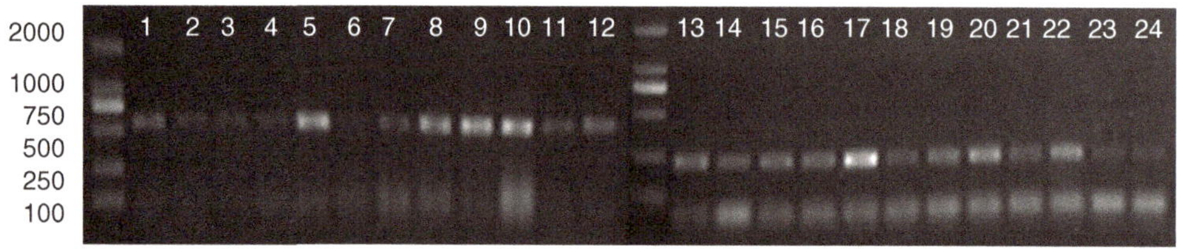


**Fig. 8.2** AT1 mRNA expression

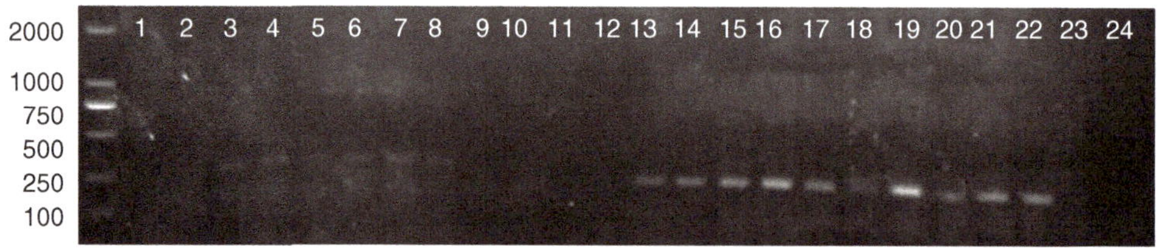


**Fig. 8.3** AT2 mRNA expression

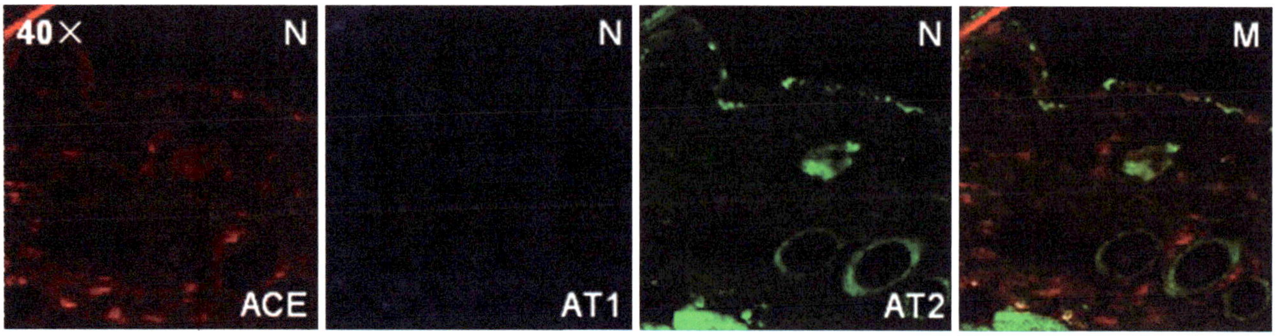


**Fig. 8.4** Expression of ACE, AT1, and AT2 in normal skin tissue

Tips that moderate stress may accelerate wound healing. The amount of ACE, AT1, and AT2 in the local tissue RAS system during wound healing was significantly different between the stress group and the unstressed group. In short, stress affects the speed and quality of wound healing. Adjusting stress levels can help improve tissue repair. Activation of the local angiotensin system in skin tissue may be one of the stress response pathways. Reactive changes in Ang I, Ang II, and ACE in systemic and local skin tissues may occur during stress response.

In addition, important members of the Xiaobing Fu academic team also used music therapy to psychologically intervene in 62 surgical patients, 55 of whom were satisfied [2]. After the music-assisted intervention, the tension was improved, the pain was relieved, and the clinical score was based on the original score. Declined 28 people were reduced from VAS > 8 points to 6–8 points; 27 people were reduced from high (6–8 points) to good (3–5 points). Another five people felt relieved, but not obvious (no change in VAS score). Only two people reported no change; the patients were male and aged <30 years. Observing the effect of music therapy on the patient's heart rate, playing light music for the patient during the operation, the patient's heart rate decreased significantly, and there was significant statistical difference before the music treatment ($P < 0.05$). The patient's systolic blood pressure also decreased. The change in diastolic blood pressure was more pronounced and there was a statistical difference ($P < 0.05$). All patients underwent orthopedic suture removal 5–7 days after surgery, and the wounds healed well without a significant difference. It shows that patients with plastic surgery can have anxiety psychological stress before surgery, and the proportion is higher than other surgical patients. Increased responsiveness of systemic Ang I, Ang II, and ACE may occur during stress response. The blood in the preoperative and postoperative period is mainly the change of ACE content in the important components of the angiotensin system. The use of music therapy during surgery can improve the patient's anxiety state. Although there is no significant change in the time of surgical wound healing, the pain of surgery has been significantly improved.

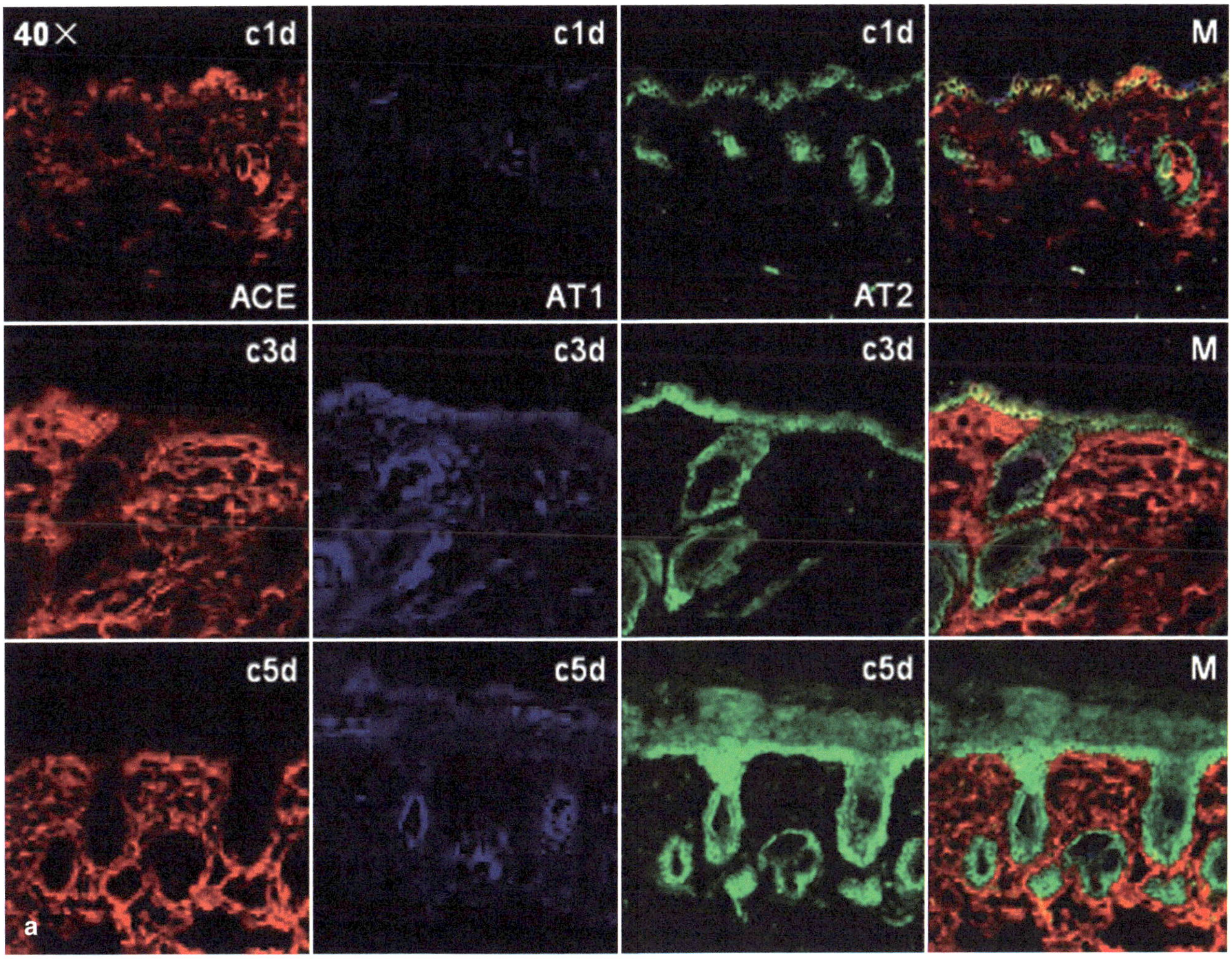


**Fig. 8.5** Expression of control group ACE, AT1, and AT2

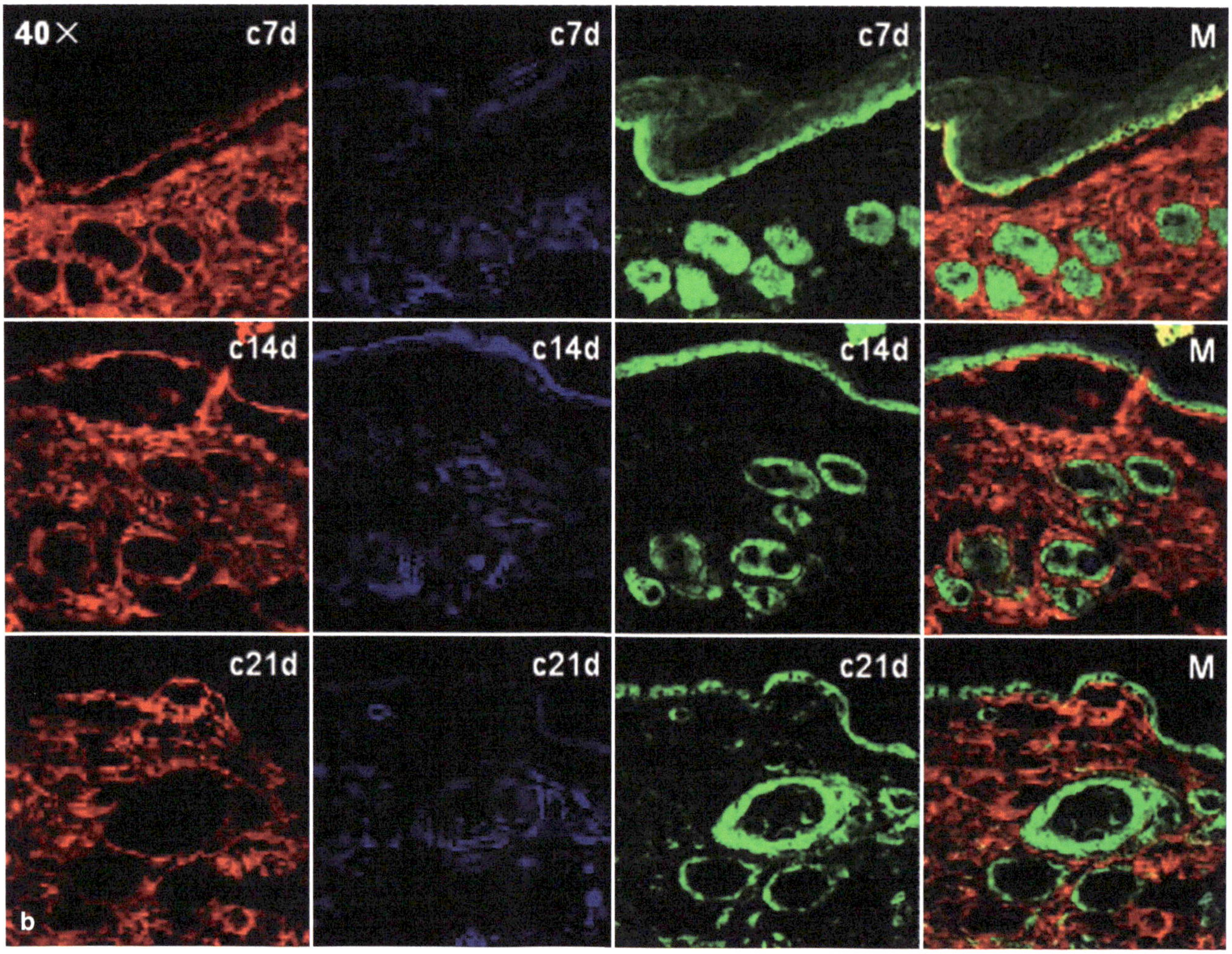


**Fig. 8.5** (continued)

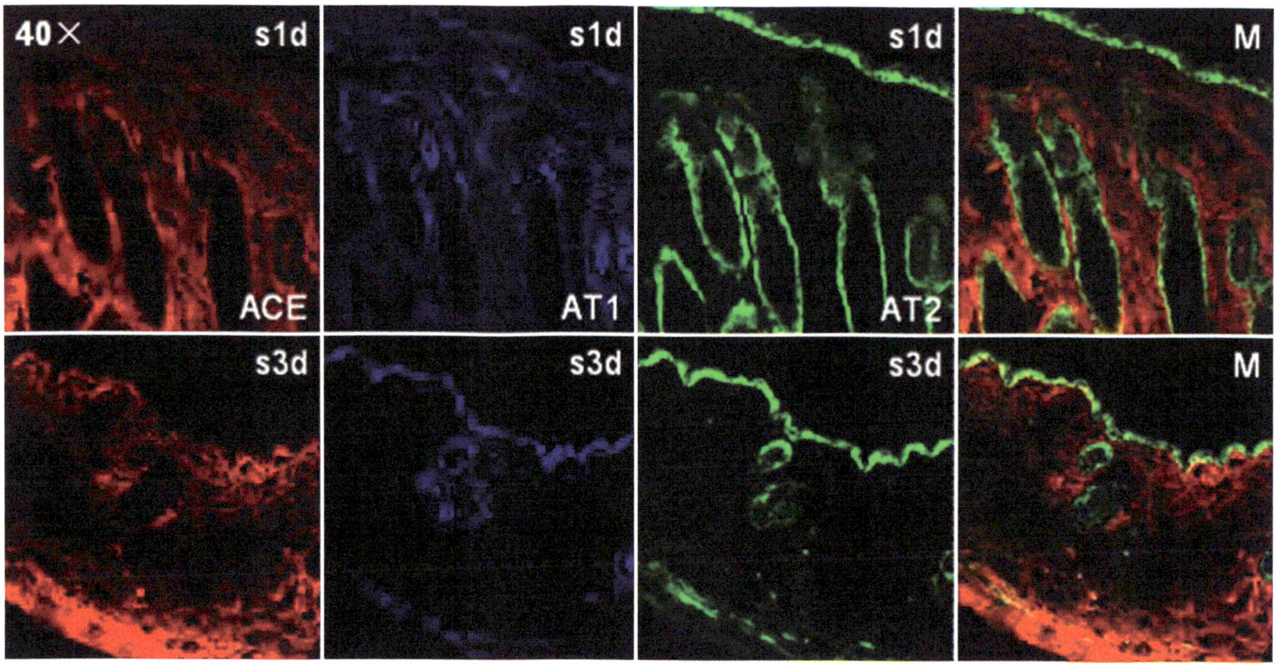


**Fig. 8.6** Expression of ACE, AT1, and AT2 in stress group

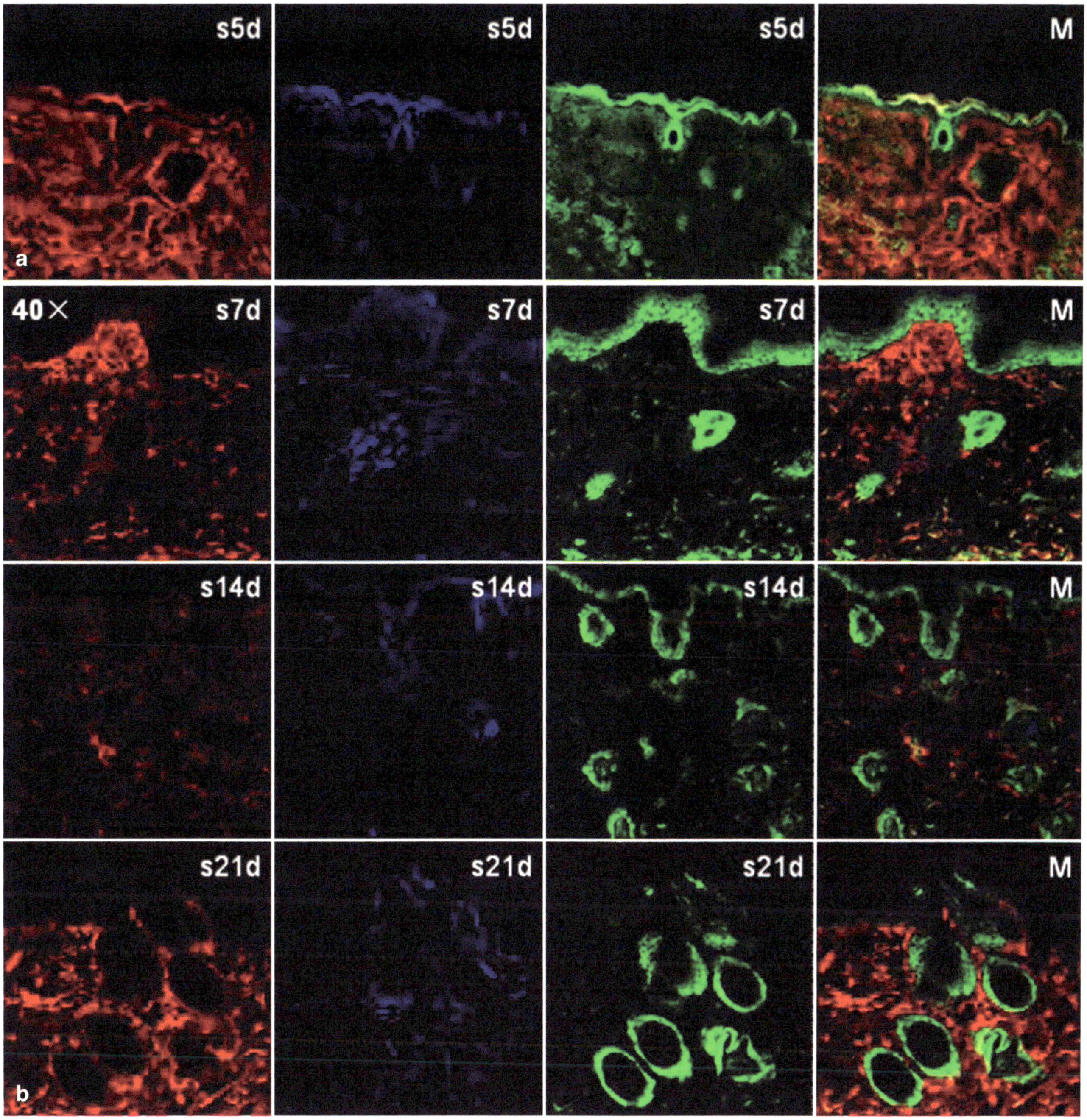


**Fig. 8.6** (continued)

The whole study suggests that the psychological stress system may have some connection with the systemic and local RAS system, that is, when the skin is damaged, the systemic and local RAS are activated, and the tissue local ACE, Ang II, and other components regulate the biological behavior of repairing cells and the producing of biologically active target proteins (neuropeptides, heat shock proteins, etc.) and changes on the phenotype of repair cells, thereby affecting cell proliferation and apoptosis, angiogenesis, and collagen synthesis activities, and ultimately regulating skin damage repair process. This study used music-assisted interventions to explore whether music can help alleviate stress during surgery. It will provide new ideas and means for improving the healing outcome of tissue fibrosis, repairing difficult wounds, and treating scars.

Psychological stress has made some progress in the study of the effects of wound healing. Psychological stress involves a complex network of the central nervous system, endocrine system, and immune system. When psychological stress changes, breaking the equilibrium state of this network will lead to the changes in body physiology and pathology, especially in skin damage repair activities, and also cause the changes in tissue healing speed and outcome. However, there are many unknowns about the detailed mechanisms of how the "psychological" becomes a "physical" physiological response, especially the changes in the number of neuroendocrine substances under stress, and the transmission pathways of stress signals. In addition, we need to study the relationship between the regularity of these substances and the levels at which the regulation of stress are mutually activated or mutually inhibited to ensure the continuity and effectiveness of the body's regulation, further research is needed. Understanding the psychological, neurological, immune, and endocrine regulation of the skin helps to provide new strategies for accelerating the speed of skin tissue repair and improving the quality of skin healing.

### 8.1.2 Age

Age is the main systemic factor that affects wound healing. As elderly patients grow with age, the body's ability to regulate is reduced, body water is reduced, and various metabolic rates slow down. After being stimulated by external damage, the stress response is weak, the immune system response is poor, and cell movement, proliferation, and maturation are significantly slowed down, which can affect wound healing. Especially in the early stage of injury, the inflammatory response is weak, the secretion of various cytokines is insufficient, the regeneration of new aging is delayed, the synthesis of collagen fibers is reduced, and the skin becomes dry, resulting in slow wound contraction. Children and young people have stronger metabolism, cell proliferation, collagen synthesis, and epithelial regeneration time are shorter than the elderly, as well so that wound healing is faster.

#### 8.1.2.1 Biological Structure and Related Functional Characteristics of Aging Skin

The biological structure and related functional characteristics of aging skin are shown in Table 8.1 [3].

1. Epidermis
   As the outermost layer of the skin, as the age increases, the size of the keratinocytes increases, the shape is irregular, the number decreases, the volume of the cells increases, and the inter-cell desmosomes gradually disappear. The nipple and corresponding protrusion of the skin are flattened, and the connection with the dermis is loose, resulting in a decrease in the skin barrier function, a decrease in hydration ability, and a dry skin. At the same time, due to aging, there are fewer basal cells or germinal cells with mitosis, and thus the production of correspond-

**Table 8.1** Major structural and functional changes in aging skin and related clinical manifestations

| Skin composition | Primary function | Changes after aging | Functional change | Clinical symptoms |
|---|---|---|---|---|
| Epidermis | Barrier between the body and the environment | Cuticle thinning, renewal of keratinocytes is slow, the lipid components of the stratum corneum are reduced, the number of melanocytes is reduced, the acidification is weakened, and the PH value changes | The integrality of the skin barrier is weakened, the recovery of the barrier after injury slows down, the wound healing slows down, the stratum corneum hickens, and the photosensitivity increases | Dry skin, increased sensitivity to bacterial, viral and fungal infections, increased incidence ofcontact dermatitis and irritant dermatitis, slow wound healing/chronic wounds |
| Dermis | To provide elasticity and tension | Thinned, the proliferation of fibroblast was decreased, the ability of collagen I and III synthesis was decreased, the collagen fiber and elastic fiber were decreased | Reduced elasticity, reduced resistance to all kinds of damage and friction | Wrinkles, delayed wound healing, blisters, ulcers |
| Subcutaneous fat | Support, insulation | Decrease | Reduced support for the dermis and blood vessels | The sensitivity to various damages increased and the heat regulation function weakened |
| Blood vessel | To provide nourishment | The structure of blood vessels atrophied, the density of blood vessels decreased and the blood vessels became thinner | Reduced blood supply, reduced nutrition, reduced response to changes in stress | Contusion, purpura, reduced heat regulation |
| Sweat gland | Sebum secretion | Decreased sebum production and secretion | Reduced sebum on the skin surface | Dry skin, hyperplasia of sebaceous glands |
| Hair follicle | Hair production | Less hair density, less melanin production | Less hair density, less melanin production | Hair removal |
| Nerve ending | Sense | Diminish | Reduced sensitivity to changes in pressure and heat | Increased risk of skin damage |

ing stratum corneum cells may be reduced. Under normal conditions, the epidermis forms cells from the basal layer and gradually proliferates, divides, and moves upward until the outermost layer of the epidermis, and the cells gradually form keratin, and the cell dynamic process from the basal layer to the stratum corneum is keratinized. With age, the ability of epidermal cells to divide and proliferate is reduced, the rate of cell renewal slows down, and the connection between the epidermis and the dermis is more toward the direction of shear. These are the causes of epidermal flattening.

2. Leather
   There are fibroblasts, various types of fibers, matrix, and accessory structures such as sweat glands, hair follicles, and sebaceous glands in the dermis. With the increase of age, the number of fibroblasts decreases, the subcellular level shows less cytoplasm, the lipid brown particles increase, and the cell viability decreases. The number of elastic fibers and collagen fibers is reduced and the arrangement is disordered. The synthesis capacity of the extracellular matrix is reduced, the activity of collagenase is increased, and the decomposition of collagen is increased, resulting in a thinning of the dermis. There is elastic tissue degeneration, mainly characterized by thickening, curling, and kinking of elastic fibers, forming amorphous, granular materials, disordered or aggregated, deposited in dermal tissue. It is generally believed to be caused by the degradation of normal elastic fibers and the abnormal expression of elastic fiber components such as elastin.
3. Blood Vessels and Nerves
   As the age increases, small blood vessels begin to degenerate, capillary vasospasm gradually disappears, and the number of capillaries decreases. The neurological structure undergoes degeneration, the pain sensitivity value decreases, the stress ability to various stimuli decreases, and the tissue regeneration ability becomes weak.
4. Skin Appendages
   The accessory organs of the skin mainly include the sweat glands, sebaceous glands, and hair. Due to the decrease in the number of skin blood vessels in the elderly, the number of viable glands is reduced, the function of the secreted cells is disordered, and even fibrosis occurs, the amount of secretion is decreased, and the response to various types of stimulation is lowered. The skin is an organ that is very sensitive to sex hormones. Therefore, sweat glands, sebaceous glands, and hair are regulated by sex hormones. As the age increases, the hormone secretion capacity decreases and the hormone level decreases, resulting in enlarged pores, whitening, reduction, and thinning of hair. Sebum production and sebaceous gland morphology cannot maintain parallel changes and balances. Human skin is smooth and sebum plays an important role. The skin evaporation ability of the elderly is mostly lost, and the heat dissipation function is obviously degraded.
5. Other
   The number of mast cells, Langerhans cells, and melanocytes in the dermis gradually decreases with age. The reduction in the number and function of such cells in the skin tissue of the elderly can cause a decrease in the mediator effect of immune cells, which affects the healing process of the wound. The number of melanocytes in aging skin decreases. The melanocytes are larger in volume and the dendrites are increased, which may also cause neuroimmune disorders and affect the wound healing.

   The skin barrier function also changes. The stratum corneum of the outer layer of the skin serves as a barrier between the body and the external environment. In the case of aging, the lipid component is reduced, resulting in a weakened barrier function and a dry skin. With aging, the pH of the skin changes. The weakening of the skin barrier function causes various external stimuli and antigens to easily enter the skin, and the incidence of skin diseases such as allergies and contact dermatitis increases.

#### 8.1.2.2 The Impact of Aging on the Healing Process

In general, the purpose of wound repair is to restore damaged tissue and ensure its original integrity. Much of the damage is caused by changes in gene expression, and when aging occurs, c-Fos expression decreases at the transcriptional initiation level. In addition, transcription factors such as NK-κB, AP-1, and Sp-1 were reduced, and several growth-related genes decreased with the activity of E2F transcription family members. At the same time, hormone levels in tissues, mitogen growth factors, and receptor changes in these factors are also responsible for delayed healing of wounds in elderly patients.

1. Infiltration of Inflammatory Cells
   After trauma, the infiltration ability of inflammatory cells (including monocytes, macrophages, and B lymphocytes) around the wound in elderly patients is reduced; these changes will cause delays in healing. In addition, the number of dermal cells in the elderly patients decreased, resulting in decreased release of histamine and decreased migration of capillary endothelial cells, which also affected the rate of healing.
2. Repair Cell Proliferation and Differentiation
   Experiments have shown that the ability of old rat mesenchymal cells to transform into myofibroblasts decreased after injury, which affected the closure time of the wound. As age increases, the number and proliferation activity of fibroblasts decrease, affecting their ability to produce and

regulate collagen, which is the key factor leading to the above performance.

3. Synthesis and Deposition of the Matrix
An important step in wound healing is the filling of the wound and the filling of the defect. The collagen in the elderly patients changes in both quantity and quality, resulting in poor filling and slowing of contraction. At the same time, the display of collagen in the elderly patients is disordered, and the decrease in the diameter and number of elastic fibers causes the tension to become smaller, which not only causes the wound healing to be hindered, but also makes the wound after healing easy to crack.
4. Epithelialization
Animal experiments have shown that the expression of matrix metalloproteinase-1, 9 and matrix metalloproteinase inhibitor-1 in aged animals is significantly lower than that of young animals, resulting in changes in the biological behavior of keratinocytes. It causes delayed reepithelization during wound healing.

#### 8.1.2.3 The Impact of Other Changes in Aging on Healing

Wound healing is a complex and orderly process. In normal healing conditions, the recovery of the skin barrier is dependent on keratinocyte migration of the skin, contraction of fibroblasts, and reconstruction of the extracellular matrix. In the elderly, wound healing is impaired, characterized by slowing of keratinocyte proliferation, decreased rate of epithelialization, decreased proliferation of fibroblasts, slowing of granulation tissue formation, and excessive inflammatory response. The nervous, endocrine, and immune systems are widely distributed in the body. The nervous system has synaptic-mediated structural continuity, and its branch ends govern various tissues and organs. Taking the skin as an example, there is a difference in the innervation of epidermal keratinocytes. In addition to keratinocytes, dendritic cells with special effects in the epidermis, Langerhans cells, melanocytes, Merkel cells, and fibroblasts in the dermis are closely related to nerve fibers. Broadly speaking, the endocrine and immune systems can be regarded as the efferent part of the nervous system reflex arc. Stress can directly or indirectly affect the functional status of the three major systems. The mode of action between the systems is not only direct or indirect, but also simultaneous and sequential. The nature of interaction between systems can be enhanced, weakened, modified, allowed, or coordinated by frequency conversion, time change, variable force, etc. The attribute of the interaction between systems, there are physiological and pathological points, is the process of mutual transformation of quality and quantity. The neural, immune, and endocrine networks more closely encompass the interactions and multiple connections between the three systems. As the age continues to grow, the internal environment of the elderly may be on the edge of a relatively "unbalanced" state or "unbalanced", manifested by decreased stress, nervous system disorders, decreased hormone levels, low immune function, the ability of the body to repair and maintain its own stability is also reduced. How to adjust the body's nervous system, hormone secretion level and immunity to the state of young people, and make the metabolism of cells (especially adult stem cells) re-energize to reverse or delay the process of aging, has become a new direction of current geriatric research [4].

1. Changes in the Nervous System of the Skin
The skin contains a dense network of sensory nerves, and the intact nervous system is essential for wound healing. Experiments have confirmed that primary afferent sensory nerves as nociceptors are extremely important for initiating inflammatory responses and successful tissue repair. With the onset of aging, this system partially loses the function of releasing factors, leading to delayed healing of wounds. At the same time, many physiological functions of the skin (such as metabolism, immunity, etc.) are also inseparable from nerve innervation. In addition, the neuropeptide released from the sensory nerves in the skin not only satisfies the requirements of innervation in the skin, but also is an important substance that directly regulates the function of keratinocytes, Langerhans cells, mast cells, microvascular endothelial cells, and infiltrating immune cells. In particular, tachykinin, substance P (SP), calcitonin gene-related peptide (CGRP), vasoactive intestinal peptide and somatostatin on the proliferation of cells, the production of cytokines, etc. have a regulatory effect. With increasing age, the release of sensory neuropeptides is reduced, and the effects on various types of cells in the skin are weakened.
2. The Effect of Hormonal Changes on the Skin
Sex hormones are another important factor in wound healing. Providing repaired patients with direct or indirect hormone replacement therapy can increase cell proliferation activity and cytokine production, affect the post-injury inflammatory response, increase matrix deposition, and promote epithelial healing in elderly patients. With age, changes in estrogen and androgen levels after menopause directly affect the phenotype of endothelial cells and fibroblasts, and play a role in wound repair by regulating their adhesion and proliferation behavior. In addition, studies have found that inflammatory response changes in male patients are significantly different from female patients, resulting in delayed healing of acute wounds. Sex hormones play an important role in the body's local and humoral immunity, which may be the main mechanism affecting healing.
3. Changes in the Immune Function of the Skin
Compared with young people, the immune function of the skin of the elderly has changed significantly. Mast cells, monocytes, and neutrophils increase, and the num-

ber of t lymphocytes also increases with skin aging, but their response to external antigens is low. In contrast, the number of Langerhans cells and the ability to migrate are reduced. A decrease in skin immune function and barrier function leads to an increased incidence of bacterial, viral, and fungal infections in the elderly.

4. Skin Blood Vessels and Blood Supply Changes
   With age, there is a certain regular change in the degradation and disorder of small blood vessels. Many capillaries and veins are missing. The nipples in the skin tissue disappear, the capillary sputum gradually disappears, and the number of capillaries is inevitably reduced. According to relevant research, the number of blood vessels in the skin of the elderly is reduced by at least 30%. As skin aging worsens, the number of vascular reductions is more prevalent and more severe. The skin damaged by light has only a few swelling and distortion of blood vessels. The blood flow of elderly patients is reduced by 35%, which leads to the failure of local perfusion, which cannot meet the oxygen and nutrients needed for wound healing, and is also the main reason for poor wound healing.
5. Changes in the Secretion Capacity of Growth Factors in the Skin
   The characteristics of aging are mainly manifested by the decrease of the overall function of the cell, and this relative effect is regulated by growth factors. The application of transforming growth factor-β1 (TGF-β1) in local and system can enhance the healing of wounds and regulate the functions of several types of repair-related cells, such as matrix production and angiogenesis. TGF-β1 plays a role in regulating cell differentiation and extracellular matrix formation in the late stage of healing. Vascular Endothelial Growth Factor (VEGF) is a polypeptide that is also a potential, special mitogen that promotes endothelial cell proliferation, migration, and endothelial surface retraction (allowing vascular penetration) and angiogenesis in living organisms and affects wound healing and tissue reshaping. Animal experiments have found that the expression level of growth factors in aged animals is lower than that of younger animals.
6. Skin Barrier Function and Dryness
   Skin barrier function and dryness refers to a series of symptoms such as tightness, desquamation, and itching caused by moisture or lipid deficiency. It is the most common skin problem in the elderly. The self-repairing ability of dry skin is weakened, and the healing rate of skin wounds (such as pressure sores, scratches, etc.) is slowed down and the skin is intact.

The main members of the team of Xiaobing's Fu academicians collected medical records of hospitalized patients with plastic surgery in a plastic surgery department in a southern hospital from July 2011 to December 2013 [5]. 120 cases of refractory wounds were screened for 2 months of non-healing of skin tissue defects. The causes of wound formation, age, location of wounds, and length of hospital stay were retrospectively investigated. 2136 inpatients were counted, including 120 patients with refractory wounds, accounting for 5.6%. The main cause of wound formation was metabolic disease (43.3%), followed by traumatic infection (20%) and tumor (20%) ($\chi^2 = 62.917$, $P < 0.01$). The high-incidence age of patients with wound healing was 40–60 years old, followed by 60–80 years old ($\chi^2 = 29.562$, $P < 0.01$).

The most difficult sites for refractory wounds were limbs (61.6%), and the most common were the feet (38.3%) ($\chi^2 = 17.546$, $P = 0.002$). Middle-aged and elderly patients with metabolic diseases become the main group of refractory wounds. Unhealthy wounds often occur in the limbs, which seriously affects the patient's actions, causing delays in hospitalization, and bringing great burdens to family members and society.

Later, the team of Academician Xiaobing Fu conducted a more in-depth study on the differential expression and correlation of autophagy in the healing process of acute wound healing in rats of different age groups [6]. Autophagy, a system involved in intracellular degradation during aging, has been shown to be closely related to the body's aging. Skin tissue, as part of the organism's organic whole, may also be associated with autophagy. The role of autophagy in age-related changes in human skin is still unclear. The changes of autophagy-related genes LC3, Beclin-1, and p62 expression during acute wound healing in rats of different age groups were studied to observe the difference of autophagy activity between the old and young rats in the normal skin and in the process of wound healing.

SPF grade SD rats (provided by Guangdong Experimental Animal Center) were selected, in which young rats were 3 months old, $n = 16$, and weighed 200–300 g. The older rat group were 18 months old, $n = 16$, weight 600–800 g. All of the above were half male and female, and the mixed feed was kept in a single cage.

They were exposed to natural light and the room temperature was controlled at around 25 °C. After 3 days of routine feeding in rats, the hair in the back area was removed with an electric razor and hair removal cream, and 10% chloral hydrate was anesthetized at a dose of 3 mL/kg. After anesthesia was successful, a skin puncher was used at each 1.5 cm on each side of the spine in the middle of the back of the rat, a circular full-thickness skin resection wound of 1.2 cm in diameter was made, the whole skin and superficial fascia were cut, and then wetted with physiological saline to wipe the wound blood, and the wound covered with aseptic dressing, and the above treatment was carried out in a single cage. The wounds of the 0th, 4th,

7th, 14th, and 21st days were taken from the two groups. All the specimens were collected under aseptic conditions. The wounds and surrounding skin specimens were cut from the outer edge of the new epithelium at 2–3 mm. Part of the specimen was fixed in a 10% neutral formalin solution and a portion was stored in a −80 °C refrigerator. The specimens were placed in a 10% neutral formalin solution for 48 h and then routinely dehydrated, embedded in paraffin, serially sectioned, and sliced 5 μm thick. Under light microscopy, in normal skin, the younger group of rats had thicker epidermis, and the subcutaneous tissue and dermis were not clearly defined. In the elderly group, the thickness of the epidermis was thinned, and the connection between the epidermis and the dermis became flat and relaxed. The amount of collagen fibers and elastic fibers in the dermis is reduced, irregularly arranged, and often broken into pieces. At 4 days, the dermis of the young group showed obvious expansion of capillaries, a large number of neutrophils and macrophages infiltrated, and a large amount of granulation tissue was formed; the neutrophil infiltration and the number of dermal capillaries in the elderly group were less than those in the young group. At 7 days, the young group showed that the wound was basically filled with granulation tissue and the inflammatory cells were reduced. The wounds in the old group were not filled with granulation tissue, and there were still a large number of inflammatory cells infiltrating. At 21 days, the young group's wounds healed basically, the granulation tissue was fibrotic, and the scar tissue was transformed. Masson trichrome staining showed that the number of collagen fibers increased compared with the old group. After 21 days, the old group was completely or nearly healed. At this time, a small amount of inflammatory cell infiltration was observed. The newly accumulated dermal collagen accumulated loosely, the number was small, the arrangement was irregular, the fragments were diffuse, and the regular accumulation of collagen was less (Figs. 8.7, 8.8, and 8.9).

Under electron microscopy, the autophagic cells can be seen in the damaged organelles, such as the swelling and degeneration of mitochondria, surrounded by a vacuole-like bilayer membrane-like structure, or a bilayer membrane surrounding the mitochondria to form auto phagosomes, also showing a remnant that ultimately cannot be degraded by autophagy lysosome, etc. In this experiment, in the keratinocytes and fibroblasts of normal skin of young and old rats, autophagic vacuoles of cytoplasmic bilayer membrane or multilayer membrane were observed, and the size was different, organelle residues such as mitochondria, endoplasmic reticulum, ribosomes can be seen, the number of autophagic vacuoles in the elderly group was higher than in the younger group (Fig. 8.10).

LC3 and Beclin-1 were expressed in the epidermis and dermis of normal skin of young and old rats. After trauma, positive expression was also observed in the epidermis, dermis, hair follicles, new granulation tissue, vascular endothelial cells, macrophages, and fibroblasts at the

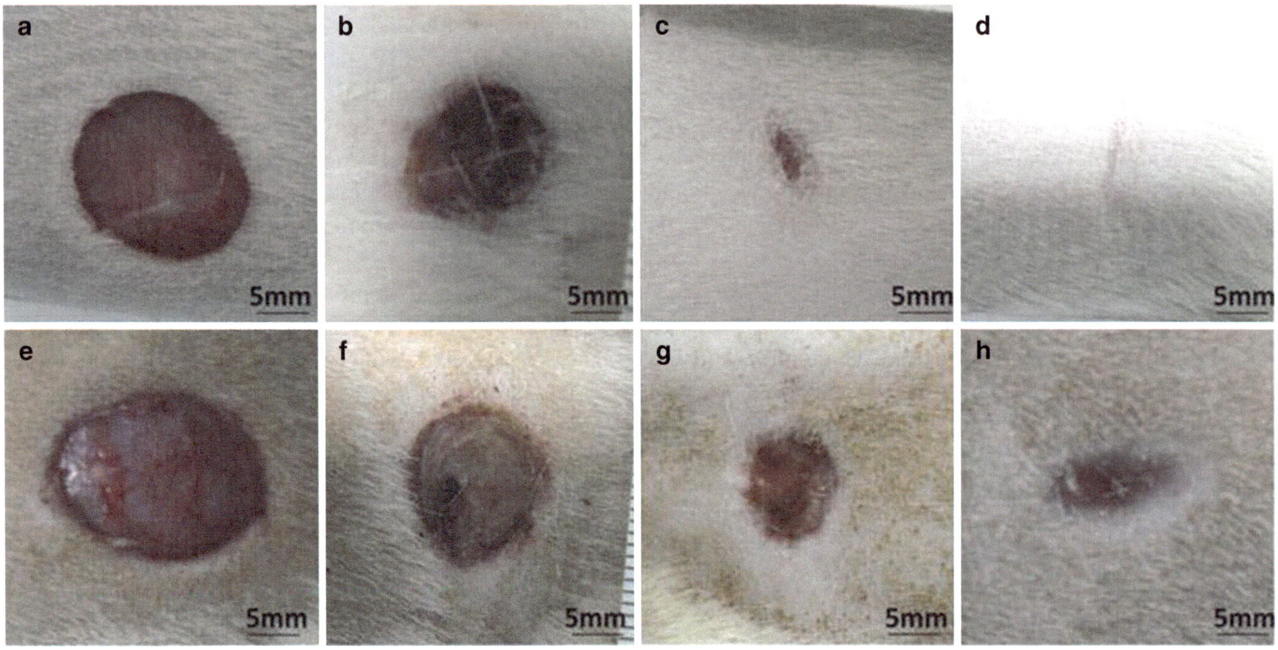


**Fig. 8.7** Wound healing in rats of different age groups

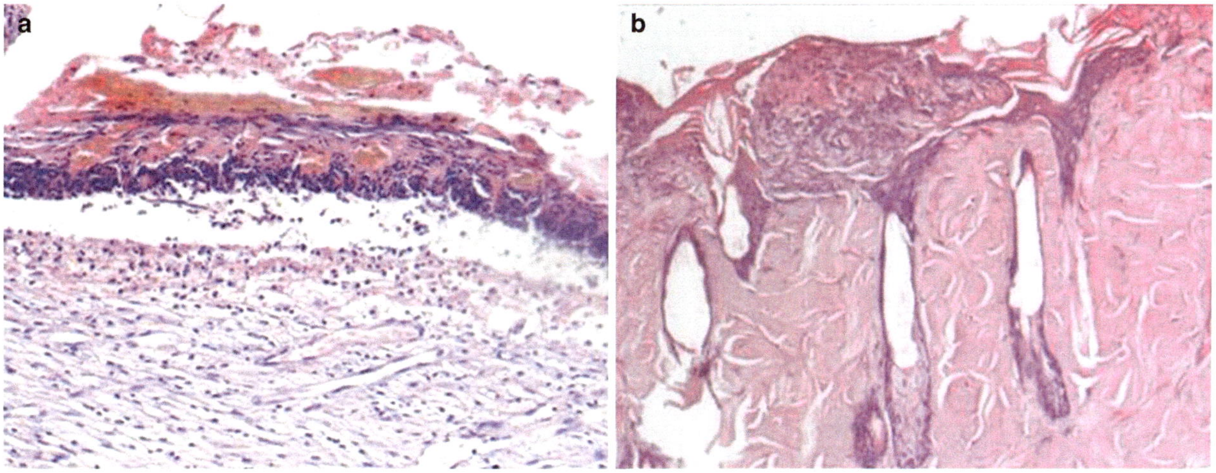


**Fig. 8.8** 4 Days' skin wounds of rats of different age groups (HE staining, ×100)

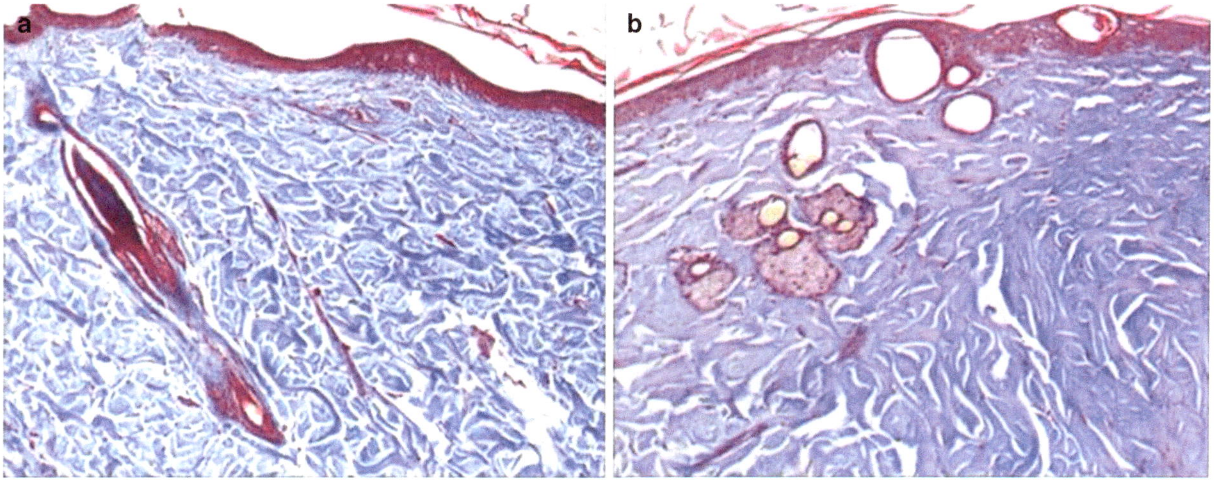


**Fig. 8.9** 21-Day wound skin in rats of different age groups (Masson trichrome staining, ×100)

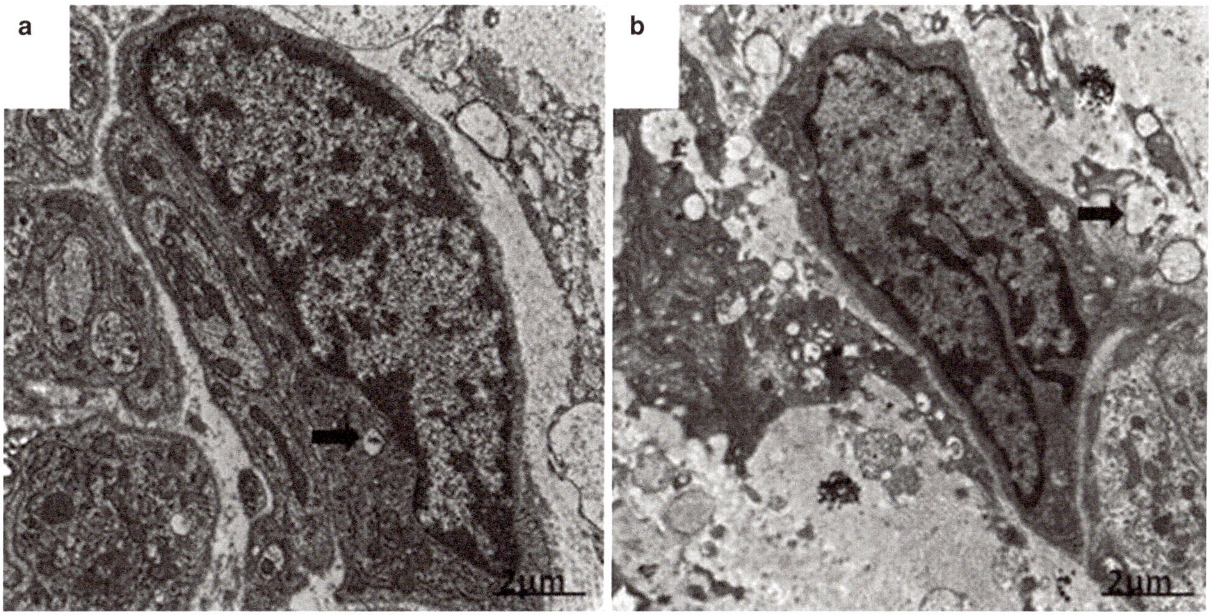


**Fig. 8.10** Autophagosome morphology and structure of normal skin fibroblasts in different age groups (electron microscopy, ×30,000)

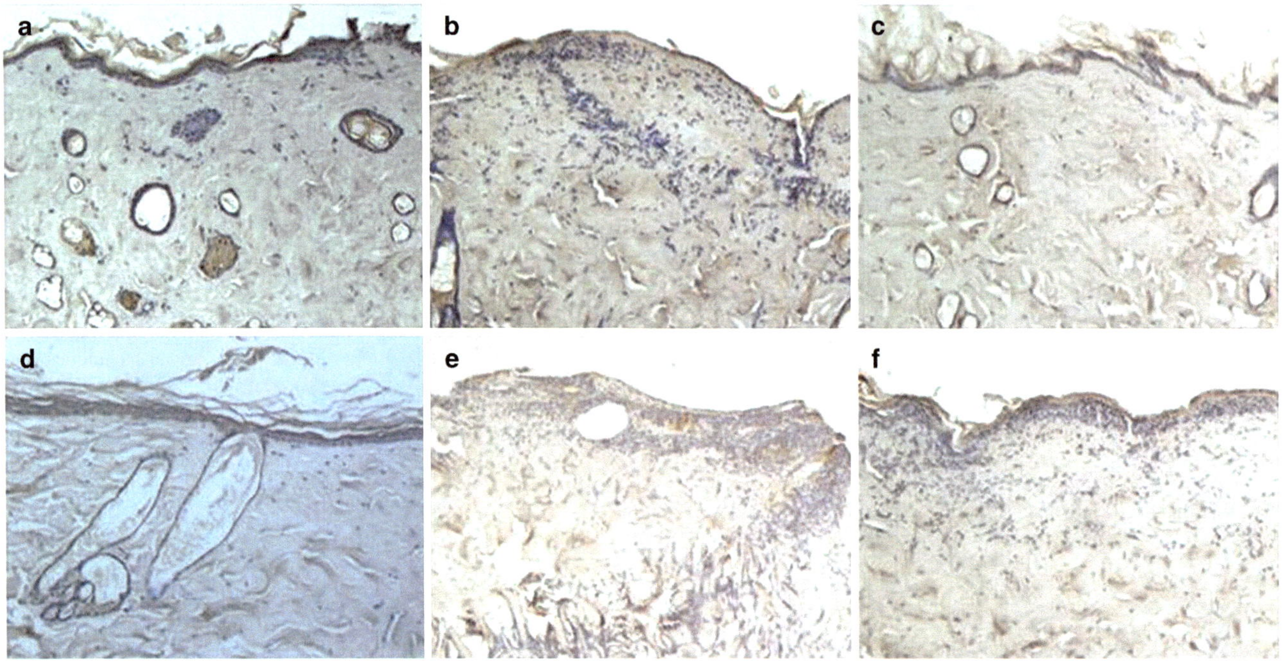


**Fig. 8.11** Expression of LC3 in skin wounds of rats of different age groups (Envison method, ×100)

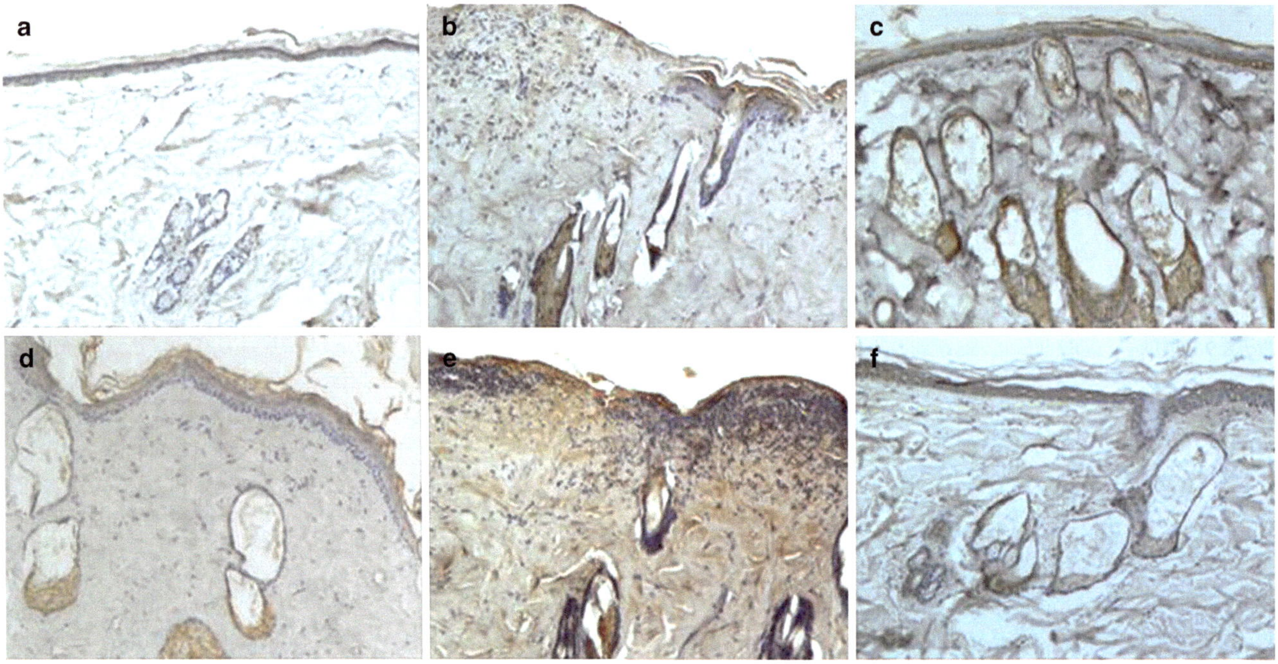


**Fig. 8.12** Beclin-1 expression in skin wounds of rats of different age groups (Envison method, ×100)

wound margin. The expression of two proteins in the pre-traumatic group was higher than that in the young group. The expression of LC3 and Beclin-1 protein increased with time. At 4 days, 7 days, 14 days, and 21 days, the expression of LC3 was more in the young group, while Beclin-1 was more expressed in the old group (Figs. 8.11 and 8.12).

In terms of individual effects, there was a significant difference in the expression of lc3 in the young rats group at 4 days, 7 days, 14 days, and 21 days ($F = 65.283$, $P < 0.001$), 4 days < 7 days < 14 days < 21 days; similarly, there was a significant difference in expression between the four phase points in the aged group ($F = 35.236$, $P < 0.001$), of which 4 days < 7 days < 14 d ays < 21 days; in 14 days, the expression of lc3 in the young murine group was significantly higher than that in the old rats ($P < 0.05$). There was no significant difference in the expression of the two groups at the other three time points. In terms of main effect, there were significant differences between the age group and the time ($P < 0.001$); however, there was no interaction between the two factors ($P = 0.072$), indicating that the two had no effect on the expression of lc3 (Table 8.2).

The expression of Beclin-1 mRNA in skin wounds of rats of different age groups: in the young rats, the expression of Beclin-1 was significantly increased in 4, 7, 14, and 21 days ($F = 166.748$, $P < 0.001$), 4 days < 7 days < 14 days < 21 days; similarly, the expression of four time points in the aged rats group was also significantly increased ($F = 38.875$, $P < 0.001$), 4 days < 14 d ays < 7 days < 21 days; at each time point, the expression of Beclin-1 in young rats was significantly lower than that in the old rats ($P < 0.05$). In terms of main effect, there were significant differences between age group and time ($P < 0.001$); and there were interactions between the two factors ($P < 0.001$), indicating that both of them affected the expression of Beclin-1 (Table 8.3).

The changes of mRNA expression of p62 in skin wounds of rats of different age groups showed that there was a significant difference in p62 expression loss in 4, 7, 14, and 21 days in young rats ($F = 12.842$, $P = 0.002$). Similarly, there was a significant difference in expression reduction at four time points in the aged group ($F = 4.257$, $P = 0.045$), and the mRNA reduction in both age groups was 4 days < 7 days < 14 days < 21 days. There was no significant difference in the expression of young rats and aged rats at 4 days and 7 days ($P > 0.05$). At 14 days and 21 days, the decrease in p62 expression in the young mouse group was significantly lower than that in the old mouse group ($P < 0.05$). In terms of main effect, there were significant differences between the group and time factors ($P < 0.001$); and there was an interaction between the two factors ($P = 0.047$), indicating that the two affected the expression of p62 (Table 8.4).

In different age groups, the expression of LC3- II/I and Beclin-1 protein increased gradually at 4, 7, 14, and 21 days after injury, while in p62 protein the expression gradually decreased ($P < 0.05$). The protein level expression of LC3-II/I, Beclin-1, and p62 was consistent with gene level expression (Figs. 8.13 and 8.14).

Through the detection of autophagy-associated marker proteins LC3, Beclin-1, and p62 during wound healing, it

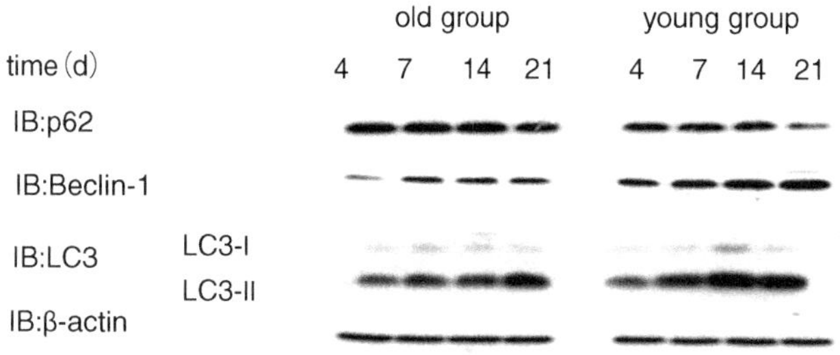


**Fig. 8.13** Protein expression of LC3, Beclin-1, and p62 in different age groups (Western blot)

**Table 8.2** Comparison of mRNA expression changes of LC3 in skin wounds of rats of different age groups

| Group | *n* | 4 Days | 7 Days | 14 Days | 21 Days | Total | *F* | *P* |
|---|---|---|---|---|---|---|---|---|
| Young | 3 | 0.40 ± 0.08 | 2.32 ± 0.19 | 5.29 ± 0.34 | 7.12 ± 1.22 | 3.78 ± 2.77 | 65.283 | <0.001 |
| Old | 3 | 0.77 ± 0.30 | 1.85 ± 0.39 | 3.55 ± 0.34 | 7.76 ± 1.69 | 3.48 ± 2.88 | 35.236 | <0.001 |
| Total | – | 0.59 ± 0.28 | 2.09 ± 0.37 | 4.42 ± 1.00 | 7.44 ± 1.36 | 3.63 ± 2.77 | 0.897 | 0.358 |
| *t* | – | 2.091 | 1.871 | 6.273 | 0.526 | 88.096 | 2.827 | |
| *P* | – | 0.105 | 0.135 | 0.003 | 0.627 | <0.001 | 0.072 | |

**Table 8.3** Comparison of mRNA expression changes of Beclin-1 in skin wounds of rats of different age groups

| Group | *n* | 4 Days | 7 Days | 14 Days | 21 Days | Total | *F* | *P* |
|---|---|---|---|---|---|---|---|---|
| Young | 3 | 0.05 ± 0.03 | 5.75 ± 0.82 | 4.81 ± 0.38 | 9.25 ± 0.47 | 4.97 ± 3.46 | 166.748 | <0.001 |
| Old | 3 | 1.39 ± 0.12 | 20.08 ± 1.56 | 27.25 ± 7.47 | 34.03 ± 1.69 | 20.69 ± 13.16 | 38.875 | <0.001 |
| Total | – | 0.72 ± 0.74 | 12.92 ± 7.92 | 16.03 ± 13.17 | 21.64 ± 13.62 | 12.83 ± 12.37 | 60.399 | <0.001 |
| *t* | – | 19.297 | 14.075 | 5.196 | 24.425 | 190.845 | 21.618 | |
| *P* | – | <0.001 | <0.001 | 0.007 | <0.001 | <0.001 | <0.001 | |

**Table 8.4** Comparison of mRNA expression changes of p62 in skin wounds of rats of different age groups

| Group | *n* | 4 Days | 7 Days | 14 Days | 21 Days | Total | *F* | *P* |
|---|---|---|---|---|---|---|---|---|
| Young | 3 | −3.03 ± 2.31 | −6.38 ± 0.95 | −8.31 ± 0.98 | −9.92 ± 1.02 | −6.91 ± 2.95 | 12.842 | 0.002 |
| Old | 3 | −2.58 ± 0.47 | −3.39 ± 0.65 | −4.62 ± 0.87 | −5.32 ± 1.36 | −4.20 ± 1.34 | 4.257 | 0.045 |
| Total | – | 2.15 ± 0.30 | 3.63 ± 0.53 | 5.54 ± 2.17 | 2.69 ± 1.41 | 3.50 ± 1.81 | 29.317 | <0.001 |
| *t* | – | 0.334 | 2.639 | 4.876 | 4.692 | 16.905 | 3.320# | |
| *P* | – | 0.755 | 0.058 | 0.008 | 0.009 | <0.001 | 0.047 | |

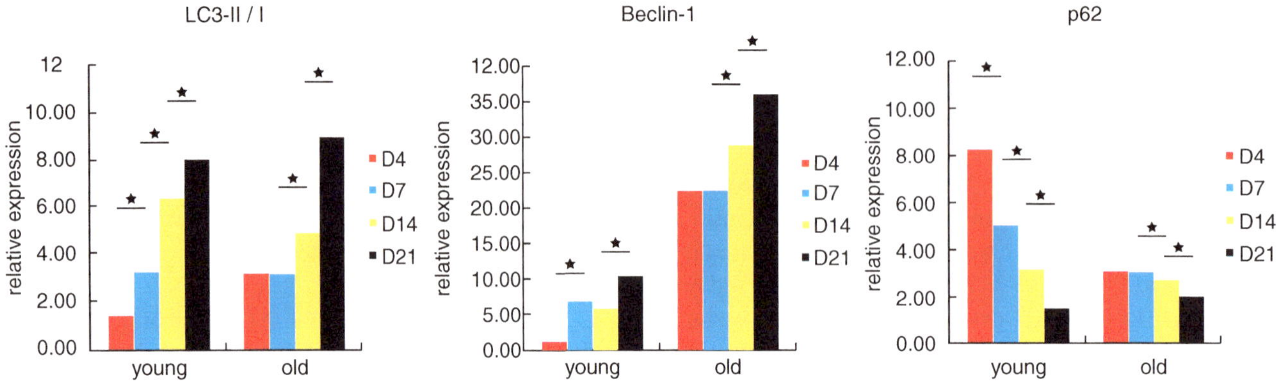


**Fig. 8.14** Protein expression of LC3, Beclin-1, and p62 in wounds of different age groups (*$P < 0.05$)

was found that the autophagy ability of skin cells in young and aged rats was enhanced, but young skin could maintain cell homeostasis and keep autophagy within the normal range, thereby promoting wound repair. Older skin may be obstructed by its own autophagy system, resulting in excessive autophagy that is incompatible with itself, causing irreversible damage to the cells and delaying the healing process.

## 8.1.3 Nutrition

Nutritional factors play an important role in wound healing. Effective energy support can provide sufficient energy and nutrients for the body to repair wounds, reduce the body's own protein degradation, enhance the body's immunity, and promote functional healing of the wound [7]. Energy, carbohydrates, protein, fat, vitamins, and mineral metabolism all affect the healing process of wounds. Under special circumstances (such as wars), due to the limitations of the conditions, nutritional imbalances often occur, and the malnutrition of the body reduces the process of wound healing. It is well known that nutrients and micronutrients are extremely important components in the process of acute and chronic wound repair. After the body is injured, the whole body tissue is in a state of decomposition, and it can last for a long time, which is easy to cause the lack of protein in the body. The entire repair process requires sufficient heat, protein supply, and sufficient vitamins A, B, C and minerals and trace elements; otherwise protein collagen fibers and granulation tissue cannot be formed. In patients with delayed wound healing after surgery, the zinc content in the skin is mostly lower than in patients with good healing. Zinc urinary excretion has been shown to increase in surgical stimulation, trauma, and burns, and zinc supplementation promotes wound healing. In addition, the lack of copper is also associated with poor wound healing.

### 8.1.3.1 Carbohydrates

Carbohydrates are the main source of energy in the healing process of wounds, and are structurally represented as monomers or multiparts of sugar. When ingested by the human body, the carbohydrate is converted into monosaccharides (mainly glucose) by the action of digestive enzymes. The role of glucose in the healing process of wounds is mainly to provide energy for various cells involved in wound repair, stimulate fiber growth, stimulate collagen production to form new tissue, and produce ATP to meet the energy required for cells to participate in wound repair to accelerate metabolism. Glucose as a source of ATP synthesis also avoids the consumption of amino acids and proteins. The body's response to energy deficiency caused by insufficient carbohydrate intake is increased mortality, decreased human albumin content, decreased muscle tissue ratio (because muscles break down to provide energy), wounds are difficult to heal, and BMI (body mass Index) is too low.

### 8.1.3.2 Protein

Abnormal protein metabolism and body nutrient disorders may be important ways to prevent wound repair. This view has been increasingly recognized since the discovery of protein detection techniques and metabolic assays. The effect of hypoproteinemia on wound repair is not directly caused by protein deficiency, but is related to the decrease of plasma colloid osmotic pressure and the accompanying tissue edema, which is also the main reason for the delayed repair in the case of war wounds. Other experiments have confirmed that chronic protein-deficient animals are affected by angiogenesis, fibroblast proliferation, collagen synthesis, and deposition.

Experiments have confirmed that the body lacks arginine, which can reduce collagen deposition and poor wound healing. Supplementing 17 g of arginine daily can not only increase the deposition of hydroxyproline, promote wound healing, and improve immune function, but also retain more skin protein under stress for healing of the incision. Arginine can also promote wound healing and promote insulin and growth hormone secretion through humoral regulation mechanisms. Supplementation with arginine was most effective 3 days before wound healing. Thus, inflammatory cells and fibroblasts are in an activated state. Therefore, patients with pressure ulcers, especially those who are at risk of protein and energy malnutrition or have occurred, need to immediately use sufficient energy and protein for nutritional intervention to meet the additional nutritional needs of patients. In addition to energy and protein, arginine and micronutrients should be supplemented to maintain optimal healing of the incision.

Other experimental studies have found that the methyl group of methionine can synthesize choline to prevent fatty liver, and methionine itself can be converted into cysteine to participate in detoxification and prevent liver poisoning. The ratio of lysine to tryptophan is also important. It is generally believed that the ratio of lysine/tryptophan is preferably (6–7):1 to improve protein utilization. Lysine is also the most important amino acid in the synthesis of proteins. It has been suggested that threonine, serine, tryptophan, tyrosine, histidine, glutamic acid, glycine, alanine, proline, and branched chain amino acids should be considered when supplementing amino acids.

Glutamate is one of the most abundant amino acids in the plasma membrane component and is a major source of energy metabolism in rapidly proliferating cells such as fibroblasts, lymphocytes, epithelial cells, and macrophages. Oral supplementation with glutamate can increase wound tension and levels of mature collagen.

#### 8.1.3.3 Vitamins

1. Vitamin C

   Vitamin C (also known as ascorbic acid) is an acidic polyhydroxy compound with six carbon atoms. It is abundant in a variety of fresh vegetables and fruits. The two enol hydroxyl groups of the 2- and 3-position carbon atoms in the molecule are easily dissociated, releasing H+ and being oxidized to dehydrogenating vitamin C. Vitamin C and dehydrogenated vitamin C form a reversible redox system in the human body, which plays an important role in biological redox and cellular respiration. Vitamin C is involved in amino acid metabolism and synthesis of neurotransmitters, collagen, and tissue interstitial cells; it can reduce capillary permeability, accelerate blood coagulation, stimulate coagulation function, promote iron absorption in the intestine; promote blood lipid decline, promote wound healing, increase resistance to infection, participate in the detoxification process, have anti-histamine, and prevent the formation of carcinogens.

   As early as 1941, foreign cooks studied the effects of vitamin C on wound healing. After more than half a century of unremitting efforts by doctors and scholars, the role of vitamin C in wound healing was affirmed. Hydrogen peroxide used in the treatment of infectious wounds has a strong bactericidal effect, but it also increases the production of oxygen free radicals. No matter what kind of disinfectant, such as hydrogen peroxide, sulfur, bleaching disinfectant, etc., poisoning will interrupt the normal function of the cells. Vitamin C is a scavenger of free radicals. It is also involved in the synthesis of tissue interstitial collagen and improves the permeability of capillaries, so it promotes the formation of fresh tissue and reduces exudation.

   Although vitamin C has an anti-infective effect, it is not very strong and therefore cannot be used as a main drug at the peak of infection, especially in the case of infectious ulcers.

   In the absence of vitamin C, wound healing stops at the stage of fibrosis, and the number of fibroblasts in the wound is normal, but not enough collagen. In severe scurvy patients, not only can new wounds not heal, but old healing scars can also rupture, as the ongoing collagen solubilization far exceeds the synthesis of new collagen. Vitamin C wet compress is beneficial to the formation of skin cells on the wound surface, promotes the growth of granulation tissue, and accelerates the healing of wounds. However, the study also found that the presence and intake of vitamin C at normal levels is usually ineffective. When patients have vitamin C deficiency or trauma, they are supplemented with vitamin C of 100–200 mg per day; when more complex trauma occurs, including stage III, IV, or severe traumatic pressure ulcers, supplementing with vitamin C of 1000–2000 mg per day can promote wound healing.

2. Other Vitamins
   (a) Vitamin A: It is an essential substance for maintaining epithelial growth. At the time of injury, the demand for vitamin A increases. Moreover, vitamin A has a positive effect in the inflammatory phase of wound healing. Vitamin A can partially reverse the adverse effects of long-term steroid treatment in patients with wound healing. If vitamin A is lacking, the wound will heal slowly.
   (b) B vitamins: B vitamins are important for wound healing and are coenzymes involved in energy metabolism. The lack of vitamin $B_2$ delays the formation of epithelia during wound repair, decreases total collagen content, and reduces the rate of wound healing. When the B vitamins are deficient, intramolecular diplomacy, collagen maturation is impaired, and the tensile force of the incision is decreased. Vitamin $B_6$ is mainly a coenzyme involved in the synthesis and decomposition of amino acids. In the absence of it, the effect on wound healing is similar to vitamin $B_2$ deficiency.

(c) Vitamin D: The Matsumoto study showed that 1,25-$(OH)_2$-Vit $D_3$ induced differentiation of keratinocytes, and inhibited the growth of the cells. Hosomi found that the differentiation of keratinocytes by 1,25-$(OH)_2$- Vit $D_3$ was accomplished by vitamin D receptor, either in vitro or in vivo. PDGF plays an important role in wound healing. It stimulates the proliferation of fibroblasts, muscle cells, promotes the synthesis of collagen and extracellular matrix, and can recruit fibroblasts, monocytes, and neutrophils. The keratinocytes in the epidermis do not have a receptor for PDGF. Studies have shown that 1,25-$(OH)_2$-Vit $D_3$ can up-regulate PDGF, and TGF-α is also affected.

(d) Vitamin E: It can promote the proliferation of capillaries, that is, micro vessels, improve the surrounding circulation, and its anti-oxidation effect has an effect on the metabolism of the body, which can promote the growth of granulation tissue and skin.

#### 8.1.3.4 Trace Elements

The lack of trace elements, such as zinc and copper, is also associated with poor wound healing. Zinc deficiency is associated with poor epithelialization and chronic wound healing. Magnesium, as a cofactor for many enzymes, is involved in the synthesis of proteins and collagen. Copper is a cofactor required for good cross-linking of cytochrome oxidase, cytosolic superoxide dismutase, and collagen. Zinc is a cofactor for RNA synthase and DNA synthetase. Iron is essential for the hydroxylation of proline and lysine, and severe iron deficiency can lead to collagen synthesis disorders.

1. Zinc
   Zinc is involved in collagen synthesis, which is a very important step in the healing process of pressure sore incision, so marginal zinc deficiency is thought to be related to delayed healing of the incision. When zinc is deficient, it affects the healing of pressure sores and other chronic incisions. When the plasma zinc concentration is less than 100 μg/mL, it is directly related to tissue repair and can be supplemented with zinc supplementation therapy.
2. Iron
   Iron is a cofactor required for the hydroxylation of proline and lysine during collagen synthesis. Chronic inflammation and infection caused by pressure sores can aggravate anemia and can be treated by iron supplementation and blood transfusion. After the occurrence of pressure sores, the body's need for certain nutrients, especially zinc and iron, increases.
3. Copper
   Copper is involved in the maturation of collagen and has an effect on wound healing. A copper- containing metalloenzyme (lysyl oxidase) catalyzes the oxidation of collagen lysyl residues to form a hydroxyl lysyl group. These groups pass through the cross-linking of extracellular collagen to increase the strength of the scar.
4. Manganese
   Many enzymes require normal participation in their function, including a lysylgalactose converting enzyme. This enzyme is involved in the glycosylation process of the original collagen fibers. Manganese also affects the production of hyaluronic acid, chondroitin sulfate, heparin, and other mucopolysaccharides, which are important factors in the healing process of the incision.
5. Selenium
   Selenium is an important component of glutathione peroxidase. The enzyme protects cells from oxidative damage by promoting hydrogen peroxide reduction. When selenium is deficient, the activity of the enzyme is reduced, and the healing of the incision can also be affected by changing the function of macrophages and multinucleated cells.

### 8.1.4 Neuro-Immune-Endocrine System

The neuroendocrine response is the earliest systemic reaction in the body after trauma. It is mainly manifested by the immediate hypothalamic–pituitary–adrenal axis (HPA) and sympathetic adrenal medullary axis, releasing hormones such as glucocorticoids and catecholamines. The heavier the injury, the stronger the neuroendocrine response. The neuroendocrine reaction can also affect the immune system. In the early stage of trauma, moderate neuroendocrine response can enhance the body's immune function, prevent or reduce secondary damage, and thus constitute a neuro-immune-endocrine regulation system, and play a regulatory role in wound healing [8].

The disorder of the neuro-immune-endocrine regulatory network can lead to disturbance of metabolic activity in the body, and the whole repair process enters a pathological stage, which affects the healing time. The effects of neurological, endocrine, and hormonal changes on skin repair and regeneration have recently received great attention.

#### 8.1.4.1 The Influence of Nerve on Wound Healing

1. The Skin Is a Nerve-Dependent Organ
   A large number of studies have shown that the skin is a very sensitive nerve-dependent organ as the largest organ in the human body. The sensory nerves from the dorsal root ganglia pass through the dermis, running parallel at the junction of the true and epidermis, penetrating the basement membrane and reaching the layer of epidermal granules vertically to form a three-dimensional network. Cells in the skin (keratinocytes, microvascular endothelial cells, and fibroblasts) can express various types of neuropeptides. Many physiological functions of the skin

(such as metabolism, immunity, etc.) are inseparable from innervation, such as sweating, immune response, thermoregulation, and DNA repair.

Skin cells can perform neuron-like functions such as the expression of neurotransmitters and their receptors. Among the myriad of neurotransmitters and neurohormones, there are currently more than 20 types of skin, most of which are neuropeptides (Table 8.5).

2. The Effect of Nerves on Wound Healing
   In the process of wound healing, the wound area will be further increased after the denervation of the wound, and the contracture will be restricted, resulting in a healing disorder; paraplegia and diabetic patients with neurotrophic disorders often lead to difficult wound healing, and even prolonged unhealed wounds; in the early stage, there is often a temporary phenomenon of excessive nerve innervation. There are indications that neurological factors have a regulatory effect on inflammation, neovascularization, granulation hyperplasia, and post-healing shaping stages in wound healing. Neurotrophic factors and neuropeptides (such as SP, CGRP, VIP, SOM, and opioid peptides) act as neuromodulators, neurotransmitters, and neurohormones to effectively regulate the function of skin cells, determine the final biological response of the cell, affecting the healing outcome and regeneration ability.

#### 8.1.4.2 The Impact of Endocrine on Wound Healing

1. The skin Is a Large Endocrine Organ
   The skin produces many important endocrine and exocrine substances (Table 8.6). Special mention is made of fat cells, which are capable of secreting leptin (LP), lipoprotein lipase (LPL), resistin, angiotensinogen (AGT), and adiponectin (Adiponectin). Among them, adiponectin, also known as GBP28, enhances insulin sensitivity and stops inflammation. Apolipoprotein E is one of the major apolipoproteins in plasma. It is polymorphic and mainly synthesized and metabolized by the liver. It plays an important role in plasma lipoprotein metabolism, tissue repair, inhibition of platelet aggregation, immune regulation, and inhibition of cell proliferation. It has been determined that leptin is involved in endocrine function, inflammatory response, and has the potential to promote vascular and granulation tissue formation and re- epithelialization, and is a new important factor in the process of wound repair. Adipocytokines are also involved in the regulation of endothelial function as inflammatory factors.

2. The Effect of Endocrine on Wound Healing
   The neuroendocrine system of the skin involves the local production of neuroendocrine mediators, which interact with the corresponding specific receptors by paracrine and autocrine.

The renin-angiotensin system (RAS) is one of several hormonal systems that regulate the function of the body, and produces an endocrine effect together with angiotensin II (AT II). In the skin, the local or tissue renin-angiotensin system affects cell proliferation and differentiation. In addition, fat cells can also secrete other peptides and

**Table 8.5** Neurotransmitters and their receptors produced by various cells in the skin

| Kinds of skin cells | Neurotransmitter and neurohormones | Neurologic receptor |
|---|---|---|
| Keratinocyte | NGF, SP, CGRP, VIP, NKA, ACh, DA, AR, NE, β-EP, CA, SOM | NGFR, VIPR, NPYR, 5-HTR, CGRPR, NK-1/2/3R, μ/ζ-opiete-R |
| Merkel cell | SP, CGRP, MEK, NGF, NKA, SOM, VIP, NPY | NGFR, NK-1R |
| Langerhans' cells | NGF, SP, CGRP, SOM, VIP, MEK, NKA | NK-1/2R, SOMR, NPYR |
| Mastocyte | NGF, CA, SP, CGRP, NKA, SOM | NK-1R |
| Fibroblast | NGF, SP, β-EP | NGFR, NK-1R, SOMR, NPYR, 5-HTR |
| Adipocyte | – | AR-β1, 2, 3 |
| Microvessel endothelial cell | ACE, Ang, NO, ET, β-EP | NGFR, NK-1/2/3R, NPYR |
| Sweat gland cell | – | NK-1R, μ-opiete-R |
| Sebaceous gland cell | – | NPYR, μ-opiete-R |

**Table 8.6** Hormones and their receptors produced by various cells in the skin

| Kinds of skin cells | Hormone | Hormone receptor |
|---|---|---|
| Keratinocyte | PTHrP, CRH, ACTH, α-MSH, corticotropin, androgens, atRA, elcosanoid | TSHR, CRH-1R, MC-1R, M-1R, VIPR-2, IGF-1R, GHR, GR, AR, PR, THR, ER-β, RAR, RXR, VDR, PPAR-α/β/γ |
| Merkel cell | Estrogens | ER |
| Langerhans' cells | GRP, PACAP, α-MSH, POMC | GRPR, PACAPR I/II/III, MC-1R/5R |
| Mastocyte | POMC | MC-1R mRNA, non-protein level |
| Melanocyte | PTHrP, CRH, Ucn, ACTH, α-MSH, epinephrine, IGF-I | TSHR, CRH-1R, MC-1R, 2R, MR, M-1R, 5-HTR, GHR, ER-β, RXR-α, VDR |
| Fibroblast | ACTH, α-MSH, IGF- I/II, IGFBP-3, Estrogens | PTHR, TSHR, CRH-1R, MC-1R, M-1R, GHR, AR, THR, ER-β/α, RXR-α |
| Adipocyte | LP, LPL, resistin, AGT, ApoE | IR, GR, GHR, TSHR, Gastrin/CCK-B R, GLP-1R, Ang II-R, VDR, THR, AR, ER, PR, LR, IL-6R, PPAR-γ |
| Microvessel endothelial cell | CRH, Ucn, ACTH, α-MSH | MC-1R, VIPR-2, RAR-2, GHR, AR, ER-β, RAR, RXR, PPAR-γ |
| Sweat gland cell | Ucn, androgens | MC-1R/5R, VIPR-2, GHR, AR, PPAR-γ |
| Sebaceous gland cell | CRH, androgens, estrogens, atRA, calcitiol, eicosanoids | CRH-1R/2R, MC-1R/5R, μ-opiete-R, VIPR-2, GHR, AR, ER-β/α, RAR, RXR, PPAR-α/β/γ |

non-peptide factors, which play a role in the axis of angiotensinogen-angiotensin II-prostacyclin, affecting the relaxation and growth of blood vessels.

The effects of hormone levels on downstream cells and tissues, including the cascade and interaction of cytokine signaling pathways, positive and negative regulation of target proteins are gradually attracting attention. Sex hormones maintain organ development, regeneration, and tissue metabolism, including normal skin, epidermal thickness, mitotic capacity, and vascularization, as well as elastin characteristics and collagen tissue content, which are important factors in the process of wound healing. It is currently believed that estrogen can down-regulate tumor necrosis factor-α (TNF-α) by binding to its receptor and affecting gene expression through the action of activator protein-1 (AP-1), increased matrix deposition, stimulated hair follicle keratinocyte proliferation, and enhanced keratinocyte growth factor (KGF) expression, affecting epithelial regeneration. In addition, estrogen affects skin healing and regeneration through inflammatory reactions, matrix deposition, re-epithelialization, and scar maturation. Studies have shown that androgen receptors (AR) expressed in the skin also affect healing by participating in inflammatory responses, cell proliferation, and matrix deposition. In short, the terminal organ of the skin acting as a sex hormone must be affected by it when it is damaged, repaired, and regenerated. Thyroid hormones also have a major impact on wound healing and regeneration.

Androgen, estrogen, corticosteroids, and their physiological and pathological signaling pathways in healing are important. Understanding the response of the cascade of signaling pathways, especially in combination with immunity, is of great importance in understanding the role of wound healing in the healing of wound healing mechanisms.

#### 8.1.4.3 The Impact of Immunity on Wound Healing

1. The Skin Is an Immunoreactive Organ

   The skin is the largest tissue and organ of the human body. Due to its special structure and function, it forms a natural barrier between the body and the external environment. Skin is often seen as a tissue organ that has a unique immune function and is closely related to the systemic immune system. It not only has nonspecific immune defense function, but also participates in the whole process of antigen recognition, immune cell activation, and skin immune response of body-specific immunity (Table 8.7).

**Table 8.7** Various cells and related immune responses in the skin

| Kinds of skin cells | Immune response |
|---|---|
| Keratinocyte | Creating a unique microenvironment for antigen uptake and recognition. There are two major features of Keratinocyte in SIS: The expression of MHC-II Antigens, which act as helper cells in T cell mediated immune responses. It produces a lot of cytokines such as IL-1, IL-2, IL-6, GM-CSF, TNF, IFN |
| Langerhans' cells | Bone marrow-derived dendritic cells are distributed in the basal layer of epidermis and adnexal epithelium, accounting for 3–8% of the total number of epidermal cells. The chemical property and surface markers are similar to those of macrophages. It is generally accepted that the Langerhans' cell, which resides in the epidermis of normal humans, is immature and has its full function only after entering the dermis or draining lymph nodes.<br>It is the main antigen presenting cell of skin and participates in skin immune reaction. It can ingest, process and present Antigen, and control T cell migration. Langerhans' cell T cells secrete important cytokines and participate in immune regulation, immune surveillance, immune tolerance, skin graft rejection, and so on |
| Mastocyte | Mainly located in the dermis around the papilla vessels, deep dermis rare, almost non-existent in the epidermis.<br>Mast cells have different membrane receptors (such as IgEFcR, which bind to IgE) on their surface. Mast cells produce and release a variety of bioactive mediators, which can be divided into vasoactive substances, chemokines, active enzymes and structural glycoproteins. They participate in delayed type hypersensitivity |
| Lymphocyte | In normal human skin, a large number of T cells (more than 90%) are localized around the dermal vessels, mainly around the dermal papilla and capillary. Only the T cells in the lymphocyte can be recycled to the skin organs |
| Dendritic cell | A specific subset of antigen presenting cells that are widely distributed in the human body. In addition to the dendritic cell of the skin, there are melanocytes, Merkel cells, tissue macrophages, unidentified cells, and dermal dendritic cells |
| Fibroblast | Dermal fibroblasts can synthesize all kinds of proteins required for activation of t lymphocyte subpopulations, which can prolong the survival time of T lymphocyte by binding adhesion molecules CD44, LFA, ICAM-1 to T lymphocyte. Cytokines produced include: IL-1/6/8, IFN-β, monocyte chemoattractant protein, B factor, C3, CSF2, TGF-α/β. The MHC-II Antigen is expressed locally and acts as an antigen presenting cell, activating T lymphocyte |
| Adipocyte | Synthesize and secrete complement D (Adipsin, which is the first complement component cloned from an Adipocyte line). Secretion of inflammatory cytokines (such as TNF-β, CRP and IL-6). It secretes Leptin, which has immunomodulatory and T lymphocyte effects on monocytes, macrophages, and natural killer cell cells. In addition, it can affect the production of cytokines by immune cells. Adiponectin reduces lipopolysaccharide induced tumor necrosis factors expression, impairs the phagocytosis of mature macrophages, and inhibits the proliferation and growth of bone marrow mononuclear cell lines, a negative regulator of the hematopoietic- immune system, to help stop the inflammation |
| Microvessel endothelial cell | In normal skin, lymphocytes are concentrated around the capillary veins, the tiny endothelial cells in the inner walls of blood vessels that promote lymphocyte circulation from the blood to the skin. In addition, it actively participates in the complex reactions between macromolecules and blood cells and extravascular substances, and participates in the immune and inflammatory processes. The activation of endothelial cells was triggered by cytokines, and the adhesion of activated endothelial cells to leukocytes was increased. Endothelial cell activation plays an important role in cellular immune response |

In the 1970s, it was suggested that the skin is a primary lymphoid organ similar to the thymus of primary lymphoid tissue. In the 1980s, the concept of skin-associated lymphoid tissue (SALT) was proposed based on the characteristics of epidermal Langerhans cell-presenting antigen, T-cell pro-epithelia, and keratinocytes producing epidermal thymic activating factor. SALT is thought to include four distinct cells: keratinocytes, lymphocytes, Langerhans cells, and endothelial cells. The SALT concept limits skin immunity to the epidermis, which is incomplete. Cells involved in the skin's immune response, such as T cells and monocytes, are mainly distributed in the dermis; cells involved in the skin's immune response include cells other than SALT cell components, such as mast cells, neutrophils, and fibroblasts and a variety of mediators involved in the immune response (such as cytokines, immunoglobulins, etc.). Therefore, in the mid-1980s, Bos proposed the concept of a skin immune system (SIS). SIS consists of two major parts, cells and body fluids. The cell components include keratinocytes, Langerhans cells, tissue cells (dendritic cells and macrophages), T cells, granulocytes, mast cells, endothelial cells, and the like. The body fluid components include antimicrobial peptides, plasmin, arachidonic acid, complement, secretory immunoglobulin IgA (SIgA), cytokines, and the like. In the mid-1990s, the concept of the dermis immune system (DIS) was proposed, which complemented and expanded SIS.

2. The Effect of Immune Response on Wound Healing
   For external damage, the skin not only has mechanical resistance, but also has immune function and can produce an appropriate immune response. In the inflammatory phase of wound healing, the infiltration of lymphocytes and macrophages, and the sources of pro-inflammatory factors are all related to stress. The degree of immunosuppression is directly proportional to the acute inflammatory response. After the rapid release of glucocorticoids and catecholamines into the blood, glucocorticoids can decrease the activity of T cells and mononuclear macrophages, and various immunosuppressions promote the synthesis of cytokines, resulting in insufficient expression of antigens in the immune response. Catecholamine inhibits the proliferation of T cells, the expression of IL-2 receptors, and the formation of immunoglobulins. Factors that cause immunosuppression are various cytokines produced by prostaglandins and inflammatory cells.

### 8.1.5 Systemic Disease Factors

#### 8.1.5.1 Metabolic Diseases

Hyperglycemia in diabetic patients can inhibit neutrophil function, and the inflammatory response of the wound is weak, which directly leads to the decrease of fibroblast growth and collagen synthesis. The hyaluronic acid of the dermal papilla of the wound surface of such patients is also reduced compared with normal, while the collagenase content is significantly increased; this phenomenon can affect the healing tissue tension strength and collagen aggregation. In addition, due to vascular pathological changes in diabetic patients, blood perfusion is low, with tissue hypoxia, and the risk of wound infection increases. The wounds of uremic patients are not easy to heal. The main mechanism may be systemic malnutrition, low blood volume, and insufficient oxygen supply. In addition, hyperlipidemia can also reduce the synthesis of collagen in fibroblasts. Diabetic patients are prone to traumatic infections. When blood glucose is >200 mg/dL, the function of leukocyte phagocytic bacteria is inhibited. Therefore, blood sugar levels in diabetic patients must be controlled during wound healing.

#### 8.1.5.2 Cardiovascular Diseases

Patients with atherosclerosis have altered vascular function, affecting blood supply to the wound and resistance to local infection. In addition, high blood pressure, high blood lipids, and other factors can affect the wound healing process.

#### 8.1.5.3 Nerve Damage Diseases

For example, ulcers caused by leprosy are not easy to heal and are caused by nerve involvement. The damage of the autonomic nerve changes the local blood supply, and the effect on regeneration is more obvious.

## 8.2 Local Factors Affecting Tissue Repair and Regeneration

### 8.2.1 Bacterial Colonization and Infection

Bacterial biofilm is a membranous structure formed by some bacteria attached to the wound surface and formed with the extracellular matrix. It consists of bacteria and its secreted products, extracellular matrix, necrotic tissue and so on. Since it is a membranous structure composed of a plurality of components present at the cellular level, it is often determined by fluorescein staining or the like in the study [9]. The formation of biofilms consists of three stages: attachment of wound microbes, secretion of EPS and formation of colonies, and maturation and spread of colony cells [10].

It is important to understand the characteristics and mode of action of this membranous structure to reveal the emergence of bacterial resistance and its role in the development of chronic refractory wounds. According to research, the formation and action of biofilms in acute wound bacteria is not obvious. Only 6% of wounds can detect the presence of this biofilm, so bacteria are not the main factor to delay wound healing. However, when the wound changes from acute to chronic, the biofilm can be detected on more than 60% of the wound surface. When the number of bacteria reaches a certain level, the bacterial biofilm may play a decisive role. Sometimes in the wounds from the acute to chronic early stage of wounds or some single factors, the types of bacteria detected may be relatively simple, but in the wounds with bacterial biofilm formation, a variety of factors and a variety of bacteria are common. As a result of mixed infection, this may be why some single-type bacteria have a higher detection rate (up to 90% or more), while in biofilm-forming wounds, the detection rate is relatively low (about 60%).

How is the biofilm of bacteria formed when chronic refractory wounds occur? It is generally believed that the wound is contaminated during the process from acute to chronic wounds. When the amount of contaminated bacteria is $<10^5$/g, the bacteria are only colonized in the wound. There is no delay in wound healing; however, when the amount of bacteria is $>10^5$/g, especially when there are multiple bacteria at the same time, the bacteria adhere to the wound and multiply on the wound to form a clone, and then embed itself in the necrotic tissue, a multi-layered matrix formed by extracellular matrix, a protective layer is formed, similar to a membrane-like structure. At this time, typical symptoms such as redness, swelling, heat, pain, and low partial pressure of oxygen are observed in the clinic. Bacteria can resist the effects of various treatments. The establishment of this biofilm allows these bacteria to escape the killing effect of antibiotics on them.

When the trauma occurs in a harsh environment, when the bacteria of the wound are transformed from pollution to infection, the exotoxin secreted by the microorganisms during the life and during the destruction, such as *Staphylococcus aureus* α toxin, not only causes the destruction of red blood cells and platelets, but also promotes small blood vessel smooth muscle contraction, paralysis, leading to capillary blood flow blockage and local tissue ischemia and necrosis.

The combined effects of a large number of bacterial exotoxin, endotoxin, and proteolytic enzymes after wound infection, and the biological effects of cytokines and free radical damage caused by their cytotoxic effects result in an increase in the number of tissue edema, hemorrhage, and purulent secretions. The protein is lost by a large amount of wounds and the electrolyte is sharply increased. The protein in the granulation tissue of the purulent wound is hydrolyzed in a large amount, and the bacteria invade the surrounding tissue in a large amount, so that the growth of the granulation tissue is slow or the epithelial formation is seriously affected by the excessive proliferation of the granulation, thereby affecting the speed of wound repair.

The mechanism by which bacterial biofilms delay wound healing may include:

1. Effect on Repairing Cells
   In the early stages of acute wound healing, neutrophils can control the extent of infection by eliminating microorganisms. When bacteria aggregate to form a biofilm, it will produce a resistance to neutrophils and affect the changes of fibroblasts and neutrophil chemotactic factors, resulting in the body's repair ability and immune function blocked, which leads to delayed healing.
2. The Role of Acetyl Homoserine Lactone
   Bacteria regulate the expression of related genes by sensing the density of peripheral cells. If the molecules of acyl homoserine lactones (AHLs) reach a certain threshold, the bacterial density sensing system is activated, and the bacteria continuously secrete the extracellular matrix to bind a single bacterium to form a biofilm, thereby hindering the penetration of the antibacterial drug. When the density of bacteria is reduced, a decrease in AHL secretion can lead to a rapid decrease in biofilm, and supplementation of exogenous AHLs can restore biofilm maturation. As a quorum sensing signal molecule, AHLs are also related to the production of bacterial virulence factors, synthesis or degradation of antibacterial drugs, plasmid binding and other biological functions, and directly affect the gene expression of host cells, which is an important molecule leading to persistent or repeated infection.
3. The Impact of the Formation of Drug Resistance Mechanisms on Wounds
   It is generally believed that bacterial infection of the wound can be eliminated by standardizing the use of antimicrobial treatment. The bacteria in the biofilm state have significantly enhanced drug resistance relative to their planktonic state. The presence of the membrane can weaken the neutrophil chemotaxis, and the inflammatory reaction of the surrounding tissue of the membrane is weakened, causing the bacteria and the organism to be in a long-term symbiotic state. The wound stays in the inflammatory phase for a long time and blocks the healing process of the wound. In addition, extracellular polymers consisting mainly of polysaccharides, proteins, lipids, metal ions, and extracellular DNA, EPS can also affect the physical and chemical properties of biofilms, leading to their resistance to antibacterial agents.

At present, the treatment methods for biofilm mainly include:

(a) Partial debridement, destroying the membrane.
(b) Negative pressure treatment.
(c) Topical drug treatment.
(d) Bioengineering alternative therapy.
(e) Hyperbaric oxygen therapy.

However, there is no better method of radical treatment, and many antigens and wound dressings are ineffective against biofilm infection. Pay attention to the following aspects in clinical work to reduce the production of biofilm:

(a) Careful and thorough debridement and local dressing change.
(b) Reasonable choice of antibiotic type and route of administration.
(c) Operating specifications for the use of various conduits and synthetic materials.

Microbiota is also known as the microbial region, the microflora. Researchers at the Stowers Medical Institute in the United States have found that there is a clear link between the composition of the microbiome and the host's immune response and the body's ability to heal itself. At present, how the microbial group changes and how the immune system responds to the regeneration and repair process is attracting more and more attention.

The immune response mainly constitutes a barrier to effective tissue regeneration and repair. When a part of the planarian population is infected, lesions appear around the eye and become larger and larger until the entire head is degraded. Under normal circumstances, the planarian can regenerate a new head, but the infection interferes with their ability to regenerate in some way.

In the future, humans may develop small-molecule interference immune pathways to improve tissue repair and regeneration, and successfully use this effective method of simple organisms only for higher organisms (such as humans).

### 8.2.2 Foreign Bodies

Among the local factors affecting wound healing, it is mainly the effect of foreign matter retention on the wound or wound in the wound, including shrapnel, warhead, and other foreign matter being carried into the body. Usually large foreign bodies can be seen by the naked eye or by X-ray, but foreign objects below the millimeter level are hard to find by the naked eye.

The effect of foreign body on wound healing mainly comes from the following aspects: First, the foreign body itself has a large number of bacteria, which easily cause local wound infection; second, some foreign bodies, such as gunpowder particles, phosphorus particles, lead particles, etc., have certain tissue toxicity, which can cause direct damage to surrounding tissues; third, foreign bodies stimulate surrounding tissues, aggravating the reaction process in the acute inflammatory phase. Therefore, the wounds caused by trauma should be removed as much as possible during debridement. Foreign bodies in deep tissues, if they do not affect physiological functions, do not need to be barely removed, so as not to cause large tissue damage. Sharp foreign bodies immediately adjacent to the nerves and blood vessels should be removed in time. Free large bone fragments should be reset as much as possible during surgery, and bone fragments that are small and lose vitality should also be removed. At the time of surgery, the ligature and the suture are also foreign bodies. The shorter and less the retention, the better, to alleviate the local inflammatory response.

### 8.2.3 Hematoma and Ineffective Cavity

Both hematoma and ineffective lumens have a tendency to increase infection and will directly or indirectly affect wound healing. A non-contaminating surgical incision should be completely stopped when the incision is closed, and the layered suture does not leave a dead space. For contaminated wounds, the use of ligation should be used to stop bleeding as much as possible. Electrocautery or compression to stop bleeding should be the first choice. A drainage strip should be placed when the incision is closed, and taken out 48–72 h after injury. If a localized hematoma is formed, it will exert pressure on the normal tissue of the wound, affecting the blood supply of the wound edge, delaying the healing of the light, and causing tissue necrosis.

### 8.2.4 Local Blood Flow Supply

Insufficient local arterial blood supply or venous return disorders can lead to a decline in the supply of oxygen and nutrients, dystrophic granulation tissue, slow growth, and impede healing. Ischemia around the wound has both systemic and local factors. Local factors include both the influence of blood vessels itself and the ischemia caused by extravascular tissue hemorrhage and edema.

Under the action of the injury factor, different degrees of cellular and tissue damage occur locally, and the inflammatory process is initiated. The arterioles are transiently contracted, ranging from a few seconds to several minutes, followed by hemodynamics and rheological changes. The three phases: high mobile phase → low mobile phase → blood flow stagnation phase. If the damage factor is too strong or long-lasting, the low mobile phase is prolonged, plasma extravasation is increased, blood viscosity is increased, and blood flow is stagnant. In addition, leukocytes swim out of the blood vessels, accumulate in large areas in the injured area, phagocytose necrotic tissue and foreign bodies, the oxygen consumption is significantly increased, and the metabolic activity is enhanced, resulting in a relative lack of blood supply in the damaged area. Hemorrhage, edema, increased tension, and compression of blood vessels around the wound are another major cause of tissue ischemia around the wound. Wound repair must have adequate blood flow, on the one hand, to provide sufficient oxygen and necessary nutrients to the wounded area, and on the other hand, to transport locally produced toxic products, metabolic waste, bacteria, and foreign bodies out of the damaged area.

The mechanical causes of local blood supply shortage are mainly local pressure, friction, and increased shear force, such as wound dressing or suture tightness, pressure ulcer formation. Vascularization caused by inflammation of local blood vessels or narrowing of blood vessel caused by small arteriosclerosis, such as venous leg ulcers and diabetic foot ulcers. In addition, smoking can also lead to dysfunction of the blood circulation system, which is mainly manifested in the following two aspects:

(a) Nicotine acts on the smooth muscle of the small arterial wall, causing the arteriole to contract and the blood flow to slow down.
(b) Inhaled carbon monoxide will compete with hemoglobin, which will reduce the oxygen carrying capacity of the blood and affect the oxygen supply of the wound tissue.

## 8.3 Other Factors Affecting Tissue Repair and Regeneration

### 8.3.1 Environmental Factors

Studies have shown that the use of moisturizing dressings to maintain a certain degree of humidity on the local wounds will help to form a local hypoxic environment, thereby stimulating fibroblast growth and capillary sprout formation. In moist, hypoxic, and slightly acidic environments, the dissolution of necrotic tissue is enhanced, and the release of various growth factors closely related to tissue repair is increased without increasing the infection rate and significantly reducing wound pain.

The climatic conditions at high altitudes often cause hypoxia in the body. After local tissue injury, when the local blood circulation of the injured tissue is subjected to certain obstacles, the wound tissue is in a low perfusion state and ischemic and hypoxic, and the repair of the injury reaction is inhibited, delaying the healing time.

Under a high-temperature and high-humidity environment, various bacteria grow and reproduce.

Therefore, it is easy to cause healing difficulties, as described in the relevant chapters.

### 8.3.2 The Impact of Ionizing Radiation on Healing

Any kind of irradiation (including gamma rays, X-rays, alpha and beta rays, electron beams, etc.) can directly cause skin ulcers that are difficult to heal, and on the other hand can indirectly affect the healing process of the wound. The mechanism is that the radiation damages small blood vessels, inhibits fibroblast proliferation and collagen synthesis and secretion. High doses of radiation can significantly delay healing wounds.

The sensitivity of different tissue cells to ionizing radiation is inconsistent. According to Bergonie and Tribondeau, the sensitivity of cell radiation is directly proportional to the ability of cells to proliferate, and inversely proportional to the degree of cell differentiation. Hematopoietic cells are sensitive to radiation damage, followed by skin cells. The effect of ionizing radiation on wound healing is closely related to the type of radiation, the dose of radiation, the way of irradiation, and the time of irradiation. Generally, the larger the irradiation dose and the longer the irradiation time, the heavier the degree of healing. For localized exposure, the same dose of soft X-rays is more effective in delaying healing than gamma rays and hard X-rays. Most of the radiation is absorbed by the superficial skin, which aggravates skin damage. For systemic radiation injury, the healing of the local wound interacts with the overall condition of the body. According to the existing literature, total body irradiation below 2 Gy has no effect on wound healing; When it comes to more than 4 Gy, wound healing is significantly delayed; and 7 Gy or more after systemic irradiation due to obvious damage of hematopoietic function, if not treated, usually not yet The wound healed and the animal has died.

The pathological process of high-dose ionizing radiation significantly delaying wound healing is mainly manifested as: hematopoietic function is inhibited, inflammatory reaction is weakened, especially inflammatory cells such as macrophages and neutrophils which are locally infiltrated by trauma are significantly reduced, and the wound initiation process is delayed; vascular damage, endothelial cell degeneration, necrosis, bleeding is obvious; granulation tissue formation and maturation are significantly slowed down, fibroblasts number and function are impaired; re-epithelialization process is delayed, healing time is prolonged. In recent years, molecular-level research has further deepened the understanding of the mechanism of ionizing radiation to delay wound healing. Studies have shown that the decrease of hematopoietic cell source and radiation-induced apoptosis is an important cause of the reduction of local inflammatory cell volume in trauma, and the radiation effect. Inhibition of cell proliferation and increased apoptosis are important reasons for the decrease in the number of fibroblasts.

The mechanism by which ionizing radiation delays wound healing is "the regulation of disorders by healing factors that are the key link of cell damage", in which "cells" include both hematopoietic cells and repair cells, while "damage" includes both quantitative and functional damage. An important principle for the healing of open wound wounds is to increase the number of hematopoietic and repair cells in the wound and promote their function.

### 8.3.3 The Impact of Drugs on Healing

1. Cytotoxic drugs: These drugs can inhibit the growth, differentiation, and collagen synthesis of fibroblasts. Theoretically, they have the effect of delaying wound healing, but they have not been fully confirmed in clinical practice.
2. Steroids: Because it is the most commonly used anti-inflammatory drug in clinical application, it has a significant inhibitory effect on wound healing. Its main mechanism is to inhibit the inflammatory process and promote protein breakdown. It has been clinically proven that the preoperative or intraoperative steroid use cases have significantly increased complications, and systemic use of vitamin A can antagonize the inhibitory effect of steroids on inflammation. Recently, studies have also shown that mastering the application time and dosage of post-traumatic steroid drugs can sometimes promote wound repair. Other anti-inflammatory drugs have less effect on wound healing, but more than the pharmacological dose of aspirin has the effect of delaying wound healing.
3. In the process of debridement, some doctors added vasoconstrictor drugs and adrenaline to local anesthetics in order to reduce wound bleeding. The further research's purpose is to determine whether this measure aggravate local tissue ischemia and secondary wound hemorrhage, and then influence the healing process.

### 8.3.4 Other

If the local fixation is poor, the adjacent joint wound is difficult to heal. This may be related to premature activity, which may cause exudation reactions in the inflammatory process, aggravate local swelling, and affect blood supply to the injured area. The new granulation tissue is very fragile, which is prone to damage bleeding, affecting the differentiation of fibroblasts and the formation of scar tissue. Premature activity of the fracture is also prone to bone disconnection and pseudo joint formation.

## References

1. Xuan L, Nie J, Cheng W. Neuro-immuno-endocrine system mediates the effects of psychological stress on wound healing. Chin J Aesthetic Med. 2009;18(12):1825–8.
2. Xuan L. The changes of systemic angiotensin system in surgical patients. Guangzhou: Southern Medical University; 2010.
3. Fu XB, Cheng W. Relationship between aging skin characteristics and wound healing. Chin J Multiple Organ Dis. 2002;1(3):229–31.
4. Fu XB, Cheng W. Pay attention to the study of the effect of aging on wound healing. J Traumatic Surg. 2005;7:383–5.
5. Chen K, Wu L, Liu YS, et al. Retrospective survey and inspiration of hospitalized patients with hard-to-heal wounds. J Pract Med. 2014;23:3849–52.
6. Xuan M. Experimental study of autophagy involved in wound healing of aging skin. Guangzhou: Southern Medical University; 2014.
7. Yao B, Liu WH, Fu Y. Research progress on nutritional factors affecting wound healing. Genom Appl Biol. 2012;31(6):640–3.
8. Fu XB, Cheng W. Emphasis on the role of neurological, endocrine and immune mechanisms in skin repair and regeneration. Chin J Rep Reconstr Surg. 2006;20:331–5.
9. Fu XB. Bacterial biofilm formation and chronic refractory wounds occur. J Traumatic Surg. 2008;10(5):416–7.
10. Wang K, Xie Y, Wang H, et al. Bacterial biofilm and chronic wound healing. Chin J Hospital Infect Dis. 2016;26(19):4554–6.

# 9 New Technologies and Tissue Repair and Regeneration (1): Stem Cells, Tissue Engineering, and 3D Technology

Nanbo Liu, Sha Huang, Bin Yao, Jing Liu, Zuguo Liu, Huiqi Xie, Jin Zhou, Hong Li, Xiaoning Yang, Changyong Wang, Quanyi Guo, Yu Zhang, and Weimin Guo

## 9.1 Tissue Engineering and 3D Technology

Since its inception, tissue engineering technology has made significant progress in many fields such as biomedicine, such as the separation of new cell sources and seed cells, the design and synthesis of high biomimetic biomaterial scaffolds, the invention of new drugs and delivery systems, and the development of flux bio-manufacturing technology. Such results have led to the rapid development of some innovative clinical treatment strategies; especially, the repair and regeneration of tissue and organ damage have achieved satisfactory clinical results. At present, tissue engineering and regenerative medicine strategies can be broadly classified into three categories: cell-based therapeutic strategies; stent-therapeutic strategies with acellular scaffolds or seeded cells; and cell-loaded structures or matrix complexes.

Specifically, cell-based therapies are allogeneic or xenogeneic cells taken from patients (autologous) or donors (same species, xenogeneic), after further processing (e.g., cell sorting and in vitro expansion) into the lesion. This therapy is relatively simple, but faces problems such as how to maintain cell activity and colonization. Therefore, a new strategy for immobilizing specific cells in biomaterial carrier scaffolds to enhance colonization and viability has emerged. Depending on the degree of damage and the biomechanical properties of the tissue, different scaffold implant materials can be selected to provide a specific environment for the cells, guiding the penetration, colonization, attachment, and proliferation of seed cells or host cells, promoting the synthesis of new extracellular matrix, thereby improving clinical efficacy. Our research team loaded gelatin microspheres containing sweat gland cells into tissue-engineered skin. It can form a full-thick skin with sweat gland structure in vitro, promote complete repair of skin in vivo, and provide a new strategy for clinical treatment of wound.

Currently, there are generally two ways to perform organ transplantation using cell 3D printing technology. Taking the liver as an example, one is to first scan the shape of the patient's liver, insert the biomaterial into the body, and then implant the cells, using the internal environment to grow the liver with sufficient nutrient solution; the species is printed directly in vitro and transplanted into the patient. The second method is more scientific and the effect will be more ideal, but to achieve a high technical content, there is still a certain distance from the application. Moreover, even if the 3D-printed artificial organs function normally in vitro, it is currently unknown whether they can be operated and what are the adverse reactions once implanted in the body. In addition, the nutrient absorption and excretion of organs after transplantation is the process of gradually repairing, adapting, and replacing the old organs in the body. If the organ support system can be constructed and studied first, the rejection reaction and relevant risk after organ implantation in the human body will be reduced [1].

On the other hand, before the real maturity of 3D printing organ technology, a series of high costs such as research and development and market development will become high-end consumption. Especially in China, 3D printing technology is still in the initial stage of development, and there are still bottlenecks in technology. If the type and performance of the material are limited, the efficiency of forming needs to be

N. Liu
Southern Medical University, Guangzhou, China

S. Huang (✉) · B. Yao · Q. Guo · W. Guo
The Chinese People's Liberation Army General Hospital, Beijing, China

J. Liu · Z. Liu
Xiamen University School of Medicine, Xiamen, China

H. Xie
West China Hospital, Sichuan University, Chengdu, China

J. Zhou · H. Li · X. Yang · C. Wang
Academy of Military Medical Sciences, Military Cognition and Brain Science Research Institution, Beijing, China

Y. Zhang
Nanjing Drum Tower Hospital, Nanjing, China


X. Fu (ed.), *Regenerative Medicine in China*, https://doi.org/10.1007/978-981-16-1182-7_9

further improved, and there is an urgent need for reinforcement in the size, precision, and stability of the process. Moreover, China's 3D printing consumables mainly rely on foreign imports. Excessive material costs may be one of the reasons hindering development, which will greatly reduce the cost performance of 3D printing technology, and to some extent weaken the market's emphasis on this technology. Therefore, at this stage, the investment in 3D printing in the field of biomedicine should focus on strengthening innovation and research and development, technology introduction and reserve, especially paying attention to the construction and maintenance of independent intellectual property rights, and strive to occupy a favorable position in the future market competition.

Currently, the biomedical field has become one of the most popular areas for 3D printing applications. In 2012, the output value of 3D printing technology in this field accounted for 16.4% of the global output value. Most of the applications focused on prosthetic manufacturing, orthodontics, and restoration. By the end of 2013, there were as many as 30,000 successful cases of using titanium 3D printing to make titanium human bones. In addition, with the advancement of technology, cost reduction, aging of the population, and the small number of donated organs, the industry is generally optimistic about the development prospects of 3D bioprinting technology in the field of regenerative medicine, especially organ transplantation. With the continuous advancement of technology, the technology of applying 3D printing to tissue and organ transplantation is not only at the theoretical level. Moreover, each person's body structure and pathological conditions are unique and differentiated; when 3D printing is combined with medical image modeling and simulation techniques, a great driving effect can be generated in the manufacture of artificial prostheses, implants, and artificial tissues. I believe that in the near future, scientists will use a research result to prove the possibility of "organized transplants." However, the regulatory mechanism for 3D printed biological organs has not yet been established, and its classification and auditing standards in biomedical products are in a state of ambiguity. These all indicate that in addition to the technical development of 3D bioprinting, there is still a long way to go to establish a review mechanism for escorting this huge future emerging industry [2, 3].

## 9.2 Stem Cells and Related Technologies and Skin Repair and Regeneration

Stem cells are one of the most rapid advances in basic research and clinical applications of life sciences in recent years. Stem cells and related technologies have shown great potential for cell therapy, tissue and organ repair, developmental biology, and pharmacology. Since stem cells have the characteristics of regeneration and differentiation, stem cells implanted in the body or tissues constructed from stem cells in vitro can be implanted into the body to differentiate and regenerate damaged organs. At present, domestic and foreign institutions have successfully tried various tissues and organ regenerations using stem cells. For example, scientists use bone marrow mesenchymal stem cells and umbilical cord mesenchymal stem cells to differentiate into muscle cells, nerve cells, and sweat gland cells in vitro and in vivo, and bring hope for the treatment of large-area trauma, such as muscle atrophy, brain atrophy, Parkinson's disease, and other degenerative diseases and burn wounds; embryonic stem cells, neural stem cells, epidermal stem cells, and dermal papilla cells are isolated from developing or adult embryonic stem cell tissues, and induced pluripotent stem cells can be obtained in vitro, and implanted in vitro after expansion and culture. The site is differentiated into neurons, astrocytes, oligodendrocytes, epidermal cells, hair follicles, sebaceous glands, and sweat glands, providing new strategies for nerve tissue and wound repair.

At present, stem cells used in stem cell therapy and tissue engineering are self-stem cells, and it is difficult to industrialize regenerative medicine results. The establishment of low-immunogenic stem cells to achieve universal seed cells across individual applications is a need to achieve tissue engineering industrialization. In addition, the safety of stem cell therapy is an important prerequisite for clinical application of stem cells. Methods for stem cells to enter the body include direct intratissue injection, as well as intravascular injection or by tissue engineering scaffold-based transport. Safe, effective, and practical route of administration is the key to the success of stem cell regeneration therapy, mainly to ensure the effective cell dose and targeting of tissue regeneration, and it is hoped that it will be less distributed in non-targeted areas and spread the blood source. The danger is minimized.

The skin is the largest in the human body, and it is also the first organ damaged after wounding (burning, war). After mild injury (burning, war), the skin and its accessory cells are destroyed, and their repair and regeneration often use their uninjured parts as a template to achieve complete repair through proliferation and differentiation. However, in the case of large-scale wounds (burning, war) in the whole layer, due to the complete destruction of the skin, the skin and its accessory cells cannot completely rely on the division, proliferation, and differentiation of the stem cells to rebuild their complex structures, thereby making the skin and the attachment regeneration difficult, and eventually there will be two aspects of healing problems, namely the formation of chronic difficult-to-heal wounds (commonly known as chronic ulcers) or excessive repair of hypertrophic scars and keloids, not only for the physical and psychological aspects of patients' serious obstacles, but also have a serious impact on the quality of life and work in the later period. The patients suffer a lot from the damage of sweat gland cells. Sweating is the main way for the body to regulate body temperature. The sweat glands are all over the body. It is difficult to regenerate and leads to a very low quality of life. It is even life-threatening in hot climates. As the most abundant gland of the body, the sweat gland can form a layered epidermis under certain conditions, and its role in skin damage repair is more important than epidermal cells. Our team used inactivated sweat gland cells to coculture with MSC and added sweat gland induction medium to induce differentiation of mesenchymal stem cells into sweat gland cells, overexpressing Eda in MSC, reprograming these two cells into sweat gland cells, and participate in skin repair by transferring NF-κB and Lef1 into fibroblasts. Liang et al. induced the differentiation of amniotic fluid stem cells into sweat gland cells by using sweat gland culture medium. Further experiments and exploration are needed to apply the above various sweat gland cell regeneration methods to the clinic. At present, the commonly used repair methods mainly include autologous free skin graft, flap transplantation, allogeneic skin, and xenograft. Autologous skin grafting is the best method for wound defect repair; but for patients with large skin defects, autologous skin sources are often insufficient to seal wounds in a timely and effective manner. Although allogeneic skin transplantation is a common clinical treatment for patients with extensive burns, the problem of immune rejection has been difficult to completely overcome, so it can only be used as a means to temporarily close the wound. In recent years, research and application of tissue engineering skin has made some progress, and it has provided new ideas and methods for solving this problem. However, there is still no ideal tissue engineering of skin that can fully meet the needs of patients with severe skin defects. One of the important reasons is the problem of the source of seed cells. Since the mature cells obtained from the patient's autologous or allogeneic cells are terminal cells and have no ability to further proliferate and differentiate to form new tissues, stem cells are the best choice for researchers in regenerative medicine [4].

So far, although there have been many breakthroughs in the application of stem cells and related technologies in skin wound repair and tissue regeneration, there are still many important problems that have not been proven, such as how to increase the proliferation of autologous cells, prolong the cells' life cycle and the ability to increase the secretion of cells; how to optimize the best cells of the same function from different tissue sources, establish a standard cell line, make the research work more comparable and scientific; the mutual interaction between cells and artificial extracellular matrix, the role and influencing factors, as well as the molecular mechanism guiding the development of pluripotent stem cells into target cells; how to accurately and efficiently transform the genome, and overcoming the immunological disorders during transplantation, will become the focus of long-term research.

## 9.3 Application of 3D Technology in Organ Tissue Engineering and Regeneration

With the development of regenerative medicine, the concept of 3D bioprinting (also known as organ printing) has received increasing attention. In 2010, 3D Bioprinters was named one of the 50 best inventions of 2010 by the Time magazine. Just like the normal 3D printing format, this biotechnology prints the tissue cells and the inner wall cells of the blood vessels layer by layer, which forms a solid organ that simulates human tissue. 3D printing technology was first proposed by Charles W. Hull in 1986. He called it "stereoscopic curing technology," which printed a thin layer of material after UV irradiation to form a solid 3D structure, which was then used to shape the biomaterial into a resin model with a three-dimensional structure. The discovery of solvent-free systems has enabled biomaterials to be printed directly to form 3D scaffolds for transplantation. 3D bioprinting as a tissue engineering technology and its further development requires the development of 3D printing technology, cell biology, and materials science. In clinical medical applications, 3D bioprinting has been used to make catheters and splints.

3D printing precisely controls the positioning of functional components such as biomaterials, biochemicals, and living cells in each layer, and prints layer by layer to form a 3D structure. Common 3D printing methods include biosimulation, autonomous self-assembly, and the construction of mini organization modules. At present, the development of new printing methods to create clinically active, biologically active 3D structures has attracted the attention of many researchers. One of the major challenges is transforming traditional printing plastic and metal technologies into new technologies that print sensitive, active biomaterials. However, the main challenge is to reproduce the microstructure of extracellular matrices and various cells with extremely high precision and to assess their biological functions (Fig. 9.1).

The main technologies used for biomaterial accumulation and molding are inkjet printing, micro-extrusion printing, and laser-assisted printing (Fig. 9.2). We discuss their differences from the most important factors of 3D bioprinting technology (interface resolution, cell activity, and biomaterials used for printing) (Table 9.1).

At first, 3D printing technology was only used in nonbiological fields, such as metal deposition, ceramics, thermoplastic polymers, and related technologies, such as organic solvents, high temperatures, and cross-linking reagents that are incompatible with biological materials and living cells. Therefore, finding materials that are compatible with both biomaterials and provide the appropriate mechanical and functional properties required for tissue scaffolding is a major challenge for 3D bioprinting.

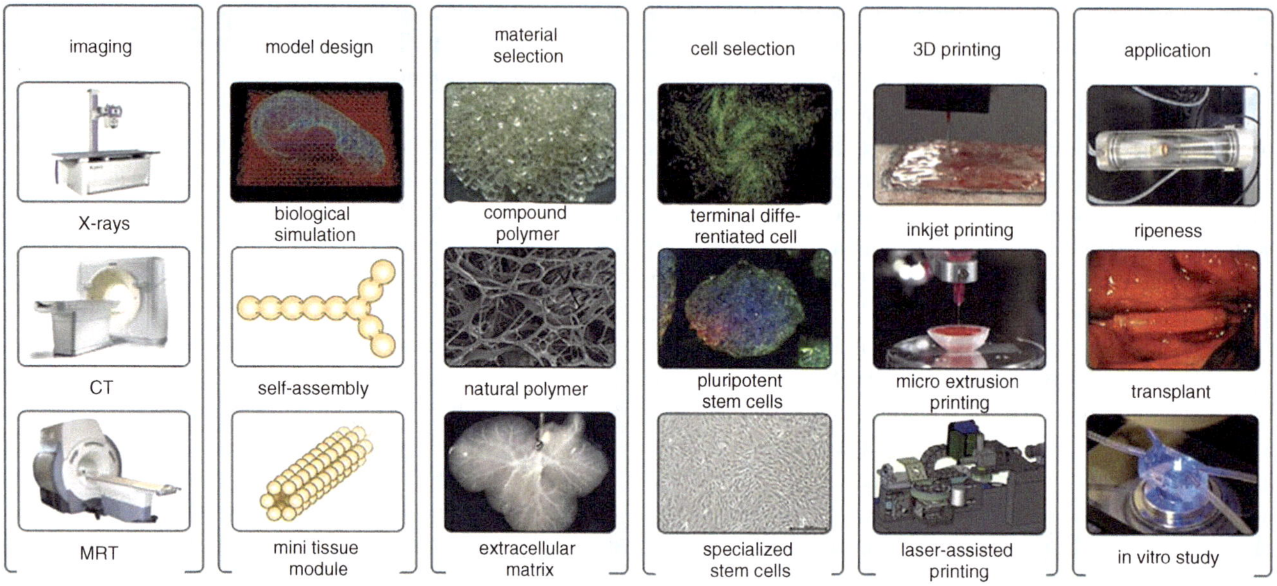


**Fig. 9.1** 3D bioprinting process

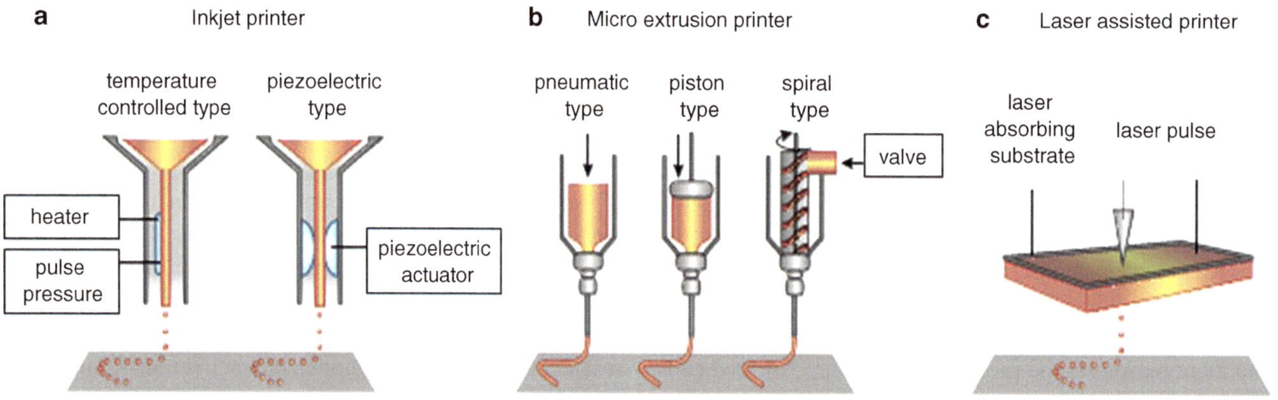


**Fig. 9.2** Composition and structure of an inkjet printer, micro-squeezing printer, and laser-assisted printer

**Table 9.1** Comparison of several bioprinters

| Bio printer type | | | | |
|---|---|---|---|---|
| | Ink Jet | Micro extrusion type | Laser assisted | References |
| Material viscosity | 3.5–12 mPa/s | 30–6 × $10^7$ mPa/s | 1–300 mPa/s | [5] |
| Molding method | Chemistry, optical cross-linking | Chemistry, temperature, optical cross-linking | Chemistry, optical cross-linking | [6] |
| Preparation time | low | Low to medium | Medium to high | [7] |
| Print speed | Quick (1–10,000 drip/s) | Slow(10–50 μm/s) | Medium to quick (200–1600 mm/s) | [8] |
| Print resolution | 50 μm | 5 μm | Microscale | [8] |
| Cell Survival | >85% | 40–80% | >95% | [9] |
| Cell density | Low, <$10^6$ cell/mL | High, cell mass | $10^8$ cell/mL | [9] |
| Print loss | Low | Medium | High | [10] |

Cellular 3D printing technology provides a new clinical medicine technology for tissue and organ repair, and also provides a very good research tool for research fields such as regenerative medicine, tissue engineering, stem cells, and cancer. In 2011, the Wake Foster Institute of Regenerative Medicine in the United States presented their human kidneys printed on a 3D printer in a TED (Technology Entertainment Design) presentation. They used the cultured kidney cells as a printed material and printed the cells layer by layer in a predesigned virtual model. The first layer is the cells and the second layer is the hydrogel used to bind the cells. Then repeat one layer until the entire kidney prints out. The initially formed kidneys are then moved to the incubator to provide nutrients for growth. By the time the cells survive, the hydrogel is degraded, leaving only the cells. At present, the laboratory said that it has been observed that this initial kidney model produced a urine-like substance, indicating that some kidney function has been obtained. Our laboratory uses the Regenovo bio 3D printer produced by a biotechnology company in Hangzhou to mix the biological hydrogel with the epidermal stem cells, construct a skin model in vitro, and successfully induce the epidermal stem cells to differentiate into skin accessories such as sweat glands, which brings hope to the perfect regeneration of the wound [11].

In 2013, Cornell University used the 3D printer to print the world's first artificial ear. Every year, tens of thousands of people lose all or part of their ears because of congenital development or illness or accident. Traditional ear replanting uses the costal cartilage as an alternative to ear cartilage, but the ear that is made out is neither aesthetically pleasing nor functional. The team used a computer to scan the normal ears of the patient's side, and then used a 3D printer to print a symmetrical ear model, in which the cell-filled collagen was injected as a scaffold for cartilage growth. The ears that are made out of this shape are suitable and beautiful in appearance. Within 3 months, these ears can grow cartilage and replace the collagen used for shaping. This research was published online in PLOS One magazine [12].

According to the May 2013 issue of the New England Journal of Medicine (NEJM), a 6-week-old boy in Ohio, USA, suffered from bronchial softening and was critically ill. The doctor used a 3D printer to create a splint that opened up a passage in the baby's airway. The baby boy finally managed to maintain his breath and survived. This is the first case of successful transplantation of 3D printed organs in medical history. According to the statistics of the US organ sharing network (UNOS), the number of patients waiting for organ transplantation is increasing year by year. However, due to the insufficient number of organ donations and the serious repulsion problems that may occur after surgery, traditional medical treatments have been unable to meet the requirements of organ transplant patients. Therefore, the application of 3D printing technology in this field will certainly bring about a medical revolution [13].

With the rapid development of 3D printing technology, the use of biocompatible materials, cells, and supporting components to print 3D functional organs is getting closer and closer to us. The future of 3D bioprinting technology will be a key technology for regenerative medicine to address tissue and organ transplant needs. Based on current trends, 3D printed tissue can be used not only for organ transplantation but also for drug delivery, analysis of chemical reagents, biological agents and toxic substances, and basic research. As we said before, 3D printing is very complex. Compared to nonbiological printing, 3D bioprinting involves many influencing factors such as material selection, cell type, cell growth, and differentiation factors, maximally maintaining cell viability and construction of tissue structure. There are many challenges that lie ahead of us, including the maturity and functionalization of the organization, the appropriate vascularization and neurochemistry. Starting from a 2D tissue such as the skin, a solid organ such as a kidney is finally formed by forming a hollow duct such as a blood vessel and a hollow tubular-free organ such as the bladder. Only by combining the knowledge of multidisciplinary fields such as engineering, biomaterials science, cell biology, physics, and medicine, can we solve these problems and realize the need for 3D bioprinting for regenerative medicine to solve tissue and organ transplants [14].

## 9.4 Tissue Engineering Cornea

### 9.4.1 The Classification of Tissue Engineering Cornea

Materials for constructing tissue engineering corneas mainly include scaffold materials and seed cells. There is no standard classification method for tissue engineering cornea in the world. At present, it is mainly classified according to the material of the scaffold and the source of the seed cells.

#### 9.4.1.1 Classification by Source of Scaffold Materials

According to the source of the scaffold material, the tissue cornea can be divided into synthetic materials and natural materials. The synthetic materials are subdivided into degradable polymer materials and nondegradable polymers. Natural materials are subdivided into natural polymer materials and biological derived materials.

A. Degradable Polymer Material

Synthetic degradable polymer materials such as polylactic acid, polyglycolic acid, and polylactic acid glycolic acid can be used as carriers for tissue engineering cornea [15]. These materials have good histocompatibility and support epithelial, stroma, and endothelial cell adhesion growth. These materials produce a large amount of lactic acid or glycolic acid during the degradation process in the body. Although they can be absorbed by the body gradually, and the metabolic mechanism is clear and biosafety is reliable, the acidic degradation products of these materials will adversely affect the activity of the cells. Therefore, it is not used as a scaffold material for tissue engineering corneal implantation, but it is tried in vitro to culture tissue engineering corneal seed cells.

B. Non-degradable Polymer

A cornea prepared using a non-degradable polymer is called an artificial cornea. Artificial corneas first appeared in clinical trials in the 1960s, initially using glass to sew directly onto the surface of the eye. Although this treatment can improve the patient's vision, due to the short-term rejection, the tissue around the artificial cornea dissolves and the artificial cornea falls off, which makes the surgery fail. With the continuous advancement of materials science, artificial corneas continue to develop, and the artificial corneas currently used in clinical practice are mainly BostonKPro [16] and AlphaCor [17], all of which have been approved by the FDA to enter the clinic.

The Boston I artificial cornea is the earliest applied artificial cornea. The optical cylindrical part is made of PMMA and has good transparency. The Boston II (Fig. 9.3) type is improved on the basis of type I, which optimizes the design of the artificial cornea, making the transplant surgery simpler, and the leakage rate of the suture is reduced. The titanium alloy fixture is added to reduce artificial corneal prolapse due to rejection (Fig. 9.4).

Osteo-Odonto-keratoprosthesis (OOKP) was pioneered by the Italian scientist Strampelli, using autologous tissue (teeth) as a peripheral scaffold and PMMA as an optical column. This special structure of the bone tooth is better for increasing corneal biocompatbility and binding to the host, which play a positive role. It has been reported that OOKP has been placed in patients for up to 20 years. Although the creative implantation of autologous tissue as part of the cornea reduces the rejection rate and visual acuity recovery after implantation, the complications are still unavoidable, and the operation is difficult and costly, which limits its wide application.

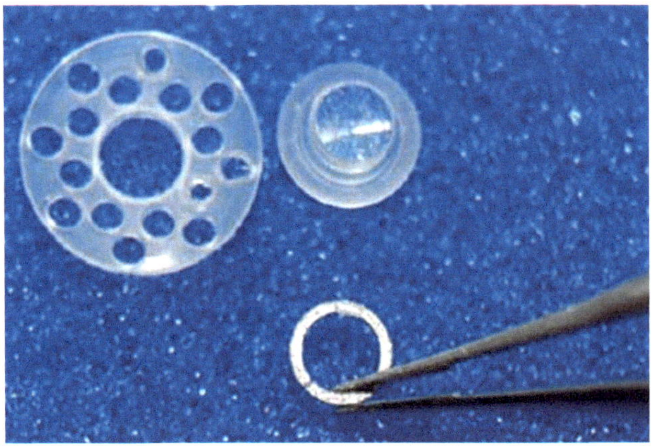

**Fig. 9.3** Boston II artificial cornea

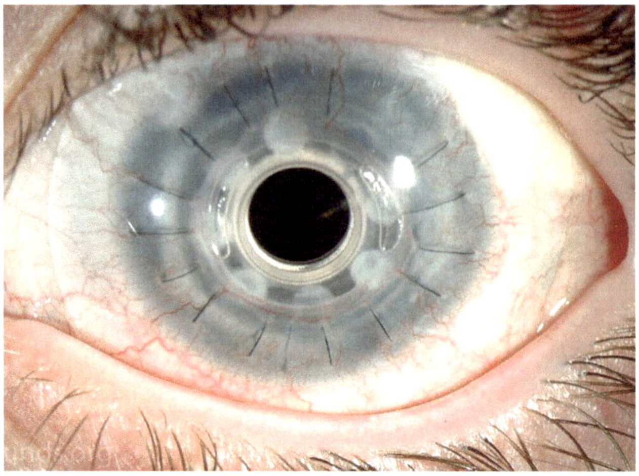

**Fig. 9.4** After Boston II artificial corneal transplantation

Due to the high rejection rate, the surgical indications for artificial corneas are relatively narrow, and patients with severe ocular surface trauma and severe damage to the conjunctival sac or tear system cannot be recovered. This is also one of the reasons why artificial cornea development is slower than tissue engineering cornea.

C. Natural Polymer Materials

Natural polymeric materials are derived from extracts of natural materials. In the early days, there were many studies on the use of natural polymer materials for tissue engineering cornea, and collagen was one of the commonly used materials. Collagen fiber is the main component of the corneal stroma, and collagen accounts for 75% of the dry weight of the cornea [18]. Collagen has no antigenicity, good histocompatibility, and contains certain specific amino acid sequences, which are beneficial to the adhesion and growth of seed cells. The shortcomings of collagen are poor stability, low mechanical strength, and rapid degradation (the degradation time of collagen produced by ordinary cross-linking method is about 1 month), and it is cross-linked by various physical or chemical methods, such as thermal cross-linking, UV and $\lambda$-ray cross-linking, and polyepoxide cross-linking, which can improve mechanical strength and resistance to degradation (the degradation time can be increased to 3 months or half a year).

Chitin is the only natural polysaccharide in the natural world that is second only to cellulose, and is widely found in insects, crustacean shells, and fungal cell walls [19]. The deacetylation reaction turns it into chitosan. Such natural polysaccharides have significant alkalinity, good biocompatibility, and biodegradability. Chitosan is hydrolyzed into oligosaccharides by the action of lysozyme and chitinase in the body. The degradation products are N-acetylglucosamine and glucosamine, which are nontoxic to the human body. The low-molecular-weight chitin or its oligosaccharide produced during the degradation process does not accumulate in the body and is not immunogenic.

Although there have been studies to continuously improve cross-linking and cross-linking methods to delay the degradation cycle of natural polymer materials, these materials cannot be transparent when used as a scaffold for corneal stroma, as a scaffold for corneal epithelium or corneal endothelium. Its biological properties are not as good as some biologically derived materials, such as amnion, so it is not widely used.

D. Biologically Derived Materials

Bioderived materials have certain advantages because their structures and biological components are closer to living tissues. The construction of tissue engineering corneas with amnion as a carrier has become a research hotspot. Amniotic membrane is a translucent membrane with no blood vessels, nerves and lymphatic vessels. It has low immunogenicity and is resistant to new blood vessels, inhibits fibrosis, and reduces scar formation. The amniotic basement membrane contains IV-type and V-type collagen, laminin, fibronectin, and various chelating proteins, which are beneficial for cell differentiation and migration. At present, amniotic membrane has been widely used in tissue engineering research, and the corneal epithelial layer, stromal layer, and endothelial layer have been successfully constructed. Amniotic membrane is considered an ideal carrier material for tissue engineering cornea [20]. However, the amniotic membrane is too thin to construct a stratified corneal tissue. The application of the amniotic membrane also has the risk of causing the spread of infectious diseases such as hepatitis and acquired immunodeficiency syndrome (AIDS).

Other tissue-derived thin carriers can be used to culture epithelial and endothelial seed cells to construct tissue engineering corneas, primarily postcorneal elastic layers, amnion basement membranes, synthetic gelatin membranes, anterior capsular membranes, and skin-derived fibrous membranes.

#### 9.4.1.2 Classification by Seed Cell Source

According to the source of seed cells, it can be divided into adult stem cells, embryonic stem cells, and induced pluripotent stem cells (iPSC). The main sources of adult stem cells are corneal epithelial stem cells and bone marrow mesenchymal stem cells. The former is mainly obtained through corneal donation and autologous biopsy, and the latter source can be obtained by sorting out bone marrow mesenchymal stem cells in the blood of the patient. Embryonic stem cells come from a wide range of sources and are mainly obtained by cord blood. The source of autologous stem cells is limited, and allogeneic stem cells have a certain rejection rate, and iPSC will be able to solve these factors that limit the development of tissue engineering cornea.

### 9.4.2 The Construction Method of Tissue Engineering Cornea

The construction of tissue engineering cornea refers to the combination of seed cells and scaffold materials to form a firm, unitary structure and functional unit by culture in vitro. The construction methods of tissue engineering corneal epithelium, stroma, and endothelium are described below.

#### 9.4.2.1 Construction Method of Tissue Engineering Corneal Epithelium

Sources of corneal epithelial seed cells: in the normal basal layer of the corneal epithelium, there are stem cells and transiently expanded cells. The corneal epithelial stem cells are small in volume, large in nucleoplasmic ratio, and positive for CK19 and CK15, suggesting that the cell proliferation ability is strong [21]. It is generally believed that corneal epithelial stem cells do not express corneal epithelial-specific surface markers CK3 and CK12, and positive markers include Importin13, p63, ABCG-2, integrin α9, and N-cadaherin. Due to the limited source of corneal epithelial stem cells, it has been found that some adult stem cells from other sources can be transformed into epithelial cells with functional properties of corneal epithelial cells by in vitro expansion and induced differentiation. Sources of tissue that have been discovered so far include bone marrow, oral mucosa, fat, skin, and circulatory systems (Fig. 9.5).

In recent years, the development and improvement of limbal stem cell culture technology has provided a platform for transplantation of cultured limbal stem cells [22]. The source of the cells may be the limbus itself or the limbus of the allograft. The carriers available for transplantation include amniotic membrane, eggshell membrane, polylactic acid membrane, contact lens, cellulose membrane, etc., in which the epithelial cell amniotic membrane has more organisms. It is suitable for the growth of stem cells and has the effect of improving the inflammatory environment of the ocular surface. Therefore, it is an ideal carrier for transplantation and lays a foundation for clinical transplantation of cultured cells. At present, the technique of in vitro-cultured corneal

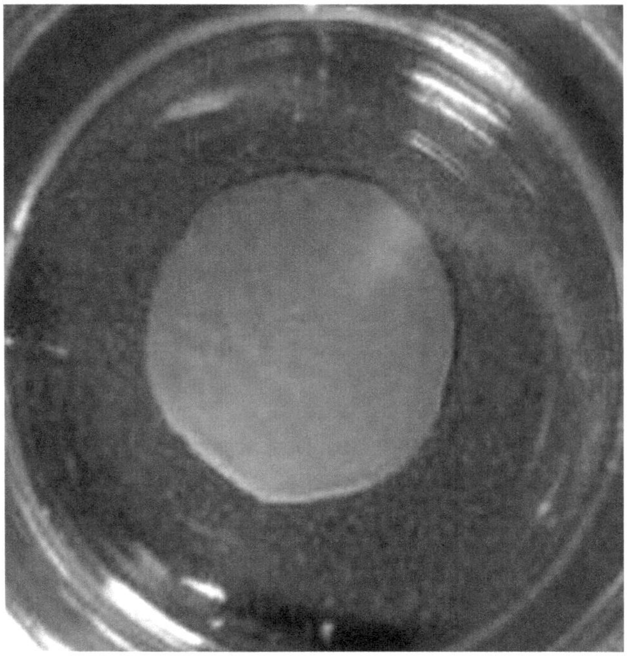

**Fig. 9.5** Amniotic membrane cocultured with stem cells

epithelial stem cell transplantation for reconstructing the ocular surface has matured, but how to shorten the culture time and maintain the characteristics of the limbal stem cells after culture still need further study.

#### 9.4.2.2 Allogeneic Corneal Decellularization Method

The allogeneic-derived cornea can be an extracellular scaffold for tissue engineering cornea by decellularization [23]. There are currently more than ten methods in the world for preparing a lamellar tissue engineering cornea by removing animal-derived corneal stromal cells. It mainly includes the following three types: a. Chemical reagent method: It destroys proteins, lipids and DNA in cells by using an acidic solution, an alkaline solution, a detergent, etc., and dissolves cell debris in a solvent to separate from the extracellular matrix. b. Biological reagents: Cells are inactivated and removed from the scaffold material by hydrolysis of catalytic nucleotides, deoxynucleotides, or peptide chains using nucleases and proteases. c. Physical decellularization method: By changing the physical temperature, pressure, osmotic pressure, and other physical factors outside the material, it will destroy the cell membrane and nuclear membrane, but cannot very effectively inactivate the cells and remove from the scaffold material.

#### 9.4.2.3 The Construction Method of Tissue Engineering Corneal Stroma

The source of corneal stromal seed cell: Some scholars believe that there are stem cells in the corneal stroma that use collagenase to decompose the corneal stroma, obtain corneal stromal cells, and select corneal stromal cells by cloning and culture. These expression stem cells have specific surface markers, such as Bmi-1, Notch-1, Six2, Pax6, ABCG2, Spag10, p62, and the like. Bone marrow mesenchymal stem cells can be used as one of the sources of corneal stroma seed cells.

#### 9.4.2.4 Construction Method of Tissue Engineering Corneal Endothelium

Sources of corneal endothelial seed cells: Human corneal endothelial cells in vivo cannot be propagated by mitosis, which is due to insufficient growth factor in the anterior chamber, and growth inhibitory factors in the aqueous humor, which block the DNA synthesis of the cells. However, the presence of various growth factor receptors on the corneal endothelium indicates that endothelial cells have potential for division. The growth and proliferation of corneal endothelial cells in vitro is also affected by cell origin. It has been shown that corneal endothelial cells in infants can be mitotic under certain conditions; the success rate of endothelial cell culture in patients over 20 years old is greatly reduced. Therefore, in the experiment of human corneal endothelial cell transplantation, the cultured endothelial cells are mostly from fetuses, infants, or young people under 20 years old [24].

Normal adult corneal endothelium does not proliferate under physiological conditions, but some endothelial cells express stem cell surface markers after trauma. McGowan believes that stem cells of corneal endothelial cells exist in the transitional region between trabecular meshwork and endothelial cells. In animal experiments, central and peripheral corneal endothelial cells have a certain proliferative capacity.

Construction of tissue engineering corneal endothelium: The method of tissue engineering corneal endothelium is to use a vector to grow into a continuous sheet of monolayer cell membrane for transplantation in vitro.

#### 9.4.2.5 Construction Method of Total Corneal Tissue Engineering

Tissue engineering of the whole cornea is constructed by cocultivating the corneal epithelium and its carrier, the corneal stroma scaffold and its seed cells, and the monolayer of endothelial cells according to the histological morphology of the normal cornea.

3D printing technology is currently being tested in the full corneal construction technology. Currently available printing materials are natural polymer materials such as agar, gelatin, collagen, and cellulose. Therefore, when the tissue engineering cornea after surgery is reconstructed, it cannot be like the corneal reconstruction after human corneal transplantation, and the transparency of the graft was decreased due to the growth of receptor cells and extracellular components into the tissue engineering cornea.

### 9.4.3 The Clinical Application of Tissue Engineering Cornea

Tissue engineering corneal epithelium progresses fastest in the direction of tissue engineering cornea. Italy, India, Japan, China, and other countries have used it in clinical practice for nearly ten years, and they initially evaluated the therapeutic effects of different culture methods and different surgical methods on tissue engineering corneal epithelial stem cell transplantation.

The clinical research of tissue engineering corneal stroma in China is at the forefront of the world. The large-scale clinical trials of tissue engineering corneal stroma in China have proved its safety and effectiveness. China's tissue engineering corneal stroma has entered the stage of industrialization, which will lay a good foundation for the development of clinical tissue engineering cornea in China.

### 9.4.4 Development Direction and Challenges of Tissue Engineering Cornea

#### 9.4.4.1 Development Direction of Tissue Engineering Cornea

Tissue engineering corneal epithelial technology has matured. With the establishment of industrialization standards such as culture, storage, and transportation of corneal epithelial stem cells, tissue engineering corneal epithelium will be widely used. At present, the most successful research on the synthesis of natural materials is the method of cross-linking type I collagen and type III collagen by aldehydes in Griffth, Canada (Fig. 9.6), and constructing a transparent corneal stroma stent with a thickness of 400 μm and transplanting it to 20 inpatients with corneal leukoplakia and keratoconus; the corneal epithelium was observed intact and the matrix was transparent 24 months after surgery [25]. The results of this research point to a new direction for the construction of tissue engineering corneal stroma for natural materials.

The tissue engineering cornea of allogeneic origin has many advantages such as wide source, low price, and simple preparation method. In animal experiments and early clinical trials, it was observed that the porcine-derived lamellar tissue engineering cornea can remain transparent for a long time. In vivo confocal microscopy revealed that 1 year after tissue engineering corneal transplantation, the subcutaneous plexus of cornea and the corneal stromal cells and nerve fibers in the stroma grow into the tissue engineering cornea. The results of this study demonstrate that pig-derived lamellar tissue engineering cornea is suitable for use as an allogeneic tissue engineering corneal scaffold with good clinical application prospects (Fig. 9.7).

The rejection rate after allogeneic corneal endothelial transplantation is higher than that of other types of corneal transplantation, so the requirements for tissue engineering corneal endothelium seed cells are higher than other seed cells. Due to the limited source of endothelial cells, the development of tissue engineering corneal endothelium technology is currently limited.

#### 9.4.4.2 The Challenge of Tissue Engineering Cornea

The ideal scaffold material has always been a bottleneck restricting the development of tissue engineering cornea. At present, although a wide range of materials have been extensively studied, there are not many scaffold materials that really meet the needs of constructing tissue engineering

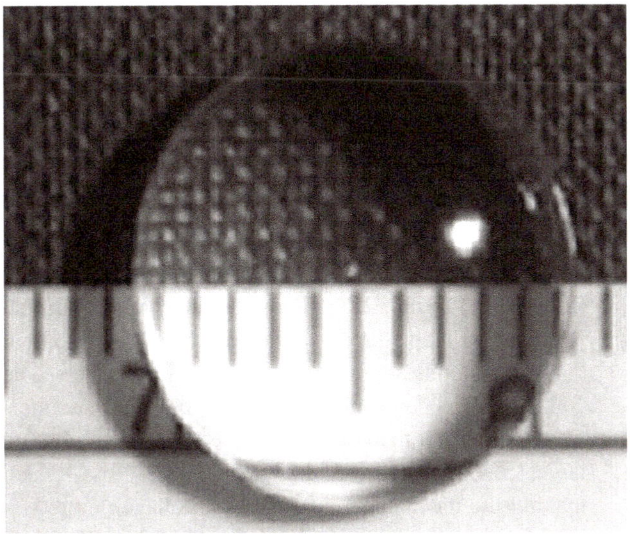

**Fig. 9.6** Tissue engineering cornea cross-linked with collagen

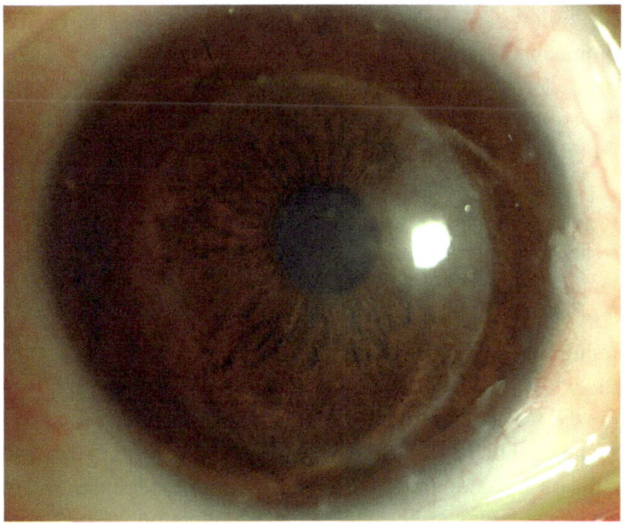

**Fig. 9.7** 3 Years after porcine-derived tissue engineering corneal transplantation

corneas, and both have certain disadvantages. Natural polymer materials, such as collagen, hyaluronic acid, chitin and its derivatives, and polysaccharide polymer materials, have good biocompatibility, but have disadvantages such as poor mechanical properties, too fast degradation, and are not conducive to the diffusion of the cellular nutrients into the material. Acidic degradation products of synthetic polymer materials tend to accumulate locally, which is not conducive to cell growth. Bioderived materials are derived from natural tissues and have certain development prospects as tissue engineering scaffold materials. However, its safety, tissue transparency, stability, and mechanicality need to be further evaluated before entering the scale of clinical trials.

In addition, the challenges faced by tissue engineering corneas include ethical restrictions, lack of relevant laws and regulations, and the lack of standardized source standards, preparation and preservation methods, and clear clinical indications.

Compared with other tissue engineering tissues and organs, tissue engineering corneas in China have developed rapidly. These clinical research advances indicate the advent of tissue engineering corneal industrialization, and the subsequent clinical research and the application will provide more choices and help for humans to cure corneal diseases.

## 9.5 Tissue Engineering Tendon

Tendon and ligament damage caused by trauma, exercise, chronic strain, and other injuries is a common clinical problem, which can lead to dysfunction and even disability. Since the advent of modern surgery, the most commonly used methods for repair of tendon are autograft, allograft, or artificial material, but they are still facing many problems.

As far as we know, the ideal tendon substitute should have the following advantages: (1) good histocompatibility and biomechanical properties; (2) does not adhere to the surrounding tissue after implantation; (3) can secure suture knots and smooth junction of tendon ends; (4) the healing speed is at or near the normal physiological healing process; (5) the tensile strength can match to the needs of the body; (6) easy to obtain or manufacture; and (7) can be assimilated by the body into a part of the body. Overall, the most important aspects of tendon substitute materials biology are able to completely replace the function of the tendon, and accept the regulation of the body and participate in the self-renewal of the body. The aim of tendon tissue engineering research is to develop a tendon substitute that meets the above requirements as much as possible. The principle is to obtain the seed cells of the tendon, and then combine with the biomaterial to form a complex after culture and amplification, and implant it into the defect site of the tendon to implant. The seed cells continue to proliferate, differentiate, and secrete the extracellular matrix to form repaired tissue, and then the biological material gradually degrades, eventually achieving complete repair in a biological sense.

In the following, we will begin with the structure and nutrition of the tendon, biomechanics, damage patterns, etc., and outline the damage and repair of tendon, the research on key technologies such as tissue engineering tendon seed cells, the study of scaffold materials, the effect of cell growth factor on tendon healing, composite culture of tendon cells and scaffold materials, as well as the practice in preclinical and clinical transformation applications, share the history of tissue engineering tendon research and development, in order to better promote the transformation of tissue engineering tendons.

### 9.5.1 The Damage and Repair of Tendon

#### 9.5.1.1 Structure and Nutrition of Tendon

The tendon is a dense connective tissue that connects the skeletal muscle to the bone [26]. Each muscle has different lengths of tendon and bone attachment. Because of the contraction of muscle belly, the tendon is pulled to drive the bone to produce movement, so that the human body can complete various activities of life and the various movements required for work. Thus tendon play a very important role in the life activities of people. It is not only the main support structure of the human body but also an important organization for accomplishing various activities, production labor, and participating in social activities.

A. Structure of Tendon

The tendon is composed of extracellular matrix and tendon cells [27]. Tendon cells belong to the class of fibroblasts, accounting for about 20%. The tendon cells are fusiform in the living body, arranged in a row, and projecting the wing-like protrusions around the collagen fibers. The extracellular matrix such as collagen, elastin, and glycoprotein secreted by tendon cells accounts for 80%, of which collagen accounts for 65–70% of the formed fraction, mainly type I and a small amount of type III collagen, but there are many other types of collagen, such as IV, V, and VI. The collagen fibers are white in color, varying in thickness, with diameters ranging from 1 to 12 μm [28]. There are alternating periodic stripes of light and dark, and the horizontal cycle is about 6.4 μm, which is a unique feature of collagen fibers. The collagen fibers have branches, and the branches are interwoven into a net to allow the collagen fibers to withstand large tensile stresses. Collagen fibers are cross-linked, making the mechanical properties of collagen more stable and the tensile strength of tissue higher. Collagen cross-linking is mainly carried out by disulfide bonds formed between cysteines. The tendon also contains a certain amount of elastin, which gives the tendon and ligament tissue a certain elasticity.

Proteoglycans are another important component of the extracellular matrix of tendons and play an important role in the formation of viscoelastic and other mechanical properties of tissues [29]. Proteoglycans are macromolecules composed of glycosaminoglycan chains covalently bound to a protein core. These branched chains with negative electrical properties form a characteristic "bottle brush" structure that attracts water molecules to hydrate tissue, while proteoglycans are embedded between collagens to provide compressive properties of tissue, hydration also enable the water-soluble molecules to rapidly disperse in the tissue.

B. Nutrition and Metabolism of Tendons

Human tendon is the kind of tissue with low blood supply and low metabolism and its nutrition is supplied by a diffusion process from the s nutrient vessels and synovial tissue [30]. In addition, metabolic activity is regulated by synovial membrane and blood vessels. Recent studies on the distribution of tendon blood vessels suggest that although tendons are less blood donor tissues, they still have an intrinsic vascular distribution, which provides nutrients and material exchange for tendons. Finally, it should be noted that further studies should pay attention to the vascularization process of engineered tendon in the research of tendon tissue engineering.

The tendons in the sheath region of the human body lies within the synovial fluid system [31]. Synovial fluid is a transparent, slightly yellow viscous liquid which is formed by the exudation of protein-rich fluid from synovial capillaries and by the addition of proteins and protein polysaccharides synthesized by the synovial lining cells. The major constituent of the proteins is mainly hyaluronic acid, the content of which is about 2 mg/mL in the normal sphincter synovial fluid. It is not only the main source of nutrients for intrathecal tendon but also provides a lubricant for the sliding of tendon. The synovial structure on the surface of the tendon plays an important role in the metabolic activities of tendons. Observation of the tendon ultrastructural found that the synovial membrane had micro pores and a network structure between the endometrium and the iliac membrane, allowing the synovial fluid to pass freely. When the muscles relax, the tendons absorb the synovial fluid like a sponge into the tendons and nourish the tendons; when the muscles contract, the internal pressure of the tendons rises, the synovial fluid is squeezed into the sheath, and the metabolites are discharged. It is suggested that the microporous structure required by this synovial nutrient should be taken into account when designing scaffold materials for tissue-engineered tendons.

#### 9.5.1.2 Biomechanics of Tendon

The structural characteristics of the tendon endow it strong tensile strength and a certain viscoelasticity [32]. The movement of the body can also cause the reconstruction of the tendon tissue structure and change its biomechanical properties. Several studies have found that proper mechanical stimulation of the tendon alters the production of collagen type I, and the synthesis of collagen I is increased when the anabolism synthesis is increased. The stress stimulation results in a series of changes in gene expression, which further lead to structural changes in tendons. Periodic stretch stress can stimulate the content of various growth factors, such as TGF-β, PDGF, bFGF, thereby promoting the proliferation, differentiation, and matrix synthesis of tendon cells, the secretion of IL-6 is also increased, and IL-6 is involved in the inflammatory response and thereby promotes tendon repair.

In growth, development, and various physiological and pathological processes, due to the change of stress, the synthesis of collagen fibers undergoes adaptive changes, including the reconstruction of various types of collagen content and spatial arrangement. Age is another important factor influencing the mechanical strength of tendons. As the age increases, the intramolecular and intermolecular cross-links of collagen increase, which makes the collagen fibers hard and brittle, and changes the mechanical properties of the tendon.

#### 9.5.1.3 Injury and Healing of Tendon

Acute and chronic injuries are the two main modes of injury to the tendon, and it varies depending on the treatment method. Tendon healing follows the classical wound closure process that is comprised of three conjunct steps, namely inflammation, formation, and remodeling [33].

The source of healing cells, the source of nutrients, and the voids present in the muscle-tendon complex rupture and conservative treatment within the tendon healing process will have an important impact on tendon healing [34]. The first is the way of the tendon healing. Endogenous healing is completely dependent on the cells of the tendon tissue itself. However, exogenous repair relies on cell infiltration of external tissues (including the tendon sheath). Normally, these two mechanisms normally act cooperatively in the repair process of the tendon: exogenous repair mainly functions in an early stage, while endogenous repair functions in the late stage. The result of exogenous healing is scar formation and it forms adhesions to the surrounding tissues in the healing process of flexor tendons, which may impede normal range of motion. Second, it is the source of nutrition. Blood vessels supply oxygen and nutrition to the most areas during the tendon healing process. While at the trochlear part, tendon nutrition is primarily dependent on the penetration of nutrients in the synovial fluid. Next, a gap between the broken ends will directly affect the range of motion of the tendon, but also the mechanical properties of the healing tendon. Finally, it is the treatment modality of choice. Generally, whether conservative treatment and/or surgical treatment are effective mainly depends on their respective indications. In comparison, surgical treatment can better promote the healing between the broken ends of the tendon; especially, the repair of the flexor tendon of the hand often requires surgery to promote a good fit between the broken ends of the two tendons and subsequent good healing and functional rehabilitation.

#### 9.5.1.4 Repair of Tendon

The most basic method of repairing tendon is direct suture and tendon transposition. If there is a tendon defect, it will require bridging between the broken ends. Bridging materials can be derived from autologous, allogeneic, xenogeneic, artificial materials, and tissue engineering materials. Among these materials, autogenous materials are the most commonly used conventional methods. The implantation autologous materials used to repair tendon defects are largely classified into autologous tendons and autologous fascia strips. Allogeneic tendon transplantation for repairing tendon defects avoids the limitation of autologous transplantation regarding materials, but the obtained materials need to special treatment, otherwise the repair effect will be reduced. Xenogeneic tendon and artificial materials to repair tendon defects are still in the experimental stage. However, some noteworthy progress has been made.

As far as we know, the ideal tendon substitute should have the following advantages: (1) good histocompatibility and biomechanical properties; (2) does not adhere to the surrounding tissue after implantation; (3) can secure suture knots and smooth junction of tendon ends; (4) the healing speed is at or near the normal physiological healing process; (5) the tensile strength can match the needs of the body; (6) easy to obtain or manufacture; and (7) can be assimilated by the body into a part of the body. Overall, the most important aspects of tendon substitute materials biology are able to completely replace the function of the tendon, and accept the regulation of the body and participate in the self-renewal of the body. The aim of tendon tissue engineering research is to develop a tendon substitute that meets the above requirements as much as possible. The principle is to obtain the seed cells of the tendon, and then combine with the biomaterial to form a complex after culture and amplification, and implant it into the defect site of the tendon to implant. The seed cells continue to proliferate, differentiate, and secrete the extracellular matrix to form repaired tissue, and then the biological material gradually degrades, eventually achieving complete repair in a biological sense.

The concept and research progress of tissue engineering tendon provides a new, more ideal treatment method for tendon injury consistent with physiological characteristics. The main contents of tissue engineering tendon include seed cells, scaffold materials, growth factors, cell and scaffold material composite culture.

### 9.5.2 The Seed Cell Research of Tissue Engineering Tendon

The tendon tissue includes the aponeurosis, the tendinous fibers, the blood vessels, and lymphatic vessels between the tendons [35]. The cell components also include fibroblasts, synovial cells, vascular endothelial cells, and tendon cells. The functional cells of the tendon tissue are tendon cells. At present, there are mainly some types of the seed cells used to study, such as tendon cells, skin fibroblasts, and stem cells, and they have their pros and cons.

#### 9.5.2.1 Tendon Cells

Tendon cells are intrinsic cells of the tendon [36]. The tendon cells, in morphological classification, belong to the class of fibroblasts. Tendon cells are highly differentiated cells. Tendon cell proliferation is relatively slow in in vitro culture conditions, and the tendon cells even lose their proliferative abilities after multiple passages. Therefore, this is unfavorable for the study of tissue engineered tendons.

Xie Huiqi et al. systematically studied the biological characteristics of human embryonic tendon cells, and found that the morphology of tendon cells and the function of secreting type I collagen were changed after 13 passages [37]. Besides, the replicative senescence phenomenon appeared. To resolve this issue, transfected human tendon cells with ptsA58H plasmid and the cell proliferation ability were enhanced after transfection. Furthermore, it can be passed on serial passage, long-term storage, and long-term recovery without alterations in growth characteristics. Thus a standard cell line was established for tissue engineering research with no tumorization tendency and relative immortalization. This cell line was used to filtrate and evaluate various tissue engineering scaffold materials of tendon.

#### 9.5.2.2 Fibroblasts

The source of fibroblasts is widely distributed compared with tendon cells, and it is easy to obtain [38]. It has the same biological characteristics as the mesoderm-derived cells of the tendon cells. They are all fusiform and can be synthesized and secrete collagen, elastin, glycosaminoglycan, and glycoprotein. Experiments have confirmed that skin fibroblasts can survive well on the surface of scaffold materials. By comparing the tissue engineered tendons constructed by skin fibroblasts and tendon cells, Chen Bing et al. observed that the gross morphology, histology, collagen orientation, and biomechanical properties were similar. After 26 weeks, the cell matrix ratio of the experimental group reached a satisfactory level and the mechanical strength reached 74% of normal tendon. It is suggested that fibroblasts can be used in place of tendon cells for tendon tissue engineering.

#### 9.5.2.3 Stem Cells

A. Bone Marrow Mesenchymal Stem Cells

Bone marrow mesenchymal stem cells (BMSCs) can be easily obtained, have multi-directional differentiation potential after in vitro culture and cryopreservation, stable genetic background, no immunological rejection in vivo, and are easy to use for clinical application [39]. Therefore, BMSCs have become an ideal seed cells in tissue engineering. Research shows that BMSCs have the ability to secrete type I collagen without induction in vitro, which is the same as the main function of tendon cells.

Young et al. seeded the proliferating BMSCs on the collagen gel and implanted the complex on the tendon defects [40]. It was found that the tendons treated with BMSCs were thicker than the control group, and alignment of collagen fibers, the quality of the joints, and biomechanical properties are better than that of the control group. Long Jianhong et al. inoculated isolated BMSCs onto type I collagen polyglycolic acid scaffolds. BMSCs grew well after 2 weeks of mixed culture, maintaining more than 89% cell viability. Transmission electron microscopy results showed that the cells in the experimental group still maintained a strong secretion function. It indicates that the collagen-polyglycolic acid has good cell compatibility with BMSCs.

Studies have found that BMSCs can lead to ectopic osteogenesis in tendon repair, suggesting that effective regulation of BMSCs specific differentiation into tendon cells is an important prerequisite for stem cell application. In addition, the cell source of BMSCs is also an important problem. Currently, there is still no perfect solution for obtaining and cultivating BMSCs to obtain a sufficient number of functionalized tendon-like cells, and the efficiency of directed differentiation is not ideal, and the related research needs to be further carried out.

B. Tendon Stem Cells

In 2007, Bi et al. successfully isolated tendon-derived stem cells (TDSCs) from mouse and human tendon tissues [41]. Later, other researchers isolated TDSCs from tendon tissues of horses, rabbits, and rats. It has been identified that these TDSCs derived from different species have the following characteristics: expression of stem cell-related markers; have the capacity to form clones; and self-renewal ability. Under suitable conditions or appropriate induction, MSCs can differentiate into a variety of tissue cells, such as osteogenesis, adipogenesis, and chondrogenesis in vitro, and muscle-like, cartilage-like, bone-like, and tendon-bone-like tissues are formed after subcutaneous implantation in nude mice.

Extensive clinical data have demonstrated that ectopic cartilage and ossification are common in the tendon healing process or tendinitis. This may be due in part to the multidirectional differentiation potential of TDSCs. However, it is because these TDSCs have these characteristics of stem cells that we can apply TDSCs as seed cells to tendon tissue engineering. PP Lui and his team found that culturing TDSCs into the lamellar structure and then wrapping them on the graft surface can help repair the anterior cruciate ligament in rats, and the TDSCs transfected with Scleraxis can better promote the repair of patellar tendon defects in rats [42]. At the same time, TDSCs can also be used in combination with other bioderived substrates, such as platelet-rich plasma (PRP), which can promote the proliferation and differentiation of TDSCs by using abundant growth factors in PRP. Lei C et al. compared the pure PRP, TDSCs, and TDSCs-PRP complexes in the treatment of rat Achilles tendinitis, and found that the repair ability of TDSCs-PRP complex was significantly stronger than that of pure PRP and TDSCs.

Currently, although TDSCs are the ideal seed cells for tendon tissue engineering, there are still many problems and deficiencies in their research. First, purification and expansion of a cell population containing only TDSCs are still difficult, because the TDSCs we have isolated also contain a part of tendon cells. Next, the research on the microenvironment of TDSCs in vivo is not thorough enough, and it is impossible to completely construct each factor involved in the microenvironment. Again, the problem of the source or quantity of TDSCs and how to meet the needs of scale clinical application of tendon repair remains to be solved. Therefore, using TSPCs as the seed cells for tendon-bone tissue engineering might need researchers' further in-depth exploration and research.

C. Other Stem Cells

It has been reported in the literature that adipose-derived stem cells (ASCs) can be used for the treatment of tendons. Whether ASCs have similar inducibility and ability to differentiate into mature tendon cells like BMSCs is also a scientific problem worthy of discussion.

Embryonic stem cells (ESCs) are also an important source of cells for tissue regeneration. Chen et al. were the first to propose the mesenchymal stem cells isolated from mouse embryonic stem cells. Cell sheets of ESCs derived MSCs were engineered into tendon-like layers under static mechanical load in vitro and used to repair a window defect in the patellar [43]. The results showed that mechanical stimulation can induce these cells into tendon-like cells, to form tendon-like structures, and to express tendon cell-associated markers. In addition, these cells can promote the regeneration of defect tendons after implantation in vivo. The results suggest that embryonic stem cells have multi-directional differentiation potential, which may be a good cell model for studying tendon cell development and stem cell-induced tendon differentiation. However, in practice, several issues need to be addressed, such as ethics, immune rejection, and biosafety.

### 9.5.3 Study on Scaffold Material of Tissue Engineering Tendon

Due to the unique structure and strong mechanical properties of the tendons, the ideal scaffold should cover a number of requirements such as: (1) It has good biodegradability, and its degradation rate should match the tissue regeneration rate; (2) The material itself or its degradation products have good biocompatibility to the cells and the tissues of the host, whether before, during, or after degradation of the material; (3) It has excellent mechanical properties and still maintains good mechanical properties during tissue regeneration; (4) It has good biological properties, which are beneficial for cell attachment, proliferation, differentiation, matrix secretion, and tissue formation; (5) It has excellent machinability, which can be easily prepared in different special structures and shapes, such as can be further knitted or woven.

#### 9.5.3.1 Scaffold Material

A. Natural Polymer Material
Silk, chitosan, and collagen are the most widely used natural polymeric materials in the biomaterials, which possess superior properties such as good tissue compatibility and can retain the normal structure of the network. However, there are still some shortcomings such as unadjusted degradation rate, residual material after disintegration, body rejection, difficult to process, and shape. Thus, more investigations are required to further research.

B. Synthetic Materials
When used as scaffolds for tendon tissue engineering, the advantages of synthetic materials are as follows: easy to obtain, stable in physical and chemical properties, nontoxic, and nonantigenicity. Therefore, it has long been used in the research of tendon tissue engineering, such as polyester, nylon, and silicone rubber.

At present, commonly used artificial polymer materials in tissue engineering are polyglycolic acid (PGA), polylactic acid (PLA), polylactic acid-polyglycolic acid copolymer (PLGA), polycaprolactone (PCL), polyvinyl alcohol (PVA), and so on. Bin et al. cultured the tendon cells in combination with PGA fibers for 6 weeks and implanted them in nude mice. It was found that cell-containing PGA fibers could become a tendon substitute [44]. Qin Tingwu et al. combined the PGA with tendon cells and implanted them into the deep flexor defect of the chicken [45]. It was found that the PGA degradation was too fast, and the biomechanical properties of the new tendon were lower than that of the normal tendon. In the study of PVA as a tendon scaffold material, it was found that PVA has good histocompatibility and mechanical properties, but pure PVA has poor cell adhesion. The PLGA was made into a film and the surface of the membrane was lined with different substances. The tendon cells were inoculated on the PLGA membrane and the adhesion of the tendon cells to the polymer film was measured. It was found that type I collagen and fibronectin mediate the specific adhesion of the tendon cells to the membrane, and this interaction can be inhibited by the corresponding antibody molecule. In addition, the synergistic effect can be produced when the concentration of the composite lining reaches a certain ratio. Moreover, the growth factor has an obvious effect in promoting tendon cells adhesion.

As a scaffold material, synthetic polymer materials have the advantages of abundant sources, easy processing, adjustable degradation rate, but their mechanical strength is low, the hydrophilicity and adhesion ability are poor, and the tissue compatibility is not ideal. However, synthetic polymer materials are still in need of further investigation and improvement, including surface modification, improving the biocompatibility of materials, reducing the body's immune response to biological materials, and reducing the impact on tendon healing.

C. Composite Materials
Due to the obvious defects of natural materials and synthetic materials, their use alone may be limited. Therefore, the combination of the two may be beneficial for improving the overall performance of the material and meeting the application requirements. The repair effect was better in the silk fibroin-collagen group than collagen alone for rabbit tendon defect. The composite material had good mechanical properties and could promote the formation of collagen fibers. Thomas et al. also found that silk fibroin/PLGA composites have good cytocompatibility, which could promote cell proliferation and collagen production, and have a certain potential in clinical application [45]. Long Jianhong et al. inoculated MSCs into the type I collagen-polyglycolic acid scaffold to observe cell growth, and found that there was no significant change in cell functional activity. The results indicated that collagen-polyglycolic acid is a good biodegradable material for carrying MSCs. The

research team led by Yang Zhiming used a variety of composite materials, such as carbon fiber combined with PGA, treated human hair combined with PGA, collagen combined with PGA, and human hair and collagen combined with PGA. It found that the collagen secreted by tendon cells was distributed along scaffold material and gradually replaced the degradable part during the PGA degradation process. In addition, the mechanical properties of the newly formed tendon and the adhesion of the tendon cells were significantly improved. After 3 months of implantation, the tensile strength of the new tendon reached 75% of that of the original tendon, and the amount of collagen secreted by tendon cells was increased.

D. Biologically Derived Materials

Bioderived materials are also a large class of natural scaffold materials, which have gradually become the focus of tendon tissue engineering research. Compared with synthetic materials, bioderived materials possess the advantages of sufficient sources, closest to the native network structure, good biomechanical properties, good biocompatibility, and so on. Typical bioderived tendon materials are derived from animal or allogeneic tendon, which are treated by a series of chemical methods to remove cellular components and retain collagen scaffolds. The obtained materials still retain all the bioactive phytochemicals and enzyme activity after rehydration. These natural scaffolds are involved in tissue development, and these molecules then interact with cell surface receptors. This signal is then transmitted across the membrane to the intracellular molecules which trigger a serious of cascade reactions from the cytoskeleton to the nucleus, and thereby lead to specific gene expression. In turn, these specific gene products affect the extracellular matrix in a number of ways. The interaction of cells with the extracellular matrix promotes cell adhesion, migration, growth, and death, as well as the regulation of cytokines and growth factors, while indirectly activating the transmission of signals between cells.

So far, it is not certain which scaffold material is the best material for tendon tissue engineering research. It involves multidisciplinary fields such as material science, chemistry, engineering, bioengineering, cytology, and medicine. It requires a close combination of disciplines, joint research, and continuous exploration to find a more ideal practical tendon tissue engineering scaffold material.

#### 9.5.3.2 Preparation Technology of Scaffold

The artificial tendon fabrication technique not only requires the prepared scaffold that can promote cell proliferation and migration but also has sufficient overall structural properties to maintain a certain shape in vivo. There are two main methods for preparing tendon tissue engineering scaffold materials.

A. Electrospinning

The scaffold material obtained by electrospinning can mimic the natural extracellular matrix at the nanometer scale, which would have the characteristics of fine size, large specific surface area, high porosity, large aspect ratio, and superior mechanical properties. Bioscaffold materials with different properties can be obtained by blending different substances. At present, the electrospinning process has made great progress in the fields of cartilage and tendon regeneration. Lucy et al. used electrospinning technology to prepare PCL nanofibers for the repair of tendon injuries. Compared to other preparation methods, electrospinning technology can easily produce nanostructured extracellular matrices and controllable mechanical properties and architecture, which can provide a better environment for cell and tissue growth [45].

B. Weaving Method

The continuous fiber woven structure can be obtained by three-dimensional weaving method, which adopts continuous interweaving of fibers to form a tight network structure, has the direction of multiaxial fibers, good mechanical strength in the weaving direction, and suitable porosity. Fang et al. wove the tussah silk and implanted it into the defect of the hind limb of the rabbit [46]. It was found that the tussah silk artificial mites can support the repair of the rabbit Achilles tendon, maintain a good mechanical strength for a certain period of time, can withstand the tendon stress required by the body, and keep the repaired tendon connected firmly at both ends.

### 9.5.4 The Effect of Cell Growth Factor on Tendon Healing

The use of growth factors that promote tissue regeneration to achieve functionalization of biological materials is of great value for the repair of tissue damage [46]. By specifically binding to receptor molecules, growth factors activate downstream signaling pathways that promote cell proliferation, inhibit apoptosis, mobilize in vivo cells chemotactically, and induce stem cell differentiation and maturation. The stimulating effect of growth factors on cells is reversible and dose-dependent. It can promote the repair of damage by controlling the types and quantity of growth factors for the physiological and pathological characteristics of different lesions. The process of tendon repair, that is, the process of proliferation, migration and secretion of extracellular matrix of tendon cells, is accompanied by the release and participation of various growth factors in the process of wound repair. Cell growth factor is a biologically active protein or polypeptide substance secreted by cells, which has the function of regulating inflammatory cell directional movement, wound cell division activation, neovascularization, and intercellular substance synthesis.

Cell growth factors associated with tendon injury repair include bone morphogenetic protein-12 (BMP-12), cartilage-derived morphogenetic protein (CDMP), platelet-derived growth factor (PDGF), vascular endothelial growth factor (VEGF), insulin-like growth factor-1 (IGF-1), transforming growth factor-β (TGF-β), basic fibroblast growth factor (bFGF), and the like [47–50]. In recent years, these cell growth factors have been applied to animal experiments to promote tendon healing, improve the mechanical properties of tendons, and reduce tendon adhesion, and have achieved positive results.

The application of cell growth factor and transgenic technology provides a new idea for tendon healing and prevention of postoperative tendon adhesion, and has important guiding significance for the clinical application of tendon tissue engineering. However, different cell growth factors play different roles at different times and different tendon healing sites, a series of questions such as how to choose the most optimal growth factor and regulate its role in the proliferation and differentiation of tendon cells, how to properly regulate the concentration of cell growth factors, when to use what kind of cell growth factor, and how to interact with each other need to be further solved. Although the single application of cell growth factor can have a positive effect on tendon repair, the effect is limited, the combined application can meet the needs of the real internal environment of the body, and help to play a synergistic effect between multigene products and improve the therapeutic effect. Therefore, the synergistic application of multiple growth factors to treat tendon injury will become a trend, and controlled release vectors and low-toxic and efficient transgenic vectors for different factors will also become the focus of future research.

### 9.5.5 Composite Culture of Tendon Cells and Scaffold Materials

#### 9.5.5.1 Non-mechanical Load Culture

Non-mechanical load culture includes three-dimensional cell tissue culture and cell coculture.

A. Three-Dimensional Cell Tissue Culture

   The scaffold material having a three-dimensional structure is cocultured with different kinds of cells in vitro, and the cells migrate and grow in a three-dimensional spatial structure of the vector to form a three-dimensional cell-scaffold complex. The technology not only retains the material and structural basis of the cellular microenvironment in vivo, but also exhibits the advantages of cell tissue culture and the controllability of conditions, and is widely used. Herchenhan et al. used tendon cell composite fibrin glue scaffold to form tendon-like tissue in three-dimensional culture in vitro for 3 weeks. The mechanical strength of the cell-scaffold complex increased with the increase of fiber diameter. The changes in cytoskeleton and cell biological behavior are crucial for its function. Three-dimensional culture makes the distribution and morphology of tendon cytoskeleton beneficial to cell proliferation and growth, and regulates cell growth to approximate living tendon. During three-dimensional culture, the cells will produce sustained tensile stress, but this tensile stress is too small to be accurately determined, or it may be a stimulatory signal that plays a role in the process of cell growth along the fibers.

B. Cell Coculture

   It can maximize the simulation of the in vivo environment and facilitate the observation of cell-cell interactions. This technique has been widely used in stem cell induction, cartilage tissue engineering, and bone tissue engineering. Wang et al. constructed an indirect coculture system of BMSCs and autologous tendon cells in vitro. The results showed that the culture environment indirectly cocultured with tendon cells could induce BMSCs to express type I collagen, but no obvious expression of tenomodulin was observed. Although the application of cell coculture technology to tendon tissue engineering conditions is not yet mature, it has certain feasibility.

#### 9.5.5.2 Mechanical Load Culture

The morphological structure, growth, proliferation, differentiation, and function of cells are closely related to the mechanical environment in which the cells are located [51]. They are mainly divided into compressive stress, tensile stress, shear stress, and microgravity. Tendon is a tissue that is subjected to tension. Mechanical stimulation can enhance the secretion of tissue collagen, which is beneficial to the directional growth of cells. It plays a positive role in the culture of cell-scaffold complex, stimulates the secretion of extracellular matrix, and promotes the directed growth and differentiation of cells. The addition of mechanical stimulation factors in the cell-scaffold complex culture has become a research trend in tendon tissue engineering.

A. Static Mechanical Load

   The tissue engineering tendon constructed in vitro tends to lose its initial strength, and it is difficult to maintain its inherent mechanical properties after transplantation in vivo. Therefore, enhancing the initial strength of tissue engineering tendon is one of the important contents in in vitro culture. Some scholars used collagen as a scaffold material to investigate the effects of porosity, length, and mechanical stimulation on the structural strength of the scaffold. The results showed that the mechanical structure was stimulated and the longer scaffold structure had better mechanical strength. Deng et al. implanted human epidermal fibroblasts on PGA scaffolds and used a spring scaffold to form a "U" shape as a static mechanical force bearing experimental group. Compared with the nonmechanical bearing group, it can form more mature tissues and form longitudinal fibers. It secretes collagen and has good mechanical properties. Some researchers have analyzed that the tensile stress causes the cytoskeleton to stretch, which is the cause of cell morphological changes. This tensile stress acts directly on cell surface receptors or ion channels, promotes cell proliferation, and improves the transport of nutrients. It has also been suggested by researchers that cells are conformed to deformation on the nonloaded scaffold in order to bond the scaffold, so that tensile stress is generated, but the loaded scaffold may cause the cells to not produce such an active action for the force of the scaffold.

B. Dynamic Culture

Dynamic culture provides periodic mechanical strain by mechanical devices, stimulates cell directional growth on scaffolds, promotes the secretion of type I collagen, and enhances the exchange of nutrients and metabolic waste. The use of intermittent dynamic culture not only retains the advantages of dynamic culture but also increases the degree of cell infiltration and maintains the formation and retention of extracellular matrix. Qin et al. found that after applying specific stress conditions to the tendon cell-scaffold complex, the number of tendon cells, DNA synthesis, and collagen secretion were significantly higher than those of the static culture control group, indicating that periodic mechanical strain can promote tissue engineering. In the construction of tendons, Abousleiman et al. encapsulated type I collagen MSCs combined with decellularized human umbilical vein stents and gave them periodic tension with a tendon stimulator. The tissue engineered tendon formed by this method has a similar natural tendon morphology and the strain value is within the range of normal human tendon.

Bioreactor is a device commonly used for dynamic culture. It can simulate the internal environment, closely control the culture and operating conditions, has high repeatability, strong control over specific conditions, and high controllability. It can provide a suitable environment for cell to proliferate, differentiate, and biochemically react. Chen et al. combined human embryonic stem cell (hESCs)-derived MSCs into scaffolds to provide in vitro mechanical stimulation through bioreactors. hESCs-MSCs were similar to tendon cells, and cell-scaffold complexes showed good mechanical properties in the experiment of tendon regeneration after in situ transplantation. Saber et al. prepared a tendon-decellular tendon complex that was stretched using a self-made bioreactor to increase its strength and modulus of elasticity. They believed that mechanical stimulation could not directly increase the strength of the scaffold and promote the formation of ordered collagen fibers. Instead, these effects are obtained by some kind of cellular reaction. The application of bioreactor can promote cell-scaffold complex to express tendon cell-related markers and some mechanically perceptible structures and molecules in vitro, and produce nonimmunogenic tendon materials with strong mechanical properties, which has certain clinical significance.

Another method of providing dynamic mechanical stimulation is to implant a cell-scaffold complex into the skin of an animal. The subcutaneous tissue environment lacks blood vessels and has low partial pressure of oxygen, which can also provide natural dynamic mechanical stimulation, simulate tendon development and internal environment, and contribute to tendinization of cell-scaffold complex. Wang et al. constructed a human embryonic extensor tendon cell-PGA scaffold complex and designed two experimental groups of dynamic mechanical load of in vitro bioreactor and natural dynamic mechanical load on the fascia of nude mice. The results showed that the internal load group formed a larger tissue volume, the collagen fibers matured and ordered, and the mechanical properties were stronger. Therefore, it is considered that the internal load is a good method to optimize the function of tissue engineering tendon, which can make it more mature and more complete.

C. Mechanism of Mechanical Stimulation

The environment in which the cells and scaffolds are located will greatly affect the biomechanical stimulation that the cells are subjected to via the scaffold [52]. The mechanism of how the specific cellular response is affected by tensile stress and the flow rate in the culture environment is still unclear. In different combinations of cells and scaffold types, different loading methods can have different effects. The specific combination of stent tensile stress and fluid shear stress may dominate the phenotype of a certain type of cells.

Stress-strain stimulate cell metabolism and affect cell function at different levels of gene transcription, translation, cell interaction [53]. Stress-strain stimulation can not only increase the cell proliferation rate but also cause calcium ion influx to enhance the sustained secretion of proteins in cells. Stress-strain stimulation leads to assembly of integrins and organization of cytoskeleton in cells. Assembly of integrins is associated with a variety of intracellular signaling pathways such as FAK and RhoA/ROCK signaling pathways, which in turn mediate cell differentiation and play a role in its function. Defining the role of stress in the cell signaling pathway can promote the modeling of mechanical stimulation and improve the tendon tissue engineering.

### 9.5.6 Clinical Trial of Tendon Tissue Engineering

Trauma, exercise, chronic strain, etc. can cause damage to the tendon (ligament), causing dysfunction and even disability. Tendon (ligament) injury is a common surgical injury. According to statistics, more than 300,000 patients in the United States need to undergo tendon (ligament) repair surgery every year. The demand for tendon (ligament) transplantation in China will be at least 3–4 times that of the United States in terms of population.

At present, the clinical application of tissue engineered tendon is still less reported in domestic and foreign literatures, and no product has been approved for listing.

We have been working on tendon repair materials and tissue engineered tendon since 1988. A large number of basic and applied research have been carried out on the ultrastructure of tendons, blood supply, biological characteristics of tendon cells, tendon repair materials, and the safety and effectiveness of tissue engineered tendon. In 2005, we signed a contract for the transfer of proprietary technology with the cooperative enterprises, and successively completed the product quality standards, the construction of the production quality system, the GMP assessment, and so on. Since 2007, a multicenter clinical trial has been carried out and the clinical trial was completed in 2013 and the new product registration technology review was conducted. In April 2016, the "Allogeneic Tendon Repair Materials" was approved in the National Class III Medical Device Product Registration Certificate, becoming the first approved tendon repair material product in China.

In summary, the repair and regeneration of tendon still has many unexplored areas, and tendon tissue engineering is one of the important methods of tendon regeneration. However, in many aspects, further research is needed, such as the optimization of scaffold materials, the degradation of materials, and the synchronization of extracellular matrix secreted by cells; exploring the source of clinically useful seed cells, rapid cell amplification techniques, prevention of cell senescence, and control of cell immunological reaction; improving the mechanical properties of tissue engineered tendon, making it closer to normal human tendon; tissue engineered tendon construction technique and timing of implantation in vivo; the outcome of tendon cell after implantation in vivo and its relationship with growth and development; preservation, transportation, and resuscitation of cell tissue engineered tendon products; and medical ethical issues in tissue engineering. It is necessary to further clarify the basic theory and mechanism of tendon tissue engineering. After strict quality testing and multicenter clinical verification, it can be promoted and applied clinically after approval by CFDA. With the development of cell biology, molecular biology, immunology, and materiology, and improvement in cell culture technology and methods, the combination of these fields will eventually provide a good way for tendon regeneration.

## 9.6 Tissue Engineered Myocardium

According to statistics, there are more and more patients with ischemic heart disease, and the incidence rate is increasing year by year [54]. Acute and chronic ischemia of the myocardium can lead to myocardial cell death, and severe damage leads to heart failure. At present, clinical treatment of heart failure is mainly based on drug treatment and interventional therapy. These treatment methods can delay the development of the disease to a certain extent, but cannot completely compensate for the dead myocardial cell. In recent years, with the continuous breakthroughs in research in the fields of stem cells, biomaterials, and bio-manufacturing engineering, the technology of engineered cardiac tissue has become increasingly mature. Artificial myocardial tissue is constructed to repair and replace necrotic myocardial tissue, providing a new treatment strategy for ischemic heart diseases.

### 9.6.1 The Selection and Application of Seed Cells

Considering the limited ability of terminal differentiated myocardial cells to regenerate, the main source of seed cells currently used for myocardial tissue engineering are mainly stem cells with different developmental stages and ability to differentiate into myocardial cells, including embryonic stem cells (ESCs) induced pluripotent stem cells (iPSCs) white adipose-derived mesenchymal stem cells (ADSCs), brown adipose-derived stem cells (BADSCs), and the like. In addition, myocardial cells obtained by directional transdifferentiation based on lineage reprogramming techniques are also a research hot spot in recent years. The following is a brief introduction to the characteristics of various types of cells and their application in myocardial tissue engineering.

#### 9.6.1.1 Embryonic Stem Cell

ESCs have multidirectional differentiation potential that can be induced to differentiate into three germ layer cells in vitro and further differentiate into a variety of terminal cells with single function. ESC can differentiate into myocardial cell. Researchers such as Wang conducted in-depth ESC-based myocardial tissue engineering studies, optimized ESC and embryoid body culture systems, and achieved ESC embryoid body batch amplification and myocardial differentiation. In recent years, researchers have found that ESC plays an important role in miRNA, transcription factors, and epigenetic modifications during myocardial differentiation [58, 59]. In addition, the researchers also found that transcriptional regulon CITED2, GATA4, SHOX2, Nkx2.5, etc. play an important role in the differentiation of ESC into myocardial cell [60]. Since ESC can be induced to differentiate into the cardiac muscle by signaling molecules, growth factors, small molecules, etc., ESC can be used as an important cell type for engineering myocardial tissue construction and in vivo transplantation studies. However, ESCs currently have significant limitations in transplantation applications. On the one hand, the source of ESC is ethically difficult to accept; on the other hand, the risk of immunological rejection and teratoma formation is also an important factor hindering the clinical application of ESC.

#### 9.6.1.2 Induced Pluripotent Stem Cells

Induced pluripotent stem cells (iPSCs) are a class of pluripotent stem cells that are reacquired by reprogramming somatic cells and have biological characteristics highly similar to ESCs. In 2006, Yamanaka first used retrovirus to overexpress four transcription factors OSKM (Oct4, Sox2, Klf4, and c-Myc) into mouse fibroblasts, and successfully induced the formation of iPSC [61]. Since then, researchers have developed a variety of safe and effective somatic cell reprogramming methods for the preparation of iPSC, such as the introduction of somatic cells into free plasmids, microRNAs, synthetic mRNA, recombinant proteins, and small molecule compounds. iPSC has the potential of multidirectional differentiation, but it avoids the ethical issues in ESC research and has better clinical application prospects. Mauritz and Zwi's research team have confirmed that iPSC can be induced to differentiate cardiomyocytes in vitro, and exhibit similar characteristics to ESC-derived myocardial cells in terms of cell morphology, molecular level, and electrophysiological function. In 2013, researchers such as Wang conducted research on the immunogenicity of iPSC in the microenvironment of myocardial infarction and the tumorigenicity of its differentiation products, and found that the immunogenicity of iPSC may increase with its differentiation in vivo, and the purification of iPSC-induced differentiation of cardiomyocytes before transplantation can effectively reduce the risk of tumorigenicity [62].

#### 9.6.1.3 Mesenchymal Stem Cells

MSCs has the advantages of abundant sources and simple methods of obtaining materials, which can better meet the needs of clinical applications. MSC can be differentiated into myocardial cells by induction in vitro. Researchers confirmed that MSC can spontaneously differentiate into myocardial cells in vitro, and further confirmed that MSC autocrine vascular endothelial growth factor (VEGF) plays a key role in spontaneous differentiation into cardiac muscle [63]. In vivo studies have shown that MSC transplantation has a significant effect on improving cardiac function [64].

#### 9.6.1.4 Brown Adipose-Derived Cardiac Stem Cells

In 2003, researchers discovered that enzymatic digestion of brown adipose can isolate stem cells with high myocardial differentiation for the first time, thereby expanding the source of seed cells constructed by tissue engineered myocardium. However, this method is less efficient. In 2009, Wang et al. established a method based on the "Cocktail" digestive enzyme to extract brown adipose CSC. This method improves the separation efficiency of CSC and the viability of isolated cells. The differentiated myocardium has similar characteristics to natural myocardium [65]. The above findings laid a good foundation for the application of brown adipose-derived CSC in myocardial tissue engineering.

#### 9.6.1.5 Myocardial Cells Derived from Somatic Cells

Lineage-specific transcription factors can reprogram terminally differentiated cells into other types of somatic or progenitor cells. By directly programming somatic cells to generate cardiovascular lineage precursor cells, the intermediate transition process of iPSC is not required, which greatly reduces the risk of tumorigenicity. This strategy has become a new model for the development of myocardial tissue regenerative medicine. In recent years, various new nongene integration pathways have been explored to achieve cell lineage reprogramming, such as free plasmids, recombinant proteins, microRNAs, synthetic mRNAs, small molecule compounds, and the like. The development of lineage reprogramming technology provides a safer and broader source of cells for the construction of engineered myocardial tissue.

### 9.6.2 The Selection and Application of Scaffold Materials

Scaffold material is another core component of constructing engineered myocardial tissue. Scaffold materials for myocardial tissue engineering studies are broadly classified into natural scaffold materials and artificial synthetic scaffold materials. In recent years, new scaffold materials such as conductive nanomaterials and polymeric conductive polymers have become the frontiers and hot spots in the field of myocardial tissue engineering.

#### 9.6.2.1 Natural Biomaterial

The natural biomaterial is derived from the extracellular matrix (ECM) component of natural tissues or organs; it has good biocompatibility and can serve as structural support of the tissue-specific microenvironment, and provides a good place for cells to grow and develop. Therefore, the natural biomaterial can be widely used in the field of tissue engineering research.

A. Collagen

Collagen is the main protein component of mammalian ECM, and it has good biocompatibility, degradability, plasticity, and porosity. In 1999, Simpson et al. first covered a layer of neutral type I collagen on the surface of the culture dish. The neonatal rat myocardial cells cultured on the collagen surface were arranged longitudinally along the collagen to form myocardial tissue like structure [66]. In addition, many researchers have grafted some chemical functional groups onto collagen in order to obtain specific functional properties and improve the adhesion or growth ability of myocardial cells on the scaffold material. In 2016, researchers such as Lin demonstrated that the stiffness of collagen scaffolds can be modulated by varying the degree of cross-linking, which in turn affects the differentiation of MSCs into cardiac progenitor cells.

B. Chitosan

Chitosan is a natural linear biopolysaccharide, which is widely used in tissue engineering research because of its excellent biocompatibility, good bioadhesion, and controlled biodegradability. In 2003, researchers such as Fujita used photosensitive chitosan hydrogel to control bFGF release to induce angiogenesis in the myocardial infarction site, protecting the damaged myocardium [67]. Due to the abundant grafting reaction of a large number of reactive functional groups on the surface of chitosan, the functionalized chitosan material has more mimic myocardial structure and functional properties. Another method for modifying temperature-sensitive chitosan is by grafting RoY peptide. The grafted chitosan-RoY can significantly promote cell survival, proliferation, and neovascularization under hypoxic condition; it is an ideal scaffold material for myocardial infarction repair (see Fig. 9.8) [68].

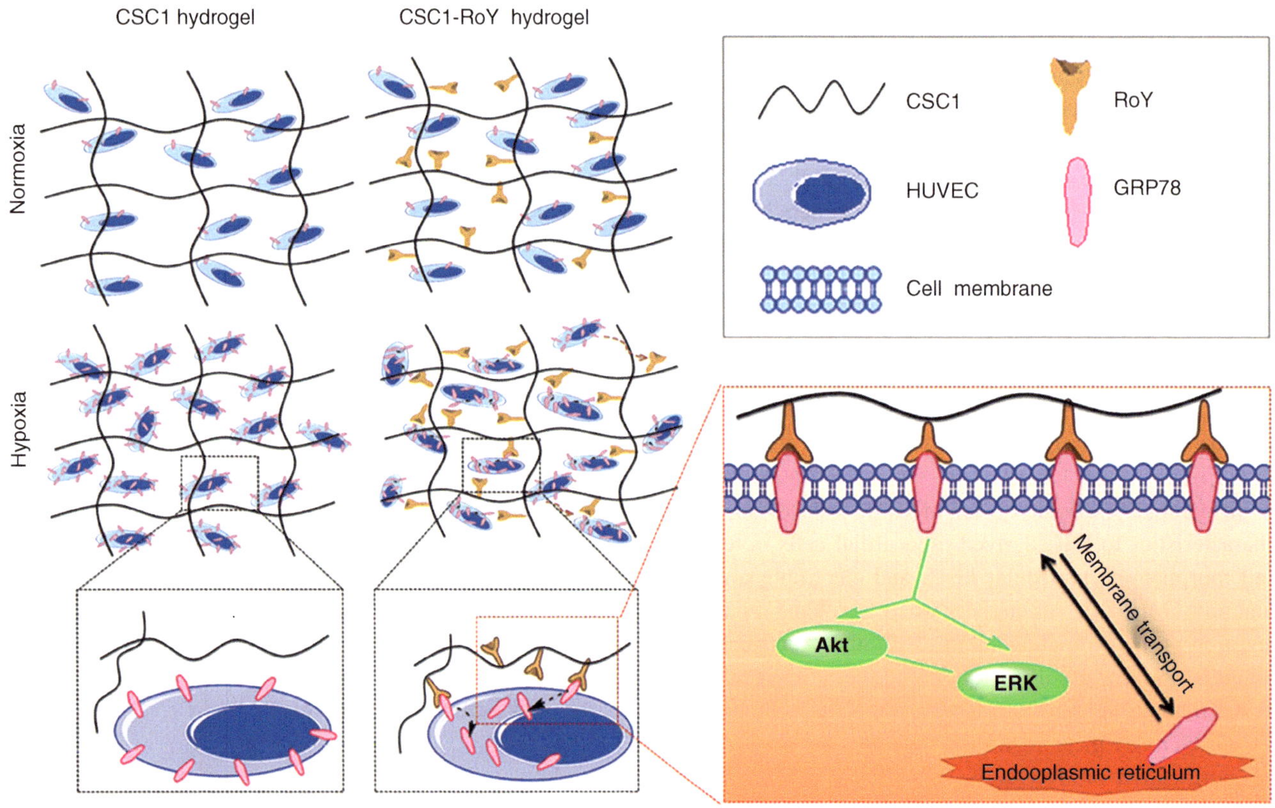


**Fig. 9.8** CSCl-RoY promotes neovascularization by stimulating the Akt-ERK1/2 signaling pathway

C. Acellular Matrix

The acellular matrix scaffold material is a three-dimensional bioscaffold material, which is obtained by acellular treatment through the combination of physical, chemical, or enzymatic methods while retaining the extracellular matrix components of tissues and organs. The main components of ECM include extracellular matrix proteins (type I collagen, mucopolysaccharide, fibronectin, and laminin) and various growth factors. In recent studies, researchers believed that ECM's ultratopological structure and 3D ultramicro conformation provide cells with "information coding" that directly or indirectly regulates cell behavior, including cell adhesion, proliferation, and directed differentiation, but specific regulation and control mechanism needs to be further studied [69].

The cardiac acellular matrix is subjected to enzymatic treatment to prepare a matrix hydrogel. In 2009, Singelyn et al. first measured the composition of the hydrogel, including type I collagen, mucopolysaccharide, fibronectin, laminin, etc., and proved its good gel-forming properties and biocompatibility, showing its enormous potential for clinical application.

#### 9.6.2.2 Artificial Synthetic New Conductive Scaffold Materials

Artificial synthetic scaffold materials mainly include traditional nonconductive and new conductive scaffold materials. Artificial synthetic traditional nonconductive materials are more focused on simulating extracellular matrix components, physicochemical properties, and spatial structure. Considering the specific structure and electrophysiological properties of myocardial tissue, it is necessary to meet the need of synchronous excitation contraction coupling of reconstructed myocardial tissue, which further supports the formation of good structural and electrophysiological integration with the in vivo myocardium after transplantation. In recent years, artificial synthetic new conductive materials have been used as scaffold for the construction of engineered myocardial tissue. A brief introduction to new conductive nanomaterials and polymeric conductive polymers is now available.

A. New Conductive Nanomaterials

Conductive nanomaterials mainly include carbon-based nanomaterials such as carbon nanotubes (CNT), graphene, and fullerene ($^{60}C$), which have become a research hot spot in the construction of engineered myocardial tissue due to their good electrical conductivity.

Carbon nanotubes are a cylindrical sheet structure with excellent mechanical strength, electrical conductivity, and thermal stability. CNTs can be prepared into composite materials by different methods and can increase the solubility of CNTs, improve biocompatibility, reduce cytotoxicity, and greatly improve the mechanical properties and electrical conductivity of composites. Compared with simple collagen, the surface roughness of collagen/SWCNT hydrogels is significantly increased, and it has excellent electrical conductivity, good cell compatibility, and tissue compatibility (see Fig. 9.9) [70].

Graphene is a hexagonal planar thin film of honeycomb lattice made up of carbon atoms with sp2 hybrid orbitals, and has the strongest mechanical properties to date. In 2013, Kim et al. reported that graphene was used to prepare thin films and evaluated the biocompatibility and cell behavior of myocardial cells. It was found that it had good biocompatibility and had the function of maintaining myocardial cell survival, promoting adhesion and contraction [71]. Researchers used the two-dimensional

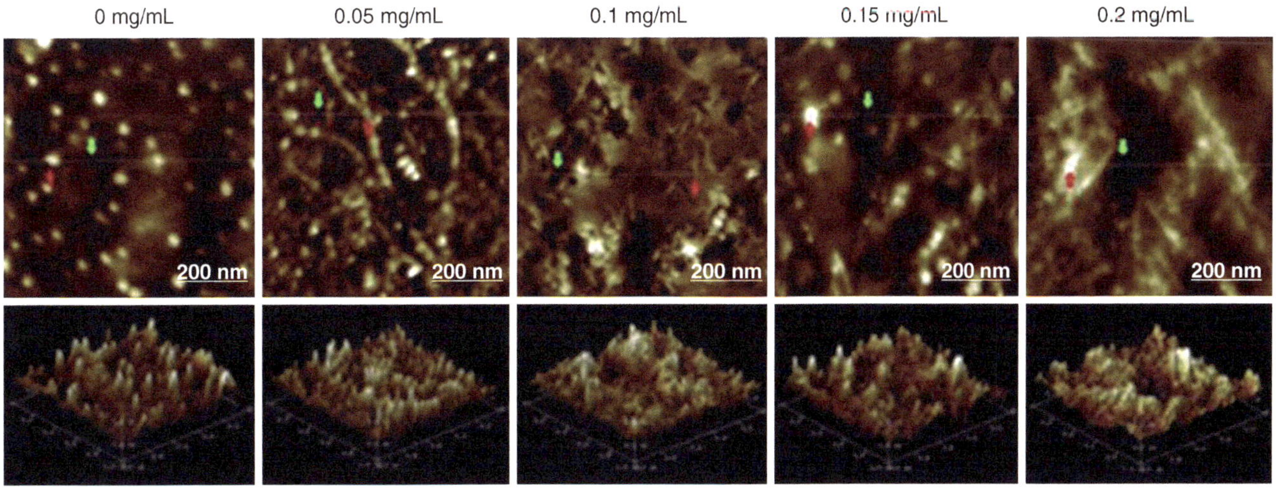


**Fig. 9.9** Development and evaluation of SWCNTs/collagen composite scaffold

sheet structure of graphene to fabricate a functionalized graphene three-dimensional tissue construct by assembly, which promoted the connection between myocardial cells and enhanced the thickness of three-dimensional myocardial tissue [72].

B. Polymeric Conductive Polymer

A polymeric conductive polymer is a type of polymer material in which a conductivity of a π bond conjugated polymer having a certain chain length is chemically or electrochemically doped to extend from an insulator to a conductor. At present, polymeric conductive polymers represented by polythiophene, polyphenylacetylene, polyaniline, polypyrrole, etc. have become one of the focuses of the field of biomaterials and tissue engineering. Polythiophene and its derivatives have good electrochemical stability, high doping level, and reversible doping and dedoping processes, which play an important role in conductive polymers.

### 9.6.3 In Vitro Construction of Engineered Myocardial Tissue and Its Role in the Treatment of Myocardial Infarction

The development of myocardial tissue engineering depends not only on the development of scaffold materials and seed cells but also on the construction techniques of engineered myocardial tissue. At present, the strategies for the construction of engineered myocardial tissue in vitro and myocardial infarction mainly include the following:

(a) In vitro construction of three-dimensional engineered myocardial tissue and treatment strategy of "band-aid" myocardial infarction.
(b) Strategy of injectable myocardial tissue engineering.

#### 9.6.3.1 Three-Dimensional Engineered Myocardial Tissue Construction Based on the Treatment Strategy of "Band-Aid" Myocardial Infarction

Engineered myocardial patch refers to engineered myocardial tissue constructed by combining seed cells with the ability to form myocardial cells and appropriate scaffold materials according to engineering principles, for in vivo transplantation to repair or replace damaged myocardium. Engineered myocardial patch can provide suitable microenvironment and structural support for seed cells, promote differentiation of transplanted cells, and prevent apoptosis.

A. Construction of engineered myocardial tissue based on dynamic mechanical stretching technique: Myocardial cells are seeded inside the material and subjected to continuous and dynamic mechanical stretching, which mimics the mechanical properties of normal myocardium and can induce myocardial cells to form a linear alignment within the material similar to that in the body. The engineered myocardial tissue constructed under this system not only has a structure similar to that of the natural myocardium, but also has mechanical strength similar to that of normal myocardial tissue, and has electrical conductivity [73]. In the same year, Wang et al. used collagen/Matrigel as a scaffold to design a mechanical device and ESC-derived myocardial cells as seed cells to successfully construct engineered myocardial tissue with spontaneous contraction in vitro.

B. Construction of Engineered Myocardial Tissue Based on Cell Layer Overlay Technology

Cell sheet technology is the use of melting membrane technology to construct a single layer of cardiomyocytes and layers of cells superimposed to form a three-dimensional cell sheet. Japanese researchers Shimizu et al. first invented a new method that did not rely on scaffold materials to support in 2002 [74]. The researchers cultured suckling mouse myocardial cells on a thin layer of temperature-sensitive polymer polyisopropylacrylamide. When the temperature was lowered, the change in the polymer separates the cell layer from the entire surface of the material. On this basis, the researchers used a variety of cell types to construct cell sheets without scaffolds, and further used for myocardial infarction transplantation studies. In the study of optimizing the technique of myocardial layer construction, in 2006, Shimizu's team successfully constructed a myocardial reconstructed tissue formed by superimposing 30 layers of myocardial slices with a maximum thickness of 1 mm. However, it is not suitable for clinical use due to thickness limitations. In order to construct a tissue that overcomes the limits of engineered myocardial thickness, it is necessary to find a way to form an adequate vasculature in vitro. In 2015, based on the layer-by-layer stacking technology, Sakaguchi developed a bioreactor perfusion vascular bed system to construct a network of blood vessels that supply oxygen and nutrient molecules similar to capillaries in natural tissues and remove waste [76].

C. Construction of Engineered Myocardial Tissue Based on Three-Dimensional Porous Scaffold Material

The three-dimensional porous scaffold material can support the adhesion and growth of seed cells.

Researchers like Roberts used collagen as a scaffold to inoculate ESC with stromal cells in collagen to construct engineered myocardial tissue [77]. Studies have shown that effective control of engineered myocardial tissue microstructure can form more complex characteristics, laying the foundation for large-scale engineering myocardial tissue regeneration.

In recent years, the construction of engineered myocardial tissue with acellular matrix as scaffold has become a research hotspot. The engineered myocardial patch based on cardiac acellular matrix-fibrin hydrogel can effectively promote the secretion of growth factors and the growth and differentiation of stem cells, and significantly promote the formation of new blood vessels in myocardial infarction. After transplanting the constructed myocardial patch into the body, the myocardial infarct size can be significantly reduced, and myocardial function after myocardial infarction can be improved.

#### 9.6.3.2 The Construction of Engineered Myocardial Tissue Based on the Treatment Strategy of Injectable Myocardial Infarction

Injectable myocardial tissue engineering refers to the local support and microenvironment improvement of myocardial infarction by injecting the injectable scaffold material alone or carrying seed cells, growth factors, etc., and further improving the cell survival rate. Therefore, it has a good therapeutic effect on myocardial infarction. This strategy has the advantages of no need to prepare special scaffold in vitro, simple operation, less trauma to patients, and is easier to be applied in clinical practice.

In case of researching, in vitro construction of injectable myocardial tissue is based on natural matrix hydrogel chemical modification and myocardial infarction transplantation repair. In 2016, Wassenaar et al. used a porcine ventricular acellular matrix to prepare an injectable hydrogel and injected it into the myocardial infarction site of rats [78]. The results showed that hydrogel injection can significantly reduce the inflammatory response and promote neovascularization in the myocardial infarction area. It has obvious therapeutic effect on the recovery after myocardial infarction, and lays a foundation for further clinical application of acellular matrix.

In addition, the strategy of compositing cells with injectable scaffold gets a lot of attention. In 2014, Wang et al. used chitosan hydrogel as a carrier to carry a BADSC for the treatment of myocardial infarction in rats [79]. In 2014, researchers like Wang used PNIPAAm/SWCNTs hydrogel as an injectable scaffold material and carried brown adipose cardiac stem cells for myocardial infarction [80]. The study showed that after transplantation, the retention rate of brown adipose cardiac stem cell can be increased, the thickness of ventricular wall can be increased, the area of ventricular infarction can be reduced, and the cardiac function after myocardial infarction can be improved.

### 9.6.4 Cardiac Reconstruction Based on Whole-Organ Acellular–Recellular Technique

At present, the method of completely treating end-stage heart failure is the orthotopic transplantation of cardiac organs. However, due to the limited supply of donor organs, the annual demand for cardiac organs far exceeds the number of donations. In addition, after a heart transplant, individuals may also face rejection reactions such as lifelong immunosuppression. The re-engineering of artificial hearts has brought hope to solve these problems. Since the acellular matrix retains tissue-specific matrix protein components, three-dimensional ultramicro conformations, vascular structures, and mechanical properties similar to those of natural tissues, it is an ideal natural scaffold material for cardiac remodeling.

Although the research on cardiac remodeling based on whole-organ acellular matrix has progressed rapidly in recent years, there is still a big gap between the functional level of reconstructed heart and the natural heart. The first problem we need to solve is to explore the regulation mechanism of the whole-organ acellular matrix microenvironment on the fate of stem cells, so as to get closer to achieving the ultimate goal of cardiac remodeling.

### 9.6.5 Prospects and Outlooks

With the aging of the world's population, the number of people dying from heart disease each year has reached 20 million, the direct cost of heart failure treatment is as high as $120 billion every year, and the 5-year mortality rate is about 50%. The treatment of heart disease has become a heavy burden on China's national economy, which has restricted the development of the country's economy and society to some extent.

The ultimate goal of myocardial tissue engineering is to produce functional healthy heart tissue in vitro, which can be directly applied to clinical treatment, replacement of damaged myocardial tissue, or drug screening. Myocardial tissue engineering is a relatively young and rapidly developing field, but it has attracted the attention of many scientists at home and abroad. We believe that further clarification of the underlying mechanisms will continue to drive clinical practice. At present, myocardial tissue engineering has made great progress in basic research, clinical application, and market transformation, and its research results have largely changed the clinical treatment ideas and benefited a large number of patients.

Compared with cell therapy, myocardial tissue engineering treatment is complex, and it is necessary to integrate multiple factors and ultimately achieve the characteristics of the natural heart in terms of function, cell, molecule, structure, and so on. Further research on myocardial tissue engineering relies on the synergistic development of seed cells, scaffold materials, in vitro construction of engineered myocardial tissue, and in vivo transplantation techniques. The in vitro construction of myocardial tissue provides great opportunities for regenerative medicine, drug screening, and myocardial disease models, as well as the enormous challenge of achieving reconstituted cardiac transplantation goals, relying on the cooperation and unremitting efforts of experts in the fields of biological sciences and engineering sciences. In short, there are still many unresolved problems in the field of myocardial tissue engineering, and we have a long way to go. We will wait and see.

## 9.7 Tissue Engineered Cartilage

### 9.7.1 Regeneration of Tissue Engineered Articular Cartilage

#### 9.7.1.1 The Histological Characteristics of Natural Articular Cartilage Tissue and the Epidemiology of Injury

Articular cartilage is widely distributed in the synovial joints of the human body and plays an important role, including counteracting mechanical load, lubricating joints, absorbing shock, endochondral ossification, and providing structural support. Cartilage tissue is a highly specialized connective tissue characterized by the lack of blood vessels, nerves, and lymphatic vessels in the tissue. The extracellular matrix is dense and solid, and the chondrocytes are surrounded by a large number of cell matrix (such as collagen fibers and proteoglycans). It is the main reason that the histological characteristics of cartilage tissue, the composition of biochemical components and the characteristics of low metabolism and low proliferative state of chondrocytes, which restricts the proliferation reaction of chondrocytes and the migration to the injured area, resulting in limited self-healing and regeneration capability after the cartilage tissue is damaged. Therefore, once the articular cartilage is damaged or partially excised, there is generally no direct cartilage regeneration, but the formation of connective tissue scar.

The incidence of cartilage damage is high, and it is harmful to individuals and society. According to the statistics of the National Health Commission of the People's Republic of China, there are more than 100 million patients with articular cartilage damage in China, and the number of patients is increasing by nearly ten million each year. About 90% of women and 80% of men over the age of 65 have different degrees of osteoarthritis, which is one of the main causes of labor loss in people over 50 years old. According to the International Arthritis Foundation, one out of every ten people worldwide is a patient with osteoarthritis. A large group of patients with osteoarthritis affects the quality of life of patients themselves, and it also brings huge economic burden to the society. Statistical data from the United States showed that the total cost of osteoarthritis in 1994 was $15.5 billion. From other developed countries, such as Canada, the United Kingdom, and France, the cost of osteoarthritis in 1997 accounted for 1–2.5% of the country's GDP for the year, and increased year by year. There is still no such statistical data in our country. Other ear cartilage defects and nasal cartilage injuries caused by burns, trauma, genetic factors, etc. affect the physiological, psychological, and social health of patients to varying degrees.

Current strategies for treating cartilage damage or osteoarthritis are limited and lack effective treatment options. It mainly includes conservative treatment and surgical intervention. The former includes reducing joint use, increasing muscle strength around the joint, local physical therapy and rehabilitation therapy, and using drug to relieve pain. The latter includes arthroscopic inflammation cleaning, microfracture surgery, and platelet factor enrichment (PRP) treatment, tibia osteotomy, autologous cartilage tissue transplantation (mosaic technique), autologous chondrocyte implantation (ACI), and artificial joint replacement surgery. Conservative treatment techniques, arthroscopic inflammatory cleaning, and tibia osteotomy can relieve symptoms and delay the development of cartilage damage to a certain extent, but cannot achieve the repair and regeneration of damaged cartilage tissue. The purpose of microfracture technology, PRP treatment, mosaic technology, and ACI technology is to repair the damaged cartilage tissue, and hope to achieve the regeneration of cartilage tissue. However, the newly obtained cartilage tissue is mostly fibrocartilage tissue, and its biomechanical strength is worse than that of normal hyaline cartilage tissue, and the surface of the tissue is rougher than normal tissue, which makes it unable to satisfy the function of long-term normal joint function. In addition, the source of autologous chondrocytes or autologous cartilage tissue is limited, and it will bring new cartilage damage to patients themselves. These are the dilemmas and problems that need to be solved by clinicians and researchers.

In recent years, with the rapid development of biomaterial science, engineering science, computer technology, and biomedical science, the exchanges of interdisciplinary information have become increasingly rich and extensive. As a new frontier interdisciplinary subject, tissue engineering has been proposed and widely used in the field of tissue regenerative medicine [81]. In 1987, the concept of tissue engineering was systematically proposed by the American chemical engineer Langer and the clinician Vacanti, meaning the combined use of cells, scaffold materials, and bioactive factors to promote tissue repair and regeneration. The specific method is to obtain a small amount of normal tissue from the human body, obtain the target seed cells through in vitro treatment, and then amplify and plant them on the scaffold material, construct the engineered tissue and implant into the body, repair the relevant tissue defects, and restore the original function. The proposal and development of tissue engineering has broken through the traditional helplessness of repairing damaged tissue at the expense of injured autologous tissue, which brings new hope for the repair and reconstruction of cartilage defects [82, 83].

The research and development of tissue engineered cartilage can be roughly divided into three historical stages. The first phase was mainly from the late 1980s to the early 1990s. The research team led by Vacanti et al. successfully constructed hyaline cartilage tissue in nude mice with isolated bovine articular chondrocytes and degradable biomaterials. The results have successfully confirmed that tissue engineering technology can be fully used for cartilage regeneration and repair. The second stage of tissue engineered cartilage development was in the mid-to-late 1990s. It mainly studied the construction of various shapes of tissue engineered cartilage and preliminary cartilage regeneration and repair in nude mice with immunodeficiency, or in mice, rabbits, and other small animals. In this phase of research, people have begun to pay attention to the selection and application of seed cells for tissue engineered cartilage. The study of tissue engineered cartilage in nude mice and small animals cannot fully and truly reflect the interaction between the microenvironment in vivo and seed cells and biomaterials. Therefore, further research and development of tissue engineered cartilage is naturally turned to tissue engineered cartilage repair and regeneration which is constructed in a large mammal with full immune function, that is, the third stage of the development of tissue engineered cartilage research. At this stage, various studies on tissue engineered cartilage have been carried out.

#### 9.7.1.2 Important Elements and Mechanisms of Tissue Engineered Cartilage Regeneration

The three major elements of tissue engineered cartilage repair are scaffold materials, seed cells, and cytokines [84]. Seed cells are considered the core of tissue engineering. The scaffold materials are the carrier of seed cells and the framework of new tissues. Cytokines are carriers of intercellular signaling and important biologically active molecules that regulate cell proliferation, differentiation, and metabolism.

A. Scaffold

As a substitute for the extracellular matrix of chondrocytes, scaffolds play an important role in cell adhesion, growth and reproduction and secretion of normal extracellular matrix during late cartilage repair.

The ideal scaffold is a temporary carrier of cells. It should have the following characteristics in articular cartilage tissue engineering:

(a) It has good biocompatibility. The scaffold material itself or degradation products are not toxic to cells, tissues, and organisms, and do not cause immunological rejection after implantation.
(b) It is biodegradable. The rate of degradation matches the rate of tissue regeneration. It is generally believed that materials with a short degradation time are more suitable for cartilage tissue engineering than materials with long time stability, because the latter inhibits the synthesis of the matrix in the later stage of the formation of new tissue.
(c) It has sufficient pore structure and porosity and generally requires a porosity of more than 90%. It can provide enough space for even distribution and growth of cells.
(d) The surface of the material has good biological activity and can promote cell adhesion and proliferation. It can regulate the adhesion and growth of seed cells through surface modification, controlled release of biomolecules, or response to environmental stimuli.
(e) It should have the ability to carry and release growth factors while ensuring that the volume of the stent remains unchanged.
(f) The scaffold has mechanical strength and elasticity matching the surrounding normal tissue, which can meet the needs of conduction stress in early joint activities.

The tissue engineered scaffold materials currently reported and studied can be mainly divided into three categories: natural biopolymer scaffold materials, artificial synthetic degradable scaffold materials, and composite scaffold materials [85].

Natural polymer bioscaffold material: Natural bioscaffold material has the advantages of good biocompatibility, high cell affinity, and high degree of degradability, and is beneficial to the adhesion and proliferation of seed cells in the later stage, but it also has shortcomings of poor mechanical properties and rapid degradation rate. The natural biomaterials currently in clinical research mainly include collagen, fibrin, chitosan (CS), silk fibroin, hyaluronic acid, acellular cartilage extracellular matrix, alginate, gelatin, agarose, chondroitin sulfate, chitin, and the like. Extracellular matrix is a macromolecule synthesized by animal cells and secreted extracellularly, distributed on the surface of cells or between cells, mainly composed of protein, polysaccharide, or proteoglycan. Acellular cartilage extracellular matrix scaffold is a better tissue engineered cartilage scaffold, which effectively removes the antigenicity of cells, mimics the microenvironment of chondrocyte growth, and makes this natural bioscaffold very beneficial to the adhesion and proliferation of cartilage cells and has superior biocompatibility and cell affinity. However, the disadvantage is that the natural conformation of the extracellular matrix of the cartilage is easily destroyed during the preparation process, and the mechanical properties of the scaffold are relatively poor. Collagen is the main fibrin component in the extracellular matrix of cartilage. It is usually divided into type I, II, III, IV, and V collagen. Its main function is to connect tissues and organs, support body weight, and protect the body. Experimental studies have shown that the collagen scaffold has the advantages of low immunogenicity, high hydrophilicity, good biocompatibility, cell affinity, and is beneficial to the growth and differentiation of the seed cells. However, the corresponding disadvantages are that the collagen scaffold degrades too fast, the toughness is poor, and the mechanical stress intensity is insufficient. It is usually used in combination with other materials to exert its performance, but how to solve its own related problems needs further research.

Artificial synthetic degradable scaffold materials: Due to the shortcomings of natural polymer materials, which cannot directly meet the corresponding requirements of tissue engineered cartilage, more and more researchers have turned their attention to artificial synthetic scaffold materials [86]. Artificial synthetic scaffold materials have been widely concerned because of their good mechanical properties, strong plasticity, controllable degradation rate, and unrestricted source. The corresponding disadvantages are that the biocompatibility is poor, the cell affinity is low, and the degradation products of scaffold materials may have certain toxicity.

Commonly used artificial synthetic scaffold materials mainly include polylactic acid (PLA), polyglycolic acid (PGA), polylactic co-glycolic acid (PLGA), polyoxyethylene, polycaprolactone (PCL), polyvinyl alcohol (PVA), polyepoxyethylene, and the like. Polylactic acid (PLA), also known as polylactide, belongs to the polyester family. It is a synthetic polymer material with good biocompatibility, degradable, and most of the degradation products are $CO_2$ and $H_2O$. Compared with natural bioscaffold materials, polylactic acid is not only mature in processing technology, but also has a good source of raw materials and good biomechanical properties. The intermediate product lactic acid is also a normal sugar metabolite in the body and will not have harmful effects on the body. The disadvantage of polylactic acid is that the degradation rate is too slow. Usually, the degradation half-life is 6–8 weeks. Although sufficient time provides a scaffolding effect on the cartilage repair area, the long-term accumulation of lactic acid in vivo easily causes tissue swelling and inflammation reaction, and the cell surface affinity of the scaffold material is poor, which is not conducive to cell adhesion and growth, and further limits its development in cartilage tissue engineering. Polyglycolic acid (PGA) is also a commonly used artificial synthetic material, and its degradation products are mainly nontoxic glycolic acid, and the degradation products can be excreted with the renal excretion system or further involved in the metabolic cycle. Polyglycolic acid has good histocompatibility and can promote cell adhesion, growth, and induced differentiation. However, its disadvantage is that the degradation rate is too fast, which easily leads to the collapse of the whole scaffold. The local mass accumulation of the acidic degradation product glycolic acid in vivo also causes a decrease in the pH of the surrounding tissue and a certain effect on the cells. Therefore, in the experimental study, PGA often combines with PLA to form a PLGA to improve its degradation rate to the desired level.

Composite materials: The emergence of composite materials is the development of tissue engineering. In order to overcome the shortcomings of each single material, two or more materials were combined in a certain proportion or way with complementary methods of their characteristics and advantages to design an ideal scaffold which can meet the needs of cartilage tissue engineering. The composite scaffold has the advantages of each single scaffold, such as controllable degradation rate, good cell compatibility, good hydrophilicity of the scaffold, and suitable biomechanical strength. Three-dimensional porous scaffolds with specific shape and pore structure are made by particle pore method, freeze drying method, and laser pore method, such as collagen-PLGA composite scaffold, collagen-hyaluronic acid-chondroitin sulfate composite scaffold, and polylactic acid-polyglycolic acid-calcium polyphosphate fiber-collagen composite scaffold.

B. Seed Cell

Seed cells are the basic unit of cartilage tissue engineering. The selection and optimization of seed cells is the key and prerequisite for constructing tissue engineering. The ideal seed cells should ensure that:

(a) It is safe and convenient.
(b) The sources are abundant.
(c) The immune rejection caused by the body after implantation in vivo is small.
(d) Cells have strong proliferation and differentiation ability.
(e) It can maintain a stable chondrocyte phenotype.
(f) It can adapt to the microenvironment of materials and damage repair areas.

Seed cells can be roughly divided into two major categories in the construction and application of tissue engineered cartilage: adult chondrocytes and mesenchymal stem cells [87, 88]. Chondrocytes can be further divided into autologous chondrocytes, xenogenic chondrocytes, and allogeneic chondrocytes; stem cells mainly include mesenchymal stem cells derived from bone marrow blood, adipose tissue, embryonic tissue, perinatal tissues (umbilical cord tissue, cord blood, and amniotic tissue), etc.

Chondrocytes belong to terminally differentiated cells and are one of the earliest seed cells used in tissue engineered cartilage research. They are also considered to be the gold standard for repairing cartilage seed cells. The biggest advantage of autologous chondrocytes is that there is no immune rejection, which is beneficial for direct clinical application. However, due to its limited source, the process of taking the material will cause new damage to the body, and the chondrocytes are terminal cells with very weak differentiation ability. Usually after about four generations of subculture, the cell phenotype is prone to variability and instability. Type II collagen, which is highly expressed in the extracellular matrix of the cartilage, gradually becomes type I collagen, and the growth and proliferation ability of the cells is deteriorated, thereby failing to reach the number of tissue engineered cartilage requirements, which limits its application. Xenogeneic or allogeneic chondrocytes have a wide range of sources and can be obtained and proliferated in a relatively short period of time. However, since they may produce large immune rejection, they are less practical, so they are not the most ideal tissue engineered cartilage seed cells.

Mesenchymal stem cells are regarded as one of the most promising tissue engineered seed cells because of their multidirectional differentiation potential and self-replication ability, and they have received extensive attention in the field of tissue engineered cartilage research. The stem cells used in the current research are mainly bone marrow mesenchymal stem cells, adipose stem cells, and umbilical cord stem cells. There are bone marrow mesenchymal stem cells (BMSCs) with multidirectional differentiation potential in the bone marrow. BMSCs can be taken from the bone marrow of the backbone, tibia, and ribs. The source is relatively abundant, and the acquisition method is simple and easy. BMSCs can differentiate into chondrocytes under the influence of inducing factors, and it has been recognized that it may become an ideal source of seed cells for articular cartilage tissue engineering. The study found that adipose-derived stem cells can differentiate and culture chondrocytes and stably passage. However, the study also found that after ten passages, the cells showed aging, such as increased lipid droplets, synaptic elongation, and slowed cell proliferation. Only cells within five generations are suitable for cartilage repair. In addition, cells such as periosteum, synovial stem cells, and muscle-derived stromal stem cells can also be induced to differentiate into chondrocytes, but they are less used in current research due to less sources and more complicated differentiation mechanisms. Embryonic stem cells (ESCs) are mainly derived from early embryos developed by fertilized eggs, and can also be obtained from an embryo developed from a somatic cell nuclear transfer. The ability of ESCs to be versatile and immortal is expected to be a new source of tissue engineered seed cells. Since the early 1980s, some scholars have used the inner cell mass or the epiblast cells of early embryos to establish ESCs. Some scholars have confirmed that ESCs can differentiate into chondrocytes under the action of BMP-2 and BMP-4. At present, the biggest problem in the application of ESCs is how to effectively induce the differentiation of ESCs into chondrocytes, effectively establish nonimmunogenic embryonic stem cell lines, and the tumorigenicity of ESCs. In order to solve the problem of difficult source of seed cells, scholars apply transgenic technology to articular cartilage tissue engineering, and transfect the genes of TGF-β, BMP, bFGF, IGF, and other factors into the corresponding target cells by means of vectors to differentiate them into chondrocytes. The most commonly used target cells are BMSCs. It has been reported that chondrocytes are cultured from BMSCs by transgenic technology. At present, there are three methods for introducing foreign genes into a target cell: in situ method, indirect method or ex vivo method, and direct method or in vivo method. With the deepening of research, some new inducible genes have been discovered one after another. Overexpression of SOX9 gene can promote the redifferentiation of osteoarthritic chondrocytes in alginate culture medium, and transfect BMSCs by adenovirus, and can be cultured in the cartilage forming matrix to differentiate into the chondrocyte and secrete type II collagen and the protein polysaccharide. These studies offer new possibilities for culturing cartilage seed cells that meet clinical applications. However, the current transgenic research on BMSCs in China still stays in the animal experiment stage. There are still many problems in the application of transgenic BMSCs in clinical practice, such as the problems of BMSCs transplantation in cartilage microenvironment, and whether it will cause malignant transformation and whether the original organism can maintain the original biological characteristic after transgenic, etc., are for further study.

C. Cytokines

Cytokines are important elements in tissue engineering to regulate the growth and reproduction of seed cells, and are important active substances that stimulate and promote seed cells to perform their intended repair functions in a timely and appropriate amount. The application methods in tissue engineering mainly include directly adding cytokines to the culture medium, regulating cell-directed cartilage differentiation, and performing gene integration by introducing the target gene into the recipient cells to continuously express the target factor protein in the cells. At present, the growth factors studied more include TGF-β, IGF, FGF, BMP, cartilage-derived morphogenetic protein (CDMP), etc. TGF-β is considered the most important cartilage-inducing factor and plays an important role in cell proliferation and differentiation. It is widely present in the body's cells, with the largest number of osseous tissue and platelets. By regulating cell autocrine, paracrine, and other stimulation of chondrocytes to synthesize proteoglycans and collagen, and inhibiting matrix degradation, stem cells can be induced to differentiate into chondrocytes in a dose-dependent manner. IGF can promote the DNA synthesis of chondrocytes, the proliferation of chondrocytes, and maintain its phenotypic stability, and even induce the differentiation of adipose-derived stem cells into chondrocytes. After topical application of IGF-1, it was observed that the apoptosis of chondrocytes was significantly reduced, and the repair of damaged cartilage was significantly accelerated. FGF is found in many tissues such as the brain, liver, kidney, cartilage, and bone of animals and humans. The study found that the mechanism of action of FGF is to combine with the receptors of heparin mucopolysaccharide molecules in the extracellular matrix and activate cells, thereby effectively promoting cell mitosis, inducing cell morphogenesis and differentiation, and participating in the repair process of cell growth, proliferation, and tissue damage. In addition, FGF can significantly inhibit the differentiation of naive chondrocytes, reduce the synthesis of alkaline phosphatase, inhibit the absorption of calcium by chondrocytes, and thus prevent the calcification of new cartilage. BMP belongs to a subgroup of the TGF-β superfamily and has many species. Its role is to mediate early development and organ formation during embryonic formation. In the motor system, BMP promotes the development of cartilage, bone and motor system-associated connective tissue. BMP-2, BMP-4, BMP-6, BMP-7, and BMP-9 have been shown to have significant osteogenesis, while BMP-3 has an inhibitory effect on osteogenesis. Different BMP subtypes have different stimulating effects on chondrocytes, and BMP-7 and BMP-6 have important effects on the repair and regeneration of cartilage damage. CDMP includes three subtypes of CDMP-1, CDMP-2, and CDMP-3, which are very similar in terms of structure or biological characteristics. They are involved in the whole process of cartilage tissue development, growth, and damage repair. It plays an important role in the regulation of chondrocyte differentiation. Among them, people's research on CDMP-1 is the most in-depth. CDMP-1 is mainly expressed in the bone and joint areas of the extremities. It is an important regulator of early cartilage. It can promote the aggregation and adhesion of cartilage progenitor cells in a dose-dependent manner. In the late stage, it plays a role in stimulating chondrocyte proliferation and promoting its maturation.

In summary, TGF-β, IGF, FGF, BMP, and CDMP coordinate and interact with each other in the growth, development, proliferation, differentiation, metabolism, and apoptosis of chondrocytes. The repair of damaged cartilage is an extremely difficult and complicated process, and the development of cartilage tissue engineering technology can greatly promote the repair of human cartilage, and has broad application prospects. The cartilage repair process is the result of a combination of multiple cytokines. In the past, researchers paid more attention to the role of single cytokines, and often ignored the complex effects of different cytokines. The combination of different factors often showed stronger synergistic or antagonistic effects. Furthermore, the signaling pathways and dose-effect relationships of various factors also require more in-depth exploration. In addition, when cytokines have an effect on other tissues, even harmful effects, the clinical safety of cytokines needs to be further explored.

#### 9.7.1.3 Challenges in Tissue Engineered Cartilage Regeneration and the Direction of Future Conquest

Although tissue engineering research has brought new hopes for the regeneration and repair of cartilage tissue, some techniques have been applied from basic research to clinical treatment of articular cartilage damage, and have achieved gratifying therapeutic effects. However, the new cartilage tissue still has a certain gap in biochemical composition, tissue structure, and biomechanics compared with normal hyaline cartilage. However, tissue engineered neonatal cartilage tissue can relieve pain symptoms in a short period of time, filling cartilage defects and providing certain joint movement function. However, the rate of re-injury of the repaired tissue is still faster than that of normal tissue, and the long-term effect is still not satisfactory. The reasons include the following aspects:

(a) The seed cells used to construct tissue engineered cartilage did not achieve the transformation of hyaline cartilage, or lost the original hyaline cartilage phenotype after in vitro processing.
(b) The biological properties, mechanical properties, and degradation rate of the scaffold materials cannot meet the needs of the dynamic remodeling process of tissue regeneration.
(c) The cytokine's mechanism of action, added components, dose, and timing are lack of detailed and sufficient basic research evidence support.

Therefore, tissue engineered cartilage should achieve a qualitative leap, and a large number of valuable basic research and clinical transformation application research work need to be carried out. The following aspects may be the most promising and prospective research directions in the future: seed cells should be widely sourced, have low immunogenicity, have good cartilage differentiation potential and good cell biological activity, and can rapidly amplify and proliferate in vitro and maintain the phenotype of chondrocytes unchanged. In the process of biomaterial research and development, special attention should be paid to the study of the interaction between cells and biological materials to avoid the disconnection between biological materials research and seed cell research. The development of composite materials, nanomaterials, biomimetic materials, and smart materials for biological or chemical modification of materials will be an important part of future biomaterial research. The development of composite materials, nanomaterials, biomimetic materials, and smart materials for biological or chemical modification of materials will be an important part of future biomaterial research because of providing structural support and spatial guidance distribution for cells, inducing cell differentiation and promoting cell proliferation, and ultimately accelerating the regeneration and repair of functional tissues. Cytokines also play an important role in tissue engineering tissue regeneration, and play a bridge-like presentation role in signal transmission between cells [89]. In the future, more research on mechanisms may be needed to reveal its role in tissue regeneration and repair, the role of signaling pathways, and the physiological functions of cells that regulate cell development, so as to apply it more accurately and meticulously to tissue engineering to regulate the occurrence and development of target cells. The way of adding cytokines should also be presented in various ways along with the development of materials science and molecular biology, such as nanomolecular materials coated to achieve slow release, or the synthesis and release of cells with the target gene-transfected cells permanently associated with cell metabolism, so as to achieve the function of cytokines for a long time.

## 9.7.2 The Regeneration of Tissue Engineered Meniscus

### 9.7.2.1 Histological Characteristics and Physiological Functions of Meniscus

A. Anatomy of the Meniscus [90]

The meniscus is a pair of crescent-shaped fibrocartilage tissue between the femoral condyle of the knee and the tibial plateau (Fig. 9.10). The lateral meniscus covers approximately 80% of the tibial plateau, whereas the medial meniscus covers only approximately 60% of the tibial plateau. The unique shape of the meniscus fits perfectly into the different configurations of the corresponding knee femoral condyle and tibial plateau. The anterior and posterior cruciate ligaments play a very important role in the firm fixation of the meniscus, which secures the meniscus to the tibial plateau. The vascular and neural tissues of the meniscus are mainly derived from the surrounding joint capsule and synovial tissue, and there are blood vessels and nerve tissues in the adult knee joint only in the 10–25% area outside the meniscus. Therefore, according to the different distributions of meniscus blood vessels and nerve tissue, the meniscus tissue can be classically divided into three regions: vascular/neural region on the outside (red-red region), no vessel/neural region on the medial side (white-white region), and the region between the two (red-white area). Therefore, when the injury occurs in the white-white area, the meniscus injury is often difficult to heal by itself.

B. Composition and Cell Characteristics of the Meniscus

The extracellular matrix and cell distribution of the meniscus are characterized by heterogeneity. The extracellular matrix component of the meniscus is more complex than the extracellular matrix component of articular cartilage. The extracellular matrix components of articular cartilage are characterized by uniformity, mainly composed of water, collagen, and glycosaminoglycans. The extracellular matrix components of the meniscus can be classified according to different regions. Type I collagen accounts for more than 90% of the dry weight of the red-red region, and the remaining component composition is less than 1%, including collagens of type II, III, IV, VI, V, and VIII. However, in the white-white region, the total collagen content is only 70% of the dry weight, of which type II collagen and type I collagen account for 60% and 40%, respectively.

Distribution of extracellular matrix components of meniscus heterogeneity (Fig. 9.11).

The cell population of the meniscus can also be classically divided into three different species based on different

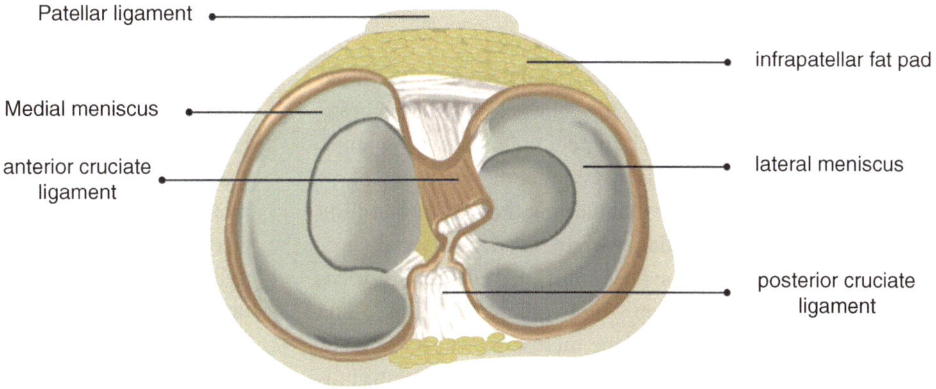


**Fig. 9.10** Anatomy of the meniscus

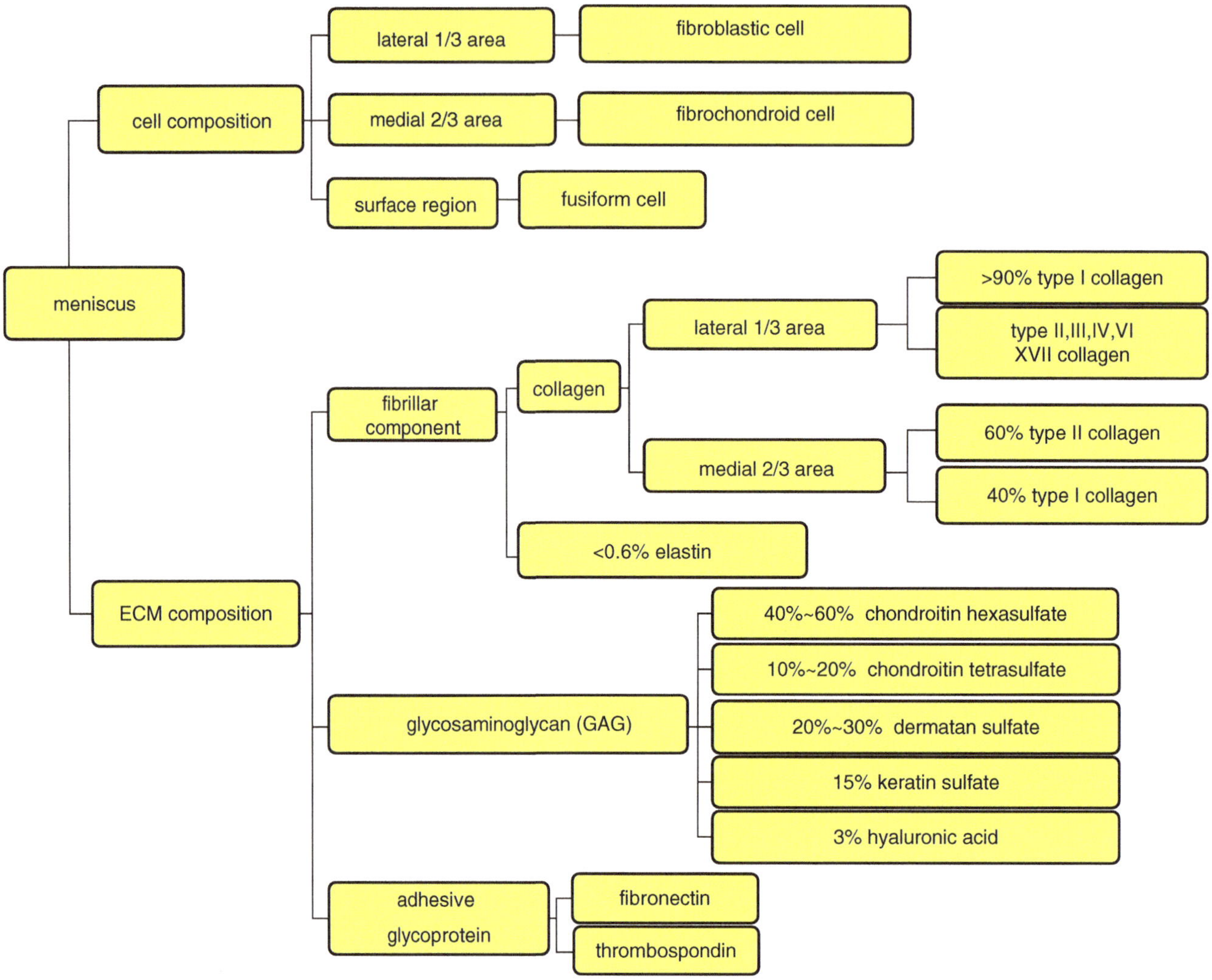


**Fig. 9.11** Composition and cell characteristics of the meniscus

regions and cell morphological features (see Fig. 9.11). The lateral one-third region of the meniscus is mainly composed of fibroblast-like cells, and mainly exhibits an elongated cell shape. The cells in the two-thirds region of the inner side of the meniscus are mainly composed of fibrocartilage-like cells and mainly exhibit circular features. The surface layer of the meniscus is composed of fusiform cells parallel to the surface of the meniscus.

C. Physiological Function of the Meniscus

The meniscus has long been considered a "non-functional residual of the origin of the thigh muscle." With the gradual deepening of the physiological function of the meniscus, people gradually discovered that the meniscus plays a very important role in maintaining the normal function of the knee joint, including weight transfer, shock absorption, stabilization of the knee joint and nutrition, lubrication of the knee joint, and other functions. The biomechanical function of the meniscus is also the basis for its physiological function. The anatomical configuration of the meniscus is closely related to the biomechanical properties of the meniscus. The special shape of the meniscus is extremely important for its adaptation to the different anatomical configurations of the corresponding femoral condyle and tibial plateau. Undoubtedly, the shape of the meniscus adapts to the increased contact area of the articular cartilage between the femur and tibial plateau in the knee joint. In daily life, while the meniscus is subjected to axial stress, it also produces cerclage stress along the semicircular direction of the meniscus, which tends to extrude the meniscus into the knee joint. However, the firm fixation of the anterior and posterior cruciate ligaments prevents the extrusion effect of the meniscus. Therefore, this ensures that a complete meniscus is located between the corresponding femoral condyle and tibial plateau and increases the contact area of the articular cartilage (60%); likewise, it can simultaneously reduce the contact stress of the tibial plateau and protect the tibial plateau cartilage. Conversely, if the anterior and posteriorcruciate ligament or the semicircular collagen fibers in the meniscus are broken, it will change the mechanism of weight transfer and damage the tibial plateau cartilage.

#### 9.7.2.2 The Damage of Meniscus Tissue and Its Epidemiology

After meniscus injury, different degrees of degeneration, edge and surrounding muscle tissue hyperplasia, hypertrophy, edema, etc., may occur. The knee joint will lose its stability and normal activity, and there will be symptoms such as quadriceps atrophy, joint pain, squeaking, shackles, and limited mobility. Long-term meniscus injury will lead to damage to the corresponding articular cartilage of the adjacent femur and tibia, induce osteoarthritis, and lead to a decline in the quality of life and viability of patients; patients with severe disease development need to undergo joint replacement therapy.

In the United States, meniscus injury is the most common intra-articular injury and is the most common disease requiring orthopedic surgery. According to reports, the average incidence of meniscus injury is 66/100,000, and 61 per 100,000 people need to undergo meniscectomy. Men are more prone to meniscus injury than women, and the ratio of male to female is (2.5:1)–(4:1), and the peak age of onset is between 20 and 29 years. In all age groups, meniscus injury most often occurs in the right knee joint, but the main etiology and pathophysiological factors vary greatly depending on the age of the patient. Meniscus injuries in young people are more common in acute injuries, but more often in the elderly population, they are secondary to degenerative changes. More than one-third of meniscus tears are associated with anterior cruciate ligament injury. From the point of view of clinical diagnosis and treatment, meniscus injury can be easily divided into two main types of damage: peripheral meniscus injury and white-white region meniscus injury.

There is relatively little content in the epidemiological study of meniscus injury in China. Yi Shouhong and others used patients with knee arthroscopy from October 2005 to November 2010 in the Joint Surgery Center of Southwest Hospital of Third Military Medical University as the research object. The clinical epidemiological characteristics of 3002 cases of knee arthroscopy were studied. It was found that meniscus injury accounted for 48.47% of knee arthroscopic surgery, indicating that meniscus injury in China is also the most common disease in knee injury.

#### 9.7.2.3 Regeneration Dilemma After Meniscal Tissue Injury

The unique blood supply and nerve distribution characteristics of the meniscus determine that the damage that occurs in the white-white region is difficult to heal by itself. Clinically, orthopedic surgeons typically perform partial meniscal resection for patients with meniscus injuries that cannot be repaired or undergo degenerative changes. However, this current major surgical treatment cannot prevent the development of knee osteoarthritis in patients with meniscus injury, which may be due to the reduction of the contact area between the femoral condyle cartilage and the tibial plateau cartilage after meniscal tissue resection. Therefore, meniscal repair or reconstruction techniques have received widespread attention. In general, repairable injuries in young patients, such as long-axis injuries or injuries that occur in the red-red region, are the best indication for meniscal repair surgery. Meniscus injury repair procedures include internal and external, external and internal repair, and enhanced repair. On the other hand, an increasing number of meniscus reconstruction strategies have also been applied to restore meniscus function, including meniscus allograft, small intestinal submucosal transplantation, and autologous ligament transplantation. However, allografts of the meniscus also have many limiting factors, including the risk of disease transmission, the decline in biomechanical properties of the graft, and graft atrophy. Similarly, small intestinal submucosal transplantation and autologous ligament transplantation did not achieve a satisfactory therapeutic effect.

#### 9.7.2.4 Proposal of the Concept of Cartilage Regeneration in Meniscus Engineering

The current strategy of meniscus injury treatment is difficult to achieve the purpose of functional regeneration of the meniscus. The idea of tissue engineering technology and the concept of regenerative medicine have brought new hope to the treatment of meniscus injury [91]. Tissue engineering technology consists of three classic parts: cells, scaffolds, and biochemistry and biomechanical stimulation. From a tissue engineering point of view, the ideal state is to construct a functional meniscus in vitro to replace damaged or degenerated meniscus tissue. The development of materials science, the advancement of medical imaging technology, and the flourishing development of 3D printing technology have brought new hopes for the realization of the regeneration of a tissue whose shape and function can completely replace the damaged meniscus.

Nowadays, a large number of strategies have been applied to the in vitro construction of meniscal tissue engineered cartilage, which can reconstruct the meniscus defect to some extent, both functionally and structurally. There is no doubt that choosing the right source of cells (autologous, allogeneic, xenogeneic, or stem) is one of the keys to successful meniscus tissue engineering. Similarly, the research and exploration of different types of tissue engineered meniscus scaffold are also extremely critical, whether applied to experimental or clinical research. There are also inevitably some problems to be solved, such as degradation by-products of the scaffold, stress shielding, and the like. In order to promote functional meniscus reconstruction and stem cell differentiation, some cytokines have also been explored. Although there are a lot of problems in the development of meniscus tissue engineering, with the development of biology, engineering, and medicine, the research of tissue engineered meniscus will continue to be promoted.

#### 9.7.2.5 Important Elements and Mechanisms of Cartilage Regeneration in Meniscus Engineering

In the field of meniscal engineering cartilage, the regeneration of the meniscus mainly includes three important components of seed cells, scaffolds, and factors. In the research of meniscal seed cells, different institutions have carried out research on adult cells, stem cells, and co-culture of various cells. Fibrocartilage cells: the team of Professor Baker subcultured the meniscus of patients undergoing knee surgery to obtain P2 fibroblasts and implanted in polycaprolactone (PCL)-oriented scaffolds, and found that with the prolongation of culture time, the dry weight, DNA, collagen, and glycosaminoglycan content of the cell-scaffold complex gradually increased. Sun-Woong Kang from Hanyang University in South Korea transplanted a meniscus with a meniscal-derived fibrocartilage-complexed polyglycolic acid (PGA) scaffold for rabbits, and found that the new tissue is similar to the original tissue in collagen content and mechanical properties. Chondrocytes: Fibrocartilage cells and chondrocytes are derived from cartilage tissue, and studies have shown that they have similar surface markers and high expression of type II collagen. Therefore, chondrocytes are also one of the most promising seed cells for tissue engineered meniscus. To this end, Hong Suk Kwak et al. repaired meniscus injury with a polylactic acid-glycolic acid copolymer scaffold treated with chondrocyte-rich platelet-rich plasma (PRP). The results showed that chondrocytes were a viable meniscus seed cell. Mesenchymal stem cells: stem cells have multiple differentiation potentials, so they are also one of the best seed cells for tissue engineered meniscus. The University of Bristol in the United Kingdom used human bone marrow stem cells and chondrocytes to grow in collagen scaffolds for in vitro culture. It was found that the collagen scaffolds combined with transforming growth factor-β-induced bone marrow stem cells had better mechanical properties. Some scholars have also carried out research on synovial cells, adipose stem cells, and mesenchymal stem cells as seed cells of meniscus. In China, Xu Qinglei and others used fibroblast growth factor and TGF to induce bone marrow stem cells to differentiate into cartilage, looking for a seed source that can replace meniscus fibrocartilage cells. Zhu Xianqi et al. used porous silk fibroin/hydroxyapatite combined with bone marrow mesenchymal stem cells to repair cartilage damage in rabbit meniscus without blood supply area. Professor Yu Jiakuo from the Third Affiliated Hospital of Beijing Medical University used peripheral blood stem cells as seed cells of tissue engineered meniscus and obtained satisfactory experimental results.

Other related research: In order to construct a tissue engineered meniscus that is more biomimetic to the natural meniscus structure and mechanical properties, some scholars have proposed the idea of cell coculture, the concept of partitioning the tissue engineered meniscus, and the high-density self-assembly culture method.

In the study of meniscus scaffold, the researchers conducted different studies mainly on scaffold materials, scaffold morphology, and 3D printing of scaffold.

A. Meniscus Scaffold Material

   In terms of tissue engineered meniscus scaffold materials, they are mainly composed of synthetic polymer materials and biological materials related to extracellular matrix components. Synthetic materials mainly include PCL, polylactic acid (PLA), and PGA. The main advantage of synthetic materials is that they provide satisfactory biomechanical properties, unlimited supply, and strong plasticity. However, there are also disadvantages such as poor hydrophilicity, lack of biological activity, and possible induction of an inflammatory response. Biomaterials related to extracellular matrix components have broader application prospects than synthetic materials, because most of the extracellular matrix component-related biomaterials are biomimetic to the natural meniscus extracellular matrix, which can create a cell adhesion for seed cells, proliferation, or differentiation of the natural microenvironment. Today's extracellular matrix-related biomaterials are mainly composed of one or two extracellular matrix components, such as type I collagen scaffolds and type II collagen scaffolds, but these scaffolds do not fully mimic the microenvironment of natural meniscus cell growth. Some domestic institutions have also carried out research on meniscus scaffold, such as Lu Huading and Cai Daozhang, who used tissue-coated polyhydroxybutyrate hydroxyvalerate to construct tissue engineered meniscus scaffold. Zhu Yunli et al. used a scaffold constructed from autologous synovial mesenchymal stem cells, a small intestinal submucosa complex, to repair rabbit meniscus injury. Zhang Yefeng and Sun Lei explored the feasibility of forming decalcified bone matrix as a substitute for prosthesis after complete meniscus defect.

B. The Shape of the Meniscus Scaffold

   Depending on the integrity of the meniscus scaffold morphology, the meniscus scaffold can be divided into partial meniscus scaffold and integral meniscus scaffold. Koller et al. constructed a partial meniscus scaffold for in vitro culture by adding polyethylene terephthalate to the hyaluronic acid/polycaprolactone scaffold. Baker et al. also produced an oriented partial meniscus scaffold by electrospinning. Mandal et al. used silk fibroin to create an integral meniscus scaffold that mimics the natural meniscus shape and internal structure. Professor Stone et al. used a cow-derived Achilles ligament to make a collagen-copolymerized whole meniscus scaffold and was used in a multicenter clinical trial. After 1 year of implantation, biopsy results confirmed the presence of a similar tissue regeneration in the chronic meniscus lesion implantation group and was well integrated with the periphery of the host meniscus, and no improvement in clinical outcomes in patients with acute meniscus injury.

C. 3D Printed Meniscus Scaffold

3D printing has also been applied to the preparation of meniscus scaffold. For example, researchers at Columbia University Medical Center used biodegradable polycaprolactone as a material to create an alternative damaged meniscus using 3D printing technology. Part of the meniscus scaffold, the connective tissue growth factor and TGF-β3 in this scaffold can stimulate the migration and differentiation of stem cells inside the body, and promote the regeneration of meniscus tissue. In addition, Australian scientists used 3D printing technology to construct meniscus fiber hydrogel scaffold.

Many different types of growth factors are also used in the field of meniscal tissue engineering. bFGF can stimulate the proliferation of meniscal cells well. A group of studies have compared the effects of nine different growth factors on the proliferation of monolayer cultured meniscus cells—epidermal growth factor (EGF), bFGF, TGF-α, platelet-derived growth factor-AB (PDGF-AB), aFGF, TGF-β1, PDGF-AA, insulin-like growth factor-1 (IGF-1), and nerve growth factor (NGF). The results showed that bFGF, PDGF-AB, EGF, and TGF-α could stimulate cell proliferation, and bFGF had the strongest stimulation. The migration of cytokines to monolayer cultured cells has also been studied intensively. PDGF-AB and human growth factor (HGF) stimulate the migration of meniscus cells in three regions, EGF, IGF-1, interleukin-1 (IL-1), and bone morphogenetic protein-2. (BMP-2) can only stimulate cell migration in specific areas. In addition to studying the effects of cytokines on cell proliferation and migration, the effects of growth factors on the synthesis of extracellular matrices in seeds have also been extensively studied. The TGF-β family, as the most important stimulator of cartilage tissue engineering, also showed strong stimulation of the synthesis of the meniscus extracellular matrix (collagen and glycosaminoglycan) in the field of meniscal tissue engineering, and can also promote cell proliferation under monolayer culture conditions. Studies have shown that TGF-β1 can also promote the secretion of lubricating protein on the surface of cartilage. Maintenance of cell phenotypes and differentiation of cells into fibrocartilage are also important research directions for meniscal tissue engineering, although relatively few studies have been conducted in this area. However, some studies have shown that FGF-2 can reverse the phenotypic changes of meniscal cells well under monolayer cell culture conditions. Similarly, TGF-β1 has also been shown to promote phenotypic differentiation of meniscal fibrocartilage cells toward chondrocytes. Because meniscus cells are in different regions and their cell phenotypes are different, research in this area has great research prospects.

#### 9.7.2.6 Challenges of Cartilage Regeneration in Meniscus Engineering and the Direction of Future Conquest

There are also many challenges in tissue engineered meniscal seed cell research. If purely from the perspective of scientific research, autologous meniscus fibrocartilage cells will be the best tissue engineered meniscus seed cells. However, it is often difficult to obtain and there is dedifferentiation in subculture. Stem cells are more satisfactory seed cells for tissue engineered meniscus, but their clinical transformation applications are often limited by laws and regulations. Existing tissue engineered meniscus scaffold research also has some problems. For example, the existing meniscal scaffold material cannot completely simulate the natural microenvironment of meniscus cell growth. Most studies only focus on partial meniscus injury repair, and overall meniscus repair research is relatively few. The existing tissue engineered meniscus scaffolds are less concerned with the reconstruction of the collagen space structure in the meniscus, especially the 3D printed meniscus scaffold is mainly concentrated in the general form of bionics, while the internal space structure has less bionic reports. In the aspect of cytokine research, the specific mechanism of action is not particularly clear. On the one hand, it is necessary to study the effects of combining various cytokines in the future; on the other hand, the culture conditions (serum, monolayer culture, scaffold, and different forms) such as self-assembly also affect the effects of cytokines on cells. Future research may focus on nontraditional cytokines, including serum-derived phospholipids and lysophosphatidic acid (LPA).

## References

1. Williams DJ, Sebastine IM. Tissue engineering and regenerative medicine: manufacturing challenges. Nanobiotechnol IEE Proc. 2006;6:207–10.
2. Dimitrov D, Schreve K, de Beer N. Advance in three dimensional printing-state of the art and future perspectives. Rapid Prototyp J. 2006;12:136–47.

3. Katari R, Peloso A, Zambon JP, et al. Renal bioengineering with scaffolds generated from human kidneys. Nephron Exp Nephrol. 2014;126(2):119–24.
4. Taylor DK, Bubier JA, Silva KA, et al. Development, structure, and keratin expression in C57BL/6J mouse eccrine glands. Vet Pathol. 2012;49(1):146–54.
5. Guillemot F, Souquet A, Catros S, Guillotin B, Lopez J, Faucon M, Pippenger B, Bareille R, Rémy M, Bellance S, Chabassier P, Fricain JC, Amédée J. High-throughput laser printing of cells and biomaterials for tissue engineering. Acta Biomater. 2010;6:2494–500.
6. Murphy SV, Skardal A, Atala A. Evaluation of hydrogels for bioprinting applications. J Biomed Mater Res A. 2013;101:272–84.
7. Peltola SM, Melchels FP, Grijpma DW, Kellomaki M. A review of rapid prototyping techniques for tissue engineering purposes. Ann Med. 2008;40:268–80.
8. Guillotin B, Souquet A, Catros S, Duocastella M, Pippenger B, Bellance S, Bareille R, Rémy M, Bordenave L, Amédée J, Guillemot F. Laser assisted bioprinting of engineered tissue with high cell density and microscale organization. Biomaterials. 2010;31:7250–6.
9. Xu T, Jin J, Gregory C, Hickman JJ, Boland T. Inkjet printing of viable mammalian cells. Biomaterials. 2005;26:93–9.
10. Jones N. Science in three dimensions: the print revolution. Nature. 2012;487:22–3.
11. Huang S, Yao B, Xie JF, et al. 3D bioprinted extracellular matrix mimics facilitate directed differentiation of epithelial progenitors for sweat gland regeneration. Acta Biomater. 2016;32:170–7.
12. Reiffel AJ, Kafka C, Hernandez KA, et al. High-fidelity tissue engineering of patient-specific auricles for reconstruction of pediatric microtia and other auricular deformities. PLoS One. 2013;8(2):e56506–14.
13. Zopf DA, Hollister SJ, Nelson ME, et al. Bioresorbable airway splint created with a three-dimensional printer. N Engl J Med. 2013;368(21):2043–5.
14. Jones N. Science in three dimensions: the print revolution. Nature. 2012;487:22–3.
15. Kobayashi H, Shiraki K, Ikada Y. Toxicity test of biodegradable polymers by implantation in rabbit cornea. J Biomed Mater Res. 1992;26(11):1463–76.
16. Ahmad S, Mathews PM, Lindsley K. Boston type 1 keratoprosthesis versus repeat donor keratoplasty for corneal graft failure: a systematic review and meta-analysis. Ophthalmology. 2016;123(1):165–77.
17. Jirásková N, Rozsival P, Burova M. Alpha Cor artificial cornea: clinical outcome. Eye (Lond). 2011;25(9):1138–46.
18. Birk DE, Lande MA. Corneal and scleral collagen fiber formation in vitro. BBA-Protein Struct. 1981;670(3):362–9.
19. Argüeso P, Herreras JM, Calonge M, et al. Analysis of human ocular mucus: effects of neuraminidase and chitinase enzymes. Cornea. 1998;17(2):200.
20. Kim JC, Tseng SCG. Transplantation of preserved human amniotic membrane for surface reconstruction in severely damaged rabbit corneas. Cornea. 1995;14(5):473–84.
21. Tsai RJ, Li LM, Chen JK. Reconstruction of damaged corneas by transplantation of autologous limbal epithelial cells. N Engl J Med. 2000;13(2):86.
22. Rama P, Matuska S, Paganoni G, et al. Limbal stem-cell therapy and long-term corneal regeneration. N Engl J Med. 2010;363(2):147–55.
23. Liu ZG, Li W, Liang LY, et al. Porcine corneal equivalent for xenographs. Science. 2012;Sup:24–6 PMID: 19819356.
24. Wang TJ, Wang IJ, Hu FR, et al. Applications of biomaterials in corneal endothelial tissue engineering. Cornea. 2016;35(Suppl 1):S25 PMID: 22941807.
25. Fagerholm P, Lagali NS, Merrett K. A biosynthetic alternative to human donor tissue for inducing corneal regeneration: 24-month follow-up of a phase 1 clinical study. Sci Transl Med. 2010;2(46):46–61 PMID: 18428020.
26. Selvanetti A, Cipolla M, Puddu G. Overuse tendon injuries: basic science and classification. Operat Techniq Sports Med. 1997;5(3):110–7 PMID: 20580082.
27. Elliott DH. Structure and function of mammalian tendon. Biol Rev. 2019;95(5):1469–185 PMID: 15193884.
28. Docheva D, Müller SA, Majewski M, et al. Biologics for tendon repair. Adv Drug Deliv Rev. 2015;84(1):222–39 PMID: 22763531.
29. Vincent C, HascallDick K, Heinegård Thomas N. Wight. Proteoglycans. Cell Biol Extracell Matrix. 1991;1991:149–75.
30. Carr AJ, Norris SH. The blood supply of the calcaneal tendon. J Bone Joint Surg. 2001;71(B):100–1.
31. Jay GD, Torres JR, Warman ML, et al. The role of lubricin in the mechanical behavior of synovial fluid. Proc Natl Acad Sci U S A. 2007;104(15):6194–9.
32. Lin TW, Cardenas L, Louis J, et al. Biomechanics of tendon injury and repair. J Biomech. 2004;37(6):865–77.
33. Sharma P, Maffulli N. Biology of tendon injury: healing, modeling and remodeling. J Musculoskelet Neuronal Interact. 2006;6(2):181–90.
34. Thomopoulos S, Parks WC, Rifkin DB, et al. Mechanisms of tendon injury and repair. J Orthop Res. 2015;33(6):832–9.
35. Song JY, Pineault KM, Wellik DM. Development, repair, and regeneration of the limb musculoskeletal system. Curr Top Dev Biol. 2019;132(5):451–76.
36. Lee KJ, Clegg PD, Comerford EJ, et al. A comparison of the stem cell characteristics of murine tenocytes and tendon-derived stem cells. BMC Musculoskelet Disord. 2018;19(116):2–9.
37. Xie HQ, Qu Y, Li XQ, et al. Reconstitution of telomerase activity in human embryonic tendon cells transfected by ptsA58H plasmid. Acta Acad Med Sinic. 2002;24(3):276–80.
38. Md Chard JK, Wright BL. Hazleman. Isolation and growth characteristics of adult human tendon fibroblasts. Ann Rheum Dis. 1987;46(5):385–90.
39. Yin Z, Guo J, Wu T, et al. Stepwise differentiation of mesenchymal stem cells augments tendon-like tissue formation and defect repair in vivo. Stem Cells Transl Med. 2016;5(8):1106–16.
40. Young RG, Butler DL, Weber W, et al. Use of mesenchymal stemcells in a collagen matrix for Achilles tendon repair. J Orthop Res. 1998;16(4):406–13.
41. Bi Y, Ehirchiou D, Kilts TM, et al. Identification of tendon stem/progenitor cells and the role of the extracellular matrix in their niche. Nat Med. 2007;13(10):1219–27.
42. Rui YF, Lui PPY, Li G, et al. Isolation and characterization of multipotent rat tendon-derived stem cells. Tiss Eng PT A. 2010,16(5):1549–58.
43. Tan C, Lui PPY, Lee YW, et al. Scx-transduced tendon-derived stem cells (tdscs) promoted better tendon repair compared to mock-transduced cells in a rat patellar tendon window injury model. PLoS One. 2014;9(5):e97453.
44. Wang B, Liu W, Zhang Y, et al. Engineering of extensor tendon complex by an ex vivo approach. Biomaterials. 2008;29(20):2954–61.
45. Xin X, Hussain M, Mao JJ. Continuing differentiation of human mesenchymal stem cells and induced chondrogenic and osteogenic lineages in electrospun PLGA nanofiber scaffold. Biomaterials. 2007;28(2):316–25.
46. Jeon SH, Chung MS, Baek GH, et al. Comparison of loop-tendon versus end-weave methods for tendon transfer or grafting in rabbits. J Hand Surg [Am]. 2009;34(6):1074–9.
47. Chen CH, Cao Y, Wu YF, et al. Tendon healing in vivo: gene expression and production of multiple growth factors in early tendon healing period. J Hand Surg [Am]. 2008;33(10):1834–42.
48. Molloy T, Wang Y, Murrell G. The roles of growth factors in tendon and ligament healing. Sports Med. 2003;33(5):381–94.
49. Hou Y, Mao Z, Wei X, et al. The roles of TGF-beta1 gene transfer on collagen formation during Achilles tendon healing. Biochem Biophys Res Commun. 2009;383(2):235–9.

50. Thomopoulos S, Harwood FL, Silva MJ, et al. Effect of several growth factors on canine flexor tendon fibroblast proliferation and collagen synthesis in vitro. J Hand Surg [Am]. 2005;30(3):441–7.
51. Nirmalanandhan VS, Rao M, Shearn JT, et al. Effect of scaffold material, construct length and mechanical stimulation on the in vitro stiffness of the engineered tendon construct. J Biomech. 2008;41(4):822–8.
52. Abousleiman RI, Reyes Y, McFetridge P, et al. Tendon tissue engineering using cell-seeded umbilical veins cultured in a mechanical stimulator. Tiss Eng Part A. 2009;15(4):787–95.
53. Stops AJ, Heraty KB, Browne M, et al. A prediction of cell differentiation and proliferation within a collagen-glycosaminoglycan scaffold subjected to mechanical strain and perfusive fluid flow. J Biomech. 2010;43(4):618–26.
54. Benjamin EJ, Muntner P, Alonso A, et al. Heart disease and stroke statistics-2019 update: a report from the american heart association. Circulation. 2019;139(10):e56–e528.
55. Maytin M, Colucci WS. Molecular and cellular mechanisms of myocardial remodeling. J Nucl Cardiol. 2002;9(3):319–27.
56. Lu L, Liu M, Sun R, et al. Myocardial infarction: symptoms and treatments. Cell Biochem Biophys. 2015;72(3):865–7.
57. Guo XM, Wang CY, Tian XC, et al. Engineering cardiac tissue from embryonic stem cells. Methods Enzymol. 2006;420:316–38.
58. Meganathan K, Sotiriadou I, Natarajan K, et al. Signaling molecules, transcription growth factors and other regulators revealed from in-vivo and in-vitro models for the regulation of cardiac development. Int J Cardiol. 2015;183:117–28.
59. Bai F, Lim CH, Jia J, et al. Directed differentiation of embryonic stem cells into cardiomyocytes by bacterial injection of defined transcription factors. Sci Rep. 2015;5:15014.
60. Pacheco-Leyva I, Matias AC, Oliveira DV, et al. CITED2 cooperates with isl1 and promotes cardiac differentiation of mouse embryonic stem cells. Stem Cell Rep. 2016;7(6):1037–49.
61. Yamada Y, Wang XD, Yokoyama S, et al. Cardiac progenitor cells in brown adipose tissue repaired damaged myocardium. Biochem Biophys Res Commun. 2006;342(2):662–70.
62. Liu Z, Tang Y, Lü S, et al. The tumourigenicity of iPS cells and their differentiated derivates. J Cell Mol Med. 2013;17(6):782–91.
63. Moon HH, Joo MK, Mok H, et al. MSC-based VEGF gene therapy in rat myocardial infarction model using facial amphipathic bile acid-conjugated polyethyleneimine. Biomaterials. 2014;35(5):1744–54.
64. Gómez-Mauricio G, Moscoso I, Martín-Cancho MF, et al. Combined administration of mesenchymal stem cells overexpressing IGF-1 and HGF enhances neovascularization but moderately improves cardiac regeneration in a porcine model. Stem Cell Res Ther. 2016;7(1):94.
65. Liu Z, Wang H, Zhang Y, et al. Efficient isolation of cardiac stem cells from brown adipose. J Biomed Biotechnol. 2010;2010.104296.
66. Simpson DG, Majeski M, Borg TK, et al. Regulation of cardiac myocyte protein turnover and myofibrillar structure in vitro by specific directions of stretch. Circ Res. 1999;85(10):e59–69.
67. Iwakura A, Fujita M, Kataoka K, et al. Intramyocardial sustained delivery of basic fibroblast growth factor improves angiogenesis and ventricular function in a rat infarct model. Heart Vessel. 2003;18(2):93–9.
68. Yao S, Tong H, Fanglian Y, et al. RoY peptide-modified chitosan-based hydrogel to improve angiogenesis and cardiac repair under hypoxia. ACS Appl Mater Interfaces. 2015;7(12):6505–17.
69. Cortiella J, Niles J, Cantu A, et al. Influence of acellular natural lung matrix on murine embryonic stem cell differentiation and tissue formation. Tissue Eng A. 2565;16(8):2010.
70. Hongyu S, Shuanghong L, Xiaoxia J, et al. Carbon nanotubes enhance intercalated disc assembly in cardiacmyocytes via the β1-integrin-mediated signaling pathway. Biomaterials. 2015;55:84–95.
71. Kim T, Kahng YH, Lee T, et al. Graphene films show stable cell attachment and biocompatibility with electrogenic primary cardiac cells. Mol Cell. 2013;36(6):577–82.
72. Hitscherich P, Aphale A, Gordan R, et al. Electroactive graphene composite scaffolds for cardiac tissue engineering. J Biomed Mater Res A. 2018;106(11):2923–29331.
73. Zimmermann WH, Schneiderbanger K, Schubert P, et al. Tissue engineering of a differentiated cardiac muscle construct. Circ Res. 2002;90(2):223–30.
74. Shimizu T, Yamato M, Isoi Y, et al. Fabrication of pulsatile cardiac tissue grafts using a novel 3-dimensional cell sheet manipulation technique and temperature-responsive cell culture surfaces. Circ Res. 2002;90(3):e40.
75. Shimizu T, Yamato M, Kikuchi A, et al. Cell sheet engineering for myocardial tissue reconstruction. Biomaterials. 2003;24(13):2309–16.
76. Sekine H, Shimizu T, Sakaguchi K, et al. In vitro fabrication of functional three-dimensional tissues with perfusable blood vessels. Nat Commun. 2013;4:1399.
77. Roberts MA, Tran D, Coulombe KL, et al. Stromal cells in dense collagen promote cardiomyocyte and microvascular patterning in engineered human heart tissue. Tiss Eng Part A. 2016;22(7–8):633–44.
78. Wassenaar JW, Gaetani R, Garcia JJ, et al. Evidence for mechanisms underlying the functional benefits of a myocardial matrix hydrogel for post-mi treatment. J Am Coll Cardiol. 2016;67(9):1074–86.
79. Wang H, Shi J, Wang Y, et al. Promotion of cardiac differentiation of brown adipose derived stem cells by chitosan hydrogel for repair after myocardial infarction. Biomaterials. 2014;35(13):3986–98.
80. Li X, Zhou J, Liu Z, et al. A PNIPAAm-based thermosensitive hydrogel containing SWCNTs for stem cell transplantation in myocardial repair. Biomaterials. 2014;35(22):5679–88.
81. Bernhard JC, Vunjak-Novakovic G. Should we use cells, biomaterials, or tissue engineering for cartilage regeneration. Stem Cell Res Ther. 2016;18(7):56.
82. Jiang S, Guo W, Tian G, Luo X, Peng L, Liu S, Sui X, Guo Q, Li X. Clinical application status of articular cartilage regeneration techniques: tissue-engineered cartilage brings new hope. Stem Cells Int. 2020;2020:5690252.
83. Campos Y, Almirall A, Fuentes G, Bloem H, Kaijzel E, Cruz L. Tissue engineering: an alternative to repair cartilage. Tiss Eng Part B Rev. 2019;25(4):357–73.
84. van der Kraan P, Buma P, van Kuppevelt T, van den Berg W. Interaction of chondrocytes, extracellular matrix and growth factors: relevance for articular cartilage tissue engineering. Osteoarthr Cartil. 2002;10(8):631–7.
85. Armiento A, Stoddart M, Alini M, Eglin D. Biomaterials for articular cartilage tissue engineering: Learning from biology. Acta Biomater. 2018;65:1 20.
86. Iulian A, Dan L, Camelia T, Claudia M, Sebastian G. Synthetic materials for osteochondral tissue engineering. Adv Exp Med Biol. 2018;1058:31–52.
87. Nakayama N, Pothiawala A, Lee J, Matthias N, Umeda K, Ang B, Huard J, Huang Y, Sun D. Human pluripotent stem cell-derived chondroprogenitors for cartilage tissue engineering. Cellul Molecul Life Sci: CMLS. 2020;77(13):2543–63.
88. Freyria A, Mallein-Gerin F. Chondrocytes or adult stem cells for cartilage repair: the indisputable role of growth factors. Injury. 2012;43(3):259–65.
89. Koseska A, Bastiaens PI. Cell signaling as a cognitive process. EMBO J. 2017;36(5):568–82.
90. Makris EA, Hadidi P, Athanasiou KA. The knee meniscus: structure-function, pathophysiology, current repair techniques, and prospects for regeneration. Biomaterials. 2011;32:7411–31.
91. Guo W, Liu S, Zhu Y, et al. Advances and prospects in tissue-engineered meniscal scaffolds for meniscus regeneration. Stem Cells Int. 2015;2015:517520.

# 10 New Technologies and Tissue Repair and Regeneration (2): Other Biotherapeutic Technologies

Xiaokun Li, Jian Xiao, Jiang Wu, Biao Cheng, Xiaobing Fu, and Hongyu Zhang

## 10.1 Growth Factors and Growth Factor Drugs

### 10.1.1 Fibroblast Growth Factor

Fibroblast growth factor (FGF) is a highly conserved polypeptide in biological evolution. It has been found that 23 FGF family members have high amino acid sequence homology. FGF has a wide range of biological effects on tissue cells derived from mesoderm and neuroectoderm. FGF promotes cell proliferation, migration, survival, and differentiation through FGF receptor (FGFR); participates in embryonic development, damaged tissue repair, neovascularization, stem cell proliferation and differentiation, nerve regeneration, calcium and phosphorus metabolism, etc.; plays an important role in wound repair, cardiovascular system diseases, nervous system diseases, and osteochondral regeneration; and have important clinical application value and broad market prospects.

FGF is such an important protein drug, which is an important endogenous functional regulatory protein in human body. The important medicinal value of FGF is reflected in wound repair and neuroprotection. International experts in this field generally believe that there are several important landmark events in the development of FGF: in 1974, American scientist Denis discovered FGF, so he was awarded the title of academician of the Academy of Sciences; in 1986, Professor Fiddes of Harvard University obtained the cDNA sequence of FGF; in 1998, our team developed the world's first new FGF drug (Fig. 10.1).

X. Li · J. Xiao · J. Wu · H. Zhang
Wenzhou Medical University, Wenzhou, China

B. Cheng
General Hospital of Southern Theater Command of Chinese People's Liberation Army, Guangzhou, China

X. Fu (✉)
The Chinese People's Liberation Army General Hospital, Beijing, China

Professor Li Xiaokun's team is the first team in China to systematically study the growth factor proteins and is one of the most influential growth factor development teams in the world. Over the past 20 years, he has developed the FGF series of drugs and developed other proteins of the FGF family as new drug candidates for major diseases such as diabetes, spinal cord injury and stroke, edited and published the first Basic and Clinical Application of Fibroblast Growth Factor in China, which has effectively promoted the application and popularization of FGF series drugs in China. Together with Academician Xiaobing Fu, we first reported the FGF series of modified proteins such as non-mitogenic hormone-like active FGF protein, transmembrane peptide fusion FGF protein, and sumo fusion FGF protein, which confirmed the role and pharmacodynamic mechanism of FGF in diabetes and its complications, spinal cord injury, stroke, corneal injury, optic nerve injury, and other important diseases in synchronization with the international community.

### 10.1.2 Fibroblast Growth Factor and Wound Repair

Studies have shown that FGF exerts its mitogenic effect mainly through the following three pathways:

A. Through activating receptor, FGF receptors have high affinity and low affinity, and high-affinity receptors are involved in tyrosine kinase activity. Low-affinity receptors may have different effects on FGF due to the variety of species.
B. Flow cytometry analysis showed that the effect of FGF on cell proliferation occurred when FGF binds to the receptor and can decrease the cells in G0 phase and G1 phase in the cell cycle, and the S phase rate is accelerated.


X. Fu (ed.), *Regenerative Medicine in China*, https://doi.org/10.1007/978-981-16-1182-7_10

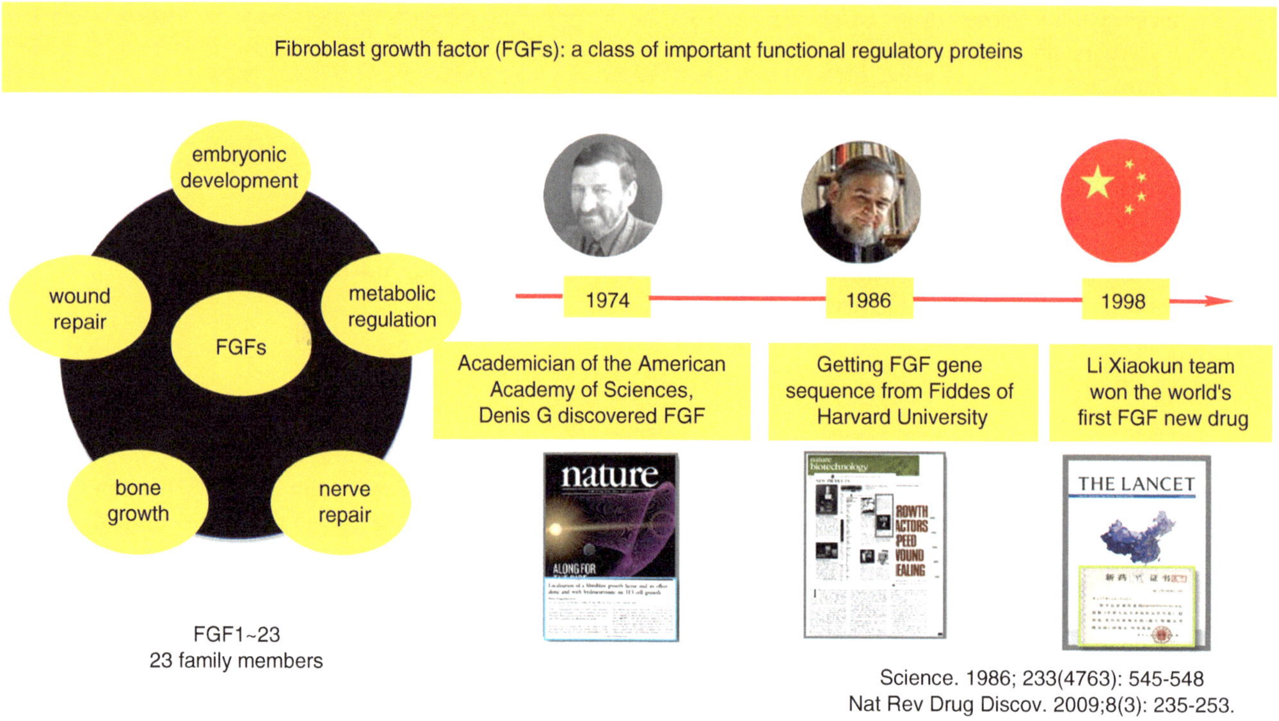


**Fig. 10.1** Fibroblast growth factor FGF family members and research process

C. By limiting enzymolysis, the inactive FGF bound to heparin is converted into a soluble, active FGF by the action of an enzyme.

The non-mitogenic hormone-like activity of FGF involved in tissue repair has the following aspects.

(a) Chemotactic activity: With the action of FGF alone or in combination with other factors, can chemotactic inflammatory cells (mainly macrophages, neutrophils, monocytes, mast cells, etc.) and tissue repair cells to the wound surface, the required concentration is only in the range of picogram (pg) to nanogram (ng). And the results can produce the following effects: first, anti-infective effect. Wound bacteria are inhibited or killed by phagocytosis and enzymatic hydrolysis of inflammatory cells. Second, the release of cell (growth) factors. After the inflammatory cells reach the wound surface, they can further release various growth factors including transforming growth factor (TGF) and epidermal growth factor (EGF) to produce a cascade effect of growth factor release [1]. Third, the role of tissue repair in the later period. Growth factors such as fibroblasts and tissue repair cells accumulate in the wound surface, and at the same time, they act on these tissues to repair the cells by autocrine means, so that they proliferate in the wound surface and reserve for repair.

(b) Hypotensive effect: this effect helps to open small blood vessels under shock and other conditions, reduces the phenomenon of no reflow, and thus reduces tissue damage caused by ischemia [2], hypoxia and reperfusion, the mechanism involves FGF affecting $Na^{+}$-$K^{+}$ ion channels and other aspects.

(c) Inhibition of gastric acid secretion, help the repair of ulcers. To this end, FGF is called "trauma hormone": through experiments in different classes and grades of mice, rats, rabbits, and miniature pigs, it has been observed that growth factors such as FGF have significant induction of angiogenesis and promote the repair of body surface [3], ischemic viscera, spinal cord, nerve, and brain tissue. In the rabbit ear trauma model, bFGF significantly increased extracellular matrix deposition and number of new blood vessels. In the surface trauma, through the superficial second-degree burn, deep second-degree burn, donor skin area, skin-cutting (except) injury, and chronic refractory wounds of diabetes, it was found that bFGF has a significant pro-repair effect in a certain dose range, which was manifested in the increased and thickened granulation tissue in wounds, accelerated epithelialization of wounds, and shortened healing time. Histological observations showed that the deposition of collagen on bFGF-treated wounds increased, fibroblasts were not only mature, but also a large number, capillary blasts increased significantly, and local circulation improved. Conversely, if bFGF antibodies are used in the experiment, the above biological effects are inhibited by 50–80%.

## 10.1.3 Fibroblast Growth Factor and Diabetes

Diabetes is one common chronic disease that is harmful to human health, and its complications are the main causes of the quality of life of diabetic patients and the ultimate death of patients. Recent studies have found that the FGF family plays a very important role in the occurrence and development of diabetes. Hart AW et al. reported that FGF and its receptors (FGFRs) are expressed in mature mouse β cells, and the weakening or blocking of the receptor FGFR1c signaling pathway leads to diabetes. FGF and its clinical application have become hotspots in the field of diabetes and its complications.

### 10.1.3.1 FGF and Diabetic Ulcer

As one of the common complications of diabetes, diabetic ulcer is a difficult skin injury. It is currently believed that its pathogenesis is mainly microvascular and peripheral neuropathy caused by hyperglycemia. When the glucose content of the skin is significantly increased, the skin has nutritional disturbance, which is prone to skin damage, and is beneficial to the growth and reproduction of bacteria, easy to secondary infection, and poor repair ability, thereby causing ulcers that are difficult to heal. The pathogenesis of wound ulcer is complex, and the pathophysiology is mainly characterized by abnormal cell metabolism of the wound tissue, immune dysfunction, especially the local macrophage and mast cell dysfunction of the wound, accompanied by impaired growth factor function in the wound microenvironment, local microcirculation perfusion disorder, tissue hypoxia, etc., resulting in long-lasting wound healing. The clinical manifestations of diabetic ulcers are local erosion, ulceration, and necrosis. How to promote the early healing of diabetic skin ulcers, shorten the course of disease, and reduce the disability rate. At present, there is still no effective prevention and treatment method, and the promotion of ulcer surface repair has become a major problem, so it is increasingly valued by medical workers and researchers.

Under normal physiological conditions, the body may release corresponding factors such as vascular endothelial growth factor and fibroblast growth factor to promote angiogenesis and cell proliferation [4], but hyperglycemia inhibits this effect, and in comparison to normal wound healing, glycosylation caused by hyperglycemia will reduce the ability of FGF to bind to the tyrosine kinase-linked receptor (RTK) and partially inhibit the signaling of growth factors, thereby reducing the mitogenic and angiogenic effects of growth factors [3]. The study found that the use of various exogenous growth factors, including FGF, in animal models or diabetic patients has significantly promoted wound healing.

Studies have shown that FGF can affect the entire process of wound repair, including early inflammatory response, granulation tissue regeneration, and re-epithelialization. As a chemokine, FGF can directly promote the accumulation of tissue repair cells at the injury site. In addition, FGF as a mitogen can directly stimulate the proliferation and differentiation of fibroblasts, vascular endothelial cells, smooth muscle cells, etc. in granulation tissue, thereby accelerating the filling of the wound by granulation tissue to and also providing the basis for epidermal cells to cover the wound. FGF can also promote the synthesis and secretion of collagen fibers in granulation tissue. Collagen constitutes an important extracellular microenvironment, which provides good conditions for cell growth and wound healing. In addition, FGF also promotes the repair of capillary network during wound repair and can directly stimulate the proliferation of epidermal cells and accelerate the covering process of wounds.

### 10.1.3.2 FGF and Diabetic Cardiomyopathy

Diabetes inhibits a variety of growth factors including FGF expression and hyperglycosylation, thereby reducing endogenous FGF expression levels and activity. Diabetes-induced oxidative stress leads to dysfunction of myocardial progenitor cells (CPC), inhibition of CPC proliferation and myocardial formation, leading to diabetic cardiomyopathy and heart failure. Our laboratory and other research groups have confirmed that FGF has a protective effect on cardiac ischemia/reperfusion (I/R) injury. The local administration of bFGF for the treatment of myocardial ischemic necrosis after coronary artery heart disease has completed Phase I clinical trials, showing good clinical application prospects. Therapeutic effects of FGF on acute myocardial injury may be related to FGF-induced angiogenesis and differentiation of cardiac progenitor and stem cells (CPC/CSC).

## 10.1.4 Basic Fibroblast Growth Factor and Brain Trauma

Basic fibroblast growth factor (bFGF) promotes tissue regeneration, participates in nerve regeneration, and promotes wound healing and tissue repair. A wide range of growth factors play an important role in the pathophysiological processes of the central nervous system. bFGF can induce proliferation and differentiation of various cells originating from mesoderm and neuroectoderm and is closely related to embryonic development, neurotrophic and regeneration, angiogenesis, wound healing, and tumorigenesis. The fibroblast growth factor family, especially basic fibroblast growth factor, is closely related to neuroprotection and repair after ischemia, metabolism, or traumatic nerve injury.

The main manifestations of brain traumatic disease are hemorrhagic necrosis in the cortex and corpus callosum; a large number of inflammatory cell infiltration in the lesion tissue, accompanied by a large number of degeneration and necrotic tissue fragments, forming obvious tissue defects; the lesion tissue arrangement is disordered, forming a glial scar. bFGF plays a role in brain trauma:

A. Directly acts on neurons. Cultured nerve cells generally die quickly in low or serum-free cultures, but after addition of basic fibroblast growth factor, not only their survival is prolonged but also axonal growth is apparent, indicating that basic fibroblast growth factor has neurotrophic effect. The neurotrophic effect of basic fibroblast growth factor is further confirmed in vivo. Treatment of basic fibroblast growth factor after optic nerve severing in adult rats can prolong the survival of retinal ganglion cells. Immunohistochemistry experiments showed that the immune response of basic fibroblast growth factor in brain tissue was significantly enhanced after artificial short-term cerebral ischemia, suggesting that basic fibroblast growth factor is associated with brain tissue damage repair.
B. Effects on glial cells. bFGF promotes the proliferation of glial cells and increases the content of myelin-related proteins and lipids. After brain injury, astrocytes can be activated by a variety of cytokines [5]. Among them, bFGF has the greatest effect on astrocytes. After injury, astrocytes begin to express bFGF and gradually increased until 2 days after injury began to decline. The dynamic changes of bFGF expression indicated that the damaged astrocytes could secrete bFGF, which is one of the early responses of astrocytes after injury. The activation of the bFGF system after injury rapidly promotes astrocyte hypertrophy, proliferation, and migration and forms reactive astrocyte gelatinization. The enhanced immunostaining of bFGF after injury was first seen in the cytoplasm of neurons and initiated a reactive astrocyte in a paracrine pathway. With the activation of astrocytes, they themselves continue to produce bFGF in large amounts, maintaining astrocyteization process in an autocrine manner. Proliferating glial cells produce more neurotrophic factors and promote the repair process after brain injury.
C. The role of the blood–brain barrier. The destruction of the blood–brain barrier after traumatic brain injury is an important cause of secondary brain injury. Within 30 min after acute injury, the blood–brain barrier is rapidly open, and secondary hypoxia and hypotension can aggravate the opening of the blood–brain barrier. The acute opening of the blood–brain barrier can cause blood components to enter the brain tissue. For example, inflammatory cells enter to enhance or induce local inflammatory reactions, exacerbate the damage, and immune cells and cytokines enter the brain tissue to initiate the brain's immune response process, which may be an important cause of sequelae of brain trauma, such as inflammatory scars, epilepsy, and multiple sclerosis. At the same time, the opening of the blood–brain barrier causes sodium and water to enter the brain tissue freely, leading to cerebral edema, which is an important cause of death from traumatic brain injury. Therefore, the increase in permeability of the blood–brain barrier is suppressed, and subsequent damage can be effectively suppressed. The blood–brain barrier is composed of brain microvascular endothelial cells, pericytes, astrocyte terminal, and basement membrane, wherein brain microvascular endothelial cells are the main structure of the blood–brain barrier, and the blood–brain barrier junction complex includes tight junctions and adhesive junctions [6]. Experiments have shown that bFGF can upregulate the expression of tight junction proteins between cells after brain injury, reduce blood–brain barrier permeability, and promote the migration of brain vascular endothelial cells.

The change of bFGF gene expression after craniocerebral injury indicates that it plays an important role in a series of cellular responses and neurological recovery after craniocerebral injury, especially bFGF promotes neuronal survival, promotes angiogenesis and glial cell proliferation, more nerve cells survive under pathological conditions [7]. The temporal characteristics of bFGF mRNA expression after different degrees of brain injury indicate that the expression of bFGF mRNA in the cerebral cortex increases with the degree of injury, and its expression also increases accordingly, indicating the ability of the central nervous system to protect the brain. The necrotic neurons in severe craniocerebral injury are significantly more than mild craniocerebral injury, which also indicates the limited ability of the central nervous system to protect itself against injury. Therefore, when the brain tissue is damaged and more nerve cells need trophic factor support, exogenous administration is necessary. However, studies have shown that exogenous bFGF can significantly reduce the infarct volume before or within a few hours after ischemia, but there is no significant difference between the administration of the brain injury and the control group 24 h after the brain injury, so the effective therapeutic window for bFGF-induced reduction of infarct volume is 2–24 h after ischemia [8], and the effect of perfusion administration is better after 3 h of focal cerebral ischemia.

Whether the expression of bFGF changes with the pathological changes of brain tissue, and whether the expression is consistent in different parts of the brain, there are few studies. Since bFGF is a polymer protein that cannot pass the blood–brain barrier, a possible therapeutic approach is to chemically modify bFGF to increase its function of crossing the blood–brain barrier. Currently, the dose, route of administration, therapeutic window, and short-term for bFGF treatment and long-term side effects need to be studied in further detail.

### 10.1.5 Fibroblast Growth Factor and Bone Disease

As the largest organ of the body, bones have important functions such as supporting the body, assisting movement and protecting internal organs, and playing a key role in regulating the body's plasma balance of calcium, phosphorus, and magnesium. The bones are always in a state of metabolism to maintain bone strength and bone integrity. In recent years, extensive and in-depth studies of FGF/FGFRs have clearly shown that FGF and its receptors play an important role in bone growth and maintenance of bone homeostasis in adulthood, and the regulation of its level and the change of relevant molecular mechanisms are closely related to the occurrence and development of bone diseases.

In the process of fracture healing, the effect of bFGF on fracture healing is similar to FGF-1, and FGF-1 and bFGF are detectable in the granulation tissue of the fracture area in the early stages of fracture repair. Subsequently, FGF-1 and bFGF are expressed in mesenchymal cells, mature chondrocytes, and osteoblasts and can increase the expression of TGF-β in osteoblasts. The combination of FGF-1 and bFGF acts as a mitogen for various mesenchymal cells, including fibroblasts, chondrocytes, and osteoblasts. However, bFGF has other special effects. bFGF knockout mice showed a reduction in bone mass and a decrease in bone mineralization deposition, suggesting an important role in the deposition and maintenance of bone mass. In addition, bFGF is also able to promote vascularization and new bone formation of transplanted bone by upregulating the expression of VEGF. In addition to its role in promoting mitosis and angiogenesis, bFGF also stimulates bone resorption. These characteristics suggest that bFGF has a potential impact on several stages of fracture repair. However, the role of bFGF in fracture healing differs in many literatures. In the dog's tibial incision model, the size of the early callus increased and the absorption rate of cartilage were accelerated after the single injection of bFGF, and finally the healing of the fracture was accelerated by stimulating the remodeling of the callus. Chen et al. established a fracture model by performing a bone metaphysis operation on the rabbit, and locally injected bFGF at the fracture site, and found that it has the effect of accelerating fracture healing and increasing the mineralization density of the fracture site. However, Nakajima et al. studied the effects of bFGF on the temporal and spatial expression patterns of chondrogenesis-related genes in a model of closed fractures in rats. It is proposed that exogenous bFGF can increase cartilage osteophytes, but it does not accelerate the rate of fracture healing. Bland et al. studied the rabbit tibia fracture model and proposed that local injection of exogenous bFGF at 4 days after fracture had no significant effect on fracture healing.

Among the many family members of FGF, FGF-23 has been closely related to blood phosphorus metabolism as a research hotspot in recent years. Phosphorus, as a very important inorganic non-metallic element, is of great significance to the health of the body. Phosphorus is present in the body in the form of inorganic phosphates and organic phosphates, of which the inorganic phosphate present in plasma is called blood phosphorus. But now there is limited understanding of its homeostatic regulation mechanism, only knowing that vitamin D3 and parathyroid hormone can affect the metabolism of phosphorus. The discovery of FGF-23 undoubtedly gives people a new understanding of the mechanism of blood phosphorus metabolism in vivo, especially the progress of genetics has shown that too much and too little can lead to the occurrence of diseases, so the corresponding research is expected to bring hope for the treatment of these diseases.

The study found that FGF-23 mice obtained by gene knockout were similar to the aging phenotype of another anti-aging protein Klotho (often abbreviated as Kl) gene-deficient mice, all of which developed skeletal dysplasia, osteoporosis and muscle aging and so on. Therefore, it was confirmed that the function of FGF-23 is closely related to Kl protein. The human Kl protein is 1012 amino acids in length (1024 in mice) and is a single transmembrane protein expressed primarily in the kidney, placenta, small intestine, and prostate. The Kl protein binds directly to the FGFR-type receptor, and the complex formed by the two forms has much more affinity with FGF-23 than the affinity of FGF-23 alone. Therefore, the Kl protein is a basic helper factor for receptors in FGF-23 signal transduction. Recent studies have shown that Kl protein itself is one of the co-receptors of FGF-23. Using kidney homogenate as a material, it was found that Kl protein itself can also specifically bind to FGF-23, and the expression of the current one is increased, which can enhance the affinity of kidney cells with the latter, and the sensitivity of cells to the latter is enhanced. When the monoclonal antibody against K1 protein was injected into mice, the induction of FGF-23 was significantly reduced. Thus, the K1 protein and the FGF-type receptor FGFR1 together constitute the FGF-23 receptor to mediate FGF-23 signal transduction.

### 10.1.6 Growth Factors and Biological Materials and Their Combined Effects

Growth factors and biological materials are an integral part of tissue engineering treatment. Tissue engineering is the use of biological materials, growth factors, and seed cells to provide a growth-recovering microenvironment for tissue damage to achieve therapeutic effects. The following describes growth factors and biological materials and summarizes the role of some biomaterials containing growth factors in treatment.

Growth factor is a kind of polypeptide factor that affects cell activity through intercellular signal transmission. It is widely distributed in various tissue cells, not only has the function of promoting angiogenesis but also its expression product is soluble, and can be secreted from cells after expression. It has strong diffusibility and easy to reach target cells, so that it can exert its biological activity well. It promotes or inhibits the proliferation, migration, and gene expression of cells and plays an important role in the development and repair of organisms. Commonly used growth factors include insulin-like growth factor (IGF), basic fibroblast growth factor (bFGF), transforming growth factor-β (TGF-β), bone morphogenetic protein (BMP), and the like.

The use of growth factors alone, due to the short half-life of growth factors, is easily degraded by enzymes and cannot meet the local and systemic therapeutic effects. Moreover, it is expensive, it is difficult to be administered in vivo, and the effective concentration of the growth factor cannot be maintained, so that the desired effect cannot be achieved.

Therefore, constructing a cell platform capable of supporting various growth factors while providing an attachment matrix for transplanted cells, guiding cell proliferation, differentiation, and accelerating the revascularization process of the transplanted vector has become an important research strategy for improving the effect of cell transplantation in academia today. A slow release platform for growth factors emerges in an endless stream. Adhesion of growth factors to biological scaffolds made of biomaterials in tissue engineering treatment has become an important achievement on our research path.

Biomaterials generally refer to materials that are used for medical purposes, alone or in conjunction with drugs, for the treatment or replacement of tissues or organs to repair damaged tissue. The purpose of using biological materials is to provide a three-dimensional scaffold for tissue cell growth, while filling and replacing the damaged parts, promoting cell adhesion, proliferation, and even differentiation.

The biomaterial can be covalently bound to the growth factor to make the release of the growth factor relatively stable, and the stem cells implanted thereon are also clearly changed with the release and local action of the growth factor. It can be speculated that the use of this platform for in vivo transplantation of cells is likely to promote revascularization of tissues surrounding the cells, creating favorable conditions for the survival of transplanted cells and reducing the loss of transplanted cells.

The role of growth-factor-containing biomaterials in applications mainly includes the following.

#### 10.1.6.1 Induced Differentiation

Xiong Gaoxin and other experimental observations found that the simple scaffold material is difficult to induce cartilage tissue by itself without the action of seed cells and growth factors. BMSCs were implanted with growth factors (bFGF and TGF-β1) and induced to differentiate into cartilage. The differentiated cells can continue to proliferate to exert cartilage activity and completely generate cartilage tissue.

Zhou Qiang et al. [9] conducted experiments and found that CPPf/PLLA materials adsorbed with BMP-2 and TGF-β1 have good osteoinductive ability, and there are obvious osteogenic reactions and new bone formation at 2 weeks after surgery, which was earlier than the osteogenic reaction with CPPf/PLLA implantation alone and the blank control, and the osteogenic ability was greatly improved. With the growth of living tissue and the gradual degradation of the material, new bone formation continued to extend to the center, and the bone defect area of the femoral head was basically repaired at 12 weeks [10]. The osteogenesis method is mainly intramembranous osteogenesis, and it is rare to see endochondral osteogenesis, thereby improving the quality of bone formation and shortening the physiological process of bone repair [11]. The simple CPPf/PLLA implantation and blank control group had low bone ability, and the bone defect could not be repaired during the experimental observation time.

#### 10.1.6.2 Slow Release of Growth Factors

To exert the biological effects of growth factors, growth factors can be added to a suitable carrier to protect them from proteolysis, controlled release for long periods of time where needed, while maintaining the activity of growth factors. The biological activity of growth factors is not only due to its own characteristics but also to the spatial and temporal nature of the presentation to cells.

The researchers found that the adhesion and proliferation of periodontal cells under the action of IGF-1 composite scaffold showed no significant difference after 1 day of culture, but on the 7th and 28th day of culture, the IGF-1 loaded chitosan collagen scaffold group was significantly higher than the normal collagen group. It can be seen that the application of IGF-1 can promote the further adhesion and proliferation of periodontal cells. At the same time, the experiment showed that the release of IGF-1-loaded chitosan collagen scaffold group was more durable for the composite recombinant human transforming growth factor β1 [2]. The normal collagen group was almost completely released after 24 h of application, while the IGF-1-loaded chitosan collagen scaffold group still had a good release effect after 1 week of application [12]. It can be seen that the application of IGF-1-loaded chitosan collagen scaffold can make the release of the drug more balanced, and the therapeutic effect is more durable, which is more conducive to the treatment of patients.

The most commonly used slow release nanoparticle, such as the polyhydroxybutyrate-hydroxyoctanoic acid copolyester-loaded growth factor sustained-release nanoparticle, it was found that the growth factor in the initial stage of release is mainly under the action of concentration gradient, with the degradation and ablation of hydroxybutyric acid and hydroxyoctanoic acid copolymer (encapsulated material), the growth factor diffuses from the pores to the tissue under the concentration gradient, with the complete degradation of hydroxybutyric acid and hydroxyoctanoic acid copolymer, the microsphere system disintegrated and the growth factor was completely released.

#### 10.1.6.3 Combined Action of Growth Factors

Most of the growth factors have been shown to have synergistic effects, and a single factor cannot mimic the complex process of bone regeneration in vivo. The traditional method of rapidly injecting growth factors into the target region also does not well simulate the transmission of signals between cells in vivo and cannot effectively regulate the release of cytokines locally according to the function of the cells.

As BMP induces the formation of the cartilage internalization bone, bFGF is a chemotactic and regulatory protein that promotes wound and tissue repair and angiogenesis and assists BMP to promote new bone growth.

It is generally accepted that the combined action of multiple growth factors in PRP stimulates osteogenesis and accelerates bone repair. The growth factors contained in PRP include platelet-derived growth factor, transforming growth factor β, and platelet-derived epidermal growth factor, which promote the regeneration and repair of bone tissue [13]. Zheng Jun and others also verified this through experiments.

Zhou Qiang et al. reported that BMP-2 is one of the most important osteogenic induction factors, which can significantly increase bone formation and increase fracture healing strength and speed. TGF-β1 is one of the important osteogenic regulatory factors. Although its ability to promote bone repair is weak, it can increase the osteogenic activity of BMP-2, increase the amount of callus formation, and increase the bone healing strength. There is a clear synergistic effect in inducing osteogenesis and promoting bone healing.

It is well known that biomaterials containing growth factors in treatment have many functions. However, there are also some questions about the structure and physical and chemical properties of biological materials, the adhesion of cells, the specificity of growth factors, etc. Therefore, in the research of tissue engineering treatment, we need to further understand the properties of various growth factors and biological materials, and whether it can be used in combination.

### 10.1.7 Clinical Application of Different Types of Growth Factors and Their Preparations

Growth factors are a class of cytokines that stimulate cell growth activity. They bind to high-affinity, specific cell membrane receptors and regulate cell growth and other cellular functions. There are a wide variety of growth factors, including epidermal growth factor (EGF), fibroblast growth factor (FGF), platelet-derived growth factor (PDGF), and growth hormone release inhibitor. In addition, cortisol and thyroid hormones are also growth factors. Different types of growth factors have different properties, and different biological agents can be selected according to different types of growth factors in order to promote their clinical application. For example, a recombinant human epidermal growth factor external solution, a recombinant human epidermal growth factor derivative external spray, a recombinant basic fibroblast growth factor gel, a nerve growth factor composite sustained release preparation, and the like.

#### 10.1.7.1 Recombinant Human Epidermal Growth Factor External Solution

Pressure sore refers to the localized damage of the skin or subcutaneous tissue that occurs at the bone prominence due to pressure or combined shear force or friction force. At present, there are many methods for clinical treatment of pressure sores, such as external application of Chinese medicine and oral administration of antibiotics, but the healing time of pressure sores is longer. The recombinant human epidermal growth factor external solution combined with the external solution of basic fibroblast growth factor can activate the directional movement of epidermal cells in the clinical treatment of pressure sores and has a strong growth promoting effect on epithelial cells and promotes the synthesis of extracellular matrix hyaluronic acid, fibronectin, collagen, glycoprotein, etc., regulates the degradation and renewal of collagen, enhances the tensile strength of wounds, and improves the complete regenerability and continuity of epithelial cells. In the anaerobic state, rhEGF can also stimulate the regeneration of epithelial capillaries and promote the re-formation of epithelium, which is beneficial to prevent and reduce the formation of scars and improve the quality of wound repair. In addition, clinical studies have shown that bFGF can promote neoangiogenesis [14], promote the formation of granulation tissue by regulating cells, promote cell division and proliferation in skin soft tissue and bone tissue, and effectively promote wound healing. The formation of scars is alleviated by partially reconstructing the basement membrane structure. The clinical occurrence of pressure ulcers is mostly stage II–IV. The regeneration of epithelial cells is the basic condition for wound healing of pressure ulcers. The combination of the two solutions meets the conditions, accelerates wound healing, and is less irritating to the wound, and is easy to be accepted by the majority of patients.

#### 10.1.7.2 bFGF Sustained Release Sponge

Basic fibroblast growth factor is an important neurotrophic factor that promotes wound healing, nerve tissue repair and protection, neurite outgrowth, and embryo development and differentiation. Studies have shown that human basic fibroblast growth factor is made into a sustained release sponge, which has a good recovery and protection effect on mouse sciatic nerve injury, and its effect is significantly better than simple human basic fibroblast growth factor. The reason for the gel in the sustained release sponge is good biocompatibility, degradability, absorbability, and enhanced penetration from the extracellular matrix, making it a good transport carrier for drugs such as proteins and sugars. Degradation of collagen in the body can be slow and can control the release of human basic fibroblast growth factor, allowing human basic fibroblast growth factor to produce a sustained action at the damaged nerve. In summary, the growth factor sustained release sponge preparation prepared by combining growth factors with spongy collagen can play a very positive role in tissue repair and tissue engineering, while the collagen sponge that controls the release of growth factors can not only promote the repair of skin wounds but also promote the reconstruction of peripheral nerves. It is an ideal controlled release material for active drugs such as proteins. The application of growth factor sustained release sponge can greatly prolong the action time of growth factor on nerve repair and protection in vivo, and at the same time maintain the high concentration of basic fibroblast growth factor in the wound, effectively solving the short half-life and low local concentration in vivo, which is a major trend in the future clinical application of growth factors.

#### 10.1.7.3 bFGF Microspheres

Basic fibroblast growth factor (bFGF) can promote the proliferation of chondrocytes and the synthesis of matrix. The bFGF can be made into a microsphere system, which can delay the degradation of drugs, reduce the toxicity and irritation of drugs in the body, and regulate the size and slowness of microspheres, release period and dissolution. Some studies have investigated and explored the preparation methods of carrier materials and bFGF microspheres, and found that poly (lactic-co-glycolic-acid), PLGA microspheres have good effects on sustained releasing of active bFGF for a long time. After clinical animal experiments, bFGF-PLGA was injected into the rabbit knee joint, and finally bFGF-PLGA microspheres were stably released in the knee joint cavity of rabbits, and the degradation effect was good. In addition to hydrolysis, the material degradation mechanism of microspheres may also be affected by local environmental factors, especially local temperature. The degradation rate of microspheres is greatly affected by temperature. The main reason is that once the local temperature exceeds the phase transition temperature of the material, obvious spherical damage will occur, and the microspheres will be in an amorphous state at the end of degradation, instead of the honeycomb shape usually presented, thereby accelerating its degradation rate. In addition, some literatures have confirmed that stress also has a certain influence on the degradation of carrier materials. Through this kind of research to find out the general law of drug release from microspheres, it has positive significance for later application in clinical treatment, making degradable microsphere technology an important way for new drug delivery.

#### 10.1.7.4 bFGF Gel

Basic fibroblast growth factor (bFGF) has a certain effect on the growth, differentiation, and function of various cells and can promote the mitosis of most cells in the source of mesoderm and neuroectoderm, and can also change the function of non-mitotic division of a large number of cells. It has a wide range of biological effects and has been applied to the repair of clinical skin wounds and corneal trauma. The bFGF aqueous solution and the lyophilized powder have obvious disadvantages, such as short expiration date, difficulty in transportation, easy contamination, inconvenient use, and poor patient compliance. In order to overcome these shortcomings, experiments were carried out with carbomer 940, glycerol and 1,2-propanediol as matrix, adding compound protective agents (heparin, human serum albumin, mannitol, and HP-β-CD) to make bFGF into bFGF gel, wherein the gel prepared by using carbomer has the advantages of quick release, spread lubrication, no grease, no irritation to skin and mucous membrane, good adhesion, and uniformity of the film. It does not pollute clothing and has suitable viscosity and stable formulation. At the same time, it is proved by experiments that when the gel acts on the wound surface, a film can be formed on the wound surface, which has a certain barrier function, can play a certain protective effect, can also reduce irritation, prevent pollution, and the fluidity is not as big as the water solution preparation, the residence time longer than the liquid preparation, produces a sustained release and long-lasting effect, accelerate wound healing. Clinically, recombinant bovine basic fibroblast growth factor external gel has been used to treat recurrent aphthous ulcer (RAU), mainly by promoting cell growth and differentiation and granulation tissue formation, inhibiting the degradation of new cells, and significantly shortening the healing time of ulcer. In comparison, the bFGF gel is more suitable for wound treatment than the bFGF aqueous solution in the dosage form.

## 10.2 Protein Peptide and Other Drugs

### 10.2.1 Protein Peptide

Polypeptides and proteinaceous drugs refer to polypeptide and proteinaceous biopharmaceuticals for the prevention, treatment, and diagnosis. Polypeptides are compounds in which α-amino acids are linked together by peptide chains, which are also intermediates in protein hydrolysis. N polypeptide chains are entangled in a certain spatial structure to form a protein. Macromolecular proteolysis produces a polypeptide. According to the structural classification of drugs, biopharmaceuticals can be divided into amino acids and their derivatives, peptides and protein drugs, enzymes and coenzymes, nucleic acids and their degradants and derivatives, sugars, lipids, cell growth factors, and biologic drugs.

#### 10.2.1.1 Platelet-Derived Growth Factor

Platelet-derived growth factor (PDGF) is a growth factor that regulates cell growth and differentiation and plays an important role in angiogenesis. Uncontrolled angiogenesis often leads to cancer. Chemically, PDGF is a glycoprotein dimer and has two different forms, A and B, which can be combined into structures such as AA, AB, and BB [15].

PDGF is a potent mesenchymal cell mitogen that regulates fibroblasts, smooth muscle, and neuroglial cells [16]. In mice and humans, the PDGF signaling network includes four ligands, from PDGFA to PDGFD, with two receptors, PDGFRA and PDGFRB [17]. All PDGF are expressed extracellularly and form homodimers by disulfide bond, but only PDGFA and PDGFB can form functional heterodimers [18].

After being synthesized, PDGF is first stored in the α particles of platelets and will not be released until it is stimulated. In addition, various cells such as smooth muscle cells, activated macrophages, and epithelial cells also produce PDGF.

Medically, synthetic PDGF can be used to accelerate the healing of chronic ulcer lesions; orthopedics and periodontology specialists also treat bone loss with PDGF.

A. Classification

Five different PDGF ligands activate cellular responses through both receptors. Known ligands include A (PDGFA), B (PDGFB), C (PDGFC), and D (PDGFD), as well as AB heterodimers. Receptors include α (PDGFRA) and β (PDGFRB).

B. Mechanism

PDGF receptor PDGFR belongs to the tyrosine kinase (RTK) receptor, a cell-surface receptor. Two types of PDGFR have been identified: α and β PDGFR. The α-type binds to PDGF-AA, PDGF-BB, and PDGF-AB, while the β-type PDGFR binds PDGF-BB and PDGF-AB with high affinity [19]. PDGF binds to the PDGFR ligand binding pocket located within the second and third immunoglobulin domains. Upon activation by PDGF, these receptors dimerize and "turn on" by autophosphorylation at several sites on their cytoplasmic domains to mediate cofactor binding and be activated through the PI3K pathway or the STAT3 pathway mediated by reactive oxygen substances (ROS). Its downstream effects include regulation of gene expression and cell cycle.

C. Function

PDGF is mitogenic during early developmental stages, driving the proliferation of undifferentiated mesenchyme and some progenitor populations. At a later stage of maturation, PDGF signaling involves tissue remodeling and cell differentiation, as well as induction events involved in patterning and morphogenesis. In addition to driving mesenchymal proliferation, PDGFs have been shown to direct migration and differentiation functions of a variety of specialized mesenchymal and migrating cell types during development and in adult animals.

PDGF plays a role in embryonic development, cell proliferation, cell migration, and angiogenesis. Overexpression of PDGF has been associated with several diseases, such as atherosclerosis, fibrotic diseases, and malignancies [20].

PDGF is an essential component in the cell division of fibroblasts, a connective tissue cell that is particularly prevalent in wound healing. In essence, PDGF allows cells to skip the G1 checkpoint for division. It has been shown that in monocyte-macrophages and fibroblasts, exogenous use of PDGF stimulates chemotaxis, proliferation and gene expression, and significantly increases the influx of inflammatory cells and fibroblasts, accelerating the formation of the extracellular matrix and collagen, thereby reducing the time of the healing process [21].

#### 10.2.1.2 Growth Hormone

Growth hormone (GH) is a peptide hormone. It promotes the development of animals and humans, as well as the proliferation of cells. It is a 191 single-chain peptide containing 191 amino acid molecules that are synthesized, stored, and secreted by growth hormone cells in the pituitary. The growth hormone produced by recombinant DNA technology is abbreviated as rhGH.

A. Gene Sequence

The human growth hormone gene is located on the q22–24 region of chromosome 17. It is very close to the gene of human chorionic prolactin (also known as placental lactogen). Growth hormone, chorionic auxin, and prolactin (PRL) are a group of homologous hormones that are involved in promoting growth and stimulating lactation.

B. Structure

The human growth hormone molecule is composed of 191 amino acid residues with a relative molecular mass of 22 124 u. The molecular structure has four α helices that allow growth hormone to bind well to its receptor. In terms of protein sequence, growth hormone and prolactin, as well as chorionic gonadotropin, are evolutionarily homologous. Human growth hormone has a certain degree of specificity, so although it is highly similar to other species, it can only be applied to humans and primates.

C. Function

Growth hormone has a high degree of species specificity. In terms of wound repair, the main functions of rhGH are:

(a) Indirectly promoting cell growth can increase the growth rate of cells. Recombinant human growth hormone promotes the growth and proliferation of whole body tissue cells by acting on the growth cell hormone receptor on the hepatocyte membrane to produce insulin-like growth factor-1.
(b) Indirect metabolic conditioning, promote protein synthesis, reduce protein decomposition, maintain nitrogen balance, increase fat decomposition and gluconeogenesis, and improve nutrient conversion rate.
(c) Immunomodulatory effects, rhGH plays an important role in triggering the production of superoxide anion and cytokines by phagocytes, increasing the activity of opsonin, and stimulating the production of immunoglobulin by B cells. At the molecular level, it has been revealed that rhGH directly stimulates the expression of protein mRNA in hepatocytes, thereby promoting protein synthesis.

## 10.2.2 Chemical Drugs and Chinese Herbal Medicines

### 10.2.2.1 Chemical Drugs

Infection is still the main factor affecting wound healing [22]. Therefore, in the design of chemical drugs, many scholars are committed to controlling wound infection, researching and developing a large number of anti-infective topical drugs, and contributing to the smooth healing of wounds [23]. In the design of chemical drugs, mainly anti-infective drugs, such as silver sulfadiazine, zinc sulfadiazine, mafenide, silver nitrate, cerium nitrate, and quinolone silver salts, have been widely used, and the anti-infection effect is obvious.

A. Mafenide [24]

Mafenide cold cream is used as a topical medicine for treating burns and is effective for certain anaerobic bacteria such as clostridium tetani and clostridium. The chemical properties of the drug are stable and suitable for suppurative necrotic wounds, but the antibacterial activity is affected by the amount of wound bacteria. When the infection is severe and the amount of bacteria in the wound is high, the application effect is poor. Mafenide is hypertonic and acidic, irritating to wounds, inhibits carbonic anhydrase, and can cause metabolic acidosis.

B. Silver Sulfadiazine [25]

Silver sulfadiazine is a weak acid with a wide range of antibacterial activity. It is effective against both Gram-positive and Gram-negative bacteria. It also has good inhibitory effects on fungi and molds. It has a significant inhibitory effect on *Pseudomonas aeruginosa*. It is also having a certain effect on methicillin-resistant *Staphylococcus aureus*. Silver sulfadiazine is formed by the reaction of silver nitrate with sulfadiazine with a penetrating power between sulfametholone and silver nitrate. In the case of aseptic wound application, it was found that the formation of the epidermis using silver sulfadiazine was faster than that of povidone iodine, and the formation of new blood vessels using silver sulfadiazine was faster than the use of silver nitrate. The application of silver sulfadiazine on the wound surface showed re-epithelialization in a few days. When silver sulfadiazine contacts the tissue, it forms a thin layer of crust, which releases silver ions, which can bind to the DNA of the bacteria. Silver ions can replace the hydrogen ions in the DNA molecule, widening the distance between purine and pyrimidine, thus inhibiting bacterial reproduction. At the same time, the released sulfadiazine can also play a certain antibacterial effect. The time of clinical application of silver sulfadiazine is decisive for efficacy.

### 10.2.2.2 Traditional Chinese Medicine

With the deepening of research on traditional Chinese medicine and the deepening of people's understanding of wound healing theory, more and more practices have been used to treat different types of clinical wounds with traditional Chinese medicine, and it has gradually become a research hotspot. There are many reports on the treatment and research of burns in the motherland medicine. The ancients have summarized many prescriptions for treating wounds. According to the effects, they are roughly divided into antibacterial and anti-inflammatory drugs, convergence scab drugs, eschar separation drugs, and promoting granulation and wound healing drugs.

A. Oriental Burn Ointment (formerly known as Oriental No. 1) is a traditional Chinese medicine ointment containing atractylodes rhizome, amur cork-tree, divaricate saposhnikovia root, common floweringqince fruit, yanhusuo, common bletilla rubber, calcined gypsum powder, calcined calamine powder, and sesame oil. The comprehensive medicine has the effects of clearing heat and eliminating dampness, promoting blood circulation and relieving pain, eliminating necrotic tissues and promoting granulation, and has a good therapeutic effect on refractory wounds.
B. Convergence and promoting granulation medicine pearl powder (water-soluble pearl powder), promoting blood circulation and granulation medicine draconis resin (dracorhodin perchlorate), promoting blood circulation and granulation medicine frankincense (frankincense aqueous extract), warming yang promoting granulation medicine pilose antler (Pilose antler polypeptides) can promote human skin fibroblast proliferation and collagen synthesis [26, 27].

There are many kinds of Chinese herbal medicines. At present, the mechanism of action is not studied enough. It is necessary to carry out in-depth and extensive experimental research to clarify the effective components and exact mechanism of various Chinese herbal medicines, and has broad prospects for the application of burns.

## 10.3 Concentrated Platelet Therapy

The main function of platelets is to participate in physiological hemostasis, promote blood coagulation, and maintain capillary integrity. In the past, the main use of clinical intravenous infusion of platelets was to treat patients with reduced or (and) dysfunction of platelets. However, platelets, as a multifunctional cell, now function not only in thrombosis and hemostasis but also in angiogenesis and tissue repair. It also plays an important role in the process of inflammation.

### 10.3.1 Historical Development

In the 1970s, platelet-rich plasma (PRP) was applied to the study of wound repair. In 1977, Harke et al. first isolated PRP and successfully used it in patients undergoing cardiac surgery. In 1993, Hood et al. proposed the concept of platelet gel (PG) for the first time. In recent years, researches on the application of platelets in wound healing aspect have been deepened and extensively developed, involving multidisciplinary surgery such as maxillofacial surgery, orthopedic surgery, plastic surgery, and aesthetic surgery, even showed unique roles in antiaging, sports medicine, and perfect healing of wound repair.

At present, platelet-rich plasma (PRP) and platelet-rich fibrin (PRF) are artificially defined as first-generation and second-generation products. In addition, there are concentrate growth factors (CGF), platelet-rich concentrate (PRC) [concentrated platelet-rich plasma (cPRP)], platelet-enriched plasma (PeRP), and so on. But too many titles are not conducive to the widespread, rational, and scientific use of concentrated platelets.

On the one hand, the concentration of biologically active ingredients (especially growth factors) contained in various types of concentrated platelet products differs several times or more. The term platelet-rich plasma (PRP) first appeared in 1965 when it focused on platelet phagocytosis and polymerization. Therefore, the definition of PRP remains in the 1960s, concentrated platelets that exceed the average value of platelets in blood by 3–5 times are called PRP, and some people set it 6–8 times. Many studies have shown that the effects of different concentrations of platelets in different cells and tissues are quite different. The current concentrated platelet product should be in a unit volume (per mL) condition, and the number of fully functional platelets (number of platelets/mL) $\geq 10^6$ or more can exert strong tissue repair and regeneration.

On the other hand, the concentrated platelet products obtained by different preparation methods contain different active ingredients and biological effects. It involves not only the composition ratio of the biologically active products contained but also the three-dimensional molecular conformation varies widely, and the biological functions played by each have their own advantages. Cellulose/fibronectin and cohesin in traditional PRP plasma components are good cell adhesion molecules and can be used as carriers of growth factors for the repair of certain types of damage. Concentrated growth factor (CGF) is rich in red blood cells, platelets, and iron, calcium, and other essential elements. CGF can accelerate the fusion and remodeling of transplanted biological materials and reduces the chance of infection. Its unique three-dimensional structure fully utilizes the synergistic effects of growth/cytokines. Fibrinogen and fibrin degradation products promote neutrophil migration and participate in phage, immune regulation, and enzymatic degradation processes. At the same time, in the case of tissue damage, it not only guides the revascularization and immune regulation of the damaged tissue but also captures the stem cells in the circulating blood and participates in tissue repair and regeneration. Even after mixing with other biological materials, it participates in the composition of the regenerated microenvironment after tissue damage.

With the deepening understanding of the factors affecting platelet count in platelet concentrate products, the difference in the composition of the components after activation, the spatial conformation and the different functions, and the continuous expansion and change of the scope and mode of application, comprehensive and innovative thinking should be given to the treatment technology of platelet concentrate. As a therapeutic technique, PRP, PRF, CGT, etc. are all according to the signaling pathways and key proteins required for tissue repair after injury, choose the appropriate form of concentrated platelet products (whether contain neutrophils or lymph, whether it is activated by exogenous or in vivo, etc.), is of great significance for further enriching treatment and improving clinical treatment.

## 10.3.2 The Mechanism of Action of Concentrated Platelets

A. Promoting wound healing: mainly by using platelets in concentrated platelets to activate and release various growth factors including platelet-derived growth factor (PDGF), transforming growth factor-β (TGF-β), and vascular endothelial growth factor (VEGF), epidermal growth factor (EGF), fibroblast growth factor (FGF), insulin-like growth factor (IGF), brain-derived neurotrophic factor (BDNF), interleukin-1 (IL-1), and platelet-activating factor to play a therapeutic role. These growth factors synergistically promote the division and proliferation of various types of tissue cells in the body, promote matrix synthesis and deposition, promote the formation of fibrous tissue and granulation tissue, increase the ability of collagen synthesis, and stimulate the involvement of posttraumatic epithelial regeneration and interstitial hyperplasia and neovascularization and so on. At the same time, PRP contains a large amount of fibrinogen to form a fibrous mesh scaffold to support the growth-factor-induced formation of new tissue, can provide a good support for repair cells, can stimulate soft tissue regeneration, promote early closure of wounds, and prevent infection. The PG prepared by PRP is gelatinous, and the gelatinous PRP can not only adhere to tissue defects, but also prevent the loss of platelets, so that platelets can slowly release growth factors for a long time, maintain high growth factor concentration, and better play the role of tissue repair. In addition to platelets, there are fibrinogen, prothrombin, various coagulation factors, complex protein components, and even cellular components such as monocytes. These proteins and cells also play a role in promoting wound healing.
B. Antibacterial effect: The study found that PRP has a good antibacterial effect and can provide a good microenvironment for wound repair. The antibacterial effect of PRP may be related to the fact that platelets themselves release some antibacterial active peptides to resist microbes. As early as 1992, Yeaman et al. found that rabbit platelets can release a small molecular weight antimicrobial protein under physiological concentrations of thrombin. Subsequent purification of this protein not only demonstrates its ability to kill *S. aureus, Escherichia coli, Candida albicans* in a dose-dependent manner but also proposes the hypothesis that platelets play an important role in host anti-infection by releasing antibacterial proteins locally against tissue damage or microbial aggregation. In 2002, the research team purified seven human antibacterial peptides from thrombin-stimulated human platelet supernatant by reversed-phase high-performance liquid chromatography: platelet factor-4 (PF-4), regulated activation of normal T cells expression and secretion factor (RANTES), connective tissue active peptide-3 (CTAP-3), platelet basic protein (PBP), thymosin beta-4 (Tβ-4), fibrin peptide B (FP-B), fiber peptide A (FP-A), demonstrating their ability to kill bacteria (*S. aureus, Escherichia coli*) and fungi (*Candida albicans, Cryptococcus neoformans*) in a dose-dependent manner, and the antimicrobial effect of platelets on staphylococcus aureus was confirmed in an animal model of infective endocarditis.

## 10.3.3 Current Application

### 10.3.3.1 Preparation of Concentrated Platelets

There are two main preparation methods, one is obtained by centrifugation of whole blood from autologous or blood donors, and the other is directly isolated from autologous or blood donors by an automatic blood cell separator. The autologous PRP preparation was separated by the former, and the allogeneic PRP was prepared by the former and the latter. Platelets have the property of being easily activated, placing higher demands on the preparation operation. Because of the limitation of conditions, PRP preparation process of clinical departments is easily polluted and requires aseptic operation in a closed, clean environment.

### 10.3.3.2 Clinical Application of Concentrated Platelets

The application methods of concentrated platelets include direct injection, addition of activators (such as calcium ions and thrombin) to PG use, extraction of PG supernatant, and application of PG to lysate by repeated freeze-thaw cycles. From the source of concentrated platelets can be divided into two types: autologous and homologous.

A. Self-concentrated platelets: for many years, the efficacy of autologous concentrated platelet therapy in various types of wound repair, such as oral and maxillofacial surgery, orthopedics, ophthalmology, burns, plastic surgery, and chronic ulcers, has been confirmed and fully affirmed by domestic and foreign scholars from experimental to clinical. Platelet concentration can improve the hemostatic effect, shorten operation time, reduce postoperative swelling, and promote wound healing, and is of great value for wound repair and tissue reconstruction. In 1997, Whitman et al. took the lead in applying autologous PRP to oral clinical research and achieved good results. Plastic surgery specialist Brown et al. found that the use of autologous PG as a sealant can reduce drainage 24 h after wrinkle resection. Clinical studies in cardiac surgery have found that the most significant effect of autologous PG is to reduce the incidence of chest infections and reduce drainage. Vang et al. found that the use of autologous PG in coronary artery bypass surgery can reduce postoperative pain, bleeding, and swelling. In the repair of bone injury, Michael et al. applied autologous PG to the exposed tissue, injected the synovial membrane, and closed the wound during total knee arthroplasty. After surgery, it was applied to the wound, which played a better hemostasis and accelerated the tissue repair, shortened hospital stay and more flexible joint activities. In China, in 2008, Ranxing Wu research group reported 142 patients with refractory skin ulcers were treated with autologous PRP, which confirmed the effectiveness of autologous PRP. Rao Zhong et al. showed that the treatment effect of autologous PRP on severe burn wounds is better than conventional treatment. Zhang Yu et al. studied autologous PRP to promote bone regeneration in oral implanted bone defect area and confirmed that PRP can promote bone regeneration in oral implanted bone defect area.

B. Homologous: Although autologous concentrated platelets have significant effects on wound repair and tissue remodeling, there are many factors (such as platelet individual differences, equipment for preparing autologous PRP, preparation conditions and preservation conditions for preparing autologous PRP are not the same, and there is a lack of uniform standards), which limit its promotion and application. The homologous platelet concentrate has the advantages of not being able to take into account the influence of collecting autologous blood on the patient, facilitating uniform and standardized preparation, low cost and ready supply; and the current research has not found any adverse reactions, which can meet the needs of more patients. Therefore, the application of homeo-concentrated platelets will become a development trend.

In 2007, Smrke et al. reported the use of PG-mixed autologous bone cancellous bones prepared by homologous allogeneic platelets (ABO and RhD blood group binding, leukocyte removal, irradiation treatment) as a graft to treat delayed fracture healing of diabetic comminuted fractures; 6 months after successful transplantation, the bone defect was completely bridged and fully loaded, no side effects occurred during the treatment, and no platelet or HLA-I antibody was detected in the patient. However, due to the problem of virus inactivation of homologous PRP has not been well resolved, its application safety needs to be studied.

Academician Xiaobing Fu studied the effect of platelet-rich plasma (PRP) on autophagy during acute wound healing in aged rats. SPF grade SD rats (provided by Guangdong Experimental Animal Center) were selected, 60 in 18 months old and weighing 600–800 g. In the male and female, 60 rats were divided into three groups according to the random number table, which were the saline group (control group), the platelet-rich plasma group (PRP group), and the platelet-poor plasma group (PPP group). An acute full-thickness skin defect model of the rat back was made. The wounds of each group were treated for 3 consecutive days. PRP was extracted with a 1 mL syringe and an average of six injection points were taken symmetrically at the skin wound edge, and 0.1 mL of PRP was injected subcutaneously at each injection site. PRP was mixed with 10% calcium gluconate solution in a volume of 10:1. After being gelled, it was evenly applied to the wound surface, and the wound was covered with a sterile 3 M film. Rats in the PPP group were treated with the PRP group. After the wound was wiped with saline gauze in the control group, the wound was covered with a sterile 3 M film. On the first, second, and third day after trauma, three groups of different treatments were given continuously. The wounds of each group were clean and rosy, and no signs of infection appeared. At 4 days, the three groups of wounds began to shrink, with less exudate, no scarring, and the edge tissue shrunk toward the center. The wound healing rate of the PRP group was the highest in the three groups (31%), the second in the PPP group, and the lowest in the control group ($F = 34.58$, $P < 0.001$). At 7 days, the wounds in the PRP group were significantly reduced, and the wound healing rate was the fastest, reaching 58%. The wound healing rate of the PPP group and the control group were lower than those of the PRP group, and there was a significant difference between the three groups ($F = 69.220$, $P < 0.001$). At 14 days, there was still a significant difference in the healing rate of the three groups ($F = 14.970$, $P < 0.001$), which showed the highest rate of healing in the PRP group, followed by the PPP group and the lowest in the control group. At 21 days, the wounds in the PRP group were basically healed, and the healing rate reached 98%, which was higher than the other two groups, and there was a significant difference ($F = 11.778$, $P < 0.001$). Immunohistochemistry was used to detect the expression of LC3 and Beclin-1 in the skin wounds of three groups of rats. The results showed that LC3 and Beclin-1 were positive for brown-yellow granules in the cytoplasm. Both proteins were expressed in the epidermis and dermis of the three groups of wounds. Positive expression was also observed in the epidermal layer, dermis and hair follicles, vascular endothelial cells, macrophages, and fibroblasts in the new granulation tissue. The expression of the two proteins in the PRP group was weaker than the other two groups (Figs. 10.2 and 10.3).

The expressions of LC3, Beclin-1, p62, and CD31 mRNA in wound healing were significantly different between the 4th, 7th, 14th, and 21st day ($P < 0.05$), and the expression level was 4 days < 7 days < 14 days < 21 days, at 14 and 21 days, the expression levels of LC3 in the three groups

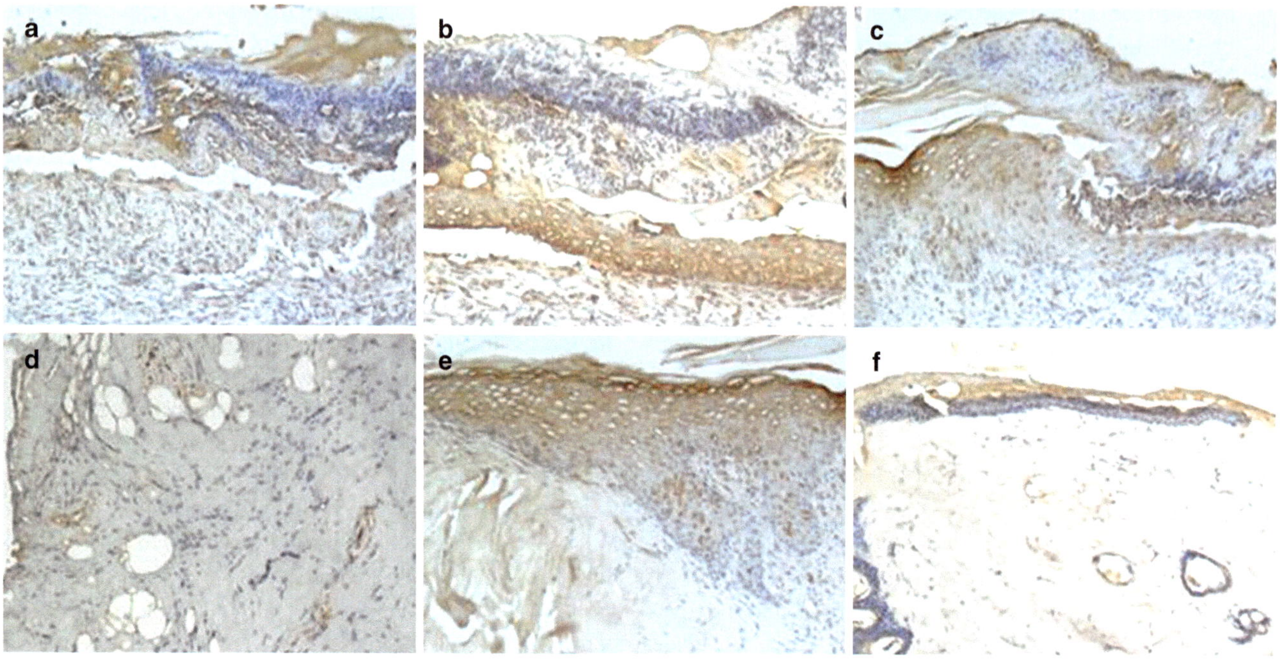


**Fig. 10.2** Expression of wound LC3 (Envison method, ×100). Note: (**a**–**c**) were stained for 14 days in the control group, PPP group, and PRP group; (**d**–**f**) were stained for 21 days in the control group, PPP-group, and PRP group, respectively; LC3 expression was expressed in the PRP group at 14 days and 21 days. Weaker than the other two groups

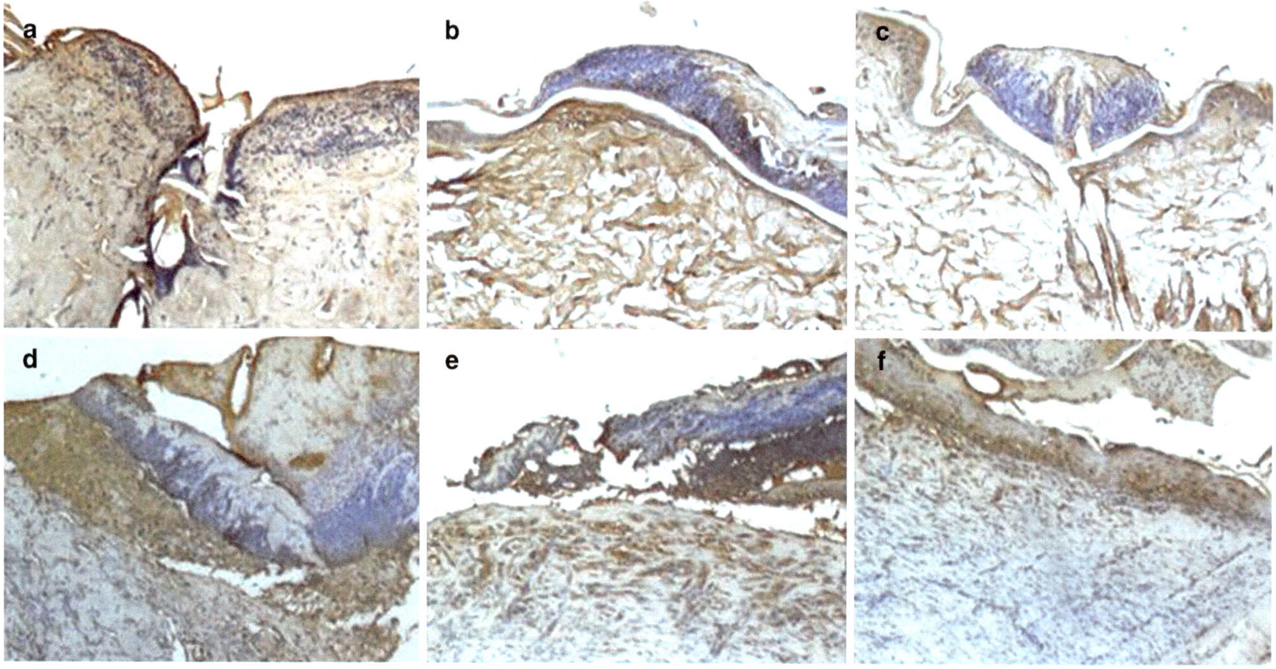


**Fig. 10.3** Expression of Beclin-1 on the wound surface (Envison method, ×100). Note: (**a**–**c**) were stained for 14 days in the control group, PPP group, and PRP group, respectively; (**d**–**f**) were stained for 21 days in the control group, PPP group, and PRP group, respectively; Beclin-1 was in the PRP group at 14 and 21 days; 1 expression is weaker than the other two groups

were significantly different ($P$ = 0.048, 0.039). In terms of main effect, there were significant differences between the two treatment groups and time ($P < 0.001$); and there was an interaction between the two factors ($P$ = 0.002), indicating that both of them affected the expression of LC3. The mRNA expression levels of Beclin-1 were significantly different at 4, 7, 14, and 21 days ($P < 0.05$), and the expression levels were 4 days < 7 days < 14 days < 21 days; in 4 days, there was no significant difference in the expression of Beclin-1 between the three groups ($P > 0.05$). At the other three time points, there was a significant difference in the expression levels between the treatment groups ($P < 0.05$), which was the highest in the control group and the lowest in the PRP group. In terms of main effect, there were significant differences between the two treatment groups and time ($P < 0.001$); and there were interactions between the two factors ($P < 0.001$), indicating that both of them affected the expression of Beclin-1. The expression of p62 mRNA was significantly different at 4, 7, 14, and 21 days ($P < 0.05$), and the expression levels were 4 days > 7 days > 14 days > 21 days. At 4 and 7 days, there was a significant difference in expression between the three treatment groups ($P < 0.05$). In the 4 days, the PPP group had the highest expression, the PRP group was the second, and the control group was the lowest. At 7 days, the PRP group had the highest expression and the control group had the lowest expression. There was no significant difference in expression between the treatment groups at 4 and 21 days ($P > 0.05$). In terms of main effect, there were significant differences between the two treatment groups and time ($P < 0.001$), but there was no interaction between the two factors ($P$ = 0.007), indicating that both of them affected p62 mRNA expression. The expression of CD31 mRNA in the control group was significantly different at each time point ($P$ = 0.009), and the expression level increased gradually from 4 days, and rose to the highest in 14 days, and then decreased. There was no significant difference in the expression of PRP group and PPP group at four time points ($P > 0.05$). At 14 days, there was no significant difference in the expression of the three groups ($P$ = 0.352). At the other three time points, the expression levels of the three groups were significantly different ($P < 0.05$), both of which had the highest PRP expression and the control group had the lowest expression. In terms of main effect, there were significant differences between the two treatment groups and time ($P < 0.001$), but there was no interaction between the two factors ($P$ = 0.447), indicating that the two had no effect on the expression of CD31. The expressions of LC3, Beclin-1, p62, and CD31 showed that the expressions of LC3-II/I, Beclin-1, and CD31 increased with time, and the expression of p62 protein decreased with time ($P < 0.05$). Protein level expression is consistent with gene level expression (Figs. 10.4 and 10.5).

In this study, the wound healing rate was higher in the PRP group than in the PPP group and the blank control group. At 21 days of trauma, the wounds in the PRP group were basically healed and the healing rate reached 98%. At the same time, the mRNA expression levels of LC3, Beclin-1, and p62 were detected. The expression levels of LC3 in each group were significantly different ($P < 0.05$). A significant difference was found between 14 and 21 days ($P < 0.05$), the expression was the highest at 14 days, suggesting that LC3 may play a more important role in the late stage of repair (proliferation, shaping). The expression of Beclin-1 was significantly different between the observation points at 7, 14,

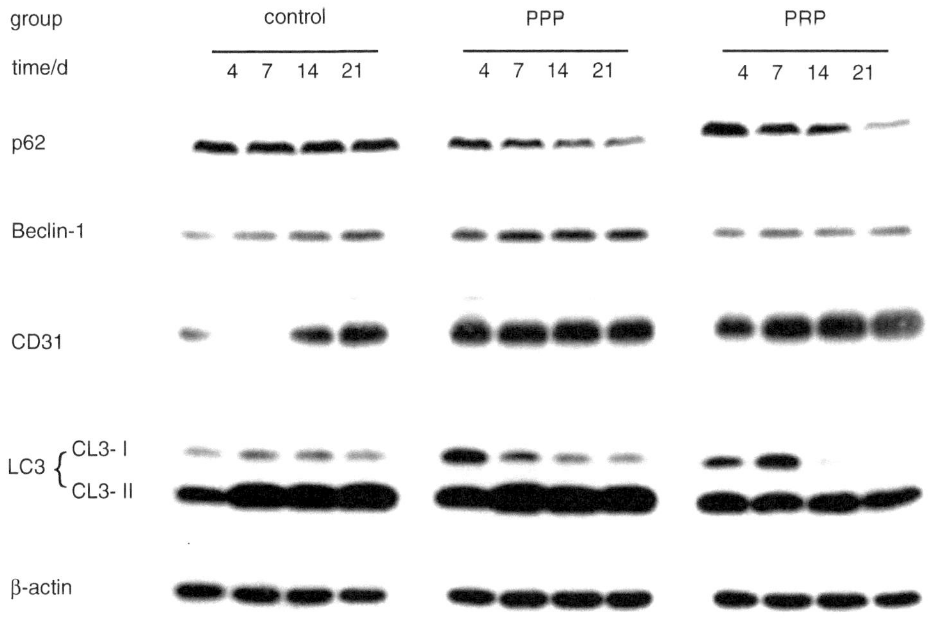


**Fig. 10.4** Expression of LC3, Beclin-1, p62, and CD31 in the three groups at 4, 7, 14, and 21 days of trauma

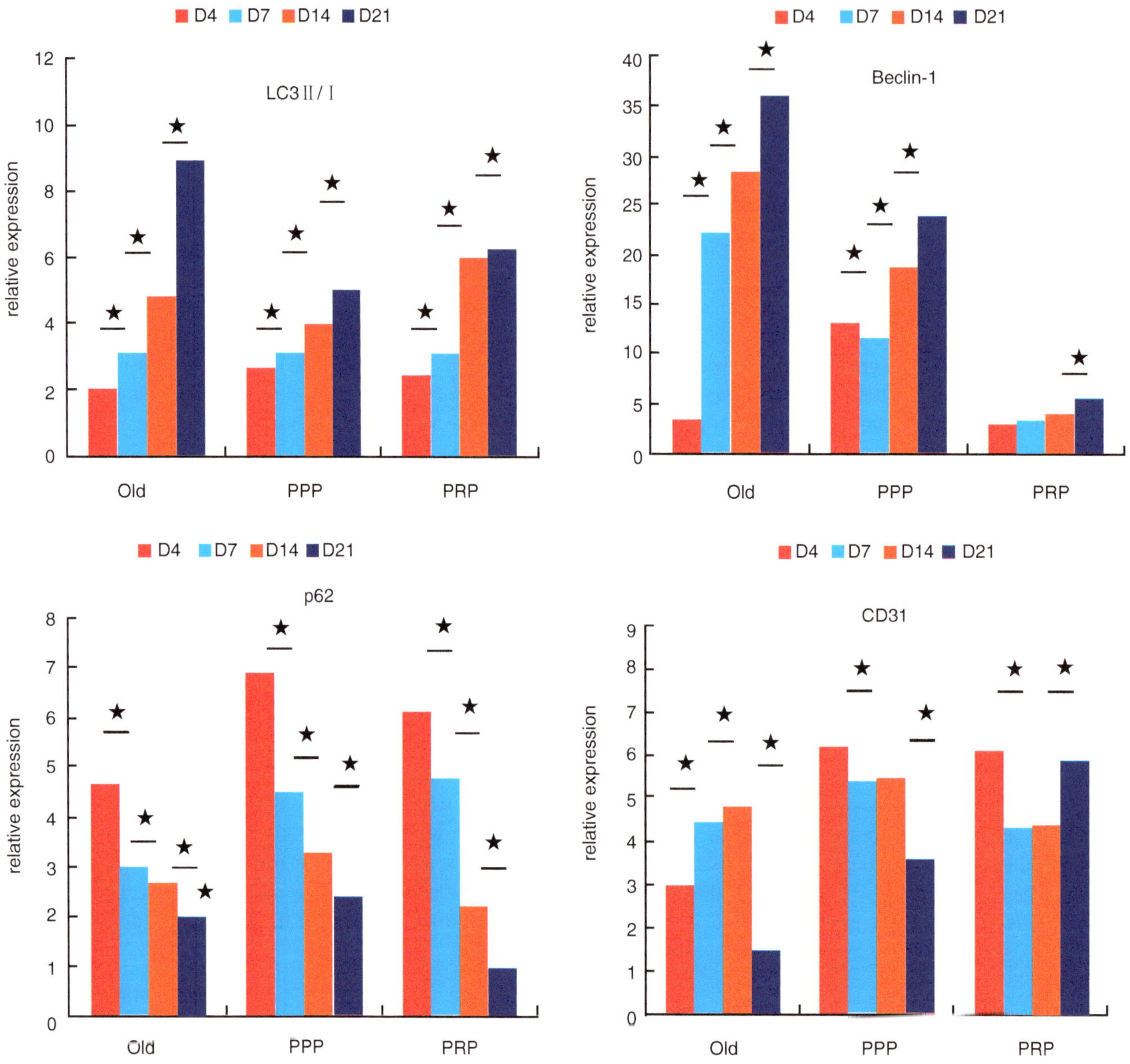


**Fig. 10.5** Protein expression differences of LC3, Beclin-1, p62, and CD31 in three groups of rats (*$P < 0.05$)

and 21 days ($P < 0.05$). The expression levels of PRP group were lower than those of the other two groups at these three time points, suggesting PRP reduced expression of Beclin-1. The posttraumatic local inflammatory response usually lasts for 3–5 days. At 4 days, the expression of Beclin-1 in the PRP group was not significantly different from the other two groups. This suggests that Beclin-1 is not significantly affected by PRP during the local inflammatory phase of wound repair, and autophagy is involved in the posttraumatic inflammatory response. The expression of p62 was decreased in all three groups. The expression of p62 in PRP group was lower than that of the normal control group at 4 and 7 days, suggesting that the autophagy substrate p62 was affected by PRP during the inflammatory reaction phase and early cell proliferation and differentiation, granulation tissue formation, PRP increases the consumption of p62.

In this experiment, the mRNA expression levels of CD31 at the four time points were higher in the PRP group than in the other two groups ($P < 0.05$). The expression of the PRP group was highest at 4 days, and the expression began to decrease at 14 days. HE staining and immunohistochemical staining showed that in the PRP group, new capillaries appeared in the PRP group, and the rohr increased. Vascular smooth muscle cells were formed and capillary network was formed initially. The capillary vascular network was rare in the other two groups. The number of proliferating endothelial cells gradually decreased after the formation of the rohr-like structure, and the expression of CD31 also gradually decreased. Correlation analysis showed that there was a correlation between CD31 and Beclin-1 and p62 expression at 4 and 7 days, which was negatively correlated with the former and positively correlated with the latter, suggesting that the expressions of autophagy genes Beclin-1 and p62 were related to the proliferation, adhesion, and connection of vascular endothelial cells during wound healing. At 14 days, there was no correlation between CD31 and Beclin-1 and p62 expression, which was consistent with the cessation of endothelial cell proliferation and the formation of blood vessels at 14 days.

In the process of promoting the healing of senile skin wounds, the expression of autophagy-related genes LC3, Beclin-1, and p62 changed with PRP, and the effects on autophagy were different in different stages of repair. In the study of human cells cultured in vitro, the expression of LC3 gene can be regulated. In view of this, future application of medical means to regulate the expression of autophagy genes related to skin aging and wound repair can regulate autophagy activity, not only for skin aging, but also may provide an effective means of accelerating healing and improving the quality of repair.

### 10.3.4 Future Development

The perfect repair, or physiological anatomical repair, advocated in recent years is the best embodiment of regenerative medicine in clinical treatment. In the 1990s, a new round of stem cell biology research laid the scientific foundation for the development of regenerative medicine, and the establishment of tissue engineering provided basic technical means and methods for the clinical application of regenerative medicine. The use of biological and engineering theoretical methods in regenerative medicine to promote the body's self-repair and regeneration or to construct new tissues and organs to repair, regenerate, and replace damaged tissues and organs not only covers stem cell technology, tissue engineering and with the continuous development of many modern bioengineering technologies, the possibility of seeking tissue and organ regeneration and functional reconstruction from various levels has been increased, so the connotation of its research is expanding, including cell and cytokine therapy, gene therapy, and micro-ecology, etc. The core content and ultimate goal of treatment are to regenerate tissue and organ that was the same as before the injury. It is precise because of the theoretical breakthrough of the major scientific problems of tissue regeneration and the establishment of innovative technologies and methods for clinical treatment. Some diseases that have been difficult to overcome in the past, such as spinal paraplegia, perfect wound repair, organ transplantation, tumor resection control, Alzheimer disease and birth defect, are re-filled with hope. Restoration of damaged tissue in regenerative medicine involves three factors: cell, chemical drug and scaffold, and the relationship between PRP and proliferation, migration and differentiation of cells (including adult stem cells and embryonic stem cells), and effects in genetic engineering and tissue engineering have become the focus of today's research. Also due to the unique role of PRP in tissue regeneration, some new mechanisms of action, such as the regulation of the immune system, have gradually received attention. With the development of microinvasive surgery (including endoscopic surgery), the physiological functions exhibited by concentrated platelet therapy show us a bright future.

### 10.3.5 Other Related Drugs

Other drugs that promote wound repair after tissue injury include:

A. Polypeptide enzymes, which are used in soft tissue trauma repair, have been paid more attention by scholars. Currently, there are more than ten kinds of enzymes listed in Europe and the United States, such as collagenase, streptokinase, streptodornase, subtilase, and krill enzyme.
B. Amino acids, cerebrolysin, dexamethasone, astragalus polysaccharide, sulfadiazine zinc, etc., either alone or in combination, have a certain effect on preventing war wound infection or promoting wound healing.
C. Reducing immune rejection drugs, and solving the rejection after traumatic organ transplantation has been one of the main problems. In recent years, the theory and practice of transplant immunity have made progress. Polymerase chain reaction (PCR)-based DNA typing technology, using in situ molecular hybridization (ISH) and reverse transcriptase polymerase chain reaction (RT-PCR) to analyze the cytokine mRNA of transplanted cells, and found that HLA molecules are highly correlated with rejection, and mismatching of amino acid residues on the folding of the DRB1 gene product may be the key to initiation of acute rejection. DNA typing technology provides a more granular analysis of HLA types and provides a reliable basis for selecting donors. Cytokine and receptor levels, such as serum interleukin (IL-2, IL-6, IL-8), tumor necrosis factor (TNF), soluble IL-2 receptor, IL-2R expression, transplantation of local cytokines or Cytokine mRNA expression; soluble adhesion molecules such as soluble intercellular adhesion molecule-1 (ICAM-1) and soluble vascular cell adhesion molecule-1 (DCAM-1) have become new indicators for monitoring rejection. It also plays an important role in the acute rejection reaction.

Cheng Biao, an important member of the Xiaobing Fu academician team, has been conducting in-depth research on concentrated platelets. The research group and others used PRP for rat bone-marrow-derived mesenchymal stem cells (BM-SCs) to phenomenon that platelet-rich plasma can resist the apoptosis of bone marrow mesenchymal stem cells and promote their survival under oxidative stress in vitro, and to explore its internal mechanism [28]. First, induce oxidative stress conditions in vitro treatment of bone marrow mesenchymal stem cells with hydrogen peroxide after serum starvation, optimal conditions for MTT toxicity detection, and optimal concentration of platelet-rich plasma; further study the antiapoptotic effect of platelet-rich plasma under optimal induction conditions on bone marrow mesenchymal, mainly by apoptosis detection, TUNEL staining method to verify apoptosis and apoptosis rate, and TYPAN blue staining method to exclude cell survival and survival rate; also study apoptosis protein Bcl-xl and p-Bad's expression. In order to further explore its antiapoptotic mechanism, immunocytochemistry and ELASA experiments were used to demonstrate whether platelet-rich plasma promotes the secretion of bone marrow mesenchymal stem cells—mainly studying growth factors VEGF and PDGF; simultaneously the effect of platelet-rich plasma on the expression of the surface receptor PDGFR in bone marrow mesenchymal stem cells was investigated; using RT-PCR, Western blot, immunocytochemistry to investigate whether platelet-rich plasma activates the signaling pathway in bone marrow mesenchymal stem cells PI3K-AKT-NF-κB or JAK/STAT3; through the proof by contradiction, block PDGFR, PI3K, AKT, (LY294002, AG1295, SC66) to study a series of effects of platelet-rich plasma on bone marrow mesenchymal stem cells, including antiapoptosis, promotion of paracrine, and other effects. Results:

(a) 10 μm/mL of $H_2O_2$ was the optimal condition for inducing oxidative stress in vitro.
(b) 10% PRP and 20% PRP are the optimal concentrations to promote proliferation.
(c) The effective antiapoptotic effect of PRP was confirmed by MTT, APOPTOSIS, TUNEL, TYPAN BLUE, etc., and the concentration was optimal at 10% or 20%.
(d) Detection of apoptotic proteins in cells, PRP pretreated MSC, Bcl-xl expression increased and p-Bad expression decreased, further demonstrating the antiapoptotic effect of PRP.

In-depth study of PRP found that it induced the paracrine effect of MSC—the expression of VEGF and PDGF increased; and the expression of GF surface receptor PDGFR was also increased; PRP pretreatment activated the signaling pathway PI3K-AKT-NF-κB; blocking the entire signaling pathway, the anti-apoptotic/promoting effects of PRP are significantly reduced or even reversed. This indicates that 10% PRP pretreatment promotes the antiapoptotic effect of MSCs under oxidative stress conditions (10 μm/mL + $H_2O_2$ serum deprivation) in vitro. This mechanism of antiapoptosis is derived from the activation of MSC intrinsic signaling pathway PI3K-AKT-NF-κB while promoting MSC secretion of VEGF and PDGF (Figs. 10.6, 10.7, 10.8, and 10.9).

Platelet-rich plasma pretreatment of bone marrow mesenchymal stem cells promotes the secretion of VEGF and PDGF, which has antiapoptosis and promotes angiogenesis of vascular endothelial cells in vitro. Anti-VEGF and anti-PDGF antibodies can reverse their antiapoptotic and angiogenic effects.

Subsequently, the research team studied the survival of bone marrow mesenchymal stem cells after platelet-rich plasma preconditioning and the repair and regeneration ability of acute full-thickness skin wound defects. Results:

(a) The survival rate of bone marrow mesenchymal stem cells pretreated with platelet-rich plasma was significantly higher than that of transplanted stem cells alone, and the apoptotic rate was decreased.
(b) Compared with the other two groups, the platelet-rich plasma group showed a significant increase in wound healing rate and a marked shortening of tissue healing time. On the 16th day after cell transplantation, the wound surface almost completely healed. The wound healing rate of the other two groups of animals was significantly lower than that of the platelet-rich plasma at each test point, and the healing time was longer. The healing state of the microstructure: in the platelet-rich plasma group, the epidermal regeneration was better than the other two groups. The dermal collagen fibers were arranged neatly and the collagen was coarse.
(c) Platelet-rich plasma group significantly promoted epidermal regeneration: enhanced angiogenesis density (immunofluorescence showed that the expression of α-SMA and CK5 was significantly higher than the other two groups); and the concentration of wound growth factor VEGF and PDGF was also significantly higher than the other two groups.
(d) Detection of signal proteins: the expression of platelet-rich plasma signaling pathway proteins was higher than the other two groups. This echoes the results of in vitro experiments, demonstrating the hypothesis of in vitro experiments: bone marrow mesenchymal stem cells pretreated with platelet-rich plasma have greater viability and regenerative capacity, And this antiapoptosis and regeneration function is closely related to the activation of PI3K-

**Fig. 10.6** Apoptosis of bone marrow mesenchymal stem cells after PRP treatment. The number of cells decreased, the expression of Bad decreased, and the expression of Bcl-xl increased, which was statistically significant compared with the other two groups, $^{*}P < 0.05$, $^{\#}P < 0.01$

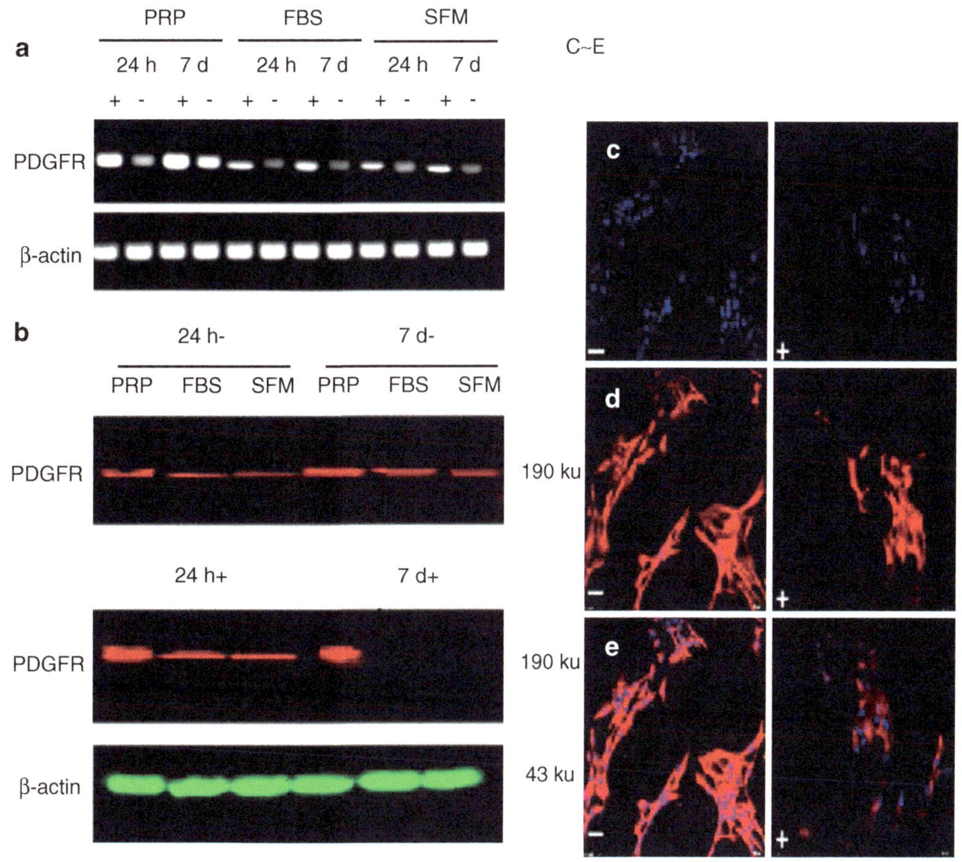


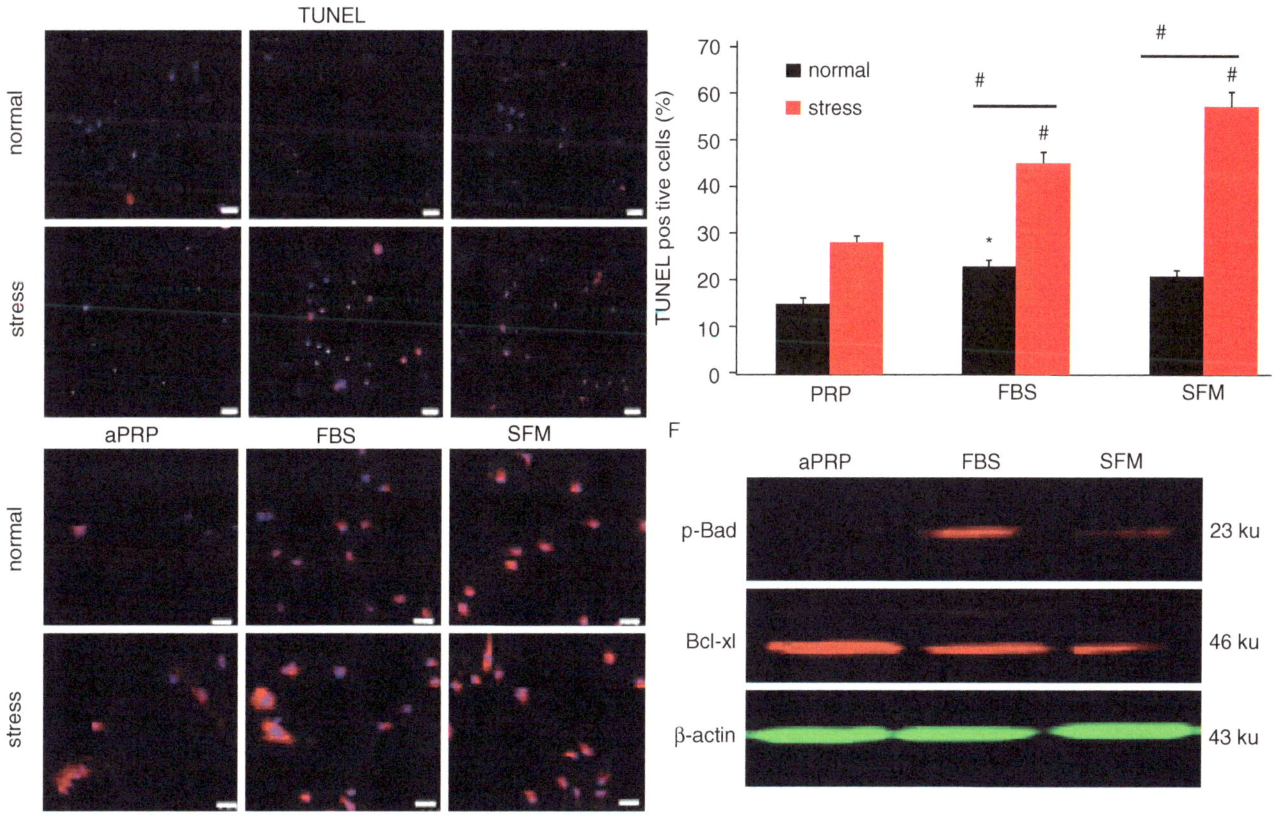


**Fig. 10.7** Platelet-rich plasma preconditioning enhances the expression of PDGFR on the surface of bone marrow mesenchymal stem cells

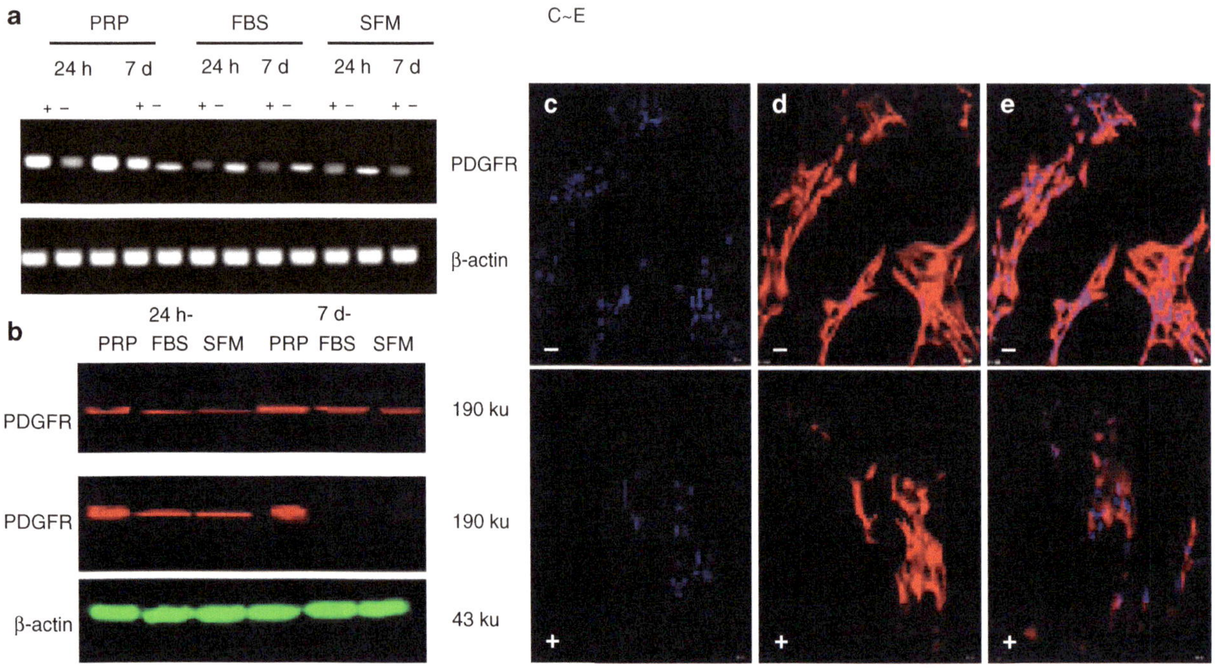


**Fig. 10.8** Pretreatment of bone marrow mesenchymal stem cells by platelet-rich plasma

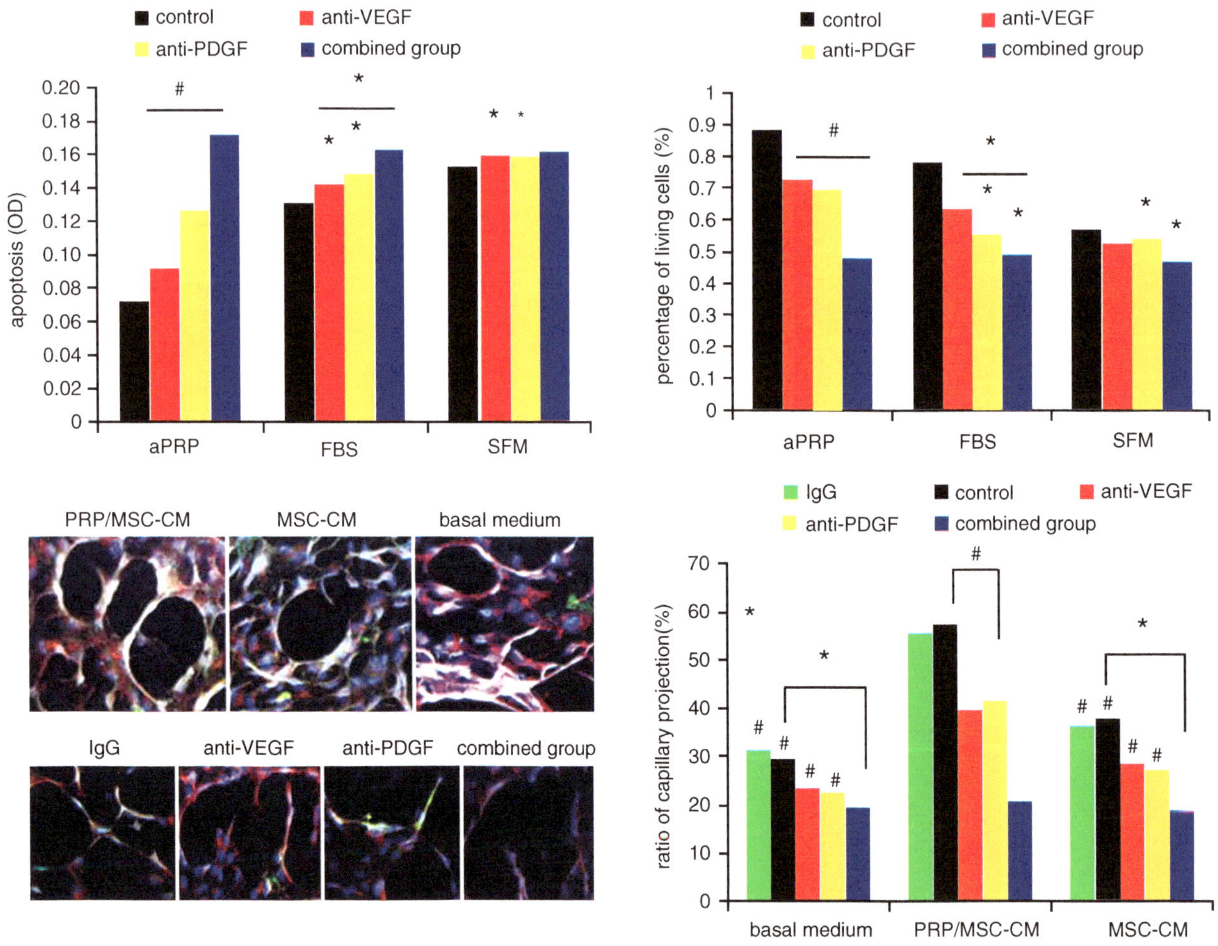


**Fig. 10.9** PRP promotes proliferation of bone marrow mesenchymal stem cells and resists apoptosis under oxidative stress. 10% and 20% PRP are optimal concentration conditions. And compared with the other groups, there are significant statistical differences. The above figures are MTT, apoptosis, and typan blue detection. $^{*}P < 0.05$, $^{\#}P < 0.01$, $n = 4$

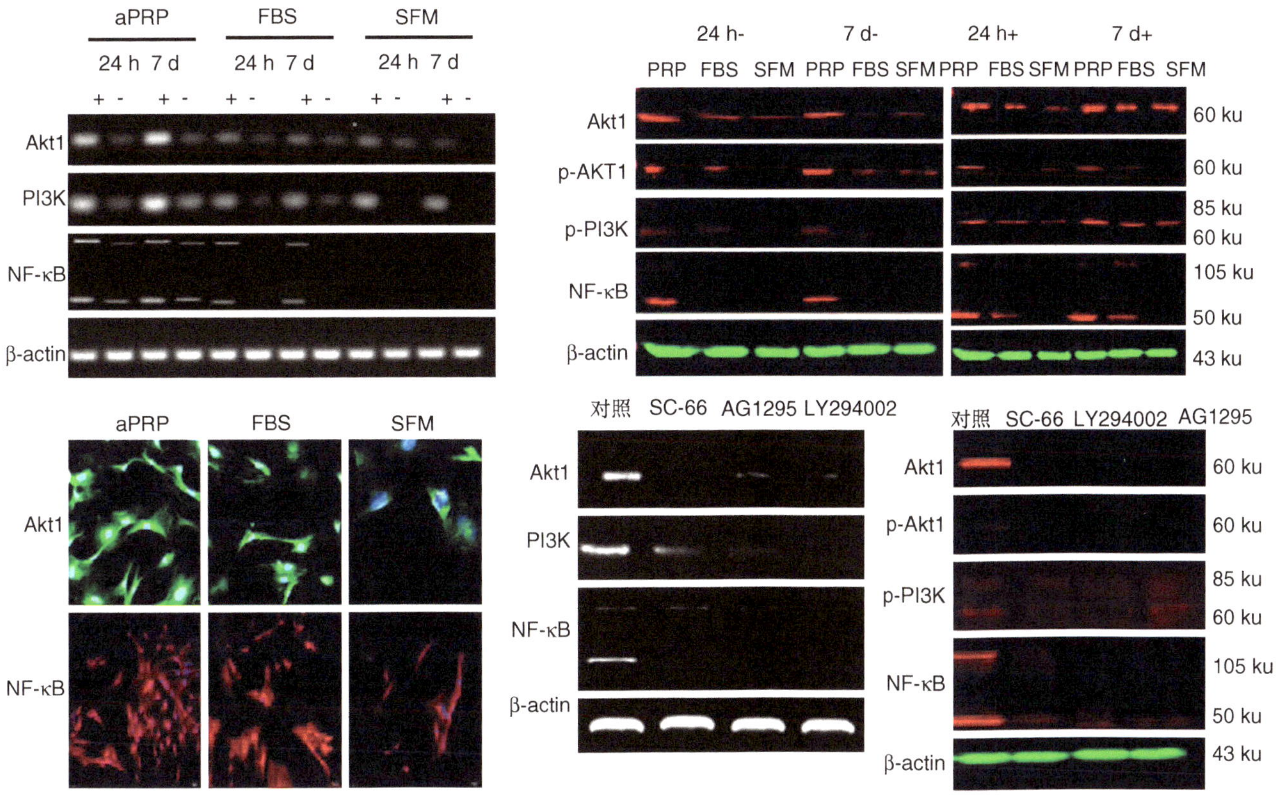


**Fig. 10.10** PI3K/Akt1/NF-κB signaling pathway is activated under oxidative stress conditions

AKT-NF-κB signaling pathway in its cells (Figs. 10.10, 10.11, 10.12, and 10.13).

At the same time, the comparison between the groups showed that the activation of this signaling pathway was stronger in the platelet-rich plasma group than in the normal or oxidative stress-induced conditions.

The pretreatment group has a promoting effect on wound healing and also has an effect on the regeneration function of blood vessels and epidermal differentiation of various layers of skin cells.

The apoptotic rate of the pretreatment group was statistically significant compared with the other two groups.

This effect is accomplished by increasing cell secretion and activation of signaling pathways within the wound.

## 10.4 Gene Therapy

Zhang Hongyu and Wu Jiang

Gene therapy is a gene transfer method at the genetic level, using genetic engineering and cell biology techniques to introduce genetic material into specific cells, allowing the introduction of gene expression to complement proteins that lack or lose normal function, or to inhibit the overexpression of a gene, to achieve gene replacement, genetic modification or gene enhancement, and ultimately the purpose of treating diseases. It is one of the most revolutionary medical technologies developed with the maturity of DNA recombination and gene cloning in the 1970s and 1980s, and it has shown unique advantages in the treatment of major diseases.

### 10.4.1 Development and Current Status of Gene Therapy Research

In the 1970s, Aposhian clearly proposed the concept of gene therapy. In 1972, Friedmann et al. proposed "the use of gene therapy to treat human genetic diseases." In 1989, gene therapy clinical studies were first approved by the FDA in the United States. In 1990, the National Institutes of Health began the world's first true gene therapy clinical trial in which they used gene therapy to repair adenosine deaminase activity in a girl with severe combined immunodeficiency (SCID) to restore its immune system. In 1999, Necker Children's Hospital in Paris, France, used gene therapy to restore several normal immune functions to infants with severe immunodeficiency. Since then, gene therapy has gradually expanded from single-gene genetic diseases to multi-gene and acquired genetic diseases such as malignant tumors, cardiovascular diseases, genetic diseases, AIDS, and other infectious diseases. In the last 10 years, gene therapy technology has made significant progress in the treatment of a series of major diseases such as malignant tumors, congeni-

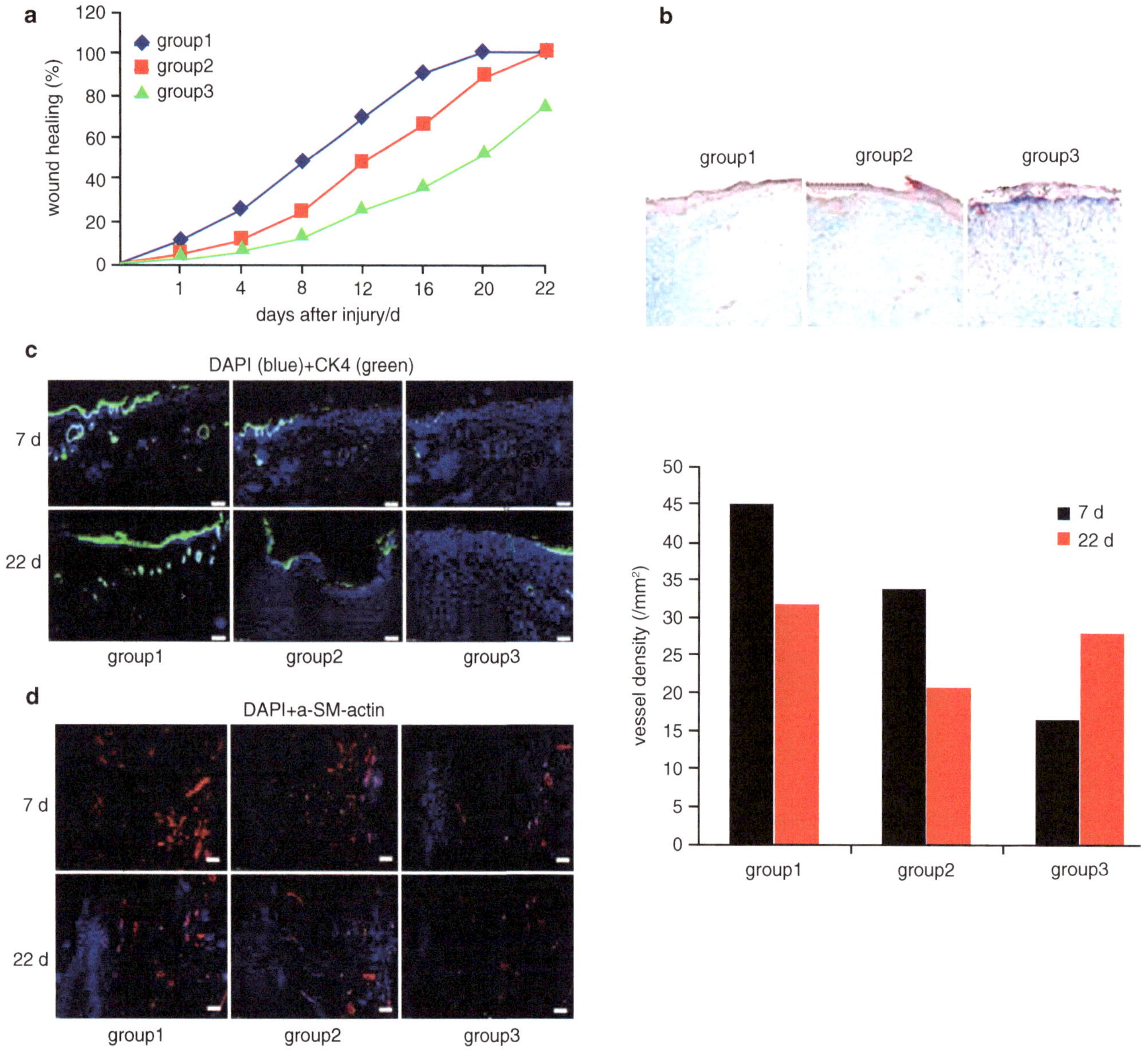


**Fig. 10.11** Effect of bone marrow mesenchymal stem cells pretreated with PRP on wound healing

tal blindness, severe combined immunodeficiency, and Parkinson's disease. To date, nearly 900 gene therapy programs in the world have been used in clinical practice, with more than 8000 cases treated. As of January 2015, 2142 gene therapy products have been approved worldwide for clinical trials, of which 461 have entered Phase II/III clinical trials, and four gene therapy products have been listed in China, the European Union and Russia.

### 10.4.2 The Use and Advantages of Gene Therapy in Tissue Repair and Regeneration

The emergence and development of regenerative medicine has provided new applications for gene therapy. Humans suffer from various forms of trauma and loss of vital organ function, and millions of people urgently need tissue and organ transplants every year. On the one hand, although transplantation has its enormous therapeutic effect, it is far more than supply, and it is difficult to meet the needs of ethics and immune rejection. On the other hand, the current tissue repair still has problems such as scar healing. There is still a distance to repair damaged tissues and organs. The emergence of regenerative medicine has solved these problems. Regenerative medicine utilizes the cell regeneration potential in human organ tissues, and with the participation of essential nutrients, regenerates and replenishes cells to maintain the structure and function of organs, and fundamentally treats diseases. Moreover, as the functions of various growth factors are gradually discovered, their cDNAs are cloned, and gene therapy is more

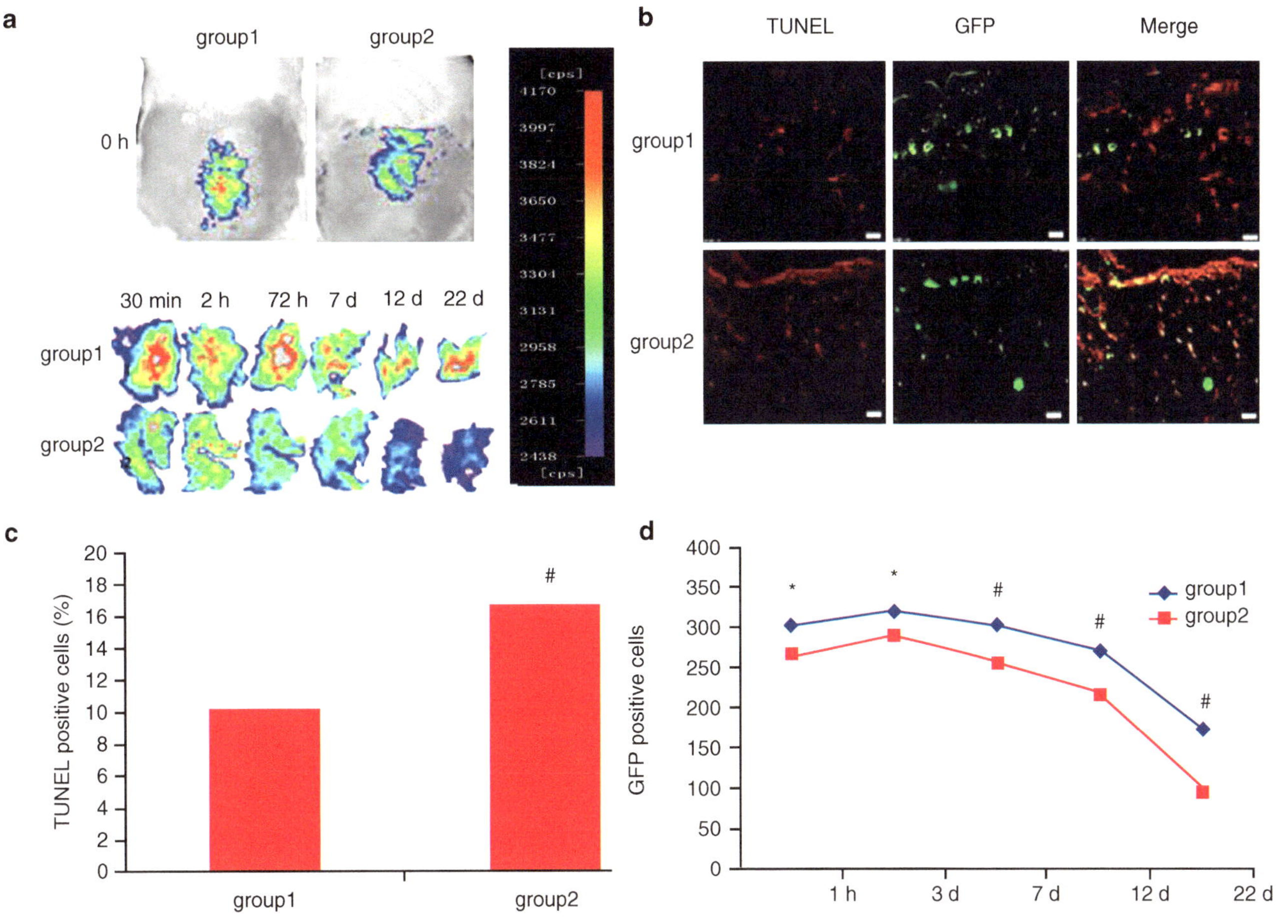


**Fig. 10.12** Pretreatment of platelet-rich plasma promotes survival of bone marrow mesenchymal stem cells in vivo and reduces apoptotic rate

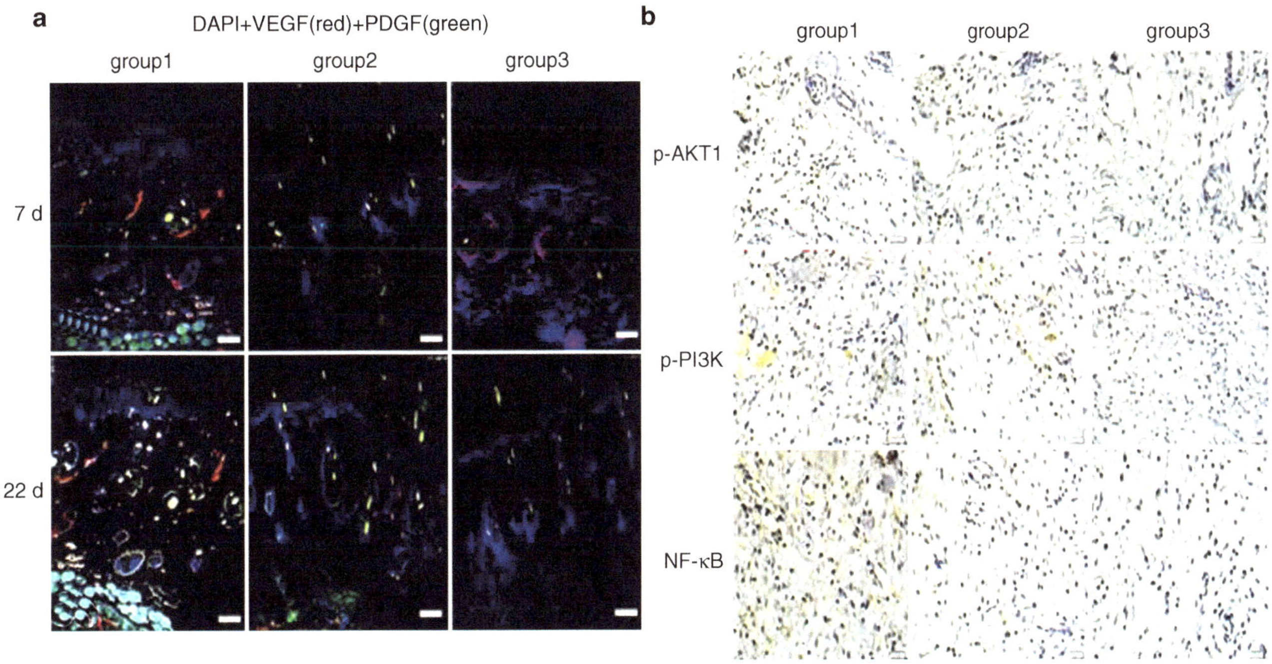


**Fig. 10.13** Bone marrow mesenchymal stem cells treated with platelet-rich plasma promote skin regeneration and enhance survival rate in a full-thickness skin defect model

applied to the field of regenerative medicine, such as promoting wound healing [29].

The target cells that receive gene therapy during gene therapy enable the body's own cells to secrete the protein of interest, and do not need to receive cytokines in the form of proteins expressed by genetic engineering. Therefore, complex processes such as protein extraction and purification are not required; and target cells are continuously secreted. The desired protein provides a stable microenvironment for tissue regeneration and improves therapeutic efficiency, thereby achieving therapeutic and repairing purposes. The current gene therapy technology still cannot make the long-term expression of the target gene and can only achieve the role of palliative, and the pathogenic gene still inherits the inherent law to the offspring. Relatively speaking, tissue repair and regeneration takes a relatively short time, and it is only necessary to express the gene for a period of time to repair the damage. Therefore, gene therapy is an ideal treatment for regenerative medicine. At present, gene therapy has been widely used in nerve tissue, bone tissue, skin tissue, heart and other tissues, islet remodeling, eye diseases and organ regeneration, and has achieved fruitful results [30].

### 10.4.3 Gene Therapy and Wound Repair

It is an indisputable fact that wound repair is regulated by genes. The incidence of scars and keloids in black and yellow wound healing is higher than that in Caucasians, suggesting that there is a racial difference in wound healing. This ethnic difference may be related to genetic factors. The phenomenon of no scar healing during fetal embryonic period and scar healing after birth, no scar healing in the hands, feet, face, and genitals of the same individual, and scar healing in other parts also suggests that the same genotype of the same individual shows different healing outcomes at different times and in different parts. Therefore, in the aspect of tissue repair, it is hoped that the gene transfer technology will affect the natural process of tissue repair, so that the time of tissue healing under normal conditions is shortened, accelerated, or wounded to heal.

Gene therapy for refractory wounds involves the introduction of exogenous DNA or RNA fragments into target cells and target tissues to correct or compensate for defects in the gene, and to shut down or inhibit abnormally expressed genes for normal therapeutic purposes. The use of gene therapy to regulate trauma, especially the repair of refractory wounds, is a hot research topic in trauma medicine. A large number of studies have confirmed that in the process of wound healing, a therapeutic gene with a certain regulatory effect is selected and introduced into cells by gene transfection technology, which can promote the repair of wounds.

### 10.4.4 Gene Therapy for Growth Factors

At present, the selection of therapeutic genes in wound healing process mainly includes the use of growth factors, cytokines, integrins, inducible nitric oxide synthase and stem cells, etc., and their effects on promoting wound healing have been confirmed and obvious curative effects have been achieved. The focus here is on the gene therapy of growth factors.

Growth factors are a series of active peptides with multiple functions that promote or inhibit cell proliferation and differentiation, and are also important substances that mediate cell-cell interactions. During the whole repair process, they affect the migration, proliferation, and differentiation of cells, regulate the growth rate of cells, and guide and adjust the response of human wound healing. Therefore, it has become the preferred therapeutic gene in wound gene therapy. The rise and development of gene therapy provides a new idea for wound healing: transfecting certain growth factor genes into cells, locally and effectively synthesizing growth factors to promote tissue repair, thereby overcoming the disadvantages of using exogenous growth factors. The gene therapy of the skin is mainly to transfect a certain growth factor gene into keratinocytes or fibroblasts to make it express a large amount, and to use the high expression of growth factors to influence the wound healing process and achieve the effect of promoting healing.

#### 10.4.4.1 Transforming Growth Factor β

TGF-β is produced by platelets, keratinocytes, macrophages, lymphocytes, and fibroblasts, and is essential for the body's inflammatory response, epithelial regeneration, and connective tissue formation, and is increased at the beginning of wound formation, and is most important for wound healing. It promotes the aggregation of inflammatory cells and enhances the tissue clearance of macrophages. At the same time, TGF-β is a major regulator of extracellular matrix production and alteration, and is involved in the regulation of wound repair and scar formation. In vitro experiments have shown that TGF-β can promote the contraction of fibroblasts in the collagen matrix, thereby promoting the contraction of the wound. In TGF-β knockout mice, the absence of TGF-β led to a delay in wound healing. Jude et al. [1] found that TGF-β was not upregulated in DFU wounds compared to normal skin, and pointed out that to some extent this may be one of the causes of DFU becoming chronic. In view of the above, Chesnoy et al. [2] used 60 μg of plasmid DNA encoding the TGF-β gene to be directly subcutaneously injected into a 1 × 1 cm skin wound of diabetic mice. The results showed that the cell proliferation and extracellular matrix formation were more significant in the gene therapy group than in the control group, and the wound healing days in the control group were 11–14 days, while the wound healing days in the gene therapy group were 7 days.

#### 10.4.4.2 Insulin-Like Growth Factor-1

IGF-1 was originally called growth regulator C, which is structurally related to proinsulin and is a growth factor with insulin-like metabolism. Under the regulation of growth hormone, IGF-1 is mainly produced in the liver and distributed in most tissues of the body. IGF-1 regulates cell metabolism, stimulates collagen synthesis in fibroblasts, and proliferates fibroblasts and keratinocytes. In acute wounds, the expression of IGF-1 was significantly increased. However, Velander et al. [3] demonstrated in experiments that the expression of IGF-1 was significantly decreased in diabetic wounds. Whether these findings can be assumed: if the expression of IGF-1 is increased in the diabetic wound, it can promote the healing of the wound. Hirsch et al. [31] cultured and transfected the IGF-1 gene in vitro with keratinocytes, and then transplanted the transgenic keratinocytes to the wound of the full-thickness skin defect of the diabetic model. The results showed that keratinocytes cultured in vitro expressed high expression of IGF-1 (740 ng/mL), and on the first day after cell transplantation, the peak of gene transfection appeared (457 ng/mL), and the wound healing rate of the gene therapy group was (83 ± 17)%, which was higher than the other control groups (57 ± 12)% and (32 ± 1)%. Moreover, IGF-1 transgenic therapy can increase wound repair speed by 25%.

#### 10.4.4.3 Platelet-Derived Growth Factor

PDGF is produced by platelets, macrophages, vascular endothelial cells, fibroblasts, and keratinocytes, and is involved in the division and chemokine action of neutrophils, macrophages, fibroblasts, and smooth muscle cells. At the same time, PDGF can also stimulate macrophage secretion of transforming growth factor beta and enhance its mediated tissue clearance and granulation tissue formation. Lee et al. [32] used a lentiviral vector to transduce the gene of PDGF-B to treat 2 × 2 cm full-thickness skin defect wounds in diabetic mice. After 21 days, the residual epithelial space, granulation tissue area, PDGF expression, collagen formation, and angiogenesis were measured. The results showed that there was no difference between epithelial formation and granulation tissue formation in the three groups, but in the PDGF gene therapy group, angiogenesis was more pronounced than in the other control groups, and the collagen fibers formed were more coherent and dense. In 2009, Mulder et al. [13] reported clinical trials of GAM501 (a combination of Ad5PDGF-B and 2.6% collagen) in the treatment of stage I/II of DFU. Of the 12 DFU patients who completed the trial, the ulcers of 10 patients healed in 3 months, and 7 of the patients received a single treatment with GAM501. GAM501 showed good biological activity in the patient and was well tolerated without toxicity. In the future, GAM501 will provide a new option for the treatment of patients with DFU, and the results of subsequent clinical trials are even more wait and see.

#### 10.4.4.4 Fibroblast Growth Factor

FGF is secreted by keratinocytes, fibroblasts, endothelial cells, smooth muscle cells, chondrocytes, and mast cells. The FGF family consists of 23 members. Currently, the most relevant gene therapy research is FGF-1 (or aFGF) and FGF-2 (or bFGF). FGF-1 is one of the mitogens of endothelial cells and vascular smooth muscle cells, which acts on every stage of angiogenesis, including proliferation, differentiation, migration, and ultimately the formation of functional blood vessels. FGF-2 plays an important role in granulation tissue formation, epithelial regeneration, and tissue remodeling. Ferraro et al. [33] used intradermal injection of a plasmid encoding the FGF-2 gene in combination with noninvasive dermal electroporation for the treatment of limb ischemic disease. Three days after surgery, Doppler perfusion imaging revealed a significant increase in blood flow in the affected limb and continued until 14 days after surgery (end point of the experimental observation). Immunohistochemistry of the gastrocnemius cross-section showed that the microvessel density was twice that of the control group. Therefore, gene therapy of FGF-1 and FGF-2 can increase angiogenesis in the limbs and increase blood perfusion in the treatment of limb ischemic diseases.

#### 10.4.4.5 Hepatocyte Growth Factor

HGF was first discovered in the serum of rats with hepatic resection and is considered to be a powerful stimulator of hepatocyte growth. Later, it was discovered that HGF is also an angiogenic factor that stimulates the proliferation and migration of endothelial cells, induces angiogenesis, enhances the migration of keratinocytes, and promotes epithelial regeneration. Therefore, HGF plays an important role in wound repair. In 2010, Ha et al. [34] conducted a study on the treatment of diabetic canine wounds with BMSCs (bone marrow mesenchymal stem cells) transfected with adenovirus-transfected HGF gene (Ad-HGF). This study showed that BMSCs transfected with HGF gene promoted the healing of diabetic wounds compared with HGF and BMSCs alone. Today, gene therapy for HGF has had important results in the treatment of severe lower limb ischemia (CLI). To assess the safety and feasibility of intramuscular injection of naked plasmid DNA encoding the HGF gene for CLI treatment, Morishita et al. performed two trials on 22 patients with CLI at doses of 2 mg and 4 mg, respectively. The trial demonstrated that this treatment is safe and feasible for the treatment of CLI and can successfully improve the symptoms of patients with CLI. It should be noted that DFU caused by lower extremity arterial disease in diabetic patients is also a type of CLI. At this stage, most scholars believe that arterial bypass is still the main treatment for the treatment of CLI.

#### 10.4.4.6 Vascular Endothelial Growth Factor

VEGF is secreted by endothelial cells, keratinocytes, fibroblasts, smooth muscle cells, platelets, neutrophils, and macrophages. It is one of the strongest angiogenic factors known to increase the permeability of venules and small veins, promotes vascular endothelial cell division and proliferation, induces angiogenesis, and plays an important role in embryonic development, wound healing, tumor growth, and metastasis. In addition, VEGF and its receptors can regulate the production of nerves, direct the growth of axons through neural progenitor cells, and regulate the proliferation of astrocytes, glial cells, and Schwann cells. It is an indisputable fact that the angiogenesis of DFU wound is poor. Experiments in the twentieth century have shown that impaired angiogenesis in diabetic mice is associated with decreased levels of mRNA and VEGF encoding VEGF. In 2009, Ropper et al. [4] conducted a randomized, double-blind clinical trial of VEGF gene therapy for diabetic polyneuropathy. The results showed that the gene therapy group improved the symptoms of patients with diabetic polyneuropathy more than the control group. Kalil et al. [35] reported that injection of 5 mL of phVEGF165-containing solution within the myocardial ischemia region can improve the symptoms of patients and myocardial perfusion, and this therapy has proven to be feasible and safe. Koyama et al. [36] transfected the VEGF gene in vitro with chopped skin particles and used it for wound healing of full-thickness skin defects. The results showed that the expression of VEGF in the gene therapy group and the number of neovascularization and epithelial regeneration were higher than those in the control group. The significance of this study is that, firstly, it changed the pattern of cell transfection. For the first time, using body tissue as a source of gene expression; secondly, for traditional flap transplantation for DFU, in the future, the treatment may well be replaced.

### 10.4.5 Gene Therapy Technology

#### 10.4.5.1 Selection of Target Genes

The target gene refers to the gene or DNA sequence that needs to be studied and can be prepared by the following method:

A. Direct separation method, also known as "shotgun method." The method mainly uses a restriction enzyme to cut the chromosomal DNA into a plurality of fragments and contains the desired gene of interest, and the operation is relatively simple and is generally used for extracting the target gene of the prokaryote.
B. Chemical synthesis of the gene of interest using a DNA synthesizer, provided that the DNA primary structure is well known.
C. Under the catalysis of reverse transcriptase, cDNA was synthesized using the mRNA strand as a template, and then replicated into a double-stranded cDNA fragment. This method is currently used for the preparation of the target gene.
D. Polymerase chain reaction (PCR) is a rapid amplification of copying technology in vitro. Commonly used target genes generally include growth factor genes, such as fibroblast growth factor gene, transforming growth factor gene, and anti-catabolic factors, such as interleukin-1 receptor antagonist gene, soluble tumor necrosis factor receptor gene.

#### 10.4.5.2 Route of Administration

A. In vitro Route

The in vitro route refers to introduction of a vector containing a foreign gene into a human body or an allogeneic cell (or a heterologous cell) in vitro and is expanded into an in vitro cell and then returned to the human body. The in vitro gene transfer pathway is currently more widely used, more classic, safe, and the effect is easier to control, but the steps are more, the technology is complex, difficult, and not easy to promote.

B. In vivo route

The in vivo route is to assemble a foreign gene into a specific eukaryotic cell expression vector and introduce it directly into the body. Such vectors may be viral or nonviral, even naked DNA. The gene transfer route in vivo is simple and easy to promote, but it is not yet mature. Its shortcomings are low gene transfection rate, short duration of efficacy, immune rejection, and safety.

#### 10.4.5.3 Gene Therapy Vector

Effective gene therapy relies on the efficient and stable expression of foreign genes in the receptor. The appropriate vector is one of the key issues in the gene transfection process, and the vector should meet the following conditions:

(a) Efficient transfection of target cells.
(b) Molecules are small in mass and can be introduced into host cells and construct recombinant genes.
(c) Lower immunogenicity.
(d) Can express functional products in target cells for a long time. In experimental research, there are two main types of carriers commonly used: viruses and nonviruses.

A. Adenovirus Vector

The main advantages of adenoviral vectors are high infection efficiency, ability to infect dividing and non-dividing cells, nonintegration into host chromosomes, no insertional mutagenicity, and the disadvantage of not being able to insert exogenous fragments larger than 8 kb, and a strong immune response is caused, and the expression time of the foreign gene is short. Adenoviral vectors are one of the most commonly used vectors.

B. Retroviral Vector

Retroviral vectors integrate the gene of interest into the genome of the target cell, which has a wide range of infected cells, a large gene capacity, and a low immune response. The transcriptional virus-mediated approach was the first vector to be used in the treatment of skin gene delivery. Breitbart et al. [36] transfected dermal fibroblasts into hPDGF-B-expressing retroviral vector in vitro and implanted them into a polyglycolic acid scaffold, which was then transplanted into a 20 × 20 mm full-thickness wound on the back of hereditary diabetic rats. The residual epithelial gap was measured 21 days after injury, which showed that the experimental group significantly accelerated the wound healing compared with the control group. Immunohistochemical staining showed that the experimental group had strong staining of hPDGF-B.

C. Adeno-Associated Virus Vector

Adeno-associated viral vectors-2 (AAV-2) can integrate human host chromosomes, can infect dividing and nondividing cells, have low immunogenicity, less toxic T cell responses, and no risk of insertional mutations and carcinogenesis. The AAV vector has a foreign gene loading capacity of less than 4.5 kb, but it is expected to be a gene therapy for wound healing by dividing the large fragment gene and its endogenous promoter into two separate vectors to form a viral DNA heterodimer, and it is expected to play a better role in gene therapy of wound healing; in addition, replication and packaging require the help of helper viruses such as adenovirus or herpes virus, and further purification is required to avoid the immunogenicity and toxicity of the helper virus.

D. Herpes Simplex Virus Type I Vector

Herpes simplex virus type I vector (HSV-I) has the property of replicating and phagocytizing nerves in epithelial cells and can be present in neuronal cells of ganglia for a long time. The newly constructed recombinant virus specific for anti-HSV-I can inhibit the parental and autoviral replicators, improve the safety of the vector, and reduce the cytotoxicity. Compared with viral carriers, nonviral vectors have the characteristics of large packaging capacity, low cost, and simple operation.

E. Naked DNA

The simplest introduction of nonviral vectors is the direct injection of naked DNA. Naked DNA cannot be transfected into cells in vitro, but transfection efficiency is higher in in vivo injection, especially in muscle and skin. The specific mechanism is unclear, and the disadvantage is poor stability and targeting.

F. Gene Gun and Microplanting Gene Gun

Gene guns and microplanted gene guns use a high-pressure helium particle stream to directly inject gold or tungsten particles carrying DNA plasmids into the target cell nucleus. This device allows DNA to be directly inserted into the nucleus to prevent degradation of the drug DNA by enzymes. The disadvantage is that the operation is complicated and has special requirements for the equipment. And the gene expression of the gene gun is different. Benn transfected TGF-β1 cDNA into a diabetic rat with a gene gun, and the tensile strength increased by 80% 14–21 days after surgery [37]. The role of TGF-β1 is partly due to chemotactic monocytes, stimulation of matrix gene expression, inhibition of protease expression, promotion of protease inhibitory factor expression, and stimulation of fibroblast contraction.

G. Electroporation

Electroporation refers to the increase of cell membrane permeability under current stimulation, and the appearance of pores in the cell membrane, thereby allowing DNA to enter the cell. Marti modeled the full-thickness of the back of the hereditary diabetic rats [38]. One group was injected with KGF cDNA and immediately stimulated with a specific parameter of current, and the other group was left untreated. RT-PCR confirmed the expression of KGF mRNA in skin samples in the treated group. At 12 days, 90% of the wounds healed in the treatment group and 40% in the control group. The researchers used a resected wound in a diabetic mouse as a model. Subcutaneous injection of a plasmid expressing hypoxia-inducible factor-1 (HIF-1) followed by electroporation, and the expression level of HIF-1 mRNA in the tissue increased. Wound healing speed is significantly accelerated. Electroporation can increase the expression of the target gene in localized wounds, but its role in humans needs further study.

H. Cationic Liposomes

Cationic liposomes with positively charged and negatively charged plasmids bind tightly to form a complex by electrostatic interaction, which protects DNA from enzymatic degradation, has low host immunogenicity, reproducible injection, large foreign gene capacity and unconformity human host and other advantages. It has been approved by the National Institutes of Health (NIH) and the Recombinant DNA Advisory Committee (RAC) as a vector for gene therapy to enter Phase II clinical trials for the treatment of certain cancers, but its shortcomings are short expression times and low targeting [12]. Jeschke injected cationic liposomes containing IGF-1 cDNA directly into rat burn wounds and transfected myofibroblasts, endothelial cells, and macrophages, which mainly occurred in granulation tissue. Compared with cationic liposomes containing LacZ, the concentration of IGF-1 in the wound was significantly increased, and the rate of re-epithelialization was accelerated.

I. Ultrasonic Microbubble Contrast Agent

Ultrasound contrast agent (UCA) is a novel in vivo gene transfection vector. UCA is a gas-containing microbubble that contains human albumin, lipids, palmitic acid, and polymers. The target gene binds to UCA by adhering to the surface of the outer shell or encapsulating it in the microbubbles. Under the action of ultrasound, the microbubbles rupture, the target gene is released to the local tissue irradiated by the ultrasonic wave, and the cavitation of the ultrasonic wave increases the permeability of the cell membrane. It is easy to absorb foreign genes. Taniyam's in vivo experiments found that simultaneous injection of plasmid and contrast agent with ultrasound was about 1000 times higher than the activity of fluorescein injected into the plasmid alone [39].

#### 10.4.5.4 Selection of Target Cells

The principle of selecting target cells is:

A. Must be strong enough to withstand handling and easily separated from the body and easily returned to the body.
B. It has the advantage of proliferation, long life cycle, can survive for several months to several years, and finally can extend to the whole life of the patient.
C. It is easy to be transformed by foreign genetic material.
D. When a retroviral vector is selected, the expression of the target gene is preferably a tissue-specific cell. More commonly used are bone marrow stem cells, skin fibroblasts, hepatocytes, vascular endothelial cells, and muscle cells. Cells, signaling factors, and scaffolds that provide a place for cell attachment are the three elements of regenerative medicine. The cells mainly use stem cells with self-renewal ability, multidirectional differentiation potential, or induced pluripotent stem cells. With the deepening of research, gene therapy has made some progress. Gene therapy brings new opportunities to clinical research and brings new hope for treatment to patients.

## 10.5 Exosomes and NETosis

Xiao Jian and Wu Jiang

### 10.5.1 Introduction to Exosomes

Exosomes were first discovered in the supernatant of sheep red blood cells cultured in vitro. They are vesicle-like bodies with uniform size, diameter of 40–100 nm, and density of 1.10–1.18 g/mL. Exosomes are by far the most defined vesicles. Intracellular endolysosomal vesicles invaginate to form a multivesicular body. Under stimulation, multivesicular bodies fuse with cell membranes, and uniform vesicles secreted extracellularly are exosomes. Exosomes are rich in cholesterol and sphingomyelin, have a lipid bilayer structure, have a variety of growth factors and cytokines (such as VEGF and SCF) on the surface, and almost all exosomes contain physiologically active lipid components such as sphingosine-1-phosphate (S1P) and ceramide-1-phosphate (C1P). Exosomes play an important role in many physiological and pathological processes, such as antigen presentation in immunization, tumor growth and migration, and repair of tissue damage. Exosomes secreted by different cells have different components and functions and can be used as biomarkers for disease diagnosis. When exosomes enter the target cells, these paracrine factors directly interact with the cells, such as S1P, C1P can inhibit apoptosis and stimulate angiogenesis. Exosomes have diverse functions, have good rejection of tumors, and have antitumor immunity and immune function inhibition. At the same time, exosome-derived miRNAs, like other signal molecules, regulate biological signal networks and participate in various physiological processes. This section focuses on the role of exosomes in tissue repair.

#### 10.5.1.1 Exosomes MEX Derived from MSCs

MSCs are widely distributed in human tissues and are a class of pluripotent precursor cells with self- renewal ability. It has a variety of functions, including multilineage differentiation, promotion of tissue repair, antiinfective therapy, immunosuppression, and neuroprotection [40]. Traditionally, it is believed that MSCs exert their biological functions mainly by targeting to damaged tissues and differentiation to replace damaged cells to play a therapeutic role. However, a series of studies have found that the colonization and differentiation of MSCs at the injury site is very inefficient and the repair effect is limited. Studies have found that MSCs decrease cell damage and enhance repair by releasing some factors [41], and the functional proteins contained in exosomal vesicles, which are the source of MSCs, can participate in some physiological processes and serve as intercellular signaling mediators. MSCs-derived exosomes (MEX) have similar effects as MSCs promote tissue repair, and mRNA in MEX is mainly involved in pro-proliferation, transcriptional regulation, and immune regulation. In addition, miRNA is also considered to be a key bioactive substance for MEX repair in tissue damage. In conclusion, in a variety of animal models, MEX showed the ideal damage repair effect, and the biological active substances such as RNA and protein contained in the exosomes did not degrade during transportation, and exosomes are not only good tissue repair materials but also ideal means of drug transportation.

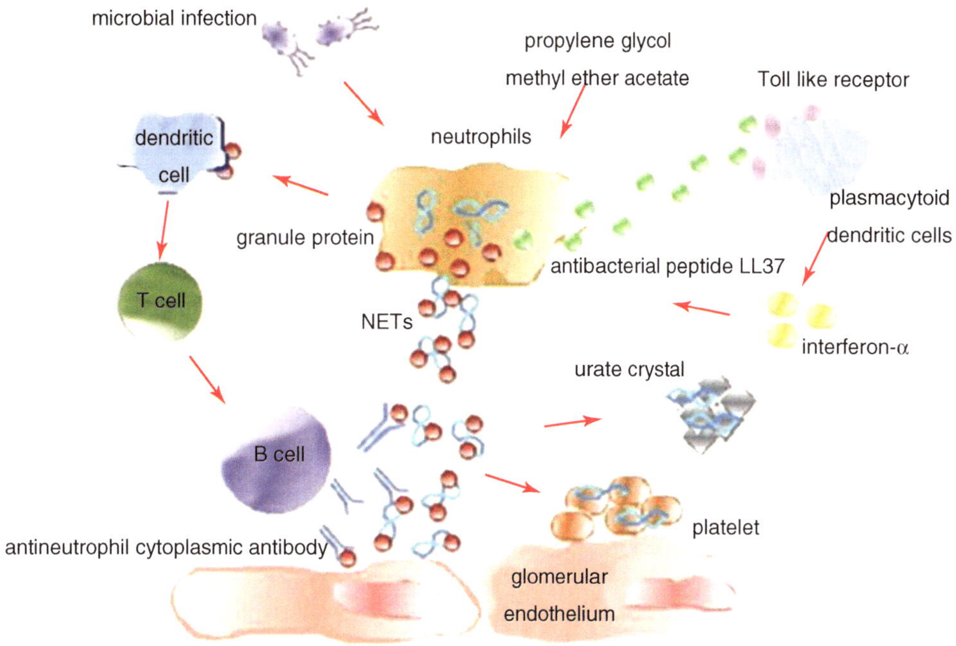


**Fig. 10.14** Schematic diagram of neutrophil NETosis formation and immune activation

#### 10.5.1.2 Exosomes from ESCs and HSCs

ESCs are multifunctional stem cells derived from undifferentiated inner cell mass of blastocyst with self-renewal ability. ESCs exosomes contain mRNA, miRNAs, and 22 proteins, including annexin A2 (ANXA2), actin-β (ACT-β), and guanine nucleotide binding protein (G-protein), enolase 1 (ENO1) and cofilin, which have the effects of inhibiting apoptosis and remodeling endocytosis, phagocytosis, and division of damaged cells. At the same time, ESCs can transport vitamin-binding protein, collagen X, apolipoprotein A, thyroxine transporter, and translation elongation factor to the recipient cells through exosomes, which plays an important role in the growth of recipient cells. Experiments have shown that ESCs exosomes are an important carrier substance that can carry a variety of active molecules to neighboring cells and participate in the regulation of cell self-renewal, growth, and differentiation.

#### 10.5.1.3 Exosomes Derived from Endothelial Progenitor Cells

Endothelial progenitor cells are precursor cells of vascular endothelial cells that are present in circulating blood, and secrete cytokines, vascular endothelial growth factor, and the like to promote angiogenesis. Exosomes are an important substance secreted by endothelial progenitor cells. Studies have shown that: endothelial progenitor exosomes are rich in miR-126 and miR-296 and other miRNAs that promote angiogenesis and antiapoptosis; in the model of ischemia-reperfusion acute kidney injury, after internalizing exosomes, the peritubular endothelial cells and tubular endothelial cells upregulate the expression of angiogenesis and antiapoptosis genes through miR-126 and miR-296, thereby promoting renal tubular cell proliferation, reducing tubular apoptosis and leukocyte infiltration, protects against acute kidney injury caused by ischemia-reperfusion. Similarly, in transplanted pancreas, pancreatic cells internalize miR-126 and miR-296 to upregulate the expression of cytokines that promote islet endothelial cell proliferation, differentiation, and angiogenesis, as well as activate PI3K-Akt and eNOS signaling pathways in islet endothelial cells, upregulates the expression of ephrin B4, EDG-1, and CD31, and inhibits the expression of TSP-1, thereby promoting islet endothelial cell migration, adhesion, angiogenesis, and inhibition of endothelial cell apoptosis, which plays an important biological role in the repair of pancreatic tissue damage.

However, the specific mechanisms by which stem cell-derived exosomes inhibit apoptosis, promote angiogenesis, and reduce inflammatory infiltration are not fully understood. The following problems must be solved before clinical use: first, the mechanism of action of various biologically active substances in exosomes and the duration of biological effects must be clarified; secondly, how to produce a large number of exosomes from cultured stem cells; thirdly, although animal experiments have initially demonstrated the safety of exosomes, further experiments are needed to prove their safety; finally, specific guidelines for the use of exosomes from different stem cell sources need to be developed.

### 10.5.2 NETosis Introduction

Neutrophils are activated by a variety of stimulating stimuli. The contained neutrophil elastase (NE) and myeloperoxidase (MPO) migrate into the nucleus and act on histones, leading to chromatin depolymerization. At the same time, the arginine residue of the three core histones is citrullinated by arginine deiminase 4 (PAD4). The depolymerized DNA filament structure together with the highly hydrolytically active enzyme particles, including various antimicrobial peptides, is rapidly released into the extracellular space after the nuclear membrane is cleaved, forming a gel-like network structure, wrapping and killing the invading pathogens. Forming a second bactericidal mechanism other than phagocytosis of neutrophils. This result is called neutrophil extracellular netting (NETs), and its process is called NETosis (Fig. 10.14). Compared with necrotic and apoptotic cells, the most significant morphological differences of NETs were nuclear envelope lysis, mixing of nucleus and cytoplasm, disappearance of intima and organelles, and no necrosis occurred throughout the process.

#### 10.5.2.1 The Existence Form of NETosis

There are two ways to find NETs: one is that the neutrophils mentioned above release the DNA in the nucleus and then lysis to death, which is suicidal NETosis; the other is vital NETosis, neutrophils still retain life activity by releasing DNA in the nucleus to become erythrocytes-like nuclear free cells. These two methods differ in the inducer and release time. Chemical reagents such as propylene glycol methyl ether acetate (PMA) induce suicidal NETs to form for hours, while microorganisms such as Gram-negative lipopolysaccharide (LPS) rapidly induce NETs release through host pattern recognition receptors. This process is regulated by platelet TLR4. In the form of release, unlike the suicidal NETosis, which release reticular matter through the cell membrane, the vital NETosis is released from the nuclear membrane to the cytoplasm through the DNA vesicle budding and merges with the membrane without penetrating the cell membrane. Neutrophil NETosis provides the host with a weapon to defend against foreign pathogens, and it also provides new clues to how systemic autoimmune diseases can expose their own antigens and break the mechanisms of self-tolerance.

#### 10.5.2.2 The Regulation Mechanism Formed by NETisos

A. Nicotinamide adenine dinucleotide phosphate oxidase (NADPHoxidase, NOX2) regulatory pathway. There is evidence that patients with chronic granulomatous disease with NOX2 deficiency or after using the NOX2 inhibitor diphenyleneiodonium (DPI). Neutrophils do not release NETs under the stimulation of PMA, suggesting that NETs formation require NOX2-dependent reactive oxygen species (ROS).

   It has recently been discovered that NOX2-mediated NETs are dependent on Akt activation, and Akt itself can block cytosolic expression by inhibiting caspase signaling as an inhibitor of apoptosis, suggesting that Akt may become a new regulatory pathway.

   However, with the deepening of the research, it was found that low concentrations of ROS such as hydrogen peroxide could not lead to the formation of NETs; neonatal neutrophils had the same ability to produce ROS as adults but could not form NETs; NOX2 potent stimulant formylmethionyl leucyl phenylanine (fMLP) does not cause NETs release; proinflammatory mediators such as IL-8 can cause NETosis but not NOX2 activity.

   These results suggest that ROS dependent on NOX2 is not the only pathway for NETs formation, but may be limited to certain characteristic diseases, suggesting that other regulatory pathways may exist during the induction of NETs.

B. Autophagy-dependent regulatory pathway.

   Mammalian target of rapamycin (mTOR) and phosphatidylinositol kinase-3 (PI3K) pathway are the two major signaling pathways in the initiation of autophagy, sirolimus and 3-methyladenine (3-MA) and wortmannin can conduct regulation by the above two steps.

   Inhibitors using mTOR increase autophagy formation and accelerate NETs formation through the histone citrullination pathway. 3-MA and Bafil A block the autophagy process and do not block NOX2 activity, but inhibit the formation of NETs characterized by chromosomal depolymerization. Interestingly, typical apoptosis occurs characterized by chromosome pyknosis. When autophagy is blocked, it causes NETs to fail to form and undergo apoptosis.

C. Regulation pathway of histone citrullination.

   Epigenetic mechanisms may also be involved in the formation of NETs. The most significant evidence is citrulline of histones, which is essential for the depolymerization of chromosomes into DNA.

   Neutrophils are capable of expressing high levels of PAD4 and initiate NETosis and subsequent responses through a citrulline-regulated pathway. Studies have shown that in rheumatoid arthritis, NETs act as important citrullinated autoantigens and stimulate inflammatory responses.

#### 10.5.2.3 NETosis and Lupus Erythematosus

Lupus erythematosus is more common in young women, and its syndrome varies from patient to patient. Its severity ranges from mild to disabling. In some patients, lupus erythematosus can be life threatening. There is currently no way to cure it. Periodic flares can affect one or more parts of the body. In the flare, the burning rash is like a scratch on a wolf's claw, often turning the cheeks red. The white blood cells that normally capture the pathogens in the joints and kidneys are a "suspect" of autoimmune diseases. Bacteria, damaged cells, and immune particles produced by the body can stimulate neutrophils to create network structure outside of them that attempt to trap offenders. Past studies have shown that these traps may also contribute to the damage of lupus to organs. The formation of neutrophil extracellular traps or NETs can lead to a form of cell death called NETosis. Abnormal NETosis or impaired NET may play a role in several autoimmune diseases, including lupus erythematosus. In mice, drugs that inhibit NETosis can improve lupus erythematosus. These drugs also reduce arteriosclerosis and abnormal blood clotting.

However, how these traps are produced, how they cause inflammation in the absence of infection, is unclear. The pockets around the heart and heart can become swollen and painful. If the brain is in an autoimmune attack, headaches, epileptic seizure, or psychotic attacks can occur. Currently, UW rheumatology professor Keith B. Elkon and a team led by Mariana J. Kaplan, head of the systemic autoimmune disease department of the National Institute of Arthritis, Musculoskeletal and Skin Diseases, found that a common RNA-protein complex in lupus patients induces cell death by NETosis in a process dependent on mitochondrial reactive oxygen species. Generally, cells have a mechanism to prevent oxidative DNA damage. In the case of immune complex-stimulated NETosis, the cell's survival pattern is disrupted. The nuclear envelope ruptures, thereby exposing the genomic DNA to reactive oxygen species. The researchers explained that mitochondrial genes are more susceptible to oxidative damage than genomic DNA. After the immune complex stimulates the neutrophils, the mitochondria of the cells rise to the cell surface. They discharge oxidize mitochondrial DNA into their environment through traps outside the neutrophils. This extracellular release of oxidized mitochondrial DNA promotes an inflammatory response. Neutrophil extracellular traps rich in mitochondrial DNA can help trigger lupus-like disease and may lead to new treatments [42].

More and more studies have found that NETs are involved in the occurrence and development of inflammation and various autoimmune diseases. Therefore, based on the role of NETs in the above pathological mechanisms, active regulation of NETs may become a new therapeutic strategy. Interventions targeting key aspects of the regulatory process, such as NOX2 and PAD4, block NETs formation or induce neutrophil differentiation to apoptosis to avoid overexposure of endogenous risk signals. In addition, the degradation of NETs by DNaseI is also expected to be a therapeutic target. With the reports of serious complications such as thrombosis in the disease, platelets have received increasing attention as an important role in the direct involvement and regulation of NETs formation. Whether NETs should be given antiplatelet therapy in the treatment of disease regulation needs further clarification.

## References

1. Hsiao CY, Hung CY, Tsai TH, et al. A study of the wound healing mechanism of a traditional Chinese medicine, angelica sinensis, using a proteomic approach. Evid Based Complement Alternat Med. 2012;2012:467–531.
2. Jude EB, Blakytny R, Bulmer J, et al. Transforming growth factor-beta 1, 2, 3 and receptor type I and II in diabetic foot ulcers. Diabet Med. 2002;19(6):440–7.
3. Chesnoy S, Lee PY, Huang L. Intradermal injection of transforming growth factor-beta1 gene enhances wound healing in genetically diabetic mice. Pharm Res. 2003;20(3):345–50.
4. Morishita R, Makino H, Aoki M, et al. Phase I/IIa clinical trial of therapeutic angiogenesis using hepatocyte growth factor gene transfer to treat critical limb ischemia. Arterioscler Thromb Vasc Biol. 2011;31(3):713–20.
5. Song LF, Meng FT, Liu XY, et al. A study of the relation between interval of the injury and the reaction of neurons, glial cells after experimental brain contusion. Fa Yi Xue Za Zhi. 2001;17(3):132–6.
6. Tao Y, Black IB, Dicicco-Bloom E. Neurogenesis in neonatal rat brain is regulated by peripheral injection of basic fibroblast growth factor (bFGF). J Comp Neurol. 1996;376(4):653–63.
7. Bethel A, Kirsch JR, Koehler RC, et al. Intravenous basic fibroblast growth factor decreases brain injury resulting from focal ischemia in cats. Stroke. 1997;28(3):609–15.
8. Fisher M, Meadows ME, Do T, et al. Delayed treatment with intravenous basic fibroblast growth factor reduces infarct size following permanent focal cerebral ischemia in rats. J Cereb Blood Flow Metab. 1995;15(6):953–9.
9. Tieline L, Puolakkainen P, Pohjonen T, et al. The effect of transforming growth factor-beta1, released from a bioabsorbable self-reinforced polylactide pin, on a bone defect. Biomaterials. 2002;23(18):3817–23.
10. Grayson AC, Cima MJ, Langer R. Size and temperature effects on poly(lactic-co-glycolic acid) degradation and microreservoir device performance. Biomaterials. 2005;26(14):2137–45.
11. Waris E, Ashammakhi N, Kaarela O, et al. Use of bioabsorbable osteofixation devices in the hand. J Hand Surg (Br). 2004;29(6):590–8.
12. Martin P. Wound healing-aiming for perfect skin regeneration. Science. 1997;276(5309):75–81.
13. Lee JA, Conejero JA, Mason JM, et al. Lentiviral transfection with the PDGF-B gene improves diabetic wound healing. Plast Reconstr Surg. 2005;116(2):532–8.
14. Kalil RA, Salles FB, Giusti II, et al. VEGF gene therapy for angiogenesis in refractory angina: phase I/II clinical trial. Rev Bras Cir Cardiovasc. 2010;25(3):311–21.
15. Hannink M, Donoghue DJ. Structure and function of platelet-derived growth factor (PDGF) and related proteins. Biochim Biophys Acta. 1989;989(1):1–10.
16. Heldin CH. Structural and functional studies on platelet-derived growth factor. EMBO J. 1992;11(12):4251–9.
17. Matsui T, Heidaran M, Miki T, et al. Isolation of a novel receptor cDNA establishes the existence of two PDGF receptor genes. Science. 1989;243(4892):800–4.
18. Heidaran MA, Pierce JH, Yu JC, et al. Role of alpha beta receptor heterodimer formation in beta platelet-derived growth factor (PDGF) receptor activation by PDGF-AB. J Biol Chem. 1991;266(30):20232–7.
19. Heidaran MA, Pierce JH, Jensen RA, et al. Chimeric alpha- and beta-platelet-derived growth factor (PDGF) receptors define three immunoglobulin-like domains of the alpha-PDGF receptor that determine PDGF-AA binding specificity. J Biol Chem. 1990;265(31):18741–4.

20. Alvarez RH, Kantarjian HM, Cortes JE. Biology of platelet-derived growth factor and its involvement in disease. Mayo Clin Proc. 2006;81(9):1241–57.
21. Kratchmarova I, Blagoev B, Haack-Sorensen M, et al. Mechanism of divergent growth factor effects in mesenchymal stem cell differentiation. Science. 2005;308(5727):1472–7.
22. Pulaski EJ, Filler RM, Dibbins AW. Local and systemic antibiotic therapy of wounds and burns. Can Med Assoc J. 1965;93(16):864–9.
23. Blaskova O, Ponfuch A, Sasko A, et al. Deviation of the genitals in nulliparae found in the material (author's transl). Ceska Gynekol. 1979;44(7):491–3.
24. Barillo DJ. Using mafenide acetate in acute and chronic wounds. Ostomy Wound Manage. 2002;Suppl:5–10.
25. Mendelson JA. Topical mafenide hydrochloride aqueous spray in initial management of massive contaminated wounds with devitalized tissue. Prehosp Disaster Med. 2001;16(3):172–4.
26. Politano AD, Campbell KT, Rosenberger LH, et al. Use of silver in the prevention and treatment of infections: silver review. Surg Infect. 2013;14(1):8–20.
27. Chak KF, Hsiao CY, Chen TY. A study of the effect of Shiunko, a traditional chinese herbal medicine, on fibroblasts and its implication on wound healing processes. Adv Wound Care (New Rochelle). 2013;2(8):448–55.
28. Peng Y. Activated platelet rich plasma precOnditioning induced P13K/AKT/NFκB signal in enhances survival and-regenerative function of rat bone marrow mesenchymal stem cells in hostile environment. Guangzhou: Southern Medical University; 2013.
29. Mckinnon RD, Matsui T, Dubois-Dalcq M, et al. FGF modulates the PDGF-driven pathway of oligodendrocyte development. Neuron. 1990;5(5):603–14.
30. Mcclintock JT, Chan IJ, Thaker SR, et al. Detection of c-sis proto-oncogene transcripts by direct enzyme-labeled cDNA probes and in situ hybridization. In Vitro Cell Develop Biol. 1992;28(2):102–8.
31. Velander P, Theopold C, Hirsch T, et al. Impaired wound healing in an acute diabetic pig model and the effects of local hyperglycemia. Wound Repair Regen. 2008;16(2):288–93.
32. Hirsch T, Spielmann M, Velander P, et al. Insulin-like growth factor-1 gene therapy and cell transplantation in diabetic wounds. J Gene Med. 2008;10(11):1247–52.
33. Mulder G, Tallis AJ, Marshall VT, et al. Treatment of nonhealing diabetic foot ulcers with a platelet-derived growth factor gene-activated matrix (GAM501): results of a phase 1/2 trial. Wound Repair Regen. 2009;17(6):772–9.
34. Ferraro B, Cruz YL, Baldwin M, et al. Increased perfusion and angiogenesis in a hindlimb ischemia model with plasmid FGF-2 delivered by noninvasive electroporation. Gene Ther. 2010;17(6):763–9.
35. Ropper AH, Gorson KC, Gooch CL, et al. Vascular endothelial growth factor gene transfer for diabetic polyneuropathy: a randomized, double-blinded trial. Ann Neurol. 2009;65(4):386–93.
36. Koyama T, Hackl F, Aflaki P, et al. A new technique of ex vivo gene delivery of VEGF to wounds using genetically modified skin particles promotes wound angiogenesis. J Am Coll Surg. 2011;212(3):340–8.
37. Breitbart AS, Laser J, Parrett B, et al. Accelerated diabetic wound healing using cultured dermal fibroblasts retrovirally transduced with the platelet-derived growth factor B gene. Ann Plast Surg. 2003;51(4):409–14.
38. Benn SI, Whitsitt JS, Broadley KN, et al. Particle-mediated gene transfer with transforming growth factor-beta1 cDNAs enhances wound repair in rat skin. J Clin Invest. 1996;98(12):2894–902.
39. Jeschke MG, Barrow RE, Hawkins HK, et al. IGF I gene transfer in thermally injured rats. Gene Ther. 1999;6(6):1015–20.
40. Katsha AM, Ohkouchi S, Xin H, et al. Paracrine factors of multipotent stromal cells ameliorate lung injury in an elastase-induced emphysema model. Mol Ther. 2011;19(1):196–203.
41. Spees JL, Olson SD, Ylostalo J, et al. Differentiation, cell fusion, and nuclear fusion during ex vivo repair of epithelium by human adult stem cells from bone marrow stroma. Proc Natl Acad Sci U S A. 2003;100(5):2397–402.
42. Nakamura Y, Miyaki S, Ishitobi H, et al. Mesenchymal-stem-cell-derived exosomes accelerate skeletal muscle regeneration. FEBS Lett. 2015;589(11):1257–65.
43. Hart AW, Baeza N, Apelqvist A, et al. Attenuation of FGF signalling in mouse beta-cells leads to diabetes. Nature. 2000;408(6814):864–8.
44. Schumacher B, Pecher P, Von Specht BU, et al. Induction of neoangiogenesis in ischemic myocardium by human growth factors: first clinical results of a new treatment of coronary heart disease. Circulation. 1998;97(7):645–50.
45. Ishibashi T. Cell biology of intraocular vascular diseases. Jpn J Ophthalmol. 2000;44(3):323–4.
46. Horner PJ, Power AE, Kempermann G, et al. Proliferation and differentiation of progenitor cells throughout the intact adult rat spinal cord. J Neurosci. 2000;20(6):2218–28.
47. Ray J, Peterson DA, Schinstine M, et al. Proliferation, differentiation, and long-term culture of primary hippocampal neurons. Proc Natl Acad Sci U S A. 1993;90(8):3602–6.
48. Yamamoto M, Ikada Y, Tabata Y. Controlled release of growth factors based on biodegradation of gelatin hydrogel. J Biomater Sci Polym Ed. 2001;12(1):77–88.
49. Vaidya R, Weir R, Sethi A, et al. Interbody fusion with allograft and rhBMP-2 leads to consistent fusion but early subsidence. J Bone Joint Surg (Br). 2007;89(3):342–5.
50. Blazevic T, Schwaiberger AV, Schreiner CE, et al. 12/15-lipoxygenase contributes to platelet- derived growth factor-induced activation of signal transducer and activator of transcription 3. J Biol Chem. 2013;288(49):35592–603.
51. Hoch RV, Soriano P. Roles of PDGF in animal development. Development. 2003;130(20):4769–84.
52. Olofsson B, Pajusola K, Kaipainen A, et al. Vascular endothelial growth factor B, a novel growth factor for endothelial cells. Proc Natl Acad Sci U S A. 1996;93(6):2576–81.
53. Maglione D, Guerriero V, Viglietto G, et al. Two alternative mRNAs coding for the angiogenic factor, placenta growth factor (PLGF), are transcribed from a single gene of chromosome 14. Oncogene. 1993;8(4):925–31.
54. Song G, Ouyang G, Bao S. The activation of Akt/PKB signaling pathway and cell survival. J Cell Mol Med. 2005;9(1):59–71.
55. Pierce GF, Mustoe TA, Altrock BW, et al. Role of platelet-derived growth factor in wound healing. J Cell Biochem. 1991;45(4):319–26.
56. Barres BA, Hart IK, Coles HS, et al. Cell death and control of cell survival in the oligodendrocyte lineage. Cell. 1992;70(1):31–46.
57. Elangovan S, D'Mello SR, Hong L, et al. The enhancement of bone regeneration by gene activated matrix encoding for platelet derived growth factor. Biomaterials. 2014;35(2):737–47.
58. Ha X, Yin Q, Dong F, et al. Study on bone marrow mesenchymal stem cells transfected with adenovirus hepatocyte growth factor gene promoting wounds repair in diabetic rats. Zhongguo Xiu Fu Chong Jian Wai Ke Za Zhi. 2010;24(12):1520–4.
59. Taniyama Y, Tachibana K, Hiraoka K, et al. Local delivery of plasmid DNA into rat carotid artery using ultrasound. Circulation. 2002;105(10):1233–9.
60. Bonafede R, Scambi I, Peroni D, et al. Exosome derived from murine adipose-derived stromal cells: Neuroprotective effect on in vitro model of amyotrophic lateral sclerosis. Exp Cell Res. 2016;340(1):150–8.
61. Xin H, Li Y, Buller B, et al. Exosome-mediated transfer of miR-133b from multipotent mesenchymal stromal cells to neural cells contributes to neurite outgrowth. Stem Cells. 2012;30(7):1556–64.
62. Caplan AI, Dennis JE. Mesenchymal stem cells as trophic mediators. J Cell Biochem. 2006;98(5):1076–84.

63. Gatti S, Bruno S, Deregibus MC, et al. Microvesicles derived from human adult mesenchymal stem cells protect against ischaemia-reperfusion-induced acute and chronic kidney injury. Nephrol Dial Transplant. 2011;26(5):1474–83.
64. Zhu YG, Feng XM, Abbott J, et al. Human mesenchymal stem cell microvesicles for treatment of Escherichia coli endotoxin-induced acute lung injury in mice. Stem Cells. 2014;32(1):116–25.
65. Xin H, Li Y, Liu Z, et al. MiR-133b promotes neural plasticity and functional recovery after treatment of stroke with multipotent mesenchymal stromal cells in rats via transfer of exosome- enriched extracellular particles. Stem Cells. 2013;31(12):2737–46.
66. Lood C, Blanco LP, Purmalek MM, et al. Neutrophil extracellular traps enriched in oxidized mitochondrial DNA are interferogenic and contribute to lupus-like disease. Nat Med. 2016;22(2):146–53.

# 11 New Technology and Tissue Repair and Regeneration (3): Application of Other New Technologies in Tissue Repair and Regeneration

Shenglin Qian, Chong Huang, Biao Cheng, and Xiaobing Fu

## 11.1 Optical Technology

The prismatic visible light can refract seven colors, red, orange, yellow, green, blue, indigo, and purple, with wavelengths ranging from 350 to 770 nm. Electromagnetic waves of different wavelengths have different color perceptions. The band of light is divided into purple 350–455 nm, blue and indigo 455–492 nm, green 492–577 nm, yellow 577–597 nm, orange 597–622 nm, and red 622–770 nm. Light is not only an electromagnetic wave but also a particle flow, which means that light waves have wave-particle duality. According to the theory of optical quantum, the quantum of light has a certain energy, which can cause thermal effects, photochemical effects, and cellular effects [1–3]. In view of the fact that the difference between monochromatic light and laser is not significant in terms of cell-generating effect, the monochromatic light effect and the laser effect are collectively referred to as photobiomodulation.

### 11.1.1 Development History

After Mester et al. [4] first discussed the role of red light in the healing of chronic wounds in 1977, the biological research on red light continued to heat up. Since the 1980s, SCI index has included many papers on wound healing by surface light therapy. With the breakthrough in power and cost of semiconductor light source technology, semiconductor photonic therapy technology has generally begun to enter the clinic. In the 1990s, NASA used semiconductor light sources to treat astronauts' various wounds, ulcers, soft tissue damage, and low immunity under microheavy conditions.

In recent years, the number of relevant research papers and the degree of influence have been continuously improved. They are published in high-end magazines such as *Science*, *Proceedings of the National Academy of Sciences of the United States of America*, *American Journal of Biochemistry*, and *The British Journal of Cardiology*. Classic papers published by Karu, Mester, Abergel, and Reddy have been cited many times. The photobiological regulation is gradually gaining the attention of the scientific community and conducting more in-depth research on the mechanism. In 2003, Zhang et al. [5] published a paper on the relationship between red light irradiation and human fibroblast cDNA gene expression, which is the most cited paper today.

### 11.1.2 Mechanism of Action

Red light refers to light with a wavelength of 600–700 nm, which can produce photochemical effects on living organisms. Red light can directly act on blood vessels, lymphatic vessels, nerve endings, and subcutaneous tissues and play a corresponding therapeutic role. In recent years, clinical research on red light is becoming more and more recognized and valued by people. Red light refers to the physical filtering of most other light, including the removal of ultraviolet ray that has a detrimental effect on the skin and the infrared portion with a significant thermal effect, leaving only the light in the 600–700 nm band. Red light is more penetrating to human body, and the penetration depth can reach more than 30 mm. It is absorbed by the human body's mitochondria After the red light is irradiated, promotes the metabolism of the substance through photochemical action, strengthens the cell activity, improves the immunity of the body and the phagocytosis of macrophages in the wound surface, and promotes the regeneration of epithelial cells, fibroblasts, and the repair of damaged capillaries, which can accelerate wound healing.

S. Qian · C. Huang · B. Cheng
General Hospital of Southern Theater Command of Chinese People's Liberation Army, Guangzhou, China

X. Fu (✉)
The Chinese People's Liberation Army General Hospital, Beijing, China


X. Fu (ed.), *Regenerative Medicine in China*, https://doi.org/10.1007/978-981-16-1182-7_11

In general, the regulation of cellular functions by external signals is mostly achieved by the activation of signal transduction pathways inside the cells. Red light (630 nm) mainly acts through light modulation. The mechanism of light modulation is thought to be the mechanism by which energy-activated switches occur at the mitochondrial level, and the absorbed energy activates cellular functions. Among them, the combination of NO and respiratory chain is the key to energy switching. Cytochrome molecules, especially cytochrome oxidases on the mitochondrial cell membrane, are chromophores that absorb light energy from mitochondria. Red light causes cytochrome oxidase to bind to oxygen molecules by causing NO to dissociate from cytochrome oxidase in the respiratory chain, causing changes in the molecular structure of mitochondrial cell membranes, and adenosine diphosphate (ADP) is converted into adenosine triphosphate (ATP), this process enables the cell battery to be charged to provide sufficient energy for cell activity to enhance cell metabolism, promotes protein synthesis and energy metabolism, changes cell function, and regulates cell gene activity, upregulates or downregulates gene expression activity, and activates or attenuates the signaling pathway of cells, stimulates the release of cytokines by macrophages, increases collagen synthesis in the dermal papilla, increases secretion of cytokine, and reduces secretion and apoptosis of MMP-1 (collagenase), so as to achieve anti-inflammatory effect and promote repair.

The effect of infrared rays on the body is mainly thermal action, which causes the tissue temperature to rise, the local capillaries and small arteries to dilate, the leukocyte infiltration around the blood vessels, and the phagocytic function of the reticuloendothelial cells to be enhanced, which has anti-inflammatory, astringent, and enhanced immunity. The thermal effects of infrared light can also improve local blood circulation, promote inflammation absorption, and eliminate edema to relieve pain. At the same time, due to the accelerated blood circulation, the tissue nutrition is improved, and the cell regeneration ability is enhanced, thereby accelerating the growth of granulation and the formation of molting, and promoting the healing of wounds.

Far-infrared rays have strong penetrating power on human skin and subcutaneous tissues, and can cause vibration of water molecules inside and outside the cell, thereby activating cells to cause the following changes: promote cytoplasmic mitochondrial metabolism and provide more energy. The energy released by ATP is in the 3 μm spectral range, and the far-infrared radiation is given in time to cause the mitochondria of the cells to oxidize to generate more ATP, to maintain all the basic activities of the organism. It can promote the synthesis, metabolism, and function of the nucleic acid along the normal pathway. The far infrared ray with a wavelength of 1–7 μm can be absorbed by protein molecules, resulting in quantum vibration of the amide bond in the molecule, thereby transferring biological energy from one place to another, keeping the living body in a normal state, maintaining the growth, development, and metabolism of the living body. The rotation of NO molecule and the stretching vibration of two atoms along the direction of chemical bond are enhanced to activate the guanylate cyclase, increase the content of cyclic guanosine monophosphate in smooth muscle cells, activate the protein kinase dependent on cyclic guanosine monophosphate, and promote more myosin to be dephosphorylated and relax smooth muscle relaxation vessels. It can maintain cell membrane integrity and permeability, increase cell excitability, and enhances deformability of erythrocyte, remove free radicals generated in metabolism, make cells in excellent condition, and better exert their effects.

Studies have shown that LED red light irradiation has a promoting effect on the radiation-burn combined injury of the wounded mice. C57BL/6 mice were divided into simple trauma group, radiation-burn combined injury group, and red light irradiation group with radiation-burn combined injury. The whole layer of skin was removed from the wound on the back. The radiation-burn combined injury group was uniformly irradiated with 5.0 Gy of $^{60}$Co ray of the whole body at one time on large wounds such as the back. The red light irradiation group with radiation-burn combined injury was exposed to LED red light after the same wound was made. After wound injury, the wound healing of each group and the general condition, body mass, and blood routine of the mice were observed dynamically. At the same time, the temperature inside the irradiated box was observed when the red light was irradiated. Compared with radiation-burn combined injury group, the average healing time of the wounds in the red light irradiation group with radiation-burn combined injury was shortened by 1–2 days ($P < 0.05$), and the white blood cell count of the peripheral blood was 25.41% higher on the 25th day and 37.98% higher ($P < 0.05$) on the 28th day. There was no significant difference in the mass growth between the radiation-burn combined injury group and the red light irradiation group with radiation-burn combined injury ($P > 0.05$).

The skin is the outermost structure of the human body and is the largest organ of the human body. It is mainly composed of epidermis, dermis, and subcutaneous tissue. The skin is not only the sensory organs of the nervous system, but also an effector. It mainly has the functions of barrier, regulating body temperature, sensing internal and external stimuli, metabolism, immunity, etc.

When the skin is damaged and the wound is formed, the healing involves multiple sequential and interdigitated pathophysiological processes: inflammation, cell proliferation, migration and apoptosis, wound remodeling, etc. Various growth factors, cells, inflammatory mediators, and extracellular matrix are involved in the wound healing process. Their interactions form a complex regulatory relationship of wound healing, so that wound healing performs histological repairs with predictable biological steps in an orderly and regular manner. After Mester proposed the role of red light in the treatment of chronic wound healing, there have been various reports on the effects of red light on animals and humans. In recent years, scholars at home and abroad have reported that red light can increase the tensile strength of wound healing tissues in experimental animals, stimulate the increase of collagen production in the wound, and accelerate the healing of skin wounds. Erdle et al. [6] found that 670 nm LED red light promoted wound healing of SKH-1 incision injury in nude mice, but failed to promote healing of burn wounds. These data may be helpful for post-operative wound repair.

Myoblasts are precursor cells that rebuild muscle tissue after trauma. Shefer et al. [7] also found that low-intensity He-Ne lasers (5305 J/m$^2$) can induce skeletal muscle myoblasts to express transcriptional regulatory proteins through the PI3K/Akt and Ras/Raf/ERK pathways. Schieke et al. [8] showed that short-wave infrared (IRA) (760–1400 nm) radiation induces the expression of metalloproteinase-1, not through thermal effects or expression of heat shock protein 70, but through activation of MAPK/ERK 1/2. Whelan et al. [9] used DNA array technology to study the process of light-emitting diode infrared light promoting wound healing in diabetic mice. It was found that tissue regeneration genes expressing integrin, laminin, gap junction protein, and kinesin superfamily molecular motor protein were upregulated. Low-intensity laser irradiation (LPLI) has been found to promote cell survival and proliferation by activating different signaling pathways, and estrogen receptors (ERs, ERα and ERβ) are transcription factors that regulate targeted gene expression, promote cell proliferation, and inhibit activation of apoptotic ligands. Studies have found that LPLI affects intranuclear redistribution and transcriptional activity in a ligand-dependent manner. Studies have shown that LPLI-mediated activation of ERs involves the PI3K/Akt signaling pathway, revealing that the PI3K/AKt signaling pathway is required for LPLI-mediated ERs activation; it was first demonstrated that LPLI relies on PI3K/AKt activity to mediate ligand-dependent ERs intracorporal redistribution and transcriptional activity, provides a direct basis for the molecular mechanism of LPLI-mediated transcription factor activation.

In the analysis of the effects of the system on the use of infrared and near-infrared laser treatment of wounds, it was found that the best results were obtained when red and near-infrared lasers were used simultaneously in the treatment of skin wounds in rats. By applying a wavelength of 400–2000 nm and an energy density of 20 or 40 J/cm$^2$ to the skin wounds of a well-nourished or malnourished mouse, it was found that the nutritional status affected the progress of the treatment and the quality of the healing of the healing tissue, and the use of positive light has a positive effect on biological regulation.

Both cell-level and in vivo studies have shown that red light promotes cell growth and proliferation, reduces inflammation, improves blood circulation, induces collagen deposition, etc. But at the same time, we should consider the choice of wavelength, energy parameters, and irradiation duration of red light, as well as the biological effects of red light on other aspects.

#### 11.1.2.1 Inflammatory Phase

In the early stage of skin healing, the occurrence of infection has a great impact on the repair of wounds. In addition, there are other factors, such as the retention of foreign bodies in the wound, the lack of blood supply, and the location of the wound, which is also one of the factors affecting healing. The previous article on the immune response of red light to wounds has been introduced.

Medrado et al. [10] found red light treatment can reduce inflammation, accelerate collagen deposition and proliferation of myofibroblasts. Nicole et al. [11] found that 1072 nm infrared light has anti-inflammatory effects on skin infections of MRSA, which not only activates the expression of related inflammatory cytokines and enhances immune function, but also promotes the involvement of other growth factors (such as VEGF) in the wound healing process. Low-energy red light at 660 nm stimulates lymphocyte differentiation and proliferation and promotes wound healing.

Experiments have shown that on exposure to low-intensity (660 nm) red light, macrophages release a series of cytokines, stimulate fibroblast proliferation and growth factor synthesis, which in turn affects inflammatory processes, healing and damage repair, resulting in important biological effects and the therapeutic effect, increase cell metabolism, promote cell synthesis, strengthen cell renewal, improve blood circulation, enhance leukocyte phagocytosis, thereby achieving analgesic effect, facilitating wound healing, and promoting hair growth. In vivo experiments found that single-dose red light (wavelength 660 nm) accelerated the repair of skin inflammatory phase in burned mice, which was associated with red light-stimulated angiogenesis and stimulation of leukocyte production. During the healing process of rat skin wounds, it was found that the two kinds of red light alternately irradiated the wound with wavelength 680 + 790 nm; the time of inflammation regression was obviously shortened, the new blood vessels were more abundant, and the collagen expression was higher than that of other groups and was mostly in mature and orderly arrangement.

Zhang et al. [5] used DNA microarray technology to show that red light can regulate gene expression. The wavelength of 628 nm red light can regulate the expression of 111 genes in HS27 fibroblasts. These genes can be divided into ten functional groups, most of which are involved in cell proliferation and inhibition of apoptosis, which involves the signaling pathway initiated by MAPK/p38 and platelet growth factor, and also includes genes related to antioxidant and mitochondrial metabolism. Studies at the genetic level suggest that red light therapy may be beneficial for accelerating wound healing.

Stachon et al. [12] found that photodynamic inactivation transiently stimulated corneal stroma to secrete FGF-β and inhibit HGF secretion (5 h) after culturing human corneal stromal cells with 670 nm red light irradiation, and inhibited the secretion of KGF after 24 h treatment. In the short term, photodynamic inactivation has no effect on the secretion of VEGF and TGF-β1 from the corneal stroma in vitro. As microbes become more resistant to antibiotics, photodynamic inactivation may become a potential treatment option. Similarly, Ankri found that blue light at 480 nm was effective in treating infected wounds, possibly related to the energy absorbed by flavin in this region. Red light at 730 nm was absorbed by cytochrome oxidase, stimulating cell growth and promoting wound closure.

#### 11.1.2.2 Proliferation Stage

This period is divided into two phases: epithelialization and granulation.

Traumatic diseases are closely related to the reduction of the number of blood vessels at the injured site. Vascular repair at the wound site is a complex physiological process. It is regulated by many cytokines and growth factors by direct or indirect regulation, among which vascular endothelial growth factor (VEGF) is the most direct versatile cytokine that promotes angiogenesis, which is essential for angiogenesis and wound repair.

In vitro experiments have shown that human basic fibroblast growth factor (bFGF) itself is both a powerful angiogenic stimulator and a regulator of cell migration and proliferation. bFGF has many biological effects such as promoting angiogenesis at the wound site and early granulation tissue formation. bFGF is a powerful mitogen and chemokine of fibroblast endothelial cells, which has a significant effect on the expression of human VEGF.

In vivo experiments also found that the use of red LEDs with a wavelength of 700 ± 20 nm and a red laser with a wavelength of 660 nm during wound healing in rats significantly increased angiogenesis. In the wound healing of the rat tongue, it was found that the stimulation with 780 nm infrared laser affected the expression of VEGF-A mRNA and shortened the healing time. Recent studies have found that red light at 635 nm promotes endothelial cell proliferation and the corresponding concentration of VEGF decreases; infrared light at 830 nm causes a decrease in TGF-β secretion.

Iron deficiency reduces the production of red blood cells and hemoglobin, and the wound healing process involves many pathophysiological processes, many of which are dependent on the presence of oxygen. In the study of the effects of 660 nm laser and 700 nm light-emitting diode (LED) on the proliferation of fibroblasts in skin wounds of iron-deficient rats, it was found that LED red light played a significant positive role in the regulation of fibroblast proliferation in anemia animals. Lasers are more effective in the proliferation of nonanemic fibroblasts.

Red light treatment also increases the efficiency of mitochondria production of cytochromes, thereby increasing the efficiency of ATP production. The results show that red light irradiation can promote the division of cells and the healing of tissues. Red light irradiation can also significantly shorten the duration of acute inflammatory response in a rat model of acute soft tissue injury, enhance the expression of local growth-promoting factor (IGF-1), and accelerate the regeneration and repair of skeletal muscle.

Susana found that LED red light from 625 to 635 nm promotes wound fibroblast growth and accelerates collagen synthesis. Hawkins et al. [13] found that when red light was used to irradiate fibroblasts and muscle cells, their growth rate was increased by a factor of five. Schindl et al. [14] found that red light at 670 nm can promote the proliferation of human umbilical vein endothelial cells. Studies suggest that promoting the formation of blood vessels or repairing endothelial cells may be one of the mechanisms of red light accelerated wound healing. Some scholars have conducted research and found that the expression of epidermal growth factor (EGF) in tissues is significantly upregulated in patients treated with high-energy red light, indicating that it can proliferate cells to accelerate wound healing.

#### 11.1.2.3 Shaping Stage

This phase is longer, and the new granulation tissue and epithelial cells need to be further divided and differentiated, transformed, matured, and finally the wound is completely healed. Collagen is the main component of the formation of fibrous tissue and promotes the healing of wound skin. Lam et al. [15] used a helium-neon laser (wavelength 632.8 nm) to irradiate human skin fibroblasts, resulting in collagen synthesis ability of fibroblast cell strain, with improved low collagen synthesis ability (up to 36 times).

Reddy and others studies found that 632.8 nm red light can significantly increase the production of collagen in diabetic rats, promote the stability of connective tissue, and accelerate the repair process of damaged tissue.

Mast cells induced fibroblast proliferation and local fiber production. Red light (685 nm) treatment did not increase the rate of fibrosis in mice, but significantly reduced the concentration of autonomous mast cells. Red light (660 nm) penetrates tissue. Local treatment of various skin mucosal erosions, ulcer wounds, and chronic skin diseases with red light can quickly stop the exudation of the wound surface and significantly reduce swelling, thereby accelerating the repair of scarring and wounds, reducing the hyperplasia of scars, and no obvious adverse reactions. Cheng Peng et al. [16] observed the pathological findings of ulcer wound surface of rats irradiated with red light. It is showed that after red light irradiation, epithelial cells and capillary proliferation were obvious, and 9–12 capillary structures were observed under high-power field, and fibroblasts were abundant and arranged neatly. Shu Bin et al. [17] used a circular drill to create a full-thickness skin defect of 6 mm in diameter on the ventral surface of the rabbit ear. He-Ne infrared laser irradiation was performed on the prominent scar 21 days after the operation. It was found that He-Ne infrared laser irradiation made the thickness of the scar thinner. Low-level (670 nm) laser treatment can effectively inhibit the proliferation of fibroblasts in vitro without changing the cell viability and has a definite therapeutic effect on scars. At the wavelength of 700 ± 20 nm, the proliferation of rat fibroblasts was effectively improved.

The main complications of diabetes are delayed wound healing, poor blood supply, and slower collagen production. Most of the complications after flap surgery are related to insufficient blood supply. Santos et al. [18] found that the range of applications for different wavelengths is different, and near-infrared light with a wavelength of 790 nm can effectively increase angiogenesis. Type I collagen is the main component of extracellular matrix and plays an important role in the process of injury repair. Studies have shown that red light at 660 nm has a biological stimulating effect on the synthesis of type I collagen in vivo and in vitro, and cell migration, survival, proliferation, collagen content, and other indicators of damaged cells in diabetic patients were all improved. In addition, studies have found that inhibition of IL-6 production can reduce the formation of scars, while red light treatment can reduce the expression of IL-6 mRNA, hence red light can reduce the formation of scars.

### 11.1.3 Current Application Status

Schindl et al. [19] treated diabetic foot with 632.8 nm red light. It was found that the skin temperature increased significantly after irradiation. Red light irradiation not only improved the blood circulation of the wound, but also enhanced the mitochondrial catalase activity of the experimental animals, increased the cell metabolism, increased glycogen and protein biosynthesis, and promote cell synthesis and wound healing. Some research showed that there was significant difference in wound healing between the two groups ($P < 0.05$). It shows that red light irradiation can promote wound healing without obvious adverse reactions. There were 88 patients with trauma, they were hospitalized in the Trauma Center of Daping Hospital of the Third Military Medical University. Of them, 68 were males and 20 females, age 18–69 (42.23 ± 13.36) years; 48 cases (54.55%) of post-traumatic wound surface, 29 cases (32.95%) after anal fistula wounds, 7 cases of chronic ulcers (7.95%), and III degree pressure sore in 4 cases (4.55%). The Carnation-22 photon therapy device produced by a certain technology company in Shenzhen was selected with a light output of >2 W and a spot diameter of >120 mm. Each irradiation time is 30 min, 2 times/day, and the interval between two exposures is more than 60 min. After the treatment, the wound condition is checked, kept clean, and properly bandaged. The effect was evaluated after 1 week of continuous irradiation. Of all, 31 cases (35.23%) were cured, 20 cases (22.73%) were markedly effective, 19 cases (21.59%) were effective, 18 cases (20.45%) were ineffective, and the total effective rate was 79.55%, and the pain has eased. In 2013, Gupta found that wavelengths of 635 and 810 nm promoted the healing of skin abrasions. The 810 nm wavelength maximized healing, significantly reduced wound area, increased collagen accumulation, and accelerated epithelialization. Compared with the other groups, the 810 nm wavelength group showed increased expression of cytokeratin-14 by immunofluorescence staining. Red light (635 nm) and near-infrared light (810 nm) indicate that the biological response of wound tissue depends on the wavelength used, which may be related to the absorption spectra of cytochrome C oxidase and mitochondria.

After reviewing the relevant literature, the team of Xiaobing Fu found that most of the previous studies on the healing of light in wounds were mostly singular or confusing. The types of cells used by different scholars in experiments were not the same, and often a researcher has studied only one type of cell in the skin. In addition, due to the large difference in cell source (human or animal), illuminating device (laser or LED), wavelength, intensity, energy, and irradiation time, the experimental results are often not completely consistent or even contradictory. The clinical treatment implications that can be provided are often limited. Therefore, the 622–770 nm red light and the 455–492 nm blue light, which have the greatest influence on the healing outcome, were selected for the three main cells (fibroblasts, microvascular endothelial cells, and epidermal cells) of the skin of same species (C57BL/6 mice) for observation at the same time, and according to a large number of literatures, three different energy densities (6, 12, 24 J/cm$^2$) were finally selected to observe their effects on the biological behaviors (migration, proliferation) of cells that mainly involved the three types of wound repair, so as to explore the role of 640 nm and 465 nm LED light in wound healing, clinically seeking the difference between two kinds of visible light in different wound surface problems (healing or overhealing) [1].

The LED light source used in the experiment is the Carnation-11 light therapy instrument provided by a certain technology company in Shenzhen (Fig. 11.1). The power density and main design of the two lamp heads pro-

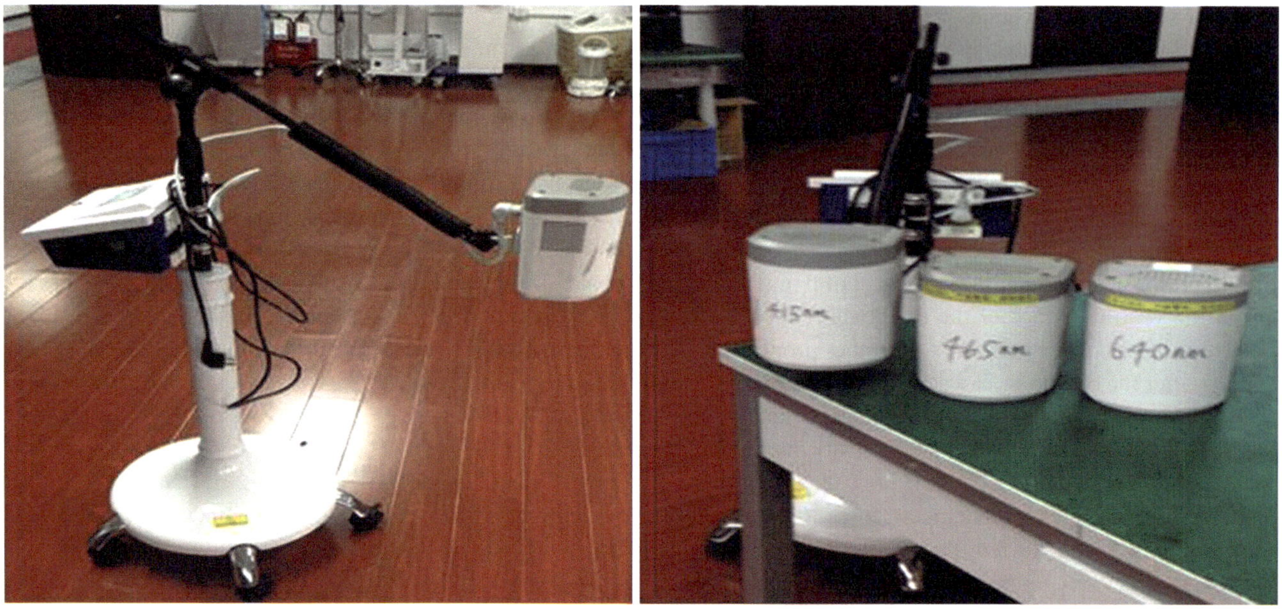


**Fig. 11.1** Carnation-11 light therapy apparatus

vided by Pumen at different distances are shown in Tables 11.1 and 11.2.

The cells in the logarithmic growth phase were seeded in a 12-well plate at a density of 6 × $10^4$/mL. Each plate was a group, and each group was set with four replicate wells and cultured in an incubator. After the number of cells has reached the required level, a syringe needle was used at the bottom of the 12-well plate to scribe horizontally along the center of the plate. A 200 μL tip was used to draw a scratch of approximately 1 mm in the center of the plate. In this way, the scratch and the underline of the orifice plate are just in the shape of "10," which is convenient for observing under the microscope and selecting the intersection as the photographing area. After the scratch, the floating cell debris is washed away with PBS.

The light energy density of 640 nm LED has no significant effect on the migration ability of C57BL/6 mouse skin fibroblasts in the range of 6–24 J/$cm^2$. After 24 h, the scratches of the control group and the experimental group are basically "healed" (as shown in the Fig. 11.2). LED light (640 nm) promoted the proliferation of C57BL/6 mouse skin fibroblasts at an energy density of 12 J/$cm^2$, but no significant impact on proliferation at energy densities of 6 and 24 J/$cm^2$(Fig. 11.3, each group of data is expressed as mean ± standard deviation, $^{**}P < 0.01$).

The 640 nm LED light promoted the migration of C57BL/6 mouse skin microvascular endothelial cells at energy densities of 6 and 12 J/$cm^2$. After 48 h, the scratch width of the two groups was smaller than that of the control group; when the energy density was 24 J/$cm^2$, it inhibited the migration of C57BL/6 mouse skin fibroblasts (Fig. 11.4, data of each group are expressed as mean ± standard deviation, $^{****}P < 0.0001$).

**Table 11.1** Optical power measurement of 465 nm and 640 nm LED lamp head

| | | |
|---|---|---|
| Test object | Microphone pole C11 (50 W LED) + voltage compatible design 465 nm, 640 nm LED | |
| | 465 nm LED: 7 strings and 6 combinations | |
| | 640 nm LED: 10 strings and 5 combinations | |
| Test tools | Fieldmax II-TO laser power meter | |
| Composition of prototype | Microphone pole version body + 465/640 nm LED lamp head rotation test | |
| Light power density values of three lamp heads (MW/$cm^2$) at different vertical distances after conversion of measurement data | | |
| Vertical distance from the front end Face of the lamp head shell (cm) | 640 nm lamp holder | 465 nm lamp holder |
| 5 | 376 | 478 |
| 10 | 178 | 207 |
| 11 | 146 | 0 |
| 12 | 121 | 0 |
| 13 | 99 | 0 |
| 14 | 86 | 0 |
| 15 | 76 | 115 |
| 16 | 0 | 89 |
| 17 | 0 | 83 |
| 18 | 0 | 76 |
| 19 | 0 | 70 |
| 20 | 45 | 64 |
| 21 | 0 | 61 |
| 22 | 0 | 54 |
| 23 | 0 | 51 |
| 24 | 0 | 48 |
| 25 | 30 | 45 |

**Table 11.2** Experimental parameter design

| Index | Red LED | | | Blue LED | | |
|---|---|---|---|---|---|---|
| Wavelength | 640 nm | | | 465 nm | | |
| Exposure distance | 25 cm | | | 25 cm | | |
| Power density | 30 mW/cm$^2$ | | | 45 mW/cm$^2$ | | |
| Irradiation time | 3 min 20 s | 6 min 40 s | 13 min 20 s | 2 min 15 s | 4 min 30 s | 9 min |
| Energy density | 6 J/cm$^2$ | 12 J/cm$^2$ | 24 J/cm$^2$ | 6 J/cm$^2$ | 12 J/cm$^2$ | 24 J/cm$^2$ |

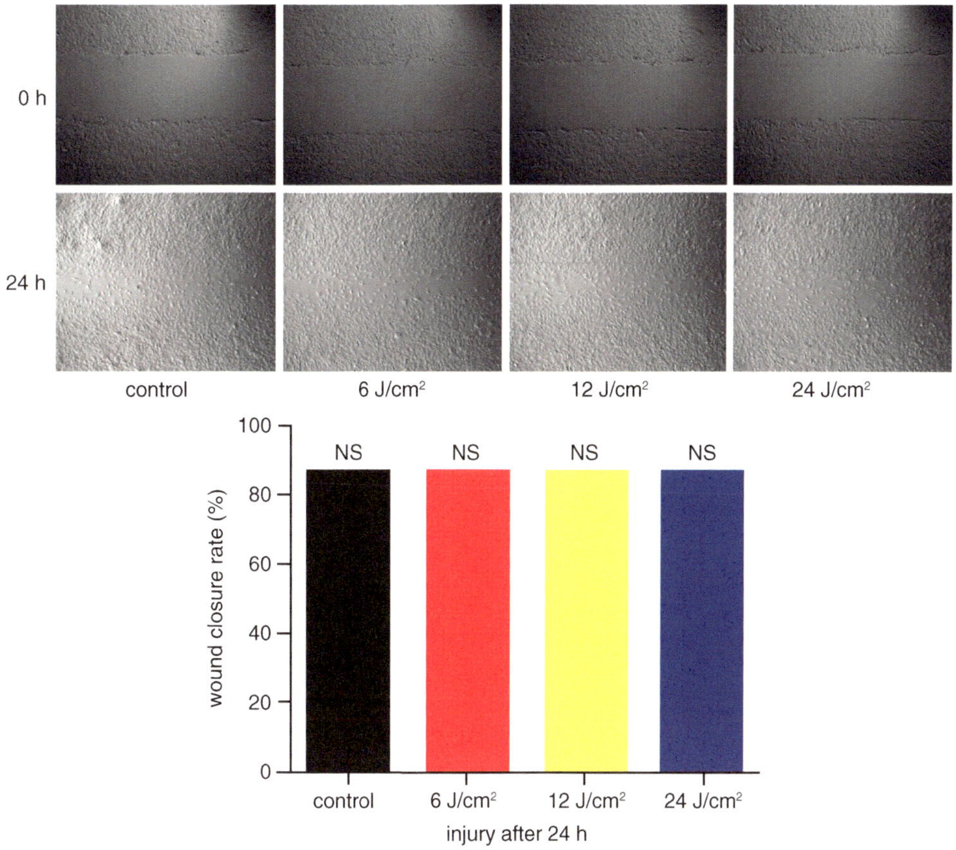


**Fig. 11.2** Effect of 640 nm LED light on migration of C57BL/6 mouse skin fibroblasts

The 640 nm LED light has a significant effect on the proliferation of C57BL/6 mouse skin microvascular endothelial cells at energy densities of 6 and 12 J/cm$^2$, but at an energy density of 24 J/cm$^2$, proliferative capacity has a significant inhibitory effect (Fig. 11.5, each group of data is expressed as mean ± standard deviation, $^{****}P < 0.0001$).

Consistent with the migration experiment results, 640 nm LED light can promote the proliferation of skin epidermal cells of C57BL/6 mice at energy densities of 12 and 24 J/cm$^2$. When the energy density is 6 J/cm$^2$, the epidermal proliferation ability of skin cells of C57BL/6 mice was not significantly different from that of the control group (Fig. 11.6, the data of each group are expressed as mean ± standard deviation, $*P < 0.05$, $**P < 0.01$).

The 640 nm LED light promoted the migration of epidermal cells in C57BL/6 mice at energy densities of 12 and 24 J/cm$^2$. As shown in Fig. 11.7, after 48 h, the scratch width

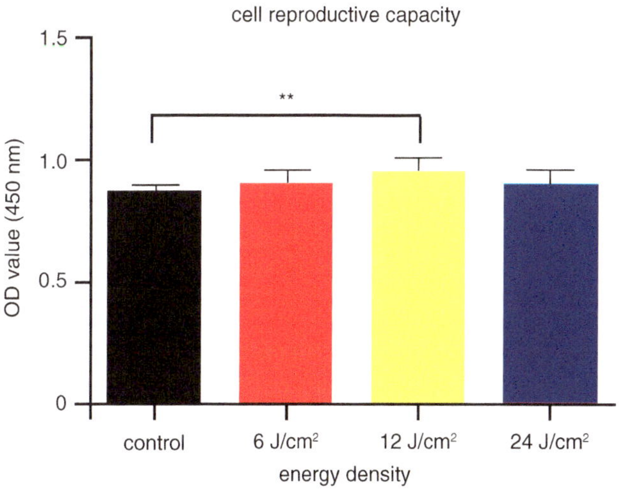


**Fig. 11.3** Effect of 640 nm LED light on the proliferation of C57BL/6 mouse skin fibroblasts

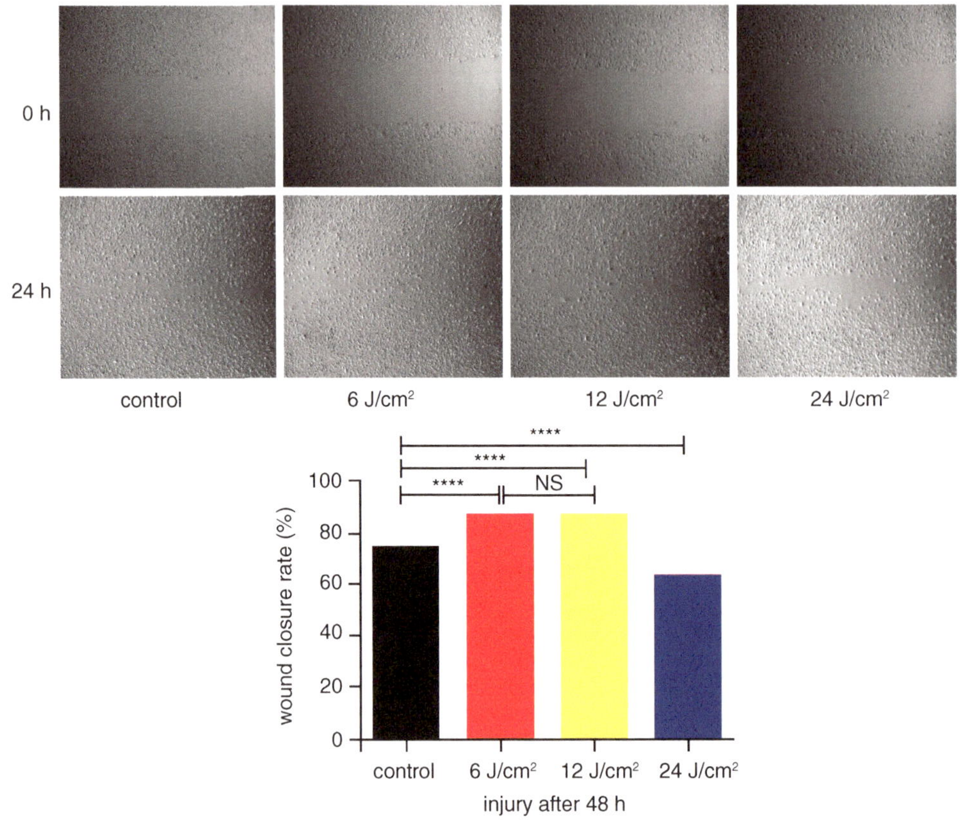


**Fig. 11.4** Effect of 640 nm LED light on the migration of skin microvascular endothelial cells from C57BL/6 mice

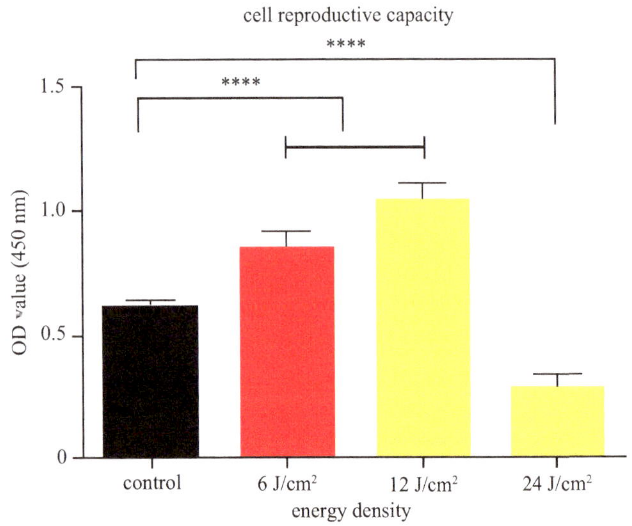


**Fig. 11.5** Effect of 640 nm LED light on the proliferation of C57BL/6 mouse skin microvascular endothelial cells

of the two groups was less than the control group; the effect of energy density of 6 J/cm$^2$ on the migration ability of C57BL/6 mouse skin fibroblasts was not significantly different from that of the control group (data of each group are expressed as mean ± standard deviation, $****P < 0.0001$).

The light energy density of 465 nm LED in the range of 6–24 J/cm$^2$ inhibited the migration ability of C57BL/6 mouse skin fibroblasts. After 24 h, the scratch width of the experimental group was greater than that of the control group (Fig. 11.8, the data of each group are expressed as mean ± standard deviation, $***P < 0.001$, $****P < 0.0001$).

The light energy density of 465 nm LED in the range of 6–24 J/cm$^2$ significantly inhibited the proliferation of C57BL/6 mouse skin fibroblasts, but there was no statistical difference between the three experimental groups (Fig. 11.9, each group of data is expressed as mean ± standard deviation, $****P < 0.0001$; NS: no significance difference).

The light energy density of 465 nm LED has an inhibitory effect on the migration ability of C57BL/6 mouse skin microvascular endothelial cells in the range of 6–24 J/cm$^2$. After 48 h, the scratch width of the experimental group is larger than that of the control group (Fig. 11.10, the data of each group are expressed as mean ± standard deviation, $****P < 0.0001$).

The 465 nm LED light inhibited the proliferation of C57BL/6 mouse skin microvascular endothelial cells in an energy-dependent manner, as shown in Fig. 11.11. The higher the energy density of 465 nm light, the more obvious the inhibition of microvascular endothelial cell proliferation

**Fig. 11.6** Effect of 640 nm LED light on the proliferation of epidermal cells in C57BL/6 mice

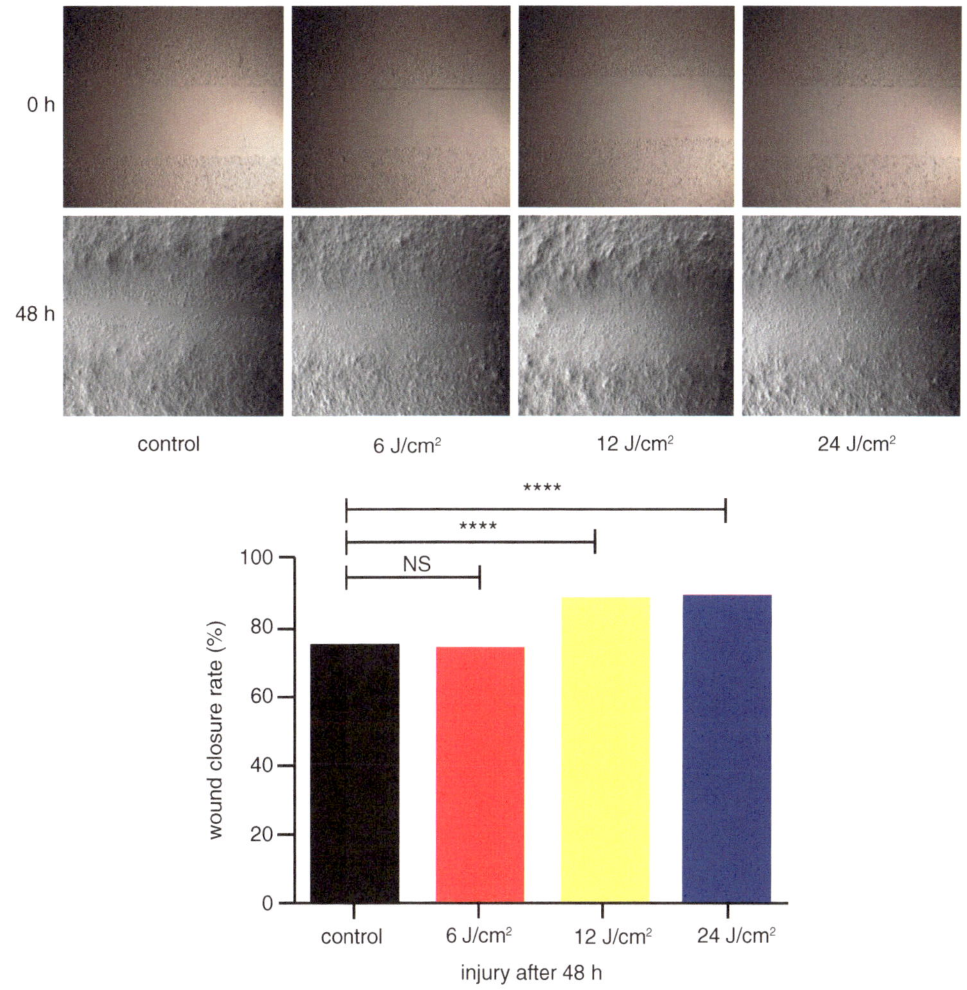


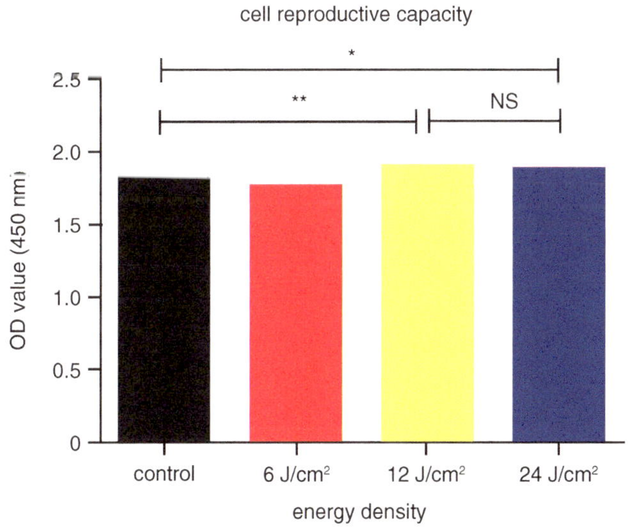


**Fig. 11.7** Effect of 640 nm LED light on the migration of skin epidermal cells in C57BL/6 mice

(data for each group are expressed as mean ± standard deviation, $****P < 0.0001$).

The light energy density of 465 nm LED in the range of 6–24 J/cm$^2$ inhibited the migration of skin epidermal cells of C57BL/6 mice. After 48 h, the scratch width of the experimental group was greater than that of the control group (data for each group are expressed as mean ± standard deviation, $****P < 0.0001$, as shown in Fig. 11.12).

LED light (465 nm) inhibited the proliferation of C57BL/6 mouse skin epidermal cells at three energy densities (data of each group are expressed as mean ± standard deviation, $**P < 0.01$, $****P < 0.0001$, Fig. 11.13).

A summary of the above results is shown in Table 11.3.

The experimental results show that the effects of 640 nm red light on the biological behavior of the three cells are not the same. Its experimental results on fibroblasts showed that the fibroblast proliferation ability was significantly promoted at an energy density of 12 J/cm$^2$, and the energy was too high

**Fig. 11.8** Effect of 465 nm LED light on migration of C57BL/6 mouse skin fibroblasts

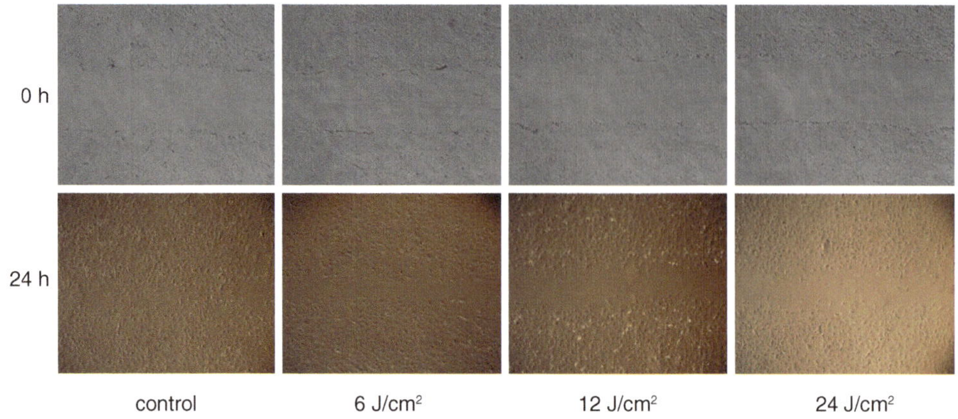


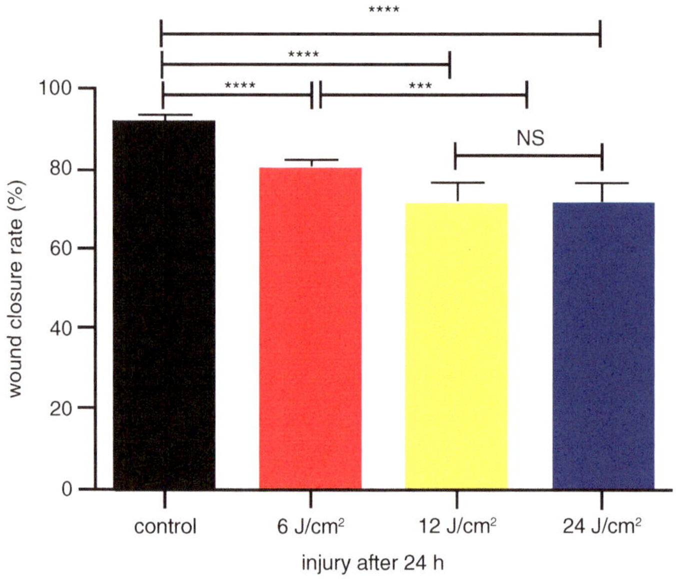


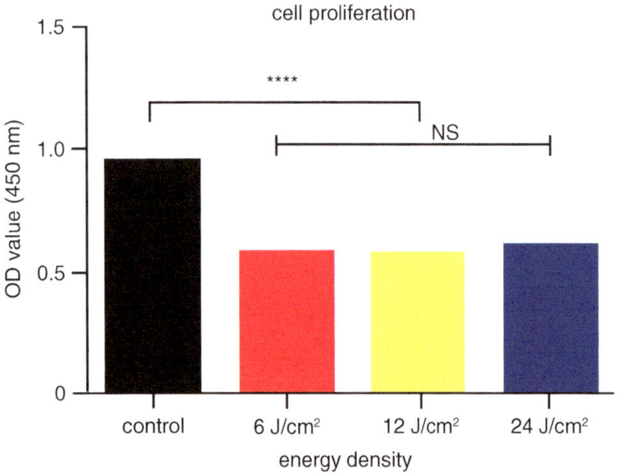


**Fig. 11.9** Effect of 465 nm LED light on the proliferation of C57BL/6 mouse skin fibroblasts

(24 J/cm$^2$) or too low (6 J/cm$^2$) and has no significant effect, and the three different energy densities had no significant effect on the migration ability of fibroblasts, suggesting that the effect of 640 nm red light on C57BL/6 murine fibroblasts is mainly concentrated on their proliferative capacity; when the wavelength of C57BL/6 mice skin microvascular endothelial cells was 640 nm and the energy density was 6 to 12 J/cm$^2$, it was shown to promote migration and proliferation. When the energy density reached 24 J/cm$^2$, the migration and proliferation ability were inhibited. When the energy density was 12–24 J/cm$^2$, the migration and proliferation of skin epidermal cells of C57BL/6 mice showed a promoting effect, but when the energy density decreased to 6 J/cm$^2$, there was no significant effect on their migration and proliferation ability.

The 465 nm blue light has a similar effect on the biological behavior of the three kinds of cells. Under the premise of no cytotoxicity, the three energy densities have a certain degree of inhibition on the migration and proliferation of the three kinds of cells.

It can be seen from the experimental results that the 640 nm LED light has different effects on the migration and proliferation of the three main cells involved in the wound repair process. This is consistent with the experimental

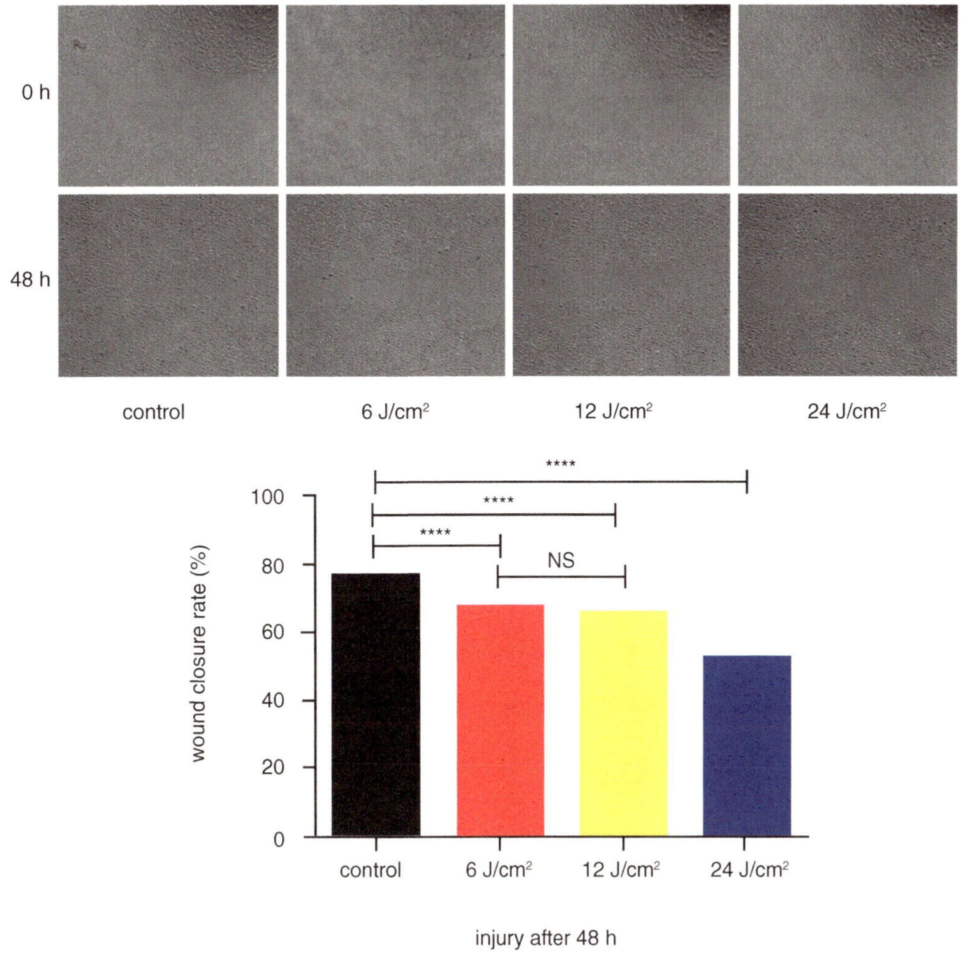


**Fig. 11.10** Effect of 465 nm LED light on the migration ability of C57BL/6 mouse skin microvascular endothelial cells

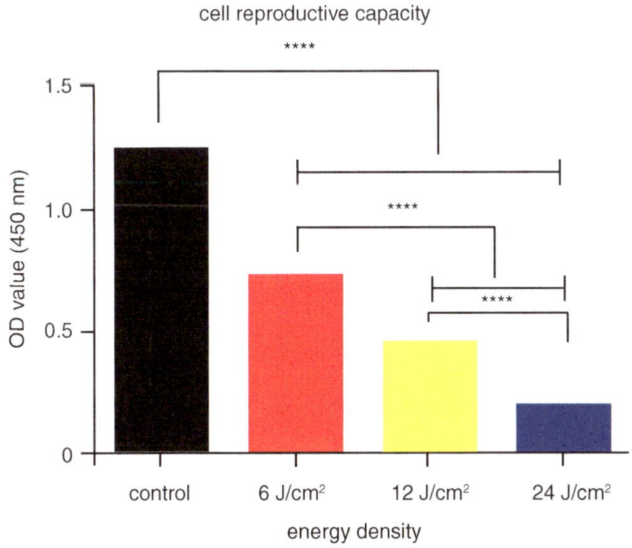


**Fig. 11.11** Effect of 465 nm LED light on the proliferation of C57BL/6 mouse skin microvascular endothelial cells

assumptions. It is confirmed that the optimal energy required for different cells to participate in wound repair is not exactly the same. If blindly irradiated with a single energy, it may be beneficial to some cells but harmful to other cells, which is not conducive to maximizing the role of different repair cells in wound healing. It should be based on the time when different cells participate in wound healing and their response to different energy densities, and select the most appropriate parameters and appropriate time to get the best healing quality.

At the same time, the specific mechanism of how light promotes wound healing is still not very clear. Only a few reports suggest that light may regulate the migration of oral epithelial cells by regulating mTOR. However, there is very little understanding of phototherapy during the re-epithelialization of wounds. Therefore, the team of Xiaobing Fu academicians focused on the role of phototherapy in the migration of human epidermal cells and its mechanism. In some cells, light can regulate changes in the

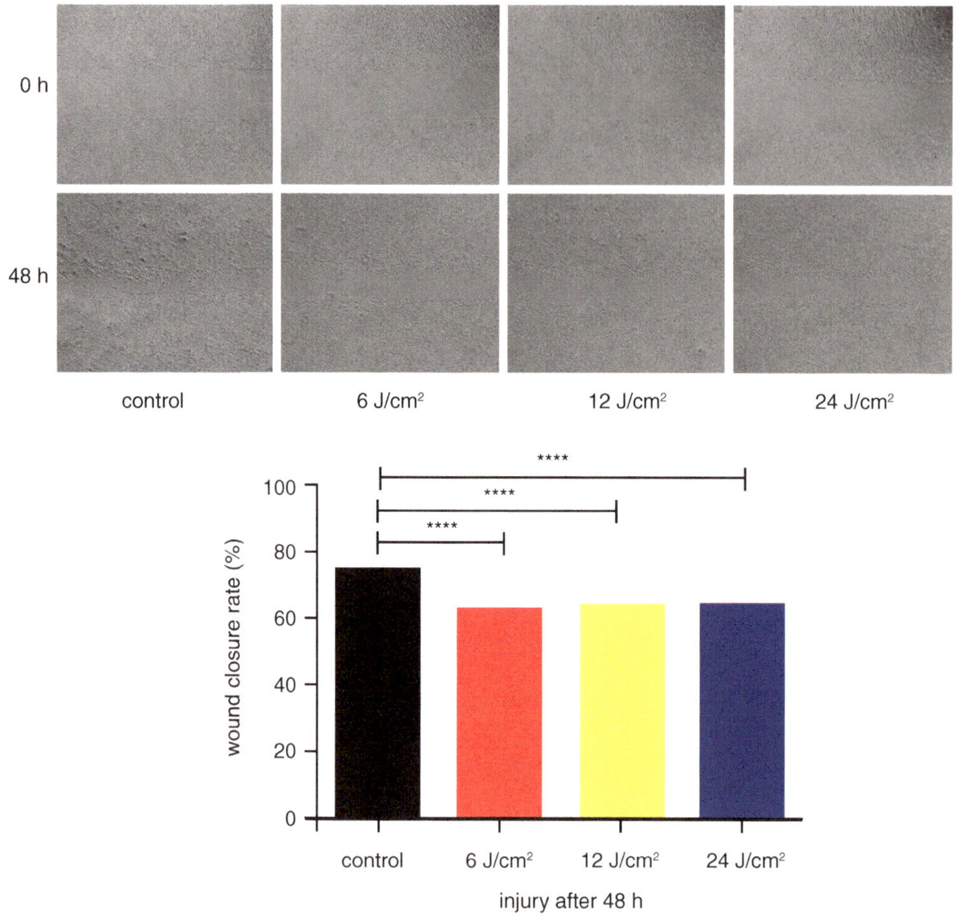


**Fig. 11.12** Effect of 465 nm LED light on the migration of skin epidermal cells in C57BL/6 mice

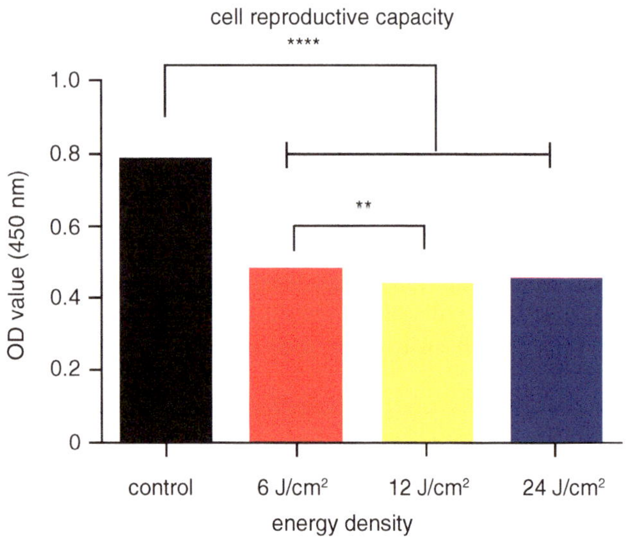


**Fig. 11.13** Effect of 465 nm LED light on the proliferation of epidermal cells in C57BL/6 mice

cytoskeleton. It is first assumed that light can regulate the redistribution of the cytoskeleton through HIF-1α, which in turn affects cell migration. [2] Thereby, to clarify the mechanism of phototherapy to promote wound healing in wound healing.After circumcision of 6–12 years old, the human tissue was taken in strict accordance with the International Ethics Guidelines for Biomedical Research in People and approved by the hospital ethics committee. Human primary keratinocytes are isolated and cultured by two-step digestion. Human keratinocyte movement was observed after red light irradiation of two different energies (12 and 24 J/cm$^2$). It was found that red light significantly enhanced the motility of keratinocytes. The parameters set on the specific red light are shown in Table 11.4. After 3 h of red light irradiation, each group is placed in a living cell workstation. Shoot once every 3 min for a total duration of 2 h. Save the recorded video after recording ends. Through software comparison analysis, it was found that the cell motility was significantly enhanced after red light irradiation, and the 12 J/cm$^2$ energy group was more obvious. Migration in the 12 J/cm$^2$ group increased by 41.9% and 24 J/cm$^2$ group increased by 18.3%. As can be seen from the results, 640 nm LED red light can significantly promote the migration of keratinocytes (Fig. 11.14).

In the living cell workstation, the 12 J/cm$^2$ energy group has a more pronounced promoting effect, so this experiment only chose to study the energy of 12 J/cm$^2$. This energy was used to observe the effect of red light on the migration of a

**Table 11.3** Effects of 640 nm red light and 465 nm blue light on cell biology

| Index | Red LED | | | | | | | | | Blue LED | | | | | | | | |
|---|---|---|---|---|---|---|---|---|---|---|---|---|---|---|---|---|---|---|
| Irradiation time | 3 min 20 s | | | 6 min 40 s | | | 13 min 20 s | | | 2 min 15 s | | | 4 min 30 s | | | 9 min | | |
| Energy density | 6 J/cm$^2$ | | | 12 J/cm$^2$ | | | 24 J/cm$^2$ | | | 6 J/cm$^2$ | | | 12 J/cm$^2$ | | | 24 J/cm$^2$ | | |
| Migration effect | FBC | mDMEC | mDEC | FBC | mDMEC | mDEC | FBC | mDMEC | mDEC | FBC | mDMEC | mDEC | FBC | mDMEC | mDEC | FBC | mDMEC | mDEC |
| | – | ↑ | – | – | ↑ | ↑ | – | ↓ | ↑ | ↓ | ↓ | ↓ | ↓ | ↓ | ↓ | ↓ | ↓ | ↓ |
| Proliferation effect | FBC | mDMEC | mDEC | FBC | mDMEC | mDEC | FBC | mDMEC | mDEC | FBC | mDMEC | mDEC | FBC | mDMEC | mDEC | FBC | mDMEC | mDEC |
| | – | ↑ | – | ↑ | ↑ | ↑ | – | ↓ | ↑ | ↓ | ↓ | ↓ | ↓ | ↓ | ↓ | ↓ | ↓ | ↓ |

**Table 11.4** Specific parameter settings for the lighting application

| Parameter setting | |
|---|---|
| Wavelength | 640 nm |
| Power output | 15 W |
| Dose | |
| Average energy | 12 J/cm$^2$, 24 J/cm$^2$ |
| Energy density | 30 mW/cm$^2$ |
| Irradiation duration | 6 min 40 s, 13 min 20 s |
| Exposure distance | 25 cm |

single layer of keratinocytes. The keratinocytes were plated on the culture plate and scratches were made by using a 200-μL tip. The photographs were taken at 0, 12, and 24 h, respectively. The light group was significantly healed 20% faster than the control group (Fig. 11.15).

LED light promotes the healing of a single layer of keratinocyte scratched wounds. A monolayer of keratinocytes was made by passing a single layer of cells with a 200-μL tip. The control group and the light group (12 J/cm$^2$) were

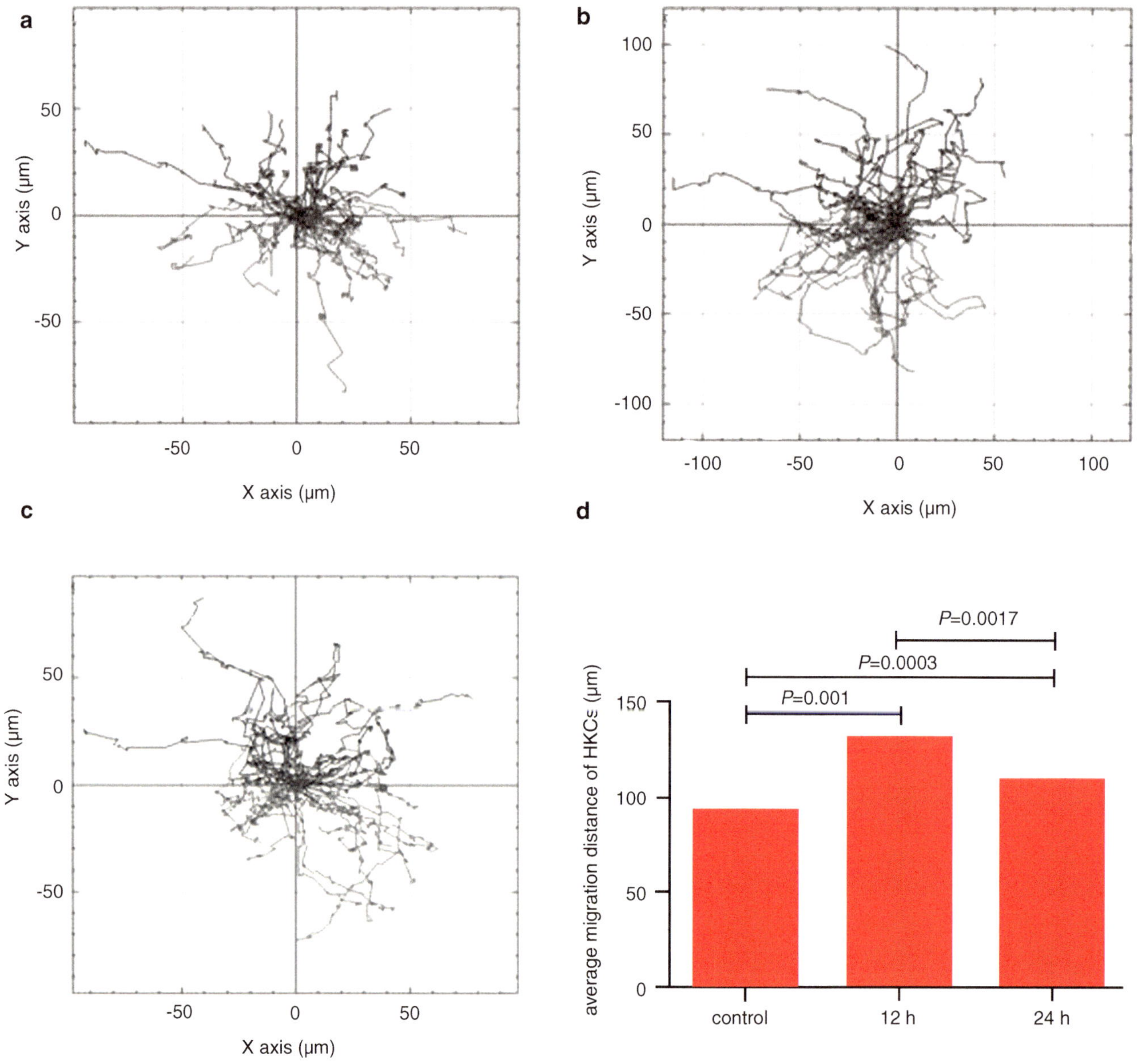


**Fig. 11.14** Effect of 640 nm LED red light on keratinocyte migration. LED light can improve the motility of human keratinocytes: it is divided into unilluminated group and 12 and 24 J/cm$^2$ light group, and measured after 3 h of illumination. (**a**–**c**) The position of each cell is recalibrated once every 3 min. In the figure, the starting position of each cell is set to be the same. (**d**) In 2 h, the travel distance of each cell was counted and analyzed. More than three independent trials, the number of cells is not less than 50. Expressed by mean ± standard deviation. $P < 0.01$ means that there is a difference in statistics.

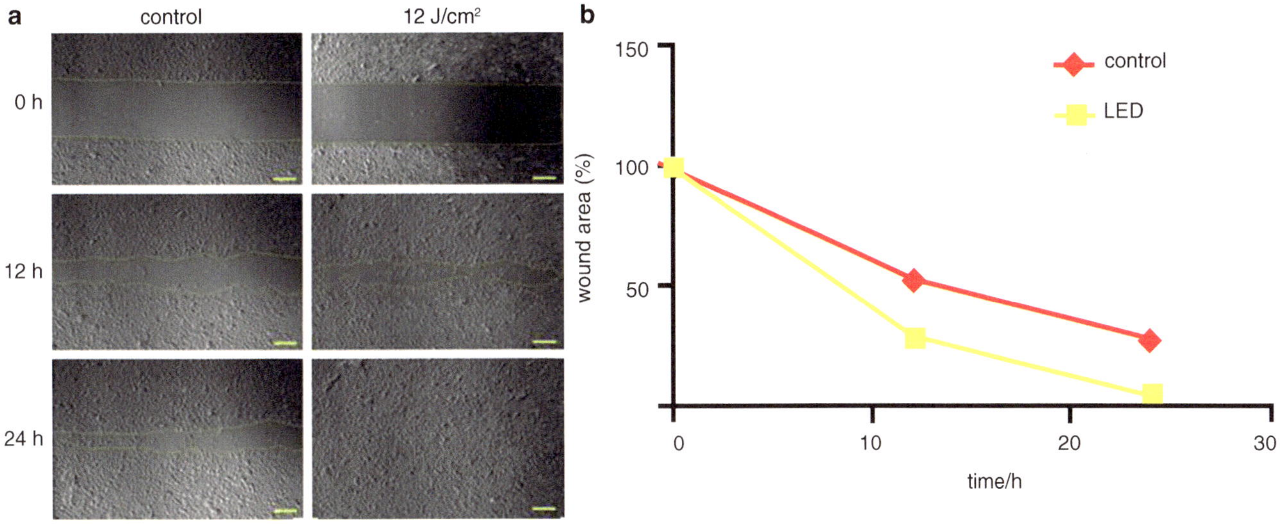


**Fig. 11.15** The effect of LED light on the healing of single-layer keratinocyte scratched wounds (**a**) photos of the scratch area (**b**) statistical graph of the scratch area

observed under the microscope. A. Photographs were taken after 0, 12, and 24 h of scratches, and the wound edges were marked with yellow marking lines. B. The wound area was measured with Photoshop CS4 software. The initial area was used as the initial wound area, and then the wounded wound ratio was calculated. The test was repeated more than three times, expressed as mean ± standard deviation, $P < 0.01$ indicating statistical difference. The yellow rule bar in the figure is bar =100 μm.

To determine whether the main effect of wound healing in the scratch test was cell migration or cell proliferation, we tested the proliferation of each subpopulation using the CCK-8 kit. Red light was not found to be effective in promoting the proliferation of human epidermal cells by analyzing the OD values in 96-well plates (Fig. 11.16).

The cytoskeleton plays an important role in cell migration, and the motility of cell migration is derived from the constant replacement of cell actin polymerization and depolymerization. In order to clarify the changes in light to the cytoskeleton, the research team further observed changes in the expression of HIF-1α in keratinocytes and changes in keratinous cytoskeleton. Protein expression changes were recorded at 0, 3, 6, and 12 h after illumination. In the case of normoxia, LED light sources can increase protein expression (Fig. 11.17).The cytoskeleton was observed by using cobalt chloride and dimethyloxallyl glycine (DMOG) to affect HIF-1α, and the effect of HIF-1α on the keratinocyte cytoskeleton F-actin was determined. The cells treated with cobalt chloride and DMOG were stained into tablets, and the state of F-actin was observed under fluorescence. It was found that F-actin in the keratinocytes of the two drug groups was spread more than the normal control group. Combined with the previous results, it is preliminarily concluded that the redistribution of the cytoskeleton by the LED light source

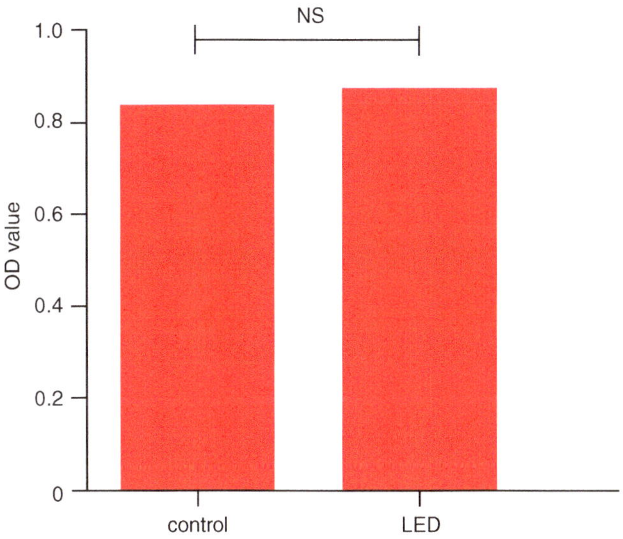


**Fig. 11.16** Effect of LED red light on keratinocyte proliferation. LED red light has no effect on keratinocyte proliferation. The OD value between the two groups of cells was measured using a CCK-8 kit under LED red light (12 J/cm$^2$) irradiation. Expressed as mean ± standard; ns: not statistically significant ($P = 0.425 > 0.05$)

may be regulated by HIF-1α. Finally, it is necessary to observe whether the regulation of HIF-1α can block the regulation of the cytoskeleton by the light source. Using the specific inhibitor YC-1 (HIF-1α specific inhibitor) to understand the downregulation of HIF-1α LED light regulation of the cytoskeleton, the results showed that YC-1 can effectively block the expression of HIF-1α. The simultaneous downregulation of HIF-1α can effectively inhibit the red light on the cytoskeleton rearrangement, with or without light treatment. After statistics, it was found that the percentage of polarized cytoskeleton in the control group was 25 ± 2%, and the percentage of cytoskeleton polarization in the illumination group was 48 ± 1%. After YC-1 treatment, the pseudopods and actin microfilaments after red light stimulation were significantly inhibited. Therefore, it can be considered that YC-1 can effectively block the regulation of red light on keratinocyte cytoskeleton by downregulating HIF-1α. Combined with previous studies, it was further confirmed that LED light can regulate cell cytoskeleton changes through HIF-1α, thereby affecting cell migration (Figs. 11.18, 11.19, 11.20, and 11.21).

In conclusion, red light can increase the expression of keratinocyte HIF-1α, while blocking HIF-1α can reverse the effect of red light on keratinocyte cytoskeleton changes and further affect cell migration.

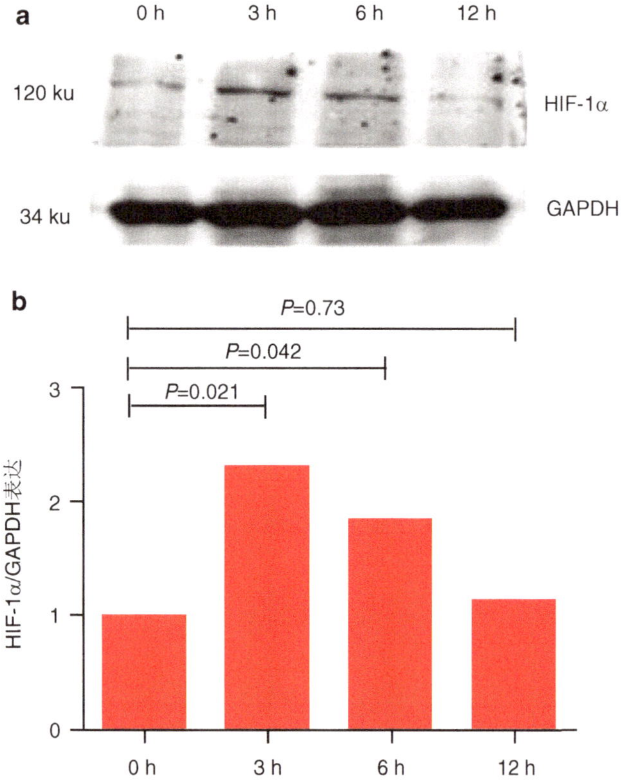


**Fig. 11.17** Illumination allows more cells to produce actin filaments and lamellipodia. The 12 J/cm² LED source increased the expression of F actin in keratinocytes by 32.9% and 42.3% ($n = 100$) after 3 h and 6 h, respectively (**a**) photo (**b**) statistical graph

### 11.1.4 Problems and Future Prospects

In summary, red light is closely related to skin wound healing. In recent years, clinical research on red light has been increasingly recognized and valued. Red light promotes cell growth and proliferation, reduces inflammation, improves blood circulation, improves the nutrition and blood oxygen supply of local tissues, promotes the proliferation of peripheral epithelium, induces collagen deposition, and so on. In addition, under the "wet healing" theory, the local moisturization of the wound surface is not formed, and the wet healing environment close to the physiological state is beneficial to the growth of the granulation tissue, which facilitates the splitting of the skin cells and promotes the complete healing of the wound. With the further understanding and research of this viewpoint, the superiority of wet healing has been confirmed and become the mainstream method of wound healing. Therefore, the "cold light" effect of "weak laser therapy" seems to be more in line with the requirements of future development and may become the mainstream direction.

## 11.2 Bioelectricity/Biomagnetism

In physics, there is a branch called "electromagnetism." In electromagnetism, there is a close relationship between electricity and magnetism. Electric energy generates magnetism and magnetic energy generates electricity. As a special type of electromagnetism—bioelectricity and biomagnetism, it

**Fig. 11.18** Effect of HIF-1α on keratinocyte cytoskeleton (**a**) photo (**b**) statistical graph

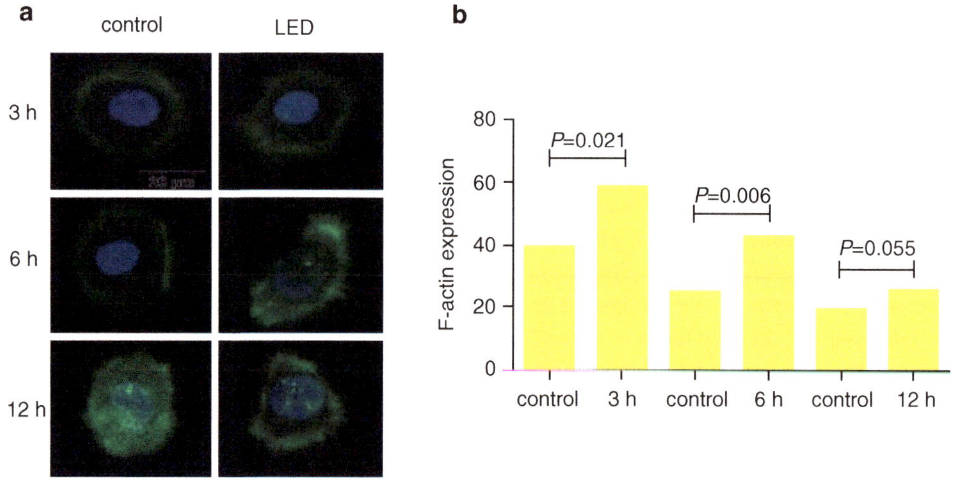

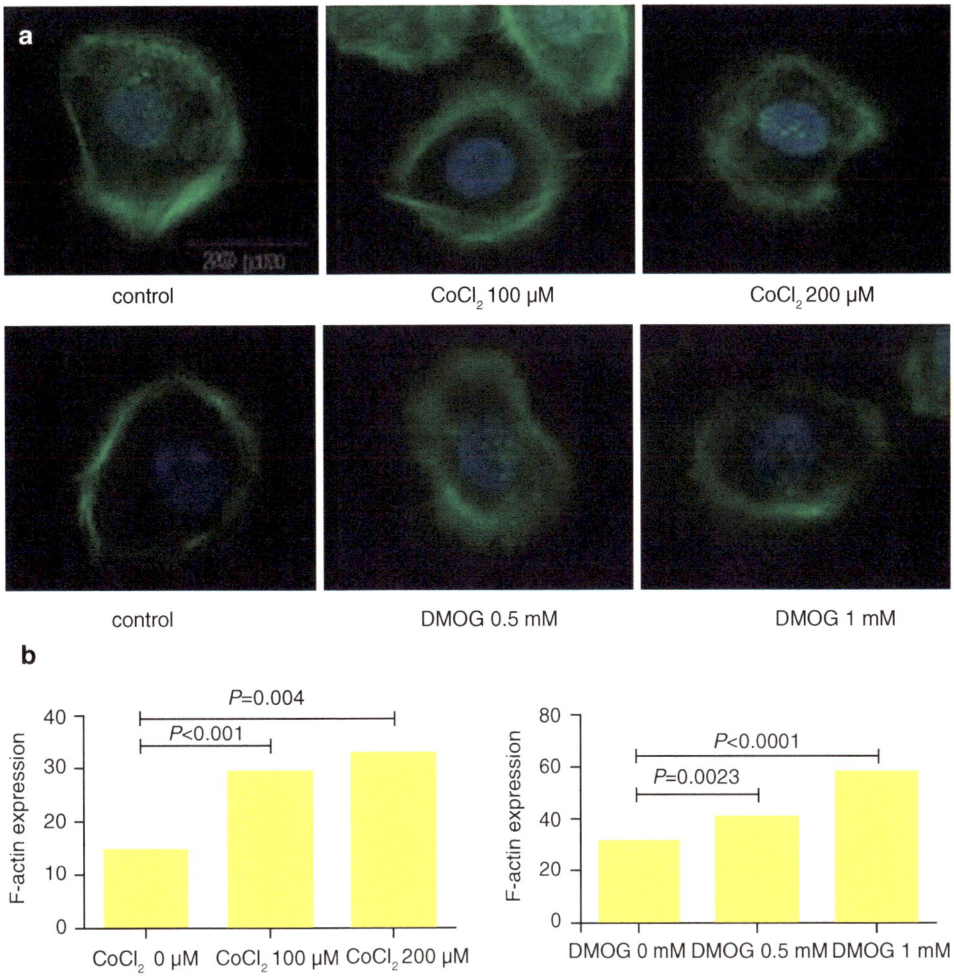


**Fig. 11.19** Effect of cobalt chloride and DMOG two HIF-1α agonists on human keratinocyte F-actin (**a**) photo (**b**) statistical graph

not only has the electrical and magnetic properties of matter, but also has the characteristics of bioelectricity and biomagnetism, namely, initiative and passiveness. Research on bioelectricity and biomagnetism is of great significance for the repair and regeneration of wound tissue.

### 11.2.1 Electrical Signals

Bioelectric phenomena are the basic attributes of life activities. Bioelectricity is produced in all life processes of the body. The so-called bioelectrical phenomenon refers to the potential change and current conduction generated in the living body and its relationship with life phenomena and functions.

Studies of intact skin and damaged wounds have shown that ion current on the surface of the skin is an important factor influencing healing. As early as 1940, Burr found that abdominal wounds produced positive transepithelial electrical through the epidermal skin. As the number of cells increased during healing, the polarity of the wound current changed. The same effect was confirmed during wound healing in guinea pig full-thickness skin defects. Illingworth also found that 10–30 μA/cm$^2$ of current appeared on the stump finger after trauma. Foulds reported that the average voltage between the human skin surface and the dermis was 23 mV after inserting the human dermis into the electrode. Barker et al. [20] found in animal models that hairless skin has a TEP of 30–100 mV and below the dermis is the negative electrode. In hairy skin, there is only 0–10 mV around the gland. TEP is reduced in the cut epidermis, creating an electric field parallel to the skin surface between the wound and the intact epidermis, which can reach 200 mV/mm.

It has been demonstrated that the transcutaneous potential energy of the basal keratinocyte plasma membrane is the result of the action of the Na ion pump. In the frog skin of amphibians, the basal and lateral membranes cross the true-skin junction through the Na ion current, producing a voltage of 80–100 mV, and the tight junctions between the epidermis prevent short circuits between the gradient energies. When this backflow is interrupted, the Na ion pump of the substrate layer produces a "wound current." An increase in the concentration of Na ions in the solution of 1.5 mmol/L produces a potential energy of 60 mV. When the embryonic epithelium

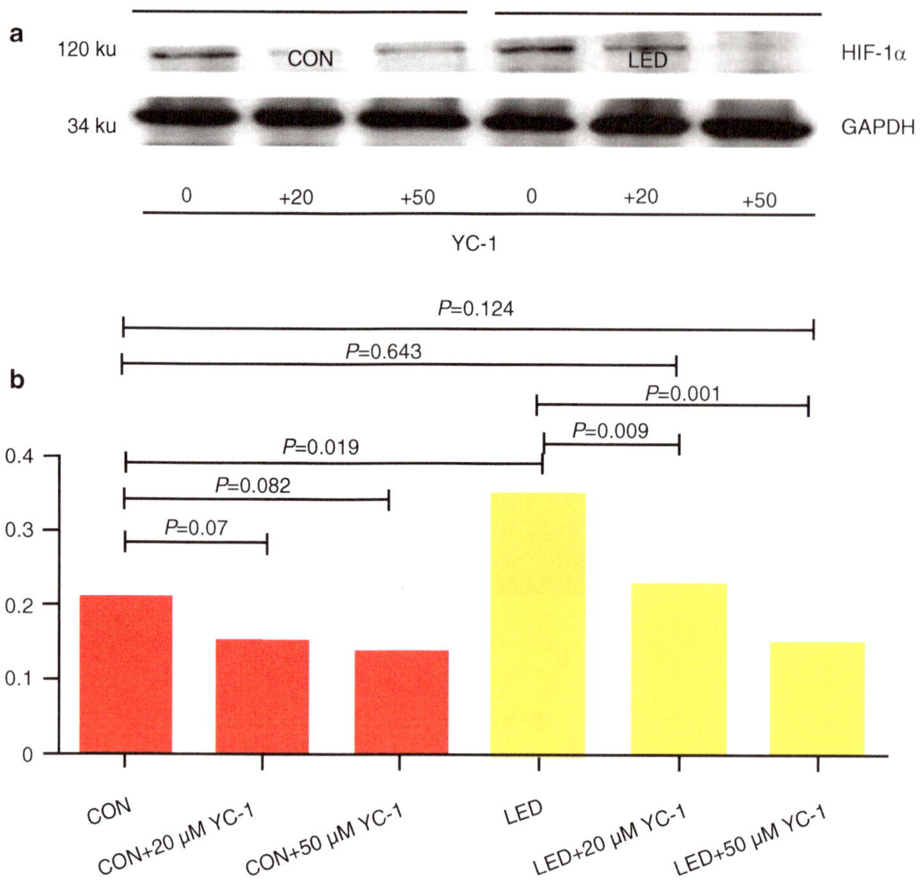


**Fig. 11.20** YC-1 reduces HIF-1α accumulation in human keratinocytes. (**a**, **b**) Cells were treated with different concentrations of YC-1 (0, 20, 50 μM) for 8 h, and each group (12 J/cm$^2$) was irradiated with red light for about 3 h. The expression of each of the grouped proteins was then examined

of the toad is cut, it produces a current of 16.7 μA/cm$^2$, which is important for healing. Other experiments have also proved that Na ion current is an important basis for the formation of mammalian potential energy. For example, the Na ion current of the fetus can reach 20–100 μA/cm$^2$.

The directed migration of cells is a guarantee of tissue formation, inflammatory response, and wound healing. Among them, chemotaxis plays an important role. Endogenous electric fields (EFs) determine the direction of cell migration. In 2002, Zhao et al. [21] found that physiological redistribution of EFs and EGFRs (epidermal growth factor receptors) resulted in increased activity of mitogen-activated protein kinases (MAPKs), which cause the polymerization of actin on the wound edge, thus in turn causes migration of epithelial cells. Antagonizing the EGF receptor-type MAPKs signaling pathway will significantly reduce actin distribution and cell migration activity.

Pulsed electromagnetic fields (PEMFs) can lead to programmed cell death in T cells. It has been hypothesized that PEMFs control the proliferation of inflammatory lymphocytes and thus affect the inflammatory process. The various cytokines produced in inflammation are important regulators in wound repair. The expression of mRNA of many cytokines was enhanced by reverse transcription polymerase chain reaction (RT-PCR).

Fibroblasts produce collagen matrices as a result of changes in cellular metabolism due to electric field prevalues. Mcleod proved that the electric field's electricity, frequency, and cell orientation determine the biosynthesis process of fibroblasts, and the cell alignment is consistent with the electric field curve. In these cells, when the electric field voltage is lower than 40 mV/cm for more than 12 h, the proline entering the extracellular matrix protein will decrease by 20%, unless the electric field voltage is increased by five times, otherwise the vertically aligned cells will not react.

In 1987, foreign scholars confirmed that human fibroblasts were inserted into a 100-Hz electrode and stimulated by a current of 40 V/cm for 20 min. Studies involving $^3$H-proline and $^3$H-thymidine deoxynucleosides indicated protein synthesis and DNA synthesis were significantly increased. This effect was frequency dependent, with proteins synthesized at 120 Hz and 16.6 V/cm maximal, and 23.3 V/cm at 60 Hz. The synthesis of DNA also has this rule.

### 11.2.2 Magnetic Signal

Biomagnetic phenomena are the magnetic fields generated in living organisms and their relationship to life phenomena. In 1963, Balule and Mefee of the University of Syracuse, USA,

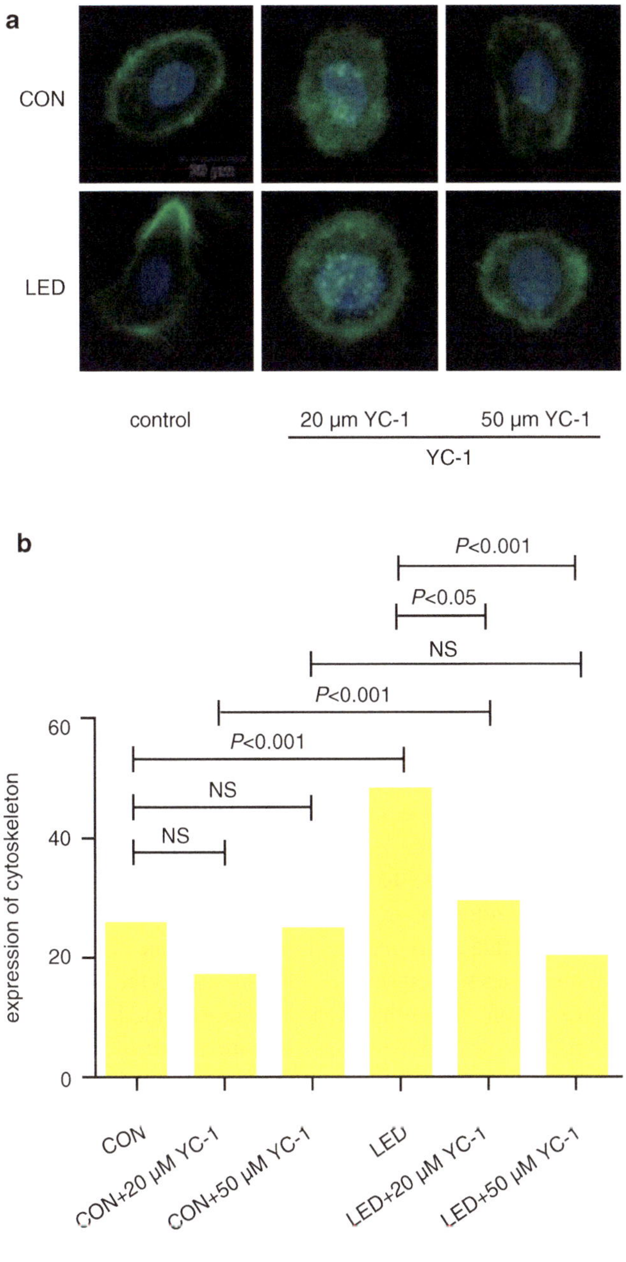


**Fig. 11.21** Effect of YC-1 inhibition of LED light on keratinocyte rearrangement. YC-1 inhibits the effect of LED light on keratinocyte rearrangement (**a**, **b**). After treatment with cells at three concentrations of YC-1 (0, 20, and 50 μM), irradiate with red light (12 J)/cm$^2$) for 3 h

recorded cardiac magnetic signals for the first time from the human body. The Biot-Savart theorem of physics "the electric charge generates a magnetic field," so a biomagnetic signal must be generated at the same time as long as the bioelectrical signal can be generated. The magnetic field generated by biological currents (produced by natural biocurrents), human organs and tissues undergo bioelectrical processes such as electron transfer, ion transfer, and neuroelectric activity during activities. These bioelectrical processes produce biological currents with different frequencies, intensities, and waveforms, resulting in a corresponding weak biological magnetic field, such as a magnetic field, a brain magnetic field, a neural magnetic field, a muscle magnetic field, and the like. The strength of biological magnetic fields is generally very weak, often buried in the environmental magnetic noise, the general detection instruments cannot be detected, with the continuous development of science and technology, the problem is gradually solved.

Strong magnetic fields have an impact on metabolism, cell differentiation, biochemical variation, and even neurophysical physics. The tissues, organs, etc., of the living body are placed in the external magnetic field, and the biological tissues, organs, and the like will have a certain biological effect under the action of the external magnetic field. The circadian rhythm of human beings is related to the distribution of the geomagnetic field. The activity of sunspots (magnetic storms) has a strong influence on the geomagnetic field. This kind of change will have certain influence on human spirit, physiology, and pathology. The biological effects of magnetic fields are multifaceted, affecting immune function, various enzyme activities, sugars, lipids, proteins, nucleic acids, and free radicals. There are many things about the biological effects of magnetic fields that are still unclear. It still needs to be further explored. Some scholars believe that the research of biomagnetic signals is more valuable than the research of bioelectrical signals, and it has wider application and greater potential. Experiments have confirmed that the low-frequency electromagnetic field (50 Hz) can increase the number of epidermal stem cells in rats with scald wounds. Pathological examination revealed that low-frequency electromagnetic field treatment not only can promote wound healing, but can also induce stem cell proliferation and differentiation. It may be because a specific pulsed magnetic field affects the signal transduction of the cell by changing the permeability of the cell membrane, thereby changing the metabolic process of the cell and promoting wound healing.

Human skin fibroblasts are exposed to an 8.4-mT (tesla) 20 Hz vibrating magnetic field and will differentiate into maturity, increase the secretion of collagen and the accumulation of cellular proteins. Cadosii found that a 75-Hz, 1.3 ms pulsed 3.5 V magnetic field increased the sensitivity of cells to phytohemagglutinin, increased the number of active lymphocytes, and significantly increased biosynthesis activity. Parallel controlled experiments were conducted to investigate the effects of constant magnetic fields on wound healing in patients after different types of surgery. In all, 260 volunteers were recruited and randomized according to the type of surgery. The results showed that the constant magnetic field can improve the wound healing rate and quality after surgery ($P < 0.01$).

In short, the method of using electromagnetic fields (EMF) to treat diseases in human body is called EMT. EMT is noninvasive, has no obvious pain and side effects, and is easy to operate. It has unique advantages in accelerating tissue regeneration and repairing wound healing, and has become an important component of many clinical treatment methods for chronic wounds in recent years. Aziz et al. [22] used a systematic review to evaluate the effectiveness of EMT on chronic wounds in a clinical randomized controlled trial (RCT) study of chronic wounds such as lower extremity vascular ulcers and pressure ulcers. In the EMF, the free charge in the electrolyte moves in a certain direction, which in turn generates an induced charge, called the electrostatic induction phenomenon of the electrolyte. The bound charge in the dielectric also moves under the action of EMF, and changes from a nonpolar molecule to a polar molecule, which are arranged regularly along the direction of the electric field, called polarization phenomena of dielectrics. The organic and inorganic molecules in the abovementioned tissues generate regular or irregular motion under the action of EMF, which will redistribute the charge in the body, thus producing a series of pathological and physiological changes, which is the biophysical basis for EMF treatment (Table 11.5).

### 11.2.3 Classification of EMT and Its Possible Mechanism for Treating Wounds

#### 11.2.3.1 Constant DC Therapy

The method of treating diseases using a low-intensity direct current electric field (LIDCEF) is called direct current therapy (DCT) and is one of the earliest applications of electrotherapy. Under the action of a DC electric field, a potential difference is generated between the two electrodes, causing the electrolyte ions and/or particles of the body to move along the direction of the current, thereby causing the cells to change from a random direction motion to a directional movement. The characteristic of directed migration under the action of an electric field is called the chemotaxis of cells and is the basis of DCT action. The pathological, physiological changes, and therapeutic effects involved in DCT mainly include:

A. Activating the cell's electrotropism, accelerating the qualitative migration of fibroblasts and keratinocytes, and promoting the growth of granulation tissue. LIDCEF stimulates the opening of L-type voltage-gated calcium channels on the cell membrane, resulting in the increase of intracellular $Ca^{2+}$ and $Mg^{2+}$ concentrations, the decrease of $Na^{+}$ and $K^{+}$ concentrations, and migration of protein molecules to the anode, which is beneficial for reducing edema and exudation. The experimental data show that under the action of low current density (0.02–0.06 mA/cm$^2$) direct current, the bactericidal effect of inflammatory cells is enhanced, and the regeneration and repair process is accelerated. At the higher current density (0.2 mA/cm$^2$) direct current, further enhances the inflammatory response in the wound and stimulates the proliferation of fibrous tissue.
B. Stimulating local microvascular dilatation and promoting blood circulation. LIDCEF's anode produces acidic substances and the cathode produces alkaline substances, which stimulate local tissues to release histamine and polypeptide, resulting in vasodilation, specifically manifested by skin congestion under the electrodes, local blood flow can be increased by about 140% and the duration can be more than 30 min. This effect is more obvious at the cathode.
C. Regulating nerve excitability. The influence of LIDCEF on the nervous system is different due to the polarity of its action. When the anode is placed in the lumbosacral region, the cathode is placed in the posterior part of the neck, and the upward current flows through the spinal cord, which increase the excitability of the nerve reflex. Conversely, the downward current passes through the spinal cord, which can reduce the excitability of nerve reflex. The role of the nervous system is one of the main physiological basis of LIDCEF in the treatment of chronic wounds in patients with spinal cord injury.

**Table 11.5** Response of repaired cells in the wound to electromagnetic fields

| Cell type | Reaction | References |
|---|---|---|
| Epidermal cells | Electrode movement | [23] |
| | Reorientation | [24] |
| Fibroblasts | Electrode movement | [25] |
| | Reorientation | [26] |
| | Increased DNA and protein synthesis | [27] |
| | Increase differentiation | [28] |
| | Increased collagen secretion | [29] |
| Lymphocyte | Increased sensitivity to migration | [30] |

DCT not only can significantly improve the exudation of plasma albumin in wounds of burned rats and reduce edema after burns, but also accelerate the re-epithelialization and revascularization of deep second degree burn wounds, improve hair growth, and reduce wound contraction and dermal fibrosis. In the process of chronic wound repair, DCT can enhance the expression of vascular endothelial growth factor and release of nitric oxide, improve the local blood supply of wounds, and promote the healing of diabetic foot ulcers. DCT is used to treat pressure ulcers in patients with spinal cord injury. As a result, DCT stimulation combined with conventional treatment can accelerate the recovery of stage IV pressure ulcer in patients with spinal cord injury.

Adunsky and Ohry et al. [31] used a multicenter, double-blind RCT study to demonstrate the clinical effectiveness of DCT in promoting pressure ulcer healing and suggested that DCT is more effective in the early stages of wound healing.

#### 11.2.3.2 Electrical Stimulation Therapy

Electrical stimulation therapy (EST) is an electromagnetic therapy that uses current to promote the structural and functional recovery of nerves, muscles, and skin tissues. The stimulation factors mainly include low-frequency pulse current and alternating current. Pathological, physiological changes and therapeutic effects caused by EST include the following points:

A. Exogenous electric field action: When the skin is damaged or wounded, the structural integrity is destroyed and the opening of intracellular calcium ion channel is stimulated to increase or the response of the cells to the electromagnetic field is complex and variable, so a large amount of research work is needed to fully and accurately understand this mechanism. When the signal transduction mechanism makes breakthroughs in wound repair research, it will have a positive impact on the final understanding of the relationship between bioelectricity and wound healing. Cell depolarization is enhanced to form endogenous electric fields (EEF) and damage currents, namely, skin cells. The presence of EEF can change cell membrane potential, enhance cell membrane permeability, stimulate cell's electrotropism, and promote fibroblasts and keratinocytes around the wound undergo directional migration in the EEF. After the wound is healed, this current will disappear. The exogenous electric field provided by EST not only enhances the cell's galvanic response, but also affect the activities of various metal ion-dependent enzymes such as choline esterase, monoamine oxidase, histamine enzyme, and cytokines.
B. Promote cell proliferation and cytokine release: EST can promote keratinocyte proliferation and vascular endothelial growth factor release, stimulating neovascularization. The wound healing rate and epithelialization degree of the keratinocyte growth factor gene-modified epidermal stem cell transplantation group with EMF intervention were better.
C. Improve the circulation effect: Low-frequency pulse current, especially 50 Hz current, promotes the improvement of local tissue blood circulation. Mechanisms include EST stimulating skin receptors causing axonal reflexes, stimulating the wall of small arteries, and dilating small arteries; EST stimulates the skin to release substance P and acetylcholine, causing arteriolar dilatation, and increased release of histamine can cause telangiectasia, leading to more persistent congestion.
D. Analgesic effect: The low-frequency current with good analgesic effect is about 100 Hz, the mechanism involves the EST through the sensory nerve crude fiber to the spinal cord after the corner glial cells cause nonpainful stimulation, through competitive inhibition, so that the pain feeling the afferent is blocked and the analgesic effect is achieved. EST stimulates the nervous system to release endogenous morphine-like neurotransmitters such as enkephalin and endorphin to cause analgesic effects.
E. Antibacterial effect: The inhibitory effect of EST on bacterial growth has also been proposed as one of the mechanisms to promote wound healing. Studies have shown that the bacteriostatic effect of cathodic current is more significant.

At present, the clinical effects of electrical stimulation to promote chronic wounds have been initially confirmed. Clinical RCT by Magnoni et al. [32] for chronic wounds of lower extremities showed that 12-week EST can relieve wound pain, improve wound status, and accelerate wound healing. Multicenter clinical studies have also shown that after EST treatment, the area of chronic wounds is significantly reduced, the granulation growth of the wound surface is obvious, and the treatment efficiency and tolerance are ideal, suggesting that EST is a safe and effective treatment for chronic and complex wounds with good tolerance and compliance.

#### 11.2.3.3 High-Frequency Electric Field Therapy

High-frequency electric field therapy refers to a method of treating diseases by using a pulse current of $>10^5$ Hz, which is called high-frequency diathermy (HFD) therapy in foreign countries. When the high-frequency electric field acts on the human body, it mainly produces two biological effects: thermal effect and nonthermal effect.

A. Thermal effect. The high-frequency electric field can cause high-frequency oscillation or movement of the electrolyte ions and dielectric particles of the tissue to generate heat, which is called endogenous thermal effect. Endogenous thermal effects can improve deep tissue microcirculation, increase the reflux of venous and lymph, promote the absorption of exudate, reduce tension pain caused by tissue swelling, and achieve pain relief and tissue repair. Compared with the exogenous transmission heat effect, the depth of action of endogenous thermal effects is significantly increased, and the chronic wounds of deep tissues have advantages that other treatment methods are difficult to reach.
B. Nonthermal effect. It means that under the action of high-frequency electric field, the vibration of electrolyte ions, charged colloids, and dipoles in the tissue occurs in

the state where the tissue temperature is not significantly increased, thereby producing a series of physiological changes of the disease. Nonthermal effects stimulate inflammatory cell function, accelerate nerve fiber regeneration, and promote inflammation absorption and tissue repair.

In clinical applications, according to the wavelength and frequency of electromagnetic waves, high-frequency electric field therapy can be divided into short wave therapy, ultrashort wave therapy, and microwave therapy.

A. Short wave therapy (SWT): The short wavelength is 10–100 m, the frequency is 3–30 MHz, the foreign application wavelength is 11 m (frequency 27.12 MHz), and the domestic application wavelength is 22 m (frequency 13.56 MHz). Short wave can promote the absorption of blood circulation and inflammation, the action site is deep, and the healing effect on chronic wounds is more obvious.
B. Ultrashort wave therapy (USWT): The ultrashort wave has a wavelength of 1–10 m and a frequency of 30–300 MHz. The therapeutic effect of ultrashort waves is roughly the same as that of short waves, but its nonthermal effects are more pronounced than short waves. For the treatment of chronic wounds, the use of microcalorie or warm-heat USWT is better, including the healing of diabetic ulcer wounds.
C. Microwave therapy (MWT): The wavelength of microwave is 1–1000 mm, the frequency is 300–300,000 MHz, clinically divided into decimeter waves (wavelength 100–1000 mm), centimeter wave (wavelength 10–100 mm), and millimeter wave (wavelength 1–10 mm). For the treatment of chronic wounds, the mechanism of MWT is more closely related to its warming effect, which can increase the temperature of local tissue, deep blood vessels dilate, promote blood circulation, enhance metabolism, promote the absorption of inflammatory exudation, and accelerate the process of tissue repair.

#### 11.2.3.4 High-Voltage Potential Therapy

The method of treating a disease using an electric field generated by a high-voltage alternating current is called high-voltage alternating current therapy (HVACT), also called high-voltage pulsed current therapy (HVPC), and its output voltage can be up to 450 V, and the current is generally no more than 3–5 mA. The therapeutic effect of HVACT is mainly based on the action of high-voltage alternating electric field, as well as air negative ion flow, ozone, and nitrogen dioxide. First, the high-voltage alternating electric field can produce obvious vascular reactions. In the initial stage, it promotes skin capillary contraction and then expands them, thereby improving local blood circulation, enhancing the process of nutrient metabolism, and accelerating wound healing. Second, the ionized air generated by the high-voltage alternating electric field is a tiny mechanical stimulus to the skin receptors, which can affect the central nervous system through nerve endings. At the same time, in the high-voltage alternating electric field, the oxygen in the air is more easily oxidized into ozone, which can increase the concentration of oxyhemoglobin, and has a bactericidal effect, and can also promote wound healing. The 30 kV alternating electric field can treat the skin purulent infection of limbs with an effective rate of 71.5%.

Compared with classic wound treatment, electromagnetic field therapy can significantly improve the symptoms of edema, pain, and other symptoms, reduce medical expenses, and improve patient compliance and tolerance. However, existing research still has problems of small sample size and low research quality. Clinical and experimental studies using EMT to treat chronic wounds may bring new ideas to the treatment of chronic wounds, and provide a scientific basis for improving and optimizing the clinical comprehensive treatment of chronic wounds, which will help improve the quality of life of patients and reduce the burden on family and society.

## 11.3 Negative Pressure Therapy

Negative pressure wound therapy (NPWT) is a new method proposed and carried out in the past decade. It includes vacuum sealing drainage (VSD), first proposed by German surgeon Fleischmann in 1993, and vacuum-assisted closure (VAC), first created by American surgeon Argenta and Morykwas in 1997. The principle of the two is the same, that is, the vacuum suction is closed, but there are differences in the selection of materials, methods, and indications. NPWT achieves the therapeutic goal of promoting debridement and wound healing by covering the wound with a special material cover and placing it under negative pressure for a period of time. Mainly used for surface acute or chronic, infectious or noninfectious wounds or ulcers, soft tissue large area damage, diabetic foot, tissue defects or organ exposure caused by war injury or trauma, even visceral inflammation of the package coverage and drainage, etc.

### 11.3.1 Development History

As early as the 1970s, the Soviet Union reported the use of negative pressure to treat wounds. In 1993, Fleischmann et al. [33] applied the negative pressure for the first time to treat wound infections in soft tissues of the extremities and obtained positive results. This method was quickly recommended for clinical treatment of various soft tissue defects and infections. Later, Morykwas et al. [34] developed a technique for the treatment of negative pressure wounds. They used animal models to compare the efficacy of negative pressure wound treatment techniques with saline gauze dressings for chronic wounds. The results showed that NPWT treatment was significantly better than the control group in increasing the local blood flow of the wound, promoting fibroblast growth, and reducing the number of wound bacteria. In 1994, Qiu Huade and others introduced the German NPWT for the treatment of general surgery and infected wounds. In 2000, Chen Shaozong and his team conducted research on hemodynamics and molecular biology in the mechanism of action of NPWT and developed a self-made closed dressing for the treatment of chronic refractory wounds with remarkable curative effect. In 2006, they also found that NPWT can promote the expression of platelet-derived growth factor (PDGF) and transforming growth factor-β (TGF-β) in chronic wound tissue, thereby promoting wound healing. As early as 2003, VSD technology has been included in the treatment guidelines for wounds in Germany and Austria. After the corresponding revisions, the scope of application has been continuously expanded. For a long time, VSD technology has gradually moved from theory to practice, and has continuously made progress in theoretical research in practice.

### 11.3.2 Mechanism of Action

The main components of NPWT are wound filling dressing, closed semipermeable membrane, drainage line, and negative pressure generating device. The wound filling dressing is a foam or sponge material with soft texture, containing microbubble pores of different sizes. It is used to buffer the wound pressure, protect the new granulation, avoid the nerve endings from being stimulated, adsorb the exudate, and the drainage material is cut and shaped under the continuous action of negative pressure, so as to be convenient to lead out through the pipeline. The most commonly used material is polyvinyl alcohol, which is a foam-type synthetic dressing. The foam has a micropore diameter of 0.2–1.0 mm. It is similar to sponge, white, nontoxic, good histocompatibility, no immunological activity, softness and has sufficient strength, excellent adsorption and water permeability, and is available in a variety of sizes. It can be trimmed as needed. The closed semipermeable membrane covers the wound surface after filling the dressing, providing a sealed environment that is permeable to water vapor but impervious to water and prevents bacterial invasion. Commonly used are the transparent dressings produced by 3 M Company of the United States. In earlier studies, wound negative pressure was obtained by some conventional methods, such as central vacuum suction devices, surgical vacuum bottles, and the like. However, these methods have inconveniences such as movement of the instrument, control and maintenance of the level of the negative pressure, and the like. Since the setting of the negative pressure mode is critical, a scale-adjustable device is recommended. A vacuum-assisted therapeutic device was introduced in 1995 that overcomes the above problems. At the heart of the instrument is a microprocessor vacuum control unit that provides a controlled continuous or intermittent negative pressure of 25–200 mmHg (1 mmHg = 0.133 kPa) for maximum effectiveness. The disadvantage is that the machine is large in size and inconvenient to move. The patient needs to use it at the bedside. It is only suitable for patients who are in bed and have severe wound exudation. Later, a portable model was developed for use in patients with less exudation and ambulatory bed. The concept of optimal pressure and negative pressure modes was not proposed in earlier studies. Until 1997, Morykwas et al. [34] conducted a series of animal experiments that focused on this issue. The study used wound blood flow and granulation tissue growth as the entry point. Laser Doppler technique was used to measure the blood flow of subcutaneous tissues and muscles around the wound. The growth of granulation tissue was determined by measuring the decrease of wound volume over time. The results showed that when the negative pressure was 125 mmHg, the blood flow in the subcutaneous and peripheral muscles of the wound was four times that of the baseline value. When the negative pressure value is 400 mmHg or more, blood flow is suppressed. The growth of granulation tissue is that intermittent negative pressure is more effective than continuous negative pressure.

The following are main mechanisms of negative pressure wound treatment technology.

#### 11.3.2.1 Promote Blood Circulation

Partial blood supply disorder or ischemia is one of the main reasons that hinder wound healing. Because the oxygen and nutrients necessary for wound repair can only be transported to the wound through blood flow, most toxic substances and metabolites generated locally are mainly transported out of the wound through blood flow. After applying vacuum suction in animal experiments, Chen et al. [35] showed a significant increase in wound perfusion through Doppler laser detection. Li Jing et al. [36] confirmed that NPWT treatment can significantly increase the number of capillaries at the wound margin, resulting in increased capillary diameter at the wound surface and increased blood flow, which promotes the recovery of normal morphology and structure of capillaries and endothelial cells, and stimulates capillary sprouting and endothelial cell proliferation, restores basement membrane integrity, and narrows endothelial cell gap. Li Xueyong and other researchers believe that there is a two-way force and two-way microdisplacement of wound tissue in NPWT treatment, that is, some tissues produce outward displacement after NPWT treatment and some tissues produce inward displacement. The blood in the tissue (positive pressure) is squeezed and accelerated to flow into the tissue under negative pressure, thereby causing the blood circulation of the wound to accelerate. This is important for explaining the effect of NPWT treatment on promoting blood circulation in wounds.

#### 11.3.2.2 Reduce Edema

Edema is one of the reasons that hinder wound healing. On the one hand, the tissue enlarges the distance between the tissue cells and hinders the exchange of substances between the cells; on the other hand, it compresses the microvessels in the wound, which is not conducive to tissue perfusion. Wound ischemia and hypoxia prevent the wound from getting the nutrients it needs for healing, thus inhibiting the healing of the wound. Under the action of negative pressure, the wound tissue fluid is attracted to the body and the tissue swelling can be resolved. Negative pressure can expand the small arteries and increase mitosis to form a new vascular bed; it can also remove excess fluid, reduce edema, and improve local blood circulation. Lu Xiaoxing et al. [37] found that NPWT treatment can effectively reduce peritraumatic edema and reduce vascular permeability. Michael et al. [38] pointed out that the NPWT treatment is beneficial to eliminate the pressure gradient caused by excessive interstitial fluid, reduce the interstitial pressure, and open the capillaries and flow to the wound tissue.

#### 11.3.2.3 Inhibit Bacterial Growth

For a long time, there has been concern about wound infections caused by bacterial growth in a relatively humid, warm environment under closed dressings, but this is not the case. Weed et al. [39] found in animal studies that the use of NPWT significantly reduced the number of bacteria, especially the number of G-bacteria. Polykandriotis and others innovatively applied NPWT to nine cases of hand trauma patients, effectively treated and prevented hand defect wound infection and reduced local pain. Wang Changjian et al. [40] used closed-label therapy in eleven patients with large-scale soft tissue infections and defects at the distal extremities, and showed no infection. The main mechanism of closed dressing to reduce wound infection may be related to the function of the immune cells in the airtight and humid environment produced by the closed dressing. Plikaitis et al. [41] conducted experiments on infected wounds of pig skin, the control group replaced the wound with a traditional dressing. The experimental group used NPWT equipment to continuously suction the wound under negative pressure, and the wound tissue was cultured daily. As a result, the number of bacteria in the wound treated with NPWT decreased and remained low level (105 microbes per gram of tissue) within 5 days after wound infection, while the control group peaked within 5 days and reached lower level at 11 days. NPWT treatment for bacterial clearance of contaminated chronic wounds is beneficial to the healing process of the wound.

#### 11.3.2.4 Remove Some Necrotic Tissue

After debridement, there may still be a large amount of necrotic tissue, which is a pathological factor affecting wound healing. Negative pressure closed drainage technique can remove some necrotic tissue while exuding the wound surface, but due to a large number of confusing factors in the data, it is difficult to obtain matched samples for accurate analysis in the study of local body fluid changes in wound surface, but there are still many studies to prove that this technology can drain various inflammatory mediators and enzymes that affect wound healing, draining a large number of toxins; local pathology factors of wounds can be reduced by the technique of closed drainage under negative pressure.

#### 11.3.2.5 Reduce Posttraumatic Immunosuppression

Posttraumatic soluble inflammatory mediators such as the release of preinflammatory cytokines are involved in immunosuppression, and continuous overdrainage of wound fluid by NPWT treatment can also inhibit wound immune response, so this technique must allow leukocytes to infiltrate and contact the wound to produce effective immunological reaction. The NPWT polyethylene foam is in intimate contact with the wound surface so that the cells can be infiltrated into the foam. Gouttefangeas et al. [42] found that after 1 week and 2 weeks of treatment with NPWT, the main cells infiltrating into the foam were granulocytes and mononuclear cells including macrophages and a small number of T and B cell populations and natural killer cells. The functional $CD4^+$ and $CD8^+$ T lymphocytes on the foam differ from the patient's peripheral blood T lymphocyte subsets, which are subpopulations of cells that are affected by wound antigens and have a heterogeneous phenotype and function. It is suggested that T lymphocytes may play a role in wound cleansing. In addition, it has been suggested that polyethylene foam may provide an advantageous environment for stimulating T cell-mediated immunological reaction.

#### 11.3.2.6 Mechanical Pulling Action

NPWT creates a shear force at the medical foam-wound interface that is believed to promote granulation tissue growth and angiogenesis. This mechanical stress promotes granulation tissue production by accelerating the production and renewal of intracellular messenger regulatory proteins. Numerous studies have shown that mechanical stress, that is, shear force, regulates the morphology, function, and gene expression of endothelial cells, and a shear-sensitive *cis*-acting element has been found in the endothelial cell gene promoter. Local shear forces also promote the production of platelet-derived growth factor (PDGF) by platelets and endothelial cells, promote the proliferation and migration of fibroblasts, smooth muscle cells, and monocytes, and promote the proliferation of glial cells. Wounds have two levels of change in NPWT treatment: tissue displacement at the edges and bottom of the wound under negative pressure and small changes in the surface of the wound that are attracted to the pores of the dressing. Tissue tension is important for tissue growth and is the basis for tissue growth. NPWT treatment causes changes in tissue tension, which promotes cell proliferation and granulation tissue formation. Penn et al. [43] believe that the mechanical force of NPWT treatment is beneficial to remove wound exudate, and the removal of exudate reduces tissue edema, thereby reducing interstitial pressure and increasing local blood flow. The removal of exudates also removes soluble factors that affect wound healing. Negative pressure sealing therapy forms a natural physical pull force on the wound edge by negative pressure, promotes the fission and proliferation of fibroblasts, and accelerates the healing of wounds.

#### 11.3.2.7 Others

With the deepening of research, many scholars have tried to explore some mechanisms of NPWT's effectiveness from a microscopic perspective. Using the pig back wound model, Kilpadi et al. [44] observed the expression of transforming growth factor-β (TGF-β), interleukin-6 (IL-6), IL-8, and IL-10 in early peripheral blood under the effects of negative pressure closed drainage and 0.9% sodium chloride solution gauze and found there was no difference in the effects of TGF-β and IL-8. Li Yuejun et al. [45] studied the dorsal skin defect of small pig as a model and found that NPWT treatment can upregulate the expression of urokinase-type plasminogen activator (uPA) and urokinase-type plasmin activator receptor (uPAR) of epidermal keratinocytes around acute wounds. The expression of the receptor allows rapid proliferation and migration and reduces the degradation of extracellular matrix by inhibiting the expression of uPA and uPAR in chronic wounds. Cao Dayong et al. [46] gave continuous NPWT treatment to five patients with chronic wounds. The results showed that before negative pressure attraction, VEGF was occasionally positively expressed in the dermal endothelial cells of the dermal tissue of the wound margin. With the prolongation of NPWT treatment, vascular endothelial cells and fibroblasts were positively expressed in dermal cells, and the microvessel density expressed by CD34 was significantly enhanced after NPWT treatment. Therefore, it is concluded that NPWT can significantly enhance the proliferation and microvessel density of vascular endothelial cells and fibroblasts in the dermal layer of the wound margin, and promote the growth of granulation tissue in chronic wounds.

### 11.3.3 Current Application Status

#### 11.3.3.1 Application Method

After routine disinfection and debridement, completely stop bleeding, properly scrape the hair within the range of 3–5 cm outside the wound edge, and use negative pressure to close the drainage under the condition of ensuring compliance with indications and no contraindications. Depending on the size of the wound, a suitable size of the wound dressing and a sufficient number of drainage tubes are selected. A thin layer of dressing is filled onto the wound surface, and then the drainage tube is wrapped with the dressing and placed in the optimal drainage position (generally placed in the central area, the number of drainage tubes is appropriately increased when the wound is large), and then covered with a thin layer of dressing. The whole dressing should be used as much as possible, and it is not recommended to cut into small pieces. Alcohol scrubs the surrounding skin removes the oil on the skin, dries the dressing, and wipes the skin, then covers the semipermeable membrane on the dressing, the edge covers 3–5 cm beyond the wound edge skin, pay attention to the tight adhesion, avoid the empty wrinkles. In particular, the formation of the pores should be avoided at the outlet of the drainage tube, and the mesangial method can be used for fixation. Adjust the negative pressure source parameters and connect the drain tube to the negative pressure source. After the operation is completed, the patient and the accompanying staff should be informed to protect the drainage system to avoid the sharp objects such as needles, nails, bed ribs, etc., piercing the sealing membrane to cause drainage failure, and avoid the compression and bending of the drainage tube. Pay attention to the characteristics and quantity of the drainage fluid, and adjust the negative pressure parameters according to the situation. At the end of the treatment cycle, when the drainage system needs to be replaced, the negative pressure should be removed first, and the semipermeable membrane and the outer layer filled dressing should be removed gently, the drainage tube should be removed, and the inner layer filling dressing should be removed. In case of dry dressing or densely attached to the wound, it should be removed after being moistened with sterile saline. If the wound is large and the replacement is bound to cause heavier pain, the operation should be performed under anesthesia.

At present, this method has been widely used in the treatment of various types of acute and chronic wounds and has achieved satisfactory results.

#### 11.3.3.2 Clinical Application

A. Acute wounds: NPWT can be used in acute skin wound types including acute burns, skin defects caused by trauma, wounds in donor sites, and surgical incisions. According to data released by the World Health Organization (WHO), the number of cases per year in the world is 187–281 million. Among them, many surgical wounds are often difficult to heal due to the specificity of the anatomical location or infection, such as skin grafts and median sternal incisions. The expansion of the NPWT technical indications has a positive impact on the treatment of the abovementioned refractory wounds, but new complications must still be prevented. In addition, NPWT can be used for joint replacement and management of skin incision after joint open reduction, which is beneficial to prevent local edema and hematoma formation, reduce the risk of infection, and accelerate wound healing. NPWT can also be used for the treatment of wound flaps in the free flaps, but the advantages of this therapy in promoting wound healing are not as obvious as those of conventional compression dressing. The application of NPWT technology in acute burn wounds is still in the exploratory stage.

   Xiaobing's Fu key laboratory of trauma repair and tissue regeneration of the PLA used negative pressure wound treatment techniques for infectious wounds of skin and soft tissue blast injuries. There are four small white pigs of 15–20 kg, half male and half female. In each animal's bilateral scapula and 2 cm posterior to the anterior superior iliac spine, an explosive wound was created (the animal model of porcine skin soft tissue explosive injury was made by Xi'an 213, Φ12 electric detonator was placed 1.0 cm away from the skin of pig's bilateral scapular and buttocks to detonate and injure them), there were 16 wounds. The wound was not treated within 3 days after the injury, and it was exposed and kept in the open air. On the third day after the injury, the animals were fixed on a self-made four-well plate, the necrotic tissue was cut off, and the wound was washed twice in the order of hydrogen peroxide, physiological saline, 0.01% bromogeramine, and physiological saline to perform wound debridement. After 16 wounds were numbered, they were randomly divided into two groups: the control group was covered with a single layer of oil yarn, and the dressing was changed once a day. The dressing was changed once every 2 days from 17 days after the injury, and five to six layers of sterile gauze covered the wound. The treatment group was treated with a negative pressure of 15 kPa, and the dressing was changed once every 1–5 days. The average area of immediate wounds after injury was (7.37 ± 1.17) $cm^2$. On the third day after the wound, the wound was stinky and there was a white turbid and sticky purulent discharge. The average healing time of the wound was 32.75 ± 1.56 days in the control group and 25.75 ± 0.96 days in the treatment group ($P < 0.01$). The wound depth was significantly shallower on the 4th day after injury in the treatment group. On the 6th and 12th days, the granulation tissue quickly filled the wound. There was a statistically significant difference in wound depth between the two groups after treatment ($P < 0.01$). In the treatment group, more fibroblasts and vascular endothelial cells appeared on the first day after treatment, the cells had no obvious edema, and the number of vascular endothelial cells increased significantly. The main reasons for the analysis are: reducing the edema of the wound, reducing the number of bacteria in the infected wound of the explosive wound, thereby reducing the range of secondary necrosis of the explosive wound, and quickly starting the wound repair process of the infected wound of the explosive wound, shortening the time for granulation tissue to fill the wound.

B. Chronic wounds: NPWT is one of the effective methods for the treatment of chronic wounds, which not only helps to reduce the wound area, but also helps shorten the wound healing time. The efficacy of NPWT for chronic wounds is often measured by the complete healing time of the wound, the change in wound size, and the preparation of the wound bed. It has been analyzed by hundreds of literatures on NPWT that NPET is one of the effective methods for treating DFU, which can improve wound healing rate, accelerate wound healing, and reduce the risk of amputation. The data show that NPWT can increase the wound healing rate of DFU by 20%. Zeng Ding et al. [47] reported the experience of NPWT in the treatment of 46 patients with refractory wounds, including 12 cases of deep burn residual wounds, 9 cases of DFU, 5 cases of poorly invasive surgical incision, 13 cases of bedsore, 4 cases of radiation ulcer, and 3 cases of other difficult wounds, achieved satisfactory results. Cheng Biao and others used negative pressure to treat chronic and difficult wounds on the buttocks and achieved good results.

C. Others: Transplantation of the wound skin graft is a common method for wound treatment. The transplantation of the wound skin graft combined with NPWT can achieve one-time healing of the wound, reduce the incidence of wound infection, and shorten the hospital stay. A retrospective study by Blume et al. [48] analyzed the effects of 262 patients receiving blade thickness grafting combined with NPWT in 10 years. The results showed that NPWT was beneficial to improve the survival rate of transplanted skin and reduce the number of reskinning. Domestic Li Jin et al. [49] reported that 46 patients with

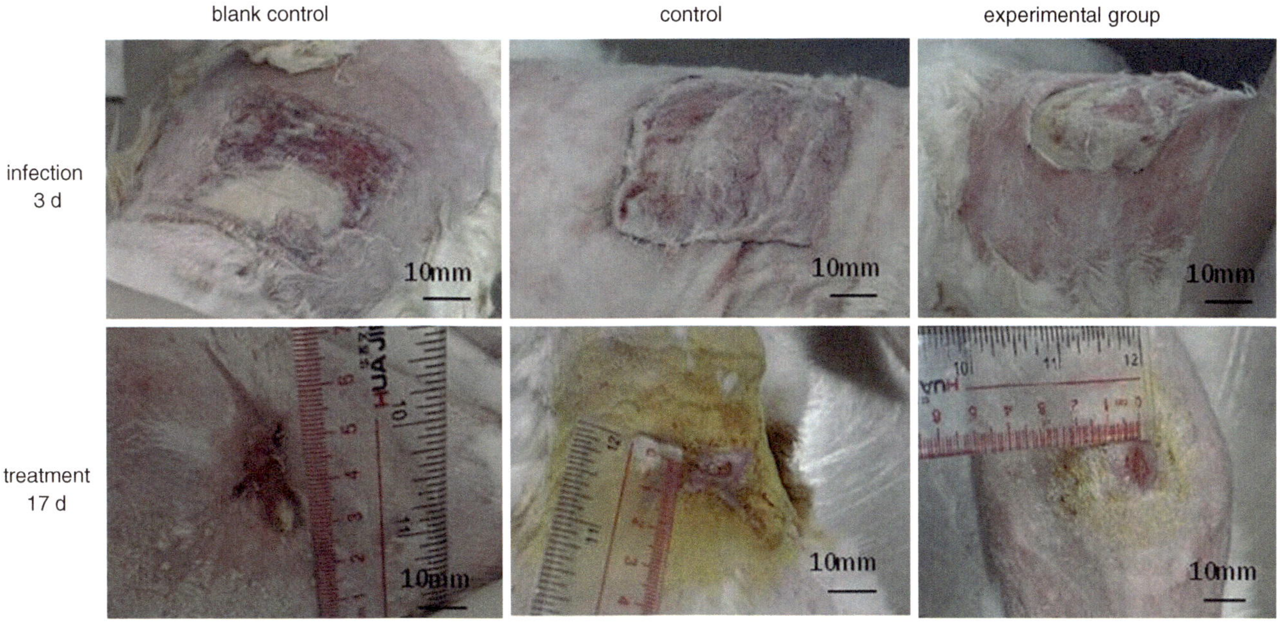


**Fig. 11.22** Treatment after infection with staphylococci

large-area skin defects underwent thick-thickness skin graft or medium-thickness skin graft combined with NPWT continuous vacuum aspiration therapy. After removing the negative pressure dressing for about 1 week, 44 patients were completely surviving and two patients were survived after active dressing change due to a little necrosis at the edge of the wound.

An important member of the Xiaobing Fu academician team has completed the preliminary animal experiment (New Zealand rabbit full-thickness skin infection with *Staphylococcus aureus* model) in cooperation with Professor Quan Daping of Sun Yat-sen University. The results show that the intelligent debridement drainage treatment system is safe and effective for infective wound treatment, promote wound healing, the results are shown in Fig. 11.22.

Gross observation and analysis showed that the wounds in the control group were basically healed, but there were still a small amount of necrotic tissue adhering to the wound surface, and the wound healing was irregular. The wound area of the blank control group was still large, the wound healing was irregular, and there were still necrotic tissue residues on the surface. There is no purulent or scab in the healing process of the experimental group, and the healing structure is flat and basically healed. Bacterial content analysis of wound tissue showed that the experimental group significantly reduced the bacterial content of the wound. The detailed results are shown in Fig. 11.23 and Table 11.6.

Histological analysis showed that there were no normal structured skin in the three groups before treatment. After treatment, the cell structure of the skin layer of the blank control group was disordered. The epidermis structure of the control group and the experimental group was intact, and the dermal papilla structure began to regenerate. The experimental group had hair follicles and sebaceous glands regeneration. As shown in Fig. 11.24.

At the same time, the team used negative pressure to treat refractory wounds and achieved better results (Figs. 11.25, 11.26, and 11.27).

### 11.3.4 Problems and Future Prospects

Although this technique has proven to be relatively effective and superior to traditional wound treatments, there is still a lack of research on the best mode of treatment for the technology itself, such as optimal negative pressure settings, how to choose the right dressing, replacement time interval, etc. Recently, Steiert et al. [50] believe that before the delayed suture, skin graft or flap transfer of complex wounds, if the early NPWT treatment is used, the time of wound closure is not limited by the fixed time of 72 h. This undoubtedly provides new development ideas for this new technology.

At the same time, however, it should also be noted that VSD technology is not applicable under certain circumstances, which may lead to risks such as intestinal fistula, and the scope of application should be strictly controlled. Any wound treatment technique or method has its limitations and uncertainties, as well as its absolute indications and relative indications. Adverse reactions caused by improper application of NPWT occur, such as local pressure sores, excessive pressure caused by peri-infectious vesicles, anaerobic infec-

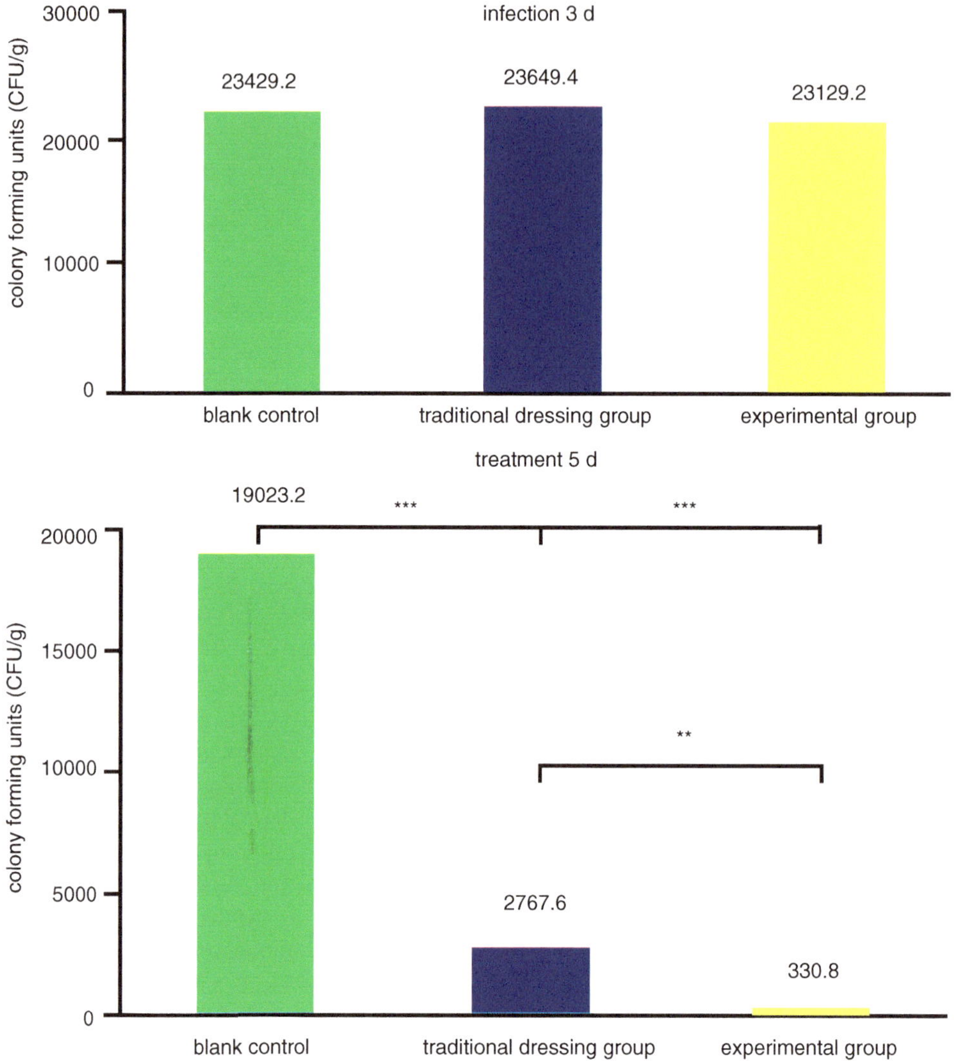


**Fig. 11.23** Comparison of bacterial content in wounds before and after treatment

**Table 11.6** Changes in bacterial culture counts of wound tissue before and after treatment

| Group | 0 Day | 5 Days | 10 Days | 14 Days | 18 Days | 21 Days |
|---|---|---|---|---|---|---|
| Blank control group | 23,429.2 | 19,023.2 | 8876.2 | 1676.2 | 348.8 | 148.8 |
| Traditional dressing group | 23,649.4 | 2767.6 | 607.6 | 327.6 | 139.6 | 31.6 |
| Experience group | 23,129.2 | 330.8 | 130.8 | 45.4 | 4.2 | 0 |

tions, due to incomplete exudation and viscous secretion resulting in poor drainage, the infection was aggravated, and even wounds sepsis and thrombosis occur, etc. In view of this, on one hand, clinicians should strictly grasp the indications of NPWT and choose appropriate treatment techniques for different wounds, which is very positive for the prognosis and outcome of patients. On the other hand, deepening the research and understanding of the mechanism of action of NPET is the basis for guiding the more rational use of NPWT, which is equally significant. With the further clarification of the principle of NPWT promoting wound healing, NPWT will be more widely and clinically applied.

Design a three-stage (existing coagulation/inflammatory phase, granulation tissue growth phase, re-epithelialization phase/tissue reconstruction phase) according to the pathophysiology of wounds, and the influence of different repair cells (inflammatory cells, fibroblasts, vascular endothelial cells, keratinocytes, etc.), completes the intelligent instrumentation of tissue regeneration and repair. It can stop bleeding and accelerate debridement in the early stage; promote

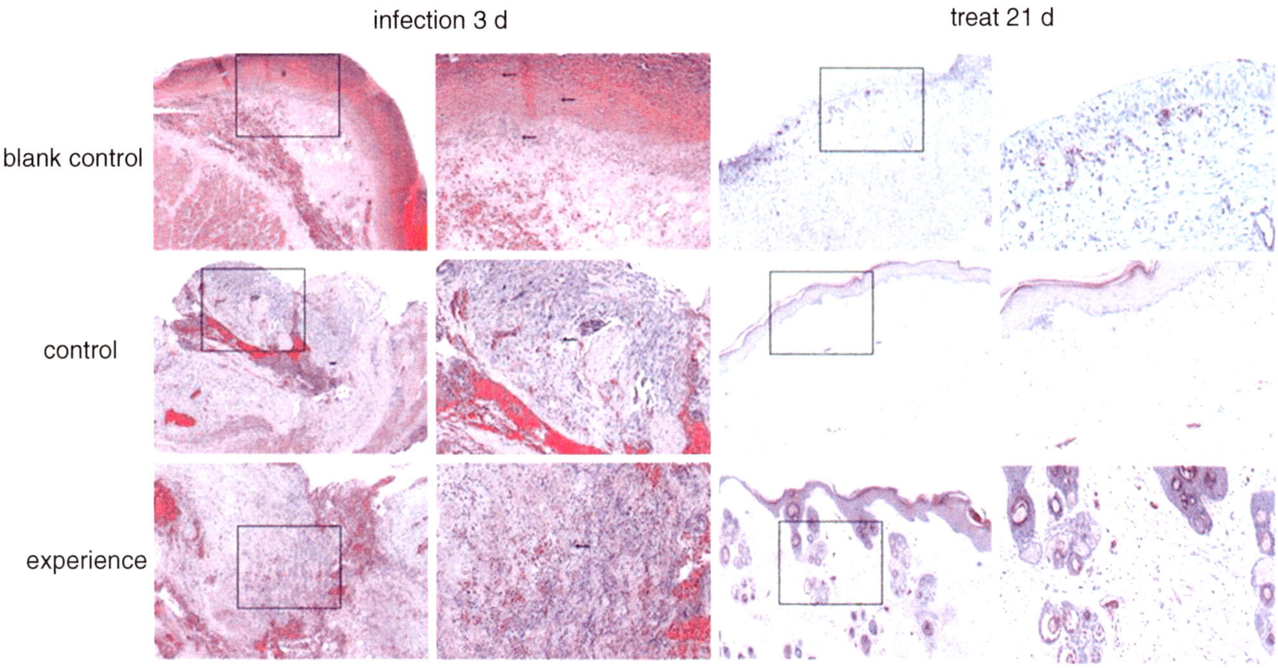


**Fig. 11.24** Results of histological analysis before and after treatment of animal experimental wounds

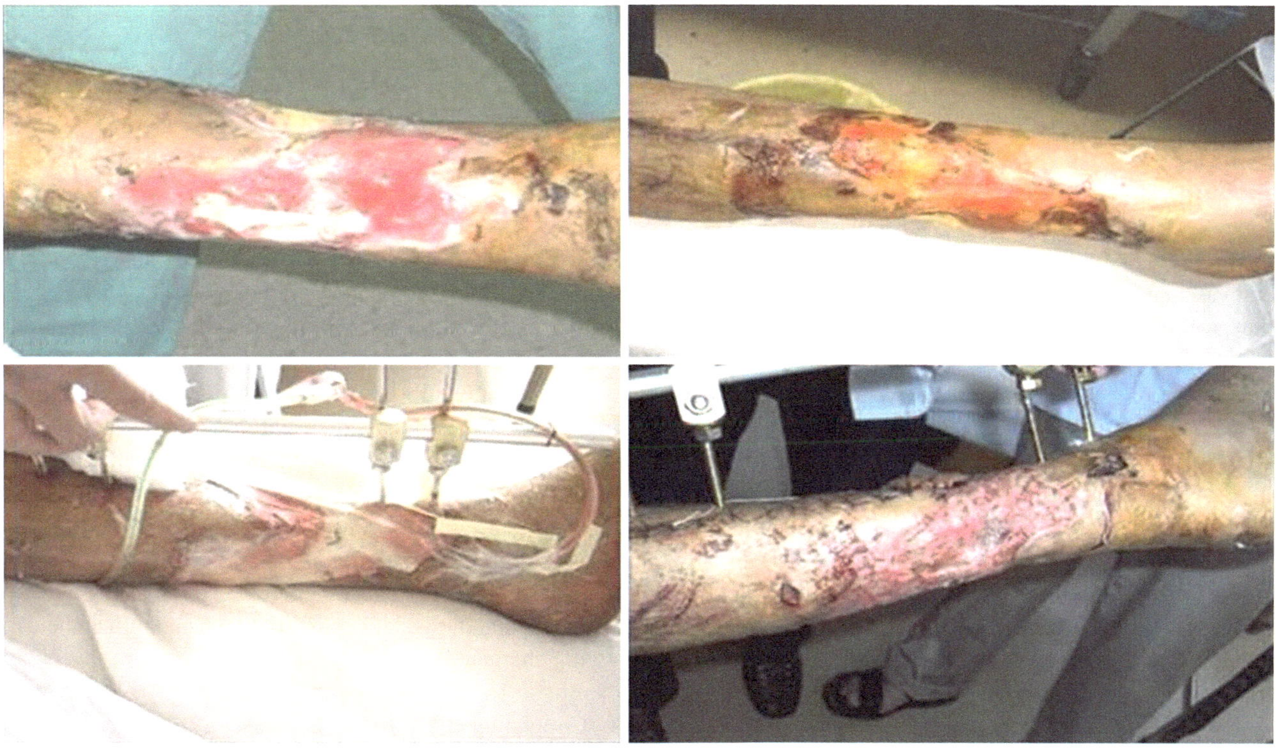

**Fig. 11.25** Negative pressure drainage and skin grafting cover the wound in the right lower extremity car accident

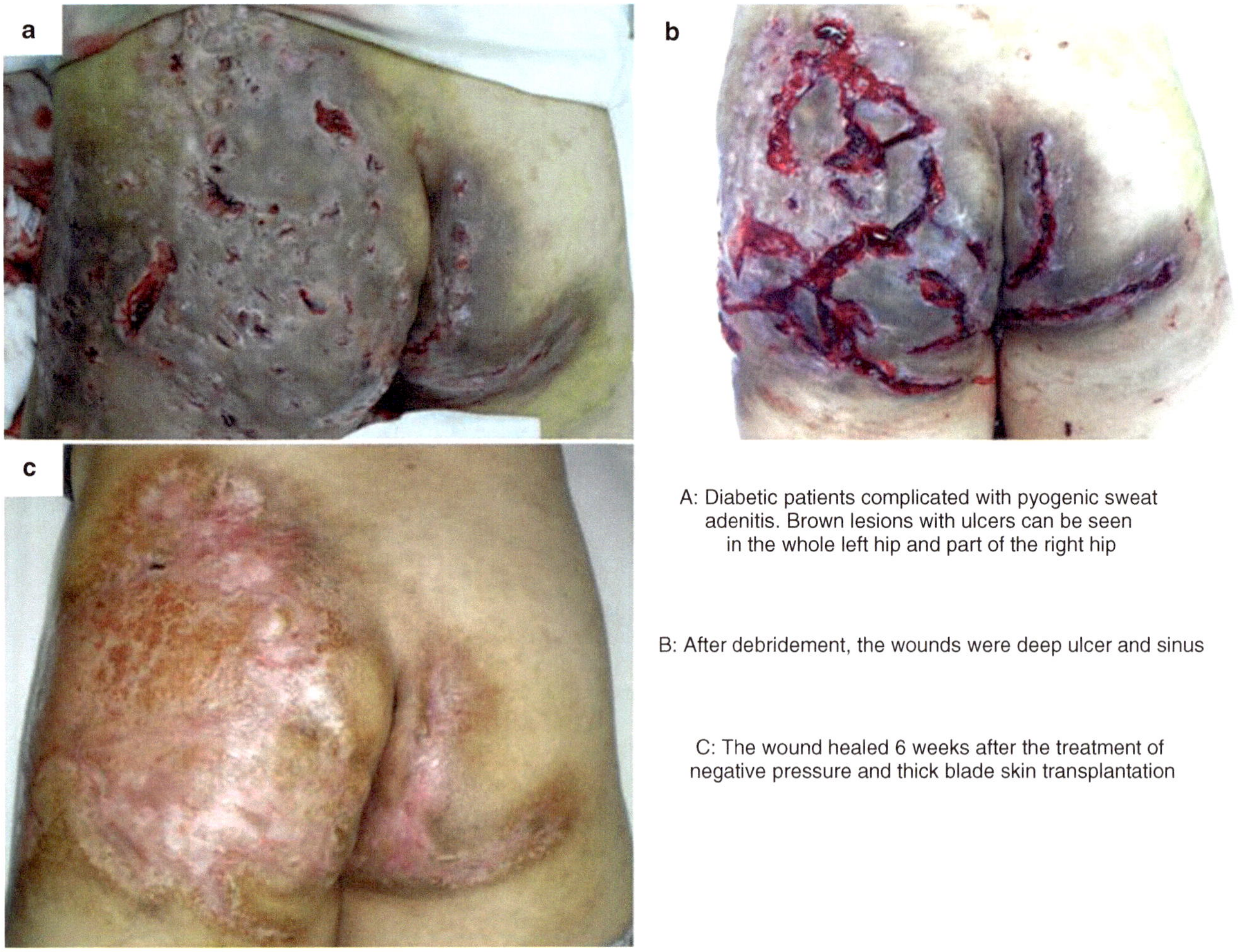


**Fig. 11.26** Inhalation treatment of infective wounds in the buttocks

the proliferation, differentiation, and migration of fibroblasts and vascular endothelial cells in the middle stage; accelerate the proliferation and migration of keratinocytes and rearrange the collagen in the later stage. In addition to the intelligent control adjustment of the attractive amount of attraction at different healing stages, and the active drug intervention in each period, coupled with the improvement of local dressings, the establishment of this system will achieve the ideal state of microenvironment in situ regeneration of skin soft tissue to prepare for perfect healing.

Further optimization of the intelligent drug-loaded skin soft tissue in situ regeneration microenvironment system, including decompression system, drug delivery system, online real-time monitoring, detection system and display system, integration of multifunction modules, portable systems, etc., to create a series of multilevel, multifunctional products to meet different clinical needs. Electromechanical and piping systems have completed product standards and entered clinical trials.

At present, Cheng Biao, an important member of the team of Xiaobing Fu, and Professor Quan Daping of Sun Yat-sen University are working on the development of intelligent negative pressure therapy devices and related materials. They will prepare new biofunctional membranes through electrospinning and decellularization techniques to study the relationship between the components, microstructure, load of growth factors and sustained release of the membrane and skin regeneration, so that the biofilm can actively promote tissue regeneration. Form 1 to 2 special skin ulcer biofunctional membrane products, establish enterprise standards, and enter clinical trials. It has the following characteristics:

A. Circulating administration, stable maintenance of local drug concentration, and solving the limitation of the current nonuniform administration of the negative pressure drainage device and the short action time of the drug. Different combinations of drugs (proportion of growth

**Fig. 11.27** Negative pressure treatment of various types of complex wounds

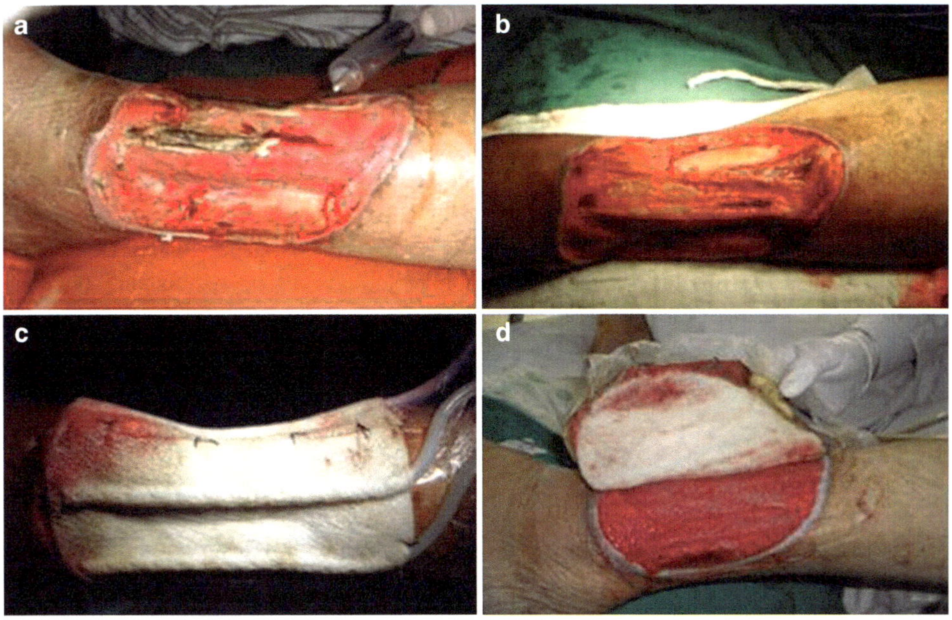


(**a**) Debridement (**b**) after debridement (**c**) negative pressure suction was used to treat the deep and periosteal open wounds of the lower extremities (**d**) After 10 days, the negative pressure device was removed, and fresh and uninfected granulation could be seen

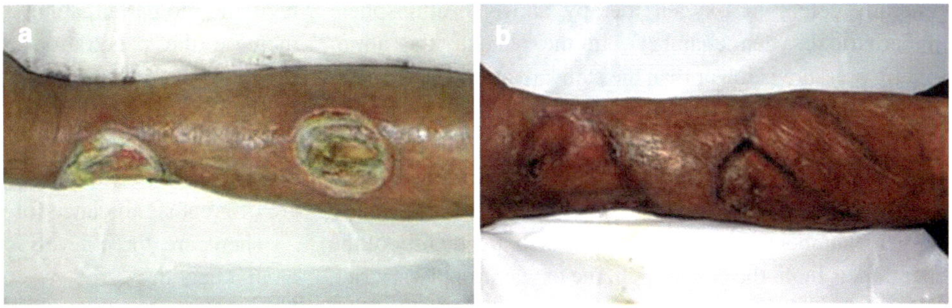


(**a**) Original wound (**b**) after debridement, negative pressure suction was used. After granulation tissue was formed, thick blade skin grafting was used to heal the wound

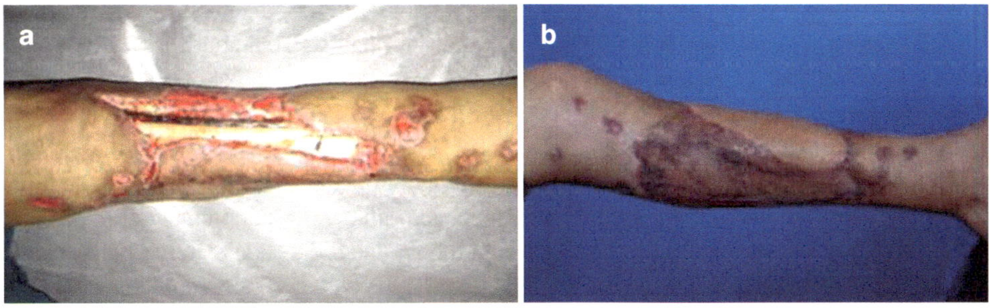


(**a**) Original wound (**b**) after debridement, the wounds were treated by suction. After granulation tissue was formed, latissimus dorsi myocutaneous flap was transplanted and recovered 2 weeks later

factors) are administered at each stage of healing to conform to the physiological and pathological processes of wound healing. Even the removal of bacterial biofilms from difficult wounds has played a technically difficult way.

B. Frequency conversion decompression: Solves the limitation that the existing equipment can only be decompressed. Promote wound healing through periodic decompression physical stimulation, so that the intelligent tissue in situ regeneration microenvironment system provides different microenvironment (continuous attraction, intermittent attraction) at different stages of wound healing to accelerate tissue regeneration and repair.

A. Skin regeneration biofilm: Based on the existing negative pressure drainage dressings using inert materials without biological functions, this topic will focus on the development of new biofilms. The surface is made of a material that mimics the structure of the skin nanofiber and is loaded with growth factors or other nutrients that promote skin regeneration, allowing it to exert a long-lasting and sustained healing effect.

## 11.4 Oxygen Therapy

The use of oxygen to promote wound healing began in the 1960s. There are two types of oxygen therapy, namely systemic oxygen therapy and local oxygen therapy. Systemic hyperbaric oxygen (HBO) refers to the pure oxygen inhaled and ambient pressure in the hyperbaric oxygen environment, generally refers to oxygen therapy above 1 atmosphere (hyperbaric oxygen chamber). In the plateau, the atmospheric pressure is lower than the standard atmospheric pressure (ATM, 1 ATM = 101 kPa = 760 mmHg), at which time HBO refers to oxygen therapy at above atmospheric pressure. Although the effect of treating wounds with HBO is very good, due to the need for special equipment (hyperbaric oxygen chamber), the conditions are harsh, the quality of the operators is high, the cost is high, the oxygen supply is strict, and there is a danger of oxygen poisoning, and it is difficult to promote the application. Therefore, topical oxygen therapy (TOT) was proposed and quickly promoted.

Adequate oxygen ($O_2$) supply is essential for normal wound healing, and it has long been recognized that when tissue oxygen partial pressure ($PO_2$) is below a certain level, the risk of chronic nonhealing wounds increases. Hypoxia occurs when oxygen consumption exceeds supply. Poor blood perfusion is generally thought to be associated with a decrease in oxygen supply leading to hypoxia in the wound, ultimately leading to wound healing disorders. Local hypoxemia is one of the key factors limiting wound healing. Supplementation with $O_2$ input to correct the presence of hypoxemia has a significant benefit to the wound healing of patients. In addition to nutritional and antibiotic bactericidal effects, $O_2$ supports life processes such as angiogenesis, cellular motility, and extracellular matrix formation. Recent studies have found that the role of $O_2$ in wound healing involves the production of reactive oxygen species (ROS). Almost all wound-related cells have specific enzymes that produce ROS, including free radicals and $H_2O_2$, which are often associated with healing damage. It is known that hypoxic pressure in wounds can jeopardize the function of these enzymes. At low concentrations, ROS acts as a cell messenger for wound healing.

In general, the basic energy needs of the human body are mainly supported by the oxygen consumption in aerobic respiration. The ROS produced by activated phagocytes consuming oxygen in respiratory bursts play an important role in the initial inflammatory response following tissue injury. $O_2$ is the most immediate requirement for the formation of new blood vessels and connective tissue in wound healing. The phagocytic NADPH oxidase (NOX-2) is required to consume $O_2$ in order for phagocytic cells to produce sufficient lactate to activate transcription factors and promote the development of angiogenic factors. The $O_2$ content available for consumption also affects the reconstitution of connective tissue as it plays a role in collagen maturation and fibroblast proliferation. In addition, the consumption of $O_2$ supports the host's strong immune response to infection, as sufficient $O_2$ ensures that the phagocytic cells produce the right amount of antibacterial ROS. $O_2$ is inhaled into halation into wound tissue, relying on local blood supply, vascular tone, arterial oxygen pressure and $O_2$ penetration distance, and immune regulation to participate in repair. Edema and necrotic tissue increase the penetration distance of $O_2$ to the wound. Peripheral vasoconstriction also significantly limits $O_2$ perfusion and oxygenation, and correcting hypoxemia and vasoconstriction can increase collagen deposition by a factor of 10. Therefore, adequate wound perfusion and oxygenation are of great significance for wound healing.

There are three levels of clinical application of $O_2$ in wound healing:

A. Diagnostic methods using percutaneous $O_2$ ($TcO_2$), but $TcO_2$ does not reflect $PO_2$ at the wound. Because the standard TcO2 determination is performed at 42 °C of the skin, the measured value is too high; and the intact skin around the wound is different from the actual situation.
B. Prophylactic applications, it has been demonstrated that supplementation of $O_2$ during the perioperative period to adequately improve wound perfusion can reduce postoperative infection.
C. Oxygen therapy for treating wounds has both systemic and local. Hyperbaric oxygen therapy (HBOT) provides 100% $O_2$ at 2–3 atmospheres, 10–30 times, 60–120 min each time, five times a week. The disadvantage is the need for equipment such as hyperbaric oxygen chambers, which is expensive, has a multiorgan oxygen poisoning crisis, and the poor blood supply of wound tissue limits its use. Local oxygen therapy does not allow $O_2$ to penetrate deep tissue, but it is beneficial for superficial wounds without intact blood supply, correcting $PO_2$ in cells at the center of the wound and improving the function of its reduced nicotinamide adenine dinucleotide

phosphate (NADPH) oxidase, the latter is related to cell dynamics, angiogenesis, and extracellular matrix formation.

## 11.4.1 Hyperbaric Oxygen Therapy

### 11.4.1.1 Development History

Hyperbaric oxygen was first used in repressurization by divers in the 1930s and was used to enhance the efficacy of radiotherapy in the 1950s. A few years later, hyperbaric oxygen was used to support patients with cardiac surgery, to treat clostridial gas gangrene and carbon monoxide poisoning. When people used hyperbaric oxygen to treat CO poisoning in coal mine explosions in 1965, it was found that hyperbaric oxygen can accelerate wound healing. Although hyperbaric oxygen has a long history in clinical applications, people are still studying its mechanism of action. As people learn more about the way oxygen interacts with living organisms, new therapeutic applications continue to emerge. The use of hyperbaric oxygen in wound therapy creates a brief pulse of oxygen every 24 h for 90 min. Although transient elevated oxygen levels do not significantly affect wound healing, hyperbaric oxygen therapy can affect the wound in a variety of ways after treatment has ceased. A typical chronic wound usually requires 20–30 hyperbaric oxygen treatments. This may reflect the amount of new blood vessels needed to maintain wound healing. Later studies have shown that for radiotherapy wounds, hyperbaric oxygen can induce angiogenesis, which becomes very noticeable after 14 oxygen treatments and will persist for several years after the end of hyperbaric oxygen therapy. Nowadays, research on hyperbaric oxygen in wound healing has continued to develop.

### 11.4.1.2 Mechanism of Action

The mechanism by which hyperbaric oxygen promotes tissue repair may involve:

A. The pressure effect of oxygen. Hyperbaric oxygen has a good effect on air bubble disease, decompression sickness, and gas embolism. Hyperbaric oxygen can reduce the damage of air bubbles to the tissue. Hyperbaric oxygen can also significantly reduce edema, and is beneficial for reperfusion injury, crush injury, chamber syndrome, burns, wound healing, and flap transplantation.
B. Superoxide synthesis of tissue. Oxygenation of hypoxic tissue is one of the key mechanisms for hyperbaric oxygen to accelerate wound healing. Many studies have shown that the oxygen obtained from the wound is related to the dose of oxygen. However, oxygen is a potent drug that, like other drugs, may be used too much or too little. The role of oxygen in wound healing is primarily related to oxygen accumulation in the tissue, rather than diffusion. However, the rate at which oxygen enters the wound is affected by its rate of outward diffusion from the capillaries. Edema can impede the enrichment of oxygen in the wound and increase the diffusion distance between the capillaries. Even mild tissue edema can significantly delay the rate at which oxygen enters the tissue, causing tissue hypoxia. Chronic wounds are usually in an oxygen-deficient state, and hyperbaric oxygen therapy corrects hypoxia. Although transient, hyperbaric oxygen therapy can still accelerate the wound healing process through specific mechanisms. Oxygenation in chronic wounds improves with the treatment of hyperbaric oxygen. In the treatment of HBOT, the oxygen dose is more than the physiological dose, and the hemoglobin is in an oxygen saturation state. At the same time, under the condition of sufficient arterial blood flow, the oxygen dissolved in the plasma has a direct proportional relationship with the oxygen pressure, and the plasma can dissolve enough oxygen to meet the tissue's need for oxygen without the need for oxygen support carried by hemoglobin. At 2–2.5 ATA, the oxygen dissolved in the plasma is increased by ten times, which is beneficial to oxygen entering the ischemic tissue, allowing the tissue to survive and maintain its activity and function. In addition to increasing the amount of oxygen in the tissue, HBOT can effectively increase the availability of oxygen. In theory, during HBOT treatment, the ability of oxygen to penetrate the skin was enhanced and the oxygen transported to the tissues was further increased. The increase in arterial oxygen partial pressure leads to vasodilation, which in turn reduces blood flow to the capillary bed, and the pressure in capillaries is reduced, allowing blood with high oxygen content to enter the tissue, promoting angiogenesis, collagen synthesis, and wound healing, the therapeutic effect lasts for 2–4 h. In addition, under ischemic conditions, the vasodilation effect of HBOT can reduce tissue blood flow, which seems to be detrimental to wound healing; however, the high oxidative effect of HBOT is sufficient to compensate for this reduction in blood flow.
C. Downregulation of cytokines and upregulation of growth factors and receptors. Hyperbaric oxygen can have a beneficial effect on many cytokines and growth factors that are important for wound healing. Hyperbaric oxygen can upregulate collagen synthesis by pro-al(I) mRNA expression. In rabbit ear wound experiments, it was found that hyperbaric oxygen can upregulate PDGF-β receptor mRNA expression. In the treatment of ischemic flaps, hyperbaric oxygen can upregulate fibroblast growth factor, producing a stronger effect than using FGF alone. In the case of FGF, ineffective, hyper-

baric oxygen can enhance its effect. In patients with Crohn's disease, hyperbaric oxygen therapy can reduce the levels of IL-1, IL-6, and tumor necrosis factor-α (TNF-α). A single hyperbaric oxygen treatment resulted in elevated levels of TNF in normal rats. Under different physiological conditions, hyperbaric oxygen can upregulate or downregulate the expression of growth factors. Hypoxia can upregulate VEGF, but hyperoxic conditions caused by hyperbaric oxygen therapy can also upregulate the factor. Hyperbaric oxygen also enhances the effects of TGF-β1 and PDGF-β.

D. Promote angiogenesis. Although hypoxia is a condition of endogenous angiogenesis, proper oxygen supplementation can maintain and accelerate the growth of blood vessels. In the murine model, HBOT directly promotes neovascularization in a dose-dependent manner, with HBOT's proangiogenic effect peaking at 2.5 ATA. It has been repeatedly demonstrated that the application of HBOT can promote the angiogenic response at the edge of the wound, and the extent of the response depends on the increase in the amount of angiogenic factors in the center of the wound.

(A) Oxygen is essential for phagocytosis and bactericidal action of neutrophils or polymorphonuclear cells (PMNs). This process involves the generation of oxygen free radicals and superoxides and is directly affected by the oxygen concentration in the tissue. When the partial pressure of oxygen is lower than 30 mmHg, the bactericidal effect of PMNs is significantly reduced. PMNs-mediated killing of aerobic bacteria, including common proteobacteria, *Salmonella typhimurium*, *Klebsiella pneumoniae*, *Serratia marcescens*, *Pseudomonas aeruginosa*, and *Staphylococcus aureus*, will disappear under hypoxia. Increasing the oxygen concentration has been shown to reduce infection. When oxygen was administered during surgery and oxygen was given 2 h after surgery, the infection rate decreased by 54%. Therefore, an increase in tissue oxygen concentration is beneficial to the bactericidal action of PMNs and prevention of infection. Hyperbaric oxygen has six ways to combat clinical infection:
   (a) To support tissue that is hypoxic due to infection.
   (b) Activate neutrophils and strengthen their effects.
   (c) Strengthen macrophage activity.
   (d) Inhibit bacterial growth.
   (e) The release of certain bacterial endotoxin is inhibited.
   (f) Strengthen the role of antibiotics and resist the hypoxia caused by antibiotic delivery and activity. In addition, the study found that free radicals in phage can inactivate pathogens, phagocytosis requires a large amount of oxygen to form a reaction medium, and HBOT can promote leukocytes to kill pathogens through phagocytic effects, reduce the inflammatory response of hypoxic tissue, hypoxia suppresses this effect.

#### 11.4.1.3 Current Application Status

Hyperbaric oxygen provides a pharmacological amount of oxygen for tissue healing. A typical wound treatment consisted of 90 min of pure oxygen treatment with a pressure of 45 ft. deep (FSW) or 13.7 m of seawater (MSW) or 1.38 bar. This is equivalent to 100% oxygen at 2.36 absolute atmospheres. In repressurization for diving-related injuries, patients may need to be exposed to 60 FSW (18.3 m/2.8 ATM/284 $kPa^{-1}$) to 0 FSW of oxygen for at least 4 h.

In vitro tests have confirmed that hyperbaric oxygen therapy promotes wound healing. Since endothelial progenitor cells participate in neovascularization in the hypoxic zone, they play an important role in wound healing. High intracellular oxygenation by hyperbaric oxygen effectively promotes mobilization of endothelial progenitor cells. However, hyperbaric oxygen therapy does not target wound sites, and serious adverse events (including epileptic seizure and pneumothorax) may be associated with this. Hyperbaric oxygen therapy is performed in a special compartment of the patient in a guardable compartment when needed. The hyperbaric oxygen chamber maintains the cabin pressure at 2.5–3 ATM using compressed oxygen or air. Treatments for nonhealing wounds are usually 1.5–2 h a day for 20–40 days.

Hyperbaric oxygen has been used as an adjunct to acute and chronic wounds. Most studies are observational, and the current small number of trials are limited by small sample sizes and low quality. A systematic review concluded that hyperbaric oxygen may be beneficial for certain types of wounds, such as the healing of diabetic ulcers.

A. Acute injury. Hyperbaric oxygen therapy may be of value to patients with extensive soft tissue injury. In one of the trials, 36 patients with crush injuries were randomized into two groups, and one group received hyperbaric oxygen therapy for 90 min once after operation, twice a day for 6 days; the other group received pseudo treatment for a total of 6 days after surgery. There were significantly more patients who completely healed in the hyperbaric oxygen therapy group, and fewer patients required flaps, transplants, vascular procedures, or amputations. Fasciotomy wounds: reperfusion animal models after acute osteofascial compartment syndrome incision suggest that hyperbaric oxygen therapy may be beneficial. Thermal injury: a systematic review of hyperbaric oxygen therapy for burns found only two high-quality trials and concluded that there is insufficient evidence to support the use of hyperbaric oxygen after thermal injury. Ischemic transplant skin and flaps: hyperbaric oxygen therapy may increase the survival of skin grafts and reconstructed flaps with impaired blood supply, thereby preventing tissue breakdown and wound development. Patients with localized vascular damage, areas that have previously received radiation therapy, or where prior transplant failures require skin grafts or reconstructed flaps may benefit from preventive treatment.

B. Chronic ulcer. Hyperbaric oxygen therapy has been used as an adjunct to chronic nonhealing wounds and ulcers caused by venous insufficiency, diabetes, and peripheral arterial disease. There is also a lack of evidence to support the use of hyperbaric oxygen therapy for venous ulcers, pressure ulcers, and wounds associated with chronic ischemia (peripheral arterial disease). Although hyperbaric oxygen therapy is associated with accelerated healing of ulcers in diabetic patients, the indications for hyperbaric oxygen for the treatment of nonhealing diabetic foot ulcers still need to be determined.

At present, the use of hyperbaric oxygen therapy in the process of chronic wound healing has shown a very significant effect. However, hyperbaric oxygen therapy has disadvantages such as being expensive, time-consuming, and side effects such as fatigue, dizziness, and even lung failure. In addition, hyperbaric oxygen (HBO) can promote wound healing, but it should be noted that (a) well-perfused wounds do not need to use hyperbaric oxygen, but effective for hypoxic or ischemic wounds, such as diabetic ulcers, venous ulcers, failed transplants, skin flap and necrotic soft tissue infection, and refractory osteomyelitis. (b) In wound healing, hypoxia refers to insufficient oxygen supply and hinders the normal healing process. Hyperbaric oxygen provides the oxygen needed to stimulate and support wound healing. (c) Hyperbaric oxygen can fight infections, such as gas gangrene. Hyperbaric oxygen can directly act on anaerobic bacteria, enhance leukocyte and macrophage activity, and enhance antibiotic effects. (d) Hyperbaric oxygen is a relatively safe, noninvasive treatment. Possible side effects include barotrauma to the middle ear and lungs and myopia. Contraindications include cardiac insufficiency and severe obstructive pulmonary disease.

## 11.4.2 Topical Oxygen Therapy (TOT)

### 11.4.2.1 Development History

Because the treatment of wounds with hyperbaric oxygen is complicated and expensive, and the oxygen pressure of 30–50 mmHg is not as effective as direct contact with wound treatment with 100% pure oxygen. In 1985, Brown used a garbage bag to insert the ulcer into the leg, fastened the bag, and used plastic tube to deliver pure oxygen to the bag for treatment. For ulcers that occur in the hips, buttocks, ankles, perineum, or other inconvenient operating areas, cut a large, sturdy trash bag at the bottom corner (a diameter slightly larger than the thigh circumference) so that the legs penetrate inside the hole and fasten the pocket at the waist. In recent years, the papers published in China on TOT treatment wounds are basically the same as Brown's method, which is similar to it, but it has played a role. Currently, there are two ways to treat wounds with TOT, namely, simple TOT and TOT combined with other therapies. In addition to plastic bags and fresh-keeping bags, simple TOT also uses disposable paper cups, treatment trays, dressing bowls, oxygen masks, and artificial anal bags. After covering the wound surface, the bag is closed with a bandage or tape on the bag. The plastic tube or the infusion tube with the scalp needle removed releases pure oxygen. It can also directly blow the wound with pure oxygen, and the effect is also very good. The oxygen supply source is mostly an oxygen cylinder, and the humidification bottle may be water or alcohol or a dry cylinder. These methods are simple, practical, and easy to popularize.

Compared with hyperbaric oxygen therapy, local oxygen therapy only supplies local oxygen to the wound, and the effects of the two on physiology and biochemistry are different. A key issue in local oxygen supply to the wound is how to effectively increase the oxygen supply to the wound. Although gaseous oxygen can diffuse to the wound surface, the skin and exudate of the wound bed prevent oxygen from diffusing, allowing only a very small amount of oxygen to enter the body through the skin and wound exudate. Local oxygen therapy needs to overcome two major problems: (a) oxygen breaks through the barrier of skin and wound exudate by diffusion. (b) Oxygen in the wound bed is transferred and diffused into cells requiring oxygen (such as fibroblasts, immune cells) and proteins that construct extracellular matrices. Increasing the oxygen concentration and oxygen partial pressure in the wound area are beneficial to both diffusion processes.

Brown, Fries, Suh, Hunt, etc., as well as many first-line wound treatment therapist in China, in the practice of a large number of cases, believed that TOT is positive effect for all kinds of wounds, including pressure ulcers, diabetic foot, wound infection, eczema, etc. After a few minutes of oxygen administration, the degenerated fat and necrotic tissue liquefaction can be seen, while the viable tissue becomes fresh. After treatment, the secretions gradually decreased, the skin edema of the wounds gradually reduced or even disappeared, and the granulation tissue gradually formed.

### 11.4.2.2 Mechanism of Action

Local oxygen supply promotes wound healing, which has many aspects and multiple levels of function, as follows:

A. Increase local tissue oxygenation, correct hypoxia, increase VEGF expression, and promote angiogenesis; promote endogenous NO production, dilate blood vessels, and increase local blood perfusion of wounds.

B. Enhance immunity, play a role in nutrition and antibiotics: (a) All cells associated with wounds can produce reactive oxygen species, oxygen free radicals, and special enzymes of $H_2O_2$, supplementing oxygen to prevent these enzymes from dying and avoiding damage to healing. (b) Tissue $PO_2$ levels are closely related to the occurrence of infection, correcting hypoxia, improving tissue oxygen content, inhibiting bacterial proliferation and producing toxins, and exerting macrophage bactericidal activity. (c) Enhance cellular oxygen metabolism, avoid white blood cells premature due to hypoxia and not play bactericidal function, increase granulocyte oxygen production capacity, reduce damage to tissues, and reduce IL-2, IL-8, reduce the amount of C-reactive protein in acute phase.
C. Improve capillary permeability of hypoxic tissue: eliminate edema, improve microcirculation, and prevent tissue from developing in the direction of degeneration and necrosis.

#### 11.4.2.3 Current Application Status

Currently there are the following application methods:

A. Local oxygen therapy classification. (a) Local pressurized oxygen therapy: at present, the local pressurized oxygen therapy products are composed of a small pressure chamber, an oxygen-permeable dressing, and an oxygen diffusion enhancer. The effectiveness of the treatment has been proved by published clinical studies and case reports. (b) Local continuous atmospheric pressure oxygen therapy: unlike local pressurized oxygen therapy, local continuous atmospheric oxygen therapy does not require increased pressure, does not contain a pressure chamber, and includes a closed dressing and an oxygen supply tube, and sometimes also includes a power supply battery. This device continuously supplies atmospheric oxygen flow. Animal experiments and clinical studies have shown that this method can promote the healing of different types of wounds. (c) Oxygen-releasing wound dressing: partial continuous atmospheric pressure oxygen therapy and pressurized oxygen therapy are directly treated with oxygen, and oxygen-releasing wound dressing is to release oxygen to the wound through the dressing. There are two methods for oxygen-releasing wound dressings. One is to store pure oxygen in the dressing (such as Oxygeneses, OxyBand), and the other is to release oxygen (such as Oxyzyme) through biochemical reactions in the dressing. In the first method, pure oxygen (>2800 mg/m$^3$ O) is stored in the dressing through the vesicles, and oxygen is released when the dressing is liquefied by the wound exudate. In vitro experiments have shown that this dressing can significantly increase the oxygen level of the wound, and the effect is obvious when dealing with larger wounds. A continuous release of oxygen can be used as a secondary dressing that releases oxygen for 5 or 6 days. In order to improve the delivery of oxygen to the wound, the wound should be cleaned regularly. The second method is to increase the oxygen concentration by a biochemical reaction (Oxyzyme). The Oxyzyme dressing is a combination of two separate gel sheets, one containing glucose oxidase and peroxidase, and the other hydrogel containing glucose oxidase. Glucose oxidase oxidizes glucose to release hydrogen peroxide, which then reacts with peroxidase to release oxygen. Studies have shown that such dressings promote the healing of different types of wounds. Oxygen release dressings can be used in the early stages of wound care, and the wound should be cleaned regularly when using this dressing. (d) Biochemical carrier oxygen supply: this oxygen therapy product uses a purified aqueous hemoglobin solution as an oxygen carrier. Hemoglobin is derived from mammals and transports oxygen molecules without the need to bind red blood cells. (e) Perfluorocarbon oxygen supply: perfluorocarbon (PFC) is a synthetic oxygen carrier that is not a source of animal. PFC is capable of binding and releasing oxygen in water. Currently, PFC has been used as a respiratory fluid, such as deep sea diving and blood substitutes, to replace hemoglobin. Davis et al. [51] reported the use of a PFC-containing emulsion as an oxygen carrier to treat second degree burn, and noted that this method can also be used to treat chronic wounds. At present, there is not enough clinical evidence to prove the safety of this technology, nor the sale of such wound care products.

## 11.5 Modern Dressing

### 11.5.1 The Development History

In ancient times, humans realized that covering the wound with leaves, fur, and stones could protect the wound. In 3000 BC, Egyptians used honey, oil, and wine to treat wounds. This is essentially a perceptual knowledge that may originate originally from an animal's instinct or mimic other animals. This is also the initial stage of human understanding of wound dressings. In the long-term evolutionary process, humans gradually found that adding some plant powder, mud, and branch secretions on the wound surface not only protects the wound, but also promotes wound healing. In the Zhou Dynasty in 1066 BC, Chinese "drug doctor" treated the wound with a medicine (external application). In the second century AD, due to advances in science, humans invented some new dressings, such as cotton and linen. The Greek scholar Galen found it necessary to keep the wound moist. He used sponge and cotton to moisten the wound. The ancient Chinese medical book *Handbook of Prescriptions for Emergencies* also used badger fat and honey to treat the wounds. In the Tang Dynasty, Sun Simiao proposed to use black plaster to treat wounds with sesame oil, yellow lead and wax in *Essential Recipes for Emergent Use Worth A Thousand Gold*. Preions for 52 diseases records the use of *Ulmus macrocarpa* Hance and lard to make ointment to treat calf burns, followed by a large number of topical plasters, the main role is to protect the wound, as well as heat and swelling, detoxification, and analgesia, detoxify the muscles, and promote healing. In 1793, Whitrey invented a cotton fiber dressing made of cotton. This type of wound dressing quickly entered due to its mature production process, wide range of raw materials, low cost, soft texture, certain adsorption capacity, reasonable price, and convenient use. In the large-scale industrialization stage, it is widely used for wound coverage of various types of wounds. In the nineteenth century, due to the advent of textile machines, dressing production techniques and techniques have made great strides, and many conceived dressings can be produced and industrialized. At the same time, the understanding and application of the disinfectant has made the application value of the dressing improve. Lister first realized that chemicals could kill bacteria and prevent the spread of bacteria. He began to incinerate bandages with carbonic acid in 1865 and invented antibacterial bandages. Inspired by Lister, Johnson has successfully produced antiseptic and bactericidal medical dressings that have greatly reduced the incidence of wound infections.

In 1962, Dr. Winter of the University of London published a famous paper in the journal *Nature*, demonstrating the healing effect of the moist environment on wounds, and the probability of re-epithelialization of wounds exposed to air is increased by 50% compared with the wounds of pig skin wounds sealed with polyethylene film. Subsequent domestic and international clinical practice and basic research support this concept. The first wet dressing is a semi-closed transparent film. The appearance of this product not only further confirms the theory of wet healing, but also promotes the development of other products. Hydrocolloid dressings appeared in the 1980s. The product contains hydrophilic colloidal particles, such as CMC, gelatin, and pectin, which can form a closed environment in local wounds. This raises new questions: whether the closed dressing is helpful for wound healing? Does pus and infection agglomerate cause more problems? Is there a risk of hematoma, seroma, or folliculitis? Wound specialists began to study the effects of local oxygen levels on wound healing. The fact that closed dressings can promote wound healing is contrary to people's long-standing understanding that people used to think that wounds need to "breathe." Another product that emerged in the 1980s was a hydrogel. The appearance of hydrogels is exciting because it makes it possible to actively add moisture to the wounds, and it allows people to better study the mechanism of wound healing. Wound dressings have seen great growth in the 1980s, and the industry is keen to promote products that accelerate wound healing and reduce pain. Polyurethane foam is another "magic" product that is popular because it not only maintains the wound's wet environment, but also manages wound exudation, does not stick to wounds, and increases patient comfort.

After the 1980s, a variety of synthetic dressings were introduced. The most important feature of these new dressings was their active participation and affecting wound healing speed and healing quality. In 2007, Xiaobing Fu, Wu Zhigu, and other editors published Modern Wound Dressing: Theory and Practice (Fig. 11.28), comprehensively introduced the development, clinical application of wound dressings, and evaluation methods for dressing performance and application effects. The content includes the research progress of tissue repair and regeneration in China, the relationship between wound dressing and wound repair, the basic types of wound dressings, the research trend and development trend of high-end products for wound repair (tissue engineering dressings), the performance and characteristics of commercially available main dressings, the preservation method of wound repair material, the clinical application of wound dressing, the relationship between wound dressing and infection, the animal model for wound repair dressing and new drug evaluation, and the evaluation index and evaluation method of wound dressing and wound healing, which can be referred to in detail.

### 11.5.2 The Mechanism of Action

The main mechanism of action of the theory of wet healing may include: (a) conducive to necrotic tissue and fibrinolysis. Clearing necrotic tissue is the first step in wound healing. In a humid environment, necrotic tissue is hydrated to release the plasmin and other proteolytic enzymes of the tissue cells themselves. These proteolytic enzymes hydrolyze the necrotic tissue, which is beneficial for absorption and debridement effect, and more importantly, in the case of venous leg ulcers, fibrous sheaths are often formed around small blood vessels, which hinder the exchange of nutrients between blood and tissues, while plasmin can dissolve the fibrous sheaths, and the nutrient exchange between blood and tissues returns to normal. In addition, protein degradation products and fibrin degradation products are also chemokines of immune cells, which can attract immune cells to move to the wound, accelerate the debridement process, and

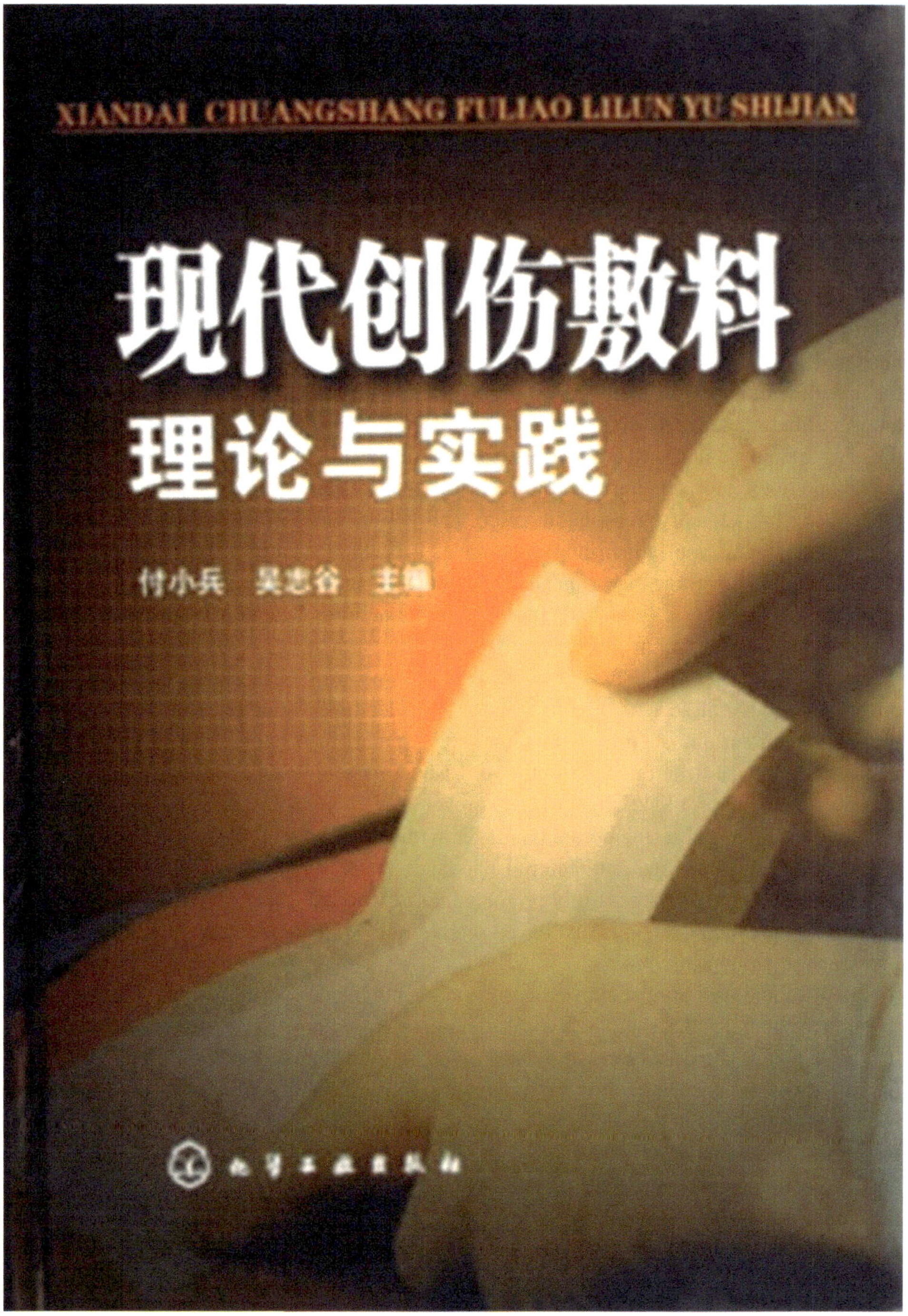


**Fig. 11.28** Modern Wound Dressing: Theory and Practice edited by academician Xiaobing Fu

promote the accelerated healing process of growth factor secretion. (b) New dressings can create a hypoxic environment and promote capillary formation. Contrary to traditional ideas, recent studies have found that fibroblasts grow fastest in a relatively low-oxygen environment and stimulate macrophages to release a variety of growth factors; capillaries are strongly stimulated, which accelerate blood vessel formation, significantly increase granulation tissue formation, and shorten wound healing time. (c) Growth factors release and upregulate their activity. The levels of fibroblast growth factor, epidermal growth factor, and platelet-derived growth factor in the exudate fluid were significantly higher than the control, and these exudates themselves promoted the growth of fibroblasts, keratinocytes, and vascular endothelium cells cultured in vitro. (d) New dressing can also reduce pain and reinjury during wound dressing change. Traditional dressings cause wound pain and reinjury to the repaired wound due to adhesion of the dressing fiber to the wound tissue, exudate, etc., and the new dressing creates a wet environment in the wound surface, which can reduce the adhesion of the dressing to the wound surface and prevent the death and exposure of the nerve endings of the wound surface. (e) New dressings reduce the chance of infection on the wound. (f) The wet environment is conducive to cell proliferation, differentiation, and migration. Both cell proliferation and differentiation and the development of enzyme activity require water as a medium. In a humid environment, the activity of the ribozyme can be maintained, and the speed of cell migration can contribute to the healing of the wound.

### 11.5.3 The Current Application Status

With the continuous deepening of wound healing research, people gradually realize that the purpose of using dressings is not only to cover the wounds and to prevent pollution or infection, but also to "actively" promote wound healing.

Conventional dressings, such as gauze and cotton pads, are commonly used dressings in clinical practice and are still widely used in various types of wounds. They have the advantages of protecting wounds, good water absorption, simple production, low price, and reusability. However, it is also easy to cause adhesion to the wound during the healing process, causing secondary damage.

In the past 40 years, a variety of temporary wound covering dressings have been developed at home and abroad. They are new dressings, also known as modern dressings. There is no definitive concept about new dressings, usually those that are different in shape from traditional dressings (gauze) and that can actively participate in the function and affect the healing speed and quality of wounds. It is gradually and widely used in clinical practice. Modern dressings for temporary wound covering in clinic mainly include natural biological dressings, synthetic dressings, and tissue engineering.

#### 11.5.3.1 Natural Biological Dressings

A. Biological dressing. Biological dressings include chitosan dressings, alginate dressings, silk fibroin materials, and the like.
   (a) Chitosan dressing: Chitin is a linear polysaccharide formed by linking *N*-acetyl-α-amino-D-glucose in the form of β-1,4 glycosidic bonds, which is second only to cellulose in nature. A large amount of natural polysaccharides can be degraded by lysozyme; chitosan is a deacetylated product of chitin. In 1976, Prudden et al. [52] pointed out that lysozyme was present in the wound, which could degrade chitin and its derivatives. Chitosan can be degraded into N-acetylglucosamine on the wound surface, which can be absorbed by epidermal cells and is an essential nutrient for the growth and reproduction of epidermal cells. Chitosan also increases the reticular formation of the wound tissue and the synthesis of collagen, thereby increasing the tensile strength of the wound. In 1983, Malette et al. [53] first reported the hemostasis of chitosan. Chitosan can increase the reticular formation of wound tissue, increase collagen synthesis, enhance the tensile strength of wounds, and have strong air permeability. It can activate macrophages and promote wound healing. It is weakly immunogenic, nontoxic, has good biocompatibility and biodegradability, and also has antibacterial, hemostasis, anti-inflammatory, good absorption of exudate, and promotes tissue regeneration and skin collagen fiber growth. Chitosan stopped bleeding quickly, but it was unstable, easy to fall off, and then added some chemicals to make it contact with blood or body fluids. It becomes extremely sticky and can quickly seal the wound surface without forming a thrombus. This kind of bandage has carried out various experiments such as spleen rupture, liver rupture, and aortic incision in pigs. The effect is satisfactory. In severe trauma test, it can stop bleeding in 1–5 min. This bandage has become the equipment of the US military. Using chitosan as a raw material, a dressing prepared by adding antibiotics and/or antibiotics with sustained release function can effectively control wound infection and accelerate wound healing. This dressing has been greatly developed at home and abroad, and has been widely used in clinical practice.
   (b) Alginate dressings: These dressings are soft, nonwoven fibers that are extracted from seaweed. Its main function is to absorb exudate, form a gel, and exchange $Na^+/Ca^{2+}$ with exudate. This product covers the wound surface after contact with the wound surface, and transforms the insoluble calcium alginate into soluble sodium alginate by ion exchange. At the same time, it releases calcium ions, so it has hemostatic function. It is used for postoperative wound filling and plays a good role in hemostasis drainage. It has good absorption performance and can absorb 20 times of its own mass (5–7 times of gauze). After absorbing liquid, it expands into a sodium alginate gel, forming a soft, moist, gel-like semisolid substance on the wound surface, so that the wound is isolated from the outside world, forming a closed atmosphere without oxygen, accelerating the proliferation of new microvessels. It is important to maintain moist environment, improve the environment, improve the regeneration ability of epidermal cells, accelerate the movement of epidermal cells, and promote wound healing.

(c) Silk fibroin protein material: Silk fibroin is a fibrous protein obtained by silk reeling and degumming from silkworm cocoons, which is rich in amino acids, nontoxic and nonirritating, and biodegradable. It promotes cell growth and has good tissue compatibility. Main advantages: silk fibroin is derived from organisms, has good cell affinity and tissue affinity; it can be easily absorbed by organisms after being degraded by bioprotease; the risk of disease transmission is small, and biosafety is reliably guaranteed; there are several methods to solve the molding problem at high porosity.

B. Mammal skin and connective tissue dressings.

(a) Natural animal dressings include autologous skin, allogeneic skin, xenogenic skin, and amniotic membrane. At present, the most ideal method for covering wounds is to transplant autologous skin, but in large-area burn patients with burns exceeding 50%, autologous skin sources are seriously inadequate.

(b) Allogeneic skin: This is one of the skin substitutes that has proven to be more effective in the past 40 years. It is an ideal wound covering. Its main source is the cadaver skin, which has a better skin barrier function. The moisture permeability and adhesion of allogeneic skin are similar to those of autologous skin, which can prevent bacterial invasion and prevent the loss of water, electrolyte, protein and heat in wounds, and have good hemostasis and promote epithelialization.

(c) Heterologous skin: Since the source of the homogeneity skin is extremely limited, research on the replacement of autologous skin and allogeneic skin by animal heterologous skin has made some progress. Although as early as 1880, there was a history of animal skin (sheep) transplantation. However, the application of this as a temporary biological dressing on burn wounds was first reported in 1965. Brember et al. [54] reported the successful use of pig skin treatment. Its greatest advantage is that it is similar to human skin in adhesion, aeration, collagen structure, and collagen content. Pigskin dressings promote the recovery of ecological tissues and reduce pain and accelerate the formation of skin attachments. In the early 1970s, China began to experiment with pigskin in clinical practice. Although it survived in the early stage after pigskin transplantation, it could not establish blood supply, and hindered the expansion of autologous skin, it falls off earlier than allogeneic skin, and it was prone to infection. In addition, there are some defects such as pain when removing pigskin and hardening after drying.

(d) Amniotic membrane: In 1910, Davis pioneered the clinical application of amniotic membrane. He first used amniotic membrane as a wound dressing for skin transplantation. The advantages of amniotic membrane: certain antibacterial effect; promote wound blood vessel growth; reduce water evaporation and electrolyte loss in local wounds; apply to cut wounds can make fresh granulation, reduce bacterial content of wounds; have certain antiangiogenic and anti-inflammatory effects; rich sources, simple production, etc. Because the single layer of amniotic membrane is brittle, easy to crack, not resistant to pressure, poor in water retention, etc., it is clinically made into a multilayer irradiated amniotic membrane or immersed in glutaraldehyde, which is nonimmunogenic, and has better adhesion and air permeability.

In 1995, Wainwright developed an acellular dermal matrix (ADM) as a permanent dermal substitute for composite skin and was successfully used in the clinic.

#### 11.5.3.2 Synthetic Dressing

Synthetic polymers have been used in medical research for burn dressings for more than 40 years. With the advancement of science and technology and the development of modern industry, especially the rapid rise of the petrochemical industry, the variety of synthetic dressings based on polymer materials is increasing, representative of film type, foam type, spray type, and composite type.

A. Film-type synthetic dressing: The dressing is formed by applying a pressure-sensitive adhesive to one side of a biomedical film. Most of the materials used to make the film are transparent elastomers such as polyethylene, polyurethane, polycaprolactone, polytetrafluoroethylene, siloxane elastomers, and the like. The film-like dressing is generally divided into two layers. The inner hydrophilic material absorbs the wound surface, the outer material has good gas permeability and elasticity, the dressing has transparent appearance and good permeability, which is convenient for dynamic observation of the wound. It absorbs the exudate of the wound to a certain extent, but it is easy to cause the accumulation of the exudate after absorption, which may induce the pathogen to breed or aggravate the wound infection, so it is not suitable for exudative and infectious wounds. Representative products are Tegaderm, Dermafilm, Oprafiex, Opsite, etc.

B. Foam-type synthetic dressing: Its structure is porous, has a large absorption capacity for liquid, and oxygen and carbon dioxide are almost completely transmitted. The synthetic raw materials are polyvinyl butyral, polyurethane, polyurethane, polyvinyl alcohol, and the like. Its treatment of wound exudate relies on sponge-type water vapor transport and absorption mechanisms to control exudate. It has a good protective effect on wounds. Due to good permeability and good water permeability, it has strong absorption to the wound exudate. In addition, the dressing is light and the patient feels comfortable. The disadvantages are poor adhesion, low dressing strength, and easy damage; another disadvantage is that the dressing is generally opaque, it is difficult to observe the wound surface, is susceptible to bacterial contamination, the dressing pores are large, the granulation tissue of the wound is easy to grow, and the dressing is easy to cause the film to be removed difficult. Representative products are Allevyn, Ivalon.

C. Spray-type synthetic dressing: The high-molecular polymer and the solvent are directly sprayed on the wound surface to form a film, which is convenient to use, and is mostly soft and transparent, which is convenient for clinical observation. Because of its good barrier effect, it is suitable for wounds after early debridement, superficial second degree burn wounds and donor areas. However, the spray film is easily dissolved by the wound surface, no anti-infection effect, and the moisturizing property of the dressing is poor, so the water loss of the wound surface is large, and it is not suitable for large-area wounds, and the adhesion and tensile strength are poor. Representative products are Hydron, Aeroplast.
D. Hydrogel-based dressings: Hydrogel-based dressings use a hydrogel material on a permeable polymer liner. Natural polymers which can form hydrogels include collagen and gelatin, hyaluronic acid and its salts, fibrin, alginate, and chitosan. This type of dressing has a water content of 96%, which can maintain the moist environment of the wound. It can undergo repeated hydration when it comes into contact with the tissue. It has a good moisturizing effect. It can closely adhere to the irregular flat wound and reduce the probability of bacterial invasion, but has poor ventilation. The treatment of the liquid is absorption, the hydrogel that absorbs the exudate does not pollute the wound, and the dressing does not have to be changed in the short term, but the absorption of the exudate causes the dressing to expand, causing the dressing to separate from the wound, and providing the opportunity for invasion of bacteria. The hydrogel itself has a temperature of only 5 °C, so it has a mild cooling effect, which can significantly reduce postoperative pain and inflammation. It is suitable for skin wounds such as skin abrasions, lasers, and chemical damage. Representative products are Duoderm, Comfeel, Span Gel Gelipem, and so on.

#### 11.5.3.3 Tissue Engineering

Human skin equivalents (HSE) is one of the most successful products of tissue engineering to date, consisting of primary cultured skin cells (including keratinocytes, fibroblasts, and/or stem cells), and ECM (mainly collagen) is an active component of skin. It is an effective strategy to cope with the lack of donor skin. It can avoid fluid loss and infection in the injured area, and can promote the secretion of cytokines and growth factors, thus accelerating wound healing.

Currently tissue-engineered skin for clinical transplantation is divided into three categories: epidermal substitutes, dermal substitutes, and whole skin substitutes.

A. Epidermal substitute. The epidermal substitute is to peel off the epidermal portion of the biopsy skin tissue of 2–5 $cm^2$ and to separate the keratinocytes and culture them on the inactivated fibroblast trophoblast to form an epidermal membrane. Currently there are several companies that offer skin substitute products, such as Epicel® made by a company using patient autologous keratinocytes for burn treatment.
B. Dermal substitutes. The dermis substitute has stronger stability, can increase skin elasticity, softness, and mechanical wear resistance after wound healing, reduce scar hyperplasia, and control spasm. The dermis substitutes currently on the market are: Transcyte®, Dermagraft®, Alloderm®, Strattice®, and Intergra® DRT.
C. Whole skin substitute. The whole skin substitute contains both an epidermis layer and a dermis layer, and forms a bilayer structure with keratinocytes and fibroblasts derived from autologous or allogeneic. Maruguchi et al. [55] implanted fibroblasts into a sponge-like matrix, and after culturing for a period of time, keratinized cells were plated and histological studies were performed 1 week later. It was found that the proliferation and differentiation of keratinocytes were very similar to those of normal human epidermis. A typical product of the whole skin substitute is Apligraf®. PermaDerm® is a promising new product for a company that can be used as a permanent covering for large burns and other wounds, made from collagen in keratinocytes and fibroblasts. Other whole skin substitute products such as Orcel® produced by a bioscience company are also composed of keratinocytes, fibroblasts, and type I bovine collagen.

Future development of wound healing and in vitro skin model development should be based on the regeneration of skin from intact human skin containing hair follicles, sebaceous glands, sweat glands, and other accessory structures. Jinan Biotechnology Co., Ltd. has achieved certain results in this area. The intact human skin regenerated on immunodeficient mice has almost no difference in tissue structure from normal skin, can spontaneously heal the wound, and the generated hair has a normal circulation cycle.

At present, there are problems: insufficient regeneration and repair performance, cell source problems, high production and storage transportation costs, and relevant regulations and management methods need to be improved. Tissue engineering skin will have broad clinical application prospects, significant social value, and great commercial value.

D. Problems and future prospects. The development of wound dressings is very rapid, and gradually presents a functional and diversified development trend. The new dressings represented by biosynthetic dressings are gradually replacing the conventional application status of traditional dressings, which has effectively promoted the progress and development of world medicine. Driven by the development of modern science and technology, the application and research of new biosynthetic dressings will surely achieve greater development, and will certainly make important contributions to the development of world and modern wound healing theories and technologies. The generation and application of new dressings represent the transformation and development of the wound dressings. It is not only a theoretical and practical breakthrough for some traditional viewpoints in the past, but also a new development for wound treatment brought by the development of the whole society, the improvement of people's living standards, and the improvement of medical treatment. In Europe and the United States, new dressings have been widely used in clinical and patient families, and have played a positive role in the repair of diabetic ulcers, arteriovenous ulcers of the lower extremities, hemorrhoids, burn wounds, and other wounds. Thanks to medical advances, the medical expenses spent by patients also showed a gradual decline during the process of wound repair.

However, until now there has not been any dressing that has all the desired features and is suitable for all stages of wounds, and there is no method or dressing suitable for all wounds. Therefore, when using new dressings, the indications of various dressings should be strictly followed, combined with the individual condition of the patient, the type of wound, the stage of wound progression, and the condition of the skin, and the wound can be comprehensively evaluated to meet the therapeutic needs of the wound under different conditions. At the same time, strict aseptic operation, strengthening nutrition, and active systemic treatment can achieve satisfactory therapeutic results.

In China, the introduction and application of new dressings began in the early 1990s and was rapidly promoted throughout the country. However, as far as the current application situation is concerned, there are still the following problems: lack of knowledge and understanding of wounds, especially chronic hard-to-heal wound treatment; lack of understanding of new dressings, especially the fear that the humid environment increases infection and delays wound repair. It hinders the promotion and application of dressings. Medical dressings are no longer limited to protecting wounds. They should also have the effect of promoting wound healing. They should have special dressings for different stages of wound healing. It is easy to use and relieves patients' pain. No scar tissue is produced after wound healing. The use of animal-derived biological dressings has safety concerns such as bacterial infections and endogenous retroviruses. The ideal wound dressing in the future should have the following characteristics: it can protect the wound, not adhere to the wound, and will not damage the wound again when the dressing is changed; it can provide a good local environment for wound healing, actively promote wound healing; no immune antigenicity, no trigger excretion reaction and inflammation; easy to make, convenient for storage and disinfection. In addition, the modification or compounding method improves the deficiencies of existing materials and enhances its various properties as a dressing. The drug is loaded with various drugs and growth factors to effectively control drug release while achieving wound healing and therapeutic effects. From the patient's point of view, try to reduce the number of dressing changes and reduce the pain caused by dressing changes. In order to meet the needs of sustainable development of society and the recycling of resources, more new types of biodegradable materials will be developed and applied to medical dressings.

With the development of tissue engineering technology and skin tissue engineering, the future will also develop appropriate three-dimensional porous structure, provide nutrient and metabolic environment for cell growth and reproduction, regulate cell growth and alignment, and finally degrade the tissue-engineered dressings for the purpose of permanent tissue replacement. At present, biological materials used for tissue damage/repair are mainly classified into synthetic polymer materials and natural biological materials. The synthetic polymer material can control the physical and chemical properties of the material by adjusting the molecular structure of the main chain, is easy to shape and mass produce, and can control the degradation rate by changing the polymerization rate of the monomer. However, its compatibility with cells is poor, which is not conducive to cell attachment and migration, and the monomeric substances formed by degradation products cannot be quickly absorbed by tissues, easily form an acidic environment, and stimulate local tissue to produce an inflammatory reaction. Compared with synthetic polymer materials, natural materials such as collagen, chitosan, hyaluronic acid, and silk protein have the advantages of low immunogenicity and good cell compatibility, which have become the focus of the research on tissue damage repairing biomaterials in the field of regenerative medicine in recent years. Among them, collagen is the main component of the extracellular matrix in tissues and is an ideal biomaterial for repairing tissue damage. At present, the extraction, purification, shaping, and cross-linking techniques of collagen have made great progress, and the degradation and mechanical properties can be controlled by cross-linking modification. However, due to the differences in mechanical properties of different tissues, the development of collagen materials with mechanical properties, structure, and regeneration characteristics is still a key issue for clinical application.

An important member of the Xiaobing Fu team collaborated with Prof. Quan Daping from Sun Yat-sen University to conduct in-depth research on the basic research of decellularized submucosal materials to accelerate wound healing and clinical trials of diabetic foot wounds. It is hopeful to transform into new dressings and scaffold products for tissue repair and tissue regeneration. The submucosal layer of pig small intestine is collected from the jejunum of pigs. It is a cell-free biomaterial with a network structure very close to human extracellular matrix. It is mainly composed of extracellular matrix (ECM). The main component of ECM is collagen, proteoglycans, glycoproteins, noncollagen glycoproteins, aminoglycans, various growth factors, and are rich in components that promote angiogenesis. The main components of collagen are type I, type III, and type V collagen fibers. The constituent proteins of collagen fibers are highly conserved in evolution, and even when xenografts are performed, they do not cause serious immune rejection. The matrix contains five kinds of mucopolysaccharides such as heparan sulfate, hyaluronic acid, chondroitin sulfate A, dermatan sulfate, and heparin. Even if the intestinal submucosa is treated with strong physical and chemical treatment and sterilization, these mucopolysaccharides can still protect the bioactivity of cytokines in the submucosa of the small intestine. There are several important glycoproteins in the collagen structure of the small intestinal submucosa, including fibronectin and laminin, which are critical for cell attachment growth. All of these features contribute to the adhesion of cells to the submucosal layer of the small intestine. Although the porcine small intestinal submucosa material has undergone a series of decellularization and other engineering processes in the preparation process, it can still retain a certain amount of growth factors, such as VEGF, PDGF, TGF-β, and bFGF. It plays an important biological activity in the repair and reconstruction process of tissues.

The submucosa of the small intestine of the pig has a unique anatomical structure. The heparin sulfate proteoglycans between the collagen fibers are mainly concentrated in the blood vessels; the bFGF is connected to the fibrous structure and diffusely distributed; the VEGF is mainly distributed around the blood vessels. This structure plays an important role in tissue regeneration. After the material is implanted into the wound area, the ordered release of growth factors can be carried out according to biological requirements, thereby guiding and inducing tissue regeneration. The study found that tissue repair and regeneration under physiological conditions are related to the regeneration of endogenous bioactive factors. Endogenous growth factors activate or "wake up" tissue cells/stem cells through specific pathways to exert tissue regeneration and repair. The porcine small intestinal submucosa has been extensively studied as a tissue engineering scaffold material. The porcine small intestinal submucosa can guide and support the growth of host cells in the body, and gradually degrade completely. The regenerated tissue structure is remodeling rather than scar formation, and is suitable for use as scaffold materials for tissue engineering. In 1998, a US company applied this material development as a soft tissue repair material to the clinic. It has been used in more than one million cases and is significantly better than other synthetic materials. At the same time, the US FDA has approved another company's OA pig small intestinal submucosa for clinical use, which has been applied to the repair of various tissues, including the treatment of diabetic skin ulcers, chronic ischemic diseases of the limbs, such as diabetic foot, thromboangiitis obliterans, arteriosclerosis obliterans, etc. However, as a natural biological scaffold, the natural structure of the material leads to difficulty in regulating the degradation time and three-dimensional structure, which limits further use. First, the submucosal layer of the small intestine of the pig is a translucent film. The thickness of the submucosa of the single-layer pig small intestine is 0.05–0.22 mm. The film-like structure lacks sufficient volume and mechanical support, and it is difficult to achieve a good repair and treatment effect. Different soft tissues have various shapes and complex shapes, and are not satisfied by a single simple structure. In order to solve the problem of thickness, the researchers used multilayer vacuum lamination technology. The thickness of the four-layer pig small intestinal submucosa was about 0.6 mm and the thickness of the eight-layer composite was about 1.2 mm. It is still impossible to build a larger size product. Moreover, it is only a simple membrane structure, and it is difficult to meet the requirements of different soft tissue repair. Therefore, it is of great significance to make the material of the porcine small intestine submucosal material into a scaffold material having a complicated shape and thickness as needed. Second, the intrinsic microstructure of the porcine small intestine submucosa is a fibrous thin layer with dense collagen fibers. As a tissue engineering scaffold tissue, it is necessary to provide a three-dimensional growth environment for the cells that migrate and proliferate, and the thin layer of the porcine small intestinal submucosa can only provide a two-dimensional growth space, which leads to slower cell growth and thus limits its application. At the same time, the dense structure leads to a low porosity of the material, and the load rate is low when the growth factor is further loaded, and it is difficult to control the release. Finally, the degradation time of the existing porcine intestinal submucosa material is uncontrollable, and its inherent structure and composition determine its degradation cycle usually 4–6 months.

However, the degradation time required for different tissue regeneration is different. Degradation too fast or too slow is not conducive to tissue regeneration. Under the premise of maintaining the activity of the submucosa of pig small intestine, it is our research purpose to construct a new type of acellular tissue matrix composite with adjustable degradation time, adjustable macroscopic size, and adjustable microscopic morphology.

Xiaobing's Fu team members collaborated with Pro. Quan Daping from Sun Yat-Sen University to remove the submucosal tissue from the pig small intestine mucosa, serosa, and muscle layers by physical (mechanical) methods, and then chemically decellularize to remove most of the cells and nuclear components (an immunogenic substance) that retains the three-dimensional structure of the extracellular matrix and maintains the biological and physical properties of the extracellular matrix. Since the remaining components of the extracellular matrix are conserved and nonimmunogenic in different species, the residual DNA is approximately 33 ng/mg, which is in line with internationally accepted standards of ≤50 ng/mg. It is lyophilized and digested into a matrix gel, and further lyophilized with a natural high molecular weight polysaccharide such as hyaluronic acid and a gel to prepare an active porous sponge-like acellular tissue matrix composite material. Acellular tissue matrix materials were used as scaffolds and implanted in situ to induce vascular growth and cell proliferation and regeneration in the host, thus promoting tissue healing. After the acellular tissue matrix composite is implanted into the body, the peripheral tissue cells can be induced to migrate, proliferate, and differentiate, and the migrated cells further transform and shape the acellular tissue matrix composite material, and finally become a part of the host tissue. Thereby achieving assimilation of the implanted tissue and completing the tissue regeneration process. Compared with similar products, the advantages are as follows. (a) The active ingredient retains better. (b) It can build brackets with complex shapes and adjustable sizes. (c) The microstructure of 10–200 μm is adjustable. (d) Degradation time can be controlled. (e) High porosity, can load growth factors and PRP, and can construct organized engineering tissue.

In short, modern dressings should have the following characteristics: extremely strong hemostatic function; strong ability to absorb wound exudate, maintain wound temperature; prevent infection, protect wounds, relieve pain; have strong biodegradability, no irritation to wounds, and promote wound healing; portable and easy to use; long shelf life, low price; can adapt to the harsh battlefield environment, such as sea water, low temperature, high temperature, etc.; no need to fix the tape, no odor. This suggests that advanced dressings in the future may be a variety of high-performance war wound dressings that can perform their respective functions or that can work synergistically. This is the new type of war wound dressing. Further research and development of China's new war wound dressings is an important task to improve our military's war wounds and first aid capabilities, save more soldiers' lives, and reduce disability and residual deformities.

## 11.6 Gene Therapy

The basic concept of gene therapy is to induce therapeutic genes into target cells, and expression of the genes can treat the disease or provide temporary benefits for tissue growth and regeneration. In order to achieve this goal, first, the therapeutic gene must be transferred to a specific target cell; second, the expression of the gene needs to reach a certain level for a certain period of time; finally, the level and timing of gene expression in the target cell can be correspondingly controlled by certain factors. Cells, signaling factors, and scaffolds that provide a place for cell attachment are the three elements of regenerative medicine. The cells mainly use stem cells with self-renewal ability, multidirectional differentiation potential or induced pluripotent stem cells. At the same time, stem cells are ideal targets for gene therapy because of their superiority in vitro. After inoculation of the target cells of gene therapy, the body's own cells can secrete the target protein, and do not need to accept the cytokines in the form of protein expressed by genetic engineering. Therefore, complex processes such as protein extraction and purification are not required; and the target cells can continuously secrete the desired protein. Tissue regeneration provides a stable microenvironment and improves treatment efficiency. Gene therapy is an ideal therapeutic platform for regenerative medicine. At present, gene therapy has been widely used in the regeneration of tissues, organs such as nerve tissue, bone tissue, skin tissue, heart, etc., and has achieved fruitful results. We mainly discuss the use of skin tissue here.

### 11.6.1 Development History

Although people have only officially carried out gene therapy research for more than a decade, the related theories and technologies that they have formed have gone through a long historical process. In 1944, Avery et al. [56] demonstrated that DNA is a substance that induces the transformation of pneumococci. In 1953, Watson and Crick proposed DNA double helix structure model, genetic code deciphering in the 1960s, and recombinant DNA technology, gene transfection technology, and selection technology appeared in the 1970s, the rapid advancement of the studies for proto-oncogenes and tumor suppressor genes in the 1980s, the development of retroviral vectors, the establishment of novel gene expression vectors and transfection techniques (including direct transfection of tissues in vivo), and the establishment of pathways, especially the discovery of new gene functions has provided a solid theoretical basis and technical conditions for the development of gene therapy.

As early as 1980, Martin of the University of California, Los Angeles (UCLA), after initial results in the transfer of drug-resistant genes to mouse bone marrow cells, attempted gene therapy for the first time in two thalassemia patients in Italy and Israel. At the "gene therapy" symposium held in Cold Spring Harbor in 1982, many people were still skeptical about the urgency, possibility, and reality of gene therapy. However, on January 22, 1985, the Federal Register published by NIH of the US Department of Health and Human Services, published the "key points to consider in the design and application of human somatic gene therapy protocols," as drafted by the human gene therapy task force. To seek public comment, in June of the same year, in the Recombinant DNA Technology Bulletin, Volume 8, Issue 2, officially announced this "point," indicating the gene therapy made a breakthrough in the short 5 years of the early 1980s. On the basis of sufficient preclinical experiments and demonstrations, in 1988, the US FDA officially approved the first application for the transfer of foreign genes into the human body. So far, gene therapy has entered the human clinical trial as a new treatment, marking the treatment of human diseases has officially entered a new stage. Gene therapy can be used to transfer genes or gene-specific substances with specific biological activities at specific times and at specific locations, so that genes can be permanently expressed. Wound healing growth factors and related substances that stimulate cell proliferation and extracellular matrix synthesis are important targets for tissue repair gene transfer.

## 11.6.2 Mechanism of Action

### 11.6.2.1 Promote Cell Activity

After tissue damage, it is necessary to fill the defect wound as soon as possible to promote cell division and proliferation. In recent years, some growth factors such as FGF, TGF, and other cytokines can promote the cell to enter the division phase from the intercellular phase, so its gene is the first choice for gene therapy.

In recent years, Eming et al. [57] reported that in soft tissue injury, PDGF was transfected into keratinocytes by retrovirus in vitro, and the cells were transplanted into the wound of thymic mice. Pathological examination revealed that the wound skin was significantly thicker than the control, with subcutaneous cell proliferation, rich blood vessel content, and increased fibronectin deposition, such as transfection of IGF. In addition to the above performance, the transfected keratinocytes divide and proliferate, quickly covering the wound surface and accelerating wound healing. However, it should be pointed out that the effects of these growth factors are not single, while promoting the increase of cell activity, some cell substrates. The secretion of collagen and fibronectin is also increased, and these combined factors contribute to the healing of the wound.

### 11.6.2.2 Promote Collagen Synthesis

Yamasak et al. [58] found that after injury to inducible nitric oxide synthase (iNOS)-deficient mice, the repair was delayed by 31% compared to the wild type, and the NO-specific synthesis inhibitor N6-ethylimine-L-arginine can prevent wound healing of wild-type mice, and the repair ability of iNOS gene-deficient mice is significantly improved, which may be due to the effect of NO. Many literatures have demonstrated that NO promotes the synthesis of collagen in damaged tissues. Thornton and other found that the collagen accumulation in the injured part of the iNOS gene transduction group was significantly increased compared with the control group. There was a significant difference ($P < 0.05$), indicating that iNOS can promote wound healing by increasing collagen synthesis, and gradually become another target for gene therapy.

### 11.6.2.3 Proangiogenesis

Blood vessels provide the growth factors, hormones, oxygen, and other nutrients required for tissue repair through blood transport. The formation of obstacles after injury will lead to a series of pathological changes such as ulcers, which directly affect the repair of tissues. It has been found that damage repair of blood vessels is involved in the interaction of three major molecular regulatory systems: the vascular endothelial growth factor system, the plasminogen system, and the hemagglutination system. Among them, vascular endothelial growth factor promotes the formation of endothelial cell channels, and the hemagglutination system contributes to the maturation of the endothelium around the blood clot, while plasminogen can dissolve blood clots on one hand and promote blood circulation; on the other hand, conducive to the formation of vascular neointima, fibrinolytic enzymes have attracted attention in gene therapy for wound repair. Carmeliet et al. [59] found that the electrical damaging of female plasminogen-deficient mice had no effect on the proliferation of perivascular smooth muscle cells, but the migration was blocked, the cells were concentrated on the edge of the necrotic area, and the neointimal formation of the blood vessels was blocked. When plasminogen activator inhibitor-1 (PAI-1) was inactivated with gene gun technology, the process is reversed and vascular synthesis tends to be normal.

### 11.6.3 Application

In the process of wound healing, gene transfer can be divided into two categories according to the different delivery methods, namely viral vector introduction system and nonviral vector introduction system. Viral vectors are mainly classified into the following four categories: retroviral vectors, adenoviral vectors, adeno-associated viral vectors, and herpes simplex virus type I vectors. For the first time, Morgan et al. [60] reported using a retroviral vector system for gene therapy of the skin. He found that human growth hormone was transfected into keratinocytes cultured in vitro and then replanted in donors, which secreted bioactive human growth hormone, and form a stratified epidermis. Eming et al. [57] introduced platelet-derived growth factor A (PDGF-A) into keratinocytes and then cultured on acellular allogeneic dermis, followed by transplantation, which significantly improved the quality of the composite skin. Fibroblasts were genetically modified with a retrovirus carrying vascular endothelial growth factor (VEGF) to overexpress VEGF, and the cells were used in skin substitutes to find an increase in the number of blood vessels in the dermis and revascularization time is shortened. After 12 weeks of implantation of human tissue-engineered skin into immunodeficient mice, Escamez et al. [61] formed a 2-mm round full-thickness wound on the dorsal skin to simulate a human skin wound model, after treatment with adenovirus vector expressing keratinocyte growth factor (KGF), the expression of KGF protein in local wounds is increased and the re-epithelialization of wounds is also significantly accelerated. The regeneration of lymphatic vessels is conducive to wound healing. Saaristo et al. [62] implanted an adenoviral vector expressing vascular endothelial growth factor (VEGF) into a full-thickness wound of diabetic rats. Compared with the control group, the number of lymphatic vessels and blood vessels increased in the Ad/VEGF group, and the time to wound healing was significantly shortened. The main potential deficiency of adenoviral vectors is that the expression time is relatively short and it is easy to cause the host's immune inflammatory response, and wound healing is a short-term process. Therefore, the short-term expression of adenovirus is beneficial in the wound healing process. After the wound is damaged, it enters the inflammatory reaction period. The transient inflammatory reaction caused by adenovirus has little effect under the promotion of growth factors. When Gu et al. [63] used the adenovirus vector expressing platelet-derived growth factor (PDGF) in the model of full-thickness skin resection, the body was observed to have an immune response to the adenoviral vector and the expressed target protein, but had no significant effect on wound healing. Bitto et al. [64] studied the role of adeno-associated virus (AAV) vector expressing angiopoietin-1 (Ang-1) in a diabetic rat model of wound healing. After 7 and 14 days of the local introduction of the treatment vector into the wound, the mRNA and protein expression of Ang-1 was increased in the experimental group, and the epithelialization and collagen maturity were significantly improved, and the muscle anti-stretching force was increased. Galeano et al. [65] transferred vascular endothelial growth factor (VEGF-A) into animal models through AAV-2. After 18 days, the wound healed 6–10 days earlier due to good granulation construction and accelerated vascularization.

The nonviral vector has the characteristics of large packaging capacity, low cost, and simple operation. However, nonviral vectors also have disadvantages such as relatively poor targeting, unstable target product content, and low infection efficiency. Mainly include: direct injection of naked DNA, gene gun and microplanting genes, electroporation, and cationic liposome cation method. Direct injection of naked DNA is one of the more practical methods for transferring naked DNA to target tissues. In 1995, Hengge et al. [66] directly injected naked plasmid DNA expressing interleukin-8 based on the similar morphology of pig skin to human skin, epidermal keratinocytes can take up plasmid DNA and express it at high levels for a short time. Eriksson et al. [67] found that the expression of epithelial growth factor in microscopic injection of skin wounds was two- to three-times higher than that of ion bombardment, four- to six-times higher than that of simple injection. The advantage is that no foreign matter is left in the tissue compared with electroporation, and can be combined with a viral vector to significantly increase the expression of vascular endothelial growth factor (VEGF). The deficiency is only expressed on the surface of the skin and less in the deeper layers of the skin. The gene gun uses 1–5 μm gold or tungsten as a probe, and is driven by helium pressure to carry various DNA plasmids to microscopically launch into skin cells. Steinstraesser et al. [68] found that in the wounds of I and II burned rats, the gene gun can introduce the target gene into the cell, but its expression ability is lower than that of the adenovirus vector. Dileo et al [69] invented a special improved gene gun to express genes in the epidermis, dermis, and muscles at a peak of 24 h, which lasted for at least 1 week and had little damage to surrounding tissues. Some people used diabetic mice to remove the wound as a model, hypoxia-inducible factor-1 (HIF-1α) plasmid was injected into the subdermis and electroporation was performed. The expression of HIF-1α mRNA was increased and the wound healing rate was significantly accelerated. In 1963, Bangham invented liposomes, but its application has been limited. In 1987, Felgner discovered that cationic lipids and DNA automatically form a single-layer shell that fuses with cell membranes. Cationic liposome-mediated transfection methods are increasingly being used more and more widely. Ferraro et al. [70] transfected VEGF plasmid into rat gastrocnemius, defect wound and random flap by direct injection and electroporation. It was observed that the expression of VEGF in electroporation gene transfection model was significantly increased, promoting angiogenesis, further promoting wound healing and reducing ischemic necrosis of the flap. Jeschke et al. [71] combined the liposome-mediated insulin-like growth factor-1 (IGF-1) cDNA and KGF cDNA to observe its role in the acute wound model of rat skin. The expression of IGF-1, KGF, VEGF, and type IV collagen were increased by immunohistochemistry, accompanied by enhanced re-epithelialization and accelerated neovascularization.

The application of cytogenetic engineering during tissue repair has the potential to provide an effective way to deliver growth factors continuously. Growth factor gene therapy avoids the cumbersome, expensive purification step of the growth factor protein and has great potential. Moreover, improvements in gene transfer measures in conjunction with traditional drugs will provide new and powerful therapeutic options for wound healing. As gene delivery systems continue to evolve, gene therapy will be more effective, safer, and more reliable. The problems that restrict clinical application mainly include safety, transfection efficiency, and economical practicability. At the same time, it takes a long time to prepare the in vitro transfection method by isolating and culturing the cells in vitro, and then introducing the target gene into the wound surface. Therefore, exploring safe and effective methods of transfection in vivo is also an important direction of current research. In addition, wound healing is a multifactor regulation process, and the effect of single gene transfection to improve wound healing process is greatly limited. (See other chapters for more information on gene therapy wounds.)

The main method used by Xiaobing's Fu team for clinical application of VEGF is protein injection, but its application is limited due to its high cost, short half-life, high concentration, and prone to side effects. By constructing the eukaryotic expression plasmid of VEGF gene and transferring it into the body cells, the VEGF factor can be efficiently, stably, and controllably synthesized, thereby overcoming the deficiency of direct use of exogenous VEGF and showing broad application prospects. First, the expression plasmid of vascular endothelial growth factor (VEGF) was constructed, and the effect of its expression product on the deep second degree burn wound of miniature pigs was observed. The cDNA sequence of the VEGF gene was cloned by reverse transcription-polymerase chain reaction (RT-PCR) and ligated into the expression vector pQE-40, the expression products were specifically identified by sodium dodecyl sulfate-polyacrylamide gel electrophoresis (SDS-PAGE) and western blotting methods. Using pig small area deep second scald model, a 1 μg/g VEGF cream was evenly applied to the wound, 200 mg of each wound, and the dressing was changed once every other day until 11 days after the injury. The wound area was measured and the wound tissue was taken for histological examination. The result showed that the cloned VEGF gene cDNA fragment consisted of 380 bp, including the translation initiation codon, coding sequence, and termination codon. The recombinant expression plasmid pQ EVEGF can be expressed in M15 bacteria, and VEGF is mainly present in bacterial inclusion bodies. VEGF was used to treat the wounds of small pigs for 7 days, the granulation tissue was proliferated, and the number of capillaries increased. After 11 days of scald, the wounds of the VEGF group had been re-epithelialized, while the wound area of the M15 group was 0.71 ± 0.23 $cm^2$, and the wounds did not heal. The difference was very significant ($P < 0.01$). It was confirmed that the constructed VEGF expression vector can encode VEGF121 protein, and its expression product can induce granulation tissue growth, accelerate neovascularization, and promote wound healing. In addition, the method of obtaining four KGF genes by RT-PCR method is as follows: preparing spel and hxof double enzyme digestion target gene and phagemid pComb3, subcloning 4 KGF genes into pComb3; using phage display technology to display inserted genes on the surface of phage; extract and purify phage DNA, identify by enzyme digestion, PCR, and sequencing; use MTT method to detect pComb3-KGF-active peptide to promote the proliferation of keratinocytes, use immunofluorescence to detect the cell affinity of pComb3-KGF-active peptide, use RT-PCR to detect the effect of pComb3-KGF-active peptide on the expression levels of KGFR, c-Fos, and c-Jun. The results showed that the target gene was obtained by RT-PCR and constructed in phagemid pComb3. The target gene was successfully expressed on the surface of the vector. The results of restriction enzyme digestion, PCR, and sequencing confirmed that the target gene was successfully constructed in the vector; MTT results showed four kinds of pComb3-KGF-active peptide can promote the proliferation of keratinocytes; the immunofluorescence assay showed that it has good cell affinity; RT-PCR results showed that KGF and two pComb3-KGF-active peptides can promote the expression of KGFR, four pComb3-KGF-active peptide have weaker effects on promoting the expression of c-Fos and c-Jun is weaker than KGF.

## 11.7 Others

### 11.7.1 Digital Medicine

Digital medical technology is a cutting-edge medical engineering technology developed in recent years. It is the product of the cross-development of traditional medicine with computers, digital information, virtual reality, biomechanics, and other related disciplines. It is also the inevitable outcome of the integration of medicine and engineering development in the digital information age. Digital medical research covers a wide range of areas, including digital engineering and human medicine, such as digital virtual human body, digital virtual surgery, surgical planning, medical simulation and training, artificial joint CAD/CAM technology, and surgical navigation. With the rapid development of computer image processing and reconstruction technology, digital medicine, a new frontier discipline between medicine and industry, has quickly become one of the most active disciplines in the world. It has received extensive attention, and has also achieved many breakthrough research results, which has promoted the leap-forward development of traditional medicine and related technologies. War wound treatment is one of the main contents of military medicine research. War wound treatment training is the main means to ensure and improve the ability of the army to treat war wounds. Due to various technical conditions, the traditional war injury treatment training is carried out through textbooks, video teaching, and onsite teaching. The trainees' lack practical onsite training, and the training results are not ideal. It is difficult to provide effective care when it is really needed. With the rapid development of digital medicine technology and virtual reality technology, the research methods, teaching methods, and training modes of traditional medicine have been deeply affected by the digital medical revolution. Many digital virtual simulation clinical medical training systems have emerged, such as SurgicalSIM surgical simulation training system, virtual computer first aid skill training system, and digital uterine simulation operating system. The emergence of these digital medicine training systems has greatly improved the effect of medical education and clinical surgical training, improved the quality and efficiency of teaching, and enabled the trainees to gain both theoretical knowledge and field operation experience, and overcome psychological barriers. These advantages of digital medicine and virtual reality technology provide an effective and convenient way to solve the problems existing in the current war wound treatment training.

At present, the commonly used digital three-dimensional reconstruction methods mainly include surface painting method and volume rendering method. The surface drawing method is to construct three-dimensional data from the slice data set output by the medical imaging device, and then extract the isosurface in the three-dimensional data to perform triangulation, and then use the primitive drawing technology to realize the surface painting. This method can effectively draw the surface of a certain value in the three-dimensional data, but cannot express the internal information of the three-dimensional volume data, and the volume rendering method is to use the "voxel" in the three-dimensional volume data as the basic drawing unit. By using each voxel in the three-dimensional volume data, the internal information of the three-dimensional object can be displayed as needed. The disadvantage is that the voxel data are computationally intensive, resulting in slower reconstruction speeds, which can be solved by increasing the computational rendering speed of the computer.

### 11.7.2 3D Bioprinting

3D bioprinting technology precisely controls the positioning of functional components such as biomaterials, biochemicals, and living cells in each layer, and prints in layers to form a 3D structure. Common 3D bioprinting methods include biosimulation, autonomous self-assembly, and the construction of mini-organization modules.

The basic process of 3D bioprinting is to first design a 3D model of an organ (such as an ear) to be printed by using a computer, and then use a 3D printing method to inject a special "bio-ink" into the model and culture it, so as to generate organs with certain physiological functions. In addition, stem cells can be induced to produce bone or cartilage tissue using this technique. In 2010, 3D bioprinters were named one of the 50 best inventions of 2010 by The Times. Compared with general tissue-engineered scaffolds, 3D biomimetic porous tissue-engineered scaffolds are mainly based on their biomimetic properties, which can simulate the microstructure and biological functions of extracellular matrix (ECM) to the greatest extent, which not only has the internal structure, surface characteristics, and mechanical properties (including elastic modulus, compressive strength, and fatigue resistance) similar to those of specific ECM, but also has gradient structures and gradient biological functions similar to natural tissues and organs, so as to guide cellular responses (including cell adhesion, movement, division, etc.) and the regulation of interactions between different cells by biological modification. The research team of Cornell University bioengineering and Weill Cornell Medical College's doctors combined with 3D printing technology and injectable glue made of living cells to create a prosthetic ear almost identical to the human ear. Within 3 months, these ears can grow cartilage and replace the collagen used for shaping. Dr. Jason Spector, the coauthor of the study, said that using human cells, especially the patient's own cell-printing organs, can reduce the probability of rejection. If the safety and effectiveness of this new technology is validated, this bioengineered prosthetic ear transplant can be implemented in humans within 3 years at the earliest. A company in Connecticut, USA, also reported the use of 3D printed skull implants, special polyetherketone (PEKK) materials, and was approved by the US Food and Drug Administration (FDA) on February 18, 2013.

At present, the development of new 3D bioprinting methods and the printing of clinically and biologically active 3D tissue structures have attracted the attention of many researchers. One of the major challenges is to transform traditional printing of plastic and metal into new technologies to printing sensitive, active biomaterials, and the main challenge is to reproduce the microstructure of extracellular matrices and various cells with extremely high precision and to evaluate their biological functions. China biomaterials 3D printer can successfully print a small proportion of human ear cartilage tissue, liver unit, and so on. This biomaterial 3D printer is characterized by many types of printed biomaterials, low cell damage rate, high printing accuracy, and easy operation. Compared with similar international printers, this 3D printer called "Regenovo" not only realizes biomaterial and cell 3D printing under aseptic conditions, but also has a new temperature control unit and print nozzle design that can support the printing of a variety of biomaterials from −5°C to 260°C molten. Live cell prints have a cell survival rate of up to 90%. The live cells currently printed have a survival time of up to 4 months. Current cell printing includes functional cell printing or stem cell printing, and stem cells can proliferate and differentiate to form the desired cell species. In addition to basic functional cells, most tissues contain cells that support and function, such as cells that participate in vascularization, provide a microenvironment for stem cells to maintain dryness and cell differentiation. The structure and function of the cells used for printing should be as close as possible to the cells in the physiological state of the body, and their function in the body can be maintained by optimizing the printing conditions.

At present, 3D printed skin still has many defects, its toughness and mechanical properties are still far from normal skin, and there are no skin accessory organ such as hair follicles, blood vessels, sweat glands, etc., and lack of melanocytes, Langerhans cells, etc. Therefore, the establishment of artificial skin similar to the normal skin structure and function, while containing the skin's accessory organs, is the problem to be solved next in skin 3D printing and biological tissue engineering.

The team of Xiaobing Fu has applied 3D printing technology to the research and development of wound burn treatment products, which has already achieved initial results [3]. The microenvironment of sweat glands in vitro was induced by 3D bioprinting technology to induce sweat gland regeneration. Using gelatin and sodium alginate as scaffold biomaterials constructed in vitro microenvironment, add mouse toe pad homogenate and epidermal growth factor to the configured bio-ink, and then mix with epidermal stem cells which contain cells. The bio-ink was printed with the set model, and the expression of sweat gland-specific markers was detected by immunofluorescence 14 days after induction. The abovementioned tissue substitute carrying sweat adenoid cells was transplanted into the mouse toe pad burn model, and the sweat gland tissue repair and partial recovery of sweat function were observed. Two 3D structures with different pore sizes were created using two different diameter print nozzles, 300 and 400 μm. There was no significant difference in cell activity and proliferative ability between the two 3D structures, but the 300 μm printed 3D structure induced the expression of sweat gland markers after 5 days of culture, and the 3D structure of the 400 μm print did not change. During the culture process, sweat gland tissue was observed in the 3D structure printed at 300 μm. The tissue blocks formed in the 3D structure were transferred to a conventional culture dish, the tissue morphology disappeared, and the cells adhered to the wall. The results of the study indicate that 300 μm printed structural pore size and geometric parameters are more favorable for cell differentiation and morphogenesis, which may be related to the pore size and geometry of the 300 μm printing structure providing suitable nutrient factor concentrations and sweat gland morphogenesis space (Fig. 11.29).

However, this technology also has limitations, and bioprinting currently does not produce the entire organ. Studies have shown that it is difficult to actually print cells while creating a scaffold structure. Several commonly used 3D printing technologies have their own advantages and limitations. The 3D material prepared by the photocuring three-dimensional printing technology has high precision and high mechanical strength, but it is necessary to avoid deformation of the molded product in the process of removing impurities such as organic solvents after posttreatment. The molded product prepared by the fused deposition molding technique has high precision and good surface quality, but requires high temperature to melt the raw material. The advantage of selective laser sintering technology is that the processing speed is fast and no support material is needed. The disadvantages are high processing temperature, rough surface of the molded product, and the like. In addition, 3D printing technology is easy to operate, rapid prototyping, and mild preparation conditions. However, the molded product has a low mechanical strength. Whether through inkjet printing or laser printing, cell membranes are damaged and cell survival rates range from 40% to 95%. Therefore, when selecting different methods for preparing three-dimensional polymer scaffold materials, it is also necessary to combine the characteristics of the raw materials and the performance requirements of the molded products.

Although bioprinted scaffold are in clinical trials, the need to transplant cell-grown scaffold into patients requires advanced techniques. The quality of this technology is currently difficult to guarantee consistently, and this is the quality necessary for medical equipment. At present, there are still many key technologies to be solved in the adjustment of mechanical strength and integrity control in the manufacture of biological frameworks; understanding and regulation of the various tissues and their microenvironments is the key to successful bioprinting; growing a good tissue tree when printing tissue, capillary, microvascular, and nerve distribu-

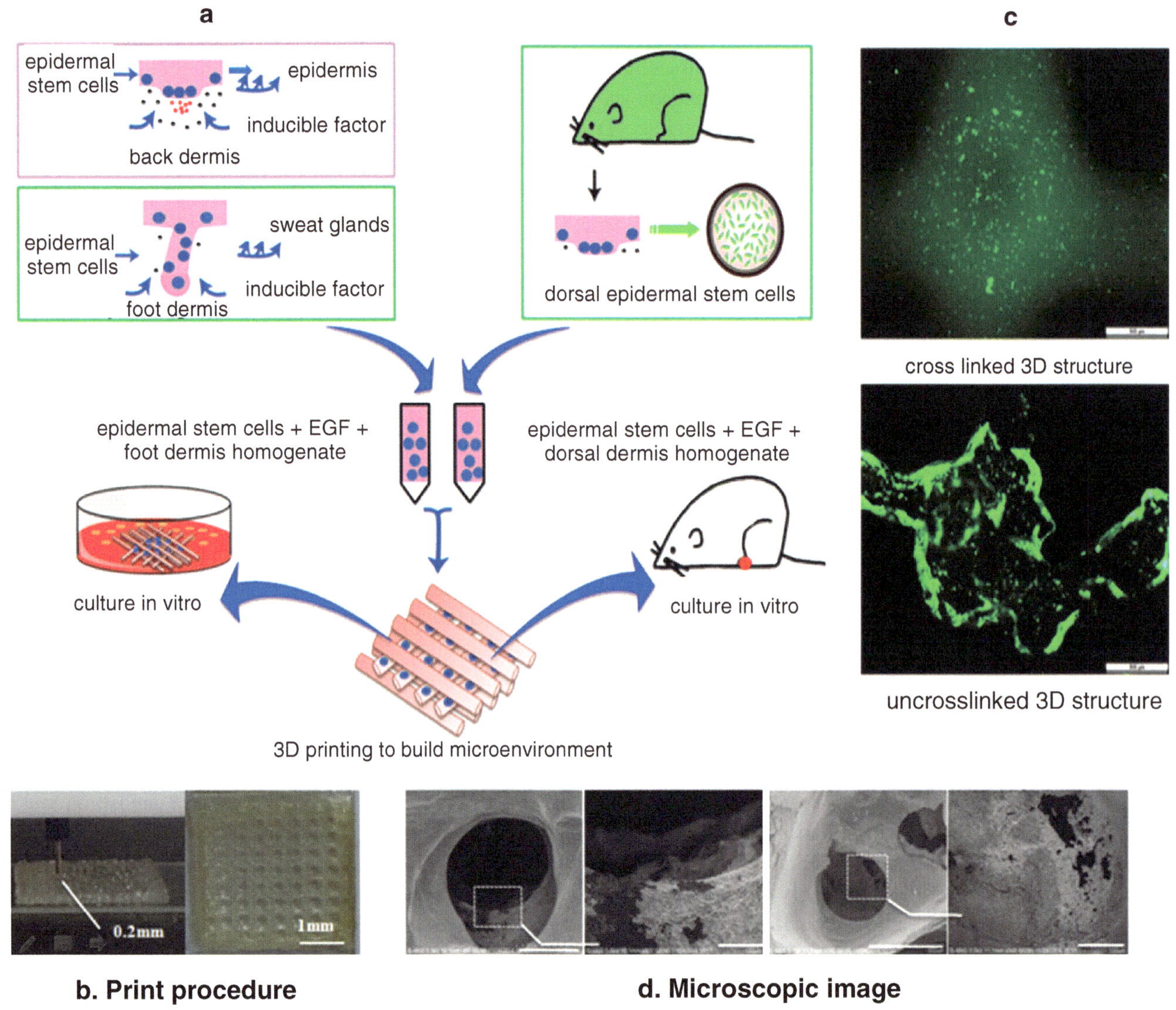


**Fig. 11.29** 3D printed extracellular matrix and orientation-induced epidermal progenitor images

tion problems in tissue irrigation, mature time required for printed tissue, printing of mature factors, and physiological stress factors are also future research fields. Bioprinting technology is still a long way from a wide range of clinical applications and requires the collaboration of scientists in multiple fields.

### 11.7.3 Telemedicine and Tissue Repair

The Internet of Things combines various information sensing devices, such as radio-frequency identification (RFID), infrared sensing, global positioning, laser scanning, with the Internet to form a huge network that enables remote sensing of items and control. Medical Internet of Things is the use of Internet of Things technology to embed and equip multiple sensors into medical devices, and integrate the Internet of Things with the existing Internet for medical, health management, chronic disease management, medical assistance, mobile health care services, and elderly health care, in order to realize the exchange and seamless connection of various medical data, real-time dynamic monitoring and continuous tracking management of medical and health care services can also help medical personnel to make accurate medical and health decisions, that is, smart medical care. However, because the word "Internet of Things" does not conform to the English abbreviation, it has not become a "buzzword" like the "Internet of Things" in China, in the United States, or abroad. The United States is more concerned about its application in specific industries, such as M2M (machine to machine or machine to mobile); using Smart Grid in the power grid; combining telecommunications with information in long distance to synthesize telematics; called telemedicine in the medical field, namely telemedicine. With the involvement of health management, preventive medicine, nursing, and especially telecare, it seems that telehealth is more relevant and richer than telemedicine.

On one hand, with gradual improvement of people's living standards, people's expectations for high-quality medical care have increased. On the other hand, the distribution of chronic diseases is more extensive, the number is increasing significantly; the mobility of personnel is increasing; medical professionals are scared; the uneven distribution of medical resources in different regions and the increasing medical costs have caused the contradiction in the medical market to be extremely prominent. In particular, China's large-scale comprehensive medical institutions are overcrowded, and the grassroots medical and health service institutions that have been established have no one to care about. It is mainly because the grassroots medical staff are subject to conditions, professional quality and service ability are not high, and patients are always worried about being delayed. Through the remote wireless health management service platform in the medical Internet of Things, large hospitals can be connected with portable devices of community hospitals or family doctors, and doctors in large hospitals can answer questions raised by grassroots hospitals and community hospitals to achieve efficient health management, reduce the cost of hospital diagnosis and treatment and the cost of medical treatment for patients, solve the problem of difficult medical treatment and expensive medical treatment, and through timely monitoring and early warning, can actively identify potential dangers and help patients achieve active treatment. Telemedicine will greatly change people's medical treatment ideas, and then change the medical model to achieve the government's requirements for "serving patients and serving the society" proposed by medical institutions.

In modern society, chronic wounds have always been a challenging problem, presenting enormous medical, economic, and social burdens related to physical and mental health and social productivity. Many developing countries, including China, have seen more and more refractory wounds caused by chronic diseases due to rapid economic growth, negative lifestyle changes (such as increased dietary fat intake and decreased physical activity), and aging problems. More than a decade ago, epidemiological studies on chronic skin wounds in China showed that trauma and infection were the main causes of refractory wounds, accounting for 67% of the total. Among them, manual workers and farmers account for the highest proportion. With the rapid development of China's economy and the significant improvement in the quality of life in the past 10 years, China's social and economic structure has undergone fundamental changes, and the disease spectrum has also undergone corresponding changes. In 2010, we participated in an epidemiological survey of chronic skin wounds and their causes in 17 tertiary hospitals in 14 provinces across the country. We found that chronic skin wounds were received in these hospitals from 2007 to 2008. Among the 2513 patients treated, the most common cause of chronic skin wounds was diabetes, and the chronic wounds caused by trauma had retreated to the second place. According to an article published in the 2010 *New England Journal*, China is currently entering a period of high incidence of diabetic ulcers. The prevalence of diabetes in adults over 20 years of age in China is 9.7% (92.4 million diabetic patients), and the prediabetes prevalence rate is 15.5% (148 million prediabetes patients). Diabetes and related diseases have become an important issue that plagues China's public health, and it is urgent to strengthen various research and prevention strategies in this field. Among them, chronic diabetic ulcers are one of the serious chronic complications of diabetes. They are characterized by "disease in the wound, co-occurrence of wound and disease," and have the characteristics of long course, difficult to cure, and high financial expenditure. The adoption of reasonable prevention, care, and treatment, coupled with the influence of factors, such as the place of residence, transportation, and expenses, often prevents patients from receiving timely and accurate treatment and care opinions, resulting in irreparable visits to hospitals. The higher amputation rate, in addition to causing physical and mental pain to the patient, also imposes a huge burden on the family and society. Treatment of chronic wounds may require a timely monitoring, presentation of treatments, care advice, and timely closure of the wound in an appropriate manner. If ulcers can be detected and treated early, better control of blood lipids, blood sugar, and stress can prevent amputation, and even reduce death from cardiovascular disease caused by long-term uncontrolled wounds. Chronic wounds require well-trained staff to properly monitor and manage the wound. Therefore, improving the management methods and techniques of wounds to properly take care of patients with chronic wounds has become a new topic facing modern society. In Europe, in 2005, Denmark's Clemensen has been found in telemedicine for diabetic foot patients.

The equipment required for operation is relatively simple. The nurse can be implemented as soon as possible after receiving the doctor's advice. The patient has reduced the burden of travel and saved the travel time to the hospital. In 2010, Bowling et al. [72] of the University of Manchester in the United Kingdom proposed using a customized camera and computer software to form a three-dimensional image of the wound of a diabetic foot, and obtained data on the length, depth, volume, and surface area of the wound. This quantitative technique can reduce the difference of doctors' judgment on the wound, and patients can receive more professional care to improve the quality of medical care. Using telemedicine to conduct expert assessments of patients in remote areas highlights the advantages of quality, convenience, low cost, and good benefits. To help remotely assess foot wounds, they studied a new type of optical imaging system that uses stereo cameras and disposable optical markers to obtain standardized forms of recording. However, imaging also has some limitations, including certain features that cannot be displayed, such as humidity or oozing, which is difficult to give doctors visual feedback on fidelity.

In 2011, the TeleDiaFoS system developed by Ladyzynski, a scholar of the Biocontrol Theory and Academy of Biomedical Engineering in Warsaw, Poland, was able to remotely scan a family doctor who delivered a foot wound to a patient, confirming the usefulness of the TeleDiaFoS surveillance system to convert the diabetic ulcer wound area into basic parameters.

In the Jutland Peninsula in southern Denmark, mobile phones with camera functions and ordinary desktop computers are connected to the Internet, and health professionals can effectively use telemedicine for data collection and communication with patients. The system can even complete the interconnection between administrative staff and local reimbursement systems.

In Asia, South Korea has reported on the use of telemedicine to monitor blood glucose in patients with type 2 diabetes, but has not yet been consulted on chronic wounds, especially in patients with diabetic foot care and related treatment reports. In India, there are only reports on the use of telemedicine for home care. Earlier in China, Chang Gung Memorial Hospital in Taiwan, China, from January to August 2003, they used a digital camera-enabled cell phone to transmit clinical images of wounds and contacted plastic surgeons online. The results of the 60 patients who were consulted were better. In 2010, China's Shanghai Ninth People's Hospital and China Mobile Shanghai Company took the lead in cooperating to build a "TOPCLASS" platform, using the "Wound Repair Telemedicine" system of wireless HD video technology, and trial operation in community health centers, with more than 100 patients have benefited. With HD video delivery, patients can truly "face to face" with experts. The telemedicine network allows community doctors to make correct judgments about difficult cases. This technology truly realizes "two-way referral"—patients who need surgery can be transferred to a large hospital for treatment immediately, and then return to the community health center for follow-up after the condition is stable.

In the developed European and American countries, due to the popularity of the Internet and the advancement of science and technology, the development of telemedicine treatment and wound care is faster, which also provides a reference for our subsequent application. However, in many areas, including Asia, the development is lagging behind and urgently needs to be broken.

The "smart medical" application has broad prospects and can make the most of experts. Achieve high speed, efficient, and personalized. Dezelić believed that telemedicine means that we are not only doing something old in new ways, but also doing something new (not only "to do old things in new ways," but also "to do new things"). The integration of the health information system enables the center and its components to provide health care to individual medical users at the same time. There are also problems with interoperability and standardization of modern medical information in these processes.

Although wound care has been practiced for hundreds of years, telewound care is a relatively new concept. Currently only a few pilot programs exist. Telewound care has not yet achieved popularity among the health care industry and the public and is recognized by other telemedicine predecessors. With the inclusion of wound care, the enormous potential of telemedicine technology is realized. The most representative feature of wound care is the need for long-term special care in chronic and diabetic conditions. Improvements in living conditions and advances in global health care have made people live longer. The rise in the proportion of elderly people in the world who need to seek medical care for chronic diseases, the rising cost of health care, and the need to promote outpatient services are only one part that requires us to pay immediate attention to the health care crisis. Using telemedicine to provide care for distant patients, we have seen positive results. In addition, in the field of radiology, the effectiveness of several programs such as technological advancement has been established. Wound care can be based on the success of these areas to create an effective care method to achieve new wound care. The goal is to create a technologically advanced, cost-effective and user-friendly process that bridges the gap between dedicated care and counseling. Storage and forwarding technologies and television play a role in telewound health care, which has a greater role in long distance consultations at home, with the former having a greater role in postoperative patients, chronic wounds, and follow-up care. We now have the ability, knowledge, and resources to develop a telewound care regimen that delivers high-quality patient care in a more concise and cost-effective manner. This is of course an easy way to prevent emotional problems and avoid the loss of material and financial resources.

From the patient side, telemedicine can provide the most valuable treatment options for those living in remote areas or having difficulty walking or transporting, eliminating travel time, stress, and travel-related costs. Long-term care facilities, fixed residents also constitute a huge traffic problem. These residents can greatly benefit from telemedicine. It can prevent residents from getting worse or worse, and take timely interventions. Using telemedicine, practitioners and experts provide counseling and treatment guidance, eliminating the need to transport patients to the emergency room, gaining more expert advice, reducing transportation costs, and reducing the relative closure of medical information for rural health care professionals.

Telemedicine can truly achieve the concept of "patient-centered care" and "medical home," avoiding the communication gaps and coordination barriers that are common in current medical systems. On one hand, computers can digitally present and visualize the knowledge and wisdom of medical experts, greatly reducing the workload of medical experts; on the other hand, using telemedicine technology to further mine massive data, we can find the laws of life activities and physical state characteristics that are not yet known, which will promote the further development of modern health medicine. The key to a good telemedicine is human factors such as convenience and ease of use, confidentiality, and reliability. In addition to the use of telemedicine for timely and correct diagnosis and reasonable treatment of chronic wounds, it can be used as a teaching mechanism in the future. For example, it is difficult for clinicians to obtain the latest treatment progress in the long-term busy nursing work of community primary hospitals, and wound treatment experts can use the built-in decision support function software to teach them.

The medical Internet of Things is one of the foundations for building a harmonious society. In the formation and development of the entire industrial structure, the government must vigorously promote and support it. It is believed that with the gradual promotion of the application of Internet of Things, the development prospects of the medical Internet of Things will be immeasurable. Of course, this evolving technology has problems and challenges, including widespread implementation, cost and reimbursement issues, patient privacy, and the quality of data transmission. These have to be further improved.

## References


1. Qian SL. Effect of 640nm and 465nm light-emitting diode irradiation on the biological behavior of cells involved in wound healing. Guangzhou: Guangzhou Medical University; 2016.
2. Huang C. Light-emitting diode irradiation (640nm) regulates keratinocytes migration and cytoskeletal reorganization via HIF-1$\alpha$. Shanghai: The Second Military Medical University; 2017.
3. Huang S, Yao B, Xie J, et al. 3D bioprinted extracellular matrix mimics facilitate directed differentiation of epithelial progenitors for sweat gland regeneration. Acta Biomater. 2016;32:170–7.
4. Mester E, Nagylucskay S, Tisza S, Mester A, Tóth J, Laczy FI. Neuere Untersuchungen über die Wirkung der Laserstrahlen auf die Wundheilung–Immunologische Effekte [Current studies on the effect of laser beams on wound healing–immunologic effects]. Z Exp Chir, 1977. 10(5):301–6. German. PMID: 303837
5. Zhang Y, Song S, Fong CC, Tsang CH, Yang Z, Yang M. cDNA microarray analysis of gene expression profiles in human fibroblast cells irradiated with red light. J Invest Dermatol. 2003;120(5):849–57. https://doi.org/10.1046/j.1523-1747.2003.12133.x. PMID: 12713592.
6. Erdle BJ, Brouxhon S, Kaplan M, Vanbuskirk J, Pentland AP. Effects of continuous-wave (670-nm) red light on wound healing. Dermatol Surg. 2008;34(3):320–5. https://doi.org/10.1111/j.1524-4725.2007.34065.x. Epub 2007 Dec 20. PMID: 18177400
7. Shefer G, Oron U, Irintchev A, Wernig A, Halevy O. Skeletal muscle cell activation by low-energy laser irradiation: a role for the MAPK/ERK pathway. J Cell Physiol. 2001;187(1):73–80. https://doi.org/10.1002/1097-4652(2001)9999:9999<::AID-JCP1053>3.0.CO;2-9. PMID: 11241351.
8. Schieke S, Stege H, Kürten V, Grether-Beck S, Sies H, Krutmann J. Infrared-A radiation-induced matrix metalloproteinase 1 expression is mediated through extracellular signal-regulated kinase 1/2 activation in human dermal fibroblasts. J Invest Dermatol. 2002;119(6):1323–9. https://doi.org/10.1046/j.1523-1747.2002.19630.x. PMID: 12485435.
9. Eells JT, Wong-Riley MT, VerHoeve J, Henry M, Buchman EV, Kane MP, Gould LJ, Das R, Jett M, Hodgson BD, Margolis D, Whelan HT. Mitochondrial signal transduction in accelerated wound and retinal healing by near-infrared light therapy. Mitochondrion. 2004;4(5-6):559–67. https://doi.org/10.1016/j.mito.2004.07.033. PMID: 16120414.
10. Medrado AP, Soares AP, Santos ET, Reis SR, Andrade ZA. Influence of laser photobiomodulation upon connective tissue remodeling during wound healing. J Photochem Photobiol B. 2008;92(3):144–52. 1016/j.jphotobiol.2008.05.008. Epub 2008 Jul 7
11. Nicole R. Traitement d'un cas de brûlure grave par les rayons ultraviolets [Treatment of severe burns from ultra-violet irradiation]. Brux Med. 1956;36(30):1475–8. French. PMID: 13374393.
12. Stachon T, Wang J, Langenbucher A, et al. IL-1$\alpha$, IL-1$\beta$, IL-6, and IL-8 secretion of human keratocytes following photodynamic inactivation (PDI) in vitro. Graefes Arch Clin Exp Ophthalmol. 2013;251(11):2585–90. https://doi.org/10.1007/s00417-013-2465-6.
13. Hawkins DH, Abrahamse H. The role of laser fluence in cell viability, proliferation, and membrane integrity of wounded human skin fibroblasts following helium-neon laser irradiation. Lasers Surg Med. 2006;38(1):74–83. https://doi.org/10.1002/lsm.20271.
14. Schindl A, Merwald H, Schindl L, Kaun C, Wojta J. Direct stimulatory effect of low-intensity 670 nm laser irradiation on human endothelial cell proliferation. Br J Dermatol. 2003;148(2):334–6. https://doi.org/10.1046/j.1365-2133.2003.05070.x.
15. Abergel RP, Meeker CA, Lam TS, Dwyer RM, Lesavoy MA, Uitto J. Control of connective tissue metabolism by lasers: recent developments and future prospects. J Am Acad Dermatol. 1984;11(6):1142–50. https://doi.org/10.1016/s0190-9622(84)80194-2.
16. Cai Y, Zhou Y, Xing L, Kang Y, Li H, Cheng P, Wang Y. Effectiveness and safety of different dressings therapy for pressure injuries: a protocol for systematic reviews and network meta-analysis. Medicine. 2021;100(3):e23520. https://doi.org/10.1097/MD.0000000000023520.
17. Shu B, Ni GX, Zhang LY, Li XP, Jiang WL, Zhang LQ. High-power helium-neon laser irradiation inhibits the growth of traumatic scars in vitro and in vivo. Lasers Med Sci. 2013;28(3):693–700. https://doi.org/10.1007/s10103-012-1127-y.
18. Martignago C, Tim CR, Assis L, Da Silva VR, Santos E, Vieira FN, Parizotto NA, Liebano RE. Effects of red and near-infrared LED light therapy on full-thickness skin graft in rats. Lasers Med Sci. 2020;35(1):157–64. https://doi.org/10.1007/s10103-019-02812-6
19. Schindl A, Heinze G, Schindl M, Pernerstorfer-Schön H, Schindl L. Systemic effects of low-intensity laser irradiation on skin microcirculation in patients with diabetic microangiopathy. Microvasc Res. 2002;64(2):240–6. https://doi.org/10.1006/mvre.2002.2429.
20. Bullock AJ, Barker AT, Coulton L, Macneil S. The effect of induced biphasic pulsed currents on re-epithelialization of a novel wound healing model. Bioelectromagnetics. 2007;28(1):31–41. https://doi.org/10.1002/bem.20267.
21. Zhao M, Dick A, Forrester JV, McCaig CD. Electric field-directed cell motility involves up-regulated expression and asymmetric redistribution of the epidermal growth factor receptors and is enhanced by fibronectin and laminin. Mol Biol Cell. 1999;10(4):1259–76. https://doi.org/10.1091/mbc.10.4.1259.

22. Raghu ALB, Parker T, Aziz TZ, et al. Invasive electrical neuromodulation for the treatment of painful diabetic neuropathy: systematic review and meta-analysis. Neuromodulation. 2021;24(1):13–21. https://doi.org/10.1111/ner.13216.
23. Luther PW, Peng HB, Lin JJ. Changes in cell shape and actin distribution induced by constant electric fields. Nature. 1983;303(5912):61–4. https://doi.org/10.1038/303061a0.
24. Cooper MS, Schliwa M. Electrical and ionic controls of tissue cell locomotion in DC electric fields. J Neurosci Res. 1985;13(1-2):223–44. https://doi.org/10.1002/jnr.490130116.
25. Erickson CA, Nuccitelli R. Role of electric fields in fibroblast motility. Prog Clin Biol Res. 1986;210:303–9.
26. Yang WP, Onuma EK, Hui SW. Response of C3H/10T1/2 fibroblasts to an external steady electric field stimulation. Reorientation, shape change, ConA receptor and intramembranous particle distribution and cytoskeleton reorganization. Exp Cell Res. 1984;155(1):92–104. https://doi.org/10.1016/0014-4827(84)90770-5.
27. Liboff AR, Williams T Jr, Strong DM, Wistar R Jr. Time-varying magnetic fields: effect on DNA synthesis. Science. 1984;223(4638):818–20. https://doi.org/10.1126/science.6695183.
28. Bourguignon GJ, Jy W, Bourguignon LY. Electric stimulation of human fibroblasts causes an increase in Ca2+ influx and the exposure of additional insulin receptors. J Cell Physiol. 1989;140(2):379–85. https://doi.org/10.1002/jcp.1041400224.
29. Löschinger M, Thumm S, Hämmerle H, Rodemann HP. Stimulation of protein kinase A activity and induced terminal differentiation of human skin fibroblasts in culture by low-frequency electromagnetic fields. Toxicol Lett. 1998;96-97:369–76. https://doi.org/10.1016/s0378-4274(98)00095-2.
30. Cadossi R, Bersani F, Cossarizza A, Zucchini P, Emilia G, Torelli G, Franceschi C. Lymphocytes and low-frequency electromagnetic fields. FASEB J. 1992;6(9):2667–74. https://doi.org/10.1096/fasebj.6.9.1612290. PMID: 1612290.
31. Adunsky A, Ohry A, DDCT Group. Decubitus direct current treatment (DDCT) of pressure ulcers: results of a randomized double-blinded placebo controlled study. Arch Gerontol Geriatr. 2005;41(3):261–9. https://doi.org/10.1016/j.archger.2005.04.004.
32. Magnoni C, Rossi E, Fiorentini C, Baggio A, Ferrari B, Alberto G. Electrical stimulation as adjuvant treatment for chronic leg ulcers of different aetiology: an RCT. J Wound Care. 2013;22(10):525–33. https://doi.org/10.12968/jowc.2013.22.10.525.
33. Fleischmann W, Strecker W, Bombelli M, Kinzl L. Vakuumversiegelung zur Behandlung des Weichteilschadens bei offenen Frakturen [Vacuum sealing as treatment of soft tissue damage in open fractures]. Unfallchirurg. 1993;96(9):488–92.
34. Morykwas MJ, Simpson J, Punger K, Argenta A, Kremers L, Argenta J. Vacuum-assisted closure: state of basic research and physiologic foundation. Plast Reconstr Surg. 2006;117(7 Suppl):121S–6S. https://doi.org/10.1097/01.prs.0000225450.12593.12.
35. Du W, He L, Wang L, Hu H, Zhou H, Bao G, Chen R, Shen F, Quan R. Experimental vascular protective shield combined with vacuum sealing drainage prevents pressure on exposed vessels and accelerates wound repair. Ann Palliat Med. 2020;9(5):3059–69. https://doi.org/10.21037/apm-20-625
36. Li XY, Li WZ, Li YJ, Lv XX, Li J, Chen SZ, Li JQ. Zhonghua Shao Shang Za Zhi. 2007;23(4):292–5.
37. Tang SY, Chen SZ, Hu ZH, Song M, Cao DY, Lü XX. Influence of vacuum-assisted closure technique on expression of Bcl-2 and NGF/NGFmRNA during wound healing. Zhonghua Zheng Xing Wai Ke Za Zhi. 2004;20(2):139–42. Chinese. PMID: 15334941.
38. Suzuki K, Michael G, Tamire Y. Viable intact cryopreserved human placental membrane for a non-surgical approach to closure in complex wounds. J Wound Care. 2016;25(Sup10):S25-S31. doi https://doi.org/10.12968/jowc.2016.25.Sup10.S25
39. Weed T, Ratliff C, Drake DB. Quantifying bacterial bioburden during negative pressure wound therapy: does the wound VAC enhance bacterial clearance? Ann Plast Surg. 2004;52(3):276–80. https://doi.org/10.1097/01.sap.0000111861.75927.4d.
40. Wang C, Yao Y. Treatment of distal extremity chronic infection and ulcerated wound with negative pressure closure and drainage. J Traumatic Surg. 2005;04:306.
41. Plikaitis CM, Molnar JA. Subatmospheric pressure wound therapy and the vacuum-assisted closure device: basic science and current clinical successes. Expert Rev Med Devices. 2006;3(2):175–84. https://doi.org/10.1586/17434440.3.2.175.
42. Gouttefangeas C, Eberle M, Ruck P, et al. Functional T lymphocytes infiltrate implanted polyvinyl alcohol foams during surgical wound closure therapy. Clin Exp Immunol. 2001;124(3):398–405. https://doi.org/10.1046/j.1365-2249.2001.01547.x.
43. Penn E, Rayment S. Management of a dehisced abdominal wound with VAC therapy. Br J Nurs. 2004;13(4):194–201. https://doi.org/10.12968/bjon.2004.13.4.12423.
44. Kall S, Kilpadi D, Reimers K, Choi CY, Jahn S, Vogt PM. Einfluss des Schwamm- und Schlauchmaterials der Vacuum Assisted Closure Device (V.A.C.) auf die Konzentration von Transforming Growth Factor beta 1 in Wundflüssigkeit [Influence of foam- and tubing material of the vacuum assisted closure device (v.a.C.) on the concentration of transforming growth factor Beta 1 in wound fluid]. Zentralbl Chir. 2004;129(Suppl 1):S113–5. https://doi.org/10.1055/s-2004-822659.
45. Li YJ, Cao DY, Chen SZ. Effect of vacuum-assisted closure on the expression of urokinase-type plasminogen activator and urokinase-type plasminogen activator receptor in acute and chronic wounds healing. Zhonghua Zheng Xing Wai Ke Za Zhi. 2006;22(4):306–9. Chinese. PMID: 17017150
46. Chen SZ, Cao DY, Li JQ, Tang SY. Effect of vacuum-assisted closure on the expression of proto-oncogenes and its significance during wound healing. Zhonghua Zheng Xing Wai Ke Za Zhi. 2005;21(3):197–200. Chinese. PMID: 16128104
47. Ding Z, Ke S, Baijiang T, et al. Application of modified closed negative pressure therapy in refractory wound. Chin J Injure Repair (Electronic Edition). 2011;006(006):46–7.
48. Blume PA, Key JJ, Thakor P, Thakor S, Sumpio B. Retrospective evaluation of clinical outcomes in subjects with split-thickness skin graft: comparing V.A.C.® therapy and conventional therapy in foot and ankle reconstructive surgeries. Int Wound J. 2010;7(6):480–7. https://doi.org/10.1111/j.1742-481X.2010.00728.x.
49. Li J, Shi JB, Hong P, et al. Combined treatment with vacuum sealing drainage, TopClosure device, and Ilizarov technique for traumatic hemipelvectomy: a rare case report of successful repairing of large-size soft tissue defects. Medicine (Baltimore). 2019;98(4):e14205. https://doi.org/10.1097/MD.0000000000014205.
50. Steiert AE, Gohritz A, Schreiber TC, Krettek C, Vogt PM. Delayed flap coverage of open extremity fractures after previous vacuum-assisted closure (VAC) therapy - worse or worth? J Plast Reconstr Aesthet Surg. 2009;62(5):675–83. https://doi.org/10.1016/j.bjps.2007.09.041.
51. Davis SC, Cazzaniga AL, Ricotti C, et al. Topical oxygen emulsion: a novel wound therapy. Arch Dermatol. 2007;143(10):1252–6. https://doi.org/10.1001/archderm.143.10.1252.
52. Prudden JF, Migel P, Hanson P, Friedrich L, Balassa L. The discovery of a potent pure chemical wound-healing accelerator. Am J Surg. 1970;119(5):560–4. https://doi.org/10.1016/0002-9610(70)90175-3.
53. Malette WG, Quigley HJ, Gaines RD, Johnson ND, Rainer WG. Chitosan: a new hemostatic. Ann Thorac Surg. 1983;36(1):55–8. https://doi.org/10.1016/s0003-4975(10)60649-2.
54. Bromberg BE, Song IC, Mohn MP. The Use of Pig Skin as a Temporary Biological Dressing. Plast Reconstr Surg. 1965;36:80–90. https://doi.org/10.1097/00006534-196507000-00011.

55. Kim BM, Suzuki S, Nishimura Y, Um SC, Morota K, Maruguchi T, Ikada Y. Cellular artificial skin substitute produced by short period simultaneous culture of fibroblasts and keratinocytes. Br J Plast Surg. 1999;52(7):573–8. https://doi.org/10.1054/bjps.1999.3162. PMID: 10658112.
56. Avery OT, Macleod CM, McCarty M. Studies on the chemical nature of the substance inducing transformation of pneumococcal types: induction of transformation by a desoxyribonucleic acid fraction isolated from pneumococcus type III. J Exp Med. 1944;79(2):137–58. https://doi.org/10.1084/jem.79.2.137.
57. Eming SA, Lee J, Snow RG, Tompkins RG, Yarmush ML, Morgan JR. Genetically modified human epidermis overexpressing PDGF-A directs the development of a cellular and vascular connective tissue stroma when transplanted to athymic miceDOUBLEHYPHENimplications for the use of genetically modified keratinocytes to modulate dermal regeneration. J Invest Dermatol. 1995;105(6):756–63. https://doi.org/10.1111/1523-1747.ep12325550.
58. Yamasaki K, Edington HD, McClosky C, et al. Reversal of impaired wound repair in iNOS-deficient mice by topical adenoviral-mediated iNOS gene transfer. J Clin Invest. 1998;101(5):967–71. https://doi.org/10.1172/JCI2067.
59. Carmeliet P, Moons L, Lijnen R, et al. Inhibitory role of plasminogen activator inhibitor-1 in arterial wound healing and neointima formation: a gene targeting and gene transfer study in mice. Circulation. 1997;96(9):3180–91. https://doi.org/10.1161/01.cir.96.9.3180.
60. Eming SA, Medalie DA, Tompkins RG, Yarmush ML, Morgan JR. Genetically modified human keratinocytes overexpressing PDGF-A enhance the performance of a composite skin graft. Hum Gene Ther. 1998;9(4):529–39. https://doi.org/10.1089/hum.1998.9.4-529.
61. Escámez MJ, García M, Larcher F, et al. An in vivo model of wound healing in genetically modified skin-humanized mice. J Invest Dermatol. 2004;123(6):1182–91. https://doi.org/10.1111/j.0022-202X.2004.23473.x.
62. Saaristo A, Tammela T, Farkkilā A, et al. Vascular endothelial growth factor-C accelerates diabetic wound healing. Am J Pathol. 2006;169(3):1080–7. https://doi.org/10.2353/ajpath.2006.051251.
63. Gu DL, Nguyen T, Gonzalez AM, et al. Adenovirus encoding human platelet-derived growth factor-B delivered in collagen exhibits safety, biodistribution, and immunogenicity profiles favorable for clinical use. Mol Ther. 2004;9(5):699–711. https://doi.org/10.1016/j.ymthe.2004.02.018.
64. Bitto A, Minutoli L, Galeano MR, et al. Angiopoietin-1 gene transfer improves impaired wound healing in genetically diabetic mice without increasing VEGF expression. Clin Sci (Lond). 2008;114(12):707–18. https://doi.org/10.1042/CS20070250.
65. Galeano M, Deodato B, Altavilla D, et al. Adeno-associated viral vector-mediated human vascular endothelial growth factor gene transfer stimulates angiogenesis and wound healing in the genetically diabetic mouse. Diabetologia. 2003;46(4):546–55. https://doi.org/10.1007/s00125-003-1064-1.
66. Hengge UR, Chan EF, Foster RA, Walker PS, Vogel JC. Cytokine gene expression in epidermis with biological effects following injection of naked DNA. Nat Genet. 1995;10(2):161–6. https://doi.org/10.1038/ng0695-161.
67. Eriksson E, Yao F, Svensjö T, et al. In vivo gene transfer to skin and wound by microseeding. J Surg Res. 1998;78(2):85–91. https://doi.org/10.1006/jsre.1998.5325.
68. Hirsch T, von Peter S, Dubin G, Mittler D, Jacobsen F, Lehnhardt M, Eriksson E, Steinau HU, Steinstraesser L. Adenoviral gene delivery to primary human cutaneous cells and burn wounds. Mol Med. 2006;12(9-10):199–207. https://doi.org/10.2119/2006-00031.Hirsch. PMID: 17225867; PMCID: PMC1770006.
69. Dileo J, Miller TE Jr, Chesnoy S, Huang L. Gene transfer to subdermal tissues via a new gene gun design. Hum Gene Ther. 2003;14(1):79–87. https://doi.org/10.1089/10430340360464732.
70. Ferraro B, Cruz YL, Coppola D, Heller R. Intradermal delivery of plasmid VEGF(165) by electroporation promotes wound healing. Mol Ther. 2009;17(4):651–7. https://doi.org/10.1038/mt.2009.12.
71. Jeschke MG, Herndon DN. The combination of IGF-I and KGF cDNA improves dermal and epidermal regeneration by increased VEGF expression and neovascularization. Gene Ther. 2007;14(16):1235–42. https://doi.org/10.1038/sj.gt.3302972.
72. Bowling FL, King L, Paterson JA, et al. Remote assessment of diabetic foot ulcers using a novel wound imaging system. Wound Repair Regen. 2011;19(1):25–30. https://doi.org/10.1111/j.1524-475X.2010.00645.x.

# Traditional Medicine and Tissue Repair and Regeneration

12

Yufeng Jiang and Xiaobing Fu

## 12.1 General Description

### 12.1.1 Concept of Regeneration in Traditional and Modern Medicine

Regenerative medicine in the modern sense mainly refers to the use of the principles and methods of life sciences, materials science, computer science, and engineering, to research and develop regenerative treatment technologies and products for replacing, repairing, improving, or regenerating various tissues and organs of the human body and for tissue and organ defects or dysfunction caused by diseases, trauma, aging, or genetic factors. The basic scientific problem of tissue repair and regeneration is actually the proliferation, differentiation, and orderly regulation of tissue repair cells [1]. The scope of regenerative medicine is not simply biology or medicine, but covers almost all areas of natural sciences and social sciences. It is a discipline that studies the mechanism of tissue and organ defects, and how to promote physiological repair for structural reconstruction and functional optimization of tissue and organ regeneration [2].

In the traditional medicine of the motherland, the concept of "regeneration" has always accompanied its development. The theory of the "mutual generation of five phases" and "mutual generation of five zang viscera" is the representative of *Huangdi Neijing*. *Bencao Beiyao* said: "Five zang viscera of human beings correspond to the five phases, mental, wood, water, fire and earth, mother offspring mutual generation." Wood generating fire, fire generating earth, earth generating metal, metal generating water, water generating wood, repeat in this way, to "Replenish the deficiency and subtract the excess." In the case of "deficiency" or "excess," there are a mutual generation of five phases of dynamic change and interpromotion and interrestraint, which are suitable for regenerating the structure and function of the damaged organs, and avoiding "virtual and reality," which is also the goal pursued by regenerative medicine. If the wound should be repaired and the rebirth is insufficient, the ulcer will form; if it is more than enough, it will form a scar. Wound repair is also in line with the theory of qi and blood, Yin and Yang balance. "Yin blood is calm, yang qi is inseparable, so that the human body can be fully refreshed. The separation and rupture between yin and yang will exhaust the essence in the body."

*Suwen • Spiritual cultivation conforming with the four seasons* said: Only the sages who know the way to keep healthy can adapt to the changes of yin and yang in the seasons, so their bodies are never seriously ill. If all things can be like the sage not to deviate from the way of health, can adapt to the change of yin and yang seasons, the life is inexhaustible. It emphasizes to enhance the regeneration ability of the body by actively adapting to the season, climate, and environment, and by strengthening the body function "inexhaustible" is the source of regeneration. The theory of essential qi in traditional Chinese medicine reflects the essence of regenerative medicine. *Lingshu • Benshen* said: "Human life comes from the combination of parents' essence." *Suwen • Jingui Zhen Yan Lun* said: "Essence is the root of life." Essence is the root of human body occurrence, development, regeneration, repair, and maintenance of life. Therefore, in the *Nan Jing Gu Yi*, it is pointed out that "There will be self--sufficiency, the pulse is fundamental, and the people have the vitality, so they do not die." From this, we can see a description similar to the modern embryo development and stem cell function. Similarly, we have seen the emphasis on the idea of inducing and enhancing tissue regeneration through adjustments to the overall and local environment.

Y. Jiang
The Chinese People's Liberation Army Strategic Support Force Characteristic Medical Center, Beijing, China

X. Fu (✉)
The Chinese People's Liberation Army General Hospital, Beijing, China



X. Fu (ed.), *Regenerative Medicine in China*, https://doi.org/10.1007/978-981-16-1182-7_12

### 12.1.2 The Modern Medical Treatment of Wound Healing

After the tissue is traumatized, local vasoconstriction, blood and cell exudation, and activation of vasoactive factors induce a blood coagulation process. The inflammatory response period occurs immediately after the injury to 48 h. Tissue changes are characterized by inflammatory reactions, edema, degeneration, necrosis, dissolution, and clearance of the wounded tissue. The essence and core of the inflammatory response period is the regulation of growth factors and their results. On the third day after injury, with the regression of inflammatory reaction and the gradual proliferation of tissue repair cells, the pathological and physiological processes of granulation tissue proliferation and epidermal cell proliferation were observed. In the future, the reconstruction of the local tissue still needs to be carried out for a certain period of time to restore the original structure and function as much as possible, mainly the transformation of granulation tissue into normal connective tissue. The formation of scars is one of the final outcomes of soft tissue wound repair [3]. In this process, a variety of cellular components (mainly macrophages), growth factors and nerves, the immune system can regulate the synthesis and degradation of connective tissue, so that collagen is repeatedly dissolved, deposited, and renewed, scars gradually disappear, and finally reach the organization the purpose of the alteration.

### 12.1.3 The Inheritance and Evolution of Wound Healing in Traditional Medicine

The traditional medicine of the motherland is specific to the field of wound repair and tissue regeneration. It has a history of 5000 years of treatment for "sore and ulcer" diseases. Wound repair is one of the oldest medical problems of human beings. Chinese medicine believes that: Too much heat will make the meat rot, the rotten meat will become pus, the pus is formed by steaming and brewing the heat and rotten flesh between the skin and the flesh, which is generated by qi and blood. *Waike Zhengzhi Quansheng Ji* said: "The poison must be made of pus, the pus must come from the blood," Xue Lizhai said: "Perhaps the generation and healing of sores are the result of blood gas action," pointed out that wound occurrence/healing has a great relationship with the body function, and is directly determined by the tissue regeneration ability, and the treatment also emphasizes the "promoting pus drainage and granulation." It was first seen in the *Waike Qixuan•Sore and ulcer•Yi Tie Gaoyao Lun* (published in 1604) by Shen Douyuan (the surgical surgeon of the Ming Dynasty), there are written records of "promoting pus drainage and granulation" to explain it.

### 12.1.4 The Traditional Medicine on the Cognition of Wound Healing

Traditional medicine on the healing of body surface ulcers is basically based on the general shape of the wound and has a unique cognition, such as "eliminating necrotic tissues and promoting granulation," "promoting pus drainage and granulation," "granulation tissue filled the tissue defect and epidermal cells grew normally," etc., and according to the healing laws of these wounds, the internal and external treatments such as "eliminating pus and removing necrosis, promoting pus drainage and granulation, nourishing blood and promoting granulation, dispelling stasis and eliminating scar." The method runs through the inflammatory reaction period, the granulation growth period, and the scar formation period.

#### 12.1.4.1 The Understanding of "Essence of Pus" in Traditional Medicine

In the inflammatory reaction phase, for "pus," traditional medicine believes that it cannot be judged as a factor to prevent wound healing, and it is necessary to dialectically consider its effect on wound healing. Traditional Chinese medicine pays special attention to the method of "discriminating pus." It is not only to distinguish the presence or absence of pus, but also to observe the shape, color, quality, and odor of pus, so as to judge the prognosis and formulate treatment measures. *Huangdi Neijing* observes the "red, swelling, hot" performance of wounds, and puts forward the idea that "too much heat and rotten flesh produce pus." The pus at this stage shows different forms depending on the type of bacteria infected. For example, for *Staphylococcus aureus*, the pus is yellow, sticky, and dirty. If it is infected with fecal bacteria, it is thin and stinking, If it is infected with streptococcus, local redness and exudation are more, and specific manifestations may be caused by multiple or special bacterial infections. Most of the pus is produced by the liquefaction of necrotic tissue, which contains more inflammatory cells and a large amount of necrotic tissue. The pus culture can have the growth of pathogenic bacteria [4].

Traditional medicine also regards "pus" as a product of qi and blood metaplasia. "Pus" is given different connotations at different stages of wound healing. In the relatively clean granulation growth period, "pus" is the exudate from the wound. After the necrotic tissue is removed, use "promoting pus method drainage," the pus turns yellowish and clear, like plasma. The pus (exudate) at this time is a product of wound metabolism, containing the wound healing indispensable white blood cells, proteins, amino acids, and various growth factors, providing a good environment for wound healing.

#### 12.1.4.2 "Promoting Pus Drainage and Granulation" and "Wet Healing Theory"

"Promoting pus drainage and granulation" is a traditional Chinese medicine external treatment method based on the summary of the causes, pathogenesis, and evolution of sores. It means that in the process of wound healing, the application of external Chinese herbal ointment (powder) through the skin and the absorption of drugs in the face promote local qi and blood patency, enhance its defensive ability, so that the pus exudation of the wound surface increases, the drug is excreted, the sinister poison is leaked out, and the purpose of wound growth is achieved, and then the "therapy of encircling lesion with drugs" and "external medicinal liquid application" are derived, which are all made after the drug acts on the body. The active ingredient is absorbed locally, and has the therapeutic effects of clearing heat for detumescence, removing congestion and relieving pain, warming channel and dissipating phlegm, that is, intercepting toxicity, restraining toxicity, and eliminating toxicity. This "pus" should be thick and should not be thin, the color should be clear, not dirty, the smell should be light, not skunk. On the basis of the other treatment methods, various medical doctors have derived such external prescriptions as "Yuhong Ointment," "Shengji Yuhong Cream," "Huanglian Jiedu Ointment," and "Shengji San," which are numerous.

In 1962, British zoologist Winter found that the wet environment significantly promoted wound healing, shortened wound healing time, and laid the foundation for modern wet wound healing theory. It was not until the 1870s that the first hermetic dressing was successfully developed, which opened the formal clinical application of the theory of wet healing [5]. The focus of "promoting pus drainage and granulation" is "promoting pus drainage," which includes two contents: first, eliminating pus and necrotic tissues, and eliminating toxicity, increase the exudation of local pus, and accelerate the shedding and decomposition of necrotic tissue of the wound; second, the pus can be turned into qi and blood and body fluid, which helps the skin to grow. In modern medicine, the stage of inflammation is also inevitable and independent of the stage of wound healing. The occurrence and healing of wound is inseparable from the participation of inflammatory reaction. Whether healing is closely related to the occurrence and intensity of inflammatory reaction, and the description and understanding between the two are consistent. In essence, the theory of "wet healing" and "promoting pus drainage and granulation" emphasizes that the growth of wounds requires a proper moist environment. It is believed that by adjusting the healing environment of the wound surface, it can promote the repair and regeneration of wound tissue and promote healing [6].

The traditional Chinese medicine "promoting pus drainage and granulation" external treatment method, because of its combination and various components, can be used for the factors of wound healing, with multi-target, multi-link, multi-level comprehensive regulation, and synergistic effect, with the advantages of simple, convenient, cheap, and effective [7]. Through basic animal experiments on traditional Chinese medicine Jingwanhong ointment, we found that Jingwanhong ointment and compound sulfadiazine zinc gel have certain effects on wound healing in the early stage of wound healing (0–7 days). The difference is not significant. The wound healing time of Jingwanhong ointment group was shorter than that of compound sulfadiazine zinc gel group. Histopathological observation also found that Jingwanhong ointment group can reduce inflammation and wound epithelialization earlier than compound sulfadiazine zinc gel, and the epithelial cells are well differentiated, the new collagen is arranged neatly, and the tissue structure of the wound surface is obviously normalized, which shows better healing quality. Jingwanhong Ointment has a large amount of pharmaceutical ingredients, which can promote blood circulation, increase the blood supply and oxygenation of chronic wounds, enhance the phagocytic ability of white blood cells, reduce local capillary permeability, reduce edema, and achieve antibacterial, anti-inflammatory effects, analgesic effect, improve the micro-circumstance of local injury are the reasons for its better curative effect. The multicenter large-sample clinical trial designed according to the RCT principle confirmed that it promotes the healing of chronic refractory wounds on the surface of the body, and has great advantages in terms of healing speed and healing quality.

## 12.2 Wound (Sore) Treated by Chinese Medicine Treatment

Commonly used external treatment methods include eliminating necrotic tissues debridement, nibbling debridement, Xi's technique of eliminating necrotic and clearing tendon, Chinese medicine fumigation and washing therapy or external medicinal liquid application, therapy of encircling lesion with drugs, etc., as follows [8].

### 12.2.1 Eliminating Necrotic Tissues Debridement

Commonly used corrosive Chinese medicines include hydrargyrum oxydatum crudum and hydrargyrum chloratum compositum. Hydrargyrum oxydatum crudum is an orange--red matt powder, or a crystalline powder with orange-red luster. It is a mercury preparation, which is a remedy for eliminating necrotic tissues. Hydrargyrum chloratum compositum is a white fine crystal or crystalline powder, which is heavy and more corrosive. It can be administered in the form of medicated thread, medicine twist, etc., and it needs to be combined with ointment for the specific application. It is especially suitable for sinus treatment with more necrotic tissue and small external cavity and deep internal.

### 12.2.2 Nibbling Debridement

It is suitable for unclear boundary between wound necrotic tissue, rotten flesh and healthy tissue is not clear, necrotic tissue is softer but difficult to fall off, that is, there are more ecological tissues, or the patient's vital signs are unstable, the systemic condition is poor, and the person who cannot afford invasive decisive debridement. The therapy can be used in combination with eliminating necrotic tissues debridement. The crust and necrotic carrion tissue is softened as soon as possible by eliminating necrotic tissues debridement. The junction of necrosis-health tissue is as clear as possible, thus selecting local rotten flesh to soften and the necrotic tissue which not closely adhered to the basal tissue, trimmed from the obvious boundary, to avoid bleeding as much as possible, from shallow to deep, small amount, many times and gradually.

### 12.2.3 Xi's Technique of Eliminating Necrotic and Clearing Tendon

It is suitable for diabetic foot non-ischemic tendon degeneration and necrosis. The clinical manifestations of the Xi's diabetic gangrene of foot tendon are red, swollen, and bulging in the back of the foot, the sole of the foot and the toe. Pressing it can cause fluctuation or breakage, the rotten tendon is exposed, the exudate is dirty and foul, and the drainage is not smooth. The rule of treatment is completely removed by walking along the direction of the necrotic tendon, thereby achieving the purpose of eliminating the lesion.

### 12.2.4 Chinese Medicine Fumigation and Washing Therapy

Traditional Chinese medicine fumigation and washing therapy is guided by the basic theory of traditional Chinese medicine. After decoction of traditional Chinese medicine, steam fumigation is first used, and then liquid medicine is used to rinse, soak the body or locally affected area. It has the effects of clearing heat and removing toxicity, cooling blood and detumescence, activating blood and expelling pus, and astringing sores and promoting granulation. It is used for the initial stage of acute suppurative infection and local redness, swelling, heat and pain, inflammation and infiltration are more obvious. The heat-toxin congestion and excessiveness can be used for fumigation and washing with honeysuckle bud and flower, dandelion, wild chrysanthemum flower, purslane herb, Tokyo violet herb, natural indigo, *Cyrtomium fortunei*, dyers woad leaf, glabrous greenbrier rhizome, heartleaf houttuynia herb, rhubarb root and rhizome, and other drugs with clearing heat and removing toxicity effects, to control local inflammation. When heat toxicity is more severe with blood stasis syndrome, it can also compatible with unprocessed rehmannia root, peony root, tree peony root bark and other cooling blood and activating blood circulation drugs, strengthen the efficacy, promote local inflammatory exudate early absorption and detumescence. If the ulcer has already formed, the pus cannot be broken or the vital qi deficiency cannot promoting toxic discharge, you can compatible with milkvetch root, Chinese angelica, Sichuan lovage rhizome, pangolin scales, Chinese honeylocust spine and other drugs for promoting pus drainage and toxic discharge, to achieve the purpose of promoting the early liquefaction of the affected area into pus, discharge of pus and toxic, swelling and pain subsided. For acute suppurative infections, such as pus, scald infection, or chronic ulcer, it can be used for clearing heat and removing toxicity drugs such as lightyellow sophora root, amur cork-tree, honeysuckle bud and flower, baical skullcap root, and unprocessed liquorice root, and it is also compatible with drugs for promoting blood circulation and dispelling stasis, promoting granulation and wound healing such as frankincense, myrrh, Chinese angelica, and milkvetch root. Decoct the decoction with these drugs and soak the affected part with heat. It can not only sterilize and eliminate inflammation, but also cleanse the wound to reduce infection. At the same time, it can make the affected part congestive, accelerate blood flow, improve blood circulation and tissue nutrition, and help the wound to heal.

### 12.2.5 External Medicinal Liquid Application

The trick is to wet the affected area with gauze or cotton wool containing the liquid, and to soak the affected area in the liquid. External medicinal liquid application is a method for achieving the therapeutic purpose by wet compressing, rinsing, soaking the physical effects on the affected part, and the pharmacodynamic effects of different drugs on the affected part, and is similar to the fumigation and washing therapy. Commonly used 6–8 layers of gauze soaked Chinese medicine liquid, to the degree of no drip, apply to wound surface. Remove every few minutes, repeat the soaking of the liquid, continue to apply, or drip the liquid frequently on the gauze to maintain certain humidity on the wound. It is used for the treatment of wet compresses with large amount of pus and red swelling wounds around the wound. The commonly used prescriptions are mainly tree yellow liquor, honeysuckle bud and flower, and lightyellow sophora root.

### 12.2.6 Therapy of Encircling Lesion with Drugs

This therapy is called "Tie Fa," "Tie Xie," and "encircling paste," that is, according to the condition of the disease, the medicine is selected and ground into a fine powder, and take vinegar, wine, medicinal juice, oil, etc., to apply around the affected area, to bundle the sore and detumescence. The redness and swelling area around the wound surface is often externally applied with encircling paste, the application range should be more than 1 cm in the whole redness, swelling, and heat area. The thickness of the medicine should be 1–2 mm, not too thick, so as not to affect the skin permeability around the wound. The commonly used encircling paste is as follows. (a) Jinhuang powder: rhubarb root and rhizome, amur cork-tree, turmeric, dahurian angelica root are 25 g each, jackinthepulpit tuber, dried tangerine peel, atractylodes rhizome, officinal magnolia bark, liquorice root are 10 g each, radix trichosanthin is 50 g. Grind the above medicines together into a fine powder and store in bottles for later use. The prescription can be applied to acute stage of carbuncle on the back, various sores, phlegm-damp and shank erysipelas, acute mastitis and erysipelas, or to patients with yang-heat excess syndrome due to persistent symptoms. (b) Yulu powder: cotton rose hibiscus leaves are not limited, grinding into fine powder and apply at any time. It can also be added to rice bean, rhubarb root and rhizome, baical skullcap root, amur cork-tree, hirsute shiny bugleweed herb, etc. It is used for carbuncle and furunculosis, acute mastitis, intestinal abscess, etc. It is especially suitable for those who have swollen red sputum and no obvious swelling with pain. (c) Chonghe powder: fried Bark of Chinese Redbud is 150 g, doubleteeth pubescent angelica root is 90 g, peony root is 60 g, dahurian angelica root is 30 g, grassleaf sweetflag rhizome is 45 g. Grind the above medicines together into fine powder and store in bottles for later use. It is used for the abscess on the back, disharmony between yin-yang, the swelling is not obvious, reddish and scorching, the pain is not very serious, and it can also treat the bone abscess and pernicious influence. (d) Hui Yang Yulong powder: kusnezoff monkshood root, roasted zingiber are 90 g each, peony root, dahurian angelica root, jackinthepulpit tuber are 30 g each; cassia bark is 15 g. Grind the above medicines together into fine powder and store in bottles for later use. It is used for the abscess, cold syndrome without swelling and pain and fever.

## 12.3 The Role of Traditional Chinese Medicine in the Healing Process of Wounds

### 12.3.1 Wound Infection

In recent years, antibacterial drug abuse and bacterial resistance have become more prominent in China. Traditional Chinese medicine has a special anti-bacterial infection mechanism, which is not easy to produce drug resistance. It can effectively control infection during wound healing. Antibacterial Chinese medicine has attracted the attention of many scholars and has gradually become a research hotspot.

#### 12.3.1.1 Mechanism of Chinese Medicine Treatment of Wound Infection

Traditional Chinese medicine treatment of infectious wounds is based on the chemical action of temperature, machinery, and drugs, and has a local therapeutic effect. For its pathogenesis, it uses clearing heat and removing toxicity, promoting granulation for hemostasis, promoting menstruation and activating collaterals, inducing diuresis and eliminating dampness. The antibacterial range and antibacterial level of Chinese herbal medicines vary. In addition, various bacteria and fungi have different sensitivities to traditional Chinese medicines, and should be targeted in the clinical application of antibacterial Chinese herbal medicines.

The common pathogens and antibacterial Chinese medicines on wounds are as follows:

A. *Staphylococcus*: honeysuckle bud and flower, medicine terminalia fruit, rhubarb root and rhizome, amur cork--tree, baical skullcap root, golden thread, siberian cocklebur grass, heartleaf houttuynia herb, snakegourd root, weeping forsythia capsule, climbing groundsel herb, wild chrysanthemum flower, purslane herb, wintergreen, garden burnet root, Taiwan beautyberry leaf, and so on.
B. *Escherichia coli*: medicine terminalia fruit, baical skullcap root, Tokyo violet herb, fried Cape jasmine fruit, common selfheal fruit-spike, purslane herb, heartleaf houttuynia herb, dandelion, etc.
C. *Candida albicans*: golden thread, peony root, Paris polyphylla, baical skullcap root, rhubarb root and rhizome, Chinese gall, garlic, etc.
D. *Neisseria gonorrhoeae*: golden thread, Chinese gall, medicine terminalia fruit, amur cork-tree, baical skullcap root, giant knotweed rhizome, honeysuckle bud and flower, weeping forsythia capsule, etc.
E. *Streptococcus*: honeysuckle bud and flower, baical skullcap root, amur cork-tree, medicine terminalia fruit, rhubarb root and rhizome, heartleaf houttuynia herb, climbing groundsel herb, Taiwan beautyberry leaf, giant knotweed rhizome, weeping forsythia capsule, wild chrysanthemum flower, Japanese climbing fern spore, stick tight, Ussurian grape, and so on.
F. *Pneumococcus*: baical skullcap root, golden thread, platycodon root, Japanese ardisia stem and leaf, giant knotweed rhizome, officinal magnolia bark, and Chinese arborvitae twig and leaf.
G. *Meningococcus*: honeysuckle bud and flower, weeping forsythia capsule, baical skullcap root, wild chrysanthemum flower, isatis root, garlic, etc.
H. *Corynebacterium diphtheriae*: honeysuckle bud and flower, weeping forsythia capsule, baical skullcap root, golden thread, dandelion, Tokyo violet herb, blackberry lily rhizome, native achyranthes root, unprocessed rehmannia root, figwort root, etc.

I. *Mycobacterium tuberculosis*: baical skullcap root, golden thread, heartleaf houttuynia herb, common andrographis herb, stemona root, garlic, ginkgo seed, realgar, danshen root, Chinese arborvitae twig and leaf, and Japanese ardisia.
J. Enterobacter: argy wormwood leaf, giant knotweed rhizome, garlic, purslane herb, heartleaf houttuynia herb, Chinese pulsatilla root, creeping euphorbia, baical skullcap root, amur cork-tree and so on.
K. Skin filamentous fungi: stemona root, radish seed, Sichuan chinaberry bark, cortex pseudolaricis, areca seed, rangooncreeper fruit, golden thread, amur cork--tree, rhubarb root and rhizome, giant knotweed rhizome, argy wormwood leaf, cassia seed, cultivated land, solomonseal rhizome, etc.
L. *Salmonella*: weeping forsythia capsule, lightyellow sophora root, heartleaf houttuynia herb, Chinese pulsatilla root, etc.

External washing of traditional Chinese medicine decoction can play the role of clearing heat and removing toxicity, promoting urination and eliminating dampness, removing stasis, and relieving pain. It is suitable for infection wounds, pus odor, and more exudation. Plaster and powder used for external application on infected wounds have the effects of eliminating dampness and astringing sores, promoting granulation for hemostasis, and are suitable for the late stage of infected wounds.

#### 12.3.1.2 Mechanism of Action of Single Traditional Chinese Medicine

The main active ingredients of Chinese herbal medicine are: alkaloids, flavonoid glycosides, anthraquinone glucosides, saponins, coumarin glycosides, volatile oils, polysaccharides, and terpenoids. The antibacterial mechanism of traditional Chinese medicine mainly interferes with the formation of bacterial cell wall, damages the cytoplasmic membrane, affects cellular protein synthesis, affects nucleic acid synthesis, and interferes with genetic code. The active ingredients of antibacterial Chinese herbal medicine can directly or indirectly kill bacteria, fungi, and viruses, inhibit the reproduction of bacteria and fungi and the replication of viruses, participate in the biochemical processes of bacteria and molds, and change the functions of enzymes and cell membranes; inducing interferon and enhancing interferon induction; enhance the phagocytosis of leukocytes and reticuloendothelial systems, enhance lymphocyte transformation rate; inhibit allergic reactions; delay the cytopathic effects caused by the virus. Although some have weak antibacterial activity in vitro, they have good curative effects. For example, mudan cortex, common anemarrhena rhizome, and golden thread can inhibit the formation of Staphylococcus aureus enzymes at a low concentration, thereby exerting an antibacterial effect. Hyun et al. studied the antibacterial effect of the methanol extract of golden thread on Salmonella. They used 26 species of Salmonella-infected chicks as animal models, and the mortality rate of chicks was greatly reduced [9]. Ban et al. used Chinese medicines such as polydatin, resveratrol, and anthracene glucoside B extracted from the root tip of Polygonum to exert anti-Streptococcus mutans by inhibiting the glycolysis pathway [10]. Mohammed et al. studied the antibacterial effect of *Podophyllum hexandrum* in Rhubarb genus in male Wistar rats. It was found that the ethanol and benzene extract of *Podophyllum hexandrum* (MIC 3.0 mg/mL) can cure *H. pylori* infection in 7 days at a relatively low concentration [11].

#### 12.3.1.3 Mechanism of Traditional Chinese Medicine Compound Prescription in Treating Wound Infection

Compared with the concentration, the antibacterial spectrum and antimicrobial MIC of the prescription were better than that of the single Chinese medicine. The MIC of the different prescriptions changes with the change of composition, and the synergistic effect of the drug appears. Zhang Hanqing et al. replicated the guinea pig skin ulcer model caused by *Staphylococcus aureus* infection, confirming that the lianyang powder has a good improvement on local redness and secretion, and the lysozyme level in the pus is also significantly improved after treatment. Zhu Zhanbo et al. used the paper diffusion method to detect the inhibitory effect of Jun Du Ling on *Staphylococcus aureus*, *Salmonella*, and *Pasteurella multocida*. Yu Keming et al. observed 60 patients with diabetes complicated with skin suppurative infection, the treatment group was treated with the homemade traditional Chinese medicine Liushen Qufu Decoction and the affected area is rinsed with physiological saline, and the gauze soaked with the traditional Chinese medicine Liushen Qufu Decoction is applied to the sore surface. After the local infection of the control group, the Vaseline gauze was applied externally, the effective rate of the treatment group was 96.67%, and the effective rate of the control group was 70%. Li Pingping used Huayu Shengji Powder external application to treat 66 cases of chronic shank ulcer of varix of lower limb. All cases were cured, the ulcer surface was completely healed. Zhou Zhaoying used 30 cases of Touhai Powder to treat 30 cases of lower limb erysipelas. 18 cases were markedly effective and 11 cases were effective. Zhao Dongrui used homemade Daqing Powder external dressing to treat 89 patients with chronic shank ulcer. The total effective rate was 96.63%.

#### 12.3.1.4 Other Mechanisms for Traditional Chinese Medicine Treatment of Wound Infection

With the increasing problem of bacterial resistance, integrated Chinese and Western medicine therapy provides a cheaper and more effective way to treat the wounds of resistant organism infections [12]. Maurer and others found that the combination of golden thread or rhubarb root and rhizome with ceftazidime can enhance the anti-infective effect on *Escherichia coli*. Que. Huafa and others applied the comprehensive treatment scheme of internal and external treatment of traditional Chinese medicine to treat chronic refractory wounds complicated with *Pseudomonas aeruginosa* and methicillin-resistant *Staphylococcus aureus*. The results showed that the negative rate of *Pseudomonas aeruginosa* was 92.21%; methicillin-resistant *Staphylococcus aureus* negative rate was 95.56% [13]. Traditional Chinese medicine has different degrees of synergistic effect on antibacterial drugs, which can improve the sensitivity of resistant organism to antibacterial drugs. Mi Wei et al. found that berberine sulfate can enhance the antibacterial activity of ceftazidime by inhibiting the β-lactamase activity of *Escherichia coli*. Bacteria are not easy to develop drug resistance to traditional Chinese medicines, especially traditional Chinese medicine compound preparations. Under the guidance of traditional Chinese medicine theory, treatment based on syndrome differentiation, and the formula is modified and applied, can successfully avoid the drug resistance of bacteria, sensitization, or reversal of resistant organism. It provides new ideas and methods for the treatment of infectious wounds with resistant organism as the main pathogenic factor.

### 12.3.2 Promote Granulation Tissue Growth

Traditional Chinese medicine has a curative effect on promoting the growth of wound granulation tissue and accelerating the healing of refractory wounds. It mainly promotes the growth of granulation of wounds by the following five ways [1].

#### 12.3.2.1 Eliminating Necrotic Tissues and Promoting Granulation

Yao Chang et al. found that Shengdan preparation can improve the hydroxyproline content and fibroblast cell count of wound granulation tissue, can eliminate wound necrotic tissue, promote wound granulation growth, and facilitate wound healing. The mechanism of Honghengdan may be at the cytological and molecular biological level by regulating growth factors such as interleukin-2, interleukin-6, and tumor necrosis factor in granulation tissue, which can improve the content of TNF and IL-6 in wound granulation, and thereby mediates the inflammatory reaction of the wound, promotes the infiltration of inflammatory cells, enhances the bactericidal effect, and at the same time mediates the production of high concentration of IL- 2R, promotes cell mitosis, and is beneficial to the proliferation of granulation to accelerate wound healing. Wei Zhendong et al. found that traditional Chinese medicine qufu shengji powder can increase the number of fibroblasts on the 12th day after the skin surgery of experimental animals, and the function is active, the cell body is enlarged. On the 15th day after surgery, the rough endoplasmic reticulum of fibroblasts is developed, and the content of free ribosome is rich, interstitial contains more fine collagen fibers, and its ointment can also reduce the wound healing integral value of sore model rats, increase the content of lysozyme in complement C3, immunoglobulin IgA, IgM and purulent secretions, increase thymus index and spleen index, thereby enhancing wound immunity and promoting wound healing.

#### 12.3.2.2 Dispelling Stasis and Promoting Granulation

Chen Jianchang and others discovered: External application of danshen root can not only accelerate the removal of necrotic tissue of the wound, reduce inflammation and edema, but also promote the growth of fibroblasts and epithelial cells and accelerate wound healing. Zhang Fengchun et al. found that: earthworm can promote the contraction of wounds in animal models, promote the proliferation of myofibroblasts in granulation tissue, and increase actin in cells, which is active in synthesis and promotes wound healing. Li Ping et al. observed the effect of Zhuxu powder, a traditional Chinese medicine for activating blood circulation and promoting granulation, on the healing of wounds with azithromycin injured rats. It was found that Zhuxiang powder can improve the blood circulation of wounds, exert the effect of promoting blood circulation for removing the obstruction in collaterals, promote local inflammatory reaction, and release cytokines, promote the proliferation of granulation tissue and collagen synthesis and have the effects of promoting granulation and consolidating skin. Fuhuang Shengji Yuchuang Ointment (hereinafter referred to as Fuhuang Ointment) is the empirical formula of Professor Tang Hanjun from Longhua Hospital of Shanghai University of Traditional Chinese Medicine. Its clinical application has been proven to have a significant effect on promoting the healing of chronic skin ulcers. Related experimental studies found that Fuhuang Ointment can significantly shorten the wound healing time of traumatic rats, and can significantly increase the content of fibronectin in serum and granulation tissue of traumatic rats, and affect the content of related amino acids in granulation tissue, it has effects in increasing hydroxyproline and deoxyribonucleic acid content in newborn granulation tissue, and can increase the levels of epidermal growth factor receptor and fibronectin in local granulation tissue of experimental wounds.

#### 12.3.2.3 Invigorating and Promoting Granulation

Qiu Ke et al. found that Astragalus injection can promote wound repair after hemorrhoid and fistula operation, accelerate the regeneration of capillaries, supplement the nutrients and trace elements necessary for wound repair, promote the proliferation of fibroblasts, and activate macrophages. Wang Zhenyi et al. found that: in the process of wound healing, the traditional Chinese medicine for invigorating and promoting granulation can inhibit the secretion of MMP-1, thereby increasing the secretion of type I and III collagen, and promoting wound healing. Cao Yongqing et al. found that Wenshen Jianpi Recipe can promote the repair of chronic refractory wounds in rats, and promote the expression of interstitial fibronectin by up-regulating the expression of epidermal growth factor and TGF-β1 cytokine protein. Zhou Yanjie et al. found that electroacupuncture at Zusanli can improve the inflammatory response caused by trauma, increase the number of mast cells and its released mediator, and increase the content of hydroxyproline, so that the gray scale of collagen fibers rises, which is beneficial to the repair of fibrous tissue of skin wounds.

#### 12.3.2.4 Benefiting qi and Removing Stasis and Promoting Granulation

Zhang Zhen et al. found that traditional Chinese medicine for benefiting qi and removing stasis can promote wound healing by increasing the level of wound TGF-β1. Que. Huafa et al. found that traditional Chinese medicine for benefiting qi and removing stasis can down-regulate the level of hypoxia-inducible factor-1α, down-regulate the expression of Smad3 and Smad4, up-regulate the expression of capillary endothelial growth factor to improve the state of ischemia and hypoxia, and can significantly promote diabetic skin ulcers. The wound healing of rats with the syndrome of blood stasis was due to qi deficiency.

#### 12.3.2.5 Other Effects

Lu Jinli et al. found that aloe vera gel can promote the formation of granulation tissue in radiation dermatitis tissue and accelerate the healing of radiation dermatitis. Zheng Xueping found that topical Zhuhuang Frost significantly increased the hydroxyproline content in the granulation tissue of the anus after surgery, increased the synthesis of the matrix, and promoted wound healing. Combination of compound Zhuhuang Frost and basic fibroblast growth factor can promote the healing of contaminated wounds on the back of rabbits and increase the filling rate of granulation tissue and the rate of re-epithelialization. Li Linggen et al. found that chitosan traditional Chinese medicine compound membrane stimulates the body to secrete a large number of phagocytic cells and promote the release of VEGF and PCNA, promote the growth of granulation tissue, reduce the proliferation of fibrous tissue, and accelerate the healing of ulcers. Wang Chunming et al. found that the myogenic ointment can make the granulation tissue of the ulcer surface healthy, with abundant capillaries, more macrophages and higher positive expression rate of VEGF and PCNA. Dong Liqiang et al. found that Shengji Yupi Ointment can increase the content of epidermal growth factor in granulation tissue of white rabbit wounds in early and middle stages, thus accelerating the healing of wounds. Yuyangling Ointment and Shikonin Oil can promote the expression of ulcerated basic fibroblast growth factor and promote the growth of granulation tissue, thus promoting the repair.

### 12.3.3 Traditional Chinese Medicine Inhibits Scar Formation

#### 12.3.3.1 Overview of Scar Modern Medicine

Scar is a general term for the appearance and histopathological changes of normal skin tissue caused by various wounds. It is an inevitable product in the process of human wound repair [14]. Superficial scars generally involve the superficial epidermis or dermis, the surface of the skin is rough or pigmented, the part is flat and soft, and generally there is no dysfunction. Over time, the scar will gradually become inconspicuous. Hypertrophic scar damage affects the deep dermis, and the scar is significantly higher than the surrounding normal skin, local thickening, and hardening. Hypertrophic scars can sometimes be as thick as 2 cm or more, but they are not tightly adhered to deep tissues and can be promoted. They generally have obvious boundaries with normal skin around them. The contractility of hypertrophic scars is smaller than that of contracture scars. Atrophic scars are generally more damaging, involving the entire layer of skin and subcutaneous fat tissue. If the disease breaks down from time to time over a long period of time, there is the possibility of malignant transformation in the late stage, pathologically mostly squamous cell carcinoma. Atrophic scars have a large contractility and can pull adjacent tissues and organs, causing severe dysfunction. Keloids generally manifested as a lump that is higher than the normal surrounding skin and grows continuously beyond the original injury site. It is hard and has poor elasticity and local itching or pain, and the early surface is pink or purple, and the early stage is mostly pale, sometimes with hyperpigmentation, has a clearer boundary with the surrounding normal skin. Inflammation necrosis may occur in the lesion due to residual hair follicle glands, or liquefaction necrosis may occur due to central ischemia. Keloids generally do not contract, except for a small number of joints that cause mild activity limitation, generally do not cause dysfunction. Keloids may be related to the following factors: cytokines released by post-traumatic inflammatory cells, immune cells, platelets, etc.; abnormal expression of related proteases, mRNAs, genes in extracellular matrix; increased free radicals in scars; microcirculation within the scar.

#### 12.3.3.2 Understanding of Scar Formation in Traditional Medicine

There are many traditional Chinese medicines for keloids, for example, called "paravertebral abscess," "meat turtles," "saw scar," and there are some other names such as "meat centipede" and "crab foot swelling." Traditional Chinese medicine believes that this disease is a pathological reaction in the process of wound healing, mainly because it originally has the syndrome of internal retention of damp-toxin or dampness-heat in the lungs and stomach, also has knife wounds, fire poison, and poisonous insect wounds, which hurts the skin, resulting in stagnation of qi and blood stasis, scars hyperplasia, and keloids over time, or due to trauma and attack of exogenous evils, disharmony between nutrient qi and defensive qi, qi stagnation, and blood coagulation. Shi Hongtai put forward a new theory of "the excess syndrome is its essence and the deficiency syndrome is its standard" on the pathogenesis of scars.

#### 12.3.3.3 Oral Decoction Treatment

Chinese medicine believes that this disease is mostly caused by qi and blood stasis and dysfunction. The internal treatment is mostly treated with promoting qi for activating blood circulation and softening and resolving hard mass. Clinically, Fuyuan Huoxue Decoction is commonly added and subtracted, regulating qi for activating blood circulation, softening and resolving hard mass, treating keloids with the syndrome of qi stagnation and blood stasis; Shengmai Powder adds flavor, benefiting qi for promoting the production of fluid, nourishing blood for moistening dryness, treating keloids with deficiency of qi and yin, blood dryness and muscular contracture. Wushuidou et al. used Wulingzhi Pills for oral treatment of 54 cases of keloids, the cure rate was 88.89%, and the difference was not significant compared with the hormone-blocked group. Liu Jianjun believes that the treatment of this disease should be activating blood circulation to dissipate blood stasis, clearing heat and removing toxicity, resolving masses and eliminating scar, and selecting Liangxue Siwu Decoction in *Jianzong Jinjian*. Xia Shiping believes that the scar is mainly caused by blood stasis, and it is treated with Shuizhi Huoxue Decoction. Ma Chuntai et al. used Quban Xiaoling Decoction, a total of 26 cases of keloid diagnosis were diagnosed and treated, the total effective rate was 96.1%.

#### 12.3.3.4 External Treatment

Because keloids occur mostly in local areas, external treatment is most commonly used.

A. Ancient Prescriptions

Mieban Ointment (the white part of domestic chicken manure is 30 g, biond magnolia flower-bud is 1.2 g, giant typhonium rhizome and manchurian wildginger are 0.6 g each), the above four traditional Chinese medicine are soaked in wine for one night, decocted with 1200 g of mutton fat over low fire for three times, the residue is removed, and the scar is washed with Gancao Decoction, and the medicine is smeared on it. Liumie Banhen Ointment (equal parts of silverfish, the white part of domestic chicken manure, eagle dung with white, Chinese peony, Japanese ampelopsis root, white bee, etc.), the above medicine are ground into powder, mixed with milk, and applied to scar three times a day. Miebanhen Prescription (limonite, pinellia tuber), the above medicine are ground into powder, mixed with hen egg yolk. First use new cloth to wipe the scar and make it red, then apply it with medicine twice a day. Do not blow the air, will recover within 10 days. People who have been ill for 10 years will also improve. Wipe the affected area with a clean new cloth to make it hyperemia, making the drug easy to penetrate and exert its effects.

B. Modern Times Prescriptions

Professor Zhao Bingnan's Heibu Ointment [old black vinegar is five jin (2.5 kg), Chinese gall is one jin and twelve liang (1.1 kg), ten golden head centipede, honey is six liang (0.3 kg), plum blossom borneol is one qian (5 g)], clean the skin before dressing change, apply this medicine 2–3 cm thick, cover with black cloth, change dressing once every 2–3 days. Compound Ai Ye Jian (30 g of old pine bark, 15 g of argy wormwood leaf and Chinese clematis root, 10 g of safflower) add external rubbing Ding Ai Oil (argy wormwood leaf is 30 g, clove is 50 g, safflower is 20 g, borneol is 6 g), compound Ai Ye Jian for 30 min, once in the morning and once in the evening, then rub the Ding Ai Oil. Wubei Ointment (smoked plum is 50 g, centipede is 5, Chinese gall and lightyellow sophora root are 30 g each, unprocessed rehmannia root is 40 g, musk is 3 g), grinding centipede and musk into fine powder, the other drugs are soaked in water for 10 h and then decoct to obtain 500 mL of juice concentrating to form a paste, then add centipede and musk powder and mix well. When using, apply the Wubei Ointment evenly on the multi-layer disinfected mulberry paper, and cover the affected part with ointment after disinfection, once a day. Xiaojin mini-pills is grinded to a powder and then add 30 g Huapu Powder (20 g of danshen root, seaweed and clam shell, 15 g of kelp, immature orange fruit, Chinese gall, zedoray rhizome and Stephania tetrandra, 10 g of borax and common aucklandia root, 5 g of cinnabar and centipede), mix with a proper amount of sesame oil and honey for external use.

C. Chinese Patent Medicine Injection for External Use

Danshen injection has an external application method and partial closed injection method, external application method is more suitable for children and skin lesions in the frontal, eyelids, breasts, etc.; local injection of ligustrazine can inhibit the synthesis of collagen in keloid fibroblasts, so that soften scar.

D. Acupuncture Therapy
   (a) Heated needle treatment, point selection in the local lesions, rapid advancement of heated needle, deep into the bottom of the scar, quickly cupping after acupuncture, leaving the tank for 5–8 min, based on mucus or blood flowing out.
   (b) Acupuncture and moxibustion and encircling needling combined with external application of traditional Chinese medicine.

E. Massage Therapy

   Generally, the wound is healed immediately after healing, and the curative effect is obvious, and the effect on the old scar is poor or ineffective. (a) Therapeutic massage, rubbing around the scar first, followed by pushing scars, grasping and lifting the scar again, and finally pushing and rubbing toward the heart, can reduce the symptoms caused by scars, improve their blood supply. (b) Ginger slice rubbing method, slicing ginger, gently rubbing scars, can prevent its granulation tissue from continuing to proliferate.

F. Combination of Internal and External Treatment of Traditional Chinese Medicine

   The combination of internal and external treatment can give consideration to both symptoms and root causes, through the overall syndrome differentiation, the treatment method can be applied separately, which can enhance the curative effect. The formula is prepared from medicines that cooling and activating blood, softening and resolving hard mass such as danshen root, Chinese gall, lightyellow sophora root, kelp, seaweed, common selfheal fruit-spike, Chinese clematis root, sulfur, coral-bean bark, divaricate saposhnikovia root, cicada slough, common buried rubber, zedoray rhizome, dahurian angelica root, pangolin scales, safflower, areca seed by addition and subtraction, oral administration, and external application.

G. Chinese Herbal Extracts

   Some of the active ingredients of traditional Chinese medicine have the effects of inhibiting the proliferation of fibroblasts, promoting apoptosis of fibroblasts, and reducing collagen synthesis. Most of them have been applied clinically, and have obvious effects on the treatment of pathological scars, and some are still in vitro. It also presents a good application prospect. (a) Asiaticoside is an extract of Chinese herbal medicine *Centella asiatica*, which is a triterpenoid saponin compound. The asiaticoside can significantly affect the ultrastructure of fibroblasts, inhibit collagen synthesis, and in a dose-effect relationship, reduce the activity of transamidase, reduce the amount of acid mucopolysaccharide and collagen, and the excessive proliferation of matrix and fiber components of connective tissue is inhibited. (b) Matrine belongs to the tetracyclic quinolizinidine and is an active ingredient of lightyellow sophora root. Matrine can inhibit the proliferation of scar fibroblasts, up-regulate bax expression, down-regulate p53 and bcl-2 expression, and promote apoptosis of scar fibroblasts by affecting cell cycle. (c) Danshensu and tanshinone are the main active ingredients of danshen root. The activating blood circulation to dissipate blood stasis drugs represented by danshen root can effectively inhibit collagen synthesis and deposition. Danshensu has the effect of inducing apoptosis of fibroblasts. The active constituents of danshen root can stimulate the up-regulation of c-Myc protein expression in fibroblasts, promote fibroblast apoptosis, and reduce collagen synthesis by inhibiting fibroblast autocrine TGF-β1. Tanshinone II A can significantly inhibit the proliferation of scar fibroblasts and induce apoptosis. (d) Ligustrazine is an alkaloid monomer extracted from the rhizome of the umbelliferous plant Sichuan lovage rhizome. Ligustrazine can inhibit the proliferation of keloid fibroblasts, reduce the collagen synthesis of fibroblasts, and change the morphology of the cells. Ligustrazine can significantly inhibit the expression of type I and III procollagen mRNA in scar fibroblasts. (e) Capsaicin is the main biological active ingredient in hot pepper and is a fat-soluble natural plant base. Capsaicin can significantly inhibit scar hyperplasia, reduce the hardness of scar, and have analgesic and antipruritic effects. Capsaicin has an inhibitory effect on fibroblasts in vitro, and has a positive effect on clinical symptoms such as itching. (f) *Tripterygium wilfordii* is a celastraceae plants, and its extract contains various active ingredients, such as diterpene lactone, alkaloid, tribasic, etc., and has anti-inflammatory and immunosuppressive effects. *Tripterygium wilfordii* extract has a negative regulatory effect on the morphology and proliferation of fibroblasts. (g) Tetrandrine is an isoquinoline alkaloid extracted from the traditional Chinese medicine mealy fangji root. It is a calmodulin antagonist with broad pharmacological activity, which can significantly reduce the proliferation activity of fibroblast, and has the effects of preventing and treating scar hyperplasia.

### 12.3.4 Problems and Prospects

Traditional Chinese medicine therapy plays a good role in the treatment of keloids, but it also has the disadvantages of poor reproducibility, high recurrence rate, difficult to control health indicators, complex and difficult extraction of single-dose and compound Chinese medicines. This disease is still a difficult problem to be solved urgently in the clinical practice of traditional Chinese medicine. Moreover, there is no uniform standard for the diagnosis and syndrome differentiation of keloids in traditional Chinese medicine, and there is no strict distinction between keloids and hypertrophic scars. The research on keloids is mostly a summary of clinical experience, and lacks a deep discussion on its pathogenesis and treatment mechanism from the perspective of traditional Chinese medicine theory. With the continuous revealing of the pathogenesis and key factors of keloids, traditional Chinese medicine treatment will play a greater role in the treatment of pathological scars in the future due to its positive curative effect, less adverse reactions and economical convenience, and comprehensive treatment based on actual conditions. The combination of surgery and medical treatment, making full use of the advantages of Chinese and western medicine, and more scientific treatment, will certainly improve clinical efficacy.

## 12.4 Traditional Chinese Medicine Wound Treatment

The three methods of "elimination, promoting, and supplementation" are based on three different stages of the initial stage of sore, pus formation, and ulceration. They are formulated under the guidance of the overall concept and the spirit of treatment based on syndrome differentiation. They are the main principles for the treatment of sores in traditional Chinese medicine. "Elimination" refers to the use of drugs that eliminate pathogen, so that the absorption of sores that have not yet become suppurated at the beginning is dissipated, which is the most ideal method for treating sores. "Promoting" means "expelling pathogens by strengthening vital qi and expelling pus." In order to tonify qi and replenish blood, to support vital qi, so that vital qi can promote pus discharge, to lead poison out and enable pathogenic factor to have a way out. "promoting" is used in the pyogenic stage, which is to use the medicine for strengthening vital qi to eliminate pathogenic factor, to accelerate the limitation of abscess and the discharge of pus, so as to avoid the method of stagnation of pathogenic toxin, but because of the different outcomes of the struggle between vital qi and pathogen, it is divided into the direct promoting method and promoting method with tonification. "Supplementation" is a kind of therapy that uses drugs to tonify deficiency and strengthen body resistance, so as to make the qi and blood in the body sufficient, eliminate various virtual images, and restore the body's vital qi. It is often used for deficiency syndrome, chronic ulcer after ulceration or not heal for a long time.

The wound has not healed for a long time, especially the chronic infection wound is the middle and late stage of the "outer ulcer" of traditional Chinese medicine. The condition is complicated and the course of disease is long. It is a clinically intractable disease. It is not treated internally or externally and cannot be cured. Its pathogenesis, because of illness and lingering, repeated symptoms, although it has been treated for a long time, the pathogenic qi have declined, but the vital qi is also damaged, cannot exorcise the pathogenic qi out, forming the syndrome of deficiency of both vital qi and pathogenic qi, and syndrome of lingering pathogen due to deficient vital qi. This syndrome cannot support vital qi without tonifying qi and replenish blood cannot exorcise the pathogenic qi out without promoting toxin and pus drainage, it is the main syndrome of the promoting therapy. The local pathogenesis of wounds is syndrome of poor health condition, especially on nutrition and immunological deficiency, fitting for local external treatment. Therefore, "expelling pathogens by strengthening vital qi and expelling pus," both inside and outside, it is necessary to take strengthening vital qi as the priority, to tonify qi and replenish blood and strengthening vital qi to eliminate pathogenic factor as the first, to restore the vital qi, to be able to promote toxin and pus drainage, and to promote the pathogenic factor out.

When the three methods are used, in addition to the cause and condition, it is also necessary to combine the pathogenesis. For example, in the early stage of sores, meridian obstruction, qi and blood stagnation, stagnation of heat is the main pathogenesis, so the syndrome is red swelling, heat and pain. In the elimination method, not only the method of clearing heat and removing toxicity should be used, but also the method of nutrient-blood-harmonizing, activating qi, dredging channels is used to eliminate heat-toxicity, unblock meridian obstruction, and regulate qi and blood stagnation to return to normal. Otherwise, "too much heat will make the flesh rot, the rotten flesh will become pus," heat is the cause of further development of the disease, pus is a pathological product of too much heat and rotten flesh. Therefore, when applying direct promoting method in the pus formation stage, it is necessary to cooperate with the method of clearing heat and removing toxicity, and the curative effect can be remarkable. After the ulcer is ulcerated, the pus and blood are discharged, and the blood and qi are damaged. Therefore, the deficiency syndrome is more common (except for the light and shallow yang syndrome). Different complementary methods should be selected according to different situations of deficiency. It can be seen that the combination of pathogenesis and syndrome differentiation plays a certain role in improving clinical efficacy.

The three methods have their own stages, but they are related to each other. Because the development and changes of the disease are intricate, it is often necessary to use the three methods in combination and cannot be separated.

## References

1. Fu XB, Wang DW. Modern trauma prosthetics. Beijing: People's Military Medical Press; 1999.

2. Fu XB, Jiang DY, Jia CY, et al. Theory and practice of prevention and treatment of chronic refractory wounds. Beijing: People's Medical Publishing House; 2011.
3. Fu XB, Han CM, Hu DH, et al. Treatment of diabetic foot and its related chronic difficult to heal wounds. Beijing: People's Military Medical Press; 2013.
4. Jiang YF, Fu XB. Analysis of pathogenic microbial characteristics of chronic refractory wounds on the surface. Infect Inflammat Repair. 2011;12(3):134–8.
5. Fu XB, Wu ZG. Theory and practice of modern wound dressings. Beijing: Chemical Industry Press; 2007.
6. Jiang YF, Xu ZR, Fu XB. The importance of holistic, systematic and multidisciplinary cooperation in the diagnosis and treatment of diabetic foot. Infect Inflammat Repair. 2012;13(2):1–3.
7. Jiang YF, Fu XB. Research progress on chronic refractory wounds on the surface. Infect Inflammat Repair. 2011;12(1):70–2.
8. Jiang YF, Xu ZR, Fu XB. Debridement in the repair of diabetic foot wounds. Chinese J Pract Intern Med. 2016;36(1):13–5.
9. Hyun AK, Yong JK, Dong YK, et al. Evaluation of antibacterial effects of a combination of coptidis rhizoma, mume fructus and schizandraefructus against salmonella. Int J Food Microbiol. 2008;127:180.
10. Ban SH, Kwon YR, Pandit S. Effects of a bio-asaay guided fraction from *Polygonum cuspidatum* root on the viability acid production and glucosyl tranferase of mutans streptococci. Fitoterapia. 2010;81(5):352.
11. Mohanmmed I, Aleem AK, Santosh KT, et al. Antimicrobial activity of sapindus mukorossi and rheum emodi extracts against H pylori: in vitro and in vivo studies. World J Gastroenterol. 2006;12(44):7136.
12. Fu XB. Bacterial biofilm formation and chronic refractory wounds occur. J Traumat Surg. 2008;10(5):416–7.
13. Tang HJ, Liu XD, Cheng YQ. Integrated TCM for therapy of refractory wound infected *Pseudomonas aeruginosa*. World J Infect. 2004;4(4):364–6.
14. Fu XB, Cheng B, Sheng ZY. Molecular study of wound healing and scar formation [J]. Chin J Clin Rehab. 2002;6(4):464–6.

# 13 Discipline Construction and Talent Cultivation of Tissue Restoration and Regenerative Medicine

Shuliang Lu, Wei Dong, Yuehong Shen, and Chunmao Han

With the development of social economy and the aging of the population, the human disease spectrum has undergone significant changes. The epidemiological data of Xiaobing's Fu team showed that as prevailing in 1998 [1], the 2008 survey showed that burn wounds accounted for only 18% of wound diseases, and the remaining 82% were chronic wounds. The survey data also estimated that nearly 100 million people in China need wound treatment every year [2]. The survey also found that wound disease brings a lot of burden to social medical resources. The first is the burden of manpower; the second is the average length of stay (ALOS). The third is the cost of hospitalization. These data show that we are not only faced with the major medical needs of wound disease treatment, but also the wound disease has brought us a major social medical burden. It can be seen that all kinds of chronic wounds have become one of the important diseases affecting people's life and health, and one of the important issues that modern clinicians and researchers must face.

Now that all kinds of chronic wounds have become a major component of wound diseases, it is necessary to establish a wound repair specialist and popularize wound treatment to meet such a huge demand for wound treatment. The current problems mainly include the following aspects:

A. There is no professional department for all kinds of wound treatment in the setting of the current clinical departments in our country, which makes the patients with wound diseases unable to find a place to seek medical treatment.
B. Wound repair specialists involve multidisciplinary intersections. Therefore, no professional has taken this business for granted, so that patients can be transferred to various subjects in disorder, without systematic treatment.
C. There is currently no uniform clinical guidelines and norms for chronic wounds.
D. The knowledge of chronic wound diagnosis and treatment in medical undergraduate teaching in China has not been extensive.
E. There is still a lack of innovative theories and techniques in the field of wound healing. Therefore, it often seems to be inadequate in specialist treatment.
F. Wound diseases have the characteristics of "small wards and large outpatients," that is, a considerable number of patients only need to change medicines in the outpatient department, and only need hospitalization when deep treatment or surgery is needed. In the current situation that there are not many wound repair specialists, it is difficult to meet the needs of patients living in different regions when the general practitioners in the primary hospital are unfamiliar with the methods of chronic wound healing.

To this end, many hospitals across the country have set up specialists in wound repair to meet the needs of the medical market. However, we realize that the establishment of the wound repair specialist is by no means a gorgeous turn of disciplines such as burns or reduction surgery. There is a need for new understanding of the theoretical mechanisms of wound repair, new methods for wound treatment techniques, new norms in clinical guidelines and diagnosis and treatment, new breakthroughs in

S. Lu (✉)
Ruijin Hospital, Shanghai Jiaotong University School of Medicine, Shanghai Burns Institute, Shanghai Wound Healing Institute, Shanghai, China

W. Dong
The First Affiliated Hospital of Jinan University, Guangzhou, China

Y. Shen · C. Han
The Second Affiliated Hospital of Zhejiang University School of Medicine, Hangzhou, China


X. Fu (ed.), *Regenerative Medicine in China*, https://doi.org/10.1007/978-981-16-1182-7_13

medical treatment models and clinical pathways, so that wound repair specialty has rich connotation.

## 13.1 Guiding Clinical Practice with Wound Repair and Innovation Theory

In addition to the huge demand in the medical market, the upsurge in the construction of wound repair specialists in China has also accumulated a certain theoretical accumulation in the past 20 years. Its landmark events were the major projects of the National Natural Science Foundation in 1992 and the three "973" projects in 1999, 2005 and 2011.Through the investment of these major projects, not only a team has been trained, but also a series of theoretical understandings of wound repair have been formed, which has played a supporting role in the construction of wound repair specialists in China [3].

### 13.1.1 Understand the Significance of Wound Repair Procedures for Wound Treatment

Wound healing is a complex and orderly biological process that involves several stages of inflammation, cell proliferation/connective tissue formation, wound contraction, and wound remodeling. The various stages of the healing process are not independent but intersect and overlap each other and involve the participation of a variety of inflammatory cells, repair cells, inflammatory mediators, growth factors, and extracellular matrices [4]. The wound healing mechanism has three characteristics, namely the regionality, time-bound, and sequential inertia of wound healing:

#### 13.1.1.1 Regional Characteristics of Wound Healing

The so-called regionality means that after the wound is formed, except for large-area wounds, a series of biological events related to repairs that occur in the body usually accumulate in the local part of the wound. It is a regional biological event, not a systemic one. Therefore, wound treatment should focus on local treatment. Wound debridement, wound dressing and adequate drainage, providing a relatively moist and suitable environment for wounds are important means of wound treatment. If the local treatment of the wound is neglected, attempts to promote wound repair by means of systemic therapy often fail to achieve the desired effect. A common clinical phenomenon is the infection of the wound and the hope to control the infection through systemic application of antibiotics, while neglecting the local treatment and drainage of the wound.

#### 13.1.1.2 Time-Bound Characteristics of Wound Healing

The so-called time-bound means that the wound repair is mainly divided into three stages, namely, the inflammation stage, the tissue cell proliferation stage, and the tissue remodeling stage. These three stages have different characteristics of cell behavior and tissue biological environment, respectively. Although the stages overlap partially, they all have their own behavioral "time window." It is necessary to take appropriate measures in the effective "time window" according to the characteristics of the phase. Taking deep burn wounds as an example, it is an important link to promote the shedding of necrotic tissue in the early stage of wound formation. There are many ways to promote the shedding of necrotic tissue, both medicated and surgical. In the medium term, it is mainly to provide suitable means for tissue cell growth and repair, such as giving the wound a relatively moist environment and drugs for promoting growth. Therefore, how to grasp the time-bound characteristics of the wound healing process in the process of wound healing, and take appropriate measures in the effective "time window" to facilitate wound repair, this is not only a technology, but also an "art", which requires long-term clinical accumulation.

#### 13.1.1.3 Network Sequential Characteristics of Wound Repair

The so-called network sequence of wound repair refers to the participation of many different cells, factors and matrix components in the process of wound repair. At different stages of wound healing, various cells, factors and matrix components increase and decrease and regulate each other, thus forming the network and sequential nature of the healing process. There are many factors affecting the sequential advancement of wound healing, including exogenous or endogenous. A variety of reasons lead to abnormal immune system in the inflammatory reaction of wound repair, affecting the repair of wounds; malnourished people can inhibit the proliferation of wound repair, affect the formation of granulation and the synthesis of related components. Therefore, in the treatment of wounds, we must give a good healing environment. At the same time, the network and sequential features of wound repair also suggest that we have different biological events at different stages of wound repair. Therefore, wound treatment is not a drug or a means to "catch the world".

### 13.1.2 The New Theory to Explain the Common Problems of Clinical Treatment of Diabetic Refractory Wounds

Diabetes mellitus combined with wound difficult to heal accounts for a considerable proportion of chronic wounds and is one of the important targets for clinical treatment. The traditional view is that the formation of refractory ulcers in diabetic foot can be divided into vascular, neurological or mixed vascular and nerve. However, we also clearly recognize that the main pathophysiological feature of diabetes is elevated blood glucose. This has led us to a series of thinking: Why is the main pathological mechanism of diabetic refractory wounds is neuropathy and vasculopathy, not elevated blood glucose? Is it possible to consider neuropathy and vasculopathy as a pathological result of hyperglycemia rather than an initial cause? Does hyperglycemia directly affect the healing process of diabetic wounds? Or does the skin tissue itself be damaged in the high glucose environment of diabetes mellitus? In response to these problems, our research group carried out a series of studies that lasted for 15 years, and through analysis and induction has formed some theoretical understanding of diabetes complicated with wound surface difficult to heal, which has reference significance for clinical practice.

#### 13.1.2.1 The Nature of Difficult Healing of Diabetes Wounds

Diabetes combined with wound healing is a pathological evolution process based on metabolic disorders of diabetes mellitus and mediated by subsequent events of metabolic abnormalities. Compared with diabetic skin vasculopathy and neuropathy, the accumulation of metabolites in local tissues is an upstream event in the development of this disease. The microenvironmental changes caused by the increase of glucose content and accumulation of metabolites in skin tissue caused by diabetic metabolic disorders, namely "cutaneous environmental disorders," are one of the initiating factors leading to the difficult healing of diabetic wounds. "Cutaneous environmental disorders" cause a series of "recessive damage" characterized by histological and cellular functional changes in noninvasive diabetic skin and continues to affect all aspects of wound healing after trauma, ultimately leading to delayed wound healing or not healed [5]. Therefore, for the prevention and treatment of diabetes mellitus complicated with wounds, it is undoubtedly the focus should be placed on the initial stage of "cutaneous environmental disorders," that is, through the intervention of the upstream element related to wound healing, to stop the occurrence or development of its follow-up effects. Therefore, it provides a means for effective and feasible prevention and treatment strategies and achieves an ideal preventive and therapeutic effect on diabetic complicated refractory wounds.

### 13.1.3 Focus on the Key Issues of Wound Repair, Explore New Entry Points for Wound Treatment

Wound repair is an old and modern medical problem. It is old, because the wound repair behavior is the body's instinct, even before humans, gorillas licking their wounds with their tongues is a proof; it is modern because human understanding of wound healing has been from the late 1980s to the early 1990s. Only from the rise of histology and cytofunctionology to the understanding of growth factors, it is gradually recognized that the wound healing process is regulated by a complex network. With the development of various related technologies, human understanding of wound repair mechanisms has made great progress: growth factors accelerate the regulation of wound repair; the role and status of inflammatory cells, especially macrophages in wound healing; role of various repair cells in wound repair; the role of extracellular matrix components and structures; and even the effects of stem cells and wound microenvironment on wound repair are gradually being recognized. The mystery of wound healing mechanisms is gradually being unveiled.

#### 13.1.3.1 The Wound Repair Process Can Be Converted from Passive to Active

Before the 1980s, the traditional view was that wound repair is a natural means of protection for the body. It has an inherent spontaneous regulation mechanism. There is a sequence of self-regulation of the network. We cannot control or accelerate the healing process of the wound. What Clinicians can do is to protect the wound environment and prevent the wound from developing in a direction that is not conducive to healing. At that time, doctors can only passively wait for the natural healing of the wound. However, since the 1980s, with the deepening of people's understanding of growth factors, it has been theoretically realized that growth factors can accelerate the healing process of wounds. In the early 1990s, a study at the Third National Burn Conference reported that the application of lymph fluid from the thoracic catheter in asthma patients to burn wounds significantly accelerated wound healing. At that time, we realized that lymph fluid may be rich in growth factors, and the effect of lymph fluid on wound healing may be related to growth factors. However, at that time, there was a lack of routine detection methods for growth factors, and the ELISA method for growth factor detection became popular in a few years. Different concentrations of cytokines and growth factors were detected in the lymph fluid, and the relationship between these growth factors and the accelerated repair of wounds was clarified. Later, a variety of commercial growth factors such as EGF, FGF, etc. were introduced one after another, widely used in clinical, and the role of growth factors in promoting wound repair was generally accepted. Since then, clinicians have no longer been passively awaiting the healing of wounds but can actively promote wound repair through the intervention of growth factors. With the gradual deepening of research on wound repair mechanism, we conclude that the wound repair process has regional, time-bound, and network sequential inertia characteristics. The three characteristics of wound healing tell us that the active repair and acceleration of the perfect restoration of the wound is not based on a means to protect the world. The perfect state of wound healing treatment should be the application of various cellular components, factors or extracellular matrix in a phased, selective or combined manner to protect the wound environment and promote wound repair. However, at present, our understanding of the wound repair mechanism and the means of promoting it are still far from perfection. There are still many scientific problems to be explored.

#### 13.1.3.2 Strive to Explore Macrophage as an Important "Regulatory" Cell Behavior Mechanism for Wound Repair

Research and understanding of the role of macrophages in wound repair has gone through three stages.

Stage 1: In the mid-1970s, Leibovich et al. [6] used systemic hydrocortisone and subcutaneous local antimacrophage serum to remove macrophages from blood circulation and cutting wound and found that the degree of fibrosis was increased in the wound, fibrin, and neutrophil and red blood cell debris clearance time prolonged; the wound fibroblasts in control group appeared on the third day after injury, peaked on the fifth day, and fibroblasts appeared on the fifth day of the experimental group, and the proliferation ability was weaker than control group. For the first time, this classic experiment confirmed that macrophages are not only an immune cell that removes pathogenic microorganisms in wound healing, but also participate in wound repair.

Stage 2: In the 1980s and early 1990s, scholars confirmed the role of macrophages in promoting fibroblast proliferation, collagen deposition, and vascularization, and in situ hybridization and cell separation techniques were used to confirm that macrophages secrete various cytokines and inflammatory mediators during wound healing. It was confirmed that the wound could not heal smoothly without macrophages.

Stage 3: Since the late 1990s, the researchers have noticed significant differences between IL-4-treated macrophages and IFN-γ-treated macrophages. Macrophages treated with IL-4 did not show strong resistance to pathogenic microorganisms, but the expression of inflammatory factors such as IL-1, IL-8, and TNF-α decreased, and the expression of mannose receptors, which mediate endocytosis and pinocytosis, was significantly enhanced. Gordon et al. referred to the high inflammatory state of macrophages against pathogenic microorganisms as classical activated macrophage (caM or M1), and the macrophages with low inflammatory state after IL-4 and IL-13 treatment are called alternative activated macrophages (aaM or M2), and for the first time define macrophage activation patterns that are quite different from the past. Since then, the differential effects of caM and aaM macrophage activation in wound repair have been paid more and more attention. Scholars have already confirmed in vitro that classical macrophages and alternative activated macrophages may have different roles of wound repair. This suggests that macrophages of different activation types may have an important impact on the outcome of wound repair.

In recent years, in vivo experiments on macrophage activation have also been carried out, confirming that different activation modes of macrophages have a certain degree of growth and decline during normal wound healing, showing that both M1 and M2 activation markers are elevated in the early stage of wound formation, but the M1 is the main one, while the M2 mark is dominant in the later stage, and the growth and decline of activated M1 and M2 suggest that they dominate the different stages of the healing process.

In clinical research, Israeli scholars have isolated mononuclear/macrophage suspensions from whole blood through ABO and Rh blood group matching, and local injection or external application for treatment of refractory wounds after stimulation with hypotonic fluid. Since 1995, More than 1000 patients have been cured by this method, 90% of which are effective only with a single use of macrophage suspension. It is further suggested that macrophages are the key cells for wound healing. Studies have shown that macrophage-activated lipopeptide (MALP-2) can be used in the full-thickness model of the back of mice, which can increase the number of wound macrophages and promote wound healing. Studies suggest that the infiltration of wound macrophages can be intervened by external means. Recently, Miao's research found that the infiltration of macrophages in the wounds of diabetic rats showed a phenomenon of "slow-in and slow-out," which was not synchronized with the inflammatory phase and the proliferative phase. At the same time, it was found that the expression of M1 was insufficient and the number of M2 was overexpressed, showing the abnormal phase of macrophage infiltration and the abnormal expression rate of M1 and M2. These abnormalities may be related to changes in the microenvironment of diabetic wounds. From the above studies, it can be found that macrophages do play an important role in wound repair and play the role of "commander." However, from the latter two studies, we can also see the infiltration of macrophages and the increase and decrease of M1 and M2 expression can be regulated by external intervention or changes in internal environment. The so-called "commander" of wound repair may be an important "executor" of wound repairs at best, not the "originator" of wound repair behavior. However, research on how to improve the wound environment, explore and create conditions conducive to the infiltration of macrophages and the orderly expression of M1 and M2 is still an important entry point to promote wound healing.

#### 13.1.3.3 Pay Attention to the Role of Dermal Template in Wound Repair

In the literature on wound repair research, a considerable part of the research focuses on cells, factors or extracellular matrix components, and these components are involved in the network regulation of wound repair, which is an important direction of research. However, some phenomena in clinical practice have led us to think more deeply about this issue. If the same incision is made, the plastic surgery technique is used to suture, and the scar formation is not obvious, but if the general triangular needle is used for suturing, a clear scar will be formed. Why the same wound is supposed to stimulate the same "strength" wound healing response, but because of the different suture skills that lead to different healing results? Then, whether we have previously described the wound repair network sequential inertia response is only a possibility "domino array"? What is the original driving force to push down this "domino array"? Similarly, deep wounds with razor graft have scars, while full-thickness skin graft has no scars, giving composite transplantation of acellular dermal matrix and razor graft also has no scar. Why does the same depth of wound and the same wound healing reaction give different thicknesses of dermal matrix for replantation, and the healing outcome is very different? Liu Yingkai and other studies have found that the degree of dermal tissue defect can affect the wound healing process [7]. The three-dimensional structure of dermal tissue has a "template-like" guiding effect on the function of repairing cells, which not only induces the growth of repaired cells, but also improves the mechanical state of wound skin tissue, regulates the function of repairing cells, and promotes tissue remodeling; and the structure of the dermal tissue has a "permissive effect" on the component. Under the nonphysiological structure, the extracellular matrix component can have an abnormal effect on the function of the fibroblast. Once the structural and mechanical properties of the extracellular matrix return to the physiological state, then the abnormal effects of extracellular matrix components on cell function will disappear. The tissue structure is a "template" that guides the cell function. The appropriate three-dimensional structure can promote the completion of the cell physiological cycle and facilitate the recovery of cell biological behavior. However, the integrity and continuity of the dermal tissue are the necessary prerequisites for the tissue structure to fully play its "template effect." The destruction of dermal tissue integrity and continuity caused by trauma may lead to the loss of dermal "template effect," which may be one of the important mechanisms affecting the function of repairing cells and leading to scar formation. Therefore, the "template defect theory" of scar formation is proposed. Jiang Yuzhi et al. constructed a cell culture system with cell adhesion points at different angles through molecular self-assembly and microprinting techniques. It was found through experiments that the same cells exhibited different cell functions under the culture conditions of cell adhesion points at different angles. It is also calculated by geometry and calculus: any unregulated shape can be fitted with a plurality of arcs of different diameters, and the surface of the substrate adhered to different arcs forms a different angle from the horizontal plane. It is inferred that the adhesion of cells at different angles is equivalent to adhesion on matrix of different morphological three-dimensional structures. Therefore, Jiang Yuzhi et al. [8] concluded that the same cells exhibited different cellular functions under the culture conditions of cell adhesion points at different angles, which indirectly proved that the morphology of the three-dimensional structure of extracellular matrix can affect the function of repairing cells and affect the outcome of wound healing. The results of this series of studies suggest that the process of wound healing is not a mere biochemical event of cell-to-cell, cell-to-factor, and the role and status of the physical factor of the three--dimensional structure of the extracellular matrix of wound tissue in wound repair cannot be ignored.

#### 13.1.3.4 The Impact of Wound Microenvironment on Stem Cells Is Worth Considering

Early studies have suggested that no matter what kind of wounds, as long as there are hair follicles remaining, the cells will have fulminant growth after injury. The reason why hair follicles can become the source of proliferation and differentiation of wound repair cells is mainly in hair follicles. At the same time, similar stem cells were also found in the basal part of epidermis. These cells differentiate into corresponding tissue cells according to their different anatomical levels, repairing defects and regenerating the skin. In recent years, the characteristics of stem cells with high self-renewal ability and multidirectional differentiation potential have been highly valued. The use of stem cells to treat various types of wounds, especially refractory wounds, has become a hot topic, and relevant basic and clinical research is continually deepening. However, in the in-depth study, many researchers have found that in addition to improving the local environment of the wound and promoting wound repair, stem cells are also susceptible to the microenvironment of the skin tissue. Various factors such as cytokines, inflammatory mediators, matrix active components, spatial structure, biochemical signals, biomechanics, etc. in this microenvironment can directly affect the differentiation direction of stem cells and their proliferative activity, this is the biological effect of so-called "stem cell niches."

Taking diabetes mellitus and refractory wounds as an example, the accumulation of advanced glycation end products (AGEs) in skin tissue is one of the main causes of diabetic wounds. Diabetic skin with severe accumulation of AGEs may appear thin; the epidermis is not clear, the collagen in the dermal tissue is slender and loose; the collagen synthesis and decomposition are dynamically unbalanced. AGEs can also affect the local cell apoptosis of wound surface to increase and proliferation to be inhibited by affecting apoptosis- related factors Bcl-2, Bax, p53, and cell cycle related factors CDK4, Ki67, and mitogenic factors. At the same time, it also glycosylates growth factors in local tissues, impaired inflammatory cell function, local abnormal inflammatory infiltration, formed a "cutaneous environmental disorders" of diabetic skin. It can be seen that the local accumulation of AGEs creates a bad tissue environment that is not conducive to wound healing. So, can stem cells also be affected by this local environment? Through the specific markers of epidermal stem cells in diabetic wounds, keratin 19 and integrin β1 immunohistochemical staining showed that the positive expression was significantly lower than normal. In the wound skin of diabetic patients, the number of epidermal stem cells is smaller than that of normal human skin, and the ability to proliferate and differentiate is lagging. It can be seen that the microenvironment of the diabetic wound makes the main force stem cells of the wound repair in a "low state," which inhibits the main driving force of wound repair and is worthy of attention. In recent years, enrichment of bone marrow mesenchymal stem cells or adipose derived stem cells has become a trend in the treatment of refractory wounds. However, whether stem cells enriched in bone marrow or adipose tissue of diabetic patients will also affect the healing of wounds due to the microenvironment of diabetes, it is worth further research and related experiments are underway. The study found that substance P acts as a stem cell synergist to increase the proliferation rate and mobilization rate of stem cells, and enhance the function of stem cells themselves to overcome adverse environmental factors; Shen et al. used degradable materials and bone marrow mesenchymal stem cells, fat marrow mesenchymal stem cells are prepared together with the biological scaffold, and the shape of the material itself changes the cell environment of the transplant, which can guide the stem cell to be repaired. It can be seen that external factors or environmental factors can effectively improve the "low state" of stem cells in the diabetic environment, which has found a breakthrough point for improving the effectiveness of the treatment of diabetic and refractory wounds, and it is worth exploring.

## 13.2 Interdisciplinary Technology to Improve the Level of Wound Healing Treatment

### 13.2.1 Improve the Accuracy of the Record of Wound History by APP

Chronic wounds belong to the category of surgery, and the history of surgical specialties requires the description of the characteristics of the wound. However, the judgment of any wound is characterized by morphology. Whether it is the existing evaluation system or classification criteria, or the description of the surgical specialty history is written, usually when the patient returns to the clinic, the doctor cannot imagine or restore the detailed characteristics of the wound surface at the time of the first visit or the previous visit according to the medical history description at the time of the first visit or the previous visit. Therefore, it is difficult to accurately determine the effectiveness of treatment or systematically review the progress of wound evolution. To this end, Shanghai Ruijin Hospital created a "mobile phone based wound information collection system" through software writing. The system photographs the wound surface through a mobile phone to record the morphological features of the wound surface, and then clicks on the drop-down menu to input the basic condition of the patient and the diagnosis and treatment plan of the wound, that is, the text can be uploaded to the database, and the information can be sent to electronic medical records and resident health records through the database. When the patient returns to the doctor, the doctor can use the mobile phone to recall the previous images and texts of the database, and visually review the medical history or the observation of the progression of the disease, making it possible to standardize and systematically diagnose the various types of wounds. Moreover, the system is also conducive to multicenter, large sample epidemiological investigations, worth promoting.

### 13.2.2 Improve the Traditional Methods to Expand the Scope of Application of Wound Treatment

Traditional methods such as debridement, expansion, dressing or skin grafting are the basic technical means of wound repair. With the development of modern science and technology, various methods for wound healing have emerged, which have greatly improved the efficacy of wound repair. Vacuum sealing continuous drainage is a clinical technique that has been widely used in recent years. Although the clinical use of this method has achieved a relatively consistent positive effect, there are still some negative reports. It is well known that wound healing is a complex biological process. Different stages have different characteristics and different clinical interventions are needed to facilitate the perfect healing of the wound. Xie Ting and Xiao Yurui of Shanghai Ninth People's Hospital, on the basis of the technology of "Vacuum Sealing Drainage, VSD," supplemented by intermittent flushing, achieved good results and expanded the indications for the application of VSD technology.

VSD has become a common technical means of wound treatment. A treatment cycle is 3–7 days. If the operation of this technique is unskilled, film leakage may occur. Therefore, patients receiving negative pressure therapy are often hospitalized. Recently, some scholars have proposed to add a pressure sensing device and a signal transmitting device to the negative pressure meter. Once the air leaks, the negative pressure meter can send a signal to the mobile doctor or nurse's mobile phone, and the doctor or nurse on duty can immediately know which negative pressure instrument is calling the alarm. This technological improvement has made it possible to treat home treatments with VSD. Once the patient's negative pressure treatment film is found to leak, the patient can be recalled for treatment. At present, the prototype of this technology has been successfully developed and is expected to be marketed in near future.

### 13.2.3 The Treatment of Sinus Wounds Under the Support of Endoscopy

The principle of surgical treatment of sinus wounds is flushing with drainage strips packing and dressing change or sinus resection. After a liver operation, the sinus was formed for more than 2 years, and the sinus was not healed after drainage strip packing and dressing change and two sinus surgeries. The sinus was about 18 cm long and the diameter was about 5 mm. It was transferred from the external hospital to our department. Our team broke the tradition and performed sinus wound treatment with the support of endoscope. This kind of wound treatment under endoscopic direct vision reduced the "blindness" of drainage strip packing and dressing change compared with traditional methods; the inside of the sinus wound is usually "dendritic" and often has many bifurcations. It is often difficult to completely remove the surgical sinus resection for such sinus wounds. The sinus wound treatment technology supported by the endoscope can overcome the deficiencies of the above traditional methods, and conveniently enter each sinus cavity, and clearly and intuitively observe the morphological features of the sinus cavity. As a result, it was found that the absorbable suture used in the proximal peritoneum of the case was not "absorbed" and became "foreign bodies," causing the sinus to be unhealed (Fig. 13.1). After removing the "foreign bodies," the sinus wound quickly healed. It can be seen that the form of wounds is diversified, and our traditional means are limited.

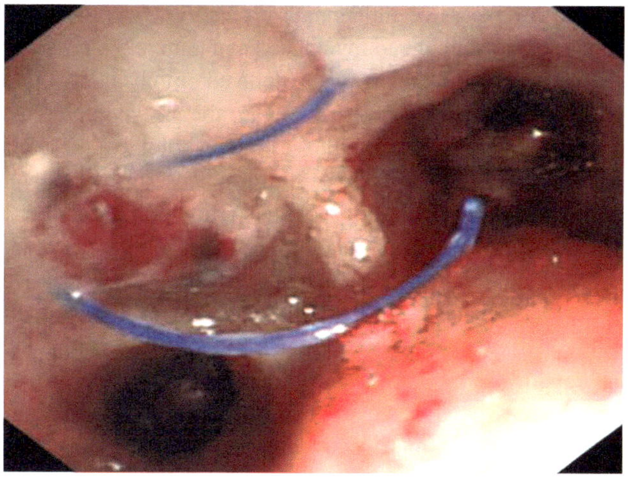

**Fig. 13.1** Case of long-term sinus failure. At the 12 cm insertion of the endoscope into the sinus, two unabsorbed "absorbable" sutures and three sinus bifurcations are seen

This requires us to innovate, improve traditional methods, and absorb interdisciplinary techniques to improve the level of wound healing.

### 13.2.4 Improve the Traditional Diagnostic System with New Ideas

The research on wound repair mechanism has accumulated in China for more than 20 years. Taking the diabetes mellitus refractory wounds as an example, the theory of diabetic skin microenvironment pollution is proposed, which is different from the traditional pathophysiological mechanism. The theory holds that: diabetes mellitus and refractory wounds are based on the metabolic disorder of diabetes mellitus, a pathological evolution mediated by subsequent events of metabolic abnormalities. The microenvironmental change caused by the increase of glucose content in skin tissue caused by diabetic metabolic disorder and local accumulation of glycosylation end products, namely "cutaneous environmental disorders," is one of the initiating factors leading to the difficulty of curing diabetic wounds. "Cutaneous environmental disorders" causes a series of recessive damage characterized by histological and cellular functional changes in non-invasive diabetic skin, and continues to affect all aspects of wound healing after trauma, including diabetic skin that has undergone histological and cellular functional changes before it is externally injured, known as "recessive damage" of diabetic skin. In addition, growth factors and their receptors are glycosylated, progressive tissue damage caused by excessive inflammatory reactions, vascular dysfunction, and damage to myelinated and unmyelinated nerve fibers, which ultimately leads to delayed or unhealed wound healing. Based on this, we can regard the vasculopathy and neuropathy of diabetes mellitus as the pathological outcome after the local accumulation of high glucose and glycosylation end products, and it is not the starting point of diabetic wounds. The local accumulation of high glucose and glycosylation end products is another upstream event of "recessive damage" of diabetic skin. It is concluded that the pathological type of diabetic wounds, in addition to vasculopathy and neuropathy, should also be included in the pathological criteria of "recessive damage" of the skin. This inference is to be established after a multicenter large sample clinical trial.

## 13.3 Establish a New Medical Treatment Mode for Wound Treatment

The treatment of wound disease has the characteristics of "small ward and big outpatient," that is, a considerable number of patients only need to change the medicine in the outpatient service and only need hospitalization when deep treatment or surgery is needed. In the current situation where there are not many wound repair specialists, it is difficult to meet the needs of patients living in different regions. The most suitable dressing change for wound patients should be at their doorstep, at the community health service center. To this end, with the support of various levels of government in Shanghai, Shanghai Ninth People's Hospital and the National Primary Medical Demonstration Unit in Shanghai, the Zhoujiaqiao Community Health Service Center in Changning District, Shanghai have established a two-way linkage mechanism between wound repair specialists and community health care, namely wound patients in the region only need to change medicines in the outpatient clinic of the community health service center. Only when deep treatment or surgery is needed, they are referred to the wound repair specialist of Shanghai Ninth People's Hospital. When the condition is stable after surgery, the patient is transferred back to the community health center for hospitalization or home treatment. The integration of this single disease vertical medical resource has made it easier for patients to seek medical treatment and reduced the medical burden. The state's investment in primary health care has been utilized, enriching the connotation of community medical care and the management index of the third-level and first-class general hospital where the wound repair specialty is located has been guaranteed, and the average length of stay in the wound repair specialist was 14 days, with the drug accounting for only 14%. But there is an urgent problem behind this gorgeous surface, that is, the general practitioners of primary care usually lack experience in wound treatment and need training and improvement. The wound restoration specialist has sent experts to meet regularly every week, but we are acutely aware that this is only a stopgap measure, because there are 232 community health service centers in Shanghai, and the limited number of wound repair specialists is obviously unable to cope with such a huge community demand. The birth of 4G communication technology brought us a solution. With the support of the Shanghai Economic and Information Technology Commission and China Mobile, the connection between the wound repair division and the community health service center was established with the high-definition video system based on 4G technology. The system enables specialists to clearly see the wounds of patients visiting a community health center through high-definition video and can direct the general practitioner to deal with the wound directly through dialogue. The system not only solves the distress of specialists running around hospitals and community health centers, but also reproducibly establishes a two-way linkage mechanism between other community health centers and specialist hospitals. At The First China-EU Wound Restoration Conference held in Shanghai in April 2011, the system was unanimously recognized by experts from various countries as a "top class" technology and an innovative wound repair medical treatment model. Government departments, medical authorities, and wound repair experts agree that this 4G HD video-based wound repair specialist integrates with the single-species vertical medical resources of community medical care to solve the problem of medical treatment for patients with chronic wounds, and meets the requirements of medical reform, has a good demonstration effect.

## 13.4 Challenge the History of Patients with "Rotten Foot Disease" Treatment

### 13.4.1 The Background

In Jinhua, Lishui, and Quzhou, Zhejiang Province, there are a number of patients with suspected biological-warfare-related foot ulcer during World War II. The number of patients is as many as hundreds. The patients' wound ulceration has not been cured for decades. Because of the inability to find direct clinical evidence related to the bacteriological warfare in the case, we refer to these patients as historically leftover patients.

In response to the call of the famous social activist Wang Xuan for the diagnosis and treatment of patients with biological-warfare-related foot ulcers, in September 2014, led by Academician of Chinese Academy of Engineering, Professor Xiaobing Fu, Professor Lu Shuliang from Ruijin Hospital, Shanghai Jiao Tong University School of Medicine, in association with the Surgeons Branch of Chinese Medical

Doctor Association and Shanghai Wound Healing Research Center and Chinese Wound Management Association, and all related experts across the country, formed a volunteer medical team to jointly carry out treatment for these patients.

### 13.4.2 Patient Characteristics

These patients have the following characteristics:

A. The patient's wound disease has been plagued for decades, many treatments have failed to heal and lose confidence in treatment.
B. Patients have limited economic conditions and are unable to bear the cost of treatment.
C. The patients are all elderly patients (70–90 years old), with varying degrees of senile diseases, and the risk of treatment is high.
D. A considerable number of patients are less likely to be cured by conventional dressing treatment, but relying on modern technology can be cured by reasonable surgical treatment.

### 13.4.3 The Treatment Plan

In response to the above situation, the medical team has carefully discussed the following:

A. Treatment Plans

Three patients were admitted to the Shanghai Traditional Chinese Medicine-Integrated Hospital with no charge. The Shanghai Ninth People's Hospital, Shanghai Jiao Tong University School of Medicine received nine patients free of charge through the Wang Zhenguo Traumatic Medicine Foundation.

The purpose of the first phase of the plan is to lay the foundation for further and more extensive treatment. At the same time, it can prove that these patients can be cured under the current medical conditions in our country using existing medical technology, thereby enhancing patients' confidence in healing the wounds. Another challenge we face is how to benefit from a limited charitable donation. This requires us to explore a safe, economical, and effective treatment.

Clinically, the fibrillar connective tissue of these patients are thick and dense, and some even have obvious calcified tissues (Fig. 13.2), which must be removed to form a wound bed with adequate blood supply, otherwise the skin grafts will not survive; elderly patients have thin skin. If the donor area is not handled properly, it is easy to form a new wound. Based on decades of experience in burn surgery, the medical team chose the scalp as the donor area. As a result, a treatment plan for these patients has been formed. By thoroughly removing the fibrillar connective tissue combined with VSD for 5–7 days, the patient's autologous scalp skin had been obtained and small size skin grafts had been used to cover the wound. It had been proved that the treatment plan's safe and effective, and all patients were cured by one skin grafting procedure. The average treatment cost for wounds was less than 20,000 yuan ($3000); it also proved that the application of TCM and medicine to cure such long-term difficult-to-heal wounds has considerable advantages.

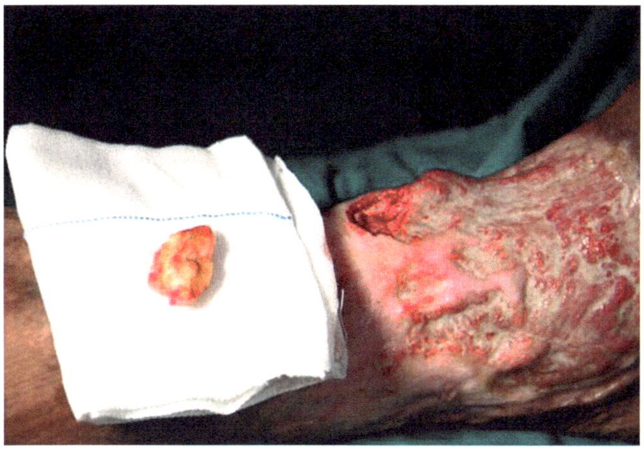

**Fig. 13.2** The thick, dense fibrous tissue of the wound surface and the removed calcified tissue

Ten out of twelve patients who received free treatment in Shanghai were cured and discharged, with one patient who requested to be discharged early due to family reasons and one patient with skin diseases who did not fall into the group.

B. The Second Phase of the Plan

Two surgical residents from Ruijin Hospital were sent to patients' local hospitals to assist local doctors. The newly developed intelligent glass was used as a communication tool to provide real-time consultation from Shanghai's senior experts as needed during operation.

The purpose of the second phase of the plan was to explore the possibility of entry-level doctors to carry out treatment plans correctly with remote help from senior experts over the internet.

After 2 months of operation, the results showed that patients can be treated according to the medical plans by the local doctors with the help of remote experts. During this period, there were a total of nearly 300 wound dressing changes, and four operations were performed on two patients, and patients were recovered and discharged.

C. The Third Phase of the Plan

Based on the successful work done during phase two, coordinated by Professor Han Chunmao, Vice Chairman of the Trauma Surgeons Branch of the Chinese Medical

Doctor Association, a two-way intelligent remote visualization system between The Second Affiliated Hospital of Zhejiang University and The First People's Hospital of Wucheng District of Jinhua City had been established in 2014. There were nine fully recovered patients who were operated by Qiu Xuguang, Director of Jinhua Hospital, through the system.

Through the implementation of the three-stage plan, we concluded that a considerable part of the patients with biological-warfare-related foot or leg ulcers can be cured; relying on high-speed visual technology, under the guidance of remote experts, doctors from primary hospitals are fully capable to carry out complex wound treatments.

At present, the Tencent Foundation and the Wang Zhengguo Trauma Medicine Foundation are collaborating to collect donations for the victims with biological--warfare-related foot or leg ulcers. The Trauma Surgeons Branch of the Chinese Medical Doctor Association is also working together with Shanghai Wound Healing Research Center to support the action and to promote the "two-way linkage model" so that more chronic wound patients can be effectively treated [9].

In summary, the wound healing specialty is an emerging discipline that has emerged due to changes in the spectrum of diseases. It involves the crossover of multiple disciplines. Many diagnoses and treatment technologies and methods need to be further improved, and there is a lot of room for innovation. Therefore, in the face of the wound repair departments that have been established today, we must emphasize: We should pay attention to the connotation construction of the wound healing specialty.

## 13.5 Construction of Wound Centers in China

The history of wound healing is also the history of surgery. From the prehistoric period, humans had already started treating wounds. Promoted by the development of human civilization, wound treatment is divided into three stages: original wound treatment, experience wound treatment, and scientific wound treatment. With the continuous advancement of the industrial revolution, scientific wound treatment has become the mainstay of wound healing. Various new technologies derived from the combination of practice and theory is continuously used for wound healing. At the same time, wound centers as the "carriers" of wound treatment developed. In modern society, with the changings of lifestyle and the aging problem, the disease spectrum changed. Chronic disease proportion increases significantly, consequently chronic wounds, which are complicated and difficult to treat, increase fast. Previous wound centers can't meet the needs of patients anymore, they need to be updated and improved, a new model of wound center was born, here let's call it modern wound center. At the end of twentieth century, many developed countries began to establish the modern wound centers, which always maintained a multidisciplinary cooperation group, and the centers grew fast. In China, modern wound centers began in the early twenty-first century and also developed rapidly. Due to different national conditions, the development of wound centers in China have their own characteristics.

### 13.5.1 The Predecessor of Wound Center in China

The predecessor of the wound center in China derived from the dressing rooms of large hospitals, some affiliated with outpatient departments or nursing departments, some belong to different clinical departments, such as burns, general surgery, and plastic surgery. In the 1950s, the population of burn patients grew rapidly because of the extensive steel-making, which made the burn departments expanded around China. Most of these burn department had separate dressing rooms which were the prototype of most wound centers in China [10].

The characteristic of the early dressing rooms was simple, simple diseases, simple conditions, simple staffs, and simple treatments as follows.

A. Single Disease

Patients needing dressing at that time were mainly acute wounds. Only a few chronic wound patients, mainly venous ulcers. It is worth mentioning that there were more intracutaneous foreign bodies injury cases at that time, because many jobs required manpower.

B. Poor Conditions, Less Equipment and Dressing

Early patients' wounds were simple, and simple treatment was enough. Otherwise because of relatively few patients the hospital paid less attentions. Therefore, the conditions of the early dressing rooms were poor. Except for some basic equipment, such as dressing trays, tweezers, scissors, there was no other equipment.

There were also very few materials only gauze, Vaseline gauze and bandages. At that time, the management of antibiotics was not strict. External application of intravenous drugs, such as gentamicin, clindamycin, and chloramphenicol, was common.

C. Simple Staff Structure and Professional Skills

In general, there were two to four nurses arranged in the dressing room. Although these nurses usually contacted with dressing changing, but they did not have formal training and knew few theory knowledge of wound. They were just arranged in the dressing room, started to work, taught by the nurse in the dressing room hand by hand. There was no doctor in the dressing room. If the patients needed doctors, they had to go to different departments.

D. Burning Department Dressing Room Was Relatively Complicated

Early in China, because of few car accidents and low proportion of chronic diseases, wounds were always simple except for burns. Dressing change was relatively complicated. That was one reason why a large ratio of wound centers in China was attached to the burn department.

### 13.5.2 The Development of Wound Centers in China

The rapid development of China's economy began in the 1980s. Meanwhile, chronic diseases became a major health problem. Consequently, chronic wounds patients increased. Farsighted experts in China begun to write relevant medical treatment norms and recommendations to promote the development of related medical treatment. Guiding Opinions on Chronic Wound Diagnosis and Treatment 2, which was started by Academician Xiaobing Fu, was the first guiding literature for chronic wound treatment in China [11]. At the same time, with the efforts of relevant experts such as Academician Xiaobing Fu, Professor Lu Shuliang and Professor Han Chunmao, the wound centers in China started a new development.

#### 13.5.2.1 The Start of the Wound Centers in China

As in other countries and regions, changes in disease spectrum and increased patients were the root causes of wound centers' construction. But the start of wound centers in China had its own characteristics. Its main feature is that they belonged to the different departments. The department that started the establishment of modern wound centers in China was the burn department. That was related to historical development as we talked. In the 1950s, the burn department developed rapidly. However, with the development of science and technology, large-scale burns were rapidly reduced. For living, burn surgeons began to look for new outlet with their rich experience in wound treatment. At the same time, general surgeons couldn't cope with the increase in chronic wounds anymore, they begun to seek help from burn surgeons. As a result, the burn department began to intervene in the treatment of various wounds rather than burns.

As mentioned above, some prospective burns departments, after analyzing the situation of foreign wound center, started to establish independent and standard wound center according to the domestic situation. They pioneered the treatment of wounds and developed into a leader in this field in China. Among them, the wound center of the second affiliated hospital of Zhejiang University Medicine College, which was established in 2004, was the first wound center led by surgeons.

In addition, some of wound centers in China were affiliated with other departments, such as endocrinology. They mainly treated diabetic foot ulcers. Diabetic foot center of Chinese People's Liberation Army 306th hospital was the most famous one. This center even equipped with its own surgeon and independent operation room. Of course, some of wound centers in China were also wound care centers affiliated with nurse department. They started earlier and developed well. Especially after the first nursing staff wound treatment school in Guangzhou, the level of wound care in China entered a new stage.

In 2015, a survey of wound centers in China was conducted which was organized by Academician Xiaobing Fu. The survey showed that most of the wound centers were derived from burns and outpatients departments [12] (Fig. 13.3).

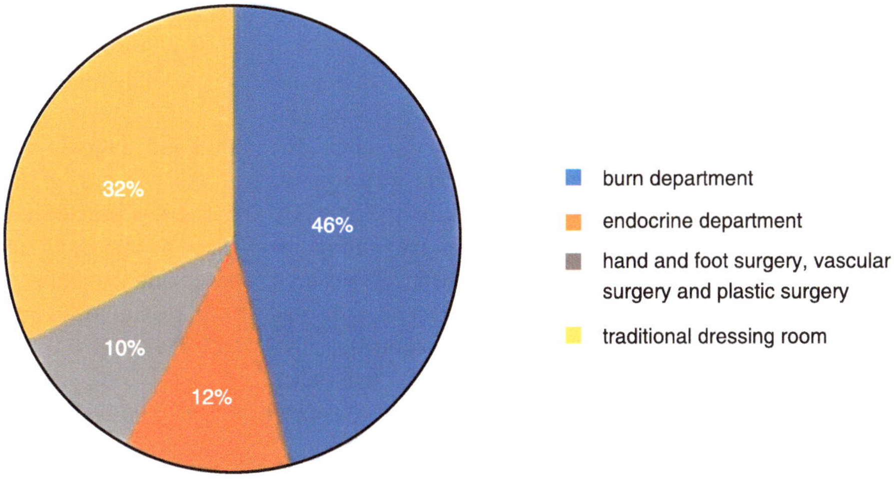


**Fig. 13.3** Predecessor of wound center and wound care center in China

#### 13.5.2.2 Development of Wound Centers in China

From the beginning of the twenty-first century, in response to the needs of social development, the wound center began to develop. Many experts have done a lot to promote its development, and their efforts have also attracted more attention from medical staff and institutions to wound centers. In the early days, the main members of the Organizational Rehabilitation Professional Committee (Group) of several Chinese Medical Association Trauma Branches, such as Xiaobing Fu, began to discuss the possibility of establishing a comprehensive wound center in China. In 2005, they proposed to build a standardized and exemplary wound center. In 2009, Academician Xiaobing Fu published an article entitled "The Construction of Wound center Is Imperative" in Chinese Journal of Burns. The article states that wound treatment is not only the basis of all trauma treatment, but also the key to prevent late complications and promotion early recovery of trauma patients, and a wound center with a certain scale and characteristics, is to promote the development of new technologies for wound healing and to benefit the trauma patients. Further calls for the establishment of a national wound center through the establishment of a demonstration wound center.

At the same time, the rapid increase of various acute and chronic wounds, especially chronic wound patients and the extremely lack of related medical resources, has formed a sharp contradiction. More and more problems caused by this contradiction have begun to become the burden of hospitals. Chronic diseases and aging of the population are two important reasons for the increase of chronic ulcers. The latest epidemiological survey shows that the incidence of chronic wounds in hospitalized patients in China is significantly increased, among which diabetic wounds, chronic wounds after trauma, and pressure ulcers are the top three chronic wounds. The contradiction between the medical needs brought about by wound diseases and the lack of medical resources in China has become increasingly prominent, as shown in the following aspects:

A. Most hospitals, including large-scale comprehensive hospitals, have few specialized departments for wound treatment. Wound patients often cannot find suitable clinics, and the difficulty of treating patients with wounds became a real problem.
B. Patients often had various basic diseases and need multidisciplinary comprehensive treatment, which also caused wound patients need to transfer in different departments, but couldn't get a more systematic and comprehensive treatment. In addition, patients with wounds often have inconvenient movements, which bring many inconveniences to patients, and even lead to unsatisfactory emotions.
C. The diagnosis and treatment of wound treatment lacked new knowledge and new technology, and a standardized diagnosis and treatment path to guide doctors to treat, which also led to the uneven effect of the current wound diagnosis and treatment.

   Wound treatment professionals are extremely scarce. At first, they were just doctors from different departments not professional. It is worth mentioning that in recent years, under the impetus of Academician Xiaobing Fu, Professor Lu Shuliang, Professor Han Chunmao, Professor Xu Zhangrong, Professor Xie Ting and other experts, the training courses for various wound treatment doctors started in China. At the same time, a wound healing association established in China to further standardize and normalize related wound medical training. In addition, some of the nursing staff trained in the wound treatment and enterostomal therapist training courses of the nursing staff in China gradually played a great role in transforming them into wound specialist nurses.
D. In some places, patients with chronic wounds couldn't get the treatment" in the outpatient clinic but could only be admitted to the hospital. These patients have long hospital stays and high medical resources, which have brought considerable influence to the management indicators of various hospitals. In fact, the treatment of wound disease has the characteristics of "small ward and large outpatient service," that is, except for some patients who need hospitalization for surgery, a considerable number of patients only need to spend time in outpatient consultation and dressing change. This feature leads to the need for our patients to have larger outpatient clinics to meet their medical treatment. The above contradictions have attracted more attention, which has become a driving force for the construction of wound centers in China.

In the 5 years from 2006 to 2010, nearly 20 hospitals established wound centers. As expected, these wound centers taken a good lead and demonstration role in China which became temples. With the establishment of the demonstration center, wound centers developed rapidly, grown by more than 10 per year [13] (Fig. 13.4).

#### 13.5.2.3 Mode of Wound Center in China

Wound centers in China have their own characteristics because of the different characteristics of each region, each hospital, and each subordinate department. However, they have some common characteristics and models in terms of their overall structure, management and norms, details as follows.

A. Doctors Were the Center

   More and more people have realized that wound treatment is not a simple dressing, and the knowledge struc-

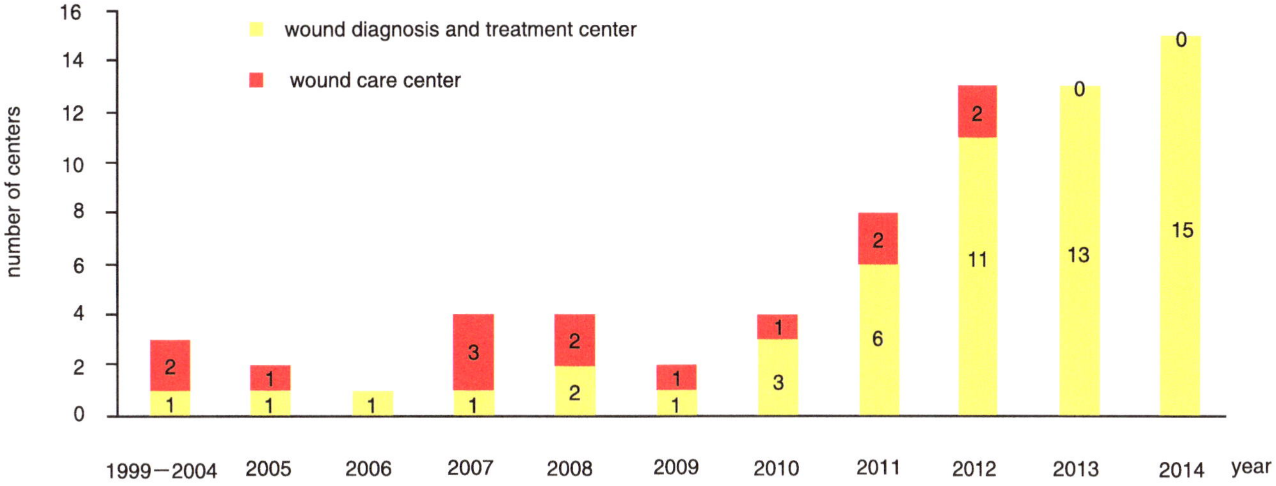


**Fig. 13.4** Established time map of wound center and wound care center in China

ture of the caregiver can no longer afford all the wound treatment. The wound centers established by academic leaders in various regions and hospitals have begun to be doctor-centered. These doctors not only have a passion for wound treatment, but also have various knowledge structures related to wound healing. In addition, they have taken the initiative to absorb the experience of foreign developed countries, take their essence, draw on their successful cases, and then establish standardized treatments for various wound centers according to their own characteristics. This kind of impetus is undoubtedly huge.

B. Multidisciplinary Cooperation, Diagnosis, and Treatment Norms

The exemplary wound centers all attach importance to multidisciplinary cooperation. For example, in the diagnosis and treatment of diabetic foot, many wound centers have established a multidisciplinary cooperation framework, focusing on the specialists of the wound center, at the same time, doctors from endocrinology, orthopedics, vascular surgery, radiology, cardiology, nutrition are involved in the and other departments intervene in the systematic diagnosis and treatment of patients through consultations and other methods. At the same time, various medical treatment norms have also received attention from everyone. For example, the Wound Diagnosis and Treatment Center of the Second Affiliated Hospital of Zhejiang University School of Medicine has established a variety of outpatient diagnosis and treatment paths for chronic wounds, and its diabetes foot clinic diagnosis and treatment path has been promoted by the whole hospital.

C. Active Use of New Technologies, New Methods, New Materials

Although there are few medical insurances for new dressings or equipment related to wound healing in China, the application of various new dressings by various wound centers has been welcomed by more and more patients. We can find a variety of advanced dressings in most wound centers, such as hydrocolloids, hydrogels, foam dressings, alginate dressings, silver ion dressings, and more. In addition, the application of various new technologies is also in full swing. For example, vacuum sealing drainage technology, China has more than ten domestically produced closed vacuum sealing drainage materials.

D. A Demonstration in a Region

Although the establishment of a wound center is growing rapidly, there is currently a wound center that can be used as a model in a region. This demonstration center will often be the core of various wound healing institutions in the region. The hospitals in this demonstration center are often large comprehensive hospitals in the area, so the equipment is relatively new and comprehensive. The general demonstration sites have equipment for ankle-brachial index, vascular Doppler, and vibration threshold inspection. There are even equipped with transcutaneous oxygen partial pressure tester, plantar pressure tester, laser Doppler, ultrasonic debridement instrument, and red light therapy instrument and so on. These demonstration sites have also begun to become training bases for wound healing personnel in the region and are beginning to play an increasingly important role.

#### 13.5.2.4 Wound Training Programs, Meetings and Organizations

A. Wound Diagnosis and Treatment Training Program

In 2010, the World Diabetes Foundation (WDF) and the Chinese Medical Association Trauma Branch Tissue Rehabilitation Professional Committee (group) jointly launched a diabetes foot and related chronic wound education program for doctors and nurses in China. The project officially launched the Chinese wound treatment training, trained thousands of medical staff, and established dozens of training bases. In addition, the training of diabetic foot is relatively early. The training of diabetes foot initiated by Professor Xu Zhangrong was started in 2005. These projects led to more comprehensive training programs. In addition, in 2014, Academician Fu Xiaobing, Professor Han Chunmao and Lu Shuliang organized an expert group to write the wound guidelines base on Chinese literature. After 1 year the first Chinese wound treatment guideline completed.

B. Related Meetings

There are a lot of relevant domestic conferences. At present, there are several conferences with influential scales.

(a) The meeting of the Tissue Restoration Group of the Chinese Medical Association Trauma Branch: The group has held several related meetings, which have received the attention of relevant experts and played the leading role in wound healing.
(b) Relevant meeting of the Association of Trauma Surgeons of the Chinese Medical Association: the association has a number of groups, including the Wound Treatment Therapy Branch, and the annual meeting brings together the nation's wound treatment experts. The first director of the club is Professor Lu Shuliang.
(c) International Diabetes Foot Forum: the conference was initiated by Professor Xu Zhangrong. It started in 2005 and held every year. The forum invites famous domestic and foreign experts from different fields such as diabetes, endocrine, vascular surgery, diabetic foot disease, orthopedics and burns, conduct academic reports and exchange of clinical experience around diabetic foot and related diseases.
(d) Sino-Europe Wound Repair Conference Wound Repair: co-organized by the Tissue Restoration Committee (Group) of Chinese Medical Association Trauma Branch, and the European Wound Technology Society, every 4 years, the first session was held in 2011 by Shanghai Ninth People's Hospital, Shanghai Jiao Tong University School of Medicine, hosted the theme of "Transformation Practice of Wound Repair."
(e) National Burns Annual Meeting and National Burn Treatment Symposium: Since most of the doctors in wound treatment come from the burn department, there are a large number of reports on wound treatment every year at burn-related meetings, and the relevant committees will also discuss issues of wound treatment.

C. Related Organizations

As the development of wound, more and more organizations founded. The earliest and most famous national organization is "Chinese Wound Management Association." On December 26, 2011, the Chinese Medical Association Trauma Brach held a special meeting in Shanghai. The chairman of the committee, Xiaobing Fu, announced the establishment of the "Chinese Wound Management Association." This Association also connected with other countries and areas' wound associations represented as Chinese wound doctors.

#### 13.5.2.5 Limitations of the Construction of Wound Centers in China

Of course, the construction of wound centers in China also has many limitations, involving systems, concepts, subject codes, and charge. The resolution of these problems requires the cooperation of government authorities and hospitals. Mainly as follows:

A. Medical Insurance Limitations

At present, medical insurance in China has not included many relevant examinations and treatments for wound treatment, such as the examination of the sputum index. Various new dressings, new technologies such as negative pressure drainage technology, stem cell therapy, etc. are often not covered by medical insurance. However, it is encouraging that medical insurance institutions have begun to pay attention to wound diagnosis and treatment and have begun to include some wound-related medical treatments and dressings in some areas and some hospitals into the scope of medical insurance. In the near future, most of the wound treatment can be included in the scope of medical insurance.

B. Concept

Although people's living standards have improved greatly, many concepts have not changed. For example, patients' perceptions, many patients are afraid to let others see their own broken skin, so there is no medical treatment! For example, doctors, many doctors often like to engage in "classic" professions, have no concept of wound healing. In addition, the concept of managers needs to be changed. At present, some hospital administrators have certain concepts about wound treatment. Compared with patient satisfaction, the relevant economic benefits are relatively low, which often affects their support for the construction of the center. The department's managers are still paying little attention to wound centers.

C. Subject Code

There is still no special discipline code for wound treatment in China, which means that many wound treatments can't be done alone, which brings us great difficulties.

D. Charge

Wound treatment is becoming more and more complicated, but the current fee system still stays for decades or even decades, which is undoubtedly counterproductive for the construction of a discipline.

E. Others

In addition, many disciplines in China are not as perfect as those in other countries. For example, there are no podiatrists and orthotists in China. The relevant decompression insoles, shoes or brace are not equipped with professional personnel.

In short, the construction of wound centers still has many limitations, which require us to pay more attention and care, and need our efforts to change and improve.

### 13.5.3 The Prospect of the Construction of Wound Center in China

The wound center in China has developed rapidly, which is closely related to the development of social economic science and technology, and has also played a role in the experience of other countries. Under the promotion and efforts of relevant experts such as Xiaobing Fu, the development of wound centers in China is gratifying. At the same time, the team of wound treatment experts in China has also begun to attract attention in the international arena. The Chinese Wound Management Association, led by Xiao Xiaobing, introduced wound diagnosis and treatment discipline in China to the world when applying for the 2020 World Union of Wound Healing Societies (WUWHS). Although it was unsuccessful, the Chinese wound diagnosis and treatment discipline began to shine on the international stage. In March 2018, at the first Asian Wound Treatment Annual Conference, Professor Lu Shuliang took over the banner of the conference from the organizers of the conference and announced that the second Asian Wound Treatment Conference will be held in Shanghai in May 2019. Looking ahead, our prospects are limitless. In order to strengthen development, we need to work harder. First, we must arm ourselves with new theories and new technologies. In the information age, we should adopt more advanced electronic processing models to better evaluate wounds, record data, and facilitate more effective, large-scale clinical research and promote the development of disciplines; second, we need to be guided by innovative ideas to promote the development of disciplines; finally, the construction of the wound center needs the support and attention of all parties. I believe that the government departments will give greater support in the near future, and medical insurance can also be included more projects. We will also serve our patients better! Wound healing: let the mind fly! [14]

## References


1. Fu X, Sheng Z, Cherry GW, et al. Epidemiological study of chronic dermal ulcers in China. Wound Repair Regen. 2010;6(1):21–7.
2. Jiang Y, Huang S, Fu X, et al. Epidemiology of chronic cutaneous wounds in China. Wound Repair Regen. 2015;19(2):181–8.
3. Fu X. Establishment of a wound care discipline system in China: the review of the construction of wound care center with Chinese characteristics in 20 years and prospect. Chin J Burns. 2018;34(12):859–63.
4. Broughton G, Janis JE, Attinger CE. The basic science of wound healing. Plast Reconstr Surg. 2006;117(Suppl):12S.
5. Lu SL, Xie T, Niu YW. A potential mechanism for impaired wound healing—cutaneous environmental disorders in diabetes mellitus. Chin J Burns. 2008;24(1):3–5.
6. Leibovich SJ, Ross R. The role of the macrophage in wound repair: a study with hydrocortisone and antimacrophage serum. Am J Pathol. 1975;78(1):71–100.
7. Liu YK, Wang XQ, Wei J, et al. Effect of tension on collagen arrangement. Chin J Burns. 2009;25(9):779–82.
8. Jiang YZ, Ding GF, Lu SL. Exploratory study on the micro-remodeling of dermal tissue. Chin J Burns. 2009;5:343–51.
9. Xie T, Ge M, Lu SL. Exploration on the linkage mechanism between wound healing department and community health system. Chin J Burns. 2011;1:43–4.
10. Shen Y, Han C, Chen G. Discussion on the model of wound center construction. Chin J Burns. 2011;27:4.
11. Han C, Sun H, Fu X. Guidance on the diakgnosis and treatment of chronic wounds. Chin J Burns. 2010;25:13.
12. Jiang Y, Huang S, Fu X, et al. Epidemiology of chronic cutaneous wounds in China. Wound Repair Regen. 2011;19:181–8.
13. Jiang Y, Xia L, Jia L, Fu X, et al. Survey of wound-healing centers and wound care units in China. Int J Low Extrem Wounds. 2016;15:274–9.
14. Han C. Facing wound healing: letting thought fly! Chin J Burns. 2012;28:2.

# 14 Problems and Prospects in Regenerative Medicine

Biao Cheng and Xiaobing Fu

## 14.1 General Description

There are still many diseases or injuries in human diseases that have not found a good way to cure or repair them. Therefore, people are looking forward to a breakthrough in the development of a new round of medical technology. Regenerative medicine based on stem cell-based repair and regeneration ability is expected to become the third disease or injury treatment method after drug therapy and surgery. Regenerative medicine mainly studies the tissues and organs that have been damaged or seriously damaged by the human body and adopts medical strategies of repairing, replacing, or reconstructing to treat diseases that cannot be cured by traditional medical means, such as trauma, cardiovascular disease, diabetes mellitus, Alzheimer's disease, and aging. On the one hand, China is the most populous country in the world, with a large number of patients. On the other hand, China's rapid economic development and modernization have caused various injuries and accidents to occur. It is estimated that about 100 million people need to be treated with rehabilitation and regeneration every year, making China the most urgent country in need of treatment. However, at present, the repair of tissues and organs of both the surface and the internal organs still remains at the level of alternative repair of scar healing, which is far from the desired "regeneration of a complete damaged organ." In short, current medical technologies and methods are difficult to meet the needs of clinical treatment.

Since the 1990s, with the rapid development of basic disciplines such as cell biology, molecular biology, immunology, and genetics, and the emergence of stem cells and tissue engineering techniques, modern regenerative medicine has adopted activity factors, gene therapy, and stem cell transplantation, tissue engineering, and cell reprogramming to support the body's ability to repair itself. It shows a good prospect in replacing or regenerating cells, tissues, or organs, and helping to complete the function of damaged organs caused by any cause (including congenital defects, diseases, trauma and aging, etc.) and going beyond traditional transplantation and replacement therapies. The role of stem cells in regenerative medicine is particularly prominent. With the deep understanding of the internal working mechanism of stem cells, stem cells and derived therapeutic cells prepared by stem cell engineering technology have been continuously found; stem cell medical technology is highly expected.

In the past 20 years, the field of regenerative medicine has maintained a growing momentum. The United States, Japan, Singapore, and European countries have invested more than hundreds of billions of dollars in research. In April 2013, researchers at the University of California, San Francisco, published an article on the prospects for cell therapy in the "Perspective" section of the *Sci Transl Med* magazine. It is believed that future cell therapy will become the "third pillar of medicine" and will be used to treat patients as well as drugs made with engineered proteins, antibodies, or smaller chemicals. Regenerative medicine research is becoming one of the most promising directions in international life science research in the twenty-first century.

## 14.2 Important Progress in the Field of Regenerative Medicine in China

Chinese scientists have achieved amazing results in pluripotent stem cells, tissue engineering, gene therapy, and active molecules. They quickly push potential treatment technologies from the laboratory to the clinic and treat difficult diseases, greatly improving the health and quality of life of patients. A number of regenerative medicine monographs have been published in the fields of tissue repair and regenerative medicine. The *Chinese Discipline Development Strategy Reproductive Medicine* published in March 2015 is

B. Cheng
General Hospital of Southern Theater Command of Chinese People's Liberation Army, Guangzhou, China

X. Fu (✉)
The Chinese People's Liberation Army General Hospital, Beijing, China



X. Fu (ed.), *Regenerative Medicine in China*, https://doi.org/10.1007/978-981-16-1182-7_14

a series of achievements jointly researched by hundreds of academicians of the Chinese Academy of Sciences. The development situation and needs of regenerative medicine were analyzed in detail, and the development proposals were put forward according to the existing layout and foundation of regenerative medicine in China.

Due to China's outstanding achievements in regenerative medicine, foreign scholars, as well as important academic journals and media, began to pay attention to the development of regenerative medicine in China in the twenty-first century. In 2002, *Nature* published a report on Chinese regenerative medicine, especially stem cell research, and introduced the medical doctor Li Lingsong from Peking University Health Science Center, Lu Guangxiu from Xiangya Hospital and Professor Sheng Huizhen from Shanghai Jiao Tong University School of Medicine, mainly the acquisition of stem cells and the establishment of therapeutic cloned embryo extraction stem cell research results. In 2002, some famous foreign media gradually paid attention to Chinese regenerative medicine. The *Wall Street Journal* of the United States and *New Scientist* and *The Times* of the United Kingdom reported on China's achievements in human cloning research. In 2009, *Nature* and its journal *Nature Reviews Molecular Cell Biology* published articles on Chinese regenerative medicine-related policies. *Cell* main publication *Cell Stem Cell*, *N Engl J Med* and regenerative medicine magazine *Regen Med*, both introduced the important progress made in the field of regenerative medicine and stem cell research in China from different perspectives, or explained the policies related to stem cells in China. The overall impression is that the Chinese government has invested a large amount of research funds in the field of regenerative medicine, making China a great advance in regenerative medicine (including stem cells, tissue engineering and clinical research). In the twenty-first century, the Chinese government has increased its investment in the field of regenerative medicine research and actively recruits high-level scientists trained overseas to seek to achieve its ambition to become a world leader in this field. In November 2012, "China's Push in Tissue Engineering" published by *Science* introduced the development of China in the field of tissue engineering in recent years, including the Chinese government strong support for the subject area, and introduced the outstanding contributions made by Gu Xiaosong from Nantong University and Cao Yilin from Shanghai Jiao Tong University in tissue engineering of Chinese regenerative medicine. In 2012, Science introduced the development of Chinese regenerative medicine in the form of a supplement, especially some progress in trauma, tissue regenerative medicine, and the foundation of embryonic development in China.

The main issue of Science also gave positive comments. According to the ISI Web of Science database, the number of published articles on global regenerative medicine continued to grow from 2000 to 2015, and China has surpassed the UK to rank second.

The research level of stem cells and regenerative medicine is an important indicator to measure the development level of life science and medicine in a country. Most developed countries in the world have listed this field research as a major national science and technology development direction. The strategic pilot science and technology project implemented by the Chinese Academy of Sciences is divided into two categories: "forward-looking strategic science and technology" and "basic and cross-cutting frontier layout." Stem cell and regenerative medicine research belong to the former. It is mainly studied in four aspects: establishment and developmental regulation of cell lineage, key technologies of functional cell acquisition, artificial tissue organ construction, and stem cell application strategy. In 2015, the Ministry of Science and Technology established "Stem Cell Research and Transformation Research" as the pilot project for the first batch of key research and development programs after the scientific and technological reform, and plans to continue to strengthen investment and layout in stem cell foundation and transformation during the "13th Five-Year Plan" period (2015–2020), so as to enhance the core competitiveness of China in the field of stem cells and their transformation applications, and accelerate the application of scientific research results as a new economic growth point in China in the twenty-first century. In 2017, the Ministry of Science and Technology of the People's Republic of China, the Ministry of Education of the People's Republic of China, the Chinese Academy of Sciences, and the National Natural Science Foundation of China jointly issued the *13th Five-Year National Basic Research Program* to clarify that stem cell and transformation research in China will be a core competitiveness project, with multiple major diseases in China as the demand for traction direction.

### 14.2.1 Stem Cells

#### 14.2.1.1 Overview

In 1956, Thomas made the world's first bone marrow transplant for a leukemia patient. In the 1960s, the medical community further expanded the cases of bone marrow transplantation, using radiation therapy and chemotherapy to overcome the allograft rejection after transplantation, and improved the therapeutic effect of leukemia. In the 1970s, bone marrow transplantation became an important clinical technology for the treatment of blood diseases including leukemia, aplastic anemia, and radiation disease worldwide. In 1990, Thomas won the Nobel Prize in Physiology or Medicine. Hematopoietic stem cell transplantation is the earliest and most mature stem cell treatment technology. At present, at least dozens of diseases can be treated with hematopoietic stem cell transplantation technology. In the late 1990s, Nature published a report on the use of adult animal cell nuclear cloning of sheep "Dolly" and cloned mice, which revolutionized the theory of developmental biology. In particular, in November 1998, Thomson and Shamblott of the United States published articles on *Science* and *Proc Natl Acad Sci USA,* respectively, successfully establishing human embryonic stem cell lines and allowing human embryonic stem cells to grow and proliferate in vitro. This development has led scientists to see the stem cell bioengineering dawn of tissue cells required to grow in vitro to replace damaged tissue in patients, which has led to a worldwide wave of stem cell research. With the emergence of new achievements in the field of basic research on stem cells in the world, even in some areas, major breakthroughs have been made, attracting attention from the scientific, industrial, and government agencies, and becoming a hot spot for research, development, and industrialization. However, due to factors such as the concept, the cultural environment and moral values of countries such as the United States and Europe oppose and hinder embryonic stem cell research. China prohibits reproductive cloning, the use of human embryos fertilized for more than 14 days, the fusion of humans with non-human gametes (cells that bind during fertilization), or the implantation of research embryos into human or animal uterus. However, in many respects, it is different from Europe and the United States. At the end of the twentieth century and the beginning of the twenty-first century, a group of Chinese scientists returned to China, and Chinese stem cell research gradually showed prosperity. The Chinese government has invested heavily in stem cell research and is concentrated in several major laboratories such as Beijing and Shanghai. Therefore, China is synchronizing with the world in the field of embryonic stem cells and certain stem cell research.

#### 14.2.1.2 Construction and Development of Stem Cell Research System in China

After the 1980s, Chinese scholars began to pay attention to the field of stem cells. At present, Chinese scholars have published more than 20 monographs in the field of stem cells in China.

In 2001, the Chinese Academy of Sciences established the Key Laboratory of Stem Cell Biology. Then gradually build a network of Chinese stem cell research, including the Shanghai Institutes for Biological Science, Chinese Academy of Sciences; the Guangzhou Institutes of Biomedicine and Health, and so on. It integrates core research strengths including 17 research institutes such as life sciences, materials, chemistry, and biomechanics, and hopes to make breakthroughs in stem cell self-renewal and directed differentiation, stem cell immune regulation and cancer stem cells, and stem cell clinical application.

(a) Key Laboratory of Stem Cell Biology, Shanghai Institutes for Biological Sciences, and so on, to establish biomedical transformation research base. Development in the field of embryonic stem cell self-renewal and directed differentiation. The human embryonic stem cell line was established and trophoblast- free culture was realized to achieve the induced differentiation of human embryonic stem cells into neural cells. The modification of important transcription factors of embryonic stem cells was found. The new mechanism of neural stem cells maintenance in early embryonic development was found.
(b) South China Institute for Stem Cell Biology and Regenerative Medicine, the Guangzhou Institutes of Biomedicine and Health, and so on, achievements have been made in stem cell pluripotency maintenance, differentiation mechanism, neural stem cell research, stem cells chemical biology, stem cell research technology platform, somatic cell reprogramming research and utilization, animal cloning technology and transgenic technology have been combined to develop and cultivate cell and tissue, organ and animal products related to stem cell therapy.
(c) Institute of Biophysics, Chinese Academy of Sciences: study on myocardial infarction of human embryonic stem cell differentiation, and study of human pluripotent stem cells and neural stem cells.
(d) Center for Stem Cell and Regenerative Medicine, Institute of Zoology, Chinese Academy of Sciences: in collaboration with Institut Nationale de la Recherche Agronomigue, it is mainly developed in the field of stem cell medicinal application and transformation, focusing on the differentiation mechanism of pluripotent stem cells into various cell lines of the nervous system, the uniqueness of human stem cell biology, and the systematic evaluation of stem cell medicinal applications.
(e) Institute of Genetics and Developmental Biology, Chinese Academy of Sciences: established "Nanjing Stem Cell and Biomaterials Research Center" in cooperation with the Affiliated Hospital of Nanjing University Medical School, focusing on the research of stem cell three-dimensional culture and self-renewal regulation network, as well as the research of stem cells and biomedical materials, tissue regeneration and wound repair products development and transformation.
(f) Kunming Institute of Zoology, Chinese Academy of Sciences: established a Key Laboratory of Animal Reproductive Biology in cooperation with Yunnan Province, established a primate stem cell (primate-based) resource bank, and used primate animal models to conduct stem cell basic research, pharmacological pharmacodynamics and preclinical safety evaluation,

promote the implementation of stem cell pilots and clinical stem cell therapy in China.

Major domestic universities and research institutes have also established or collaborated with foreign countries to establish stem cell research institutes/centers.

#### 14.2.1.3 Establishment of Chinese Stem Cell Bank

The establishment of modern stem cell banks is critical for basic research and clinical transformation of stem cells. In 2007, the Ministry of Science and Technology of the People's Republic of China took the lead in setting up and establishing four stem cell resource banks. Relying on the complementary stem cell resource bank, we have established a platform for 3–4 key stem cell technologies. On December 25, 2002, the network system of Chinese hematopoietic stem cell donor database was officially established.

#### 14.2.1.4 Basic Research on Stem Cell Research in China

Prior to 2007, the research basis of stem cells in China was mainly focused on bone marrow and embryonic stem cells. In 2009, the *Oxford Journals' Science and Public Policy* pointed out that China is a new entrant to the bioeconomy and is gradually leading the world in stem cell basic science research. As predicted, in December 2008, Professor Deng Hongkui's laboratory at Peking University reported on the *Cell Stem Cell* that the rhesus iPSC system was first established. In April 2009, Professor Wu Ji of Shanghai Jiao Tong University and others first isolated germline stem cells in the world and cultured germline stem cell lines that could be self-renewing for a long time. In July, *Nature* published on its website: Chinese scientists used iPSC to breed mice for the first time in the world and for the first time in the world proved the versatility of iPSC. This achievement was selected by *The Times* "2009 Global Top Ten Biomedical Progress" and considered the study "marking an important advance in stem cell research." *Nature* reported that Chinese scientists "opened a new path for cloning adult mammals" and pointed out that "this method is more efficient and safer than traditional cloning methods and will cause interest in therapeutic cloning." At the beginning of 2010, the research team led by Pei Duanqing from Guangzhou Institutes of Biomedicine and Health, Chinese Academy of Sciences, increased the iPSC induction efficiency by ten times by adding vitamin C. In February 2012, *Proc Natl Acad Sci USA* published the latest research results of several collaborations, including the Institute of Zoology, Chinese Academy of Sciences, and so on, People's Liberation Army: the new function of the stem cell factor receptor c-Kit and its application in translational medicine. In September of the same year, researchers from the Institute of Zoology, Chinese Academy of Sciences and Northeast Agricultural University, published an article on *Nature*, successfully established a haploid embryonic cell line from the orphan male blastula, and obtained breakthrough results in embryonic stem cell research. In July 2013, the research team led by Professor Deng Hongkui and Dr. Zhao Yang re-issued in *Science*, using small molecule compounds to induce somatic cell reprogramming into pluripotent stem cells, which brings the possibility of the application of regenerative medicine in the treatment of major diseases in the future. In 2013, *Cell* launched a "Spotlight on China," which focused on the rapid development of immunology research in China in recent years, especially the evaluation of immunological research results in stem cell use in clinical treatment.

The basic research of stem cell in China is consistent with the mainstream of iPS and embryonic stem cells, cancer stem cells and stem cell differentiation potential. However, in the study of adult stem cells such as neural stem cells and hematopoietic stem cells, the basic research work is not comprehensive enough. There are still quite a lot of basic works to do in areas such as stem cell regulatory networks, stem cell self- renewal and differentiation mechanisms.

#### 14.2.1.5 Clinical Application of Stem Cells in China

The clinical application of stem cells is the key to the desire of countries to convert basic medicines as quickly as possible. Chinese stem cell therapy practices can be traced back to the bone marrow transplant in the 1960s, which is the transplantation of bone marrow stem cells. In March 2009, China announced the third legalization of stem cell treatment as a third-class medical technology after the United Kingdom and the United States.

At present, stem cell technology applications are still mainly hematopoietic stem cells, mainly for the treatment of acute heart failure, liver failure, and lower limb ischemia. However, studies have begun on the clinical application of other stem cells. The exploratory work done included: in 2006, Zhu Jianhong and his research team at Fudan University published a paper on *N Engl J Med*, recording Huashan Hospital Affiliated to Fudan University, Shanghai to help a woman who was inserted into the brain by chopsticks. The woman's prefrontal cortex was damaged because chopsticks were inserted into the brain from the eye. After taking out the chopsticks, Zhu Jianhong decided to cultivate the brain tissue attached to the chopsticks in order to find stem cells that repair the loss of the living body. Zhu Jianhong's team decided to continue the experiment, extracting the intermediate stem cells, repairing the damaged tissue, and avoiding the attack from the patient's immune system because the cells are from the patient itself. This research on the ability to utilize and mobilize self-healing is the focus of stem cell field. In 2009, Xiaobing's Fu team used autologous bone marrow mesenchymal stem cells to regenerate skin sweat glands [1]. More than 30 cases have been completed so far, followed up for more than 4 years, and have been praised as "milestone research" by international peers. In 2013, doctors from the Third Medical Center of Chinese People's Liberation Army General Hospital transplanted umbilical cord mesenchymal stem cells to treat patients with posttraumatic brain syndrome. Forty cases of posttraumatic brain syndrome were randomly assigned to the stem cell treatment group or the control group. Patients in the stem cell treatment group underwent stem cell transplantation. Six months later, the evaluation group performed fugl-meyer assessments (FMA) and functional independence measures (FIM) tests on all patients who used stem cell transplants and those who did not receive any treatment. The FMA and FIM scores (upper limb and lower limb movement) in stem cell transplantation group were better than the control group ($P < 0.05$). It was confirmed that umbilical cord mesenchymal stem cell transplantation can improve the neurological function of patients with posttraumatic brain syndrome. However, this result requires a multicenter large sample prospective randomized clinical trial. In many areas of clinical concern, such as heart disease, it also depends on further in--depth and standardization. According to the website of the State Food and Drug Administration (search date: 2013-08--01), the stem cell related products currently approved for clinical research are as follows.

#### 14.2.1.6 Comparison with Foreign Stem Cell Research

In the field of stem cell research, the United States maintains an absolute leading position. Stem cell research has been in the United States for more than 30 years since the initial bone marrow transplant. There are also significant gaps between China and the United States in stem cell research related policies (Fig. 14.1). The United States started early on stem cell research policy and has implemented strict management since 1998. China started late in this area. The Ministry of Science and Technology of the People's Republic of China and National Health Commission of the People's Republic of China began to formulate regulations and policies related to stem cells in December 2003. But so far, China is still constantly improving various policies and hopes to have practical execution. Stem cell research management regulations vary widely among European countries. Although the European Union (EU) announced in 2007 that it will continue to fund research on human embryonic stem cells, the introduction of regulations prohibiting the cloning of humans and the destruction of human embryos is important for the development of regenerative medicine in the EU and globally. In particular, the ethical questioning of research on stem cells, including human embryonic stem cell lines.

In terms of establishing a stem cell bank, the United States started early in this field, far exceeding China. In 1993, researchers at the New York Blood Center established the first federally funded modern cord blood hematopoietic stem cell bank. In 2004, the US government plans to establish an embryonic stem cells bank. In 2006, the first baby dental bank was established. In 2008, the US National Stem Cell Bank was established.

According to statistics, there were more than 100 important stem cell centers in the world in 2009, and 50 advanced centers in the United States and Canada. In 2004, Harvard University invested millions of dollars in a stem cell research center, the most important stem cell research base in the United States. In 2008, Stanford University School of Medicine planned to establish the largest stem cell research center in the United States.

In addition to formulating relevant policies to pave the way for the development of the stem cell industry, many governments and research institutions have invested heavily or supported the stem cell industry through policy orientation. From the perspective of government and private investment, in April 2002, the National Institutes of Health decided to allocate \$3.5 million to fund four institutions for human embryonic stem cell research. This is the first large sum of money the US government has invested in this field since President Bush announced his limited support for human embryonic stem cell research. In October 2005, the US Food and Drug Administration (FDA) also approved the transplantation of neural stem cells into the human brain.

In 2009, for the first time, French scientists succeeded in using human stem cells to create a complete epidermis. In October 2010, the UK's first stem cell human trial was approved. In May 2012, Health Canada approved the sale of Osiris's (Prochymal) stem cell drugs. This is a breakthrough in the field of stem cell drugs worldwide and has an extraordinary social significance and immeasurable economic benefits for the development of the clinical stem cell therapy industry. In addition, the Australian Therapeutic Goods Administration (TGA) has approved Mesoblast's production and supply of autologous mesenchymal precursor cell (MPC) products for sale in Australia. In 2013, the Japanese Ministry of Health, Labor, and Welfare's review committee approved clinical studies using iPSCs for retinal regeneration.

The United States has not only banned embryonic stem cells in basic research. In 2009, the US Food and Drug Administration (FDA) approved a California biotechnology company to conduct the world's first clinical trial based on human embryonic stem cells, which is a milestone in medical history. Subsequently, the FDA approved another company (Advanced Cell Technology) to conduct clinical trials of human embryonic stem cells. In the coming years, there will be more clinical trials based on human embryonic stem cells worldwide.

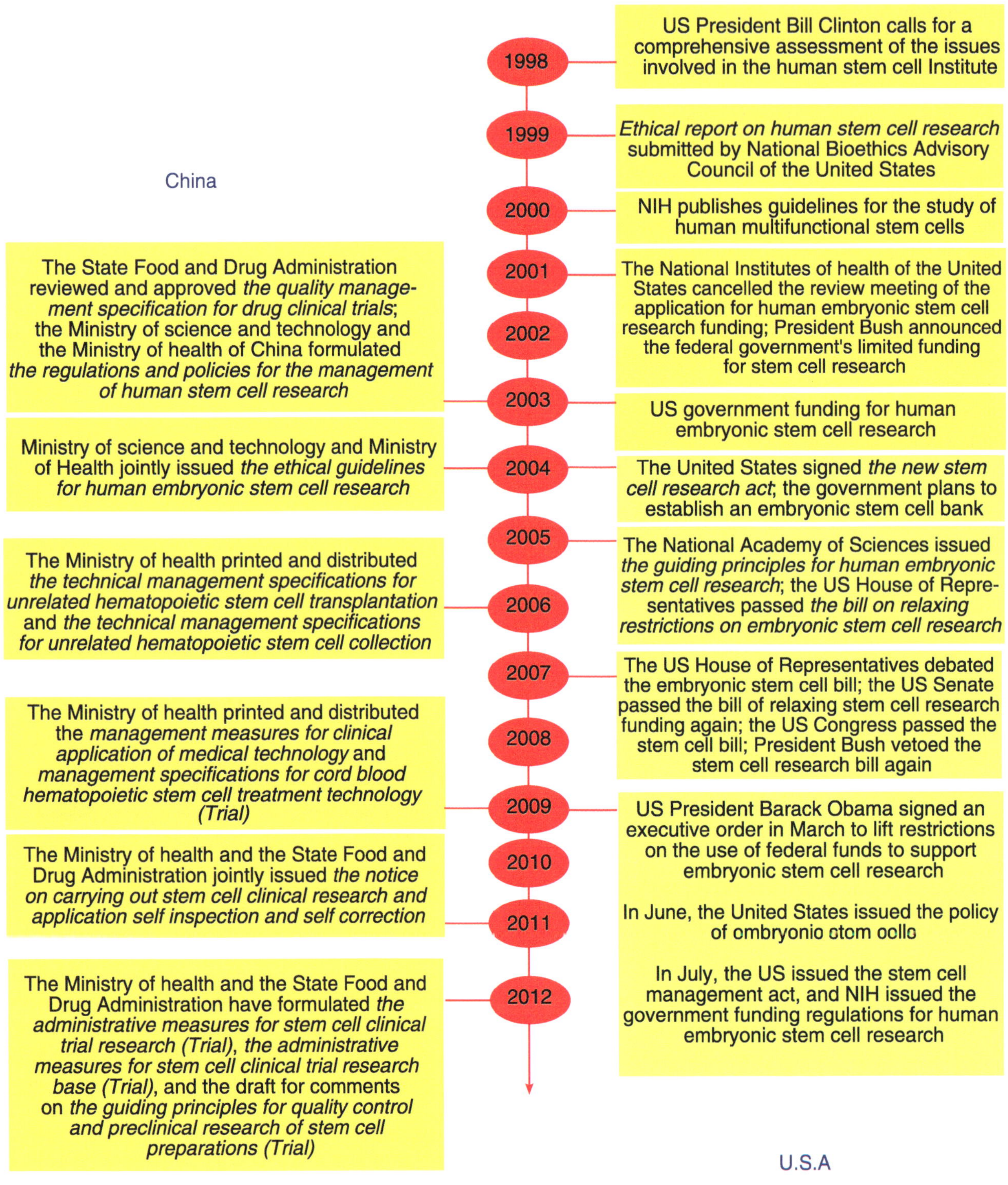


**Fig. 14.1** Comparison of stem cell research policies between Chinese and US government agencies

From the perspective of patents, the first patent application for stem cells appeared in 1980. From 1993 to 2000, the number of patent applications increased slowly, and it showed a rapid growth trend after 2000. Organizations that apply for more stem cell-related patents include the University of California, Massachusetts General Hospital, and the Japan Science and Technology Agency. Of the top ten organizations, there are eight US agencies and two Japanese institutions, and research institutes account for 50%. From the perspective of countries, the main countries/

regions/organizations that accept patent applications related to stem cells are World Intellectual Property Organization, the United States, the European Patent Office, Japan, Australia, China, etc.; the countries that have applied for more patents as patent priority countries include the United States, Japan, China, etc. The policy bias of stem cells in various countries/regions can be divided into research models that firmly ban embryonic stem cells, strictly restrict stem cell research, and actively develop relevant regulations and ethical guidelines to promote stem cell research. In 2007, the United States Patent and Trademark Office rejected the basic patent for human embryonic stem cells. In 2008, the European Patent Office (EPO) rejected a technology-related patent developed by James Thomson, a researcher at the University of Wisconsin, to culture primate embryonic stem cells from preimplantation embryos. In September 2011, the UK drug regulatory authority approved a biotechnology company to conduct human embryonic stem cell trials, and Europe first approved human embryonic stem cell clinical trials. However, in 2011, the European Court of Justice announced that it still prohibited stem cell research from entering the patent application process. The number of patent applications related to stem cell technology in China has also increased significantly, and the proportion of patent applications has increased from 14.35% in 2011 to 26.12% in 2015.

Chinese stem cell therapy practices can be traced back to the bone marrow transplant in the 1960s. In March 2009, China became the third country to declare stem cell treatment as the legalization of three types of medical technology after the United Kingdom and the United States. In the United States, after the FDA approved clinical trials of embryonic stem cells, the Chinese SFDA will gradually open the limits of clinical trials using human embryonic stem cells. Stem cell clinical research has also entered a period of vigorous development. Due to the lack of rules in the corresponding regulations, the stem cell market is chaotic driven by profits. From 2009 to 2010, *N Engl J Med* and *Nature* both reported the chaotic phenomenon of stem cell therapy in China. They expressed concern about the safety of stem cell therapy in China and hoped that there would be stronger enforcement measures to protect patients. If these immature and unsafe methods of stem cell treatment are rampant, it will not only bring health concerns, but also make the public misunderstand stem cell therapy. On December 16, 2011, National Health Commission of the People's Republic of China issued the *Notice on Conducting Stem Cell Clinical Research and Applying Self-examination and Self-correction Work*. The notice clearly stipulates that "the clinical research and application activities of stem cells that have not been approved by National Health Commission of the People's Republic of China and the National Medical Products Administration will be stopped. No report will be accepted until July 1, 2012." Since this notification is a one-size-fits-all measure, stem cell clinical research has also been affected by stem cell treatment disorder, and the current state of freezing has not been lifted. However, this rule seems to have little effect, and some agencies have turned a blind eye to the regulations. In June 2012, the Institute of Medical Information of the Chinese Academy of Medical Sciences presided over the *Stem Cell Technology and Industry Development Report*, which was respectively management, science and industry articles, mainly tracking and analyzing the research and development strategies of the international stem cell field, and in-depth introduction to the research progress of stem cell technology. Looking forward to the development direction of the global stem cell industry. On this basis, the paper puts forward suggestions for stem cell research in China and provides reference and information support for policy formulation and stem cell research direction and industrial development in stem cell field in China. The National Stem Cell Clinical Research Leading Group is working on a new set of stem cell management systems, and stem cell clinical application research will be managed in comparison to a new class of drugs in developed countries. On March 30, 2015, the National Health Commission of the People's Republic of China and the National Medical Products Administration jointly organized the *Stem Cell Clinical Research Management Measures (Trial)*, *Stem Cell Preparation Quality Control and Preclinical Research Guidelines (Trial)*, and other documents. Published on the official website of the Science and Technology Education Department of the National Health Commission of the People's Republic of China. This *Management Measures*, which is a milestone in the history of the development of stem cell industry in China, has attracted strong attention from hospitals and industry companies. On May 30, 2016, the official website of the National Health Commission of the People's Republic of China issued an announcement to publicize the first batch of stem cell clinical research institutions that have been filed. The first batch of hospitals that have passed the record are 30, including six hospitals in Beijing, four hospitals in Shanghai, three hospitals in Guangdong, three hospitals in Tianjin, two hospitals in Jiangsu, and two hospitals in Guizhou. There are one hospitals in Guizhou, Hebei, Liaoning, Jilin, Jiangxi, Zhejiang, Hubei, Hunan, Sichuan, Shandong, and Henan.

In accordance with the requirements of the *Stem Cell Clinical Research Management Measures (Trial)*, the National Stem Cell Clinical Research Expert Committee reviewed the filing materials of the stem cell clinical research institutions submitted by the local authorities. According to the opinions of the expert committee, a list of recommendations for the first batch of stem cell clinical research institutions has been formed.

From the research stage of clinical trials in the field of stem cells, most of the clinical trials are concentrated in the clinical stage I and phase II, that is, to study the metabolic characteristics of the stem cell-related drugs in the human body and the efficacy of the drugs and to evaluate the safety of drugs at the same time. From the countries (regions) where clinical research is conducted, the United States and Europe are countries and regions with more stem cell-related clinical trials, and there are more clinical studies in Canada and Australia, while clinical studies in Asia are relatively rare.

With the rapid development of stem cell and regenerative medicine industry, its industrialization and marketization have also advanced by leaps and bounds. At present, dozens of stem cell research and development (or) sales companies of different scales have been formed nationwide, engaged in stem cell product development and establishment of stem cell bank, cell storage (mainly cord blood hematopoietic stem cells and adult stem cells of different tissue origin) and sales of related accessories. In addition to establishing stem cell banks in Beijing, Shanghai, and Guangzhou, important stem cell resources for basic research and clinical transformation are reserved. In Shenzhen, China has established the first national gene bank to effectively protect, develop, and utilize precious genetic resources in China, improve the level of life science research in China, promote the development of bioindustry in China, and safeguard national bioinformation security. This is the first national-level gene bank in China, which will break the monopoly of foreign strategic resources, and has important strategic significance.

The gap between China and the United States and Europe in the field of stem cell therapy is mainly reflected in the fact that a unified quality inspection standard and quality inspection acceptance unit have not been established and cannot be used on a large scale; the approval procedures and regulatory requirements for stem cell clinical research and application have not been formed, and the long-term mechanism needs to be improved. In short, in the fiercely competitive frontiers of stem cell research, the Chinese government is working hard to improve various rules and regulations, and Chinese scientists are making unremitting efforts to shorten the gap with the United States and Japan. Whether it is basic research or clinical application of stem cells, the achievements China has made are obvious to all.

### 14.2.2 Tissue Engineering

#### 14.2.2.1 Overview

Since the concept of tissue engineering was proposed in the 1980s, many achievements have been made in basic research and clinical applications, and the construction of physical organs has been carried out from the construction of structural organization.

#### 14.2.2.2 The Construction and Development Process of Organizational Engineering Research System in China

Tissue engineering research in China started a little later. In 1994, the Science and Technology Commission of Shanghai Municipality regards the tissue engineering research as a key funding direction. The establishment of this major research project marked the official start of tissue engineering research in China. In 1997, the tissue engineering project was officially established in the National Natural Science Foundation of China. In the same year, Shanghai established first tissue engineering laboratory in China, the Shanghai Key Laboratory of Tissue Engineering Research. In 1998, the National "973" Key Basic Research Program formally established the research project "Basic Scientific Issues in Tissue Engineering," Shanghai Jiao Tong University School of Medicine; West China Hospital, Sichuan University; Tianjin University; Institute of Mechanics, Chinese Academy of Sciences and Institute of Chemical, Chinese Academy of Sciences are co-sponsors of the project, which indicates that the country has listed the research of organizational engineering as a key development project in the high-tech field. In 1999, the first national conference on tissue engineering in China was held in Shanghai. In 2001, Shanghai Tissue Engineering Research and Development Center and National "863" Program Biological Field Tissue Engineering Research and Development Base were established in Shanghai Caohejing Hi-Tech Park. This is the first and currently the only national-level tissue engineering research and development base in China. In 2001 and 2002, the National "863" High-tech Research and Development Plan continued to provide funding for the application research and product development of tissue engineering, marking that the country has officially adopted tissue engineering as the national industrial development direction in the biological field. At present, tissue engineering research has been carried out in different degrees in colleges and universities, research institutes and research institutes affiliated to the Chinese Academy of Sciences. A number of unique tissue engineering laboratories have been established, covering research in clinical medicine and cell biology, molecular biology, polymer biomaterials and related fields, and is gradually shortening the gap with foreign countries. In some projects, research has reached or exceeded the world's advanced level, forming a high-level professional tissue engineering research team. On March 26, 2013, the Secretariat of the Subcommittee of Tissue Engineering Medical Device Products of China received the notice from the International Organization for Standardization (ISO), China has completed its registration as an active member (P member) of the International Organization for Standardization/Technical Committee for Standardization of Surgical Implants and Orthopedic Devices/Tissue

Engineering Medical Products Sub-Technical Committee (ISO/TC150/SC7), and have obtained international voting rights for ISO/TC150/SC7 standardization activities. Academician Xiaobing Fu is the chairman of the committee of China. The International Tissue Engineering Medical Products Subcommittee was established in 2007 with 12 member states, China is the 13th and the first member of the Asian developing countries. This indicates that the standardization work in the field of tissue engineering in China will officially go to the international arena and participate in the standardization activities in relevant international fields. China is no longer just an unconditional executor of international standards in this field, but a member of the rules-making. From tissue engineering to regenerative medicine, the logo is a merger of the Tissue Engineering and Regenerative Medicine International Society to form a unified academic organization. Since 2002, Chinese regenerative medicine scholars have published a total of eight monographs on tissue engineering.

In 1997, after the Shanghai Ninth People's Hospital, Shanghai Jiao Tong University School of Medicine first established the Shanghai Key Laboratory of Tissue Engineering Research, a large number of institutions in China established a tissue engineering research center, such as the Stem Cell and Tissue Engineering Research Center of Sun Yat-sen University (2003.01), Tissue Engineering Center of China Academy of Medical Sciences (2003.12), Tissue Engineering Center of the Fourth Military Medical University (2003.12), Biomedical Materials and Tissue Engineering Research Center of Peking University (2007.03), Zhejiang University established Zhejiang Provincial Key Laboratory of Tissue Engineering and Regenerative Medicine (2011). In addition, the Institute of Chemistry, the Chinese Academy of Sciences; the Institute of Basic Medical, Academy of Military Medical Sciences; the Institute of Polymer Science, Tianjin University; West China Center of Medical Sciences, Sichuan University, and Tsinghua University have also established key laboratories for tissue engineering research. In June 2012, 39 universities, research institutes, and industrial enterprises in the field of domestic tissue engineering and regenerative medicine, jointly organized the "organization of tissue engineering and regenerative medicine. Innovation Center."

The National Medical Products Administration issued the *Notice on Issuing the Relevant Requirements for the Research and Declaration of Tissue Engineering Medical Products* (National Food and Drug Administration [2007] No. 762). National Health Commission of the People's Republic of China issued the *Technical management specification for tissue engineered tissue transplantation therapy (Trial)*, in November 2009, which puts forward requirements for the tissue engineering technology production environment. In November 2009, National Health Commission of the People's Republic of China issued the *Management Specifications for Three New Medical Technologies for Cell Transplantation and Tissue Engineering Organizational Transplantation*.

#### 14.2.2.3 Research on Tissue Engineering in China

In 2007, former State Food and Drug Administration (SFDA) approved ActivSkin, the first tissue engineering product in China. This makes China the second country in the world to hold artificial skin technology after the United States. And continue to develop acellular dermis tissue engineering (recombinant human acellular dermal matrix), tissue engineered skin products: fat-containing tissue engineered skin, pigmented tissue engineered skin, microvascular tissue engineered skin, hair follicle tissue engineered skin and tissue engineered leather. In 2010, Cui Fuzhai, a tissue engineering expert at Tsinghua University, also developed a bone repair stent that was also approved by the former SFDA. This material is currently used on 30,000 patients and is being rolled out to other parts of the world. The Third Military Medical University used compound chitosan and animal-derived materials (heterogeneous acellular dermal scaffolds, gene transfected pigskin, and pig embryonic skin precursor tissues) to construct tissue engineered skin. The world's first bioengineered corneal "Ai Xin Tong" clinical trial, independently developed in China, was successful in April 2015, with a total effective rate of 94.44%, and obtained the medical device registration certificate issued by the former State Food and Drug Administration. This means that China has become the first and only country in the world to complete high-tech bioengineered corneal products for clinical trials. The National Engineering Research Center of Tissue Engineering (Shanghai) has initially established an epidermal cell bank and a skin fibroblast cell bank to solve the problem of seed cell source of the product. The seed cell and chitosan-gelatin film material are being used to construct tissue engineered skin containing sweat glands in vitro. There are also tissue engineered tendon, tissue engineered (soft) bone, tissue engineered neural tube, and other products (Table 14.1). For more than 10 years, China has achieved a series of landmark achievements represented by the industrialization of tissue engineering "artificial skin" and the clinical application of individualized tissue engineered cartilage in the field of tissue engineering and regenerative medicine research. A number of high-tech enterprises engaged in tissue engineering and regenerative medicine have emerged, initially formed a situation of joint innovation of production, education, and research.

**Table 14.1** Main domestic tissue engineering production enterprises and products

| Company | Time | Product name | Constitute | Application situation | Progress |
|---|---|---|---|---|---|
| Beijing jieyalaifu Biotechnology Co., Ltd | 2006 | J-1 acellular allogenic dermis | After special physical and chemical treatment, the allogeneic skin can remove all the cells that cause host immune rejection and preserve the same extracellular matrix as the original tissue | Extraction wound filling, plastic and filling, repair of various kinds of hernia | GSYJX (Z) Zi 2000 No. 346027 and 2006 No. 3460430 |
| Beijing Qingyuan Weiye biological tissue engineering technology Co., Ltd | 2007 | Acellular allogenic dermal matrix for medical tissue patch | Extracellular matrix formed by acellular treatment of allogeneic skin tissue | Repair of oral mucosa and soft tissue defects caused by various reasons; wound closure during dental implantation; hernia repair; urethra repair | GSYJX (Z) Zi 2007 No. 3461290 |
| Chongqing Zongshen Junhui Biotechnology Co., Ltd | 2007 | Artificial skin gene transfer pigskin | Human CTLA4Ig gene was introduced into the skin of Bama miniature pig by gene transfer technology | Therapeutic coverage of burn and other wounds to promote wound healing and prevent microbial infection | GSYJX (Z) Zi 2007 No. 3461287 |
| Qidong Oriental Medical Research Institute Co., Ltd | 2010 | Dongci dermal matrix | Pig skin is the extracellular matrix of pig dermis | The treatment of superficial second degree burn (scald) wound, donor area wound, deep burn cut scab wound and granulation wound | GSYJX (Z) Zi 2010 No. 3641111 |
| Shaanxi Erfu Tissue Engineering Co., Ltd | 2007 | Tissue engineering skin | Double layer artificial skin substitute: the epidermis is composed of human epidermal cells, and the dermis is composed of human fibroblasts and bovine collagen | Deep second degree burn wound; third degree burn wound not more than 20 $cm^2$ | GSYJX (Z) Zi 2007 No. 3461110 (changed) |
| Yantai Zhenghai Biotechnology Co., Ltd | 2007 | Haiao oral repair film | Bovine acellular cell | Removal of oral soft tissue defect and tumor | GSYJX (Z) Zi 2007 No. 3630062 |
| | 2009 | Skin repair membrane | A series of different acellular dermal matrix was prepared from bovine skin tissue after a series of treatment, the main component of which was collagen | Wound repair of dermis defect caused by various reasons | GSYJX (Z) Zi 2009 No. 3460425 |
| | 2009 | Artificial dural patch | Collagen is the main component of acellular dermal matrix | Repair of dura mater caused by trauma, tumor and vascular disease | GSYJX (Z) Zi 2009 No. 3460602 |
| Guangdong Guanhao Biotechnology Co., Ltd | 2009 | Sterile biological wound protection membrane | The visceral membrane of pig is made by a series of biochemical treatment such as antigen removal and virus inactivation. The basic component is collagen in the form of membrane, which can keep the basic structure of biological membrane, and has flexibility and permeability | Treatment of deep and shallow wounds caused by skin burn, scald, trauma and skin defect | GSYJX (Z) Zi 2009 No. 3640426 |
| | 2011 | Type B dural patch product | The membrane tissue of pig was made by cross-linking treatment with epoxy chemical reagent and biochemical modification | The repair of tension defects of part of dura (spinal cord) or dura (spinal cord) plays the role of repair, fixation, tension reduction and isolation | GSYJX (Z) Zi 2011 No. 3461355 |
| Beijing Daqing Biotechnology Co., Ltd | 2011 | Allogeneic bone repair material | Healthy human bone tissue selection, low temperature storage, thawing, processing and molding, crystal soaking, cell removal, freeze-drying, vacuum packaging, irradiation, sterilization packaging | Filling, fusion, repair, reinforcement and reconstruction of non-load bearing bone for spinal injury, degenerative disease and other clinical needs | GSYJX (Z) Zi 2011 No. 3460627 (changed) |

#### 14.2.2.4 Comparison of Chinese Tissue Engineering Research with Foreign Countries

The concept of organizational engineering was formally proposed by the National Science Foundation in 1987. As early as 1988, the United States funded a series of research projects in tissue engineering in the form of funds. Therefore, the United States is also in an absolute world leading position in the field of tissue engineering. In 1995, the Tissue Engineering Society was established. In 2001, the Tissue Engineering Society was formally established and a global academic organization was gradually formed. The United States has a large number of research institutions (including NASA, DOE, NIH), universities (including MIT, HMS, GIT, UCSD, etc.), companies (such as Sandoz, Organogenesis, AdvancedTissue, etc.). According to statistics, from 1995 to 2002, the United States invested a total of 4.5 billion US dollars in the field of tissue engineering, and the annual comprehensive expansion rate of the industry is 11%. A $6 billion tissue engineering industry has been formed and is growing at a rate of 25% per year.

The US FDA has approved the listing of nearly ten products including tissue engineered skin and cartilage. China has also approved the listing of tissue engineered skin, and the industry of tissue engineering products has begun to take shape. An aseptic polymeric carrier wound covering produced by a cell tissue engineering company in Jiangsu has also been used for clinical treatment of burns. However, there are standard lag problems in the field of tissue engineering medical product technology, which limits the clinical application and industrialization of such products. The technical level in the field of tissue engineering in China has basically been in line with international standards, and it is at the international advanced level in the technical field of cartilage regeneration. Being a member of ISO/TC150/SC7 not only enables our country to win the right to speak in the international standardization activities in this field and the opportunity to participate in the revision of international standards but also to promote the development of tissue engineering medical device industry in China. The public will soon use high-tech tissue engineering medical device products. Tissue engineered bone has entered clinical trials in the United States, Germany, Italy, and China; tissue engineered cartilage has entered clinical trials or trials in the United States, Singapore, Australia, and Germany; tissue engineered tendons have been reported in clinical applications in China. In addition, tissue engineered oral mucosa, bladder, artificial liver, artificial kidney, artificial heart valve, myocardial patch, blood vessel, nerve, urethra, testis, thyroid, etc. have basic research or clinical trials, showing tissue engineered implants in an important role in tissue regeneration and repair. The list of tissue engineering products such as skin and bone in the United States is as follows (Table 14.2).

### 14.2.3 Growth Factors

#### 14.2.3.1 Overview

Tissue repair and regeneration under physiological conditions are related to the regeneration of endogenous bioactive factors. Such as angiogenesis is related to VEGF, PDGF, bFGF, etc.; BMP is related to bone regeneration; bFGF, EGF, and others are related to epithelial regeneration; NGF, ciliary neurotrophic factor, and others are related to nerve regeneration. Endogenous growth factors activate or "wake up" tissue/stem cells through specific pathways, acting as tissue regeneration repairs. However, due to the limited amount of endogenous bioactive factors and the influence of in vivo microenvironment, its regeneration and repair function is not perfect. In some cases, it is necessary to supplement the exogenous biological activity factors. Currently, bFGF, NGF, and BMP have been approved for clinical use, showing good clinical results. The problem of exogenous bioactive factors is that there are few types of clinical application, and the dose- effect relationship is obviously affected by individual differences. At the same time, the microenvironmental factors in the body have a great influence on its effect, and the time to maintain activity in vivo and in vitro is short. In vivo action is often multifactor orderly action, but it is still difficult to achieve multifactor order addition. At present, how to regulate biological activity factors to promote tissue regeneration and avoid excessive regeneration has not yet found an effective method, which needs further study.

#### 14.2.3.2 Development Status of Growth Factor Research in China

In 1991, Xiaobing Fu edited and published the first academic monograph on the development of growth factors and wound repair in China (Table 14.3). In 1998, he published a clinical article on growth factor accelerated wound repair at *Lancet*. The team's early main research direction was the effect of a series of active molecules such as growth factors on the repair and regeneration of tissues and organs.

#### 14.2.3.3 Foundation and Clinical Research of Chinese Growth Factors

In the mid-1990s, some scholars reported that some adult tissue stem cells can differentiate into other series of cell types that are not related to development, that is, adult tissue stem cells have "plasticity," "trans-differentiation," or "cross-line differentiation" potential. Around 2002, there was a divergence of understanding of adult stem cells in the inter-

**Table 14.2** Status of tissue engineering products approved by the US FDA for skin and bone

| Company | Time | Product name | Constitute | Application |
|---|---|---|---|---|
| Genzyme Tissue Repair | 1981 | EpicelTM | an artificial epidermis formed by in vitro culture of autogenous cells as a permanent skin substitute | Wounds of moderate and severe burn patients |
| Bertek Pharmaceuticals | 1989 | Biobrane | The outer layer is silicon membrane, and the inner layer is nylon fiber mesh partially embedded in it. The mesh is filled with crosslinked collagen, which is non degradable | Donor and superficial burn wounds |
| LifeCell, Biohorizons | 1996 | Alloderm | The removal of epidermis and cells, leaving the extracellular matrix of dermis and the acellular dermal matrix of intact basement membrane complex | Repair and replace damaged and defective dermis, burn wounds, periodontal and plastic repair |
| LaJolla advanced organization science, Inc.; Smith & nephew, UK | 1997 | TransCyte (Dermagraft-TC) | Polylactic acid was used as scaffold material, in which fibroblasts isolated from neonatal prepuce were cultured to form active artificial dermis | Prevent the water loss of wound and bacteria invasion in the environment for the second and third degree burns |
| Genzyme Surgical Products | 1997 | Carticel | Autogenous cartilage tissue implanted in patients | repair of cartilage defect |
| Organogenesis | 1998 | Apligraf (Graftskin) | Collagen extracted from bovine tendon collagen was used as scaffold material to culture fibroblasts with double-layer structure. And then inoculate keratinocytes to fuse into pieces | Venous ulcer and diabetic ulcer |
| Smith & Nephew, UK; Advanced Tissue Science, USA | 2001 | Dermagraft | Culture of fibroblasts on the net of absorbable PLA fiber | Treatment of diabetic foot ulcer |
| Ortec International Inc | 2001 | OrCel | The double collagen matrix was composed of upper collagen gel and lower cross linked multipore bovine collagen sponge. The keratinocytes and fibroblasts were respectively inoculated into the upper and lower layers of cultured artificial skin | Burn donor site, reduce scar formation and dystrophic epidermolysis bullosa |
| Integra LifeSciences | 2002 | Integra | The lower bovine collagen and aminopolysaccharide porous membrane, the upper silicone rubber membrane, the permanent dermal substitute of different origin | For the treatment of third degree or more burns and burn scars |
| Wright Medical Co. | 2002 | Graftjacket Regenerative Tissue Matrix | Allogeneic source, removing epidermis, preserving basement membrane, preserving elastin, collagen, and polysaccharide skeleton of dermis | Repair skin, Achilles tendon, ligament and periosteum |
| Tulsa Dental Co. | 2006 | PerioDerm | Acellular collagen matrix of human skin | Parotidectomy, reconstruction of lower eyelid, cleft palate repair, vestibuloplasty, mastectomy and repair |
| Obagi | 2000 | Cymetra Hans Biomed | Acellular dermal allografts | Scaffold for regeneration of various tissue cells |
| Davol | 2006 | CollaMend FM Implant | Acellularization of pig epidermis | Soft tissue repair |
| TEI Bioscience | 2002 | TissueMend | Fetal bovine dermal matrix | Repair of various hernias, chest wall, urethra and pelvic floor |
| | 2006 | Durepair Dura Regeneration Matrix | Acellular bovine matrix products | Replacement of automeninges in the repair of dura mater |
| | 2007 | SurgiMend Collagen Matrix | Acellular bovine matrix products | plastic reconstruction, myocutaneous flap repair and hernia repair |
| | 2008 | PriMatrix Dermal Repair Scaffold | Acellular bovine matrix products | Local full-thickness skin defect, diabetic ulcer and second and third-degree burn |
| Tissue Science Laboratories | 2006 | Zimmer Collagen Repair Patch | Acellular porcine dermal matrix | Plastic reconstruction, myocutaneous flap repair and hernia repair |

national academic community. In April 2002, *Nature* and *Science* published a series of questionable articles on the theory of stem cell "plasticity" in adult tissue. Among them, the core question is: Is there really "plasticity" of adult tissue stem cells in nature? Reports on the "plasticity" of stem cells in various adult tissues have appeared frequently in *Nature*, *Science*, and *Cell*, especially around 2000, when the report reached its climax. In the field of tissue repair and regeneration, Professor Xiaobing Fu has published articles in *Lancet* [2] and *J Cell Mol Med* [3] to explain the role of growth factors in tissue testing in the skin repair of epidermal stem cells in vivo. In particular, he found that under living conditions, growth factors have significant dedifferentiation effects on cells. This innovative theory immediately caused controversy among scholars at home and abroad. But this groundbreaking thinking has important implications for the later reprogramming of adult cells into active stem cells using active factors. The growth factor products approved by the National Medical Products Administration are as follows (Table 14.4).

**Table 14.3** Monographs published by Chinese scholars on growth factors

| Time | Monograph | Author | Press |
|---|---|---|---|
| 1991 | *Growth factors and wound healing* | Xiaobing Fu | People's Military Medical Press |
| 1992 | *Peptide growth factor foundation and clinical* | Zhou Tingchong | China Science and Technology Press |
| 1994 | *Basic and clinical application of cell growth factor* | Qi Yanchao | Henan science and Technology Press |
| 2003 | *Polypeptide growth factor and spinal cord injury* | Wang Yanhua, Feng Zhongtang | Xinjiang science and Technology Health Press |
| 2007 | *Research on the basis and application of fibroblast growth factor* | Li Xiaokun, Gong Shouliang | Jilin University Press |

In 2004, a product Chuang Bi Fu from Liaoning Green Valley Pharmaceutical Machinery Co., Ltd., research and developed by Biopharmaceutical Research and Development Center of Jinan University, [National Food and Drug Administration (quasi) word 2004 No. 3640131]. After special treatment, the modification of collagen and fibroblast growth factor (FGF), while exerting the sustained release and absorption of collagen, FGF uses collagen as a carrier to bind its specific receptor. Maintains ideal concentration and activity around the damaged tissue and matches with normal cell differentiation to achieve a unique therapeutic effect, maximizing its biological function and overcoming the adverse effects and shortcomings of the individual use. Suitable for diabetic ulcers, radiation ulcers, bedsore, fistula, mucosal ulcers, and erosions. However, the current

**Table 14.4** Topical growth factor products approved for tissue repair in NMPA

| Company | Time | Product | Effect | Approval Status |
|---|---|---|---|---|
| Zhuhai Yisheng biopharmaceutical Co., Ltd | 1998 | Recombinant bovine basic fibroblast growth factor for external use | Promote the healing of burn and scald, wound, refractory sore, recurrent oral ulcer, chronic cervicitis, plastic and cosmetic surgery, and reduce the formation of scar | Country medicine accurate character S10980077 |
| | 1999 | Recombinant bovine basic fibroblast growth factor eye drops | Corneal epithelial defect and punctate keratopathy, mild to moderate dry eye, bullous keratopathy, corneal abrasion, mild to moderate chemical burn, corneal surgery, and poor postoperative healing caused by various reasons | Country medicine accurate character S19991022 |
| | 2005 | Recombinant bovine basic fibroblast growth factor ophthalmic gel | Corneal epithelial defect, punctate keratopathy, corneal abrasions, mild to moderate burns, and poor postoperative healing caused by various reasons | Country medicine accurate character S20050100 |
| Beijing Shuanglu Pharmaceutical Co., Ltd | 2002 | Recombinant human basic fibroblast growth factor for external use | It can promote wound healing and be used to repair chronic wounds (including chronic granulation wounds, ulcers, and bedsores) and fresh wounds | Country medicine accurate character S20020025 |
| Guilin huanuowei gene Pharmaceutical Co., Ltd | 2002 | Recombinant human epidermal growth factor gel | The treatment of skin burn wounds (superficial to deep), residual, donor, and chronic ulcer wounds | Country medicine accurate character S20020111 |
| Nanhai Langtai Pharmaceutical Co., Ltd | 2004 | Recombinant human basic fibroblast growth factor for external use | Promote the healing of burn and scald, wound, refractory sore, chronic cervicitis, plastic and cosmetic wound, reduce scar formation | Country medicine accurate character S20040052 |
| Shanghai Wanxing biopharmaceutical Co., Ltd | 2006 | Lyophilized Recombinant human acidic fibroblast growth factor for external use | Promote the healing of burn and scald, wound, refractory sore, chronic cervicitis, plastic and cosmetic wound, reduce scar formation | Country medicine accurate character S20060102 |
| Wuhan Haite biopharmaceutical Co., Ltd | 2006 | Nerve growth factor for injection | Peripheral nerve disease, trauma (peripheral nerve injury, craniocerebral injury, spinal cord injury), cerebrovascular accident (cerebral hemorrhage, cerebral infarction), degenerative disease (AD, PD) | Country medicine accurate character S20060051 |

research in this field is not broad enough and is not deep enough, and it is one of the important research directions in the future.

#### 14.2.3.4 Comparison of Growth Factor Research in China and Foreign Countries

For the admission of clinical application of growth factors, the United States is more cautious. Currently, only Chiron's genetically recombinant human platelet-derived growth factor, approved by the FDA in 1998, is used for debridement healing and repair of diabetic advanced extremity ulcers, severe burns, dermatosis, and bone and tooth defects; and Amgen's recombinant human keratinocyte growth factor, Palifermin, was approved in 2004 for the treatment of severe oral mucositis due to radiotherapy and chemotherapy.

### 14.2.4 Other: Gene Therapy, Therapeutic Cloning, and Xenotransplantation

At present, gene therapy has important prospects in nerve cell, cardiovascular, and islet cell regeneration. In 2012, *FASEB J* reported that PDGF and VEGF were introduced into mouse muscle at a certain rate to promote neovascularization. The recombinant human hepatocyte growth factor (HGF) independently developed in China is the first gene therapy product to enter the clinical trial stage for the treatment of cardiovascular disease and is currently undergoing phase II clinical trials. In addition, China also has pcD2/hVEGF121 gene therapy for limb arterial infarction, which has been approved by SFDA for special clinical trials. It is the second country to conduct such research after the United States.

The field of "therapeutic cloning" has been listed as a national key basic research project. The overall goal is to transplant the patient's somatic cells into the enucleated oocytes and to develop them into blastocysts after certain treatment, and then use the blastocysts to establish embryonic stem cells to induce differentiation into specific tissues or organs in vitro.

With the solution of the immune rejection problem of allogeneic organ transplantation, the transplantation of some important organs has saved the lives of many patients. However, because the donor system is not perfect and the donor source is limited, allogeneic organ transplantation cannot be widely carried out. In addition to the tissue engineering and stem cell technologies mentioned above, the feasibility of xenotransplantation is gradually being recognized. Using gene knockout, gene knock-in and somatic cell cloning techniques to transform donors into animal organs, overcoming heterogeneous rejection is becoming the main means to solve the problem of allogeneic organ transplant shortage. At present, the problems of animal organ transplantation mainly overcome hyper acute rejection/acute rejection, and the cultivation of animals without specific pathogens. The Pan Deng Group of the Institute of Animal Science of Chinese Academy of Agricultural Science has established the pure Wuzhishan minipigs in China with the first batch of GT-KO (homozygous deletion of the double copy of the GGTA1 gene). SFDA has approved several pigskin excipients that treat immunogenicity reduction in different ways. This allogeneic skin has a good effect on the coverage of burn wounds. In addition, α-galactosidase-treated pig cardiac valves, pericardium, ligaments, and the like have also been patented. In 2010, Kobayashi implanted rat iPS cells into the blastocyst cavity of Pdx1 knockout mouse embryos. These embryonic mice grew normal pancreases, derived almost entirely from rat cells, to save mice that had died after birth and kept them alive. If the same strategy can be achieved in large animals in the future, it will be possible to obtain functional cells for human transplantation, as well as various humanized organs. This solves the immune rejection of xenobiotic organs and obtains a well-functioning organ.

## 14.3 National Development Strategy of Chinese Regenerative Medicine

### 14.3.1 The Development Strategy of National Regenerative Medicine

In 2006, the State Council issued the *Guidelines for the Medium- and Long-Term National Science and Technology Development Program (2006–2020)*, which included stem cells as one of the five biotechnologies as the key research areas of cutting-edge technology in the next 15 years in China. At the same time, local governments have also made stem cell research a priority for science and technology and actively supported it. Relevant government departments and academia have paid close attention to and strongly supported the development of regenerative medicine. Recently, the relevant departments have further strengthened the management of stem cell therapy. The academic community held two "Reproductive Medicine" Xiangshan Science Conferences in 2005 and 2010, fully discussing the concept, scope, key breakthrough directions of regenerative medicine development in China, and key scientific issues that need to be solved. The future development has laid a good foundation and provided relevant guarantees. The Xiangshan Science Conference also be held focus on "Stem Cell Biology and Cloning," "Strategy for Gene Therapy Research and Development," and "Biomedical Materials and Tissue Engineering." It is enough to show that China attaches importance to the research of regenerative medicine.

### 14.3.2 Policy on Regenerative Medicine Research in China

From the perspective of policies and regulations, China is gradually strengthening its management of stem cell research and clinical applications. Since December 2003, the Ministry of Science and Technology of the People's Republic of China and former State Food and Drug Administration jointly formulated the first *Ethical Guiding Principles for Human Embryonic Stem Cell Research*. In 2013, a number of regulations were promulgated by the Ministry of Science and Technology of the People's Republic of China, former State Food and Drug Administration, and National Medical Products Administration. On October 25, 2011, the first National Stem Cell Research Coordination Committee was established. In December 2011, *the Notice on Conducting Stem Cell Clinical Research and Application Self-examination and Self-correction Work* was issued. Medical institutions and research institutes engaged in clinical research and application of stem cells should be in accordance with the requirements of the *Quality Management Regulations for Clinical Trials* reviewed and approved by the former State Food and Drug Administration on June 4, 2003, and the *Administrative Measures for the Clinical Application of Medical Technology* of the No. 18 document issued by the Health and Medical Administration in 2009. In March 2013, the Ministry of Science and Technology of the People's Republic of China and former State Food and Drug Administration's Leading Group for Stem Cell Clinical Research and Application Regulations organized the development of the *Methods for the Management of Stem Cell Clinical Trials (Trial)*, *Management Methods for Stem Cell Clinical Trials and Research Bases (Trial)*, and *Guidelines for Quality Control and Preclinical Research in Stem Cell Preparation (Trial)*.

### 14.3.3 Capital Investment in Regenerative Medicine in China

The Chinese government attaches great importance to stem cell technology and has given strong support in policy. The increased support for applied research indicates that the country is accelerating the promotion of stem cells from basic research into preclinical and clinical research. In addition, the National Natural Science Foundation of China, as an important mechanism to support free exploratory research, has also paid great attention to stem cell research with high risk. The following is the annual investment in regenerative medicine by the National Natural Science Foundation of China after 2000. Both the amount of funds and the number of projects are increasing year by year.

Regenerative medicine also plays an important role in military medicine. In March 2008, the US Department of Defense (DOD) announced that it will raise $250 million in the rapidly growing field of regenerative medicine to form the Armed Forces Institute of Regenerative Medicine (AFIRM) in the next 5 years. The research fund of the Chinese military has also invested heavily in the field of regenerative medicine.

In the "973" project in basic science, China has funded many projects related to stem cell research. In the "863" project, a major project of tissue organ engineering was launched, covering all the key technologies supported. More than ten clinical trial licenses have been approved by the former State Food and Drug Administration.

### 14.3.4 The Results of Chinese Regenerative Medicine

In 2012, China completed a phase I clinical trial of "Mesenchymal stem cell myocardial infarction injection," one of the three stem cell drugs approved for clinical trials 6 years ago. "Mesenchymal stem cell myocardial infarction injection" is a stem cell drug developed by the Research Center for Stem Cell Application Engineering in Hebei Province. Prior to this, former SFDA also approved two stem cell drugs into clinical trials, namely, "bone marrow primitive mesenchymal stem cells" and "autologous bone marrow mesenchymal stem cell injections." In addition, no new stem cell drugs have been approved for clinical trials in China for the past 6 years. In 2012, three new stem cell drugs were approved for production in the market. From the perspective of stem cell drugs, the stem cell industry in China has lagged behind other stem cell research powers.

In addition to the United States with strong scientific research strength, the research results of China and other countries in the field of stem cell research are not too different. In 2009, *Med Sci Monit* published an article that Chinese medicine is making more and more contributions to international biomedical research. The search by ISI Web of Knowledge shows that both Chinese papers have increased in quantity and quality, and some of them have been published in magazines with high international influence. On June 20th, 2012, the *Nature* Supplement released the *2012 Global Natural Publishing Index*, which ranks 100 countries in the world in terms of scientific research output in 2012. The top 20 of the world's top 200 research institutions, the United States has 12 seats. In addition, there are Germany (3, 19), France (5), the United Kingdom (8, 14), Japan (9), Switzerland (10), and China (12). According to the article, the high-quality scientific research output is rapidly increasing in China, and it has the strength to rank among the top five scientific powers in the world. In 2011, China published more literature in the field of stem cells than Germany, Japan, and the United Kingdom, ranking second; 2012 is even more obvious. In terms of tissue engineering, it has surpassed Germany, Japan, and the United Kingdom in 2000. After 2008, it is even more open to these countries.

In terms of patent applications, as of March 2010, the number of Chinese inventions related to stem cell-related inventions and the number of patents in countries with patent priority were ranked sixth and third, respectively, in the world. In addition, there is no research institution in China that has the top 20 papers or patents in the world, lacking new products, and the industry is not large. China has applied for a batch of patents in stem cell research. Although it has become one of the world's foremost in some technologies, it has also achieved certain effects in stem cell clinical treatment. However, due to the relatively weak basic research, the original innovative results are less. In addition, the stem cell industrialization in China still lacks institutional guarantees, clinical research methods and efficacy evaluation standards are still irregular and not rigorous, and the lack of industrialization and stamina greatly limits the development of industrialization. In the stem cell treatment market, China does not need to develop standards, regulations, and management methods that are suitable for the characteristics of stem cell technology to guide its healthy development.

In May 2005, at the second World Regenerative Medicine Conference held in Leipzig, Germany, Prof. Pei Xuetao, the head of the overall expert group of the "Tissue Organ Engineering Project of "863" Project in China and the Director of the Institute of Transfusion Medicine of the Academy of Military Medical Sciences, was awarded conference "Best Scientific Contribution Award." In 2008, Prof. Xiaobing Fu, an academician of the Chinese Academy of Engineering, won the "Lifetime Achievement Award" from the World Wound Healing Alliance for his achievements in the repair and regeneration of wounds. All of these indicate that China has a place in the field of international regenerative medicine.

### 14.3.5 Industrialization of Regenerative Medicine in China

In 2004, the first national-level stem cell industrialization base in China was officially opened. In 2005, Tianjin's national stem cell engineering product industrialization base passed the acceptance test. In 2006, the China-US Stem Cell and Regenerative Medicine Center of Qingdao University was unveiled. In 2007, the Tianjin National Engineering Research Center for Cellular Products launched a library of mesenchymal stem cells (MSC). In December 2011, the first academician of the stem cell life science industrialization base in China was launched in Inner Mongolia. During the "the 12th Five-Year Plan" period, Inner Mongolia will create and develop a stem cell industry and build a comprehensive development base for stem cell production, learning, and research that is leading domestically and internationally. Saiye (Guangzhou) Biotechnology Co., Ltd. and Hangzhou Baitong Biotechnology Co., Ltd. specialize in the development and sales of stem cell products. In November 2009, Shenzhen Beike Biotechnology Co., Ltd. and Japan's Yokohama Biomaster Company reached an agreement on their technology investment. Under the agreement, the investment will help Biomaster advance the development of stem cell-based hair regeneration, spinal cord repair, and organ regeneration therapy. In addition, on June 15, 2009, NeoStem also announced an exclusive agreement with Shanghai companies to strengthen biomedical cooperation. The purpose of this agreement is to use NeoStem's proprietary technology in Shanghai, Jiangsu, Zhejiang, Fujian, Anhui, Jiangxi, and other provinces in China create a network of stem cell collection and build treatment centers to boost the rapid development of the Chinese stem cell industry. On May 18, 2006, the Institute of Zoology of the Chinese Academy of Sciences, the Institute of Genetics and Developmental Biology of the Chinese Academy of Sciences, and the Tianjin Central Hospital of Gynecology Obstetrics jointly established the Stem Cell and Regenerative Medicine Research Center. Guided by national needs, the center integrates the strength of the Chinese Academy of Sciences in stem cell and regenerative medicine and complements the strength of Tianjin. Under the framework of the Advanced Biotechnology Innovation Base of the Chinese Academy of Sciences, it promotes interdisciplinary research, faces the frontier of science, faces the market demand, attracts world class talents, opens up a new way of combining scientific research and industrialization, persists in independent innovation, and promotes the development of stem cell and regenerative medicine research in China. In January 2010, Beike Biological Stem Cell Bank and Stem Cell Preparation Laboratory successfully passed the ISO9001 quality management system certification and obtained the qualification certificate issued by China Quality Certification Center (CQC), becoming the first comprehensive stem cell library certified by ISO9001 quality management system in China. In November 2012, the Beijing Institute of Life Science, Chinese Academy of Sciences and the Jingmeng Stem Cell Strategic Cooperation Signing Ceremony were held in Beijing. The Beijing Institute of Life Sciences, Chinese Academy of Sciences, and Beijing Jingmeng High-Tech Stem Cell Technology Co., Ltd. jointly established the "Translational Medicine Research Center, Beijing Institute of Life Sciences, Chinese Academy of Sciences." At the same time, Beijing Jingmeng High-Tech Stem Cell Technology Co., Ltd. officially became the "Stem Cell Translation Medical Research Base" of the Beijing Institute of Life Sciences, Chinese Academy of Sciences; it indicates that the research and application of stem cells in China have been accelerated in the competition of industrial transformation strategy. In the industry chain of Zhongyuan Union, stem cell genetic engineering is the main feature. They signed a letter of intent with British Cell Therapy Co., Ltd. (CTL), which is intended to carry out technical development and commercialization cooperation in the field of "development and commercialization of autologous mesoderm stromal cells for the treatment of heart failure technology." At present, Zhongyuan Union is the only biopharmaceutical company in securities market that truly uses stem cells as its main business in China.

At present, China has established a number of industrial bases. At the end of 2010, the National Stem Cell and Regenerative Medicine Industry Technology Innovation Strategic Alliance was established, with 27 leading research institutes in the field of stem cell and regenerative medicine, well-known top three hospitals, 211 key engineering universities, and leading enterprises in the industry as the initiators and council member units. The purpose is to promote stem cell and regenerative medicine technology innovation, results transformation and industrial development. It promotes the transformation of stem cell-related technologies and genetic engineering drug research results into actual productivity and gradually promotes the formation of new stem cell research and new industrial landscape.

The clinical trials of stem cell therapy are registered at the US http://www.clinicaltrials.gov/ website and the registration of clinical studies on active factors. The search revealed that before 2005, China registered 0 on the website. Since 2005, Chinese scholars have paid more and more attention to this issue. The number of projects registered on this website has increased year by year, reaching 138 in 2012, and as of our search (August 20, 2013), in 2013, there were 28 projects. Although there is still a big gap compared with developed countries in Europe and America, substantial progress has been made.

From the perspective of the distribution of the research and development stage, the clinical transformation process of China and international stem cell therapy is basically the same, and they are all in the study of the characteristics of drug efficacy and safety. In addition, stem cells used in these clinical studies and types of treated diseases mainly use hematopoietic stem cells and mesenchymal stem cells, and the types of diseases are mainly concentrated in blood diseases, vascular diseases, and diabetes.

### 14.3.6 Cooperation Between China and Other Countries in Research on Regenerative Medicine

At present, China has cooperated with countries with more advanced stem cell research in the world. In November 2007, the Ministry of Science and Technology of the People's Republic of China and the Australian Department of Education, Science and Training jointly funded the "China-Australia National Stem Cell Science Excellence Research Center" jointly established by the Peking University Stem Cell Research Center and the Monash University Stem Cell Research Institute. In March 2009, the Ministry of Science and Technology of the People's Republic of China and the Canadian Institute of Health Research (CIHR) signed a memorandum of understanding to establish a China-Canadian Health Research Cooperation Program to support research institutions in the two countries to cooperate in common priority research areas to strengthen health and medical research capacity building, promote mutually beneficial research partnerships. The first of the ten projects supported by the 2009 China-Canada Health Research Cooperation Program is collaboration between basic and applied research (including clinical and population health research), and item ten is Nano pharmaceuticals, stem cell biology, and tissue engineering. In April 2013, the cooperation between China and Canada further deepened. On April 10, 2009, the Scottish Center for Regenerative Medicine (SCRM) at the University of Edinburgh and the Peking University Stem Cell Research Center (PKUSCRC) signed a cooperation agreement on stem cell research. The agreement lasts for 5 years. In October 2009, China and the United States will jointly fund the research on stem cell cooperation between the two countries, and the Ministry of Science and Technology of the People's Republic of China and California will sign a memorandum of understanding on joint research on stem cells. In 2009, the National Natural Science Foundation of China also published the "National Natural Science Foundation of China and the German Science Foundation Collaborative Research Project (Molecular Principles of Stem Cell Biology)" through its official website. In the same year, seven well-known institutions at home and abroad, including Peking University, Chinese Academy of Sciences, and the famous Roslin Institute in the UK, participated in the establishment of the International Consortium of Stem Cell Research (INCOSC). In January 2012, the Medical Research Council (MRC) and the National Natural Science Foundation of China jointly funded a collaborative stem cell research project. The British Medical Research Council has invested 400,000 pounds and the National Natural Science Foundation of China has invested 3.6 million yuan. In April 2012, the

China-US Center for Regenerative and Translational Medicine was established by the Key Laboratory of Neuroregeneration of Nantong University and the Institute of Regenerative Medicine of Wake Forest University. In May of the same year, six world-renowned comprehensive regenerative medical research institutions from Germany, the United States, Canada, Spain, and the Netherlands signed a contract to establish the Regenerative Medicine Coalition (RMC) to jointly promote the research and development of regenerative medicine treatment methods at the cellular level. The six regenerative medicine centers that initiated the alliance are the core members of the alliance, but the alliance is an open network, and high-level scientific research institutions are welcome to participate in the cooperation (Table 14.5). Even some large foreign pharmaceutical companies, such as GE and Sanofi-Aventis, have invested in stem cell-related research in China and have produced relevant results.

**Table 14.5** Cooperation between China and countries in regenerative medicine

| Country | Time | Partners and contents |
|---|---|---|
| China–France | 2005.11 | Institute of zoology, Chinese Academy of Sciences and INRA began to cooperate |
| | 2007.09 | The Institute of zoology, Chinese Academy of Sciences and INRA, French National Center for Agronomy, jointly formed the Sino French Joint Laboratory of embryonic stem cell biology |
| China–Australia | 2007.11 | Jointly funded by the Ministry of science and technology of China and the Ministry of education, science and training of Australia, and jointly established by the stem cell research center of Peking University and the stem cell research institute of Monash University of Australia, "China Australia National stem cell science research center of excellence" |
| China–Canada | 2007 | The two governments signed an agreement on scientific and technological cooperation |
| | 2009 | Memorandum of understanding between the Ministry of Science and Technology and the Canadian Institute of health |
| | 2013.04 | Cooperation between the Ministry of Science and Technology and the Ministry of economic development and innovation of the government of Ontario, Canada |
| China–UK | 2005.10 | Memorandum of cooperation between NSFC and BMRC |
| | 2009.04 | The Scottish Regenerative Medicine Center (SCRM) of the University of Edinburgh and the Stem Cell Research Center (PKUSCRC) of Peking University jointly set up a national level international joint research center, and signed a 5-year cooperation agreement on stem cell research |
| | 2009 | Boya stem cell group, together with Peking University, Chinese Academy of Sciences, and the famous Roslin Institute in the UK, established the international stem cell joint research center (INCOSC) |
| | 2012.01 | The Medical Research Council (MRC) and the National Natural Science Foundation of China jointly funded the cooperative stem cell research project |
| China–USA | 2009.10 | Collaboration between California Institute of Regenerative Medicine (CIRM) and Ministry of science and technology of China (MOST) researchers in stem cell research |
| China–Germany | 2009 | The National Natural Science Foundation of China and the German Science Foundation jointly set up the molecular principle research project of stem cell biology |

## 14.4 Existing Problems and Prospects

The core and ultimate goal of regenerative medicine is to repair or regenerate various tissues and organs to address tissue and organ defects and dysfunction caused by disease, trauma, aging, or genetic factors. In theory, stem cells can be used for the treatment of various diseases, but its application is restricted by social ethics. Although stem cell research has done a lot of work, there are still many problems in stem cell research that need to be solved.

### 14.4.1 Several Aspects of Regenerative Medicine in China That Need to Be Strengthened

#### 14.4.1.1 Perfect Systems, Regulations, Technical specifications, Guidelines

There is still much work to be done to improve the health of stem cell research and applications. The first thing that should be solved is the establishment and improvement of systems and regulations. It can be said that China has not really established a management system for clinical application research of adult stem cells. Based on the current development status of China, we will formulate long-term development plans for stem cells, strengthen top-level design, and improve the established stem cell research network or center to make the development of the whole industry clear, effective, scientific, and standardized, and promote the effective and coordinated development of stem cell applications. In 2011, the Chinese Academy of Sciences launched the Strategic Pilot Science and Technology Project for "Stem Cell and Regenerative Medicine Research." Stem cell specialization focuses on three major aspects: major theoretical breakthrough, key core technology, and clinical application of stem cells, focusing on major scientific issues and core key technologies.

#### 14.4.1.2 Pay Attention to the Cultivation and Reserve of Stem Cell Research Talents

China has become an important member of the regenerative medicine research competition. However, the existing problems are also quite prominent. Compared with the international advanced level, there is still a gap between the research on stem cells and regenerative medicine in China, both in scale and overall level. There are not many original things, especially some innovative ideas and research directions that can lead the trend. In the field of tissue regeneration (including stem cells, tissue engineering, etc.), China still lacks influential scientists around the world.

#### 14.4.1.3 Reasonable Allocation of Resources and Breakthroughs in Key Areas

The research and development in China spending on technology has grown from $5.9 billion in 1996 to $44 billion today. Stem cell research, tissue engineering, and gene therapy are key areas for priority funding and are largely concentrated in universities, hospitals, and research institutions in major central cities in China, particularly in Beijing and Shanghai. However, only 5.2% of research and development budget in China is allocated to basic research, compared with 13–19% in Japan, Korea, and the United States. In the future, China will use limited funds to focus on research on regenerative medicine in stem cell differentiation and simultaneous repair and regeneration of various damaged tissues, construction of large organs in tissue engineering, and tissue engineering products from basic research to large-scale application. A large number of studies, represented by the study of the induced pluripotent stem cells and human embryonic stem cells and the mechanism of cell reprogramming, have made some breakthroughs. The series won the second prize of the 2014 National Natural Science Award. In addition, the preparation of collagen biomaterials for guiding the regeneration of uterine wall tissue damage, on the basis of animal experiments, the researchers, and the Nanjing Drum Tower Hospital cooperated in the clinical treatment of 13 cases of autologous bone marrow stem cell composite biomaterials for the treatment of severe intrauterine adhesions. Seven of them were pregnant and three were born healthy (2014/7/17, 2014/10/31, 2014/11/2). The project leader Dai Jianwu was awarded the "Top Ten Technology Figures" by CCTV in 2014. Furthermore, 168 large animal (dog) experiments were performed to repair spinal cord injury. After 9 months of long-term observation, the results showed that the biomaterial can effectively promote the recovery of motor behavior and electrophysiological function of spinal cord transected dogs and promote the regeneration of nerve fibers. At present, it has cooperated with the Chinese People's Armed Police Brain Hospital (Tianjin), the First Affiliated Hospital of Suzhou University (Suzhou), and the First Affiliated Hospital of the People's Liberation Army General Hospital (Beijing) to complete five clinical trials, and follow-up clinical evaluation work is underway. It will provide a possible treatment plan for patients who are currently clinically incurable.

#### 14.4.1.4 Extensive International Cooperation

Although there are extensive cooperation between multi-units and multicountry, multiregion, and multiresearch institutions in China, it is not enough. It should continue to be strengthened, especially in cooperation with well-known foreign universities, research centers, and key laboratories. A planning, systematic, and open research team should be established at the national level to avoid waste of resources and to concentrate on overcoming difficulties. At present, China is seeking opportunities for cooperation with international organizations. China has abundant sources of human embryonic stem cells and has policy support. The only thing that lacks is research experts. Therefore, it is necessary to strengthen cooperation to improve the level of stem cell research.

#### 14.4.1.5 Diversification of Inputs

Stem cell technology is attracting scientists and entrepreneurs from all over the world with its huge market potential. Facing the huge business opportunities revealed by the stem cell industry, it encourages drug research and development companies to participate in the translational medicine research of regenerative medicine, integrating with basic researchers, doctors, and medical developers to participate in research and promote the transformation of stem cell technology.

### 14.4.2 The Issues That Need Attention in the Research of Tissue Engineered Scaffold Materials

The research focus of tissue engineered scaffold materials is mainly to enhance the adhesion of synthetic scaffold materials to cells through surface biomimetic technology; physical or chemical methods are used to improve the mechanical properties and permeability of natural scaffold materials. In the future, the research direction of scaffold materials is to further study the surface modification of synthetic scaffold materials, improve its function of guiding cell behavior, promote the adhesion of materials to cells, further improve the microscopic permeability and biological activity of natural scaffold materials, and promote capillary vessels to grow in. The preparation of structural bionic scaffold materials and high-activity composite scaffold materials to promote their application in actual production is the focus of future skin tissue engineering development.

The major breakthroughs in stem cell research and its wide application in tissue engineering have basically solved the bottleneck problem of seed cell sources. Various new biodegradable bioscaffold materials have emerged, and various unique bioreactors have been developed successfully, the internal and external construction techniques and defect repair experiments of various organizations are basically completed. These advances have led to the maturity of biomaterial research and tissue construction techniques, and a variety of tissue engineered tissues have entered the preclinical research phase. Despite this, we must always be aware that there is still a long way to go before tissue engineering can be applied to the repair of clinical traumatic defects. Many more complicated problems have yet to be overcome. The source of seed cells of most other tissues is still under investigation. It is far from being solved. Biomaterials research cannot really meet the different requirements of various organizations. In terms of tissue construction, the development of bioreactors has just started, and it will take some time to finally use it for tissue engineering product development. In general, most of the current research is still limited to single tissue construction and defect repair, composite tissues, and organs.

### 14.4.3 Closely Integrate with Industrialization to Strengthen the Transformation and Application of New Technologies and New Products

Due to the close integration of genetic engineering technology and trauma medicine, the research and development of genetic engineering drugs for wound repair and tissue regeneration has become possible, and it has become one of the most rapidly developed areas of wound and burn medicine and has achieved remarkable results in clinical application in recent years. Since the 1990s, several gene-pharmaceutical companies in our country and the basic departments of wound repair have been closely integrated with clinical research units to produce several genetically engineered new drugs in this field, including epidermal growth factor (EGF), basic fibroblast growth factor (bFGF), acid fibroblast growth factor (aFGF), and transforming growth factor (TGF), some of which have been approved for use in patient treatment by the former State Food and Drug Administration, and some are still undergoing preclinical and clinical research. Preliminary statistical results show that genetic engineering drugs represented by EGF and bFGF not only significantly accelerate the healing time of acute wounds and significantly improve the healing quality. Moreover, it has a significant healing effect on radioactive ulcers, diabetic ulcers, varicose ulcer of the lower limb, and bedsore, which have been difficult to heal by conventional methods. In addition, the development of new genetic engineering drugs within growth factors has also provided conditions for research in the field of tissue engineering. So far, nearly ten genetic engineering drug companies in China have been engaged in the production of drugs in this field. From the current basic research and clinical application at home and abroad, it is suggested that the future development of genetic engineering drugs for wound repair and tissue regeneration should pay attention to the following points: further attention and in-depth study of the mechanism of genetic engineering drugs on wound repair and tissue regeneration. In particular, the polygenic mechanism and network regulation mechanism that they may involve in wound healing should be further identified. Objectively evaluate the short-term and long-term effects of genetic engineering drugs on wound repair and tissue regeneration, it is necessary to pay close attention to and monitor its possible adverse reactions. Further rational development and broadening of the application of genetic engineering drugs in the field of wound repair and tissue regeneration, including anatomical repair to functional repair, active repair of severe visceral injuries, active repair of central and peripheral nerve injuries, and the regeneration and repair of the damaged tissue in degenerative diseases, etc., should pay special attention to the effects of different dosage forms, dosages and application methods on the repair outcome, in order to maximize the therapeutic effect of these drugs on trauma. Pay close attention to the latest research trends in this field in the world, especially the possible impact of international similar genetic engineering drug research on the production of domestic related enterprises after China's accession to the WHO, and take corresponding measures. It is emphasized that the genetic drug companies engaged in research and development in this field will fully communicate between research and development and market development to achieve strong alliance and participate in international competition.

### 14.4.4 The Development of Basic Research and the Emergence of New Technologies Will Bring New Dawn to Regenerative Medicine

#### 14.4.4.1 In-depth Study on the Mechanism of Wound Repair and Tissue Regeneration

Tissue engineering and stem cell research have generated a strong interest in some special biological phenomena, that is, a fertilized egg forms a fully functional newborn from the time of implantation to 38 weeks, what mechanism is indicating a group of embryonic stem cells proliferate and differentiate into tissue cells and organs of different germ layers. During the 38 weeks of pregnancy, the proliferation and differentiation speed of various cells is several times or dozens of times that of normal cells and even tumor cells, but why is there so little tumor formation in this highly proliferating and differentiated tissue? What factors are controlling or monitoring this biological process? From the biological process, wound repair and tumor formation are the result of cell proliferation and differentiation and angiogenesis, only that the former is controllable and the latter is out of control. In the past, it was suggested that the formation of tumors is a result of mutations in some genes, which in turn leads to overexpression and action of proto-oncogenes such as c-Fos and c-Jun. However, many studies have suggested that proto--oncogenes or their proteins are also highly expressed or upregulated in different stages of embryonic development and in some important organ tissues, and these tissues have no tumor formation. Conversely, during the rapid proliferation of such cells, the healing of the wound is scar-free. Therefore, the scar-free, cancer-free, and tumor-producing phenomena of embryonic tissues highly expressed in these proto-oncogenes also suggest that cell proliferation and differentiation are controlled, and normal cell proliferation, differentiation are out of control (such as uncontrolled growth of cancer cells). There may be similar and different regulatory mechanisms in terms of embryonic development and postnatal repair. An understanding of this regulatory mechanism may lead us to find a switch that regulates wound healing.

An interesting phenomenon is the recent understanding of the tumor suppressor gene p53, which has undergone three stages: tumor antigen, proto-oncogene, and tumor suppressor gene. But now it seems that it is not only a gene that inhibits cancer, but also a gene involved in development and regulation of aging. Some scholars have suggested that the high expression of p53 inhibits the growth of cancer cells, which leads to the occurrence of aging, which is the result of tumor suppression. At the same time, p53-mediated aging can be reversed by the induction of other proto-oncogenes. Therefore, linking the biological processes of development, growth, repair, and aging to think and study may find new ideas for people's wound repair and tissue regeneration research. Recently, when studying some biological characteristics of sweat gland development, we found some interesting phenomena, that is, at the age of 16 weeks, the primary epidermal ridge basal cells are affected by certain factors, closely arranged in multiple parts, and are in a focal shape, aggregate to form a hillock (basal lamina formation). By 18–20 weeks, these focal agglomerated cells formed cylindrical cell cords and began to cut deep into the skin. By 24 weeks, the end of the cell cord formed a sickle-like shape, which was characteristic of mature sweat glands. Because the cells of the sweat gland duct and the secretory cells can express β1 integrin, keratin 19 (K19) and K8, and the focal growth time of cells is later than the appearance time of embryonic epidermal stem cells. Therefore, epidermal stem cells can be considered to be the source of sweat glands. What is of interest is what is the mechanism in the process of sweat glands from epidermal stem cells that directs some epidermal stem cells (but not all) to produce sweat glands while others do not occur? What causes the sweat gland cells to "cut in" deep into the skin, rather than non-horizontal growth? Although we have studied the effects of EGF, MMP2, MMP7, LN, and Fn on this, the basic biological problems are still unclear. It can be said that the lack of understanding of these basic problems is the main reason that prevents people from reconstructing sweat glands and performing functional wound repair after extensive burns.

The understanding of wound repair and tissue regeneration related to genetic factors is gradually being accepted. This understanding comes first from some strange biological phenomena in nature. Lower animals, such as the damaged tissue of newt or earthworm, can be completely regenerated, and the lizard-cut tail can re-grow, while humans cannot. Another example is that after the animal is injured, it is generally scar-free and humans are mainly scar healing. As human beings, the probability of scarring between different races varies greatly. The body in the embryonic period is generally no scar healing and generally scar healing process occured after birth. These phenomena strongly suggest that ethnic and genetic factors have an important impact on the outcome of the repair. In the case of embryonic stage scar-free healing, in the past, people mainly thought that it was related to the environment in which the embryo is located, especially after the injury. Recently, we have found from immunohistochemistry, in situ hybridization, and PCR studies that the genes, proteins, and receptors of growth factors such as bFGF, EGF, TGF-β3 isomers (β1, 2, 3), and PDGF in embryonic skin tissues of both rats and humans are low or no expression, but their content or activity begins to increase and increase in the late embryo and after birth. This result led us to think that the main growth factors that are closely related to scarring, such as the silence or closure of embryonic tissue, may be an important cause of scar-free healing. But the question is what mechanism is not clear in determining the closure and activation of these factors. Therefore, the original and lower animals can be completely regenerated after being injured, and the biological phenomena such as incomplete regeneration of rats and pigs and human scar repair suggest that studying repair from the perspective of comparative biology may find the key to solve the problem for us. The completion of the Human Genome Work Framework provides us with a potential for comparative biological research in wound healing. The study found that the human genome consists of 316,647 million base pairs, with a total of 30,000 to 3.15 million genes, only 10,000 more than nematodes, and 20,000 more than fruit flies. There are 99.99% identical genetic codes shared by humans on earth. The difference between human and chimpanzees is only 1–2.3%, while 61% of human proteins are homologous to fruit fly and 43% are homologous to nematode; 46% is homologous to yeast, and almost all of the genes on human chromosome 17 can be found on mouse chromosome 11. Therefore, if we make full use of the research results and gene technology of human genomics and compare the differential genes between different repaired animals, it will be possible to find a basis for the "repair genes" we envision. The "repair genes" or "repair-related genes" that have been looking for in recent years are gradually beginning to make a good start. By knocking out mice, it was found that the healing time of knockout Smad3 mice can be cut in half, and whether Smad3 is a repair gene? Swiss scientists claim that they found a gene called "PPAR-β" that heals in skin wounds. It plays a key role and is considered a repair gene. In foreign countries, the difference of gene response after skin injury was studied by 4000 point gene chip. It was found that there were 124 genes with increased expression (accounting for 3%) after 30 min of injury, involving posttranscriptional and transduction genes. At 1 h of injury, 46 of the 4000 genes increased, but 264 of them decreased, and the factor signal suppressor gene, rho Hp1, and BB1 genes may be involved in early injury. Domestically reported more than 120 genes that are normal and scar tissue detected by chip technology, including apoptosis, cytoskeleton, and signal transduction genes. From these results, it can be seen that the "repair gene" or "repair related gene" that determines the outcome of repair may not be a single gene, but may be the result of the participation of multiple genes under the influence of internal and external environment.

#### 14.4.4.2 The Impact of 3D Bioprinting Technology on Regenerative Medicine

Known as "one of the important signs of the 3rd industrial revolution," 3D printing is developing into a popular research technology in medical engineering, and its related research has set off a new wave of development at home and abroad. 3D bioprinting is a branch of 3D printing technology. It is currently the forefront of 3D printing technology research and the most dynamic and promising direction of 3D printing technology. In 2010, 3D bioprinter was named one of the 50 best inventions of 2010 by The Times. The bioprinting technology uses a computer design to print out a model and then injects a special "bio-ink" into the model and cultures it to produce an organ with certain physiological functions. This technique can also be used to induce stem cells to produce bone or cartilage tissue. The use of human cells, especially the cells of the patient's own cells, can reduce the probability of rejection. If the safety and effectiveness of this new technology is proven, then this bioengineering transplant can be implemented in humans within 3 years at the earliest. OPM (Oxford Performance Materials) of Connecticut, USA, also reported approval from the US Food and Drug Administration (FDA) on February 18, 2013, using the 3D printed skull implant, special polyether ketone (PEKK) material. Xu Mingen, the head of the China Biomaterials 3D Printer research and development team and a professor at Hangzhou Dianzi University, independently developed the first domestic biomaterial 3D printer. At present, this printer has successfully printed a small proportion of human ear cartilage tissue, liver unit, and so on. This biomaterial 3D printer features many types of printed biomaterials, low cell damage rate, high printing accuracy, and easy operation. Compared with similar printers in the world, it not only realizes biomaterials and cell 3D printing under aseptic conditions, but also has a new temperature control unit and print nozzle design that can support printing from a variety of biomaterials from −5 °C to 260 °C. Printed cells have a survival rate of up to 90%.The longest survival time of live cells printed is 4 months. Kang Yujian, a special expert in the "Thousand Talents Program" in China, aims to break through the trauma signal system and repair cardiovascular function, solve key theoretical and technical problems in regenerative medicine, and realize the clinical application of regenerative medicine. His team used Rollosesseller 3D printing platform, with "bio-ink" composed of seed cells, growth factors and nutrients, combined with other materials to print out the product, printed and cultured to form a physiologically functional organization \structure; and invented bioprinting core technology biobrick patent, a new, accurate, biomimetic stem cell culture system. Domestic 3D bioprinting technology has developed rapidly and has been developed in many applications such as cells, organs, and medical implants.

3D printing technology has limitations, and bioprinting currently does not produce the entire organ. Studies have shown that it is difficult to actually print cells while creating a scaffold structure. The cell membrane is damaged during the printing process, and the cell survival rate is unstable (40–95%). In addition, it is important to improve the resolution of 3D printing; lack of mechanical strength and integrity in the manufacture of biological frameworks, and the ability to improve the use of high-viscosity biological materials is one of the problems; a better understanding of the microenvironment of tissues, organs, and their structures that contain a variety of cells is also key to the success of 3D bioprinting.

#### 14.4.4.3 The Impact of the Development of Nano-Intelligent Materials on Regenerative Medicine

Nanotechnology is one of the top ten high-tech technologies in the twenty-first century. The medical community at home and abroad has always attached great importance to the research of nano-biotechnology. Through the improvement of material characteristics and functions, many new generations of smart materials have been created and applied in the field of regenerative medicine. Intelligent biological materials undergo molecular modification on degradable materials, cause cell integrin interaction, induce cell proliferation, differentiation, and synthesis and assembly of extracellular matrix, thereby initiating the body's regeneration system.

In short, multidisciplinary, multidisciplinary integration, and collaboration will greatly promote the development of regenerative medicine. In the preface to the Supplement to Chinese Regenerative Medicine in May 2012, Xiaobing Fu, academician of the Chinese Academy of Engineering and director of the Institute of Basic Medical Sciences of the Chinese People's Liberation Army General Hospital, mentioned in his outlook for the next 10 years that Chinese regenerative medicine is expected to make substantial progress in the following areas: the use of induced stem cells for simultaneous repair and regeneration of multiple tissue types after injury, the reconstruction of large organs through tissue engineering, and the large-scale clinical application of tissue engineering products. These results will bring hope to improving health care and building a healthy society.

## References

1. Fu X, Qu Z, Sheng Z. Potentiality of mesenchymal stem cells in regeneration of sweat glands. J Surg Res. 2006;136(2):204–8.
2. Fu X, Sun X, Li X, et al. Dedifferentiation of epidermal cells to stem cells in vivo. Lancet. 2001;358(9287):1067–8.
3. Zhang C, Fu X, Chen P, et al. Dedifferentiation derived cells exhibit phenotypic and functional characteristics of epidermal stem cells. J Cell Mol Med. 2010;14(5):1135–45.

GPSR Compliance

*The European Union's (EU) General Product Safety Regulation (GPSR) is a set of rules that requires consumer products to be safe and our obligations to ensure this.*

*If you have any concerns about our products, you can contact us on ProductSafety@springernature.com*

In case Publisher is established outside the EU, the EU authorized representative is:

Springer Nature Customer Service Center GmbH
Europaplatz 3
69115 Heidelberg, Germany

Batch number: 10731661

Printed by Printforce, the Netherlands